Essential Surgery

Problems, Diagnosis and Management

SIXTH EDITION

Edited by

Clive R. G. Quick MBBS(London), FDS, FRCS(England), MS(London), MA(Cantab)

Emeritus Consultant Surgeon, Addenbrooke's Hospital, Cambridge University Hospitals NHS Foundation Trust;
Associate Lecturer in Surgery, University of Cambridge; Former Examiner in Basic Sciences and Clinical Surgery for FRCS and
Current Examiner in Basic Sciences for MRCS(England), London, UK

Suzanne M. Biers BSc, MBBS, MD, FRCS

Consultant Urological Surgeon, Addenbrooke's Hospital, Cambridge University Hospitals NHS Foundation Trust;
Honorary Lecturer, Anglia Ruskin University, Cambridge, UK

Tan H. A. Arulampalam MBBS, MD, FRCS

Visiting Professor of Surgery, Anglia Ruskin University, Chelmsford;
Consultant Surgeon, Colchester Hospital, Colchester, UK

Illustrations by
Philip J. Deakin BSc(Hons), MBChB(Sheffield)

General Medical Practitioner, Sheffield, UK

Foreword by
Conor P. Delaney, MCh, PhD, FACS, FRCSI, FASCRS(Hon)

Chairman, Digestive Disease and Surgery Institute, Cleveland Clinic;
Victor W. Fazio MD Endowed Chair in Colorectal Surgery and Professor of Surgery,
Cleveland Clinic Lerner College of Medicine, Cleveland, Ohio, USA

ELSEVIER   Edinburgh   London   New York   Oxford   Philadelphia   St Louis   Sydney   2020

First edition 1990
Second edition 1996
Third edition 2002
Fourth edition 2007
Fifth edition 2014
Sixth edition 2020

Notices

ISBN: 978-0-7020-7631-2

978-0-7020-7632-9

Content Strategist: Laurence Hunter
Content Development Specialist: Helen Leng
Project Manager: Louisa Talbott
Design: Bridget Hoette
Illustration Manager: Narayanan Ramakrishnan
Illustrator: Dr Philip Deakin

Printed in the United Kingdom

Last digit is the print number: 9 8 7 6 5 4 3

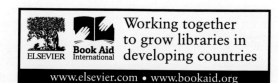

Contents

It is a sincere honour to be asked to write the Foreword for the sixth edition of *Essential Surgery*, written and edited by an esteemed and experienced editorial team. *Essential Surgery* was first published in 1990, and since that time has been singularly focused on being a concise, readable text for medical students and junior surgical trainees around the world. The chapters were formerly written by junior consultants and trainees, bringing perspective on the issue that mattered most to those in training. Now more senior clinicians are providing guidance; however, each has a particular interest in surgical education. Mr Clive Quick continues as senior editor—a steadying hand present since the first edition. New additions are Professor Tan Arulampalam and Miss Suzanne Biers. Professor Arulampalam is an experienced and passionate educator, establishing the ICENI centre in Colchester, and has taught surgical skills and knowledge around the world. Miss Biers is clinical lead for the Cambridge Urology Masters Degree Programme and directs surgical and operative skills training courses.

A quick review of this book shows why it is so popular. The mixture of simple, yet high-quality tables and illustrations, and carefully selected superb clinical photographs brings an easy readability. Equally important is the imaging, with a mixture of standard radiography and cross-sectional imaging, useful for readers in many styles of practice around the world. The summary boxes are particularly useful, highlighting key content.

The way the book is structured is also very approachable for readers. Initial sections on surgical principles and perioperative care give excellent and highly relevant perspective on topics such as immunity, screening, preoperative assessment and management of complications. Principles of accident surgery receives its own section, and reviews topics from set-up of trauma bays, to management of blunt and penetrating abdominal trauma. The final section on symptoms, diagnosis and management makes almost two-thirds of the book, and provides a comprehensive review of all surgical topics with chapters for each anatomic area and disease process. In each, there is a thorough discussion of clinical problems and management, emphasising history and physical findings, and frequently using a problem-based learning approach.

All in all, this is just a great book, with appropriate detail for the student and junior trainee, written and presented in a style that is easy to read, providing rapid access to the most important information. It is no surprise then that it has been so successful, and is back for a sixth edition, which I am sure will be even more successful than prior editions!

Conor Delaney
Cleveland, Ohio

Preface

When we first set about writing this book, we felt we had something worthwhile to say about how surgery worked. If readers could acquire this knowledge and implement it, we believed surgical practice would improve, as would outcomes for patients. We wrote the book in an entirely different way from most medical books, determined to avoid propagating myths and giving inadequate explanations. To achieve this, the authors discussed each topic in depth before writing an agreed version. Many original ideas came in the form of diagrams from Dennis Gatt. We have continued this method for each new edition, and now have the advantage of rapid internet access to check facts and investigate trends. We believe our approach has helped us understand the subjects better and put them across with exceptional clarity.

The original authorship was unusual in that only Clive Quick was a consultant surgeon: George Burkitt was a junior doctor-cum-medical author; Dennis Gatt was a junior surgical trainee (later consultant surgeon); whilst Phil Deakin was a family practitioner. This mix enabled us to address surgical problems from the viewpoint of the student and junior doctor and to this end, trainee doctors have assisted in every edition.

For this edition, Clive Quick has continued in his role as author and managing editor. Two other authors/editors have joined the editor team for this sixth edition: Tan Arulampalam from Colchester Hospital brings his contemporary knowledge of general surgery, laparoscopic techniques and experience as clinical director of the ICENI Surgical Skills Centre; Suzanne Biers, a urology consultant from Addenbrooke's Hospital, Cambridge, has extensive experience in the teaching and training of clinical and operative skills to students and surgical trainees at all levels. Our overall concept has always been to produce an authored rather than an edited book, so as to retain control over content, to give uniformity of style and apply our own high standard of elucidation so readers could grasp the main ideas easily and effortlessly in one reading. Nevertheless, an enormous amount of help has been generously given over the years by colleagues in specialist areas. Their invaluable contributions have been integrated and edited to emphasise lucidity and fluency (see detail in the Acknowledgements section).

When completed, the whole text is then reread several times by the editors and given a concluding 'polish'. Writing in this manner is time consuming, but if the text proves enjoyable to read and draws the reader in as we intend, we feel it will have been worthwhile.

The book covers general surgery, trauma, orthopaedics, plastic surgery, cardiothoracic surgery, vascular surgery, neurosurgery and urology in detail, with sufficient basic science for modern clinical courses, and we have endeavoured to present sometimes complex ideas in ways accessible to anyone with a moderate understanding of human biology, and yet still prove valuable to readers at more advanced levels.

The continuing enthusiasm of students and teachers for this book has highlighted the need for this updated edition. The book has been written for clinical medical students seeking a comprehensive understanding of surgical principles and practice, as well as for junior surgical trainees (particularly those preparing for MRCS and equivalent examinations). We have tried to build on the quality and content of the original without increasing its length. The content of each chapter has been carefully revised, often with input from colleagues, with a few sections relocated to facilitate navigation. At the same time, we have used the opportunity to continue to match the book's content with the UK Intercollegiate MRCS examination curriculum, rendering the book appropriate for junior surgical trainees. Other major changes represent the evolution and refinement of surgery and our approach to it over the 5 or so years since the previous edition. Throughout, we emphasise the importance of surgical safety with World Health Organization (WHO) checklists, avoiding cross infection and thorough auditing of complications.

All of the text has been brought up to date, adding new concepts where medical understanding has advanced. Major changes in surgical infection and recognition of the microbiome have been included and the section on vascular interventional treatment has been completely updated. The section on major trauma has been entirely reworked in line with current ATLS guidelines. Covering the MRCS curriculum has required updating several sections, including surgical ethics and consent, audit and research, and a new chapter dedicated to elective orthopaedic surgery. New consensus guidelines for managing common disorders have been incorporated where appropriate. We emphasise the new understanding of frailty and prehabilitation, and insights from the UK National Emergency Laparotomy Audit (NELA) have informed our text. We believe that *Essential Surgery* will continue to have the greatest appeal for readers who want to understand surgery rather than merely pass examinations.

Previous editions have demonstrated a broad appeal beyond medical students and junior surgeons, from surgical nurses and trainees in professions allied to medicine, to dentists. In addition, the book was designed to be a continuing reference text for doctors in other specialties, including family practice. We have used a problem-solving approach to diagnosis and treatment where practicable, believing that understanding how diagnoses are made and why particular treatments are used is more memorable than rote learning. With this in mind, we have tried to view the practical management of patients through the eyes of the trainee or student. In particular, the pathophysiological basis of surgical diseases and management is presented to bridge the gap between basic medical sciences and clinical problems.

Throughout the book, we have used original illustrative material to emphasise important concepts, avoid unnecessary text and assist revision for exams. This includes photographs of clinical cases, operations and pathological specimens, radiographs, anatomical and operative diagrams, and tables and box summaries of the text. We believe the illustrations are one of the particular strengths of the book, and all have been reviewed and updated or replaced as necessary. The clinical material is largely drawn from our day-to-day practice and we have generally chosen typical rather than gross examples, so the reader can see how patients present most commonly. Whilst we have tried to teach in a problem-oriented way, we believe descriptions of individual diseases are also required and these have been covered in a more conventional manner.

We make no apology for including outlines of common surgical operations. This is to enable students and trainee surgeons to explain operations to patients, to gain informed consent, to participate intelligently in the operating department, to understand and thereby prevent complications, as well as to help them perform certain operations themselves.

We hope our readers will continue to enjoy the book and will appreciate the continuing efforts we have made to keep pace with change. Above all, it remains our ambition to stimulate the reader to a greater enjoyment and understanding of the practice of surgery.

C. R. G. Q.
T. H. A. A.
S.M.B.

List of Contributors

In addition to those listed, the editors would like to acknowledge and offer grateful thanks for the input of all previous editions' contributors. Without their solid base, this new edition would not have been possible.

Hemantha Alawattegama, MBBS, BMed Sci, FRCA
Lead Clinician for Transplant and Hepatobiliary Surgery Anaesthesia, Cambridge University Hospital, Cambridge University Hospitals NHS Foundation Trust, UK
2. Managing Physiological Change in the Surgical Patient
4. Shock and Resuscitation

Tariq Ali, MBBS, MRCP, MSc, MRGP, AFHEA FRCS
Interventional Radiology Consultant, Norfolk and Norwich University Hospitals NHS Trust, Norwich, UK
5. Imaging and Interventional Techniques in Radiology and Surgery

Tan H.A. Arulampalam, MBBS, MD, FRCS
Visiting Professor of Surgery, Anglia Ruskin University, Chelmsford; Consultant Surgeon, Colchester Hospital, Colchester, UK
Editing throughout the book
1. Mechanisms of Surgical Disease and Surgery in Practice
10. Principles and Techniques of Operative Surgery Including Neurosurgery
12. Complications of Surgery
18. Nonacute Abdominal Pain and Other Abdominal Symptoms and Signs
26. Appendicitis
32. Hernias and Other Groin Problems

Suzanne M. Biers, BSc, MBBS, MD, FRCS
Consultant Urological Surgeon, Addenbrooke's Hospital, Cambridge University Hospitals NHS Trust; Honorary Lecturer, Anglia Ruskin University, Cambridge, UK
Editing throughout the book
1. Mechanisms of Surgical Disease and Surgery in Practice
12. Complications of Surgery
18. Nonacute Abdominal Pain and Other Abdominal Symptoms and Signs
33. Disorders of the Male Genitalia
34. Symptoms, Signs and Investigation of Urinary Tract Disorders
35. Disorders of the Prostate
36. Tumours of the Kidney and Urinary Tract
37. Stone Disease of the Urinary Tract
38. Urinary Tract Infections
46. Disorders of the Skin

Tony Booth, FRCR
Consultant Radiologist, Everlight Radiology and Hinchingbrooke Hospital, Huntingdon, UK
5. Imaging and Interventional Techniques in Radiology and Surgery
And major contributions to radiology throughout the book

Colin Borland, BA, MB, BChir, MD, FRCP
Formerly Consultant Physician, Hinchingbrooke Hospital, Huntingdon, UK
7. Preoperative Assessment and Management of Postoperative Problems
8. Medical Problems

Malcolm G. Cameron, MBBS, BDS, FRCS(Eng), FDSRCS(Eng), FRCS(OMFS)
Consultant Oral and Maxillofacial Surgeon, Addenbrooke's Hospital, Cambridge University Hospitals NHS Foundation Trust, Cambridge, UK
16. Head and Maxillofacial Injuries
47. Lumps in the Head and Neck and Salivary Calculi
48. Disorders of the Mouth

Dan Carroll, BM BCh, BA, MA, DM, MRCS, FRCS (Paed)
Director, Senior Lecturer and Consultant in Paediatric Surgery, James Cook University, Townsville, Australia
50. Acute Surgical Problems in Children
51. Nonacute Abdominal and Urological Problems in Children

Aman S. Coonar, BSc (Hons), MBBS, MD, MRCP(UK), FRCS (CTh)
Consultant Surgeon, Royal Papworth Hospital NHS Foundation Trust, Cambridge, UK
31. Thoracic Surgery

Patrick Coughlin, MB ChB, MD, FRCS(Eng)
Consultant Vascular Surgeon, Addenbrooke's Hospital, Cambridge University Hospitals NHS Foundation Trust, Cambridge, UK
40. Pathophysiology, Clinical Features and Diagnosis of Vascular Disease Affecting the Limbs
41. Managing Lower Limb Arterial Insufficiency, the Diabetic Foot and Major Amputations
42. Aneurysms and Other Peripheral Arterial Disorders
43. Venous Disorders of the Lower Limb

Aimee N. DiMarco, MA(Cantab), PhD, FRCS
Specialist Registrar in Endocrine & General Surgery, Hammersmith Hospital, Imperial College NHS Trust; Academic Clinical Lecturer, Department of Biosurgery, Imperial College, London, UK
49. Disorders of the Thyroid, Parathyroid and Adrenal Glands

Gary Doherty, MB, BChir, MA, PhD, MRCP
Consultant Medical Oncologist, Cambridge University Hospitals
  NHS Foundation Trust; Director of Studies in Medicine,
  Robinson College, University of Cambridge, Cambridge, UK
  6. *Screening for Adult Disease*
  13. *Principles of Cancer Management*
  45. *Disorders of the Breast*

Alexander Durst, BSc (Hons), MRCS
Speciality Registrar, Trauma & Orthopaedics; East of England
  Rotation, Addenbrooke's Hospital, Cambridge, UK
  11. *Elective Orthopaedics*
  15. *Major Trauma*

**David A. Enoch, BSc, MBBS, MSc, MRCP(UK), FRCPath,
DTM&H**
Consultant Medical Microbiologist, Clinical Microbiology &
  Public Health Laboratory, Addenbrooke's Hospital, Cambridge
  University Hospitals NHS Foundation Trust, Cambridge, UK
  3. *Immunity, Inflammation and Infection*
  10. *Principles and Techniques of Operative Surgery Including
    Neurosurgery*

Helen Fernandes, MBBS, FRCS(Sn), MD
Consultant Neurosurgeon, Addenbrooke's Hospital, Cambridge
  University Hospitals NHS Foundation Trust, Cambridge, UK
  10. *Principles and Techniques of Operative Surgery Including
    Neurosurgery*
  16. *Head and Maxillofacial Injuries*

Theodora Foukaneli, MD, FRCPath
Head of Department, Blood Transfusion, Cambridge University
  Hospitals NHS Foundation Trust; Patient Blood Management
  Team, NHS BT, Cambridge, UK
  9. *Blood Transfusion*

Fay J. Gilder, BSc (Hons), MBBS, FRCA
Consultant Anaesthetist, Cambridge University Hospitals NHS
  Foundation Trust, Cambridge, UK
  7. *Preoperative Assessment and Management of Postoperative
    Problems*

Ashley Groves, BSc (Hons), MBBS, MRCP
Professor of Molecular Imaging, Institute of Nuclear Medicine,
  University College Hospital, London, UK
  5. *Imaging and Interventional Techniques in Radiology and
    Surgery*

Simon Harper, MB ChB, BSc, MD, FRCS
Consultant Transplant and Hepatobiliary Surgeon, Cambridge
  University Hospitals NHS Foundation Trust, Cambridge, UK
  20. *Gallstone Diseases and Related Disorders*
  24. *Tumours of the Pancreas and Hepatobiliary System; the
    Spleen*
  25. *Pancreatitis*

C. Elizabeth Hook, MB/BChir, PhD, MA
Honorary Consultant Paediatric Histopathologist, Cambridge
  University Hospitals NHS Foundation Trust,
  Cambridge, UK
  Important contributions on pathology throughout

**Muhilan Kanagarathnam, MBBS, MRCP, FRCA, MBA (Health
Executive)**
Consultant Anaesthetist, Cambridge University Hospitals NHS
  Foundation Trust, Cambridge, UK
  2. *Managing Physiological Change in the Surgical Patient*
  4. *Shock and Resuscitation*

John Kiely, BM, BCh
Registrar in Plastic and Reconstructive Surgery, Cambridge
  University Hospitals NHS Foundation Trust, Cambridge, UK
  17. *Soft Tissue Injuries and Burns*

James Kinross, PhD, MBBS, FRCS
Senior Lecturer, Imperial College Healthcare NHS Trust,
  St. Mary's Hospital, London, UK
  3. *Immunity, Inflammation and Infection*
  10. *Principles of Operative Care*

**Roderick Mackenzie, PhD, BSc, MB, BChir, FRCEM, FRCS,
FRCP**
Consultant in Emergency Medicine and Pre-hospital Emergency
  Medicine; Clinical Director of the Major Trauma Centre,
  Addenbrookes Hospital, Cambridge University Hospitals
  NHS Foundation Trust, Cambridge, UK
  A large contribution on trauma
  15. *Major Trauma*
  16. *Head and Maxillofacial Injuries*
  17. *Soft Tissue Injuries and Burns*

Charlotte Beth Miller, BSc (Hons), MBChC, MRCS
Registrar in Plastic and Reconstructive Surgery, Cambridge
  University Hospitals NHS Foundation Trust, Cambridge, UK
  46. *Disorders of the Skin*

**S. Ramani Moonesinghe, MD(Res), FRCA, FFICM, FRCP,
BSc(Hons)**
Professor of Perioperative Medicine, Division of Targeted
  Intervention, University College London, London, UK
  7. *Preoperative Assessment and Management of Postoperative
    Problems*

Krishna Moorthy, MS, MD, FRCS
Senior Lecturer and Honorary Consultant Surgeon, Imperial
  College, London, UK
  19. *The Acute Abdomen and Acute Gastrointestinal
    Haemorrhage*
  21. *Peptic Ulceration and Related Disorders*
  22. *Disorders of the Oesophagus*
  23. *Tumours of the Stomach and Small Intestine*

Fausto Palazzo, MD, MS, FRCS
Consultant Endocrine Surgeon, Thyroid & Endocrine Surgery,
  Imperial College Healthcare, London, UK
  49. *Disorders of The Thyroid, Parathyroid and Adrenal Glands*

Animesh J. Patel, MA, MB, BChir(Cantab), LLM, FRCS(Plast)
Consultant in Plastic and Reconstructive Surgery, Cambridge
  University Hospitals NHS Foundation Trust, Cambridge, UK
  10. *Principles and Techniques of Operative Surgery Including
    Neurosurgery*
  17. *Soft Tissue Injuries and Burns*
  46. *Disorders of the Skin*

Clive R.G. Quick, MBBS(London), FDS, FRCS(England), MS(London), MA(Cantab)
Emeritus Consultant Surgeon, Addenbrooke's Hospital, Cambridge University Hospitals NHS Foundation Trust, Cambridge; Associate Lecturer in Surgery, University of Cambridge; Former Examiner in Basic Sciences and Clinical Surgery for FRCS and Current Examiner in Basic Sciences for MRCS (England), London, UK
Managing author/editor of entire book
  1. *Mechanisms of Surgical Disease and Surgery in Practice*
  3. *Immunity, Inflammation and Infection*
  6. *Screening for Adult Disease*
  10. *Principles and Techniques of Operative Surgery Including Neurosurgery*
  12. *Complications of Surgery*
  16. *Head and Maxillofacial Injuries*
  17. *Soft Tissue Injuries and Burns*
  18. *Nonacute Abdominal Pain and Other Abdominal Symptoms and Signs*
  19. *The Acute Abdomen and Acute Gastrointestinal Haemorrhage*
  20. *Gallstone Diseases and Related Disorders*
  21. *Peptic Ulceration and Related Disorders*
  22. *Disorders of the Oesophagus*
  23. *Tumours of the Stomach and Small Intestine*
  26. *Appendicitis*
  27. *Colorectal Polyps and Carcinoma*
  28. *Chronic Inflammatory Disorders of the Bowel*
  29. *Disorders of Large Bowel Motility, Structure and Perfusion*
  30. *Anal and Perianal Disorders*
  32. *Hernias and Other Groin Problems*
  39. *Congenital Disorders and Diseases Secondarily Involving the Urinary Tract*
  40. *Pathophysiology, Clinical Features and Diagnosis of Vascular Disease Affecting the Limbs*
  41. *Managing Lower Limb Arterial Insufficiency, the Diabetic Foot and Major Amputations*
  42. *Aneurysms and Other Peripheral Arterial Disorders*
  43. *Venous Disorders of the Lower Limb*
  46. *Disorders of the Skin*
  47. *Lumps in the Head and Neck and Salivary Calculi*
  48. *Disorders of the Mouth*
  49. *Disorders of the Thyroid, Parathyroid and Adrenal Glands*

Kourosh Saeb-Parsy, MA, MB, BChir, PhD, FRCS
Lecturer, Department of Surgery, University of Cambridge, Cambridge; Consultant Transplant Surgeon, Cambridge University Hospitals NHS Foundation Trust, UK
Consultant Transplant Surgeon, Cambridge University Hospitals NHS Foundation Trust, UK
  14. *Principles of Transplantation Surgery*
  24. *Tumours of the Pancreas and Hepatobiliary System; the Spleen*

Arun Sebastian, MBBS, MRCP, FRCR, EBIR
Consultant Radiologist, East Suffolk and North Essex NHS Foundation Trust, Colchester Hospital, Colchester, UK
  5. *Imaging and Interventional Techniques in Radiology and Surgery*

Neil Smart, PhD, MBBS (Hons), FRCSEd
Consultant Surgeon, Royal Devon and Exeter Hospital, Exeter, UK
  32. *Hernias and Other Groin Problems*

Alexandra Sutcliffe, MBBS
  10. *Principles and Techniques of Operative Surgery Including Neurosurgery*
  16. *Head and Maxillofacial Injuries*

Chloe Swords, MA(Cantab), MBBS, MRCS(ENT)
Registrar in Otolaryngology, Peterborough City Hospital, Peterborough, UK
  10. *Principles and Techniques of Operative Surgery Including Neurosurgery*

Nagendra Thayur, MBBS, DMED, DNB(RD), MRCP, FRCR
Consultant Radiologist, East Suffolk and North Essex NHS Foundation Trust, Colchester Hospital, UK
  28. *Chronic Inflammatory Disorders of the Bowel*
  29. *Disorders of Large Bowel Motility, Structure and Perfusion*

Steven Tsui, MA, MD, FRCS (Eng), FRCS (C-Th), FHFA
Consultant Cardiothoracic Surgeon, Royal Papworth Hospital, Cambridge, UK
  44. *Cardiac Surgery*

Keith Tucker, MBBS, FRCS
Consultant Orthopaedic Surgeon (Retired), Norwich, UK
  Major revision of orthopaedics
  11. *Elective Orthopaedics*
  15. *Major Trauma*

Helen Weaver, MB ChB, BSc, MRCS
Cardiothoracic Registrar, Glenfield Hospital, Leicester, UK
  31. *Thoracic Surgery*

James Wheeler, MBBCh, MD, FRCS
Consultant Surgeon, Colorectal Surgery, Addenbrooke's Hospital, Cambridge University Hospitals NHS Foundation Trust, Cambridge, UK
  26. *Appendicitis*
  27. *Colorectal Polyps and Carcinoma*
  28. *Chronic Inflammatory Disorders of the Bowel*
  29. *Disorders of Large Bowel Motility, Structure and Perfusion*
  30. *Anal and Perianal Disorders*

Acknowledgements

As in all previous editions, the editors are deeply indebted to contributing authors for helping us keep the book up-to-date and accurate. Some have contributed a large amount of material and others in lesser ways, but without them all, the book would not be what it is.

A continuing debt of gratitude is owed to all who have contributed to each of the editions of *Essential Surgery*, including of course, any whose names are not mentioned here. A substantial part of the book's success is due to them.

In previous editions: we gratefully acknowledge the huge contributions made by Dennis Gatt, now a surgeon in Malta, the late Leonard Beard, medical photographer, Dr Graham Hurst, radiologist, Michael Williams, oncologist and the late Andrew Higgins, urologist. We also owe a tremendous debt to Jane Hailey, then a junior trainee and now a paediatrician in Canada, who helped turn our first edition prose into accessible and fluent text. We owe grateful thanks for contributions from Prof Ted Howard, Stephen Large, the late Grant Williams, Mark Farrington, Richard Miller, John Benson, Neville Jamieson, Jeffrey Brain, Madan Samuel, Nimish Shah, Sue Clark, Paul Perkins, Adrian Harris, Dr Anita Gibbons, Dr Suzanna Lishman, Dr Helen Smith, David Adlam, Nick Skelton, Paul Hayes, Roger Gray, Elizabeth Ambler, Howard Smith, Catherine Hubbard, Paul Siklos, Katie Hoggarth, Paul Hage, Joanna Reed and Alban Bowers.

For this edition we are once again grateful for the substantial and unstinting help we have received from colleagues and friends. Most are based at Addenbrooke's Hospital Cambridge or Hinchingbrooke Hospital, Huntingdon, and are acknowledged individually in the list of contributors.

SECTION A

Principles of Surgical Care

1

Mechanisms of Surgical Disease and Surgery in Practice

CHAPTER OUTLINE

Approaches to Surgical Problems

What Do Surgeons Do?

Surgeons are perceived as doctors who do operations, that is, cutting tissue to treat disease, usually under anaesthesia, but this is only a small part of surgical practice. The range individual surgeons undertake varies with the culture, the resources available, the nature and breadth of their specialisation, which other specialists are available, and local needs. The principles of operative surgery—access, dissection, haemostasis, repair, reconstruction, preservation of vital structures and closure—are similar in all specialties.

A **general surgeon** is one who undertakes general surgical emergency work and elective abdominal gastrointestinal (GI) surgery. In geographically isolated areas, such a surgeon might also undertake gynaecology, obstetrics, urology, paediatric surgery, orthopaedic and trauma surgery and perhaps basic ear, nose and throat, and ophthalmology. Conversely, in developed countries, there is a trend towards greater specialisation. GI surgery, for example, is often divided into 'upper' and 'lower', and upper GI surgery may further subdivide into hepatobiliary, pancreatic and gastro-oesophageal cancer surgery.

Surgeons are not simply 'cutting and sewing' doctors. The drama of surgery may seem attractive but good surgery is rarely dramatic. Only when things go wrong does the drama increase, and this is uncomfortable. Surgery is an art or craft as well as a science, and judgement, coping under pressure, taking decisive action, teaching and training and managing people skilfully are essential qualities. Operating can be learnt by most people, but the skills involved in deciding when it is in the patient's best interests to operate are essential and must be actively learnt and practised.

Surgeons play an important role in diagnosis, using clinical method and selecting appropriate investigations. Many undertake diagnostic and therapeutic endoscopy including gastroscopy, colonoscopy, urological endoscopy, thoracoscopy and arthroscopy. Indications for laparoscopic surgery, supported by good quality clinical trials, continue to broaden as equipment and skills become more sophisticated.

A SHORT HISTORY OF SURGERY

There is no doubt that the first surgeons were the men and women who bound up the lacerations, contusions, fractures, impalements and eviscerations to which man has been subject since appearing on Earth. Since man is the most vicious of all creatures, many of these injuries were inflicted by man upon man. Indeed, the battlefield has always been a training ground for surgery. Right up to the 15th century, surgeons dealing with trauma were surprisingly efficient. They knew their limitations—they could splint fractures, reduce dislocations and bind up lacerations, but were only too aware that open wounds of the skull, chest and abdomen were lethal and were best left alone, as were wounds involving major blood vessels or spinal injuries with paralysis. They observed that wounds would usually discharge yellow pus for a time; indeed, this was regarded as a good prognostic sign and was labelled 'laudable pus'.

The 15th century heralded a new and dreaded pathology—the gunshot wound. These injuries would stink, swell and bubble with gas. There was profound systemic toxicity and a high mortality. Of course, we now know that this was the result of clostridial infection of wounds with extensive anaerobic tissue damage caused by shot and shell. The surgeons of those times were shrewd clinical observers but surmised that these malign effects were caused by gunpowder acting as a poison, for it was not until centuries later that the bacterial basis of wound infection became evident. At that period, the remedy was to destroy the poison with boiling oil or cautery. Boiling oil was the more popular since it was advocated by the Italian surgeon Giovanni da Vigo (1460–1525), the author of the standard text of the day, *Practica In Arte Chirurgica Compendiosa*. These treatments not only produced intense pain but also made matters worse by increasing tissue necrosis.

The first scientific departure from this barbaric treatment was by the great French military surgeon Ambroise Paré (1510–1590) who, while still a young man, revolutionised the treatment of wounds by using only simple dressings, abandoning cautery and introducing ligatures to control haemorrhage. He established that his results were much better than could be achieved by the old methods.

Ignorance of the basic sciences behind the practice of surgery was slowly overcome. The publications of *The Fabric of the Human Body* in 1543 by Andreas Vesalius (1514–1564) and of *The Motion of the Heart* by William Harvey (1578–1657) in 1628 were two notable landmarks.

Surgical progress, however, was still limited by two major obstacles. First, the agony of the knife: patients would only undergo an operation to relieve intolerable suffering (e.g., from a gangrenous limb, a bladder stone or a strangulated rupture) and, of course, the surgeon needed to operate at lightning speed. Second, there was the inevitability of suppuration, with its prolonged disability and high mortality, often as high as 50% after amputation. Amazingly, both these barriers were overcome in the same couple of decades.

In 1846, William Morton (1819–1868), a dentist working in Boston, Massachusetts, introduced ether as a general anaesthetic. This was followed a year later by chloroform, employed by James Young Simpson (1811–1870) in Edinburgh, mainly in midwifery. These agents were taken up with immense enthusiasm across the world in a matter of weeks.

The work of the French chemist Louis Pasteur (1822–1895) demonstrated the link between wound suppuration and microbes. This led Joseph Lister (1827–1912), then a young professor of surgery in Edinburgh, to perform the first operation under sterile conditions in 1865. This was treatment of a compound tibial fracture in which crude carbolic acid was used as an antiseptic. The development of antiseptic surgery and, later, modern aseptic surgery progressed from there.

So at last, in the 1870s, the scene was set for the coming enormous advances in every branch of surgery whose breadth and successes form the basis of this book.

Prof. Harold Ellis, CBE MCH FRCS

What Sort of Patients Come to Surgeons?

Different types of surgeons practise in very different ways. In the United Kingdom, most patients are referred by another doctor, for example, GP, accident and emergency (ER) officer or physician. The exceptions include trauma patients who self-refer or arrive by ambulance. In some countries, patients can self-refer to the specialist they consider most appropriate. Regardless of the route, surgical patients fall into the following categories:

- **Emergency/acute**, that is, symptoms lasting minutes to hours or up to a day or two—often obviously surgical conditions, such as traumatic wounds, fractures, abscesses, acute abdominal pain or GI bleeding
- **Intermediate urgency**—usually referrals from other doctors based on suspicious symptoms and signs and sometimes investigations, for example, suspected colonic cancer, gallstones, renal or ureteric stones
- **Chronic conditions** likely to need surgery, for example, varicose veins, hernias, arthritic joints, cardiac ischaemia or rectal prolapse

The Diagnostic Process

To manage surgical patients optimally, a **working diagnosis** needs to be formulated to guide whether investigations are necessary and their type and urgency, and to determine what intervention is necessary. The process depends upon whether immediate life-saving intervention is required or, if not, the perceived urgency of the case. For example, a patient bleeding from a stab wound might need pressure applied to the wound immediately whilst resuscitation and detailed assessment are carried out. At the other end of the scale, if symptoms suggest rectal carcinoma, a systematic approach is needed to obtain visual and histologic confirmation of the diagnosis by colonoscopy and radiologic imaging. **Tumour staging** (see Ch. 13, p. 185) aims to determine the extent of cancer spread to direct how radical treatment needs to be. Treatment may be **curative** (surgery, chemotherapy, radiotherapy) or **palliative** if clearly beyond cure (stenting to prevent obstruction, local tumour destruction using laser, palliative radiotherapy).

Formulating a Diagnosis. The traditional approach to surgical diagnosis is to attempt to correlate a patient's symptoms and signs with recognised sets of clinical features known to characterise each disease. While most diagnoses match their 'classical' descriptions at certain stages, this may not be so when the patient presents. Patients often present before a recognisable pattern has evolved or at an advanced stage when the typical clinical picture has become obscured. Diagnosis can be confusing if all the clinical features for a particular diagnosis are not present, or if some seem inconsistent with the working diagnosis.

This book seeks to develop a more logical and reliable approach to diagnostic method than pattern recognition, by attempting to explain how the evolving pathophysiology of the disease and its effect on the anatomy bring about the clinical features. The overall aim is to target investigations and management that give the best chance of cure or symptom relief with the least harm to the patient.

Principal Mechanisms of Surgical Disease

Surgical patients present with disorders resulting from inherited abnormalities, environmental factors or combinations in varying proportions. These are summarised in Box 1.1, as a useful 'first principles' framework or *aide-mémoire* upon which to construct a

• BOX 1.1 The Surgical Sieve

When considering the causes of a particular condition, it may be helpful to run through the range of causes listed here. This should only be a first step and not a substitute for thought. This approach gives no indication of the likely severity, frequency or importance of the cause.

Congenital
- Genetic
- Environmental influences in utero

Acquired
- Trauma—accidents in the home, at work or during leisure activities, personal violence, road traffic collisions
- Inflammation—physical or immunological mechanisms
- Infection—viral, bacterial, fungal, protozoal, parasitic
- Neoplasia—benign, premalignant or malignant
- Vascular—ischaemia, infarction, reperfusion syndrome, aneurysms, venous insufficiency
- Degenerative—osteoporosis, glaucoma, osteoarthritis, rectal prolapse
- Metabolic disorders—gallstones, urinary tract stones
- Endocrine disorders and therapy—thyroid function abnormalities, Cushing syndrome, phaeochromocytoma
- Other abnormalities of tissue growth—hyperplasia, hypertrophy and cyst formation
- Iatrogenic disorders—damage or injury resulting from the action of a doctor or other healthcare worker; may be misadventure, negligence or, more commonly, system failure
- Drugs, toxins, diet, exercise and environment
  - Prescription drugs—toxic effects of powerful drugs, maladministration, idiosyncratic reactions, drug interactions
  - Smoking—atherosclerosis, cancers, peptic ulcer
  - Alcohol abuse—personal violence, traffic collisions
  - Substance abuse—accidents, injection site problems
  - 'Western diet'—obesity, atherosclerosis, cancers
  - Lack of exercise—obesity, osteoporosis, aches and pains
  - Venomous snakes, spiders, scorpions and other creatures—local and systemic toxicity
  - Atmospheric pollution—pulmonary problems
- Psychogenic— factitious disorder, unspecified (Munchausen syndrome) leading to repeated operations, problems of indigent living, ingestion of foreign bodies, self-harm
- Disorders of function—diverticular disease, some swallowing disorders

differential diagnosis. This is useful when clinical features do not immediately point to a diagnosis. This approach is known as the *surgical sieve*; however, it is not a substitute for logical thought based on the clinical findings.

Congenital Conditions

The term **congenital** defines a condition present at birth, as a result of genetic changes and/or environmental influences in utero such as ischaemia, incomplete development or maternal ingestion of drugs such as thalidomide. Congenital abnormalities of surgical interest range from minor cosmetic deformities such as skin tags through to potentially fatal conditions such as congenital heart defects, posterior urethral valves and gut atresias.

Congenital abnormalities become manifest any time between conception and old age, although most are evident at birth or in early childhood. Some are diagnosed *antenatally*, for example, foetal gut atresias with grossly excessive amniotic fluid (polyhydramnios). There are expanding specialist areas involving *intrauterine* or foetal surgery, for example, for urinary tract obstruction. During infancy, conditions such as congenital hypertrophic pyloric stenosis come to light. In childhood, incompletely descended testis may become evident. Finally, some disorders may present at *any stage*. For example, a patent processus vaginalis may predispose to an inguinal hernia even into late middle age.

Whilst many congenital abnormalities give rise to disease by direct **anatomical effects**, others cause disease by **disrupting function**, with the underlying disorder revealed only on investigation. For example, ureteric abnormalities allowing urinary reflux predispose to recurrent kidney infections.

Acquired Conditions

Acquired surgical disorders result from trauma or disease or from the body's response to them, or else present as an effect or side-effect of treatment. For example, bladder outlet obstruction may result from benign prostatic enlargement, from urethral stricture after gonococcal urethritis or from damage inflicted during urethral instrumentation. The classification detailed here is a framework, but conditions may fit more than one heading, and the mechanism behind some disorders is still poorly understood.

Trauma

Tissue trauma, literally injury, includes damage inflicted by any physical means, that is, mechanical, thermal, chemical or electrical mechanisms or ionising radiation. Common usage tends to imply blunt or penetrating mechanical injury, caused by accidents in industry or in the home, road traffic collisions, fights, firearm and missile injuries or natural disasters, such as floods and earthquakes. Damage varies with the causative agent, and the visible injuries may not indicate the extent of deep tissue damage.

Inflammation

Many surgical disorders result from inflammatory processes, most often stemming from infection. However, inflammation also results from physical irritation, particularly by chemical agents, for example, gastric acid/pepsin in peptic ulcer disease or pancreatic enzymes in acute pancreatitis.

Inflammation may also result from immunological processes, such as in ulcerative colitis and Crohn disease. Autoimmunity, where an immune response is directed at the body's constituents, is recognised in a growing number of surgical diseases, such as Hashimoto thyroiditis and rheumatoid disease.

Infection

Primary infections presenting to surgeons include abscesses and cellulitis, primary joint infections and tonsillitis. Typhoid may cause caecal perforation, and abdominal tuberculosis may be discovered at laparotomy. Amoebiasis can cause ulcerative colitis-like effects. Preventing and treating infection is an important factor in surgical emergencies, such as acute appendicitis or bowel perforation. Despite the rational use of prophylactic and therapeutic antibiotics, postoperative infection remains a common complication of surgery.

Neoplasia

Certain **benign tumours**, such as lipomas, are common and are excised mainly for cosmetic reasons. Less commonly, benign tumours cause mechanical problems, such as obstruction of a hollow viscus or surface blood loss, for example, leiomyoma. Benign endocrine tumours may need removal because of excess hormone secretion (see *Endocrine disorders* later). Finally, benign tumours may be clinically indistinguishable from malignant tumours and are removed or biopsied to obtain a diagnosis.

Malignant tumours may present with signs and symptoms from the primary, the effects of metastases ('secondaries') and sometimes, systemic effects, such as cachexia. Malignant tumours are responsible for a large part of the general surgical workload.

Vascular Disorders

A tissue or organ becomes **ischaemic** when its arterial blood supply is impaired; **infarction** occurs when cell life cannot be sustained. **Atherosclerosis** progressively narrows arteries often resulting in **chronic ischaemia**, causing symptoms, such as angina pectoris or intermittent claudication. It also predisposes to **acute-on-chronic ischaemia** when diseased vessels finally occlude. Other common causes of acute arterial insufficiency are thrombosis, embolism and trauma. Arterial embolism causes acute ischaemia of limbs, intestine or brain; emboli often originate in the heart. If blood supply is restored after a period of ischaemia, further damage can ensue as a result of **reperfusion syndrome**.

When a portion of bowel becomes strangulated, the initial mechanism of tissue damage is venous obstruction, and this progresses to arterial ischaemia and infarction.

An **aneurysm** is an abnormal dilatation of an artery resulting from degeneration of connective tissue. This may rupture, thrombose or generate emboli.

Chronic **venous insufficiency** in the lower limb causing local venous hypertension is responsible for the majority of chronic leg ulcers in the West.

Degenerative Disorders

This is an inhomogeneous group of conditions characterised by deterioration of body tissues as life progresses. In the musculoskeletal system, **osteoporosis** decreases bone density and impairs its structural integrity, making fragility fractures more likely. Spinal disc and facet joint degeneration is common, causing back pain and disability, and osteoarthritis is widely prevalent in later life: the almost universal musculoskeletal aches and pains are probably caused by degeneration of muscle, tendon, joint and bone.

Other degenerative disorders include age-related retinal macular degeneration, glaucoma, the inherited disorder retinitis pigmentosa, and certain neurological disorders (Alzheimer, Huntington and Parkinson disease, bulbar palsy). Atherosclerosis and aneurysmal arterial diseases are often nonspecifically labelled degenerative.

Metabolic Disorders

Metabolic disorders may be responsible for stones in the gall bladder (e.g., haemolytic diseases causing pigment stones) or in the urinary tract (e.g., hypercalciuria and hyperuricaemia causing calcium and uric acid stones, respectively). Hypercholesterolaemia is a major factor in atherosclerosis and hypertriglyceridaemia is a rare cause of acute pancreatitis.

Endocrine Disorders and Hormonal Therapy

Hypersecretion of hormones, as in thyrotoxicosis and hyperparathyroidism, may require surgical removal or reduction of glandular tissue. Endocrine tumours, benign and malignant, may present with metabolic abnormalities, such as hypercalcaemia caused by a parathyroid adenoma, Cushing syndrome resulting from an adrenal adenoma or episodic hypertension caused by a phaeochromocytoma.

Diabetes mellitus, particularly when poorly controlled, causes a range of complications of surgical importance, for example, diabetic foot problems, retinopathy and cataract formation, as well as predisposing to atherosclerosis.

Hormone replacement therapy in postmenopausal women brings mixed benefits: it slows osteoporosis and reduces colorectal cancer risk whilst slightly increasing risk of breast and endometrial cancer. There is also evidence of an increased rate of thromboembolism, as with higher oestrogen-containing oral contraceptive pills.

Other Abnormalities of Tissue Growth

Growth disturbances, such as **hyperplasia** (increase in number of cells) and **hypertrophy** (increase in size of cells) may cause surgical problems, in particular benign prostatic hyperplasia, fibroadenosis of the breast and thyroid enlargement (goitre).

In surgery, the term **cyst** imprecisely describes a mass which appears to contain fluid because of characteristic fluctuance and transilluminability. A cyst is defined as a closed sac with a distinct lining membrane that develops abnormally in the body. A variety of pathological processes produce cysts. Most are benign but some cysts may be malignant.

Iatrogenic Disorders

Iatrogenic damage or injury results from the action of a doctor or other healthcare worker. It may be an unfortunate outcome of an adequately performed investigation or operation, for example, perforated colon during colonoscopy or pneumothorax from attempted aspiration of a breast cyst. These are termed **surgical misadventure**. However, if the damage results from a patently incorrect procedure, for example, amputation of the wrong leg or removal of the wrong kidney, then **negligence** is likely to be proven. Such wrong site surgery is termed a **never event** and is now rare because of mandatory preoperative site marking and comprehensive theatre staff briefing (World Health Organization [WHO] checklist). Other never events include retained foreign objects postprocedure (i.e., surgical swab, guidewire), transfusion of incompatible blood products or administration of medication via the wrong route. Prescription or administration of the incorrect drug or dose is usually iatrogenic. It is unusual for iatrogenic problems to be caused simply by one person's failure. More often it is a **system failure**, with inadequate checks and balances in the system. Complications of bowel surgery, such as anastomotic leakage may result from poorly performed surgery but can occur in expert hands; audited results can demonstrate whether the surgeon is proficient.

Drugs, Toxins and Diet

Problems with prescribed drugs include unavoidable **toxic effects** of certain chemotherapeutic agents, for example, neutropenia, and the **side-effects** of drugs, such as nonsteroidal anti-inflammatory drugs (NSAIDs) causing duodenal perforation, or codeine phosphate causing constipation. Drug **allergy, idiosyncrasy** or **anaphylaxis** may result from individual responses to almost any drug, and **interactions** between drugs cause adverse effects; in this respect warfarin is a prime culprit. Maladministration of drugs may also cause problems with, for example, the wrong drug given for intrathecal chemotherapy causing paralysis (a never event).

In many countries, venomous creatures, such as spiders, snakes or scorpions cause toxic and sometimes fatal harm.

Although major advances have now been made to discourage it, cigarette **smoking** has been the biggest single preventable cause of death and disability in developed countries. Cigarette smoke is highly addictive and contains an array of carcinogens in the tar, the vasoconstrictor nicotine, and carbon monoxide that binds preferentially to haemoglobin. Not surprisingly, smoking is a powerful factor in a huge range of diseases including cardiovascular disorders of heart, limbs and brain, dysplasias and cancers of lung, mouth and larynx, respiratory disorders, such as pneumonias, chronic obstructive pulmonary disease (COPD) and emphysema via small airways inflammation, stillbirth and peptic ulcer disease. Smoking compounds the atherogenic effects of diabetes and is also strongly associated with premature skin ageing. Environmental pollution adversely affects health: for example, microfine particles produced by diesel engines cause pulmonary inflammation.

Alcohol and substance abuse may have a surgical dimension: alcohol can lead to personal violence or road traffic collisions; cannabis smoke is carcinogenic and causes dysplasias and premalignant lesions of the oral mucosa, as well as contributing to mental health problems. Misdirected injection of opioids and other drugs may cause abscesses, false aneurysms and even arterial occlusion. Misuse of ketamine can cause intractable bladder pain, cystitis and urinary symptoms.

The so-called Western diet, rich in fat and calories and low in vegetables, fruit and fibre, is linked with a range of diseases including colorectal and breast cancers, obesity, dyslipidaemias, diabetes and hypertension. This is particularly so when combined with a lack of exercise. Dietary fibre protects against colorectal adenomas and carcinomas as well as diverticular disease.

Psychogenic Disorders

Psychogenic disorders are not often a source of surgical disease but factitious disorder (previously referred to as *Munchausen syndrome*) patients may present with abdominal pain and become subjects of repeated laparotomies, psychiatric patients living rough may suffer from exposure and frostbite, and others may repeatedly cause self-harm or swallow foreign bodies, even such items as razor blades or safety pins.

Disorders of Function

A range of common disorders are defined by the functional abnormalities they cause, although their pathogenesis often remains ill understood. The GI tract is particularly susceptible, with conditions, such as idiopathic constipation, irritable bowel syndrome and diverticular disease.

Medical Ethics and Confidentiality

The term *medical ethics* refers to the universal principles upon which medical decisions should be based, and governs the beliefs and actions that influence the day to day judgements of doctors. Whilst benevolence should govern all medical practice, other factors, such as self-interest, money, the distribution of resources and individual technical skills are important motivating factors.

To some extent, the practice of surgery is influenced by the need for self-protection but in trying to avoid litigation, a surgeon may overtreat or overinvestigate in ways that are unnecessary and may even be unethical. A degree of self-interest is inevitable but the guiding principle should be that the patient's interests are paramount. Desirable attributes in a surgeon are listed in Box 1.2.

Surgeons generally aspire to practise their craft in line with the principles of the **Hippocratic Oath**. This originated from the

---

• BOX 1.2	Desirable Attributes in a Surgeon

After Professor George Youngson, Emeritus Prof. of Paediatric Surgery, University of Aberdeen.
- Technical knowledge and clinical experience
- Listening and communication skills with patients, secretary, colleagues and managers
- Qualities of leadership and the ability to work in a team
- Personal attributes—kindness and empathy
- The ability to make reasoned judgements and decisions under pressure, often with incomplete information
- Situation awareness—the ability to collect and synthesise information rapidly
- Problem solving ability—often in situations not previously encountered
- Insight into one's own practice and a willingness to change plans or behaviours if shown to be incorrect. Being prepared to listen and to learn from constructive criticism
- Organisation and planning ability to cope effectively with a heavy workload
- Professional integrity and honesty
- A genuine desire to continue learning and professional development
- Reliability in fulfilling responsibilities and commitments
- The ability to recognise one's own values and principles and understand how they differ from others

---

Greek School of Medicine around 500 BC and its essence is as follows:
- Doctors must be instructed and then registered to protect the public from amateurs and charlatans.
- Medicine is for the benefit of patients, and doctors must avoid doing anything known to cause harm.
- Euthanasia and abortion are prohibited.
- Operations and procedures must be performed only by practitioners with appropriate expertise.
- Doctors must maintain proper professional relationships with their patients and treatment choices should not be governed by motives of profit or favour.
- Doctors should not take advantage of their professional relationships with their patients.
- Medical confidentiality must be respected (see later).

Confidentiality

Patients allow the National Health Service (NHS) to gather sensitive information about their health and personal matters as part of seeking treatment. They do this in confidence and legitimately expect staff will respect this trust.

In the United Kingdom, patient information is held under legal and ethical obligations of confidentiality. This information must not be used or disclosed in a way that might identify a patient without their consent. *Caldicott Guardians* are senior staff in the NHS and social services appointed to protect patient information locally. The doctor's duty of confidence is a legal obligation derived from case law and is a requirement in professional codes of conduct. Even if a patient is unconscious, the duty of confidence is not diminished.

Whilst cases are often discussed over lunch and elsewhere with colleagues, this should not be done in a public place. When patients are discussed at meetings, identification data should be concealed and written notes about patients should not be left lying around or taken from the hospital except using official channels, for example, during patient transfer.

Do Not Resuscitate Orders

A do not resuscitate (DNR) order on a patient's file means that doctors are not required to resuscitate a patient if their heart stops. It is designed to prevent unnecessary suffering and potential side-effects such as pain, broken ribs, ruptured spleen or brain damage. The British Medical Association and the Royal College of Nursing say that DNR orders can be issued **only** after discussion with patients or family, difficult though this may be. Decisions should not be made by junior doctors alone but in consultation with seniors. The most difficult cases are those involving patients who know they are going to die and are suffering pain or other severe symptoms but who could live for months.

All adult patients who are admitted to hospital should have documentation of their resuscitation status. A DNR order does not mean that patients cannot be offered any active treatment. Discussion should take place with the patient and family to set boundaries on acceptable treatment of potentially reversible factors (such as antibiotics for infection), but it may be agreed that it is not appropriate to escalate care to a high dependency unit if the condition significantly deteriorates.

Guidelines for When a DNR May be Issued

- If a patient's condition is such that resuscitation is unlikely to succeed.
- If a mentally competent patient has consistently stated or recorded they do not want to be resuscitated.
- If an advance notice or living will says the patient does not want to be resuscitated.
- If successful resuscitation would not be in the patient's best interest because it would lead to a very poor quality of life.

In the United Kingdom, NHS Trust Hospitals must agree explicit resuscitation policies that respect patients' rights and are readily available to patients, families and carers; policies must be regularly monitored.

Communication

With Patients

Doctor–patient relationships are best learnt by following good examples in the clinic and ward in an apprenticeship model. Patients are vulnerable, often with unpleasant symptoms and usually with little understanding of anatomy, physiology or pathology. They rarely understand the likely progress of a disease or its treatment and may have been conditioned by the media to expect miracle cures or to believe that the latest technology is what they need. Patients take in only about 10% of what is said during a consultation, but this can be improved in the right setting and with reinforcement. Important messages need to be given in comfortable surroundings, without giving the impression the doctor is in a rush, perhaps with family present and with a nurse who can later ensure messages have been understood.

Doctors are in a privileged position, able to make decisions on a patient's behalf that can have dramatic effects on their life and that of their family. Patients these days generally wish to know more about their condition, but can then take greater responsibility for it than in the old days of the paternalistic doctor. Thus an effective doctor–patient relationship involves not only taking an accurate history but also intelligent listening to discover what patients know, or think they know, about their health and likely treatments, and responding to their concerns in ways they can understand. A good interview also involves imagining 'the third eye', how both sides of the consultation might appear to an observer. Patients frequently complain, with good reason, that they 'don't know what is going on'. They pick up bits of information that may be inaccurate, so doctors should anticipate what they should explain to patients and families and give information in a timely fashion.

During the process of diagnosis and treatment, there is often uncertainty and incomplete information, so it is valuable to explain at intervals the stage reached, both to the patient and, with the patient's permission, to relatives. Where there are different treatment options, a balanced view of the alternatives should be given, perhaps with some statistics, but when the doctor has reason to prefer one approach, this should be explained too, and then the patient can make a considered choice. It can be easy to persuade patients to undergo treatment—after all, you are the expert in their eyes—but trust, respect and empathy teach that patients may wish to reflect at leisure. Except in emergencies, patients should be able to go away and consider options rather than having to sign a consent form just before treatment. They may even wish to take a second opinion if choices are uncertain or potentially life-changing; this should be welcomed rather than discouraged. By helping patients understand their condition, their self-management will be more effective. Similarly, key factors such as diet or smoking habits can be discussed in an atmosphere of trust with more hope of success.

Palliative Care

Sometimes cure is not possible. Then quality of life may become the goal, with palliative treatment being offered. Patients generally want to know what will happen, including their mode of dying. Whilst this can be hard to predict, they need to know their symptoms, particularly pain, will be managed effectively and that they will be looked after. Experience teaches it is usually impossible to say with accuracy when a patient will die except a few days before it will happen, so it is unwise to predict life span except in general terms.

Breaking Bad News

All doctors in clinical practice experience the need to break bad news, such as an unfavourable outcome, unsatisfactory care, a cancer diagnosis or a poor prognosis. It is an event doctors tend to remember and a moment in the patient or relative's life they will never forget.

Ideally, bad news should be conveyed by the most senior member of the team but in reality, bad things often happen at night, often in the A&E department, and the most junior doctor is the one on the spot. Discuss what is to be said with your seniors even under these circumstances wherever possible. The following general points apply:

- Bad news is private. Find a quiet space, preferably an office with chairs (you do not need a desk).
- Avoid hiding behind jargon: 'the metastatic nature of the neoplasm makes it inoperable' is useless. 'I'm sorry to say that the cancer has spread and an operation won't help' is better.
- Give time and space; turn off pagers and phones if possible.
- Do not be defensive and do not be afraid to express regret.
- Avoid filling the silence of grief with continuous chatter.
- Allow time for questions. If you do not know the answer, say so and try to find out.
- Always offer another meeting, ideally with the head of the team.

- Many patients/families will wish to discuss what has been imparted with their family doctor, so it is vital that you get all information to the GP before that visit.

Communicating With Colleagues

Communicating with colleagues involves speaking, both face to face and on the telephone (Box 1.3), and writing (handwriting, dictating, typing, emailing) patient notes, information letters to patient or family practitioners, for example, after an outpatient consultation, referral letters, discharge summaries, reports and presentations for local or larger scale medical meetings. All of these need to be honest, accurate and timely, particularly when communicating patient information. Remember, recipients are entitled to rely on what you have written in their later treatment of a patient. Also any written information may be called in evidence in a court of law should something go wrong later. Patient notes must *never* be altered later, although rarely, amendments may be *added* provided they are signed and dated.

Hospital doctors work in teams where it is important to know one's responsibilities and those of everybody else, and to understand when to call for help in good time. Changes in a patient's condition usually need to be passed on to other team members. If you have made a mistake, admit it early and do everything you can to mitigate it.

With diminishing junior doctors' hours, it is vital to have structured *handover* of patients to the incoming team at the end of shifts and at weekends and holidays, including especially details of ill patients and those with complex management problems and any agreed plans for them.

Communication via the Clinical Record

Reduced junior hospital doctors' hours make it imperative to keep the written records for every patient up to date, including management plans and what to do if predictable changes occur. Date and legibly sign each entry giving your name in capitals and grade,

record important test results and write instructions for antibiotic and deep vein thrombosis (DVT) prophylaxis. In high operative risk patients, seniors should document discussions before surgery. After operation, write or type an operation note with clear postoperative instructions so these are immediately available to recovery and ward staff.

Document details of any discussions with patient and relatives—particularly about poor prognosis or withdrawal of active treatment and who has been told about this or about a diagnosis of malignancy. Regarding a discharge summary, ensure all investigation results have been checked and the diagnosis and future plans have been recorded and send it immediately on discharge. If the patient died, record the cause of death in the notes as it is written on the certificate and inform the family doctor.

Evidence-Based Medicine and Guidelines

History

Evidence-based medicine (EBM) as now understood really began when Professor Archie Cochrane, a Scottish epidemiologist, published his book *Effectiveness and Efficiency: Random Reflections on Health Services* in 1972 and continued with his later advocacy of its principles. EBM has gradually gained political support and acceptance within the medical profession. EBM calls into question the traditional belief that 'we've always based our practice on science'. Cochrane's work has been recognised by the proliferation of Cochrane Centres and the international Cochrane Collaboration, all devoted to meticulously evaluating evidence and promoting its use.

The aim of EBM is to apply best scientific evidence to clinical decision making. It relies on critical assessment of published evidence about risks and benefits of treatments (or lack of treatment) and of diagnostic tests. Only between 50% and 80% of the volume of medical treatments are evidence based, with better evidence available for more common treatments. Statements by medical experts are seen as the least valid form of evidence, but evidence-based practice is not relevant where imponderables, such as quality of life judgements are involved. **Evidence-based guidelines (EBG)** have an appeal to health economists, policymakers and managers as they help to measure performance and perhaps justify rationing or centralising resources.

Austin Bradford Hill, the grandfather of modern medical research, who was fundamental in discovering the link between smoking and lung cancer, produced a set of guidelines, as given in Box 1.4, for assessing *causality*, that is, the relationship between an exposure and an outcome, and these remain the foundation of EBM today.

• BOX 1.3 Effective Telephone Consultation and Handover

When you need to consult a consultant or colleague by telephone about a patient, particularly during unsocial hours, you must clarify details yourself before phoning. Think through the case, pinpointing key elements listed subsequently:

- On phoning, state your name and status (on-call SpR for instance) and say at the outset what you think you want—whether advice or for the consultant to come in.
- Summarise the case succinctly, visualising how your description appears to the listener.
- When did the problem start (day, time)?
- What circumstances necessitated the patient coming to hospital?
- What was the patient's state on arrival (conscious/unconscious; wounds or bleeding; level of pain; resuscitation status)?
- Did you examine the patient and establish the signs or were they reported to you?
- Is there any relevant past history?
- What has progress been since arrival?
- What investigations have been ordered and what results do you have so far?
- Are any other specialists involved, for example, plastics or orthopaedics?
- Finally, indicate again what you want the consultant to do.

• BOX 1.4 Guidelines for Assessing the Relationship Between an Exposure and an Outcome

- A strong and consistent association, specific to the problem being studied
- The supposed cause must come before the possible effect
- There should ideally be a biological gradient or dose-response effect
- The association should be consistent with what is already known or at least not completely at odds with it
- It should be biologically plausible

Cherry-Picking the Evidence Versus Systematic Review

Cherry-picking is a dubious means of reinforcing what you already believe, the very opposite of systematic review. It involves relying only on published work that supports your view and finding reasons to ignore what goes against it. The solution is a process of systematic review as conducted by the Cochrane Collaboration. Their methodologies were largely established at McMaster University. The term EBM first appeared in 1992 and journals devoted to the subject have included the British Medical Journal's *Clinical Evidence*, the *Journal of Evidence-Based Healthcare* and *Evidence Based Health Policy*, all co-founded by Anna Donald, an Australian pioneer.

EBM encourages clinicians to integrate valid and useful scientific evidence into their clinical expertise. Using systematic reviews, meta-analyses, risk-benefit analyses and randomised controlled trials (RCTs), EBM aims that health professionals make 'conscientious, explicit, and judicious use of current best evidence' in everyday practice. Systematic review of published research studies is a very important method of evaluating treatments. An explicit search strategy is used finding relevant data, both published and raw and unpublished. The methodological quality of each study is evaluated, ideally blind to the results. Alternative treatments are compared, and then a critical, weighted summary is given. This thorough sifting of information often reveals large knowledge gaps and sometimes grossly flawed 'best practices'; it has saved numerous lives without undertaking new research studies. Sir Muir Gray, an internationally respected authority on healthcare systems, has commented 'advances will be made through clean, clear information'.

The Cochrane Collaboration is perhaps the best known, most rigorous and respected organisation providing systematic reviews. Once the best evidence has been assessed, treatment is rated as 'likely to be beneficial', 'likely to be harmful', or 'evidence did not indicate benefit or harm'. A 2007 analysis of 1016 systematic reviews from all 50 Cochrane Collaboration Review Groups found 44% of the interventions beneficial, 7% harmful and 49% where the evidence did not support benefit or harm. Ninety-six percent recommended further research.

When it comes to new or radical ideas, well-trained experts using clinical common sense should be able to make rational judgements about what is likely to be true; the more unlikely the claims for a new treatment, the higher must be the standard of proper evidence.

Longitudinal or Cohort Studies

For predicting prognosis, the highest level of evidence is a systemic review of *inception cohort studies*, that is, groups of patients assembled near the onset of the disorder. These groups are followed over years to determine how variables, such as smoking habits, exercise, occupation and geography may affect outcome. Prospective studies take years to perform but are valued more than retrospective studies, which are more likely to generate bias.

Ranking the Quality of Evidence (Box 1.5)

The strongest evidence for therapeutic interventions is by systematic review of randomised, double- or triple-blind, placebo-controlled trials with allocation concealment and complete follow-up, in a homogeneous patient population and medical condition. In

---

• BOX 1.5   How Cochrane Centres Evaluate Evidence

Note that the hierarchy of evidence relates to the strength of the literature and not necessarily to its clinical importance.
1. Strength of evidence
   a. *Level of evidence*: that is, is the evidence a true measure of the benefit of an intervention? In descending order of reliability:
      • Cochrane (or equivalent quality) systematic reviews of all relevant randomised controlled trials (RCTs).
      • At least one well-conducted RCT.
      • A nonrandomised trial assigning participants to a treatment group alternately or by date or time of arrival, for example.
      • Nonrandomised studies where a control group ran concurrently with an intervention group.
      • Nonrandomised studies where intervention effects are compared with historical data.
      • Single case studies.
      • Opinion of experienced experts—'conventional wisdom'.
   b. *Quality of evidence*: determined by how well the study methods minimise bias.
   c. *Statistical precision*: the degree of certainty about whether a measured effect truly exists.
2. Size of effect
   For clinically relevant benefits or harms, how far away is the outcome of the intervention from 'no apparent effect'?
3. Relevance of the evidence
   How appropriate is the outcome for the healthcare problem studied, and how useful is it for measuring the benefits (or harms) of the treatment? To which groups or subgroups of patients may the results apply?
4. The likely range of the true effect
   Studies that are well designed and carried out can show unreliable results because of chance. **Confidence interval** (CI) describes the likely range of the true effect. For example, a study may show that 40% (95% CI, 30%–50%) of people appear to be helped by a treatment; we can thus be 95% certain the true effect lies between 30% and 50%.

---

contrast, patient testimonials, case reports, and even expert opinion have lesser value because of the placebo effect, biases inherent in observation and reporting, and personal and institutional biases.

A series of classifications of the strength of different types of evidence have been fashioned, grading them according to their freedom from biases that plague medical research; all are based around the same descending hierarchy:
• Systematic reviews of RCTs
• Individual RCTs
• Controlled observational studies—cohort and case control studies
• Uncontrolled observational studies and case reports
• Established practice and expert opinion (not to be confused with personal experience, sometimes dubbed eminence-based medicine). Expert opinion may be the best guide in the absence of good research evidence

Other Classifications of Quality of Evidence

For a review of classifications of evidence, see:
https://patient.info/doctor/Different-Levels-of-Evidence
For access to the GRADE system of assessing the strength of recommendation and quality of evidence in systematic review see:
https://www.jclinepi.com/article/S0895-4356(10)00330-6/abstract

Quality and Limitations of Clinical Trials

Trials must now be registered in advance: the *Declaration of Helsinki 2008* requires that every clinical trial be registered in a publicly accessible database before recruitment of the first subject. The International Committee of Medical Journal Editors refuses to publish clinical trial results if the trial was not recorded in this way. This should eliminate the bias inherent in the failure to publish negative trials.

In 1993 30 medical journal editors, clinical trialists, epidemiologists and methodologists met in Ottawa to develop a new scale to assess the quality of RCT reports. This eventually resulted in the Consolidated Standards of Reporting Trials (CONSORT) Statement, published in 1996 and now largely adhered to by respected medical journals (http://www.consort-statement.org/). Cochrane adheres to similar standards and uses software 'RevMan' to help reviewers evaluate published studies.

Resources

- Cochrane Library: http://www.cochranelibrary.com/
- UK National Institute for Health and Care Excellence (NICE): https://www.nice.org.uk/
- NHS search engine for Evidence in Health and Social Care (from NICE): https://www.evidence.nhs.uk/

Guidelines

Clinical guidelines, practice policies, protocols and codes of practice are locally or more widely published mechanisms aimed at harmonising processes of care using best practice. Some are produced by surgical societies, such as the Association of Surgeons of Great Britain and Ireland (ASGBI). Guidelines should be just that—providing a structure rather than absolute ways to proceed in every case; they may be varied if clinical conditions dictate. Guidelines should have an evidence basis or be of proven clinical effectiveness and need regular review as evidence accumulates. Local guidelines are a natural outcome of clinical audit studies (see p. 11, later).

Keeping Up to Date: Continuing Professional Development (CPD)

Clinicians are quite properly expected to keep up with current developments and to demonstrate this to be revalidated. Surgical knowledge and wisdom can be acquired by reading, from seniors in clinic and on ward rounds, by discussion at local and regional meetings and by attending courses. Meetings may include journal clubs, case presentations, reviews of specific topics, and presentation of research or audit projects. Broad national update meetings are valuable and in the United Kingdom, include the ASGBI and speciality meetings, such as the Vascular Society and the British Orthopaedic Association. Meetings are a forum for trainees to present their work, learn from other presentations and find out what is current from colleagues. Surgeons in the United Kingdom are required to keep a log-book record of their educational activities to demonstrate their continued learning and this document forms part of regular appraisal and revalidation.

Consent to Treatment

Treatment against a patient's will is only rarely justifiable. Clearing the airways of someone about to choke to death who is irrational because of impaired consciousness can easily be justified on the grounds that the patient would have wanted it if fully rational. UK common law holds that an adult of sound mind has the right to determine what is done with his body and a surgeon who performs an operation without consent commits an assault in the eyes of the law. The General Medical Council (GMC) guidance on consent can be accessed via: https://www.gmc-uk.org/ethical-guidance/ethical-guidance-for-doctors/consent

When Is Consent Necessary?

Ideally, medical treatment should not proceed without first obtaining the patient's consent. Consent may be *expressed*, or it may be *implied*, as when a patient presents for examination and acquiesces in the suggested procedure. Expressed permission can be based on an oral or a written agreement. Most invasive investigations (such as upper GI endoscopy or arteriography) and any surgical operation should be preceded by written consent, ideally well in advance to give the patient time to think it over. If oral consent alone has been obtained, then a note should be made in the patient's record.

A doctor may proceed without consent if the patient's balance of mind is disturbed or if the patient is incapable of giving consent because of unconsciousness. The same principles apply if the patient is a minor, but it is sensible to seek consent from responsible relatives or to check with colleagues that the planned action is in the patient's best interest. Opinions should be recorded in the notes before action is taken.

The Unconscious Patient

Under the *necessity principle*, a surgeon is justified in treating a patient without expressed consent if what he seeks to protect is more valuable than the wrongful act, that is, treating without consent, provided there is no objection to treatment. Treatment must be no more extensive than is essential and procedures not needed for the patient's survival must not be performed. For example, a diseased testis could be removed during a hernia repair but sterilising a patient during a Caesarean section without consent constitutes assault.

Ambiguous wording on consent forms requiring a patient to agree to any operation the surgeon considers necessary is regarded by the courts as completely worthless. For this reason, a model consent form was produced by the NHS Executive in 1990 to be used throughout the health services.

Practical Aspects of Consent for Treatment

In British law, there is no such thing as informed consent. Surgeons like to feel they obtain informed consent after explaining to the patient in nontechnical language the nature, purpose and risks of the proposed investigation or treatment, together with alternatives and the likely outcome of treatment. It is good practice to provide a printed information leaflet on the specific operation detailing the procedure, alternatives, risks and recovery. The patient must be capable of understanding the explanation and if this is not the case then informed consent has not been obtained. It follows that consent cannot be obtained from patients who are unconscious or of unsound mind.

Obtaining Consent (Box 1.6)

There has been a significant change in UK law following the case of Montgomery versus the East Lanarkshire Health Board whereby the process of consent must stand the test that a reasonable body of patients and relatives would understand the benefits and disadvantages of all possible treatments for the particular condition.

• BOX 1.6   The Informed Consent Process

The informed consent process should include:

- a description of the procedure or operation and anaesthetic;
- why the procedure is recommended and the risks and benefits;
- the degree of severity and likelihood of complications;
- treatment alternatives with related risks and benefits;
- probable consequences of declining the recommended or alternative therapies;
- name of doctor conducting the procedure and the anaesthetic;
- other doctors performing tasks related to the procedure.

This now supersedes the Bolam test in law, which relied only upon a reasonable body of medical opinion supporting a particular course of treatment. Consent should be obtained by a doctor sufficiently knowledgeable to explain the treatment, any alternatives, the likely outcome and any significant risks. Sometimes trained nurses obtain a first-stage consent, which is confirmed by a doctor later.

The types and level of risk that have to be discussed are not well defined, but a risk of complication or potential failure to treat the condition of 5% to 10% should certainly be discussed. Operation-specific or disease-specific risks must be explained (e.g., facial nerve damage in parotid surgery, hypoparathyroidism following thyroid surgery) and the discussion detailed in the records. General risks, such as DVT or pneumonia are not usually discussed but this does place doubt on whether such consent is truly informed.

Discussion before consent should occur in an unhurried manner, giving the patient time to absorb the information, to question the doctor obtaining consent and to indicate treatments he/she does not want. The patient may wish to discuss aspects of what is proposed with family or friends before consenting. In patients incapable of giving consent, it is customary to obtain consent from a near relative, and for the doctor to complete a consent form 4 (for adults who lack capacity). Whilst not essential in law, this represents good practice.

Most patients do not read the forms they sign before undergoing treatment; more than half do not understand them; and only a quarter of forms include all the data needed to make an informed decision. The US Department of Veterans Affairs has adopted an electronic informed-consent software program with a digital pad to sign, with details stored in their medical record. The program, known as *iMedConsent*, includes a library of anatomical diagrams and explanations at easy reading level for 2000+ procedures in 30+ specialties. The process was initially slow to perform, but soon became quick. Patients having elective procedures could now gain all the information they needed in advance and it was easy to check they had understood it. The main disadvantage is that these privately produced programs are expensive.

Consent in Children

Consent can be obtained from children aged 16 years and over and occasionally in those under 16 years. It is always sensible to liaise with parents wherever possible in young people aged 17 and 18 years. In the absence of parents, another relative or person 'in loco parentis' can give consent for children.

For children in care, the local authority usually has full parental rights and the director of social services or deputy needs to sign the consent form. If the child is in voluntary care, the parents still act as guardians and their consent should be obtained.

Jehovah's Witnesses

Adult Jehovah's Witnesses usually refuse blood or blood product transfusion even in an extreme emergency because of their interpretation of part of the Bible. If permission to transfuse is withheld, then blood should not be given. Failure to respect the patient's wish may result in an accusation of battery. The moral dilemma of allowing a patient to die when blood transfusion is likely to prevent death is uncomfortable but the law is clear. General advice is that a surgeon cannot refuse to treat simply because the patient imposes conditions on that treatment, although it may be possible to transfer the patient to a compliant surgeon's care. In these circumstances, it is wise to interview the patient in the presence of a witness and explain the risks. The discussion should be noted and the witness should sign the hospital record.

In elective cases where anaemia needs to be treated to optimise the patient preoperatively, they may accept synthetic (recombinant) erythropoietin, which stimulates bone marrow to replace red blood cells. Some may consider the use of a cell saver during major surgery (anticipated to experience high blood loss) to harvest blood, process it and then reinfuse back into the body if required.

In children of Jehovah's Witnesses the position is different. If a blood or blood product transfusion is needed to save the life of a child or to prevent harm, the transfusion can be given and defended in law by claiming that the decision was taken in the best interests of the child. If parental consent is withheld and there is ample time, the child can be made a ward of court, but this is not essential to obtain consent. If the decision to give blood is made, a second medical opinion confirming the need should be obtained if time allows. It is important to realise that a child subjected to transfusion against parental wishes may be rejected by the parents.

Clinical Governance and Clinical Audit

Clinical governance is a systematic approach to preserving and advancing the quality of patient care within a health system. Since the 1970s, there has been a growing realisation that looking critically at the way we run our clinical practice, and then taking active steps to move ahead, is much more effective than simply following time-honoured practices or even opening new avenues of research. In the United Kingdom, this movement is now universal but with varying degrees of success. Clinical governance starts with the mindset that the *quality of care* matters; it embodies a range of activities described here and elsewhere in this chapter.

Management Attitude to Quality of Care

Health service managers have to keep quality of care high on their long list of priorities and facilitate clinicians' initiatives.

Education and Training of Clinical Staff

Thorough and well-rounded teaching in medical and nursing school, including anatomy and surgery, is the starting point. Training posts then need to offer a wide range of experience in an apprenticeship model, including step-by-step learning of procedures to back up continuing medical education, as well as specific courses, such as Advanced Trauma Life Support (ATLS). During training, good behaviours, attitudes and judgement can be acquired (see attributes of a good surgeon, earlier). All clinicians need to remain open-minded to change and remember it is their professional duty to remain up to date.

Clinical Audit

Clinical audit reviews clinical performance against agreed standards, refining clinical practice and then reauditing—a cyclical process of improving quality.

Clinical Effectiveness

Clinical effectiveness studies evaluate the extent to which an intervention works, its efficiency, safety, appropriateness and value for money. Studies of this type can be instructive and worthwhile for trainees to undertake.

Research and Development

Professional practice can change in the light of good research evidence, provided it can be implemented effectively. EBM involves critical appraisal of the literature and development of EBGs, protocols and implementation strategies from research.

Clinical Performance

Poor performance and poor practice often thrive behind closed doors but can be revealed by a local climate of openness; this also demonstrates the organisation meets the needs of its population. In surgery, trouble may come to light through morbidity and mortality meetings, clinical audit, via patient complaints or by 'whistle blowing', and these should provide the motor for change. Critical incident meetings, for example, can thoroughly examine particular adverse events and recommend change.

Nationally in the United Kingdom, the National Patient Safety Agency (http://www.npsa.nhs.uk/) 'informs, supports and influences healthcare organisations and individuals' by handling patient safety incidents, by running national independent Confidential Enquiries (NCEPOD in surgery and anaesthesia), by encouraging ethical research, and by developing and implementing safety recommendations, advice and strategies. Through the Practitioner Performance Advice, formerly the National Clinical Assessment Service (https://resolution.nhs.uk/services/practitioner-performance-advice/), it endeavours to solve concerns about the performance of health practitioners short of referral to the General Medical Council.

Risk Management

This is a prospective process to identify hazards that could cause harm, decide who might be harmed and how, then evaluate the risks and decide on precautions. Risks in a health service include risks to patients, risks to practitioners and risks to the organisation itself. Recognising in advance where particular risks lie is the first step to minimising those risks. Areas of potentially high risk include:

Older people: surgeons deal with an increasingly elderly population. The likelihood of comorbid disease is higher, although chronological age by itself is less important than biological age
Emergency surgery: this carries a higher risk of complications and death than elective surgery. Patients may be more physiologically disrupted or not fully resuscitated, intervention may be required out-of-hours when the ideal mix of staff is not available; investigations, such as computed tomography (CT) scanning may also not be so readily available
Day surgery: preoperative assessment can preselect patients for day surgery and minimise risk

Critically ill patients: these patients need optimising before surgery, often with shared care with a senior anaesthetist, physician or other specialist. More preoperative investigations and resuscitation may be needed, perhaps in an intensive care unit or high dependency unit. The initial surgical approach may become a damage limitation exercise with more realistic expectations about outcome
Operative risk assessment: the American Society of Anaesthesiologists grade scheme gives anaesthetist and surgeon a subjective idea of how sick the patient is and the likely outcome.

Information Management

Information management is vital to facilitate good, effective and economic practice. For example, high quality and available patient notes, systems for ordering laboratory and imaging tests and receiving results, accurate and prompt discharge summaries, easy outpatient booking, good feedback to family practitioners and reliable A&E systems. Hand-written methods have been used for many years in the United Kingdom, however because of advances in many hospitals, electronic ('paperless') systems are now flourishing, following success in the United States. In addition, the use of individual smart cards for patients to hold their own records, and easily portable devices, such as the iPad, hold promise for the future use in patient care, provided clinicians take sufficient interest in their development.

Surgical (Clinical) Audit

Research is concerned with discovering the right thing to do; audit with ensuring that it is done right.

RICHARD SMITH, FORMER EDITOR BMJ

There is a tendency to be overoptimistic or even defensive about one's own practice. Yet patients, referring doctors, medical defence organisations (who defend the professional reputations of members when their clinical performance is called into question) and those paying for health care (governments and their agents and private insurers) are entitled to know that the quality of care provided in a given unit is up to standard. Examining morbidity and mortality at regular meetings within a unit ('significant event' reviews) are important but suffer from inherent weaknesses, such as defensiveness, incomplete data and rivalry. These meetings usually fail to address overarching problems, such as wound infection rates, or aspects of care from the patient's point of view, such as delayed treatment, off-hand consultations, poor pain control and failure to give explanations. It is well established that medical errors are generally more likely to be caused by a system failure than an individual error and system errors are unlikely to be discovered by these morbidity and mortality meetings.

Clinical audit is a means by which clinicians can be collectively accountable for the care they provide and demonstrate its quality to outsiders. It requires a mechanism for scrutiny of each other's work in a nonthreatening and constructive manner or else it would not function. In brief, a group of clinicians examines a topic of concern and agrees in advance what are acceptable standards of practice or outcomes, ideally based on published norms ('the gold standard'). In other words, they establish and sign up to a set of standards for **indicator based audit**. The process embodies specific objectives, accepting peer review and being committed to change should weaknesses be revealed.

Once a topic is agreed, an **audit cycle** can begin with a pilot project on a small number of subjects, perhaps 20. A questionnaire is designed which ideally is capable of being completed retrospectively by nonclinical staff from hospital notes. With the pilot results, methods are refined and a larger scale project undertaken. Results are analysed by the group and necessary changes, and how these should be implemented, agreed. This is the most thorny aspect of clinical audit and the most difficult to achieve. Once the necessary changes have been implemented, the same audit needs to be repeated after a defined interval (completing the audit cycle) to bring the process up to a quality assurance mechanism.

Clinicians do need to be trained in audit methods and helped to design audits that are useful and sound. It is best to start with a simple project, such as, for example, what proportion of the entries in the notes is clearly signed.

Medical Research Versus Medical Audit

Medical research is used on a one-off basis to determine scientifically how interventions affect outcomes. Clinical audit measures how effectively aspects of good health care are put into practice. Every doctor can improve the way patients are cared for by critically examining local practices against current standards using audit methods.

Clinical audit and research share common features including defining explicitly what is to be measured and analysing and interpreting the data without bias. Audit can improve understanding of system failures, help develop guidelines and identify areas for education and training.

Carrying Out an Audit (Box 1.7)

Selecting topics for audit means taking into consideration how frequent the condition or treatment is, how high the risk to patients is, whether there is doubt about which treatment is the best, where care crosses specialty boundaries and finally, any topics of particular concern to clinicians or professions allied to medicine.

Single subject audits usually require no more than 50 patients to reveal problems and plan improvements. Subjects focus on aspects of the process of care (including resources used), appropriateness of tests or treatments or outcomes of treatment. They may include subjects, such as adequacy of pain relief from the patient's point of view or, from the family doctor's point of view, how long a discharge summary takes to be received.

The group then develops an audit indicator, which has objective, measurable standards of care and specifies a percentage of cases expected to reach the standard. For example, perhaps 100% of patients referred for palliative radiotherapy for lung cancer should receive their first treatment in less than 10 days after referral, or wound infection rates after appendicectomy should be no more than 3%. These indicators (known as **criteria**) can be based on published results, on previous local results or on standards the group hopes to achieve after running a pilot study.

Deficiencies usually turn out to be caused by **system failure**, such as poor coordination between departments (e.g., preassessment between anaesthesia and surgery) or poor communication between clinicians, with people not being informed about what is happening when. These factors are usually more important than lack of resources or personnel or poor individual performance. Improvements may result from simple organisational changes.

Peer Group Review of Medical Audit Data

Using audit indicators has advantages over raw data analysis or informal morbidity meetings. As standards have of necessity been agreed, any numbers of cases can be screened to select out for

---

• BOX 1.7 Key Elements of Criterion-Based or Indicator-Based Audit

- Looks in a structured way at a small problematic aspect of care
- Criteria need to be agreed in advance by all clinicians involved
- Time is needed to plan and pilot the audit, discuss the results, implement change then reaudit after a period
- Whether criteria have been met must be reliably retrievable by nonmedical audit officers
- Recognition that there may be more than one valid way of achieving a solution

---

further discussion only those that vary from the standard. In itself, the process of refining and employing audit indicators is an educational experience that encourages self-analysis by individuals, departments, units or regions.

Examples of How Clinical Audit Can Improve the Quality of Care

- Reduction of risk of morbidity or mortality
- Improved effectiveness of care, such as streamlined processes of treatment
- Improvement in diagnosis—availability, appropriateness or quality
- Improved timing of care—reduced delay, better planning, efficient use of facilities
- Better use of resources—equipment, beds, support services, money
- Consumer satisfaction—patients and referring doctors
- Access to care—availability of diagnostic services and treatment
- Documentation and records—improved recording of the process of care
- Identifying educational needs by audit activity—for example, pain management

Confidential Enquiry Into Perioperative Deaths (CEPOD)

The pilot study was designed in 1983 jointly by the ASGBI and the Association of Anaesthetists to examine perioperative deaths and the delivery of surgical and anaesthetic care in Britain. This was followed by a review of all deaths within 30 days of surgery (all specialties) in three English Regions for the whole of 1986: 500,000 operations were reviewed with 4000 deaths (0.8%); 79% of deaths occurred in patients over 65 years of age. More information is available from: http://www.ncepod.org.uk/, including all published reports from 1987 onwards.

Educational Lessons From CEPOD

Many of the substandard practices identified could be put down to a lack of education or training in particular fields. These included:
- when and how to investigate
- when to give prophylaxis against infection and thromboembolism
- when to delay operation to resuscitate
- when not to operate
- when to call the consultant
- management of head injuries
- managing comorbid disease and the elderly
- keeping accurate records
- safe use of local anaesthetics
- local protocols for referral, handover and transfer
- organising effective audit or morbidity and mortality meetings

Research in Surgery

How Are Potentially Improved Methods Evaluated?

When new surgical techniques appear, they must be dispassionately evaluated and compared with existing practices, ideally by people with no vested interest. For a new technique to be introduced, it must be at least as good as existing methods or better in some way, for example, in achieving oncological clearance. New methods should be easily and quickly learnt—an operation that requires a learning curve of 500 patients is of little use to those 500. Methods need to be reasonably economical in equipment and in operating time and high-level hazards should be no greater than existing operations. While this may seem utopian, 'the greatest uncontrolled medical experiment of all', namely the introduction of laparoscopic cholecystectomy, was undoubtedly at the expense of a massive increase in common bile duct injuries. The proper view should be that the safety of the many outweighs the foibles of the few.

It was encouraging that laparoscopic hernia repair was not allowed to escape peer review in the same way, with multicentre trials comparing the existing standard of Lichtenstein open repair with the prospective standard of laparoscopic repair. Laparoscopic colorectal surgery has now been shown to give improved short-term outcomes with evidence of reduced pain, more rapid discharge from hospital and return to normal activities. However, recent multicentre noninferiority trials from Europe, the United States, Korea and Australasia have questioned long-term oncological outcomes. The response of the global surgical community to these data will be a watershed moment for the way clinical conduct is properly scrutinised, and research evidence is applied. Similar clinical scrutiny of outcomes applies to other new developments in surgery including robotic-assisted laparoscopic surgical techniques which are rapidly gaining popularity and wider-spread clinical use.

Design of Research and Experiments

All British health authorities have to establish an Ethics Committee charged with examining and sanctioning each research project before it is launched. They help ensure that all projects are ethical and can be justified and that the methodology is sound. Among medical members, these committees generally include lawyers, ethicists, statisticians and lay members.

Clinical Trials

Drug Trials

Once a potential drug has been identified, say from a likely plant molecule, a cell receptor that might be influenced or a modification of an old drug, it is tested for toxicity in animals and to see if it works. Then Phase I trials 'first in man' are performed on a few healthy young people. This is for toxicity, excretion rates and pathways, etc. If this works, Phase II trials in perhaps 200 people with the relevant illness are performed as 'proof of concept' to see if the drug is effective and to work out the dose. Many drugs fail at this point. Then Phase III trials are performed in hundreds or thousands of patients. These are randomised, blinded trials comparing the new drug against placebo or comparable treatments. More data on efficacy and safety is collected. Once successful trials are complete, the company applies for a licence to sell the drug. After it reaches market, the company and others usually conduct further trials and studies to look out for unnoticed side-effects.

However, trials do not tell the whole story: in the 1960s thalidomide, a very effective drug for morning sickness, had not been tested in pregnancy, and this led to many avoidable birth deformities in countries where it had been licensed.

Trial Design and Conduct

For a surgical trial, background work establishes the depth of current knowledge and the need for a trial. The hypothesis to be tested should be defined before designing the study and perhaps the need for a pilot study.

In general, *prospective studies* ensure that data are accrued chronologically and that patients are entered into the trial as they become available. However, it may take months (or even years) to recruit enough patients to make the data meaningful.

Retrospective analyses of previously recorded data are open to criticism because of the lack of an appropriate control group and the difficulty of extracting complete data from case notes. Despite flaws, a retrospective study may show the need for a prospective study, give some idea of the likely results and allow the trial design to be streamlined.

Longitudinal studies examine the effects of therapy on a predetermined population or epidemiological changes in a population.

Cross-sectional studies take a 'snap shot' at a particular time and place; these are most commonly used to monitor the incidence and location of diseases and treatment.

For most trials, computer randomisation removes the natural tendency for bias to affect results and is particularly relevant when comparing new treatments with tried and tested techniques. This is often 'blinded' such that neither the patient (single blind), or neither the patient nor the investigator (double blind), knows which arm an individual has been allocated to. Any therapeutic effect of placebos is maximised if patients are unaware of the nature of their treatment. The double-blind technique attempts to eliminate personal preferences of the doctor for a particular treatment. To study the effects of a treatment in a particular environment, like must be compared with like and a case control study used. Matching of individuals for characteristics, such as weight, sex, age and disease severity allow comparisons to be made when looking for small differences between groups.

Once the study design has been established, an achievable cohort size must be identified which has sufficient power to show differences between treatments and organise data collection, storage and analysis. After that, it is necessary to establish inclusion and exclusion criteria, the population size and characteristics to be studied and then to determine how the data will be analysed and presented statistically.

Specialised personnel, equipment and training must be funded. Worthwhile research is expensive and should not be undertaken simply for the sake of the CV.

Patient Safety

Dealing With an Adverse Event

- Apologise to the patient for the failure as soon as the error is recognised.
- Report to your consultant and other responsible people.
- Take steps to correct the error and make sure you see the patient often.
- If an official complaint is made, patient letters are usually sent to the patient advice and liaison service then to the department managers.

- If asked to comment, provide full and honest detail.
- If legal action is threatened, contact your medical insurance society.
- Adverse outcomes should be discussed at local meetings to seek system problems.

Introduction

'First do no harm', an aphorism attributed to Thomas Sydenham, an English physician in the mid-1600s, is sound advice for surgeons too. All surgical treatments should be thought of in terms of their potential harm as well as benefit.

Some hazards are intrinsic to the surgical procedure or disease and are unavoidable. Other hazards are avoidable, and systems need to be designed to assist. Furthermore, the surgeon's prime responsibility is to the patient so, for example, prioritising an operation should be based on need not on financial or managerial grounds, although surgeons have responsibilities to balance demands as far as possible.

To Err is Human is an influential report published by the US Institute of Medicine in 1999 that is well worth reading. It called for a national effort to make health care safer. The recent impetus given to **Human Factors** training by governments, surgical regulatory bodies and commissioners is a welcome move to protect both patients and surgeons. Human factors are, in short, all the things that make us unpredictable individuals. The scope of Human Factors is broad and includes team working, communication, risk management, situational awareness and self-management (stress and fatigue).

General Hazards

The two most common sources of error leading to patient harm are communication failures and drug prescribing errors. Some 26% of 100 consecutive cases referred to the Medical Protection Society resulted from communication failure. There need to be explicit systems for dealing with risky situations, for example, informing seniors about sick patients, handing over properly to staff coming on duty, knowing who to call about patients that have 'gone off' during unsocial hours. This applies especially to anyone not familiar with the patient's current state, particularly locums, who are unlikely to be familiar with how things work locally.

Drug prescribing is fraught with dangers: illegible prescription, wrong drug, wrong dose, unexpected drug interactions or failure to elicit a history of allergy or idiosyncrasy. Electronic prescribing systems with built-in warnings of interactions help, but so does the regular presence of a ward pharmacist.

Theatre Safety

The period between a patient entering the operating department and leaving the recovery unit is potentially hazardous for both the patient and the staff (Boxes 1.8 and 1.9). A fully conscious patient has automatic defence mechanisms to avoid injury but when anaesthetised or recovering, relies on the care of trained staff.

All operating theatres have safety protocols, with patients' identities, nature and type of operation, allergies, etc., being repeatedly checked—but errors still occur. The WHO has developed a well-tested tool for minimising errors using a simple three-stage checklist for each case: before induction of anaesthesia (with at least nurse and anaesthetist), before the skin incision (with nurse, anaesthetist and surgeon) and before the patient leaves the operating room (with nurse, anaesthetist and surgeon). This is now used extensively around the world; see Box 1.8 and http://www.who.int/patientsafety/safesurgery/en/

• BOX 1.8   World Health Organization Surgical Safety Checklist 2009 (Revised 1/2009 WHO, 2009)[a]

Checks Before Induction of Anaesthesia (With at Least Nurse and Anaesthetist)

- Has the patient confirmed his/her identity, site, procedure and consent? Yes
- Is the site marked? Yes/Not applicable
- Is the anaesthesia machine and medication check complete? Yes
- Is the pulse oximeter on the patient and functioning? Yes
- Does the patient have a known allergy? No/Yes
- Difficult airway or aspiration risk?
  - No
  - Yes, and equipment/assistance available
- Risk of >500 mL blood loss (7 mL/kg in children)?
  - No
  - Yes, and two intravenous lines, central access and fluids planned

Before Skin Incision (With Nurse, Anaesthetist and Surgeon)
All Team Members

- Confirm all team members have introduced themselves by name and role.
- Confirm the patient's name, procedure and where the incision will be made.
- Has antibiotic prophylaxis been given within the last 60 minutes? Yes/Not applicable
- Anticipated critical events.

To Surgeon

- What are the critical or non-routine steps?
- How long will the procedure take?
- What is the anticipated blood loss?

To Anaesthetist

- Are there any patient-specific concerns?

To Nursing Team

- Has sterility (including indicator results) been confirmed?
- Are there equipment issues or any concerns?
- Is essential imaging displayed? Yes/Not applicable

Before Patient Leaves Operating Room (With Nurse, Anaesthetist and Surgeon)
Nurse Verbally Confirms

- The name of the procedure
- Completion of instrument, swab/sponge and needle counts
- Specimen labelling (read specimen labels aloud, including patient name)
- Whether there are any equipment problems to be addressed

To Surgeon, Anaesthetist and Nurse:

- What are the key concerns for recovery and management of this patient?

[a]http://www.who.int/patientsafety/safesurgery/en/

• BOX 1.9   Avoidable Hazards in the Operating Theatre

- Wrong procedure (including wrong side)
- Anaesthetic mishaps
- Surgical mishaps
- Handling injury (patient or staff)
- Equipment failure
- Cross-infection (patient or staff)

Anaesthetic incidents can be substantially reduced by good anaesthetist training, by having trained anaesthetic assistant staff so that more than one pair of hands is available, by standardised patient monitoring including pulse oximetry, and by 'preflight' checking of anaesthetic equipment. Professional recovery nurses and equipment further increase safety.

Surgical Mishaps

Surgical mishaps in the operating theatre range from dramatic uncontrolled haemorrhage to the harder to define inadequate surgery leading to complications, slow recovery or avoidable recurrence of cancer. Surgeons have long had clear evidence of poor results of surgical treatment and at last, improvements are occurring with audit, specialisation, national audit databases, training and continuing medical education after specialist accreditation. Governments eager to save money sometimes mandate excessively short training and this is likely to impair outcomes and, in the end, do more damage and cost more.

Injuries and Hazards of Moving and Positioning Patients

Damage to the cervical spine may occur if the unsupported head is allowed to fall backwards or sideways in unconscious patients, particularly those with rheumatoid arthritis of the cervical spine.

Falls to the floor usually occur only if several things go wrong simultaneously.

Damage to upper limbs can occur during transfer and positioning, and lower limb damage can occur when placing diseased hips into flexed abduction.

Traction on infusion lines, tubes and catheters can cause tissue injury or interfere with monitoring or intravenous therapy, or both.

Drains and catheters are at similar risk. *Chest drains* require special attention as detachment allows air to enter the pleural cavity causing pneumothorax.

Acute compartment syndrome is a rare complication of patients placed in lithotomy position for prolonged periods. It is good practice to monitor the leg elevation time and ensure the legs are lowered at set intervals during a long operation.

Peripheral Nerve Injuries

Peripheral nerve injuries after anaesthesia are probably caused by nerve ischaemia and can occur after as little as 30 minutes in an adverse position. Examples include ulnar nerve compression at the elbow, facial nerve damage from face mask pressure, radial nerve injury from a post clamped to the operating table. The brachial plexus is vulnerable to traction. If the arm is to be placed at right angles, the hand should be *pronated* and the patient's head turned towards the arm.

Eye Injuries

Irritant fluids such as antiseptics, sprays or gastric acid may be spilled on the cornea causing chemical injury. The eyelids are usually taped gently shut during operation to prevent direct trauma and drying which causes damage after 10 minutes.

Direct Pressure Effects

Under anaesthesia, the weight of parts of the body may cause pressure necrosis of skin over the occiput, sacrum and heels. The heels of patients with lower limb ischaemia are particularly at risk.

Pressure on calves on the operating table may cause DVT by compression of veins, trauma to the vein wall and stagnation of blood. Elevation by pads under the ankle, graduated compression stockings and pneumatic compression devices all reduce the risk.

Burns

Burns on the operating table are often caused by faulty positioning. Diathermy burns occur if the patient comes into contact with bare metal of the operating table. Other diathermy burns result from poor earth plate contact.

Hypothermia

Unintentional hypothermia is a danger to children and to adults undergoing prolonged surgical procedures and is largely avoidable. Reduced core temperature causes changes in drug metabolism, impaired coagulation and an increase in tissue oxygen requirement during the postoperative period and consequent acidosis. This has been shown to predispose to serious postoperative complications. Maintaining normothermia is a mainstay of enhanced recovery protocols. Trauma patients are particularly vulnerable as are patients undergoing laparoscopy for prolonged periods. Efforts to maintain normothermia with foil blankets, warmed fluids, warm air blankets and insufflation of warmed, humidified carbon dioxide are simple, but effective measures for minimising hypothermia and its associated complications.

Infection Risks

These are dealt with in Chapter 3.

Hazards During Immediate Postoperative Recovery

Twenty percent of all deaths and serious neurological damage caused by anaesthesia are believed to occur in the recovery room, and full monitoring and observation needs to be continued in the recovery area.

Radiation Hazards

In the United Kingdom, all healthcare workers who use or prescribe X-irradiation (X-ray) undergo mandatory radiation protection training courses to learn the risks and safeguards needed.

2

Managing Physiological Change in the Surgical Patient

CHAPTER OUTLINE

- **Haemorrhage and fluid infusion** including blood; fluid and electrolyte abnormalities
- **Infection, inflammation and sepsis**
- **Hypoxia and hypotension**

The way the body responds to major systemic insults depends on several factors: the **physiological reserve** of the patient's vital organ systems (i.e., basic fitness), the nature of the injurious process, the severity of physiological disruption, the duration of delay before resuscitation and the virulence of any microorganisms involved. Most patients are remarkably resilient given good basic care but in a deteriorating patient, several physiological systems are likely to be impacted upon simultaneously, evoking a range of complex homeostatic mechanisms.

Managing the Deteriorating Patient

The aim is always to recognise problems early by regular clinical observation, and to correct abnormal physiology rapidly and accurately to prevent intrinsic compensatory mechanisms becoming overwhelmed. If this happens in one organ system without correction, escalating decompensation of other organ systems follows.

Management requires careful monitoring, often in a high-dependency or intensive care unit, with repeated investigations of organ function and dysfunction. In most elective operations, many of the responses discussed subsequently can be mitigated by good preoperative assessment, preoperative optimisation, appropriate perioperative fluid management, ensuring oxygenation, adequate analgesia, reducing psychological stress, preventing infection and using best operative technique to minimise tissue trauma, blood loss and complications. **Enhanced recovery programmes** (Enhanced Recovery After Surgery Programmes [ERAS] have been introduced which give special attention to these factors before, during and after operation and benefits accrue with attention to each of many small details (Table 2.1). A list of ERAS society guidelines is given at: http://erassociety.org.loopiadns.com/guidelines/list-of-guidelines/. 'Prehabilitation' exercise training has been used but has so far failed to translate into improved outcomes.

The individual variables responsible for potentially excessive systemic responses to severe injury or major surgery are summarised in Box 2.1.

Systemic Responses

Factors Responsible for Systemic Responses (Box 2.1)

Surgical patients are subject to a variety of major stressors that make massive demands on the body's ability to maintain physiological equilibrium and sustain life. Examples of such stressors include:

- **Major operations**—tissue trauma, blood and fluid loss, anaesthesia (particularly Trendelenburg head-down position + pneumoperitoneum for laparoscopic surgery), healing and repair
- **Major trauma** including fractures and burns; head, abdominal and chest injuries
- **Major cardiovascular events,** for example, myocardial infarction, pulmonary embolism, stroke

BOX 2.1   Factors Responsible for Systemic Responses to Severe Injury or Major Surgery

- Direct and indirect tissue trauma
- Fall in intravascular volume, leading to a fall in cardiac output and reduced peripheral perfusion and hypoxia
- Excess intravenous fluids, particularly 0.9% NaCl, causing interstitial oedema
- Local and spreading inflammation and infection
- Systemic inflammatory responses and sepsis
- Pain
- Psychological stress
- Excess heat loss
- Secondary effects on the blood
- Starvation

Stressors in the Surgical Patient

Direct and Indirect Tissue Trauma

Tissue disruption (whether surgical or traumatic) leads to activation of local cytokine responses more or less in proportion to the damage. Responses are exaggerated if wounds are contaminated (e.g., debris, foreign bodies, faeces) or there is tissue ischaemia.

Fall in Intravascular Volume

This is a key factor in initiating systemic responses. Hypovolaemia results from:
- **Excess fluid loss** (Box 2.2)
- **Interstitial sequestration** of fluid as oedema in damaged tissues, and generally as a result of systemic hormonal responses. This process is amplified in systemic sepsis
- **Restricted oral intake** during any perioperative period or whilst in intensive care

Falling intravascular volume stimulates sympathetic activity by removing baroreceptor inhibition in an attempt to maintain blood pressure by increasing cardiac output and

TABLE 2.1   Factors in Enhanced Recovery Protocols

When	ENHANCED RECOVERY PROTOCOLS	
	Component	Rationale
Well in advance	Structured preoperative information, education and counselling, including psychological assessment and treatment for depression and anxiety	Reduce fear and anxiety
	Stopping smoking and excessive alcohol consumption	Reduce complications
Day of surgery	No prolonged fasting. Preoperative fluid and carbohydrate loading	Reduce insulin resistance and improve recovery
	No routine bowel preparation	Reduce dehydration and ileus
	Prophylaxis against thromboembolism	Reduce thromboembolic complications
	Preoperative antibiotic prophylaxis against infection	Reduce rate of infection
	No premedication	More alert patient postoperatively
Intraoperative	Short-acting anaesthetic agents	More rapid recovery
	Midthoracic epidural for analgesia	Reduce need for opioid analgesics
	No drains or rapid removal	Less discomfort and greater mobility
	Goal directed fluid therapy	Avoid water and salt overload
Postoperative	Epidural analgesia continues postoperatively	
	No nasogastric tubes	Less discomfort and greater mobility
	Anticipate and treat nausea and vomiting	Improve comfort
	Continue goal directed fluids	Avoid overload
	Early oral nutrition to stimulate gut motility	Improved nutrition and recovery of bowel function
	Early removal of urinary catheter	Improve comfort
	Nonopioid analgesics (e.g., NSAIDs)	Avoid complications of opioids
	Early mobilisation	Restore strength; vary pressure on pressure points
	Regular audit of compliance and outcomes	Ensure ERAS is maintained

ERAS, Enhanced Recovery After Surgery Programmes; *NSAIDs,* nonsteroidal anti-inflammatory drugs.

• BOX 2.2   Sources of Excess Fluid Loss in Surgical Patients

- **Blood loss**—traumatic or surgical
- **Plasma loss**—burns
- **Gastrointestinal fluid loss**—vomiting, nasogastric aspiration, sequestration in obstructed or adynamic bowel, loss through a fistula or an ileostomy, diarrhoea
- **Inflammatory exudate into the peritoneal cavity**—generalised peritonitis or acute pancreatitis
- **Sepsis (septicaemia)**—massive peripheral vasodilatation and third space losses caused by increased capillary permeability causing relative hypovolaemia
- **Abnormal insensible loss**—fever, excess sweating or hyperventilation

---

peripheral resistance. Restricted oral intake also explains the mild tachycardia commonly seen in postoperative patients. Compensation is most effective in young fit individuals, but decompensation can be sudden and rapid. **Catecholamines** also have profound catabolic effect, increasing the turnover of carbohydrates, proteins and lipids. Falling renal perfusion activates the **renin–angiotensin–aldosterone** system, increasing renal reabsorption of sodium and water. A centrally mediated increase in antidiuretic hormone (ADH) secretion promotes further conservation of water.

Reduced Cardiac Output and Peripheral Perfusion

Circulatory efficiency may be impaired by hypovolaemia, and myocardial contractility may be depressed by anaesthetic agents and other drugs. Anaesthetic drugs generally cause peripheral dilatation and positive-pressure ventilation impairs venous return. Head-down positioning and artificial pneumoperitoneum for laparoscopic surgery further stress cardiovascular physiology by affecting venous return, systemic vascular resistance, and particularly cause myocardial dysfunction in elderly patients with cardiac disease. Major events, such as sepsis (septic shock), pulmonary embolism or myocardial infarction may precipitate cardiovascular collapse.

Pain

Pain causes increased catecholamine and adrenocorticotrophic hormone (ACTH) secretion. Perioperative blockade of pain (e.g., by regional anaesthesia, such as thoracic epidurals) greatly reduces the adverse systemic effects.

Stress

Psychological stress associated with injury, severe illness or elective surgery has an effect similar to pain on sympathetic function and hypothalamic activity.

Excess Heat Loss

This can occur during long operations and after extensive burns. Heat loss imposes enormous demands upon energy resources. If body core temperature falls, physiological processes, such as blood clotting are impaired. Small babies are particularly vulnerable to heat loss. Heat loss in the operating theatre is counteracted as far as possible by raising the ambient temperature, insulating exposed parts of the body, covering the head (especially in babies as they lose heat more through the head), using warm air 'bear-huggers' and by warming fluids during intravenous infusion.

Blood Coagulation Changes

General metabolic responses to injury activate thrombotic mechanisms and initially depress intrinsic intravascular thrombolysis. Thus the patient is in a **prothrombotic state** and may suffer intravenous thrombosis and consequent thromboembolism.

If substantial haemorrhage occurs, clotting factors eventually become exhausted, causing failure of clotting. The systemic inflammatory response syndrome (SIRS, see Ch. 3, p. 48) may initiate widespread intravascular thrombosis, using up clotting factors and precipitating **disseminated intravascular coagulation (DIC)**, with failure of normal clotting.

Starvation and Stress-Induced Catabolism

Patients with major surgical conditions are often malnourished before operation (see *Nutritional management,* later). Many are starved for 6 to 12 hours preoperatively and often do not start eating for 12 to 24 hours after surgery. After major gastrointestinal (GI) surgery, starvation may be prolonged for several days, or much longer with complications such as anastomotic breakdown or fistula formation.

Systemic Inflammatory Responses and Sepsis (See Ch. 3)

Metabolic Responses to Pathophysiological Stress

In severe trauma or extensive operative surgery, particularly if complicated by sepsis, the key factors in the systemic response are **increased sympathetic activity** plus increased **circulating catecholamines** and **insulin**. Cytokine responses signal other cells to prepare for action (e.g., polymorphs, T and B cells), to compensate for starvation, provide additional energy and building blocks for tissue repair, and conserve sodium ions and water.

Glucose production is massively increased by **gluconeogenesis** under the influence of catecholamines. There is also enhanced secretion of ACTH, glucocorticoids (cortisol), glucagon and growth hormone, all contributing to the general **catabolic response. Insulin** acts as an antagonist of most of these and is secreted in increased amounts from the second or third day after injury.

The sum of these factors is to cause inevitable catabolism and potentially extreme changes in fluid balance and electrolytes. These metabolic changes are shown in Fig. 2.1.

Effects on Carbohydrate Metabolism

The overall effect is rising blood glucose (levels may reach 20 mmol/L); often resulting in **hyperglycaemia** and a pseudo-diabetic state, and glucose may appear in the urine. This is in marked contrast to simple fasting, in which glucose levels are normal or low and glycosuria does not occur.

Effects on Body Proteins and Nitrogen Metabolism

In a normal healthy adult, nitrogen balance is constantly maintained. Protein turnover results in daily excretion of 12 to 20 g of urinary nitrogen which is made good by dietary intake. In a hypercatabolic state, nitrogen losses can increase three- or fourfold. Most importantly, this metabolic environment prevents proper use of food or intravenous nutrition. There is therefore huge destruction of skeletal muscle. This state of **negative nitrogen balance** contrasts markedly with simple starvation in which body protein is preserved.

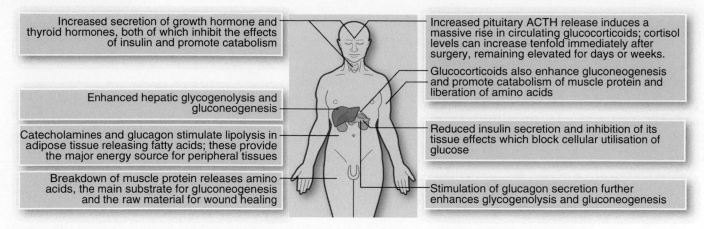

Increased secretion of growth hormone and thyroid hormones, both of which inhibit the effects of insulin and promote catabolism

Enhanced hepatic glycogenolysis and gluconeogenesis

Catecholamines and glucagon stimulate lipolysis in adipose tissue releasing fatty acids; these provide the major energy source for peripheral tissues

Breakdown of muscle protein releases amino acids, the main substrate for gluconeogenesis and the raw material for wound healing

Increased pituitary ACTH release induces a massive rise in circulating glucocorticoids; cortisol levels can increase tenfold immediately after surgery, remaining elevated for days or weeks.

Glucocorticoids also enhance gluconeogenesis and promote catabolism of muscle protein and liberation of amino acids

Reduced insulin secretion and inhibition of its tissue effects which block cellular utilisation of glucose

Stimulation of glucagon secretion further enhances glycogenolysis and gluconeogenesis

• **Fig. 2.1** Metabolic Responses to Major Systemic Insults. *ACTH,* Adrenocorticotrophic hormone.

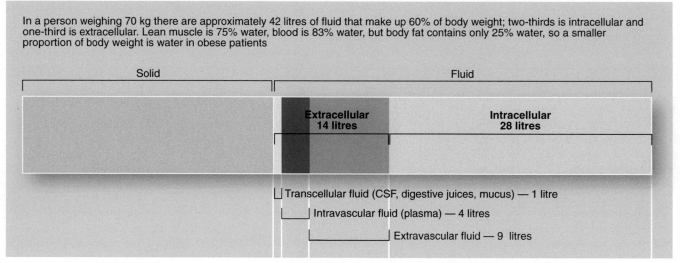

In a person weighing 70 kg there are approximately 42 litres of fluid that make up 60% of body weight; two-thirds is intracellular and one-third is extracellular. Lean muscle is 75% water, blood is 83% water, but body fat contains only 25% water, so a smaller proportion of body weight is water in obese patients

Solid

Fluid

Extracellular 14 litres

Intracellular 28 litres

Transcellular fluid (CSF, digestive juices, mucus) — 1 litre

Intravascular fluid (plasma) — 4 litres

Extravascular fluid — 9 litres

• **Fig. 2.2** Distribution of Fluid Content in the Body Compartments. *CSF,* Cerebrospinal fluid.

Effects on Lipid Stores and Metabolism

The effects of major body insults on lipid metabolism are little different from simple starvation; most of the energy requirements are met from fat stores.

Surgical catabolism reverses only as the patient recovers from the illness and therefore early parenteral nutrition has little effect, although carbohydrate administration may spare some protein loss.

Note that when patients have been severely ill, carbohydrate metabolism is minimal and energy comes from catabolism of protein and fat. Once feeding recommences, there is a danger of **refeeding syndrome** which should be anticipated (see later).

Fluid, Electrolyte and Acid–Base Management

Introduction

Fluid, electrolyte and acid–base derangements can be minimised if high-risk patients are assessed before operation and closely monitored before, during and after operation. If abnormalities do develop, the diagnosis and management can be worked out with reasoning and common sense. Plasma urea and electrolytes should

be checked at least daily in patients undergoing major surgery or those receiving intravenous fluids for more than a day or two.

In general, patients who are unable to meet their fluid or electrolyte needs require maintenance replacement therapy equivalent to 25 to 30 mL/kg per day of water, 1 mmol/kg per day of sodium, potassium and chloride, and 50 to 100 g/day of glucose (noting that 5% glucose contains 5 g glucose per 100 mL).

Severely ill patients with abdominal infection, sepsis and fistulae, and patients with severe burns are likely to suffer major problems of fluid balance (and nutrition, see later). These are best managed with the help of experienced anaesthetists and intensivists in high dependency or intensive care units, where monitoring and therapy can be rigorously managed.

Normal Fluid and Electrolyte Homeostasis

The body of an average 70 kg adult contains 42 L of fluid, distributed between the intracellular compartment, the extracellular space and the bloodstream (Fig. 2.2). Fluid input is mainly by oral intake of fluids and food but about 200 mL/day of water is produced during metabolism. Normal adult losses are between 2.5 and 3 L/day. About 1 L is lost insensibly from skin and lungs, 1300 to 1800 mL are passed as urine (about 60 mL/h or 1 mL/kg per h) and 100 mL are lost in faeces. About 100 to 150 mmol

TABLE 2.2	Summary—Normal Daily Fluid and Electrolyte Input and Output	
Normal Daily Intake	**Normal Daily Output**	
Water		
Diet 2300 mL	Urine 1400 mL (minimum obligatory	
Metabolism 200 mL	volume = 400 mL)	
	Skin loss 500 mL (obligatory diffu-	
	sion and vaporisation)	
	Note: sweating in pyrexia or a	
	high ambient temperature can	
	cause several litres extra loss	
	each day	
	Lung loss 500 mL (obligatory)	
	Faecal loss 100 mL	
Sodium		
Diet 150 mmol/day (range	Stool 5 mmol/day	
50–300 mmol)	Skin transpiration 5 mmol/day (in	
	the absence of sweating)	
	Urine 140 mmol/day (can fall down	
	to 15 mmol/day if required)	
Potassium		
Diet 100 mmol/day (range	Stool 10 mmol/day (obligatory)	
50–200 mmol)	Skin <5 mmol/day	
	Urine 85 mmol/day (rarely falls	
	below 60 mmol/day)	

of sodium ions and 50 to 100 mmol of potassium ions are lost each day in urine and this is balanced by the normal dietary intake (Table 2.2).

Maintenance of Water and Sodium

For most patients, the daily water and sodium requirements are best met by using appropriate balanced quantities of normal saline solution (0.9% sodium chloride) and 5% dextrose (glucose) solution. Normal saline contains 154 mmol each of sodium and chloride ions per litre. One litre will thus satisfy the daily sodium requirement of uncomplicated patients. The additional requirement for water is made up with 2 to 2.5 L of 5% glucose (Box 2.3). The small amount of glucose this contains contributes little to nutrition but renders the solution isotonic. This prescription is altered for patients with electrolyte abnormalities by varying the volume of normal saline given.

Note that **Hartmann solution** (or similar balanced electrolyte solutions, such as Ringer lactate) is often used as the sole fluid for intravenous infusion. This is more physiological and contains somewhat less chloride (111 mmol/L), some potassium (5 mmol/L) and insignificant amounts of calcium and lactate.

In children, water excretion is markedly reduced in the postoperative period as a result of increased ADH secretion. Maintenance fluids requirements can be based on published guidelines and formulae for example, https://www.nice.org.uk/guidance/ng29/ and https://www.mdcalc.com/maintenance-fluids-calculations

Maintenance of Potassium

Basic potassium requirements are met by infusing 60 to 80 mmol of potassium chloride in divided doses over each 24-hour period. Premixed intravenous fluids are generally available with 20 or 40 mmol of potassium chloride per 1000 mL infusion bags. If concentrations of potassium chloride greater than 40 mmol in 500

• BOX 2.3	Example of Daily Intravenous Fluid Regimens as a Substitute for Oral Intake in Uncomplicated Cases

Prescription (1) for 24 hours (each bag to be given over 8 hours):
1. 1000 mL 0.9% sodium chloride + 20 mmol KCl
2. 1000 mL 5% dextrose + 20 mmol KCl
3. 1000 mL 5% dextrose + 20 mmol KCl
   Total: 154 mmol sodium and 60 mmol potassium

Prescription (2) for 24 hours (each bag to be given over 8 hours):
1. 1000 mL dextrose–saline (i.e., 4% dextrose + 1.8% NaCl) + 20 mmol KCl
2. 1000 mL dextrose–saline + 20 mmol KCl
3. 1000 mL dextrose–saline + 20 mmol KCl
   Total: 90 mmol sodium and 60 mmol potassium

Also refer to NICE CG174 on intravenous fluid therapy in adults in hospital (https://www.nice.org.uk/guidance/ng29/).

mL are required, they should be given via a central venous infusion in a critical care unit, with cardiac monitoring. Bolus injections of potassium chloride must *never* be given because rapid increases in plasma potassium can cause cardiac arrest.

Limits of Compensatory Mechanisms

Healthy kidneys are normally able to maintain fluid and electrolyte homeostasis in spite of large variations of fluid intake. The same also applies to fluid and electrolytes given intravenously.

The total blood volume in an adult male is about 5 L, of which about 55% to 60% is water (about 3.5 L). Falls in blood volume which are not too rapid or extensive can be compensated by fluid movement from the extracellular compartment, which has a volume of more than 10 L. A deficit of more than 3 L in whole body fluid volume cannot be sustained and intravascular volume inevitably becomes depleted. This is reflected in compensatory cardiovascular changes. Vasoconstriction causes cold peripheries: this is an important warning sign of hypovolaemia and more reliable than the early mild tachycardia, particularly in fit children and young adults as they compensate for a long time owing to good physiological reserves, before abrupt decompensation. When overall fluid deficit reaches about 3 L, the pulse rate becomes very rapid and **hypotension** and shock develop. Note that patients on beta-adrenergic blocking drugs or with cardiac conduction defects may not be able to increase heart rate and will therefore decompensate earlier. With 4 or more litres fluid deficit, the limit of cardiovascular compensation is reached and the patient develops **hypovolaemic shock**.

In neonates, children, the elderly and the chronically ill, cardiovascular compensation capacity is greatly reduced. A relatively small fluid and electrolyte imbalance may cause life-threatening complications.

Physiological Changes in Response to Surgery and Trauma

The stresses of trauma or surgery cause a rise in circulating catecholamines. Stress also stimulates the hypothalamo–pituitary–adrenal axis, which increases secretion of **cortisol** and **aldosterone**. These hormones promote renal conservation of sodium and water and cause a reduction in urine volume and urine sodium concentration.

Effects of a Fall in Renal Perfusion

Any substantial reduction in effective circulating volume may cause a fall in renal perfusion. In addition, aortic surgery involving aortic clamping may alter the dynamics of renal artery flow, whilst raised intraabdominal pressure (see *Abdominal compartment syndrome*, later) disrupts renal blood flow.

A fall in renal perfusion activates the renin–angiotensin–aldosterone mechanism to sustain blood pressure. As glomerular filtration falls, **renin** release is stimulated from the renal juxtaglomerular apparatus and this catalyses the conversion of **angiotensin I** to **angiotensin II** in the lungs. Angiotensin II has a powerful pressor effect on the peripheral vasculature, counteracting hypotension, as well as stimulating **aldosterone** release from the adrenal cortex. Aldosterone promotes active **reabsorption of sodium** ions from the distal convoluted tubules of the kidney, accompanied by passive reabsorption of water. Sodium reabsorption is linked to increased excretion of potassium and hydrogen ions.

The net effect is that in conditions causing renal perfusion to fall, the urine output falls by several hundred millilitres per day, and the urine produced is low in sodium (less than 40 mmol/L), high in potassium (greater than 100 mmol/L) and acidic. The loss of hydrogen ions causes a degree of **metabolic alkalosis**.

Other Factors in Water Conservation

Water conservation is further enhanced by stress-mediated secretion of **ADH**, also known as *vasopressin*, from the posterior pituitary. Loss of water alone increases the plasma osmolality, stimulating ADH release, mediated by osmoreceptors in the hypothalamus. ADH binds to receptors in the distal renal tubules and promotes reabsorption of water. Release of ADH is also stimulated by falls in blood pressure and volume, sensed by stretch receptors in the heart and large arteries. Changes in blood pressure and volume are not nearly as sensitive a stimulator as increased osmolality, but are potent in extreme conditions (e.g., loss of over 15% volume in acute haemorrhage). Stress and pain probably also promote ADH release via other hypothalamic pathways.

Postoperative Situation

At the site of trauma or major surgery, fluid is effectively removed from the circulation in the form of inflammatory oedema (isotonic local third space losses). This displaced volume is compensated by fluid retained by the hormonal changes described earlier. More potassium is released from damaged cells than the excess lost by exchange in the kidney. Thus the postoperative plasma **potassium level tends to rise** in the first day or two. This is particularly true if stored blood has been transfused as this releases potassium from elderly red cells. This means potassium supplements are not usually needed for the first few days after operation provided preoperative plasma potassium is normal and potassium-losing diuretics are not prescribed.

It is important to recognise the normal phase of relative oliguria and sodium retention that inevitably occurs for up to 48 hours after major injury or surgery as this influences fluid management. Like surgical catabolism, these effects are resistant to external manipulation but resolve with recovery of the patient.

Abdominal Compartment Syndrome

Abdominal compartment syndrome is the term used to encompass the pathophysiological consequences of raised intraabdominal pressure. In normal circumstances, intraabdominal pressure is less than 5 mmHg, but after surgery or trauma it may rise as high as 15 mmHg. Cardiac output begins to fall off at 10 mmHg, and hypotension and oliguria are likely between 15 and 20 mmHg. Anuria occurs with pressures over 40 mmHg.

The causes of abdominal compartment syndrome are often multifactorial and include fluid accumulating as a result of retroperitoneal haemorrhage, for example, in ruptured abdominal aortic aneurysm, postoperative haemorrhage (particularly if clotting is disordered), organ trauma, pancreatitis, and interstitial oedema in sepsis or zealous fluid resuscitation. When abdominal pressure exceeds the capillary pressure, perfusing abdominal organs, dysfunction and eventually infarction of these organs becomes likely.

Adverse effects include:
- Oliguria caused by renal hypoperfusion and collapsed renal veins.
- Respiratory decompensation caused by restriction and elevation of the diaphragm, and compression of alveoli. This results in increased peak airways pressure, decreased tidal volume, hypoxaemia and hypercarbia.
- Decreased venous return leading to falling cardiac output and hypotension.
- Bowel ischaemia causing GI bleeding.

In patients with a distended and taut abdomen, measuring abdominal compartment pressure can help early recognition. Treatment involves conservative management to reopening the abdomen and leaving it open until the risk of rising pressure subsides.

Problems of Fluid and Electrolyte Depletion

Loss of Whole Blood or Plasma

Rapid and copious blood loss in traumatic injury or operative surgery initially depletes the intravascular compartment. Loss of only 1 L may cause hypotension or even hypovolaemic shock. When haemorrhage is less rapid, there is time to replace fluid from the extracellular compartment, so greater volumes can be lost before the cardiovascular system becomes compromised, although losses still need to be restored physiologically or by transfusion.

If blood loss has ceased, the need for transfusion is based on estimated or measured volume lost and on known haemoglobin concentration. Acute blood loss of 500 to 1000 mL is usually treated by transfusing crystalloids. Larger volume losses are best replaced by transfusion of whole blood or packed red cells supplemented by normal saline. Slow chronic blood loss, for example, from a peptic ulcer or hookworm infestation, does not cause fluid balance problems but may cause symptoms and signs of anaemia; transfusion is not usually required.

In **severe burns**, the amount of plasma likely to be lost is easily underestimated and should be calculated using a standard formula based on the burnt area to guide fluid replacement (see Ch. 17).

Gastrointestinal Fluid Loss

Between 5 and 9 L of electrolyte-rich fluid is normally secreted into the upper GI tract each day as saliva, gastric juice, bile, pancreatic fluid and succus entericus (small bowel secretions; Table 2.3). Most of the fluid is reabsorbed in the large intestine.

Huge volumes of water and electrolytes may be lost as a result of vomiting, nasogastric aspiration, diarrhoea, sequestration of fluid in obstructed or adynamic bowel or drainage to the exterior via a fistula or an ileostomy. If there is widespread **bowel inflammation** causing diarrhoea as in gastroenteritis or ulcerative colitis, inflammatory exudate may greatly increase the total fluid lost.

TABLE 2.3	Daily Gastrointestinal Secretions and Electrolyte Composition				
Secretion	Volume (L)	Na⁺ (mmol/L)	K⁺ (mmol/L)	Cl⁻ (mmol/L)	HCO₃⁻ (mmol/L)
Saliva	1–1.5	20–80	10–20	20–40	20–160
Gastric juice	1–2.5	20–100	5–10	120–160	Nil
Bile	Up to 1	150–250	5–10	40–60	20–60
Pancreatic juice	1–2	120	5–10	10–60	80–120
Succus entericus (small bowel secretions)	2–3	140	5 (increases up to 40 in inflammatory diarrhoea)	Variable	Variable

Cholera and other infective diarrhoeal diseases can cause the loss of up to 10 L of electrolyte-rich fluid in 1 day and this fluid loss is the usual cause of death, particularly in children.

Abnormal fluid losses in hospital must be measured or estimated accurately and recorded on a fluid balance chart. In addition, observations should be regularly made for signs of fluid depletion including pulse rate, blood pressure, periodic urine output and, if necessary, central venous pressure (CVP). Oesophageal Doppler can be used to guide fluid therapy by measuring stroke volume and its response to 250 mL infusions of fluid. These measures enable accurate intravenous replacement and prevent the adverse consequences of fluid and electrolyte depletion.

From Table 2.3, it can be seen that vomitus, nasogastric aspirate and diarrhoea are variably rich in sodium and potassium. As a general rule, GI fluid losses should be replaced by an equivalent volume of normal saline, with potassium chloride added as needed. In intestinal obstruction or adynamic ileus, fluid sequestrated in bowel is replaced in a similar manner, although volume requirements have to be estimated. Fistulae and overactive ileostomies cause chronic loss of fluid that is high in chloride and bicarbonate.

Intraabdominal Accumulation of Inflammatory Fluid

Severe intraabdominal inflammation may cause several litres of fluid rich in plasma proteins and electrolytes to be lost into the peritoneal cavity. This typically occurs in peritonitis or acute pancreatitis and often in the context of the **systemic inflammatory response syndrome (SIRS)**. This is best replaced (as well as can be estimated) by physiological saline or other suitable crystalloids.

Systemic Sepsis (SIRS and Multiple Organ Dysfunction Syndrome)

Systemic sepsis is associated with widespread endothelial damage and a large increase in capillary permeability mediated by a range of cytokines and other circulating mediators. The result is extensive loss of protein and electrolyte-rich fluid from the circulation into the extravascular space ('third space loss'), which, combined with loss of peripheral resistance, results in cardiovascular collapse and shock (see Sepsis, Ch. 3, pp. 48–49).

The required fluid volume is difficult to estimate and replacement is usually given so as to maintain cardiovascular stability (pulse rate and blood pressure) and urinary output (at least 0.5 mL/kg body weight per h) whilst avoiding fluid overload and cardiac failure. In the severely ill patient, in whom the volume requirements are particularly difficult to judge, a central venous pressure line or transoesophageal Doppler provide a more accurate method of assessing precise fluid replacement needs (see *Enhanced recovery programmes*, Table 2.1 and p.24).

Abnormal Insensible Fluid Loss

Abnormal insensible fluid loss can greatly increase overall fluid loss, particularly in the seriously ill or elderly patient and must be included in the fluid balance equation. **Pyrexia** increases insensible loss by approximately 20% for each degree Celsius rise in body temperature, mainly in the form of exhaled water vapour. A pyrexia of 38.5°C for 3 days would therefore cause an extra litre of fluid loss. **Sweating** causes loss of sodium-rich fluid which can be easily overlooked in patients with fever and when the ambient temperature rises.

Preventing Acute Kidney Injury

Maintaining fluid balance in surgical patients depends on anticipating problems before they cause adverse effects and risk acute kidney injury (AKI), which is a serious complication with a high mortality in surgical patients. Prevention involves similar strategies in all patients at risk, namely:
- observing changes in vital signs—pulse rate, blood pressure and CVP if appropriate;
- checking hourly urine output is adequate;
- measuring fluid losses to guide replacement;
- seeking clinical signs of fluid imbalance (dehydration or overload);
- regularly estimating plasma urea and electrolytes.

In patients with cardiac failure or shock, monitoring and treatment is best carried out in a critical care unit, using invasive monitoring to determine the volume of fluid replacement.

Common Fluid and Electrolyte Problems

Intermediate Elective Operations and Uncomplicated Emergency Operations

Most operations fall into this category. Patients are generally in fluid and electrolyte equilibrium before operation, although diuretic therapy (for cardiac failure, hypertension or chronic renal failure) may cause problems. For these, plasma urea and electrolytes should be checked before operation. Note that loop and thiazide diuretics may cause **hypokalaemia** whilst potassium-sparing diuretics, such as spironolactone, may cause **hyperkalaemia**. If serious abnormalities are found, operation must be postponed until the problem is corrected. Hypokalaemia can usually be treated by oral potassium supplements or by adding a potassium-sparing diuretic. Hyperkalaemia is usually corrected by substituting a loop or thiazide diuretic.

Mild renal dysfunction (plasma urea up to about 15 mmol/L and creatinine up to about 170 mmol/L) is not usually a contraindication to surgery. These patients tend to be mildly dehydrated, however, and as a general measure oral fluid intake should be encouraged.

Introduction to Fluid and Electrolyte Management

For elective surgery, the patient is often kept 'nil by mouth' for 6 to 12 hours before operation, although most can take clear fluids by mouth up to 2 hours before operation. The patient is likely to take very little oral fluid for up to 6 hours after operation and a fluid deficit of 1000 to 1500 mL is therefore common. Mild fluid deficits can usually be quickly made up once the patient is drinking normally and intravenous fluid replacement is rarely required. Early oral fluids help in this regard. For patients with mild renal impairment, an infusion should be set up at the outset of the nil by mouth period to prevent acute-on-chronic kidney failure. Occasionally, and despite the use of antiemetics, patients vomit after operation; intravenous fluids should be used if vomiting is prolonged.

Children and especially infants and neonates are much more vulnerable to fluid deprivation because of their small total body fluid volume and disproportionate insensible losses. Even relatively minor operations can cause dehydration and intravenous fluids may be necessary, with the rate and volume calculated according to body weight and measured blood loss.

As a rule, the sooner the body can assume control over its own fluid and electrolyte homeostasis the better. Intravenous fluids should be discontinued as soon as normal oral intake has resumed and urine output is satisfactory to prevent fluid overload.

Major Operations

Major elective or emergency operations, especially those involving bowel, pose particular problems with fluid management. The principal reasons are:
- Patients are often elderly and are likely to have a diminished cardiovascular reserve. They may have preexisting fluid and electrolyte abnormalities.
- Preoperative vomiting and restricted fluid intake may have caused dehydration and electrolyte abnormalities.
- Blood loss during and after operation may be substantial.
- Operations may take several hours with consequent insensible losses from the open wound.
- Third space losses of 500 to 1000 mL can occur as a result of systemic responses to trauma after major surgery or trauma.
- The recovery period when oral intake is nil or restricted may become extended—several days following complicated bowel surgery or peritonitis (e.g., perforated diverticulitis or an anastomotic leak).

Careful pre- and postoperative assessment of patients is crucial so problems can be anticipated. This should include clinical examination for **dehydration** (dry mouth and loss of normal skin turgor) or **overhydration** (elevated jugular venous pressure or cardiac failure). Plasma urea and electrolytes, creatinine and full blood count should be measured daily. Elevated urea concentration with little elevation of creatinine is characteristic of dehydration. An abnormally high haemoglobin concentration (providing polycythaemia is not present) also indicates dehydration, especially if it was normal beforehand.

Enhanced Recovery After Surgery Programmes

Enhanced recovery regimens (see Table 2.1) aim to shorten hospital stays and reduce complication rates after major surgery by developing structured systems that reduce the stress response to enhance recovery in multiple, often small, ways. These involve attention to all facets of surgical care, so-called **multimodal optimisation** or **fast track recovery**. This includes special attention to perioperative fluid management, the use of minimal access surgical techniques and mechanisms to preserve postoperative organ function, including:
- Thorough preoperative assessment.
- Educate and prepare patients for the planned early discharge, and ensure appropriate home arrangements are in place.
- Calculation of fluid replacement to ensure the patient remains normovolaemic, preventing central hypovolaemia and fluid overload. The National Institute of Clinical Excellence (NICE) have recommended the use of transoesophageal Doppler ultrasound monitoring of left ventricular stroke volume to enable intraoperative assessment of fluid status and provide **individualised goal-directed fluid therapy**. Trials have shown this can reliably shorten hospital stays and reduce complication rates.
- Planned and assisted early postoperative mobilisation.
- Early enteral nutrient challenge and the use of gut-specific nutrients, such as glutamine, antioxidants and symbiotics (nutritional supplements that improve the balance of intestinal microflora). Methods that enable earlier return of gut function may be fundamental to rapid recovery. GI gut-associated lymphoid tissue forms more than half the body's immunologic cell mass and is believed to play a key role in stress responses to surgery. Sustaining nutrition of the small bowel wall from within the lumen may prevent breakdown of intestinal barrier function. Healthy bowel function enables earlier tolerance of food, less postoperative ileus and less postoperative nausea and vomiting.
- Avoiding opiates by using epidural or regional analgesia.
- Delivering high concentrations of inspired oxygen.

Abnormalities of Individual Electrolytes

See Table 2.4 for a summary of causes and effects.

Abnormalities of Plasma Sodium Concentration

Plasma sodium abnormalities are usually discovered incidentally on regular measurement of electrolytes.

Hyponatraemia

A low plasma sodium level may be real or spurious. Spurious results commonly arise when blood is taken from an arm receiving an intravenous infusion; less commonly, false laboratory results can occur if there is lipaemia resulting from parenteral nutrition. If in doubt, the test should be repeated with appropriate precautions.

In hyponatraemia (except in severe hyperglycaemia or infusion of mannitol), the plasma becomes **hypotonic**. This causes cellular overhydration which in severe cases results in cerebral oedema. Mild hyponatraemia is symptomless but when the plasma sodium falls below about 120 mmol/L, patients become confused. Convulsions and coma occur when concentrations fall below about 110 mmol/L. If hyponatraemia is confirmed biochemically, the next step is to clinically assess the state of hydration (i.e., the extracellular fluid volume) and this will guide therapy.

There are three possibilities:
- *Water deficit but with a larger sodium deficit* (clinical signs—dry mouth, poor skin turgor, poor urine output, high urine osmolality): sodium insufficiency is usually caused by diuretic therapy, vomiting, diarrhoea or other excessive losses of body fluids with inadequate replacement. Treatment involves rehydration with appropriate sodium-containing intravenous fluids.
- *Normal sodium with a larger water excess* (clinical signs—weight gain, ankle swelling, raised jugular venous pressure): this

TABLE 2.4	Causes and Effects of Sodium and Potassium Deficiency and Excess	
Electrolyte Abnormality	Causes	Adverse Effects
Hyponatraemia	Diuretics (especially thiazides) Water excess (ingested or intravenous) Diarrhoea Vomiting Losses from intestinal fistula Renal failure Syndrome of inappropriate antidiuretic hormone secretion (SIADH) Addison disease Nephrotic syndrome Liver failure	Confusion Seizures Hypertension Cardiac failure Muscle weakness Nausea Anorexia
Hypernatrae-mia	Fluid loss without water replacement (e.g., diarrhoea, vomiting, burns) Saline excess (usually iatrogenic) Diabetes insipidus Diabetic ketoacidosis Primary aldosteronism (Conn syndrome)	Thirst Dehydration Confusion Coma Seizures
Hyperkalaemia	Sampling artefact (haemolysis of sample or delayed processing) Drugs (e.g., ACE inhibitors, spironolactone, suxamethonium) Digoxin poisoning Excess potassium chloride (iatrogenic) Massive blood transfusion Burns Rhabdomyolysis Tumour lysis syndrome Renal failure Aldosterone deficiency Addison disease Metabolic acidosis	Cardiac arrhythmias Sudden death
Hypokalaemia	Vomiting Diarrhoea Losses from intestinal fistula Diuretics Purgative abuse Renal tubular failure Cushing disease, exogenous steroids or ACTH Metabolic alkalosis Primary hyperaldosteronism (Conn syndrome) Secondary hyperaldosteronism	Cardiac arrhythmias Muscle weakness Hypotonia Muscle cramps Tetany

ACE, Angiotensin-converting enzyme; *ACTH,* adrenocorticotrophic hormone.

usually results from organ dysfunction. Cardiac failure is the most common cause, followed by renal, liver and respiratory failure. Overhydration is compounded by excessive intravenous fluid administration. Management is based primarily on treating the organ failure, for example, diuretics for cardiac failure.

• *Water excess:* this is uncommon and is usually caused by **inappropriate ADH secretion.** It can occur following head injury or neurosurgery, or may occur in pneumonia, empyema, lung abscess or oat-cell carcinoma of the lung. Excess ADH increases water reabsorption by the renal tubules independently of sodium. The result is water overload and dilutional hyponatraemia. Inappropriate ADH secretion is the most likely diagnosis if the urine osmolality is found to be high and the plasma osmolality low. Hyponatraemia caused by inappropriate ADH secretion is managed by restricting fluid intake to 1 L per day. Transurethral resection (TUR) syndrome is a rare surgical cause of iatrogenic 'water intoxication'. It is a potential complication of endoscopic procedures, such as TUR of prostate irrigated with glycine solution. The risk can be decreased by limiting operating duration and using a bipolar or laser technique which uses saline irrigation.

Hypernatraemia

This is uncommon and is often iatrogenic in the surgical patient. The usual cause is either excess administration of sodium via intravenous fluids or inadequate water replacement. Hypernatraemia is more likely to occur after operation because increased aldosterone secretion causes sodium to be conserved by the kidney. Very rarely, hypernatraemia is caused by Conn syndrome (primary hyperaldosteronism).

Treatment involves encouraging the patient to drink more water, or infusing fluids with a low sodium content.

Abnormalities of Plasma Potassium Concentration

Acid–base abnormalities (see later) can have a profound effect on plasma potassium concentration but are likely to correct spontaneously as the acid–base problem is treated.

Hypokalaemia

In the preoperative patient, hypokalaemia usually results from poor dietary intake, diuretic therapy, chronic diarrhoea, losses from a malfunctioning ileostomy or, rarely, excess mucus secretion from a rectal villous adenoma. Rarely, hypokalaemia may be caused by **primary hyperaldosteronism** (Conn syndrome).

Postoperatively, hypokalaemia is usually caused by inadequate potassium supplementation in intravenous infusions. The lack of intake is compounded by increased urinary losses from stress-induced **secondary hyperaldosteronism**.

Hypokalaemia causes skeletal muscle weakness and reduces GI motility, with paralytic ileus in extreme cases. When severe, there is also a risk of sudden cardiac arrhythmias or even cardiac arrest. Hypokalaemia can usually be corrected with oral potassium supplements (effervescent or slow-release tablets). For patients on intravenous fluids, potassium supplements are added as appropriate. The infusion rate should not generally exceed 15 to 20 mmol per hour, but larger quantities may be required following operations involving cardiopulmonary bypass.

Hyperkalaemia

This is less common than hypokalaemia in surgical patients but requires urgent correction. In the preoperative patient, it is most commonly caused by chronic renal failure, high doses of angiotensin-converting enzyme inhibiting drugs or potassium-sparing diuretics. Occasionally, nonsteroidal anti-inflammatory drugs cause hyperkalaemia. Postoperative hyperkalaemia is usually iatrogenic, caused by excessive intravenous potassium administration, although it may be associated with AKI or blood transfusion.

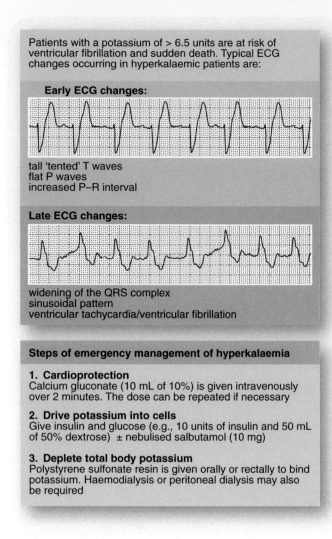

Patients with a potassium of > 6.5 units are at risk of ventricular fibrillation and sudden death. Typical ECG changes occurring in hyperkalaemic patients are:

Early ECG changes:

tall 'tented' T waves
flat P waves
increased P–R interval

Late ECG changes:

widening of the QRS complex
sinusoidal pattern
ventricular tachycardia/ventricular fibrillation

Steps of emergency management of hyperkalaemia

1. Cardioprotection
Calcium gluconate (10 mL of 10%) is given intravenously over 2 minutes. The dose can be repeated if necessary

2. Drive potassium into cells
Give insulin and glucose (e.g., 10 units of insulin and 50 mL of 50% dextrose) ± nebulised salbutamol (10 mg)

3. Deplete total body potassium
Polystyrene sulfonate resin is given orally or rectally to bind potassium. Haemodialysis or peritoneal dialysis may also be required

• **Fig. 2.3** Emergency Management of Hyperkalaemia. *ECG,* Electrocardiogram.

Hyperkalaemia is asymptomatic in its early stages but there is a high risk of sudden death from asystole when plasma potassium concentration reaches about 7.0 mmol/L. The emergency management of hyperkalaemia is shown in Fig. 2.3.

Acid–Base Disturbances (Fig. 2.4 and Table 2.5)

Major acid–base abnormalities are rare in uncomplicated surgery and usually arise in seriously ill patients. In a nutshell, when breathing is inadequate, carbon dioxide builds up and combines with water to produce carbonic acid ('respiratory acid') which contributes to an acidic pH. Treatment is to lower the partial pressure of carbon dioxide (PCO_2) by assisted breathing. In addition, when normal metabolism is impaired, oxidative metabolism declines and lactic acid accumulates. Treatment is directed at the cause of metabolic impairment, for example, sepsis, together with organ support therapy, for example, oxygen, intravenous fluids and antibiotics.

Metabolic Acidosis

Metabolic acidosis usually follows an episode of severe tissue hypoxia resulting from hypovolaemic shock, myocardial infarction or sepsis. The most common cause is inadequate tissue oxygenation leading to accumulation of lactic acid. In surgical patients, the onset of metabolic acidosis is often an indicator of serious intraabdominal problems, such as an anastomotic leak. Metabolic acidosis is also seen in AKI and uncontrolled diabetic ketoacidosis. Clinically, patients have rapid, deep, sighing 'Kussmaul' respirations as they hyperventilate to blow off carbon dioxide (a respiratory compensatory mechanism). Arterial blood gas estimations show the characteristic picture of raised hydrogen ion concentration and low standard bicarbonate with a low arterial PCO_2. Plasma potassium concentration is elevated because of a shift from the intracellular compartment to the extracellular compartment. Urgent treatment is directed at the underlying cause.

Respiratory Acidosis

This results from carbon dioxide retention in respiratory failure. The usual causes in surgical patients are underlying chronic respiratory disease made worse by postoperative chest complications or prolonged respiratory depression caused by sedative, hypnotic or opioid drugs. Plasma hydrogen ion concentrations and PCO_2 are elevated but standard bicarbonate is initially normal. A degree of metabolic compensation may occur as the kidneys excrete excess hydrogen ions and retain bicarbonate. Treatment is directed at the underlying cause and providing assisted ventilation until the underlying cause is corrected.

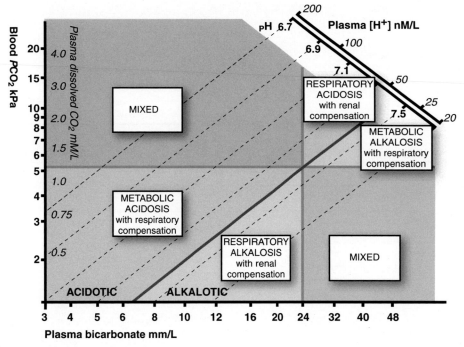

• **Fig. 2.4** Interpretation of Blood Gas Analyses in the Patient with Acid–Base Disturbances. PCO_2, Partial pressure of carbon dioxide.

TABLE 2.5   Acid–Base Disorders

Acid–Base Status	BLOOD GAS ANALYSES		
	pH	PCO_2	HCO_3^-
Respiratory acidosis	↓ or normal (if compensated)	↑↑	↑ (if compensated)
Respiratory alkalosis	↑ or normal (if compensated)	↓↓	↓ (if compensated)
Metabolic acidosis	↓ or normal (if compensated)	↓ (if compensated)	↓↓
Metabolic alkalosis	↑ or normal (if compensated)	↑ (if compensated)	↑↑

HCO_3^-, Bicarbonate; PCO_2, partial pressure of carbon dioxide

Metabolic Alkalosis

Metabolic alkalosis is usually caused by severe and repeated vomiting or prolonged nasogastric aspiration for intestinal obstruction. Pyloric stenosis causes persistent vomiting and an associated loss of gastric acid. The patient becomes severely dehydrated and depleted of sodium and chloride ions; the condition is thus known as ***hypochloraemic alkalosis***. The kidney attempts to compensate by conserving hydrogen ions but this occurs at the expense of potassium ions lost into the urine. Patients become hypokalaemic not only from excess urinary loss but also because potassium shifts into the cells in response to the alkalosis. Treatment of hypochloraemic hypokalaemic alkalosis involves rehydration with normal saline infusion with potassium supplements; large volumes (up to 10 L) are often required. Renal excretion of bicarbonate ions eventually corrects the alkalosis.

Respiratory Alkalosis

This is unusual and occurs when carbon dioxide is lost via excessive pulmonary ventilation. The cause in surgical practice is prolonged mechanical ventilation during general anaesthesia or in the intensive care unit without adequate monitoring.

Nutritional Management in the Surgical Patient

Essential Principles

Malnutrition is a wasting condition resulting from deficiencies in energy (i.e., calories), protein and sometimes vitamins and trace elements. Recognising and treating preexisting malnutrition and preventing postoperative starvation are often neglected but important aspects of management. Basic evaluation for malnutrition should be a standard part of assessing surgical patients (Box 2.4), because untreated malnutrition predisposes to a range of problems that substantially increase morbidity and mortality rates and delay recovery (Box 2.5).

Causes of malnutrition include **reduced food intake** (anorexia, fasting, pain on swallowing, physical or mental impairment), **malabsorption** (impaired digestion or absorption, or excess loss from gut) and **altered metabolism** (trauma, burns, sepsis, surgery, cancer or cachexia). Patients with any of these predisposing factors need to be scrutinised more thoroughly for malnutrition.

Clinical Assessment

- Lack of nutritional intake for 5 days or more.
- Clinical appearance —does the patient look malnourished?
- Unintentional weight loss of more than 10% from usual body weight within previous 6 months indicates malnutrition. More than 20% is likely to represent severe malnutrition.
- Body mass index (BMI)—less than 18.5 suggests malnutrition.

Anthropometric Assessment

- Triceps skin fold thickness—technically difficult to perform but provides a good proxy for body density and hence overall fat content.

Blood Indices

- Reduced plasma albumin, prealbumin or transferrin. In critically ill patients, plasma albumin of less than 35 g/L is associated with a fivefold increase in complications and a 10-fold increase in death rate. Note that low plasma albumin alone is not an accurate marker of malnutrition but may be caused by other metabolic abnormalities.
- Reduced lymphocyte count. If plasma albumin and lymphocyte count are both low, there is a 20-fold increase in death rate.

• **BOX 2.5** **Adverse Effects of Protein/Calorie Depletion in Surgical Patients**

- Protein deficiency leads to impaired wound healing and higher rates of wound breakdown.
- Protein depletion seriously impairs immune function and the ability to combat infection.
- Skeletal muscle mass is lost, reducing muscular strength and general physical activity as well as causing fatigue. This increases the risk of thromboembolism and pressure sores.
- Thoracic muscle mass depletion depresses respiratory efficiency and increases risk of pneumonia.
- Albumin becomes depleted leading to generalised oedema.
- Small bowel mucosal atrophy reduces its ability to absorb nutrients and may lead to bacterial translocation into the bloodstream because of loss of mucosal integrity.
- Impaired mental function leads to apathy, depression and low morale.
- Postoperative complication rates are higher—twice the rate of minor complications, three times the rate of major complications and three times the mortality compared with well-nourished patients.
- Combinations of these factors lead to prolonged recovery times and longer hospital stays.

In practice, most surgical patients have no special nutritional requirements and easily withstand the short period of starvation associated with their illness and operation. All hospitalised patients should be screened using a recognised screening tool and their nutritional state recorded and optimised preoperatively as far as is feasible. In any case, optimal nutritional support should be provided after operation.

Nutritional support in hospital is usually provided by a dedicated team. Strategies include encouraging the patient to eat regularly, providing nutritionally complete high-protein or high-energy supplements to drink (e.g., Fortisip), supplementary enteral nutrition given via nasogastric tube, and long-term total parenteral nutrition (TPN) for patients unable to absorb nutrients from the GI tract.

Recognising the Patient at Risk

Malnutrition is common in surgical patients and often goes unrecognised. Studies have shown that as many as 50% of surgical inpatients suffer from mild malnutrition and 30% from severe malnutrition. Simple clinical assessment is the best determinant of the state of nutrition, although other indices can also be used (see Box 2.4). The duration of starvation should be kept as short as possible and appropriate nutrition provided. This contributes to healing, improves resistance to infection and reduces complications caused by muscle weakness (see Box 2.5).

Effects of Starvation

Simple Starvation

During simple starvation (i.e., in the absence of illness or trauma), blood glucose concentration is maintained by lowering of insulin secretion and increasing glucagon production. Liver glycogen becomes exhausted within 24 hours but **gluconeogenesis** in liver and kidneys is enhanced, using amino acids from protein breakdown and glycerol from lipolysis as substrates. Much of the glucose thus produced is used by the brain, as most other tissues are able to metabolise fatty acids and ketones derived from adipose tissue. Overall energy demands fall in simple starvation and energy is obtained largely from body fat. Protein is conserved until a late stage.

Trauma, Surgery or Sepsis

In severe trauma or major surgery and particularly in sepsis, energy requirements increase by 20% to 100% of normal. As in simple starvation, lipid becomes a major fuel source; this decreases glucose use, but fatty acids other than glycerol cannot be used for glucose synthesis. Hepatic glucose **production** increases, but peripheral glucose **utilisation** is impaired, often leading to hyperglycaemia.

Skeletal **muscle proteolysis** and urinary nitrogen excretion increase enormously compared with the fasted state. Protein from skeletal muscle is catabolised to release amino acids (particularly alanine), lactate and pyruvate. The stimulus for proteolysis is likely to be macrophage cytokines (e.g., interleukin [IL]1, IL6, tumour necrosis factor [TNF]). IL1 reduces hepatic albumin synthesis in favour of more urgently needed **acute-phase proteins** and gluconeogenesis. Amino acids are also used directly in wound healing and in haemopoiesis.

In sepsis, there is a progressive inability at mitochondrial level to fully oxidise substrates for energy generation, leading to a fall in oxygen consumption as sepsis worsens. Fatty acids are increasingly mobilised from adipose tissue, manifesting as hypertriglyceridaemia; mobilisation is governed by raised levels of glucagon, catecholamines, cortisol and TNF. Fatty acids are oxidised for adenosine triphosphate (ATP) production to fuel synthesis of new glucose and proteins. If liver failure develops, amino acid clearance deteriorates and plasma concentrations rise. Some amino acids are then metabolised into false neurotransmitters which promote the vasodilatation and hypotension seen in sepsis and cause septic encephalopathy.

Supplementary Nutrition

Supplementary nutrition other than liquidised diets and sip feeds is a complicated and sometimes expensive process with distinct risk of complications. It should not be undertaken without proper assessment. Deciding whether a patient is likely to benefit from supplementary nutrition depends on determining:

- that the patient is malnourished or will be deprived of nutrition for at least 5 days;
- that the patient is likely to benefit—certain conditions make supplemental nutrition ineffective (e.g., enteral feeding in high output enterocutaneous fistula);
- whether there is an appropriate route for administration, for example, suitable gut function.

Nutritional support is generally recommended in well-nourished patients who are unable to tolerate oral feeding for more than 7 days, or less than 5 days if already malnourished.

Methods of Giving Supplementary Nutrition

Box 2.6 summarises the range of nutritional regimens and their main surgical indications. The GI tract should be used whenever possible because any form of enteral feeding is intrinsically safer than parenteral nutrition and is more effective and much cheaper. In addition, the small intestinal mucosa tends to atrophy when not used. Enteral feeding supports the gut-associated immunologic shield and prevents microorganisms translocating into the circulation, reducing the chances of blood-borne infection. Contraindications to enteral feeding include intestinal obstruction, high-output intestinal fistula, intractable vomiting or diarrhoea, and severe malabsorption.

Sip Feeds

If the patient is able to eat, fluid diets (total or supplementary) can be given orally. Proprietary sip feeds containing easily absorbed calories, protein, minerals and vitamins are available in a variety of formulations and flavours and are well tolerated.

Tube Feeds

Certain patients are unsuitable for sip feeding but can be fed by one of several tube feeding routes. Indications include patients with swallowing difficulties, anorexia, lack of palatability of liquid feeds, the need for a higher volume of feed than the patient can comfortably manage and anticipated substantial delay in resuming oral feeding after operation.

Even if the patient is unable to swallow (e.g., because of bulbar palsy, unconsciousness or facial fractures), complete enteral nutrition can be delivered by means of a **fine-bore nasogastric** or **naso-jejunal tube**, the latter for those who require postpyloric enteral feeding, (e.g., in acute pancreatitis). An individual fluid diet is formulated and is delivered at a controlled rate using a pump, often overnight.

Feeding tubes can also be placed percutaneously into stomach or jejunum, either at operation (if feeding problems are anticipated) or with endoscopic or laparoscopic help. Gastrostomies are often used in patients after stroke or in those with upper GI anastomoses or obstructing lesions. The usual technique nowadays is by **percutaneous endoscopic gastrostomy (PEG)**, combining gastroscopy and percutaneous placement. PEG tubes are contraindicated in peritonitis, ascites and prolonged ileus.

For jejunostomy placement, the tube is tunnelled submucosally for a distance before entering the bowel lumen using a wide-bore needle; this minimises the risk of leakage. Jejunostomy tubes must be placed under direct vision at operation or laparoscopically.

Certain patients not requiring full enteral or parenteral feeding may benefit from vitamin supplements, for example, folic acid

> ### • BOX 2.6 Special Methods of Nutrition and Their Indications
>
> 1. **Selective diets for specific indications**, for example, diabetic, low-protein (renal and liver failure), low-fat (gallstones), high-fibre (constipation, diverticular disease) or weight reducing (obesity).
> 2. **Liquidised normal diet**—for patients with partial oesophageal obstruction (e.g., stricture, tumour or oesophageal intubation for cancer).
> 3. **High-protein, high-calorie dietary supplements 'sip diet'**—for chronically malnourished patients capable of a normal diet or debilitated convalescent patients.
> 4. **Polymeric liquid diet** via tube—short chain peptides, medium chain triglycerides and polysaccharides plus vitamins and trace elements. These contain the full range of nutritional requirements often including fibre. Used for nutritional support of patients unable to eat or drink, such as the unconscious, ventilated and seriously ill patient in intensive care or patients unwilling to take adequate nutrition following major surgery or trauma.
> 5. **Elemental diet** via tube, containing L-amino acids and simple sugars requiring no digestion and minimal absorptive capacity—for patients with minimal remaining bowel after massive resection. These are expensive and unpalatable and the high osmolarity can cause diarrhoea.
> 6. **Peripheral parenteral nutritional support** for patients unable to have tube feeding but needing specific energy or protein supplementation.
> 7. **Total parenteral nutrition (TPN)**, that is, comprehensive intravenous nutrition—for patients with prolonged ileus or a very proximal fistula.

and thiamine for alcoholics, or vitamin K injections for patients on prolonged antibiotic therapy where disturbed gut flora may impair absorption of vitamin K.

Total Parenteral Nutrition

Parenteral nutrition should be reserved for appropriate cases of intestinal failure (see later) and should not be embarked upon lightly.

TPN formulations principally contain a mixture of glucose, amino acids, lipids, minerals and vitamins. Nonnitrogenous sources of energy in the form of glucose and lipids have a protein-sparing effect and minimise the consumption of amino acids as energy.

The osmolality of the mixture is usually high, so the most common route of administration is via a dedicated central venous line, peripherally inserted central catheter line or Hickman catheter to minimise the risk of venous thrombosis; formulations for peripheral infusion are also available but this route should only be used for a limited time. The usual aim of TPN is to provide sufficient nitrogen and energy to offset the catabolic demands of surgery and/or trauma and their complications and, if possible, compensate for any preexisting malnutrition.

In calculating requirements, protein intake should be matched to estimated nitrogen losses; this can be calculated by measuring urinary nitrogen losses as urea or else a standard formula (which also estimates other requirements) can be used. For example, basic adult daily requirements are 100 g protein (as amino acids), 350 g glucose and 50 g lipid to provide energy. These quantities are adjusted for individual requirements.

Excessive nutrition can be a problem. Hyperglycaemia can be corrected with modest doses of insulin but in the longer term, disturbances of liver function may reflect intrahepatic cholestasis caused by fatty infiltration. In intrahepatic cholestasis, blood tests show elevated plasma alkaline phosphatase and gamma glutaryl transferase.

Indications for Total Parenteral Nutrition. Parenteral nutrition should be reserved for patients who are already malnourished (or are likely to become malnourished), in whom the GI tract is not functional or is inaccessible and is likely to remain so for a substantial period of days or weeks. Note that in major sepsis, the metabolic changes described earlier mean that TPN brings little benefit.

Indications may include:
- enterocutaneous fistula
- intraabdominal infection
- short bowel syndrome where there is insufficient residual absorptive capacity after massive small bowel resection
- multiple injuries involving viscera

Methods of Giving Total Parenteral Nutrition. Parenteral nutrition is usually delivered into the superior vena cava via the internal jugular or subclavian vein so that high venous flow rapidly dilutes the hyperosmolar solution, minimising thrombosis risk. If long periods of nutritional support are anticipated, a designated tunnelled line is usually used, with the skin access point remote from the venous entry point to minimise risk of line infection.

The choice and quantity of nutrients starts from a standard baseline for body weight and is varied (with specialist advice) according to individual needs.

Parenteral nutrition is costly in materials and staff time and is prone to complications; it should be discontinued as soon as nutrition can be supplied by an enteral route. Patients on TPN need close and regular monitoring for a range of problems including line problems, local and systemic infection, fluid balance and deficiencies of electrolytes (Box 2.7). Complications of TPN are detailed in Box 2.8.

Refeeding Syndrome

Refeeding syndrome was first described in prisoners in the Far East after the Second World War who developed cardiac failure when starting to eat after prolonged starvation. With reduced carbohydrate intake, insulin secretion falls and fat and protein are catabolised in place of carbohydrate. This results in loss of intracellular electrolytes, particularly phosphate, which becomes depleted. Phosphate is essential for generating ATP and for other vital phosphorylation reactions.

When enteral or parenteral feeding is restarted after starvation, there is sudden reversion from fat to carbohydrate metabolism. Insulin secretion rises and cellular uptake of glucose, phosphate, potassium and water increases. This can lead to profound hypophosphataemia, often with hypokalaemia and hypomagnesaemia. Note that all extracellular fluid is affected by declining levels of these electrolytes. In the starved state, there is total body depletion of electrolytes but plasma concentrations can be misleadingly normal because of renal compensation.

Refeeding syndrome occurs when plasma phosphate falls to less than 0.50 mmol/L. Clinical features include cardiac and respiratory failure, arrhythmias, rhabdomyolysis, white cell dysfunction, seizures, coma and sudden death. Early signs may go unrecognised; the plasma phosphate may not be measured or the significance of grossly abnormal results not appreciated.

• BOX 2.7   Monitoring of Parenteral Nutrition

8-hourly
- Blood glucose (finger-prick sticks) two to four times daily
- Temperature and pulse rate

Daily
- Fluid balance charts and body weight
- Inspection of line entry site (blood cultures on any sign of local or systemic infection)
- Plasma urea, electrolytes until stable

Twice-weekly
- Creatinine and liver function tests

Weekly
- Plasma calcium, phosphate, magnesium (if risk of refeeding syndrome, should be measured daily until stable)
- Zinc and selenium can be measured initially and then every 2–4 weeks

---

• BOX 2.8   Complications of Parenteral Nutrition

Catheter Problems (10% of Central Lines Develop Substantial Complications)
- Central venous line placement problems, for example, failure to cannulate, trauma to great arteries or veins, pneumothorax, haemothorax, brachial plexus injury, loss of Seldinger wire into vein
- Line infection—a common cause of fever and tachycardia likely to progress to systemic sepsis. If suspected, blood cultures should be taken from the line. If positive, line must be removed and tip cultured
- Blockage, breakage or leakage of catheter
- Air embolism
- Central venous thrombosis

Metabolic Problems (5% Develop Metabolic Derangements)
- Hypophosphataemia (PO_4 <0.5 mmol/L)
- Hypernatraemia (Na >150 mmol/L)
- Hyponatraemia (Na <130 mmol/L)
- Hyperglycaemia
- Overnutrition
- Long-term—fatty degeneration of the liver
- Trace element and folate deficiency
- Deranged liver function tests
- Linoleic acid deficiency

Malnourished patients at risk of refeeding syndrome should start artificial feeding with a quarter to half of the expected calorie requirements. Plasma phosphate, magnesium, calcium, potassium, urea and creatinine concentrations should be measured daily and deficiencies corrected. If required, 50 mmol of intravenous phosphate is given over 24 hours and may need repeating. Thiamine must also be replaced in these patients.

3

Immunity, Inflammation and Infection

Immune Responses

Introduction

The **innate immune response** constitutes the first line of defence against invading microorganisms. The key mechanism is the body's recognition of pathogen-derived molecules by Toll-like receptors (TLRs) found on the surface of dendritic cells. This triggers inflammatory responses to limit infection. The **adaptive immune system,** involving T and B cells, is much more organism specific. It evolves during the course of an infection to deal optimally with the microorganism(s) involved. Once created for a specific infection, some memory T and B cells remain, priming the body for any later attack by the same organism. Vaccines operate by promoting this adaptive system.

Innate Immunity

The innate system produces a semi-specific response to newly encountered organisms. It is also essential to triggering adaptive responses via signalling cytokines. **Macrophages** and **dendritic cells** patrol the tissues for foreign proteins likely to indicate infection. Invaders bearing foreign proteins are engulfed and destroyed by antimicrobial molecules and the **complement system** is activated. Once engaged, the TLRs on the cell surface prompt the cells to unleash particular suites of cytokines, which then recruit additional macrophages, dendritic cells and other immune cells to contain and destroy the infecting organisms. **Dendritic** cells containing engulfed protein then transit to lymph nodes, where they present fragments of the pathogen's protein to an array of T cells and release more cytokines. **Lipo-polysaccharide** (LPS) produced by gram-negative bacteria is a particularly powerful immune stimulator. It prompts inflammatory cells to release **tumour necrosis factor alpha (TNF-alpha), interferon** and **interleukin-1 (IL1)**. These cytokines are probably the most important in controlling the inflammatory response, and also, if unchecked, in causing autoimmune disorders, for example, rheumatoid arthritis.

At least 10 human varieties of TLRs are known. They act in pairs and each pair binds to a different class of protein characteristic of a type or group of organisms, for example, gram-negative bacteria, single-stranded deoxyribonucleic acid (DNA) viruses or flagellin. The released cytokines generate the typical symptoms of infection—fever and flu-like symptoms.

Overactivity of this innate system can lead to potentially fatal **sepsis**. TLRs may also be implicated in **autoimmunity** by responding inappropriately, for example to damaged cells. A range of **drugs** that activate particular TLRs are in advanced stages of testing, for example, as vaccine adjuvants or antiviral agents. Inhibitors are also under development for treating sepsis, inflammatory bowel disease and autoimmune diseases, so far with limited success.

Adaptive Immunity

Macrophages and other antigen-presenting cells, having 'processed' a pathogen, display fragments on their surface. This ultimately activates B and T cells that recognise that fragment to proliferate, and thereby initiate a powerful and highly focused immune response. Activated B cells secrete antibody molecules that bind to unique antigen components and destroy the target or else mark it for destruction. T cells recognise antigens displayed on cells. Some activate more B and T cells whilst others directly attack infected cells. Following the initial infection, enough memory T and B cells remain to deal effectively with the organism, should it return. This can occur so quickly that inflammation may not occur.

The Gut Microbiome

Introduction

The microbiome describes the combined genomic composition of microorganisms in an ecosystem. Several projects have investigated the human microbiota including skin, oral, vaginal and nasal cavities, but most research is focused on gut microbiota, where the greatest numbers reside. Data is derived from faecal samples and some from mucosal biopsies.

The gut microbiome is vast, containing thousands of species and over 20 million genes, dwarfing the human genome. The small intestine contains a very different composition with more dynamic variation. The colonic microbiota is largely driven by the efficient degradation of complex indigestible carbohydrates.

The Microbiome and Surgical Disease

The gut microbiome is now believed to play a critical role in the aetiology of some chronic disease states. The microbiome implies a network effect of interacting organisms rather than a direct relationship between single organisms and disease states as in Koch postulates. The gut microbiome is highly individual and varies through age, reaching its adult structure by the age of 3 years. Abnormalities have been incriminated in a range of conditions including cancer, obesity, diabetes, autoimmune diseases and neuropsychiatric disorders. Widespread use of antibiotics and proton-pump inhibitors changes the structure and function of the gut microbiome, thereby influencing health in adult life, although the extent and mechanisms of the changes are as yet ill understood.

For surgeons, the gut microbiome appears involved in the aetiology of colonic diseases such as diverticulosis(itis), inflammatory bowel syndrome and cancer. Sporadic colorectal cancer (CRC) is the third most common cause of cancer-related death worldwide and its incidence is increasing. There is strong epidemiological evidence that diet is a major risk factor (high in red meat and fat, and low in fibre), but data now suggest the colonic microbiota and its metabonome is an important driver of CRC risk. One mechanism is through its modulation of dietary fibre, resulting in upregulation of butyrate metabolism and reduction in secondary bile acid metabolism. Another idea is that certain microbiome members may produce prooncogenic carcinogens and promote a mucosal immune response and colonic epithelial cell changes that initiate colorectal carcinogenesis.

Supersystem and Surgery

The gut microbiome is a complex supersystem, and all surgically related interventions that disturb it have implications for the host. For example, the microbiome may play a critical role in anastomotic healing, postoperative ileus, surgical nutritional status and the systemic inflammatory response syndrome (SIRS).

The gut microbiome probably also plays a fundamental role in the host response to chemotherapeutic drugs for tumour types anywhere in the body, by facilitating drug efficacy, compromising anticancer effects and mediating toxicity. The modern surgeon needs to be aware of the potential impact of bowel preparation, antibiotics and surgical resection on the oncological function of the gut.

Inflammation

Acute Inflammation

Introduction

Acute inflammation is the principal mechanism by which living tissues respond to injury. The purpose is to neutralise the injurious agent, to remove damaged or necrotic tissue and to restore the tissue to useful function. The central feature is formation of an inflammatory **exudate** with three principal components: **serum**, **leucocytes** (predominantly neutrophils) and **fibrinogen**.

Formation of inflammatory exudate involves local vascular changes collectively responsible for the four 'cardinal signs of **Celsus'**—rubor (redness), tumour (swelling), calor (heat) and dolor (pain)—as well as loss of function. These vascular phenomena are described in Fig. 3.1. The outcomes of acute inflammation are summarised in Fig. 3.2.

Resolution

If tissue damage is minimal and there is no actual tissue necrosis, the acute inflammatory response eventually settles and tissues return virtually to normal without evidence of scarring. A good example is the resolution of mild sunburn.

Abscess Formation (Fig. 3.3)

An abscess is a collection of pus (dead and dying neutrophils plus proteinaceous exudate) walled off by a zone of acute inflammation. Acute abscess formation particularly occurs in response to certain **pyogenic** microorganisms that attract neutrophils but are resistant to phagocytosis and lysosomal destruction. Abscesses also form in response to localised tissue necrosis and to some organic foreign bodies (e.g., wood splinters, linen suture material). The main pyogenic organisms of surgical importance are *Staphylococcus aureus*, some streptococci (particularly *Streptococcus pyogenes*), *Escherichia coli* and related gram-negative bacilli ('coliforms'), and *Bacteroides* species (spp.).

Without treatment, abscesses eventually tend to '**point**' to a nearby epithelial surface (e.g., skin, gut, bronchus), and then discharge their contents. If the injurious agent is thereby eliminated, spontaneous drainage leads to healing. If an abscess is remote from a surface (e.g., deep in the breast), it progressively enlarges causing much tissue destruction. Sometimes local defence mechanisms are overwhelmed, leading to runaway local infection (**cellulitis**) and sometimes sepsis.

Even with small, well-localised abscesses, showers of bacteria may enter the general circulation (**bacteraemia**) but are mopped

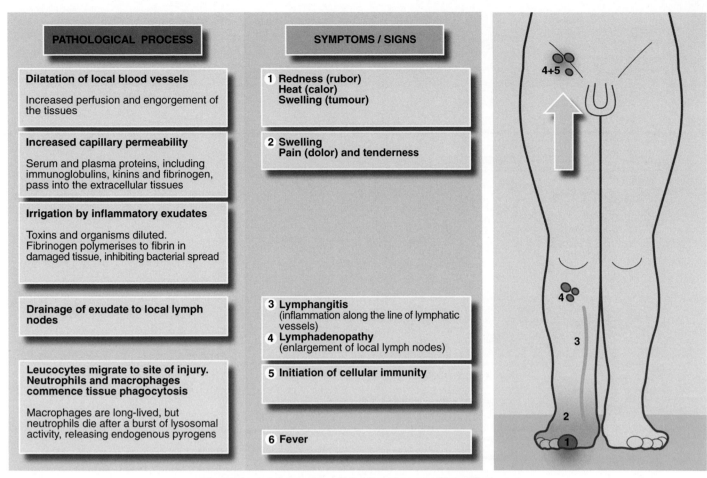

PATHOLOGICAL PROCESS	SYMPTOMS / SIGNS
Dilatation of local blood vessels Increased perfusion and engorgement of the tissues	**1** Redness (rubor) Heat (calor) Swelling (tumour)
Increased capillary permeability Serum and plasma proteins, including immunoglobulins, kinins and fibrinogen, pass into the extracellular tissues	**2** Swelling Pain (dolor) and tenderness
Irrigation by inflammatory exudates Toxins and organisms diluted. Fibrinogen polymerises to fibrin in damaged tissue, inhibiting bacterial spread	
Drainage of exudate to local lymph nodes	**3** Lymphangitis (inflammation along the line of lymphatic vessels) **4** Lymphadenopathy (enlargement of local lymph nodes)
Leucocytes migrate to site of injury. Neutrophils and macrophages commence tissue phagocytosis Macrophages are long-lived, but neutrophils die after a burst of lysosomal activity, releasing endogenous pyrogens	**5** Initiation of cellular immunity
	6 Fever

• **Fig. 3.1** Acute Inflammation—Pathophysiology and Clinical Features.

up by hepatic and splenic phagocytic cells before they can proliferate. This is responsible for the **swinging pyrexia** characteristic of an abscess. The abscess site may not be clinically evident if deep-seated (e.g., subphrenic or pelvic abscess) and the patient may be otherwise well. In the presence of an abscess, circulating neutrophils rise dramatically as they are released from the bone marrow; thus a marked **neutrophil leucocytosis** (i.e., white blood cell [WBC] greater than 15×10^9/L with more than 80% neutrophils) usually indicates a pyogenic infection. Severe infection causing excessive cytokine responses spilling over into the systemic circulation causes **sepsis** and rapid clinical deterioration (see Chapters 2 and 3).

The Chronic State
(see *Chronic inflammation*, p. 34)

The essence of managing any abscess is to establish complete **drainage**, usually by incision or aspiration. Any residual necrotic or foreign material needs to be eliminated by curettage or excision. If drainage of an abscess does not eliminate the injurious agent, the neutrophil response persists and pus continues to be formed, resulting in a **chronic abscess**.

Antibiotics and Abscesses
If appropriate antibiotics are given early enough, organisms can be eliminated before abscess formation. In surgical operations with a particular risk of infection, therefore **prophylactic antibiotics** dramatically reduce abscess formation and other infective complications. However, once an abscess has fully formed, antibiotics seldom effect a cure because pus and necrotic material remain and the drug cannot gain access to the bacteria within. Nevertheless, antibiotics may halt expansion or even sterilise the pus; the residual sterile abscess is known as an ***antibioma***.

Organisation and Repair
The most common sequel to acute inflammation is **organisation**, in which dead tissue is removed by phagocytosis and the defect filled by vascular connective tissue known as ***granulation tissue***. This tissue is gradually 'repaired' to form a **fibrous scar**. Sometimes the original tissue regenerates, that is, rebuilds its specialised cells and structure.

Wound Healing

Healing by Primary Intention
The simplest example of organisation and repair is healing of an uncomplicated skin incision (Fig. 3.4). There is no necrotic tissue and the wound margins are brought into apposition with sutures. An acute inflammatory response develops in the vicinity of the incision, and by the third day, granulation tissue bridges the dermal defect. In the meantime, epithelium proliferating rapidly from the wound edges restores the epidermis. Fibroblasts invade the granulation tissue, laying down collagen so the repair is strong enough for suture removal after

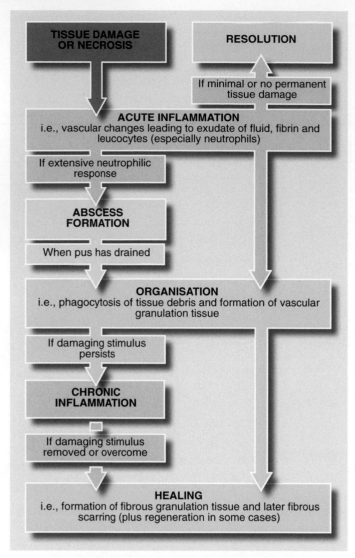

• **Fig. 3.2** Acute Inflammation and Its Sequelae.

5 to 10 days. The scar is still red but blood vessels gradually regress and it becomes a pale linear scar within a few months. This is known as ***healing by primary intention***.

Healing by Secondary Intention

If tissue loss prevents the wound edges from coming together, healing has to bridge over the defect, which is initially filled with blood clot. This later becomes infiltrated by vascular granulation tissue from the healthy wound base. Inflammatory exudate solidifies, forming a protective scab. Fibroblasts invade and lay down collagen in the extracellular spaces; after about a week, some fibroblasts differentiate into **myofibroblasts** and contraction of their myofibrils eventually shrinks the wound defect by 40% to 80%, beginning about 2 weeks after the injury. Over the weeks and months, blood vessels regress and more collagen is formed, leaving a relatively avascular scar; gradual contraction of the mature collagen (cicatrisation), combined with wound contraction, ensures the final scar is much smaller than the original defect. The epidermal defect is gradually bridged by epithelial proliferation from the wound margins. Epithelial cells slide over each other beneath the edges of the scab on the granulation tissue surface and the scab is eventually shed. This

whole process is known as ***healing by secondary intention*** (see Fig. 3.4).

Factors Impairing Wound Healing
The rate and success of wound healing may be impaired by a variety of local, regional and systemic factors (Fig. 3.5).

Chronic Inflammation

Sometimes an injurious agent persists over a long period causing continuing tissue destruction. The body attempts to deal with the original and the continuing damage by acute inflammation, organisation and repair, all at the same time. The damaged area may display several pathological processes at once, that is, tissue necrosis, an inflammatory response, granulation tissue formation and fibrous scarring. This is known as *chronic inflammation* and is characterised histologically by a predominance of **macrophages** (sometimes forming giant cells), responsible for phagocytosis of necrotic debris. Lymphocytes and plasma cells are also present, indicating immunological involvement in chronic inflammation.

Chronic inflammation represents a tenuous balance between a persistent injurious agent and the body's reparative responses. Healing only occurs if the injurious agent is removed and then proceeds in the usual manner but often with much more scarring.

A range of agents can lead to chronic inflammation. The clinical patterns can be grouped into three categories:
• Chronic abscesses
• Chronic ulcers
• Specific granulomatous infections and inflammations

Chronic Abscesses

A chronic abscess arises if the agent causing an acute abscess is not fully eliminated. Pus continues to be formed and the abscess either persists, discharges continuously via a **sinus** or else 'points' and discharges periodically with the sinus healing over between times. A chronic abscess wall consists of fibrous scar tissue lined with granulation tissue.

Causes of chronic abscesses include:
• **Infected foreign bodies**—probably the most common cause in modern surgical practice. Foreign bodies implanted deliberately may become infected (e.g., synthetic mesh for inguinal hernia repair, prosthetic hip joint); others become embedded during trauma (e.g., wood fragments)
• **Dead (necrotic) tissue** can act as a foreign body, forming a nidus for infection. For example, diabetes may be complicated by deep foot infections with necrosis of tendon and bone leading to chronic abscesses and ulcers. Hairs deeply implanted in the natal cleft skin may cause a pilonidal sinus or abscess. An infected dead tooth or root fragment may intermittently discharge via an associated 'gum boil' (Fig. 3.6). Chronic osteomyelitis is associated with remnants of dead bone known as *sequestra*
• **Deep abscesses.** A chronic abscess can arise without a foreign body if the acute abscess is so deep as to prevent spontaneous drainage. A good example is a subphrenic abscess

Chronic Ulcers

An ulcer is defined as a persistent defect in an epithelial or mucosal surface. Except for malignant ulcers, ulceration usually results from low-grade mechanical or chemical injury to epithelium and supporting tissue, together with an impaired reparative response. For example, elderly debilitated patients

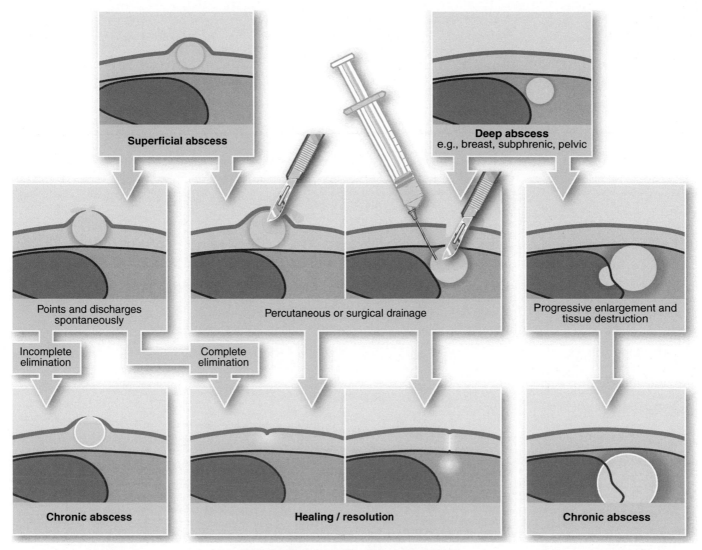

Superficial abscess

Deep abscess
e.g., breast, subphrenic, pelvic

Points and discharges
spontaneously

Percutaneous or surgical drainage

Progressive enlargement and
tissue destruction

Incomplete
elimination

Complete
elimination

Chronic abscess

Healing / resolution

Chronic abscess

• **Fig. 3.3** Outcomes After Abscess Formation.

are susceptible to **pressure sores** ('bed sores') which develop over bony prominences, such as the sacrum and heels. In these cases, immobility or diminished protective pain responses prevent the patient regularly shifting position to relieve the pressure of body weight. Tissue necrosis results and healing is impaired by the presence of necrotic tissue and continuing pressure ischaemia. Other contributing factors may include poor tissue perfusion (from cardiac or peripheral vascular disease) and malnutrition.

Another common ulcer is the longstanding leg ulcer in chronic venous insufficiency; this fails to heal because of local nutritional impairment induced by high venous pressure and oedema and is often exacerbated by secondary infection. Ischaemic leg ulcers fail to heal because of insufficient arterial blood flow.

In summary, a chronic ulcer represents an unresolved balance between persistent damaging factors and inadequate reparative responses. The principle of managing ulcers is to remove damaging factors and promote healing mechanisms.

Specific Granulomatous Infections and Inflammations

Certain microorganisms excite a minimal acute inflammatory response whilst stimulating a chronic inflammatory response almost from the outset. These include *Mycobacterium*

tuberculosis, *Mycobacterium leprae* and *Treponema pallidum* (causing tuberculosis [TB], leprosy and syphilis, respectively). Lesions are characterised by accumulation of macrophages forming **granulomas**, and the diseases are known as *granulomatous infections*.

A tuberculous **cold abscess** is a pus-like accumulation of liquefied caseous material containing the occasional mycobacterium. In contrast to a pyogenic abscess, the lesion is cold to the touch since there is no acute inflammatory vascular response. Cervical lymph node TB ('scrofula') often produced a 'collar-stud' abscess, that is, a superficial fluctuant abscess communicating with a deep (and often larger) lymph node abscess via a small fascial defect. TB of the thoracolumbar spine causes local destruction and deformity and may track down beneath the inguinal ligament within the psoas sheath, presenting as a '**psoas abscess**' in the groin. TB, and infection caused by nontuberculous mycobacteria (NTM), is increasing in frequency in the United Kingdom. Many are immigrants, particularly from India/Pakistan and Eastern Europe (e.g., Lithuania, Latvia). It is important to consider TB in the differential diagnosis as specialist techniques are required to grow mycobacteria. Culture (and subsequent sensitivity testing) is of increasing importance in view of the rising incidence of drug resistance in TB.

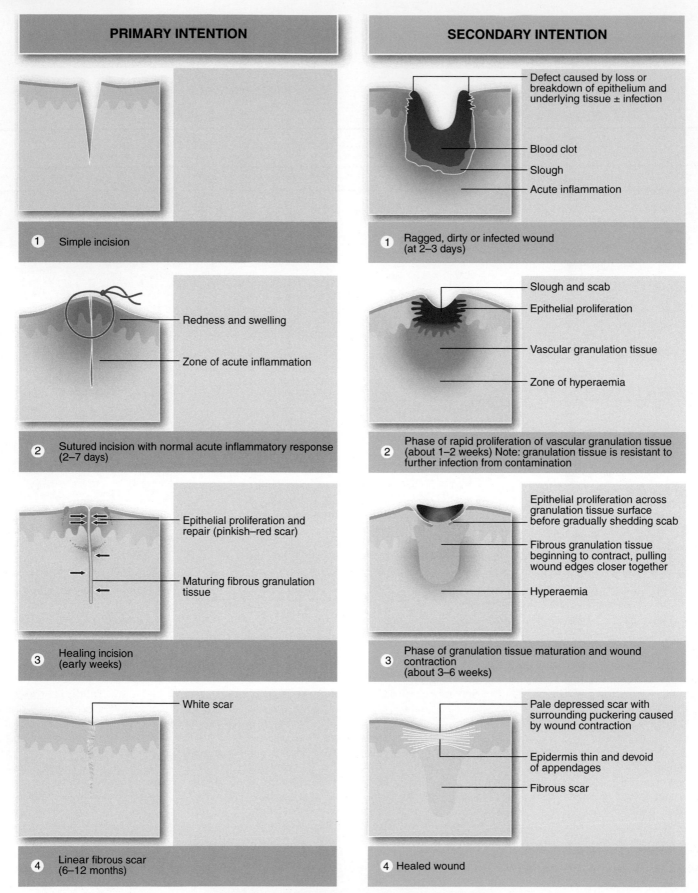

PRIMARY INTENTION

1 Simple incision

2 Sutured incision with normal acute inflammatory response (2–7 days)
- Redness and swelling
- Zone of acute inflammation

3 Healing incision (early weeks)
- Epithelial proliferation and repair (pinkish–red scar)
- Maturing fibrous granulation tissue

4 Linear fibrous scar (6–12 months)
- White scar

SECONDARY INTENTION

1 Ragged, dirty or infected wound (at 2–3 days)
- Defect caused by loss or breakdown of epithelium and underlying tissue ± infection
- Blood clot
- Slough
- Acute inflammation

2 Phase of rapid proliferation of vascular granulation tissue (about 1–2 weeks) Note: granulation tissue is resistant to further infection from contamination
- Slough and scab
- Epithelial proliferation
- Vascular granulation tissue
- Zone of hyperaemia

3 Phase of granulation tissue maturation and wound contraction (about 3–6 weeks)
- Epithelial proliferation across granulation tissue surface before gradually shedding scab
- Fibrous granulation tissue beginning to contract, pulling wound edges closer together
- Hyperaemia

4 Healed wound
- Pale depressed scar with surrounding puckering caused by wound contraction
- Epidermis thin and devoid of appendages
- Fibrous scar

• **Fig. 3.4** Wound Healing by Primary and Secondary Intention.

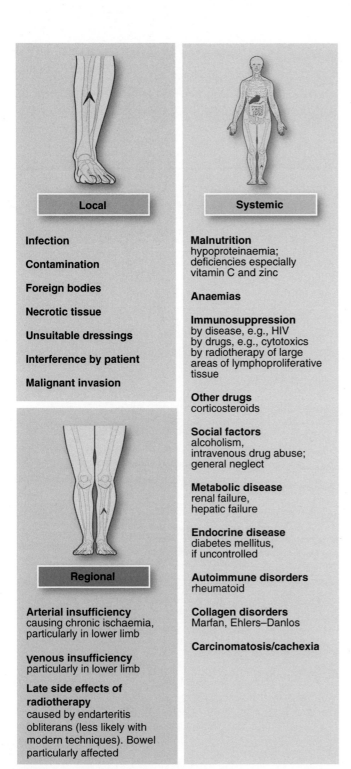

Local	Systemic
Infection	**Malnutrition** hypoproteinaemia; deficiencies especially vitamin C and zinc
Contamination	
Foreign bodies	**Anaemias**
Necrotic tissue	**Immunosuppression** by disease, e.g., HIV by drugs, e.g., cytotoxics by radiotherapy of large areas of lymphoproliferative tissue
Unsuitable dressings	
Interference by patient	
Malignant invasion	
	Other drugs corticosteroids
	Social factors alcoholism, intravenous drug abuse; general neglect

Regional

Arterial insufficiency
causing chronic ischaemia,
particularly in lower limb

Venous insufficiency
particularly in lower limb

Late side effects of radiotherapy
caused by endarteritis
obliterans (less likely with
modern techniques). Bowel
particularly affected

Metabolic disease
renal failure,
hepatic failure

Endocrine disease
diabetes mellitus,
if uncontrolled

Autoimmune disorders
rheumatoid

Collagen disorders
Marfan, Ehlers–Danlos

Carcinomatosis/cachexia

• **Fig. 3.5** Factors Influencing Wound Healing. *HIV*= Human immunodeficiency virus.

A tuberculous ulcer overlying tuberculous inguinal nodes is shown in Fig. 3.7.

Certain extremely fine particulate materials, such as talc and beryllium produce similar granulomatous reactions known as *foreign body granulomas*. Talc was traditionally used as a lubricant powder in surgical gloves and sometimes caused severe peritoneal granulomatous reactions. For this reason, when body cavities are opened, best practice is to use gloves without powder.

Infection

General Principles

It is important to distinguish between colonisation, infection and sepsis:

- **Colonisation** is when bacteria are present in or on a host but do not cause an immune response or signs of disease
- **Infection** occurs when microorganisms provoke a sustained immune response and signs of disease, for example, when normal commensal bacteria in the colon such as *Escherichia coli* contaminate the peritoneal cavity
- **Sepsis** (systemic sepsis) is the result of an excessive and inappropriate production of cytokines in response to severe infection or tissue necrosis (e.g., a gangrenous limb) that causes organ dysfunction and progressive organ failure

Clinically significant infection arises when the size of an inoculum or the virulence of a microorganism is sufficient to overcome the innate and adaptive immune responses and lead to symptoms. The **virulence** of an organism depends on its qualities of adherence and invasiveness and its ability to produce toxins. **Tissue invasion** of microorganisms may be enhanced by their secretion of enzymes (e.g., hyaluronidase and streptokinase), by mechanisms to avoid phagocytosis (e.g., encapsulation or spore formation), by inherent resistance to lysosomal destruction or by their ability to kill phagocytes. Toxins may be secreted by the organism (**exotoxins**) or released upon the death of the organism (**endotoxins**). In either case the toxin may produce local tissue damage (e.g., gas gangrene), cause distant toxic effects (e.g., tetanus), or activate cytokine systems to cause sepsis (e.g., disseminated intravascular coagulopathy).

Infections may be **community-acquired** (e.g., pneumococcal lobar pneumonia in a fit young adult) or **hospital-acquired**. The latter are also known as *nosocomial* infections and are defined as infections not present or incubating at the time of hospital admission. A third category is **healthcare–associated infection** (HCAI) in patients making frequent contact with healthcare institutions or in long-term care. Nosocomial and HCAI may be acquired by cross-infection from infected patients, from contaminated furnishings, or from 'carriers' among staff by inhalation, ingestion or through contamination of medical equipment and devices, such as intravenous cannulas or urinary catheters. These infections are often caused by antibiotic-resistant bacteria, such as methicillin-resistant *Staphylococcus aureus* (**MRSA**). Risk of such infections can be drastically reduced by the simple measure of everyone in contact with patients washing their hands with soap and water or using alcohol-based gel between **every patient contact**. Patients or carriers of multiresistant organisms should be isolated when in hospital. Patients having operations where infection carries very high risk should ideally be treated in areas separated from sick patients, especially emergency admissions from long-term care institutions. Particular risk is associated with eye surgery, joint replacements and prosthetic vascular grafts.

Postoperative patients are at particular risk of nosocomial infections (e.g., pneumonias, urinary tract infections) as host defences are impaired by the surgical assault, and physiological **protective mechanisms** are disrupted allowing infection to gain ascendancy. For example, neutropenia predisposes to infection, and smokers are more liable to develop bronchopneumonia following general anaesthesia. The surgical patient's **general**

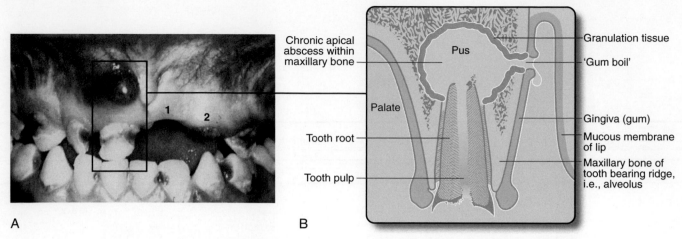

Chronic apical abscess within maxillary bone

Pus

Granulation tissue

'Gum boil'

Palate

Tooth root

Tooth pulp

Gingiva (gum)

Mucous membrane of lip

Maxillary bone of tooth bearing ridge, i.e., alveolus

A   B

• **Fig. 3.6** 'Gum Boil' as an Example of a Chronic Abscess. (A) Grossly neglected mouth showing widespread dental caries. There is an inflammatory swelling on the buccal (cheek) aspect of the alveolus *(G)* caused by a chronic apical dental abscess on the upper right incisor. Note the left central incisor *(1)* is missing and the left lateral incisor *(2)* has fractured at gum level because of caries. (B) Sagittal section through gum boil of upper incisor tooth. The gum boil is in fact a sinus on the gum which discharges either chronically or intermittently. Exposed to infection, the tooth pulp has become necrotic while the apical abscess is slowly expanding because of the continued presence of infected necrotic tissue (i.e., the tooth pulp). The tooth root is all that remains after the crown has fractured because of dental caries.

CASE HISTORY

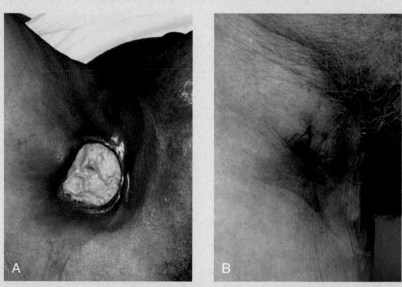

A   B

• **Fig. 3.7** Tuberculous Ulcer. (A) This patient had lived in South Africa and had developed this painless and slowly enlarging ulcer about 3 months earlier. It originates from nearby infected lymph nodes and shows the typical appearances of a 'wash leather' base and an undercut edge. Diagnosis was based on a biopsy and treatment involved draining the involved lymph nodes visible above the ulcer and a course of antituberculous chemotherapy. (B) The healed lesion 2 months later.

resistance may be further impaired by malnutrition, malignancy, rheumatoid disease, corticosteroids or other immunosuppressive drugs.

In **postsurgical** ('surgical site') infections, organisms enter the tissues via an abnormal breach of epithelium. This may be surface damage (such as a surgical or traumatic wound or an injection) or result from a perforated viscus. The infecting organisms are often part of the patient's normal skin, bowel or respiratory tract flora or are normally present in the external environment. For example, *Staphylococcus epidermidis* is commonly present on skin but causes serious chronic infection of implanted arterial grafts.

Methods of Control of Nosocomial Infection
Environment
Patient areas in hospitals must be clean and free from contaminating bacteria, including *Clostridium difficile* and MRSA, especially

where invasive procedures occur, such as operating theatres and high-dependency units. Special precautions are taken in theatres (see Ch. 10, p. 125).

Staff

Staff must be vaccinated against hepatitis B. Human immunodeficiency virus (HIV)-positive individuals should discuss their status with occupational health before undertaking invasive procedures. Open wounds must be securely covered and staff with infective skin lesions should avoid patient contact. **Universal blood and body fluid precautions** should be taken to prevent viral transmission (see later) and guidelines followed for dealing with needle-stick injuries. Risk of MRSA and other infections can be drastically reduced by the simple measures, such as washing hands with soap and water or an alcohol-based gel between **every patient contact**.

Patients

Bacterial swabs should ideally be taken for MRSA from elective patients before admitting them to hospital and MRSA-positive patients should receive topical decolonisation therapy and have follow-up bacterial screening cultures to assess MRSA status before surgery. Patients known to have transmissible infections or to be carriers, for example, of MRSA, should be nursed in isolation. Surgery should ideally be deferred on patients with acute respiratory or urinary tract infections. Some units also screen for other multiresistant organisms, such as CPE (Carbapenemase Producing Enterobacteriaceae) or VRE (vancomycin resistant enterococci).

Procedures

Equipment—including instruments, needles, theatre gowns and drapes—must be sterile, in secure packaging or as single-use disposable items.

Universal Blood and Body Fluid Precautions

Increasing awareness of blood-borne viral infections, such as hepatitis B and C and the prevalence of HIV led to the concept of **universal blood and body fluid precautions** in combating cross-infection between patients and staff. Staff often try to be vigilant with high-risk patients but relax at other times and this extra care soon lapses. For this reason, every patient should be assumed to be a potential carrier of blood-borne viral infection and precautions used whenever skin is likely to be breached and whenever instruments contaminated with blood or other body fluids are handled. Transmission of infection occurs in obvious situations, such as needle-stick injury (see later) and with less obvious events, such as splashes of infected material into the eye.

Disposable gloves should be worn for all medical procedures and physical examinations except for palpating skin with no obvious open lesion in patient or examiner. Staff with broken skin should apply occlusive dressings. Protective **eyewear** should be worn during invasive procedures to prevent conjunctival splashes.

Hepatitis B Vaccination

Staff directly involved in patient care should be vaccinated against hepatitis B. Hepatitis B serology should be checked 2 months after completion of vaccination. Around 5% of healthy young people fail to seroconvert and should be revaccinated. Half of these will seroconvert and the remainder are genetic nonresponders.

Needle-Stick and Other Penetrating Injuries

Sharps injury, especially from a contaminated hollow needle (needle-stick injury), may lead to transmission of infection if the patient carries a blood-borne virus. Such injuries are capable of transmitting hepatitis B and C, but the risk for HIV is much lower because the viral concentration in HIV-positive fluids is much lower and the volume transmitted is small.

Needle-stick injury is common but is largely avoidable: resheathing of used needles causes about 40% of needle-stick injuries and should be avoided. Venepuncture is a high-risk procedure and should be performed with caution. Needles, scalpel blades and other disposable instruments contaminated with blood should be handled with care and disposed of immediately into special plastic 'sharps' containers.

Viral Infection Following Sharps Injury

If a definite sharps injury that involves blood being transmitted from an infected person has occurred, the risk of hepatitis B infection to a recipient with no or only partial immunity to hepatitis B (i.e., not completely vaccinated or a nonresponder) is about 30%. For hepatitis C, the risk is 3% and for HIV 0.3%. There is also a very high risk after sharps injury in a recreational environment (e.g., needles left on the beach by intravenous drug users) since hepatitis B and HIV survive well in warm, moist conditions, especially in serum and tissue debris. Thus all sharps injuries should be treated with the utmost concern. A recommended protocol is shown in Box 3.1.

After a significant exposure to HIV, antiretroviral drugs should be given promptly for postexposure prophylaxis, ideally within 24 hours. A combination of antiretroviral drugs (typically Truvada with Kaletra or raltegravir) is given for 4 weeks. Side-effects are often very unpleasant and include nausea and other gastrointestinal (GI) symptoms, and headache. For health care workers exposed to hepatitis C, no vaccination or preventative treatment can yet be recommended. Guidelines for postexposure management are to enable early identification of infection and specialist referral.

Use of Microbiological Tests in Managing Surgical Infections

Surgical infection should be diagnosed clinically and the laboratory used to define its nature and guide antibiotic therapy. Inexperienced junior staff often take swabs which grow organisms in the laboratory, without realising this may be from **colonisation** and not a clinically important infection. The clinical picture should always determine decisions to treat, although organisms such as *Strep. pyogenes* may require treatment to prevent cross-infection even if the lesion is mild.

Results of specimens from contaminated sites must be interpreted with caution. Superficial slough or discharge often contains only colonising organisms. For example, in *Staph. aureus* osteomyelitis, the sinus opening may be colonised by *Proteus* spp. or *Pseudomonas* spp. The infecting organism may not be grown unless the wound is cleaned with saline and then swabbed deeply. If possible, a syringe of pus or excised infected tissue should be sent for culture. Samples should ideally be taken before antibiotics are given.

For best results, microbiological specimens should be transported to the laboratory within 2 hours or kept at 4°C.

Microbiological testing for TB and nontuberculous mycobacteria (NTM) requires specific techniques which include prolonged

1. Wash injured area immediately and encourage blood to flow from wound
2. Record names of people involved and all details of incident and report the incident according to local protocols
3. Take a serum sample from the injured person (the recipient) which is stored (and available later on for HIV, hepatitis B and hepatitis C testing if needed).
4. Test person whose blood/body fluids contaminated the sharp (the donor) for HIV, hepatitis B and hepatitis C
5. If hepatitis B status of recipient or donor is uncertain and cannot be determined reliably within 48 hours of injury (e.g., over a weekend), administer the following to the recipient as soon as possible:
   — hepatitis B immunoglobulin
   — hepatitis B vaccine—first dose
6. The immune status of donor and recipient dictates further management as follows:
   — recipient hepatitis B immune—no further action (or may give hepatitis B booster)
   — recipient hepatitis B nonimmune (or nonresponder) and donor positive or unknown—give hepatitis B immunoglobulin and start course of hepatitis B vaccination
   — recipient hepatitis B nonimmune and donor negative—start course of hepatitis B vaccination
   — donor HIV antibody-antigen positive or in high-risk group (e.g., homosexual, intravenous drug user, prostitute, heterosexual patients from high HIV incidence countries)—consult infectious diseases physician for postexposure prophylaxis
   — counsel recipients on safe sex procedures to prevent possible infection of their sexual partners
7. Follow up recipients with testing after 6 weeks (HCV PCR), 3 months (hepatitis B, hepatitis C, HIV serology) and 6 months (hepatitis B and C serology); ensure completion of hepatitis B vaccination courses instituted earlier

HCV, Hepatitis C virus; *HIV,* human immunodeficiency virus; *PCR,* polymerase chain reaction.

culture. As described earlier, culture and subsequent sensitivity testing is increasingly important in the era of increasing resistance. Polymerase chain reaction (PCR) can be used but the sensitivity and specificity are still not 100%. New technologies are becoming a reality: MALDI-ToF (matrix assisted laser desorption/ionisation—time of flight) enables same-day microbe identification, and molecular techniques, such as 16S PCR allow identification of microbes from culture-negative samples. In general, the microbiology laboratory works most effectively when all relevant clinical information is provided.

Principles of Treatment of Surgical Infection

Removal of Infected Foci

A poorly vascularised infected area is effectively isolated from humoral and cellular defence mechanisms and from circulating antibiotics. Retained infected material may overactivate cytokine mechanisms and thus precipitate sepsis. A vital first step is to remove infected necrotic tissue and drain collections of pus. This applies even if the patient appears too ill for operation because the very ill patient may recover dramatically after this type of surgery. Common examples include draining abscesses, amputating infected necrotic limbs, removing infected foreign bodies (e.g., cannulae, prostheses, trauma debris) and draining the infected contents of hollow viscera, such as bile ducts, kidneys and ureters.

Antibiotic Therapy (See Table 3.1)

Empirical Antibiotic Therapy. If treatment is urgent, antibiotics are chosen according to the most likely pathogens and local antibiotic sensitivity profiles. A Gram stain on material from a usually sterile site can guide initial therapy until detailed results are available. In abdominal wound infections where hollow viscera have not been opened, *Staph. aureus* is the likely organism and flucloxacillin can be commenced. If the patient is a known MRSA carrier, vancomycin may be indicated. If bowel has been opened, gram-negative organisms (e.g., Enterobacteriaceae) and anaerobes are likely and an antibiotic regimen is chosen to include these.

Specific Antibiotic Therapy. Once microbiological results are available, therapy is modified to deal with the organisms and their sensitivities. 'Narrow-spectrum' therapy is more effective and has fewer side-effects than broad-spectrum 'empirical' therapy. It also minimises superinfection with organisms, such as *C. difficile* and yeasts. *C. difficile* infections have become a major scourge of hospitals in North America and Europe, mainly caused by an ageing population more susceptible to infection and the emergence of a highly virulent clone. Extreme measures to control its spread have been required including strict isolation of patients, high level environmental cleaning and strict antibiotic controls.

Nutritional Support. Major infection and sepsis result in severe catabolism (see Ch. 2, p. 19), often associated with hypoalbuminaemia and malnutrition. In these cases, nutritional support, such as nasogastric tube feeding or (rarely) parenteral nutrition may be appropriate.

Bacteria of Particular Surgical Importance

Staphylococci

Pathophysiology

Staphylococci are **gram-positive cocci** that appear in grape-like 'clumps'. *Staph. aureus* is the main pathogenic species. It is part of normal human bacterial flora, with about 30% of the population being nasal carriers and 10% carrying it on perineal skin. *Staph. aureus* typically produces pustules, boils, breast abscesses, wound infections and osteomyelitis. They are capable of causing bacteraemia and are now the commonest cause of infective endocarditis. They can also cause pneumonia in ventilated patients or postviral infection (e.g., postinfluenza). Their virulence is partly caused by the enzymes and toxins they produce. All staphylococci produce an enzyme, catalase, an enzyme that destroys hydrogen peroxide. Neutrophils typically use hydrogen peroxide to kill bacteria so staphylococci are comparatively resistant to this form of immune attack. A few patients harbour virulent strains that produce the **toxic shock syndrome** toxin (TSST-1). This has serious systemic effects, such as hypotension, shock and multiorgan failure (MOF). Another toxin of importance is **Panton-Valentine leucocidin** (PVL). This toxin has the ability to destroy leucocytes, so staphylococci harbouring this toxin are also comparatively resistant to neutrophil attack. PVL-producing *Staph. aureus* strains typically present with recurrent boils and abscesses or necrotising pneumonia. Coagulase negative staphylococci (e.g., *Staph. epidermidis*) are typically skin commensals. They rarely cause significant infection except when exogenous materials become infected. This includes prosthetic implants (e.g., hip replacements and heart valves), where infection often requires the major step of implant removal, and also intravenous catheters.

Some *Staphylococcus* strains, including MRSA, can be passed from patient to patient via the hands of staff if scrupulous hand washing is not performed after every patient contact.

TABLE 3.1	The Main Surgical Infections, Their Common Microbial Causes and Suggested Empirical Therapy

Clinical Condition	Common Pathogen	Commonly Used Antibiotics
Gastrointestinal Tract		

Gastroenteritis	**Bacterial:**
	  Salmonella
	  Shigella and others
	  Campylobacter
		Antibiotics not normally required.
		If severe or lasting >48 h, consider:
		  ciprofloxacin
		  clarithromycin

	Viral:
	  Norovirus
	  Adenovirus
	  Rotavirus
		Supportive therapy

	Travel associated: Entamoeba histolytica	Metronidazole
Pseudomembranous colitis (hospital-acquired)	Clostridium difficile	Metronidazole orally (or IV if nil by mouth) Vancomycin orally for severe cases Fidaxomicin

Peritonitis
Biliary tract
	Enterobacteriaceae
	  • E. coli
	  • Klebsiella spp.
	Anaerobes
	  • Bacteroides spp.
	  • Clostridium spp.
	  • Enterococcus spp.
	  • Pseudomonas spp.
		Co-amoxiclav ± gentamicin
		  (ciprofloxacin + metronidazole for penicillin allergy)
		  or amoxicillin + gentamicin + metronidazole
		Piperacillin-tazobactam (for Ps. aeruginosa)

Oesophageal perforation	Candida albicans and Enterobacteriaceae	Fluconazole + co-amoxiclav
Superficial and Wound Infections		
Breast abscess or mastitis	Staphylococcus aureus	Flucloxacillin or clarithromycin
Carbuncle, furunculosis	Staphylococcus aureus	Avoid antibiotics unless signs of systemic infection Flucloxacillin or clarithromycin If recurrent, consider mupirocin nasal cream and consider testing for PVL toxin

Cellulitis	Staphylococcus aureus, Streptococcus pyogenes
	  (group A Strep.)
		Flucloxacillin or clarithromycin. If diabetes mellitus,
		  add ciprofloxacin or gentamicin

Gas gangrene	Clostridium perfringens and other spp. Bacteroides spp. and other anaerobes Coliforms	Surgery essential Benzylpenicillin + clindamycin

Infected surgical wound
  6–72 hours
  3–7 days
  >7 days
	Streptococcus pyogenes (group A)
	Clostridium spp.
	Staphylococcus aureus
	Streptococcus pyogenes (group A)
	Pseudomonas aeruginosa
	Coliforms
		Surgery essential
		Co-amoxiclav
		Co-amoxiclav
		Drainage/debridement if necessary. Antibiotics if
		  spreading infection

Infected traumatic wound	Staphylococcus aureus Streptococcus pyogenes (group A)	Cefradine or erythromycin
Necrotising fasciitis	Streptococcus pyogenes (group A) Mixed infection with anaerobes and coliforms	Surgery essential Piperacillin-tazobactam + clindamycin

Bites (cat, dog, human)	Anaerobes
	Pasteurella spp.
	Streptobacillus moniliformis
		Co-amoxiclav or doxycycline
		  (note: Pasturella are resistant to macrolides,
		  such as clarithromycin)

Lungs		
Pneumonias Community-acquired	Pneumococcus Staphylococcus aureus Chlamydia psittaci Mycoplasma Legionella pneumophila	Co-amoxiclav + clarithromycin

Continued

TABLE 3.1	The Main Surgical Infections, Their Common Microbial Causes and Suggested Empirical Therapy	
Clinical Condition	Common Pathogen	Commonly Used Antibiotics
Hospital acquired pneumonia	Pseudomonas aeruginosa Staphylococcus aureus Enterobacteriaceae	Piperacillin-tazobactam Meropenem Vancomycin and ciprofloxacin
Neurosurgery	Staphylococcus aureus Coagulase negative staphylococci Rarer: Pseudomonas aeruginosa Enterobacteriaceae	Vancomycin* +/- ceftazidime OR meropenem
Orthopaedics	Staphylococcus aureus Coagulase negative staphylococci	Vancomycin* +/- gentamicin
Cardiothoracic	Staphylococcus aureus Rarer: Pseudomonas aeruginosa Enterobacteriaceae	Vancomycin* +/- gentamicin

*can be switched to flucloxacillin once susceptibility testing results available

Antibiotic Sensitivities

Most *Staphylococcus* strains were once sensitive to penicillin but more than 90% in family practice and hospital are now resistant. Resistance is largely caused by production of the enzyme beta-lactamase (also known as **penicillinase**). Most strains remain sensitive to a range of common antibiotics, for example, **flucloxacillin**, **erythromycin** and some **cephalosporins**. **Gentamicin** also usually retains activity.

MRSA. Some strains of *Staph. aureus* are resistant to flucloxacillin, co-amoxiclav and cephalosporins; these are **MRSA**. Methicillin is used in the laboratory to predict flucloxacillin resistance. These organisms are often also resistant to macrolides (e.g., clarithromycin) and fluoroquinolones (e.g., ciprofloxacin). MRSA accounted for about half of all *Staph. aureus* isolates in hospitals in the 1990s/2000s but this has declined following intensive infection control interventions. Ward areas at greatest risk are burns units, intensive care units (ICUs) and cardiothoracic, neonatal, orthopaedic and geriatric wards. The public often erroneously believes that MRSA is more pathogenic than other strains. In fact, the organisms excite similar inflammatory responses but MRSA infections are more difficult to treat. Glycopeptides (e.g., vancomycin and teicoplanin), daptomycin, dalbavancin, linezolid, tetracycline, co-trimoxazole or a combination of rifampicin and fusidic acid have activity against most strains; the combination prevents rapid development of resistance to each agent alone.

A worrying development is the emergence of vancomycin-insensitive *Staph. aureus* (**VISA**). Inappropriate use of vancomycin must be avoided to prevent selection of such mutants.

Streptococci

Pathophysiology

Streptococci are **gram-positive** cocci that appear in chains. They were first described in infected surgical wounds by Billroth in 1874. Streptococci are classified by their oxygen requirements into **aerobic**, **anaerobic** and **microaerophilic** and subdivided by their **haemolysis** patterns on blood agar culture plates. They do not express the catalase enzyme. **Alpha-haemolytic streptococci**

cause partial haemolysis on blood agar plates with green discolouration; important pathogens include the **viridans** group and *Streptococcus pneumoniae*. **Beta-haemolytic streptococci** produce complete (clear) haemolysis on blood agar plates and can be grouped serologically into **Lancefield groups** A to O. The important human pathogens are group A (*Strep. pyogenes*—of major surgical importance) and group B (*Strep. agalactiae*—a common cause of serious neonatal sepsis). Group C and G streptococci are occasional causes of cellulitis and bacteraemia. Microaerophilic streptococci, such as *Strep. milleri* carry a group F antigen.

Streptococci of Particular Surgical Significance

Streptococcus pyogenes (**Group A** *Streptococcus* **and Other Beta-Haemolytic Streptococci**). This is the main human pathogenic *Streptococcus* and is carried in the upper respiratory tract by about 10% of children but less often by adults. It can cause cellulitis and is a common cause of sore throat as well as poststreptococcal syndromes, such as rheumatic fever (which predisposes to cardiac valvular damage and risk of infective endocarditis). Outbreaks frequently occur.

Acute **cellulitis** is a locally spreading infection of the dermis and hypodermis, facilitated by production of hyaluronidase and streptokinase. In limb infections, organisms draining towards lymph nodes can produce perilymphatic inflammation and painful red streaks along the limb, that is, **lymphangitis**. Regional nodes react vigorously, becoming enlarged, painful and tender, that is, **lymphadenitis**. This may also occur in staphylococcal infections.

Highly invasive strains of *Strep. pyogenes* may cause **necrotising fasciitis,** a deep-seated infection of subcutaneous tissue that rapidly and progressively destroys fascia and fat. Exotoxins produced by certain strains can lead to a life-threatening **streptococcal toxic shock syndrome**, with fulminant soft tissue infection, shock, acute respiratory distress syndrome (ARDS) and renal failure; 30% to 70% of patients die in spite of aggressive modern treatments.

Viridans **Streptococci.** The *viridans* group are oral commensals of low virulence but are capable of causing infective endocarditis. The subject is described in Chapter 8, p. 107.

Streptococcus pneumoniae (*Pneumococcus*). This is the most common cause of lobar pneumonia and can cause bronchopneumonia in susceptible postsurgical patients, as well as middle ear infections (otitis media) and acute exacerbations of chronic bronchitis. Pneumococcal meningitis may occur in the young and elderly and may complicate head injury. Severe pneumococcal sepsis is particularly likely after splenectomy but may be prevented by planned vaccination and penicillin prophylaxis.

Other Streptococci. Many of the *Strep. milleri* group have microaerophilic culture requirements. They are often found in abscesses in the appendix area, the liver, lung and brain. *Strep. gallolyticus*, (formerly *Strep. bovis*) is commonly grouped as a Lancefield Group D and is associated with endocarditis and CRC. It is not yet known whether the association with CRC is causative or opportunistic.

Anaerobic Streptococci
These are bowel commensals and may form part of the mixed flora in intraperitoneal abscesses or infections associated with necrotic tissue, for example, diabetic foot ulcers.

Antibiotic Sensitivities
Penicillin is the drug of choice for most streptococcal infections. In seriously ill patients, **benzylpenicillin** is given parenterally. For less serious infections in patients able to tolerate oral therapy, **penicillin V (phenoxymethylpenicillin)**, or **amoxicillin** are the drugs of choice. Many streptococci are also sensitive to **macrolides** (e.g., **erythromycin**, **clarithromycin**). Some pneumococci are now partially resistant to penicillin. Most infections, however, are still cleared with high-dose benzylpenicillin although meningitis needs alternative antibiotics, such as ceftriaxone or vancomycin.

Enterococci

Pathophysiology
The enterococci are **gram-positive cocci** closely related to streptococci. *Enterococcus faecalis* (formerly *Strep. faecalis*) and *E. faecium* are the most commonly identified species. Enterococci are part of the normal bowel flora and may cause infection where bowel has been opened or else infect urinary, biliary or genital tracts. They are also capable of causing infective endocarditis.

Antibiotic Sensitivities
Penicillin, **amoxicillin** and **vancomycin** have activity against *E. faecalis* whilst *E. faecium* is resistant to penicillin and amoxicillin (and therefore piperacillin-tazobactam and carbapenems, such as meropenem). In serious infections, such as endocarditis, a combination of high-dose benzylpenicillin and gentamicin ensures bactericidal activity. The cephalosporins and fluoroquinolones are all ineffective. In hospitals where broad-spectrum cephalosporins are used empirically for bowel-related infections or septicaemia, enterococci are a frequent cause of nosocomial (hospital-acquired) infection. **Vancomycin-resistant enterococci (VRE)** are now being found. They are usually low-grade pathogens infecting intravascular lines in transplant and haematology patients and on ICUs. VRE endocarditis is difficult to treat, but newer antibiotics linezolid, daptomycin and tigecycline are active against most strains.

Enterobacteriaceae

Pathophysiology
The Enterobacteriaceae are a large family of **gram-negative bacilli** (rods) and usually make up about 1% of intestinal flora

TABLE 3.2	Bacteria of the Family Enterobacteriaceae	
Organism	**Clinical Infection**
Primary Gut Pathogens	
Salmonella (e.g., *S. typhi*, *S. enteritidis*)	Typhoid fever Gastroenteritis
Shigella (e.g., *S. dysenteriae*, *S. sonnei*)	Dysentery Traveller's diarrhoea
Some *Escherichia coli* strains (e.g., O157:H7)	Haemolytic uraemic syndrome
Gut Colonisers That Can Cause Infections	
Escherichia coli	Peritonitis and intraperitoneal abscesses (usually mixed infection with anaerobes)
Klebsiella	
Proteus	
Enterobacter	Septicaemia
Morganella	Urinary tract infections
Citrobacter	Ascending cholangitis (may also cause hospital-acquired infections, [e.g., after instrumentation, central venous catheters, pneumonia in intensive care])
Gut Colonisers That Rarely Cause Infection	
Enterobacter	Usually hospital-acquired infections (e.g., after instrumentation, central venous catheters, in intensive care)
Serratia	
Morganella	
Citrobacter	

(see Table 3.2); they are known as *coliforms* and can be cultured under aerobic and anaerobic conditions and, like other bowel flora, grow in bile salt-containing media, such as MacConkey agar; this helps identification.

Infections of surgical importance are usually opportunistic with the bacteria originating from the patient's bowel. Infection results from direct contamination (perforated or surgically opened bowel), perineal spread (to nearby wounds or urinary tract) or haematogenous spread. These and other gram-negative organisms contain the sugar **LPS**, a powerful stimulator of inflammation and macrophage production of TNF-alpha and IL1 cytokines.

E. coli is the most common pathogen of the group and causes many surgical infections, often in synergy with other bacteria. *E. coli* causes **gram-negative sepsis** and about 80% of urinary tract infections. Bronchopneumonia caused by Enterobacteriaceae occasionally occurs in debilitated, immunosuppressed or seriously ill patients. *Klebsiella*, *Enterobacter* and *Serratia* are found more often in surgical bowel-related infections. *Proteus* is a common cause of urinary tract infections but occasionally causes other surgical infections, usually originating from the urinary tract. *Proteus* spp. have the ability to produce the enzyme urease, which splits urea. This raises the pH of urine, creating conditions in which renal stones may form. These may then become a nidus for further infections.

Antibiotic Sensitivities
Many coliforms are now resistant to amoxicillin and first-generation cephalosporins, for example, cefalexin, but most are sensitive to **second- and third-generation cephalosporins**, for example, **cefuroxime**, **cefotaxime/ceftriaxone**. Gentamicin is still a very effective agent. Many are sensitive to

fluoroquinolones (ciprofloxacin, levofloxacin, moxifloxacin) but resistance is emerging. For prophylaxis in bowel and biliary tract surgery and for related local and systemic infections, gentamicin or an amoxicillin–clavulanate combination (co-amoxiclav) is recommended for its additional anaerobe activity. Beta-lactam and beta-lactamase inhibitor combination antibiotics, such as co-amoxiclav or piperacillin–tazobactam are very active against bowel flora with good activity against anaerobes. Anaerobes are the main colonisers of the bowel and often accompany Enterobacteriaceae in infections.

Resistant strains of Enterobacteriaceae are much more frequent in hospitals (often on ICUs) than in the community. They often cause urinary tract infection in catheterised patients after repeated courses of antibiotics. Multidrug resistant strains of *E. coli* and *Klebsiella* spp. have emerged in hospitals all over the world since the 1980s and are now common in community settings. Some Enterobacteriaceae produce an extended spectrum beta-lactamase (ESBL) enzyme that is encoded on a plasmid that is highly transmissible. ESBLs destroy second- and third-generation cephalosporins, and are often resistant to quinolones and most aminoglycosides. This severely restricts number of active antibiotics. Urinary tract infections caused by ESBL-producing Enterobacteriaceae may be treated by nitrofurantoin, pivmecillinam or fosfomycin but systemic infections (e.g., bacteraemia) require treatment by **carbapenems** (meropenem, imipenem, ertapenem), temocillin or amikacin.

The carbapenems are very broad spectrum, but must be given parenterally. Hospital use is restricted to prevent development of resistance. The emergence of CPE (there are a variety of different types: KPC, OXA-48, VIM, IMP and NDM) is a growing problem as treatment is largely limited to old and toxic antibiotics, such as colistin (though resistance to colistin is now emerging). Some CPE are even resistant to recently introduced antibiotics, such as ceftolozane-tazobactam or ceftazidime-avibactam. CPE, like ESBL, also spread on plasmids and so are readily transmissible. Some countries have high rates of CPE that are responsible for serious infections and have a high mortality rate. Resistant bacteria have now spread around the world and pose the greatest current infection threat to patients in hospital.

'Nonsurgical' Enterobacteriaceae

Other members of the family cause primary bowel infections. *Salmonella typhi* causes **typhoid** which may cause bowel perforations and *Shigella* causes **bacillary dysentery**. Rarely, *Salmonella* is incriminated in acute appendicitis and primary 'mycotic' aneurysms. An increasingly important cause of **acute haemorrhagic colitis** is *E. coli* O157:H7 and other verotoxin-producing *E. coli*. This is indistinguishable from acute haemorrhagic ulcerative colitis and should be sought bacteriologically in all cases. These strains have also caused large outbreaks of food-borne disease and produce a verotoxin (Shiga-like toxin) responsible for haemolytic uraemic syndrome (HUS) resulting in acute renal failure. *Yersinia* sometimes produces an acute ileal inflammation which may mimic acute appendicitis and has a similar appearance to Crohn disease at laparotomy. *Campylobacter jejuni*, the most common cause of food-borne infection, can also cause a pseudo-appendicitis by initiating terminal ileitis and mesenteric lymph node inflammation.

Pseudomonas

Pathophysiology

The main pathogen in this group of **aerobic gram-negative rods** is *Pseudomonas aeruginosa*, an uncommon cause of surgical infection except in debilitated, hospitalised patients. It is found in a wide variety of habitats including soil, water, plants and animals, reflecting its predilection for moist environments. It is commonly found on hospital and cleaning equipment and even in chemical disinfectants and antiseptics. In about 10% of the population, *Ps. aeruginosa* is a normal intestinal commensal and is primarily an in-hospital (nosocomial) pathogen. The organism is resistant to many antibiotics and so tends to proliferate when other flora are suppressed by broad-spectrum antibiotics.

Pseudomonas is a common colonising organism in long-standing wounds, such as compound fractures, chronic leg ulcers and indwelling urinary catheters but its presence is not always clinically significant. In wounds and ulcers, it can be recognised by its characteristic blue-green discharge. It colonises burns and may become pathogenic in patients with extensive burns, giving rise to fatal sepsis. *Pseudomonas* infection can be serious in ophthalmic surgery and may lead to loss of the infected eye and is often responsible for chronic and recurrent external ear infections (otitis externa). Finally, *Ps. aeruginosa* may be responsible for hospital-acquired pneumonias in ventilated patients or for fatal systemic sepsis in terminally ill patients.

Antibiotic Sensitivities

True infection must, as ever, be distinguished from colonisation where treatment is not indicated and would encourage development of resistance. *Ps. aeruginosa* is intrinsically resistant to most antibiotics; those that have activity include the **aminoglycosides** (**gentamicin, amikacin** and **tobramycin**), some extended-spectrum beta-lactam antibiotics (**ceftazidime, cefepime, ceftolozane-tazobactam;** note that ceftriaxone has no activity against *Ps. aeruginosa*), **piperacillin-tazobactam** and the carbapenems (**imipenem** or **meropenem;** note that ertapenem, a once daily carbapenem has no activity against *Ps. aeruginosa*). The quinolones, **ciprofloxacin** and **ofloxacin**, are the only orally effective antipseudomonal agents.

Acinetobacter

These are gram-negative coccobacilli that are strictly aerobic nonfermenters and are generally not pathogenic to healthy individuals. Their importance lies in causing infections in vulnerable patients, especially on ICUs and burns units, and their high rate of intrinsic antibiotic resistance, including to carbapenems; treatment options are usually limited to amikacin, tigecycline or colistin. The most commonly identified species is *Acinetobacter baumanii*.

Anaerobes

Anaerobic bacteria form a major part of the GI tract flora, outnumbering *E. coli* and related coliforms by 1000 to 1. Many parts of the body are colonised by anaerobes, even those exposed to air, including skin, mouth, upper respiratory tract, external genitalia and vagina. These colonising organisms become important because surgery disrupts anatomical barriers to allow contamination and infection. Other important factors that promote anaerobe growth include intestinal obstruction, tissue destruction and hypoxia (as in burns and vascular insufficiency), and foreign bodies. Anaerobic infection can be life-threatening and surgical management is often required. Some anaerobes cause toxin-related diseases including tetanus. The most commonly encountered anaerobes are:

- **Gram-negative bacilli**—*Bacteroides fragilis* and other *Bacteroides* species (spp.), *Porphyromonas* spp., *Prevotella* spp., *Fusobacterium* spp. and *Bilophila wadsworthia*
- **Gram-positive cocci**—*Peptostreptococcus* and microaerophilic streptococci
- **Gram-positive bacilli**—*Clostridium* spp. (spore forming), *Actinomyces* spp., *Propionibacterium* spp. and *Bifidobacterium* spp.

Antibiotic Sensitivities

Most anaerobes are highly sensitive to **metronidazole**. Metronidazole can be given orally, intravenously or rectally, with the rectal route resulting in plasma levels equivalent to intravenous administration. Metronidazole is standard prophylaxis before appendicectomy and large bowel surgery, and has dramatically reduced peritoneal and wound infections. Other antibiotics with broad anaerobic activity are co-amoxiclav, piperacillin/tazobactam (Tazocin), clindamycin, tigecycline, the carbapenems (imipenem and meropenem) and chloramphenicol.

Bacteroides

Pathophysiology

Bacteroides cause pyogenic infections after faecal contamination of the peritoneal cavity, along with other gut commensals, and occasionally cause sepsis in debilitated patients. *Bacteroides* were not identified as pathogens until the early 1970s because their strict anaerobic culture requirements were unrecognised. Indeed *Bacteroides* spp. were probably responsible for many so-called sterile intraabdominal abscesses. The importance of *B. fragilis* as a cause of surgical infection is probably still underestimated.

Clostridia

Clostridia are gram-positive rods widely distributed in soil and as intestinal commensals. Clostridia form **spores** resistant to drying, heat and antiseptics and can survive for long periods. They are mostly **obligate anaerobes** which can only proliferate in the absence of oxygen; they cause much of the putrefaction and decay of animal material in nature. The main pathological effects are caused by powerful **exotoxins**. Those of surgical importance are **gas gangrene**, **tetanus** and *C. difficile* **pseudomembranous colitis**.

Gas Gangrene

Gas gangrene results when *Clostridium perfringens* (formerly *C. welchii*) and other anaerobes (e.g., *Bacteroides* spp. and streptococci) proliferate in necrotic tissue, secreting powerful toxins. Toxins spread rapidly and destroy nearby tissues, generating gas which causes the characteristic sign of crepitus ('crackling') on palpation and the typical x-ray appearance (see Fig. 3.8). Deep traumatic wounds involving muscle, and wounds contaminated with soil, clothes or faeces are most susceptible. The condition is very common in battle wounds—gas gangrene was responsible for vast numbers of deaths during the First World War.

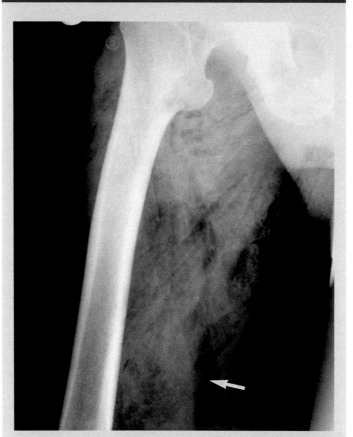

• **Fig. 3.8** Gas Gangrene. This 46-year-old man sustained extensive contaminated lacerations of the medial right thigh *(arrowed)* in a road traffic collision. Gas gangrene developed, rapidly involving all the muscles of the thigh because the condition was not recognised early and necrotic muscle was not excised immediately and completely. Note the widespread streaks of radiolucent gas bubbles tracking along the muscle planes. This patient died of toxaemia despite antibiotics, surgery and hyperbaric oxygen therapy

In surgical practice, the highest risk of gas gangrene is in **lower limb amputations** for ischaemia (infection from the patient's bowel) and in high-velocity **gunshot wounds** (from perforated bowel or by external contamination). Gas gangrene occasionally occurs in surgical wounds when ischaemic tissue is contaminated with bowel flora. The area of muscle necrosis may initially be small. Gas gangrene is recognised when the overlying skin turns black, and spreads at an alarming rate. Within hours, necrosis rages along muscle planes. Later the skin breaks down and a thin, foul-smelling purulent exudate leaks out. Toxins are absorbed and cause rapid clinical deterioration and death within 24 to 48 hours unless the process can be halted by timely and vigorous intervention.

C. perfringens is very sensitive to **benzylpenicillin** which should be given prophylactically by injection as soon as possible after a traumatic injury involving muscle, or less than an hour before ischaemic limb amputation (metronidazole is suitable for patients allergic to penicillin). In the surgery of contaminated wounds, preventing clostridial infection requires meticulous excision of all necrotic tissue followed by packing of the wound rather than suturing. Further excisions are likely to be needed and delayed primary closure performed when risk of infection is over, a few days later.

Treatment of Gas Gangrene. Treatment of established gas gangrene is urgent and must proceed vigorously for any hope of survival. Treatment is with high doses of intravenous benzylpenicillin to kill organisms in viable and vascularised tissue, and emergency radical excision of all necrotic tissue. This involves carving back the necrotic muscle to healthy bleeding tissue; affected muscle is recognised by its brick-red colour and failure to contract on cutting. In the surgery of contaminated wounds, preventing clostridial infection requires meticulous excision of all necrotic tissue followed by wound packing rather than suturing. Further excisions are likely to be needed and delayed primary closure performed a few days later.

Hyperbaric oxygen therapy can raise oxygen tension in necrotic tissues, inhibiting organism growth. The patient is placed in a high-pressure chamber with pure oxygen at about 3 atmospheres for several hours daily. However, gas gangrene may still spread, necessitating further heroic surgical interventions. Even with intensive treatment, the prognosis for established gas gangrene remains bleak.

Tetanus

Tetanus is caused by *Clostridium tetani*, which also infects dirty wounds. The entry wound may be minute, perhaps caused by a rose thorn or splinter. The organism produces an **exotoxin** with little local effect but, even in minute quantities, with powerful neuromuscular effects causing widespread muscular spasm. The first signs are often **acute muscle spasms** and **neck stiffness** or **trismus ('lockjaw')**. If untreated, these progress to **opisthotonus** (arching of the back caused by extensor spasm), generalised convulsions and eventually death from exhaustion and respiratory failure several days later.

Tetanus is now rare in developed countries because of immunisation with **tetanus toxoid** during childhood, followed by boosters at 10-year intervals. In the United Kingdom, boosters are no longer needed if an initial five-dose vaccination schedule has been completed. In Australia and New Zealand, a single booster is recommended at age 45 to 50 years. In developed countries, the annual incidence of tetanus is about one per million and is most common following trivial gardening injuries in the elderly. If the immunisation status following a major contaminated injury is unknown, **benzylpenicillin** should be given plus passive immunisation with **tetanus immune globulin (TIG)**. Treatment of established tetanus usually requires artificial ventilation with drug paralysis, antibiotics and passive immunisation. Debridement of the wound is also useful for diagnostic purposes (culture and PCR), and therapy (i.e., source control). Tetanus serology should also be taken before TIG is given, if possible, for diagnostic purposes. Mortality remains high, especially in the elderly.

Globally, tetanus after trauma remains a massive problem. In some developing countries, neonatal tetanus results from the practice of applying cow dung as a dressing to the umbilical stump.

Pseudomembranous Colitis

Pseudomembranous colitis can be the most serious form of **antibiotic-associated diarrhoea** (see Ch. 12) and is caused by overgrowth of a toxigenic *C. difficile*. The organism gets its name from the difficulty of growing it in culture. Infection produces a thick fibrinous 'membrane' on large intestinal mucosa, within which the organism proliferates. Its toxins cause a profound watery and sometimes bloody diarrhoea, leading to dehydration and electrolyte loss.

Pseudomembranous colitis may develop after only a single dose of any antibiotic. Cephalosporins and ciprofloxacin are the most commonly implicated antibiotics, but any antibiotic that is used frequently will cause it. Diagnosis can be made by sigmoidoscopy and biopsy in the 50% of patients with left-sided colonic involvement, but beware of the increased risk of bowel perforation when harvesting biopsies from patients with active *C. difficile* infection. Cases of pseudomembranous infection are increasingly recognised in patients after total colectomy and *C. difficile* should be suspected in cases of large unexplained stoma output and rising white cell count. Diagnosis is best made by **detecting the specific toxin in the stool**. *C. difficile* can also be cultured from the stool. Mortality rates are high, as are recurrence rates. Although the organism is sensitive to penicillin, this fails to penetrate the pseudomembrane. Oral vancomycin is now the treatment of choice and should be used if severe disease is suspected (suggested by raised inflammatory markers, deteriorating renal function, toxic megacolon, low albumin); the intravenous formulation can be given by rectal tube in patients unable to take oral treatment, especially on ICUs. Fidaxomicin, has recently been licensed for *C. difficile* infection and appears to have a lower relapse rate than traditional treatment. Other recently introduced therapeutic options include bezlotuxumab (a monoclonal antibody that has been shown to reduce recurrences) and faecal transplantation (which can be used to treat recurrences).

Mycobacteria

Mycobacteria (e.g., *M. tuberculosis*, NTM) are, as described earlier, increasing in frequency owing to increased travel and increased immunosuppression. These should be considered the 'great mimic' as they can infect any site in addition to the lungs (e.g., lymph nodes, abdomen, bone and joint) and cause many conditions. Swabs are not appropriate samples—biopsies are usually required (e.g., peritoneum, lymph node) and culture for TB/NTM should be requested. Treatment is prolonged (minimum of 6 months) with multiple drugs and usually requires a multidisciplinary approach. HIV coinfection should also be excluded. Culture and sensitivity testing is even more important now because of the development of resistant strains.

Viruses of Particular Surgical Importance

The chronic blood-borne viral infections **hepatitis B** and **C** and **HIV** are important in surgical practice because of the risk of virus transmission from patient to surgeon during operation and vice versa, as well as cross-infection between patients. Patients may also need surgical intervention for complications of hepatitis or HIV infection.

Human Immunodeficiency Virus (HIV)

Classification of HIV Infections

HIV causes a chronic infection that may progress to **acquired immune deficiency syndrome (AIDS)**. The illness evolves through several stages or groups, classified by the US Centers for Disease Control, in 1986, as:

- (Group I) the **acute seroconversion illness.** Seroconversion occurs as long as 3 months after infection, and as many as 70% of infected patients are asymptomatic at the time of seroconversion. Patients usually test negative for antibodies against HIV before and during the seroconversion illness. Most modern diagnostic kits used in the United Kingdom test for antigen AND antibody so 'false negative' results are now much less likely
- (Group II) the **asymptomatic period** during which patients usually feel completely well

- (Group III) as the disease progresses, the patient may develop generalised lymphadenopathy and wasting (**AIDS-related complex**)
- (Group IV) **AIDS** is manifest by development of unusual opportunistic infections (e.g., *Pneumocystis* pneumonia, cytomegalovirus [CMV] infections, cerebral toxoplasmosis, atypical mycobacterial infections), certain malignant diseases (Kaposi sarcoma, generalised or cerebral lymphoma, aggressive invasive uterine cervical cancer) and neurological disease (**AIDS dementia complex**)

The use of combinations of antiretroviral drugs ('high activity antiretroviral therapy') has dramatically affected the natural history, with a large sustained drop in mortality from opportunistic infections.

Surgical Involvement in HIV Cases. Surgeons may be involved in diagnosing bowel-related problems (e.g., oesophageal candidiasis) by oesophago-gastro-duodenoscopy (OGD). In late-stage disease, CMV infection may involve any part of the GI tract, ranging from mouth ulcers, to ulcers in the jejunum that may perforate, to colitis. For AIDS colitis, colonoscopy and biopsy are often required for diagnosis. Treatment involves intravenous antiviral drugs.

AIDS patients may develop severe perianal herpes with secondary anal fistula or abscess formation. In a patient with known AIDS, perianal lesions should be assumed to be herpes until proven otherwise as the presentation is often atypical. Kaposi sarcomas (see Ch. 46, p. 596) may require local excision. Other examples of surgical involvement with HIV-infected patients include insertion of long-term central venous catheters (e.g., Hickman line), insertion of percutaneous endoscopic gastrostomy tubes for feeding, or joint replacements in HIV infected haemophiliacs.

Viral Hepatitis

Viral hepatitis manifests with anorexia, nausea and sometimes abdominal discomfort in the right upper quadrant followed by jaundice. Many viruses cause acute hepatitis, often with different modes of transmission, incubation times, prognosis and complications. These include CMV, Epstein–Barr virus (EBV) and the hepatitis viruses.

Hepatitis A

Hepatitis A is transmitted by the faecal–oral route and has an incubation period of 2 to 6 weeks. It rarely causes fulminating disease and never leads to chronic hepatitis or cirrhosis. Its only surgical importance is in the differential diagnosis of jaundice. A vaccine for hepatitis A is available.

Hepatitis B

Hepatitis B is transmitted by blood or body fluids, including sexual intercourse, or from mother to foetus or baby (termed *vertical transmission*). Incubation is 6 weeks to 6 months. Hepatitis B infection leads to chronic hepatitis and cirrhosis in 5% to 10% of cases; this variety of cirrhosis may progress to **hepatocellular carcinoma** (the most common cause worldwide). Hepatitis B is preventable by vaccination and this is indicated for neonates of mothers who carry the virus, all healthcare workers and people living in high-risk areas.

Exposure to hepatitis B virus has several possible outcomes:
- Acute fulminant hepatitis—rare but fatal (or may require liver transplantation)
- Acute hepatitis—clearing of the virus leads to lifelong immunity

- Chronic infection—may lead to chronic hepatitis/cirrhosis (and hepatocellular carcinoma)
- Chronic carrier state—mainly caused by infection at birth but can occur later with development of immune tolerance and no obvious active disease

Diagnosis of Hepatitis B. The hepatitis B surface *antigen* (**HBsAg**) can be detected in blood in the early stages. Patients later develop *antibodies* to the viral core (**anti-HBc**) which is a marker of exposure to the virus but does not confer immunity. Later still, with clearance of the virus, patients develop surface *antibodies* (**anti-HBs**) which confer lifetime immunity. Patients who do not clear the virus remain surface *antigen* (HbsAg) positive and may become **chronic carriers**, that is, remain infectious to other people and prone to risk of complications themselves.

HBsAg-positive patients may transmit the virus if there is recipient exposure to sufficient material, for example, by blood transfusion. The special case of **e antigen positivity** (HBeAg) indicates patients with higher infectivity.

Hepatitis B vaccines contain recombinant inactivated surface *antigen* and induce immunity by stimulating production of surface *antibody*; this is the only positive serological marker in vaccinated people.

Treatment of Hepatitis B. Hepatitis B DNA can now be detected in blood, giving a definitive diagnosis and an estimate of the quantity of virus in the bloodstream (viral load) to guide treatment. Therapy with interferon (typically pegylated forms which are better tolerated) and antivirals (e.g., lamivudine, entecavir, adefovir or tenofovir) has been partially successful in treating chronic infections, reducing infectivity and the risk of hepatocellular carcinoma. Chronic carriers failing therapy should be monitored for hepatocellular carcinoma by annual estimation of **serum alpha-fetoprotein** and undergo liver ultrasound scanning every 2 years, as partial hepatectomy can sometimes cure early cases.

Hepatitis C

Hepatitis C is transmitted via the same routes as hepatitis B but sexual transmission is believed to be less common. The incubation period is approximately 2 months. Chronic liver disease develops in a higher proportion of cases (30% to 50%) but is often of low grade. Hepatitis C is also an important cause of hepatocellular carcinoma worldwide.

Serological diagnosis is troublesome because hepatitis C virus (HCV) antibody tests often give false positives. Seroconversion occurs late, often weeks to months after the acute illness. Definitive diagnosis is made by detecting hepatitis C ribonucleic acid in serum. As in hepatitis B, viral load assays are used to monitor response to therapy and infectivity. Treatment varies by genotype but options include interferon with ribavirin, simeprevir, sofosbuvir, daclatasvir, a combination of ledipasvir and sofosbuvir, a combination of ombitasvir, paritaprevir and ritonavir, taken with or without dasabuvir, and a combination of sofosbuvir and velpatasvir are now available. In most cases a positive hepatitis C antibody test is likely to mean continuing infection.

Hepatitis D

This is a defective virus that requires hepatitis B surface antigen for full expression; it occurs only as a coinfection with hepatitis B and can be prevented by vaccination for hepatitis B.

Hepatitis E

Hepatitis E is transmitted by the faecal–oral route and is usually self-limiting. However, it may cause fulminant liver failure, particularly in pregnant women.

• **BOX 3.2** Definitions of SIRS, MODS and Sepsis

Systemic Inflammatory Response Syndrome (SIRS)
Present if two or more of the following are present:
- Temperature >38°C or <36°C
- Heart rate >90 beats/min
- Respiratory rate >20 breaths/min or $PaCO_2$ <4.3 kPa
- White cell count >12,000 or <4000 cells/mm³ or more than 10% immature forms
- Serum lactate >4 mmol/L

Multiple Organ Dysfunction Syndrome (MODS)
Present if SIRS is associated with organ dysfunction (e.g., oliguria, hypoxia)

Sepsis (or Systemic Sepsis)
Defined as SIRS in association with bacterial infection proven by culture

Severe Sepsis
Defined as sepsis associated with signs of organ dysfunction (e.g., renal failure)

Septic Shock
Defined as SIRS associated with hypotension refractory to volume replacement and requiring vasopressors

Bacteraemia
Presence of bacteria in the bloodstream

Septicaemia
Presence of bacteria in the bloodstream with the presence of sepsis

PaCO₂, Partial pressure of carbon dioxide in arterial blood.

Sepsis

See also http://www.survivesepsis.org/.

Multiple Organ Dysfunction and the Systemic Inflammatory Response Syndrome

Multiple organ dysfunction syndrome or MODS (multiorgan failure or MOF) was recognised as a clinical entity in the mid-1970s when it became recognised that any major physiological insult could lead to failure of organs remote from the initiating disease process. Later, the underlying condition was found to be an unrestrained systemic inflammatory response (**SIRS**), initiated by adverse events, such as trauma, infection, inflammation, ischaemia or ischaemia–reperfusion injury. MODS is the most common reason for surgical patients to stay longer than 5 days in intensive care (see Box 3.2).

Sepsis (also known by or incorporated in the terms **septic shock**, **systemic sepsis**, **septicaemia** and **sepsis syndrome**) describes the clinical features when infection is the initiating factor of MODS. Early on, the condition may be reversible. Note that sepsis is *not* synonymous with infection. In MODS, the sequence of individual organ failure often follows a predictable pattern with **pulmonary failure** first, followed by hepatic, intestinal, renal, cerebral and finally cardiac failure. Pulmonary failure is associated with acute (formerly 'adult') respiratory distress syndrome (**ARDS**). In hepatic failure, patients have a rising bilirubin level, impaired clotting (rising prothrombin time), low albumin (caused by impaired hepatic synthetic function), thrombocytopenia and rising serum alanine transaminase, and lactate dehydrogenase (caused by liver damage). Intestinal failure is recognised by **stress bleeding** requiring transfusion, renal failure by rising

plasma creatinine and low urine output, and cardiac failure by low cardiac output and hypotension. Altered mental states, such as confusion also occur (cerebral failure), as may disseminated intravascular coagulopathy.

The mortality of MODS is related to the specific organ involved, the number of failing organs, the duration of the insult and the presence of concomitant sepsis: mortality is around 20% with one organ; 45% with two; 65% with three organs; and more than 75% with four or more.

Pathophysiology of SIRS and MODS

SIRS involves widespread changes, including inflammatory cell activation leading to cytokine release, endothelial injury, disordered haemodynamics and impaired tissue oxygen extraction. It thus represents grossly exaggerated activation of innate immune responses intended as host defences. An unregulated release of inflammatory mediators causes widespread microvascular, haemodynamic and mitochondrial changes that eventually lead to organ failure.

Following initial tissue injury, a local inflammatory response occurs with cytokine induction (see *Immunity* at the start of this chapter). The response to this is mobilisation of inflammatory cells including macrophages and neutrophils which diapedese into the tissues. In addition, cytokines provoke systemic elements of inflammation, including activation of endothelium, the complement system and blood coagulation, amplifying the primary inflammatory response. This sequence is part of the normal and appropriate inflammatory response. However, if the injury is severe or persistent, the local reaction may extend excessively into the systemic circulation producing a systemic inflammatory response or, if initiated by infection, the sepsis syndrome.

Mediators of SIRS and MODS

SIRS and MODS involve complex interactions of endogenous and sometimes exogenous mediators. A range of cytokines is released from activated macrophages and from endothelial and other reticulo-endothelial cells. The suite of cytokines released depends on the nature of the provoking agent and is governed by the specific type of TLR that recognises the aggressor. Cytokines released include **TNF-alpha,** the **interleukins** (particularly IL1 but also IL2, IL6) and **platelet activating factor**. Pharmacological attempts to suppress excess cytokine responses have thus far been ineffective.

Sepsis

The classic septic response, with a hyperdynamic circulation, systemic signs of inflammation and disrupted intermediary metabolism, can be induced in healthy volunteers by injecting **LPS** (from the cell walls of gram-negative bacteria) or the cytokines TNF-alpha or IL1. In gram-negative sepsis, the LPS component of the organisms powerfully activates TLRs on dendritic cells and hence the whole inflammatory cascade. This results in endothelial activation which increases vascular permeability and neutrophil–endothelial interaction. The final common pathway may involve activated neutrophils migrating into the interstitial space of the affected organ and tissue hypoxia. In sepsis, these and other circulating factors working in synergy bring about the devastating effects of MODS.

Clinical Conditions Leading to SIRS and MODS

These include infection and endotoxaemia (gram-negative sepsis) in 50% to 70% of cases, retained necrotic tissue and shock.

Any of these can initiate distant organ failure by the following mechanisms:

- Inducing excessive release of endogenous cytokines
- Disrupting oxygen delivery to the tissues
- Impairing intestinal barrier function allowing **translocation** of intestinal bacteria and endotoxin to the portal and systemic circulations
- Damaging the reticulo-endothelial system

Organ failure induced by acute pancreatitis is caused by a combination of these factors.

Infection

The infection source that leads to MODS may be **acquired** (e.g., intraabdominal abscess) or **endogenous**, that is, from the patient's bowel. Local infection, especially with gram-negative bacteria, stimulates the release of inflammatory cytokines. A similar response is provoked by a substantial volume of necrotic tissue, for example, gangrenous leg, and is worse if the tissue is infected. These **paracrine responses** are beneficial in a local sense, combating infection by increasing blood flow and vascular permeability to allow influx of dendritic cells and macrophages, and activating neutrophils to degranulate and release cytotoxic oxygen radicals. If the stimulating factor is great, a cascade is initiated which leads to sepsis and MODS. Superoxide radicals and other circulating factors then damage cells elsewhere, causing widespread vasodilatation and increased vascular permeability leading to hypotension and circulatory collapse. The myocardium is depressed and cellular metabolic functions are disrupted.

Endogenous Sources of Infection. The large bowel is a reservoir for bacteria and endotoxin which are normally safely contained. If the **intestinal barrier** is breached (e.g., by splanchnic ischaemia, impoverished luminal nutrition of enterocytes or altered intestinal flora), **translocation** of bacteria into the portal circulation can occur in as little as 30 minutes. If the liver Kupffer cells are also impaired, intestinal bacteria and endotoxin are not prevented from reaching the systemic circulation in the normal way. This may explain the potential for renal failure in jaundiced patients undergoing operation *(hepatorenal syndrome)*. This endogenous source probably explains the 30% of patients who suffer organ dysfunction without an obvious source of infection. Typically, such patients become affected after prolonged hypotension (hypovolaemic or cardiogenic shock) or hypoxaemia (e.g., multiple trauma victims), or as a result of direct visceral ischaemia (e.g., prolonged aortic clamping and hypotension in a patient with a ruptured aortic aneurysm).

Prevention of Sepsis and MODS

Prevention and early treatment of MODS is summarised in Box 3.3.

Surgical Aspects

In surgical patients, multiple organ dysfunction often results from a complication, such as a bowel anastomotic leak, or from severe acute pancreatitis (which may be sterile but becomes devastating if infected). Tissue necrosis following trauma, or death of an ischaemic limb may also precipitate the syndrome.

Organ dysfunction often begins insidiously. At an early stage, dysfunction can be confirmed by investigation and active resuscitation and treatment of causative factors are likely to have beneficial effects. By 7 to 10 days without effective treatment, pulmonary failure (ARDS) and hepatic and renal failure appear; MODS is now present and the prognosis becomes substantially worse.

• BOX 3.3   Prevention and Early Treatment of Sepsis and Multiple Organ Dysfunction Syndrome

General Prevention

- Rapid resuscitation and early definitive treatment of major injuries
- Good surgical technique
- Appropriate use of prophylactic and therapeutic antibiotics
- Early diagnosis and treatment of infective surgical complications (e.g., leaking anastomoses)
- Early and thorough excision of necrotic and infected tissue

Prevention for At-risk Patients and Treatment of Early Signs

- Rapid cardiovascular resuscitation and prevention of shock (minimise splanchnic ischaemia)
- Optimisation of oxygen delivery (measure arterial PO_2 and pH and correct metabolic acidosis)
- Nutritional support via an enteral route (to nourish enterocytes)

The Sepsis Six (http://www.survivesepsis.org/)
All within 1 hour:
1. Give high-flow oxygen via non-rebreathe bag
2. Take blood cultures and consider source control
3. Give IV antibiotics according to local protocol
4. Start IV fluid resuscitation with Hartmann or equivalent
5. Check lactate
6. Monitor hourly urine output; consider catheterisation

IV, Intravenous; *PO_2,* partial pressure of oxygen.

Preventing sepsis and early management of major gut-related infection before it provokes the SIRS–MODS cascade is vital. Appropriate use of **prophylactic antibiotics** in bowel surgery or trauma helps, but intraoperative and postoperative **errors in technique**, particularly anastomotic leakage or clinical judgement, are major factors in more than 50% of patients with multiple organ dysfunction. Good clinical judgement, effective resuscitation, good operative technique, effective excision of necrotic tissue, minimising bacterial contamination and preventing accumulation of postoperative fluid collections (serum or blood) are all necessary for prevention. The purpose is to eliminate environments in which bacteria multiply and improve the delivery of host antibacterial defences.

Surgical complications with septic potential should be treated early, usually by definitive surgery, for example removal of necrotic tissue, drainage of abscesses and control of peritoneal contamination by exteriorising leaking anastomoses. This helps reduce the circulating level of inflammatory mediators and limits the period of stress. It is often better to perform a laparotomy on suspicion and find it normal than to 'wait and see' and risk rapid deterioration and death.

Other Preventive Factors in At-Risk Patients

Adequate and early **fluid resuscitation** is vital in patients with hypovolaemia, including in trauma victims, acute pancreatitis or bowel obstruction, because the loss of intravascular volume leads to deficient tissue perfusion (i.e., shock) and splanchnic ischaemia. Maintaining tissue oxygenation is also vital; at-risk patients must have arterial blood gases and pH estimated and receive supplemental oxygen or assisted ventilation as required. To help prevent intestinal bacterial translocation, enterocytes and colonocytes are best supported by **enteral feeding**, if necessary, by a feeding jejunostomy or a fine-bore nasogastric tube. Glutamine, arginine and omega-3 fatty acids are believed to be important.

4

Shock and Resuscitation

The Pathophysiology of Shock

The term 'shock' can be defined as **acute circulatory failure of sufficient magnitude to compromise tissue perfusion**, which if untreated, proceeds rapidly to irreversible organ damage and death of the patient.

Circulatory failure and subsequent hypotension in the shocked patient results in cellular and tissue hypoxia. This occurs when there is either reduced oxygen delivery to tissues or inadequate oxygen use. Reduced delivery may be caused by mechanical airways obstruction, chest trauma, impaired gas exchange (e.g., pneumonia or pulmonary embolism) or hypoventilation (e.g., respiratory depression caused by opioids), for example. When not treated, tissue hypoxia results in systemic effects (including activation of both inflammatory and anti-inflammatory pathways) leading to tissue damage, intracellular oedema, and cell membrane dysfunction. These eventually lead to worsening acidosis, end-organ damage and potentially death.

There are four mechanisms of shock
1. **Hypovolaemic shock**
2. **Cardiogenic shock** occurs when the pump function of the heart is impaired
3. **Distributive shock** arises as a result of severe peripheral vasodilatation (e.g., septic shock, anaphylactic shock)
4. **Obstructive shock**

The classical symptoms and signs of shock include hypotension, hyperventilation, a rapid weak pulse, cold clammy cyanotic skin and oliguria. Mental changes also occur, most commonly anxiety, confusion and combativeness. Investigations reveal metabolic acidosis, low oxygen saturation and low central venous pressure (CVP). Notably, in **septic shock,** there is peripheral vasodilatation rather than vasoconstriction.

Shock has been described as progressing through three stages. In stage I, there are attempts at **compensation** with skin and splanchnic vasoconstriction. Symptoms and signs are minimal but recognisable. In stage II, **decompensation** occurs, with body mechanisms unable to sustain tissue perfusion despite working at full capacity. Urgent intervention is needed at this stage. By stage III, the changes are essentially **irreversible**, with prolonged shock having caused severe damage to major organs. Successful treatment depends crucially on **early recognition** of shock and its precursors, prompt diagnosis and treatment of the underlying cause and effective support of vital organ function.

Early Recognition of Shock

When surgical patients deteriorate catastrophically, it is often found on retrospective examination of charts that vital signs had been deteriorating for some time and that clinical staff had failed to respond. Early recognition and intervention is crucial because failure of one organ leads to synergistic failure of other organs and an escalating risk of irreversible damage and death.

To help recognise these patients early, structured scoring systems have been developed, seeking to emulate the simplicity, reliability and clinical value of the Glasgow Coma Scale (Table 16.1, p. 246). These generally use routinely recorded physiological data and most are modifications of the **Early Warning Score** (Table 4.1). These have proved very useful for spotting those at risk of deterioration and needing urgent medical attention and have become part of standard care for surgical patients. However, they are not a substitute for frequent clinical observation by doctors of sick patients.

Score	3	2	1	0	1	2	3
TABLE 4.1 **Modified Early Warning Score (MEWS)**[a]							
Respiratory rate (breaths per min)		<9		9–14	15–20	21–29	≥30
Heart rate (bpm)		<40	41–50	51–100	101–110	111–129	≥130
Systolic blood pressure (mmHg)	<70	71–80	81–100	101–199		≥200	
Temperature (°C)		<35		35–38.4		≥38.5	
AVPU score				Alert	Reacting to **V**oice	Reacting to **P**ain	**U**nresponsive

[a]MEWS is one form of bedside scoring that can help early identification of patients likely to need urgent assessment (score 3 or more). A score of 5 or more indicates that the patient is likely to require critical care, usually in a high-dependency or intensive care unit.

Types of Shock

Hypovolaemic Shock (Preload Insufficiency)

This is the most common cause of shock encountered in hospital. **Preload** is defined as the rate of venous return of blood to the heart. Preload insufficiency reduces the diastolic filling pressure and volume and leads to low cardiac output. The underlying problem is inadequate intravascular volume and underfilling of the venous compartment. This can be caused by haemorrhagic or nonhaemorrhagic causes.

Haemorrhagic Hypovolaemic Shock

This can be further subdivided into:
- 'Revealed' haemorrhage—visually acknowledged blood loss, commonly seen in trauma, upper gastrointestinal (GI) and lower GI bleeding. Also occurs intraoperatively and postoperatively (from drains, etc.)
- 'Concealed' haemorrhage, for example intraabdominal bleeding from ruptured spleen or aortic aneurysm, haemorrhage from a duodenal ulcer into small intestine, intramuscular blood loss from fractures, or intracavity haemorrhage after operation.
In concealed haemorrhage, estimating blood loss is difficult. Even in the revealed form, a large proportion of blood loss may also be concealed. Fig. 15.1 (p. 211) shows the changes in vital signs associated with increasing amounts of blood loss.

Nonhaemorrhagic Hypovolaemic Shock

This is caused by loss of intravascular volume other than blood, for example:
- Loss of plasma in extensive burns, resulting in massive loss of serum into blisters or from the skin surface.
- Loss of body sodium and water resulting from severe vomiting or diarrhoea, prolonged fluid loss from a small bowel fistula or ileostomy, or third space loss secondary to acute pancreatitis or bowel obstruction.

Distributive Shock (Vasodilatory Shock)

Relative hypovolaemia occurs if there is inappropriate expansion of the circulatory capacity in relation to blood volume. It may result from failure of normal peripheral resistance and/or vasodilatation of large veins. Peripheral resistance normally maintains cardiac **afterload** and is controlled by the tone of smooth muscle arteriolar and capillary sphincters. About 80% of capillaries are normally closed, and any mechanism that causes inappropriate opening greatly expands circulatory capacity. Molecules that mediate this initiation of vasodilatation vary between causative factors, but all result in severe peripheral vasodilatation. Causes are described subsequently.

Septic Shock

This is the most common form of distributive shock and occurs in response to an infective cause, resulting in impaired tissue perfusion in the setting of an uncontrolled immune response. Patients with septic shock will most likely have all the criteria for the systemic inflammatory response syndrome (SIRS, see later). Septic shock is a combination of distributive shock and organ dysfunction induced by mediators of the host inflammatory response (e.g., cytokines, complement) and sometimes directly by bacterial toxins, especially certain staphylococci or gram-negative bacilli, for example, from a colonic anastomotic leak. Bacterial toxins and cell wall components activate defensive mechanisms and the net result of this **immune burst** is that oxygen usage declines, metabolic acidosis and lactaemia develops and multiple organ dysfunction ensues. Failure of oxygen usage is the result of cardiorespiratory impairment, microcirculatory imbalance and, at cellular level, mitochondrial dysfunction. Septic shock itself can be thought of in three phases. In phase 1 there is extensive vasodilatation, causing relative hypovolaemia. In phase 2 there is widespread endothelial damage causing greatly increased capillary permeability and massive fluid leakage into the interstitial space. This manifests clinically as inadequate blood pressure in the presence of normal or increased cardiac output, until phase 3, when depression of myocardial contractility ensues.

The inflammatory burst also upsets normal blood coagulation by downregulating normal anticoagulants such as alpha-1-antitrypsin, and stimulating procoagulants such as **tissue factor,** as well as inhibiting fibrinolysis. The result may be **disseminated intravascular coagulation** (DIC) with microvascular occlusion, large vessel thrombosis and ischaemia, all contributing to organ dysfunction.

Toxic shock syndrome is a particular form of septic shock associated with staphylococcal or streptococcal infection associated with the use of superabsorbent tampons.

Systemic Inflammatory Response Syndrome

SIRS is characterised by an uncontrolled inflammatory response to an insult which provokes a complex cellular response and mediator cascade that leads to progressive abnormal clinical manifestations (see Box 3.2, p. 48). As mentioned earlier, septic shock is a SIRS response mediated by an infective cause. Non-infective triggers of SIRS include ischaemia, acute pancreatitis, blunt trauma, burns and embolic events (amniotic, air and fat). Mediator responses involve the complement system, acute phase proteins and cytokines (particularly tumour necrosis factor alpha and the interleukins [IL]1-beta and IL6); once triggered, the inflammatory response cascade is difficult to control or suppress.

Anaphylactic Shock

This is an immunoglobulin E (IgE) mediated type 1 hypersensitivity response to a specific antigen resulting in release of mast cell mediators. The predominant effect is extensive **dilatation of the venous compartment** and rapid movement of fluid into the tissues. In addition, there can be bronchospasm, laryngeal oedema, rash and GI signs. Death can occur in minutes and prompt recognition is vital. First-line treatment is removal of potential causative agent, administered epinephrine (IM initially, but may need IV) and volume resuscitation.

In surgical practice, anaphylactic shock usually results from drug administration, particularly via the intravenous route. **Antibiotics**, particularly penicillins, and radiological contrast are the most common culprits. Anyone administering a drug must first check the patient is not sensitive. Insect bites (wasps, bees and hornets) and ingested nuts are also important causes and may be encountered in the emergency department.

Pump Failure (Cardiogenic Shock)

Cardiogenic shock describes a drastic reduction in cardiac output resulting from any form of 'pump failure' caused by direct myocardial damage, mechanical abnormality or malfunction of the heart. This most commonly arises from an **acute myocardial infarction** (MI) or an **acute ventricular arrhythmia**. MI may cause ischaemia or infarction of papillary muscles, which produces acute mitral regurgitation. Another cause is when a large **pulmonary embolus** obstructs blood flow through the lungs and causes secondary cardiac failure. Other causes include cardiac (pericardial) tamponade and tension pneumothorax.

Obstructive Shock

This is caused by extracardiac causes of cardiac failure and circulatory flow. This can be caused by pulmonary problems (and consequent right-sided failure) or mechanical disruption resulting in reduced preload.

Pulmonary associated shock can be caused by:
- pulmonary embolism
- pulmonary hypertension
- valvular stenosis

Mechanical shock can be caused by:
- tension pneumothorax
- pericardial tamponade
- constrictive pericarditis
- restrictive cardiomyopathy
- abdominal compartment syndrome

Clinical Features of Shock

The essential feature of any type of shock is a **precipitate fall in arterial blood pressure**. The immediate homeostatic response is **intense sympathetic activity** and catecholamine release. The heart rate increases dramatically in an attempt to increase cardiac output. Except in septic shock, there is intense cutaneous and visceral vasoconstriction to restore intravascular volume by increasing peripheral resistance. Sudomotor activity causes profuse sweating. Hypoxic tissues revert to anaerobic respiration, producing lactic acid sufficient to cause a metabolic acidosis and compensatory tachypnoea. The clinical picture is a cold, pale, clammy, hypotensive patient with a rapid thready pulse and increased respiratory rate.

Septic shock presents a contrasting clinical picture in which cytokine-mediated peripheral vasodilatation is unresponsive to circulating catecholamines. The patient's skin is flushed and hot and cardiac output is increased to fill the dilated periphery. The pulse is typically 'bounding' in quality. Temperature may be above normal or below normal ('cold sepsis').

In all forms of shock, the circulatory system cannot support the main organ systems without treatment, and organs fail (i.e., decompensate) one by one in a synergistic manner. Pulmonary failure leads to **acute respiratory distress syndrome (ARDS)**, and cerebral hypoxia soon causes confusion and eventually coma. Inadequate renal perfusion causes oliguria which, if not rapidly corrected, leads to acute tubular necrosis and kidney failure. If shock persists, reduced coronary flow and heart failure cause death. In septic shock, organ damage is exacerbated by an intense inflammatory burst and deterioration is inevitable unless the source of infection can be rapidly eliminated and effective support instituted.

Because of the nature of the process, early detection, rapid assessment and treatment is paramount. For all forms of shock, immediate assessment of airway, intravenous access and fluid therapy (with the addition of antibiotics in septic shock) are the first response.

Specific Treatments for Shock

Hypovolaemic Shock

Identifying the cause of the fluid loss is the top priority. Immediate measures should be taken to control blood loss, for example, pressure on a swab over a bleeding wound, endoscopic injection of bleeding peptic ulcer. Fluid replacement should be equivalent to estimated fluid loss but adjusted according to the response of pulse rate, blood pressure, observed jugular venous pressure (or CVP) and urine output. In trauma cases, focused assessment with sonography for trauma (FAST scan) can show evidence of intraabdominal mischief, which would not otherwise be revealed. Where possible, fluids of similar composition to those lost should be used: whole blood for haemorrhage, colloids after major burns. Fluids should be titrated in rapid boluses, for example, 250 mL at a time, and the response to each observed.

Cardiogenic Shock

Rapid diagnosis and resuscitation is key. Escalation to an enhanced care unit, respiratory support, correction of electrolyte and acid-base abnormalities, and prompt drug therapy to maintain blood pressure and cardiac output, along with urgent treatment of the underlying cause, are essential steps in optimising the outcome.

The management of pulmonary embolism (which may present as cardiogenic shock) is discussed in Chapter 12. Fluid overload is a significant hazard in cardiogenic shock.

Septic Shock

(see *Sepsis—MOD and SIRS*, Ch. 3, p. 48)
Systemic sepsis leading to septic shock usually originates from a specific focus of infection or bacterial translocation from the patient's own intestine. In general surgical practice, septic shock most commonly results from **faecal peritonitis** following large bowel **perforation** or **anastomotic breakdown**. Infection in sites unrelated to the primary surgical pathology, such as bladder, chest or 'venous line' (usually central venous cannula) infection, are often the cause. Debilitated patients, uncontrolled diabetics and infants are particularly vulnerable to acute sepsis; a clear source of infection is not always found. Gangrene (necrotising fasciitis) is also a potent cause. The damaging effects of the underlying poor organ perfusion are increased by direct and indirect bacterial exotoxic and endotoxic tissue damage.

Treatment of septic shock is urgent and involves fluid resuscitation, oxygenation, administration of appropriate antibiotics and the tracing and eliminating of the source of infection. Blood cultures must be taken and intravenous broad-spectrum antibiotics administered on a 'best-guess' basis following local protocols (see Box 3.3 'The Sepsis Six', p. 49). Because of interstitial losses, plasma expanders are often needed in large volumes, but should still be titrated against clinical measures (e.g., pulse, CVP). Volume expansion helps to sustain cardiac output and tissue perfusion but addition of inotropes to induce peripheral vasoconstriction, in particular noradrenaline (norepinephrine), may be required. Corticosteroids are known to stabilise cell membranes and low dose administration has been shown in *some* clinical trials to prolong survival in patients with refractory shock.

If the diagnosis of septic shock is correct, resuscitative measures should produce dramatic improvement in the patient's condition within 1 to 2 hours. By that time, the patient should be ready for immediate operation if an abscess, bowel perforation or other surgically remediable cause needs treatment. It is important to emphasise that the source of infection must be urgently eliminated if the septic cascade is to be reversed.

Disseminated Intravascular Coagulation

A major problem in sepsis is generalised activation of the clotting cascade causing DIC. This exhausts the supply of platelets and clotting factors V, VIII and fibrinogen (**consumption coagulopathy**), and activates intrinsic fibrinolytic mechanisms. DIC manifests as spontaneous bleeding or bruising and uncontrollable haemorrhage from operation sites. Diagnosis is made by finding low **fibrinogen** levels and high levels of **D-dimers**, cleaved from fibrin by plasmin and providing evidence of fibrin lysis. Treatment includes managing the initiating cause, giving intravenous heparin to arrest the coagulation process and transfusing appropriate clotting factors, for example, fresh frozen plasma, cryoprecipitate under haematological guidance.

Anaphylactic Shock

Immediate treatment of anaphylactic shock includes removing the causative agent, securing the airway and giving oxygen. Lay the patient flat, raise the feet and start an intravenous fluid challenge (stop intravenous colloid if suspected of being the causative agent). Administer 500 μg of intramuscular adrenaline (epinephrine), that is, 0.5 mL of 1:1000 solution. This dose may be repeated at 5-minute intervals if necessary. An antihistamine (e.g., chlorphenamine 10 mg) should be given by slow intravenous injection (up to a maximum of four doses per day), and continued for up to 48 hours to stabilise mast cells. Hydrocortisone 100 to 300 mg should also be given intravenously, but takes several hours to block histamine receptors and so should not be regarded as contributing to emergency treatment. Intravenous fluids may also be needed to treat hypovolaemia. Be aware of a biphasic response, in which patients stabilise after treatment but relapse later.

Resuscitation of the 'Collapsed' Nontrauma Patient

Principles of Managing Shock by Resuscitation

The aim is to restore tissue perfusion and oxygenation by resuscitative measures, whilst establishing the underlying diagnosis to guide further specific treatment. Early management, ideally within 24 hours of acute deterioration, can be summarised as follows:

- *Clinical volume assessment*—dryness of mouth, peripheral perfusion, pulse rate, blood pressure (compared with normal), jugular venous pressure observation, peripheral and pulmonary oedema (lung bases), measured urinary output, fluid balance charts and trends in body weight.
- **Treat the cause of shock**—this can shut down the inflammatory response. Treatment may mean an operation to exteriorise a leaking anastomosis (i.e., bring the bowel ends to the skin surface) or to excise infected and necrotic tissue or drain pus.
- **Treat infection**—if infection is apparent or suspected, institute antibiotic therapy using potent agents chosen on clinical suspicion until definitive microbiological results are available—remember to take blood cultures as early as possible.
- **Support vital organs** during the time it takes surgery or antibiotics to work. Airway and breathing support (e.g., oxygen administration, intubation, ventilation) benefits most patients, but the critical concern is to optimise the cardiovascular and haemodynamic system, aiming for a CVP between 8 and 12 mmHg, a mean arterial pressure over 65 mmHg and a urine output of at least 0.5 mL/kg per hour.
- **Monitor and assess the response**—clinically, by urine output and, ideally by ultrasonographic assessment of stroke volume.

A Scheme for Managing the Acutely Ill or Shocked Patient

This scheme is given in note form as an *aide-mémoire* for clinicians.

Recognition of the Acutely Unwell Patient

(see Table 4.1)
The cardinal signs in a patient likely to need critical care in a high-dependency or intensive care unit include:

- substantially increased or decreased respiratory rate
- bradycardia or tachycardia
- low blood pressure (compare with usual)
- hypo- or hyperthermia
- decreased level of consciousness

Sequence for Action in the Patient at Risk

In summary, this includes the following steps, which are detailed subsequently:

A. Initial assessment
B. Broad diagnosis
C. Immediate care
D. Monitoring and reassessment
E. Investigation to narrow the diagnosis
F. Definitive treatment

A. Initial Assessment

The aim is rapidly to establish the urgency and severity of the situation. If vital signs are unsatisfactory and the patient unresponsive, a cardiac arrest or 'crash call' may be needed to bring more hands to assist. If an early warning score (such as Modified Early Warning Score) is above a predetermined threshold, consultation is needed to arrange transfer to a critical care unit.

History

As much history should be gleaned as time permits, for example, the context of the acute deterioration, medical state before deterioration, past medical history including allergies, and recent treatments including operations. Check drug charts.

Vital Signs

Nurses can help gather information while assessment continues; vital signs should be monitored at frequent intervals. Observations include respiratory rate, temperature, pulse rate, systolic blood pressure and level of consciousness (the AVPU descending scale is simple and reproducible—A means the patient is fully **A**lert, V means responds to **V**oice, P means responds to **P**ain and U is **U**nresponsive).

Initial tests include oxygen saturation, blood glucose estimation, blood gas analysis and electrocardiogram (ECG) for evidence of MI. Note that new onset atrial fibrillation or flutter on ECG is often an indicator of sepsis. A bounding pulse and flushed extremities may suggest septic shock.

Examination—the Initial Survey

General Impression Including Skin
- Intravenous lines and fluids, drug treatments being given via syringe driver, catheters, etc.
- Peripheral perfusion, hydration, oedema, anaemia, jaundice, bruising, rashes, nutritional state.

Head and Neck
- Stridor—obstruction of upper airway, for example, oedema, bleed into thyroid lesion/mediastinal mass or postoperatively, inhaled foreign body, inhaled vomitus
- Mouth and throat—evidence of abscess, for example, peritonsillar abscess (quinsy), Ludwig angina

Chest
- Localised poor air entry—infection, atelectasis, pneumothorax
- Generalised poor air entry—asthma, large pleural effusions
- Expiratory wheeze—anaphylaxis or cardiac failure
- If acutely breathless, consider thromboembolism

Heart
- New onset chest pain—MI
- Cardiac murmurs—infective endocarditis, MI, acute valve prolapse
- Elevated jugular venous pressure—acute cardiac failure caused by MI

- If cardiac problem suspected, check ECG for changes of ischaemia, arrhythmias

Abdomen Including Rectal and/or Vaginal Examination if Necessary
- Localised tenderness—localised intraabdominal infection, renal colic (loin)
- Generalised tenderness—peritonitis
- Distension—bowel obstruction, intraperitoneal or retroperitoneal bleed, ascites
- Melaena or fresh blood per rectum—GI bleed
- Lump—strangulated hernia, intraabdominal mass

Limbs
- Unilaterally (or bilaterally) pale and cold with or without necrosis—acute ischaemia
- Globally pale, cold—peripheral shutdown caused by shock
- Swollen and blue—deep venous thrombosis (in patient with suspected pulmonary embolism)
- Red—cellulitis, diabetic foot infection with systemic sepsis

Neurology
- Conscious level
- Signs of unilateral palsy—stroke

B. Broad Diagnosis

Priorities for immediate treatment and further investigation need to be decided following initial assessment, if necessary from a single major finding. Priorities change as evidence is collected and depending on the response to treatment.

Examples are:
- *Respiratory*—upper airways obstruction, for example, thyroid enlargement/haemorrhage into nodule
- *Vascular events*—abdominal aortic aneurysm rupture, aortic dissection, pulmonary embolism, acute coronary syndromes including MI, stroke and lower limb gangrene (usually causes insidious rather than acute development of shock)

Abdominal Problems

- *Blood loss*—upper or lower GI bleeding, intra- or retroperitoneal bleed
- *GI obstruction including strangulation*—gastric, small bowel or large bowel, hernia, volvulus
- *Generalised peritonitis*—perforation of an abdominal viscus (appendix, peptic ulcer, diverticular disease); acute pancreatitis
- *Abdominal colic*—ureteric, biliary, intestinal
- *Intraabdominal infection*—gastroenteritis, acute appendicitis, diverticulitis, cholecystitis; urinary tract infection
- *Obstetric and gynaecological*—ruptured ectopic pregnancy/ovarian cyst/pregnancy/salpingo-oophoritis
- *Other infections*—infected central venous line, abscesses, cellulitis, diabetic foot, limb gangrene, gastroenteritis including antibiotic-associated colitis
- *Metabolic*—surgical disease can precipitate or be complicated by hypoglycaemia in diabetics; consider Addison disease (adrenal insufficiency) if the patient is hypotensive

C. Immediate Care

Inform a senior doctor about the urgency of the case.

Oxygen

Immediately secure a mask delivering 100% oxygen. The comatose patient may need to be intubated and positive pressure ventilation commenced.

Fluid Management

Haemodynamic optimisation is very important and is based on clinical signs and monitoring of CVP and urine output.

- Take **venous blood** for haemoglobin, haematocrit, urea and electrolytes, glucose, amylase and blood grouping/ordering of blood for transfusion if necessary. Take an arterial sample for blood gas estimation and acid–base status; get blood cultures if septic shock is suspected
- Set up an **intravenous infusion** and administer intravenous fluids/drugs, guided by vital signs and findings. For example, if the patient is hypotensive, give crystalloid or colloid solutions (at least 1 litre rapidly); if cardiogenic shock is likely, the circulating volume must not be expanded rapidly
- Blood transfusion if necessary
- Urinary catheter to monitor hourly output; urine dipstick

Drugs

- Infection—antibiotics
- Analgesia if in pain—morphine intravenously
- Low blood glucose—dextrose

D. Monitoring and Reassessment

Monitoring

The most useful guides to the success of resuscitation are respiratory rate (unless ventilated), CVP, hourly urinary output and plasma lactate.

- Central venous line—often required to monitor central pressure and response to fluids
- Arterial line if necessary
- Nasogastric tube if vomiting; include fluid aspirated on the fluid balance chart
- Request a cardiac ECG monitor if a cardiac problem is suspected

Reassessment

Check the response to therapy: respiratory rate, pulse rate, blood pressure, CVP and plasma lactate. Consider moving the patient to a critical care bed and surgical intervention if the response to therapy is inadequate.

E. Investigation to Narrow the Diagnosis

Consider the most likely diagnosis and quickest route to confirming the initial 'best guess':

- Check blood results
- If there is infection: blood culture, sputum culture
- Chest problems: chest x-ray, computed tomography (CT) pulmonary angiogram if pulmonary embolism is suspected
- Cardiac problems: troponin blood levels, echocardiogram
- Abdomen: plain x-ray/ultrasound or CT scan/endoscopy if the clinical diagnosis is equivocal

F. Definitive treatment

Give definitive treatment as required according to the diagnosis.

5

Imaging and Interventional Techniques in Radiology and Surgery

Introduction

This chapter gives an overview of imaging, endoscopic, interventional and biopsy procedures used to make a diagnosis and treat patients. **Interventional radiology** describes minimal access procedures using image guidance to treat conditions whilst causing least trauma. It is usually performed by radiologists or specialist clinicians. Examples include angioplasty, nephrostomy and endoscopic placement of biliary stents.

Plain Radiology

Body tissues absorb x-rays in proportion to their electron density, which is determined by the atomic number of their elements and their physical density. A plain radiograph is a shadow of the summated densities along the line of the x-ray beam and a computed tomography (CT) scan is a plan of electron density in a section of the body. Calcium is a large atom contained in bone, and has many electrons, so bones absorb x-irradiation very well. Conventionally, bones are displayed white on radiographs or CT. **Contrast media** also absorb x-rays well as they contain iodine or barium, both are large atoms with many electrons. Low-density tissues made up of atoms with a low atomic number, such as air in lungs, absorb few x-rays and are displayed as black. Intermediate densities, such as water in muscle or organs are displayed as grey. The electrons in fat are more widely spaced than in water and so it does not absorb as much x-radiation as water. Remember, fat floats on water because its physical density is less than water. This is why fat (subcutaneous fat) appears darker than water (gallbladder) on a CT scan.

Some **foreign bodies** in wounds are radiopaque, including metal and most glass fragments, but wood and plastic are radiolucent and invisible. Gauze swabs used in operating theatres are radiolucent but have a radiopaque strand allowing them to be located radiographically if left in a wound (Fig. 5.1).

CASE HISTORY

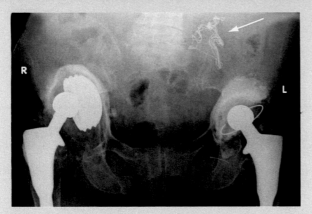

• **Fig. 5.1** Plain abdominal x-ray showing retained surgical swab. This 83-year-old woman had persistent pain in the left iliac fossa after a left hip replacement. This pelvic x-ray was taken to investigate the new joint. However, a radiopaque marker was spotted *(arrowed)* indicating a surgical swab that had been left in the abdomen after a laparotomy for perforated duodenal ulcer, 8 years previously. The swab was removed uneventfully at a second laparotomy.

Safety in Departments of Medical Imaging

Radiation Safety

Ionising radiation is both mutagenic and carcinogenic and irradiation of patients and observers must be minimised. This is achieved by:

- Giving training in radiation protection to all staff using and working near x-ray equipment.
- Ensuring every investigation potentially helps with management and none is performed merely as 'routine'.
- Improving design of x-ray equipment to minimise radiation dose and scatter whilst preserving diagnostic detail.
- Low energy radiation which would be absorbed by the body is removed by thin copper or aluminium filters. This radiation would cause harm and not contribute to formation of the image.
- Physical barriers are built into radiology suites or provided to protect staff. These include barium plaster in walls, lead-glass windows and lead-rubber aprons.
- Workers involved with x-rays should keep away from the direct beam line and maintain a good distance from the x-ray source during exposure. Note that the inverse square law determines the fall-off of radiation with distance.
- All involved in radiography should be monitored and wear x-ray-sensitive **film badges** which need to be regularly assessed for excess radiation exposure.

Contrast Media Safety

1. **Iodinated contrast**—intravenous iodinated contrast can occasionally cause **hypersensitivity** reactions and rarely **anaphylaxis.** It is also potentially **nephrotoxic** in patients with impaired renal function. Risk factors should be specified in requests to help the radiologist plan the safest investigation. Alternatives, such as ultrasound, unenhanced CT or magnetic resonance (MR) may be considered.

Important risk factors for hypersensitivity are:
- known previous reaction to iodinated contrast
- history of asthma
- previous significant allergic reactions or eczema

Risk factors for nephrotoxicity:
- diabetes mellitus
- renal insufficiency (include results of renal function tests in requests for CT). Patients with estimated glomerular filtration rates (EGFR) greater than 45 mL/min/1.73 m^2—do not require any precautions. EGFR 30 to 45 mL/min/1.73 m^2—consider precontrast hydration with intravenous normal saline. EGFR less than 30 mL/min/1.73 m^2—give precontrast hydration. Contrast can be given if the patient is on dialysis or is planned to have dialysis.
- multiple myeloma
- heart failure

Further information can be obtained at:

https://www.ranzcr.com/college/document-library/ranzcr-iodinated-contrast-guidelines

2. **Gadolinium chelates**—gadolinium compounds used for intravenous contrast enhancement for magnetic resonance imaging (MRI) can cause allergic reactions, although the risk is lower than with iodinated contrast. The main risk is of inducing **nephrogenic systemic sclerosis** (a fibrotic skin disorder) in patients with impaired renal function. Particular compounds are less risky than others and should be used if enhancement is essential in a patient with renal impairment.

Magnetic Resonance Imaging Safety

MRI is safer than ionising radiation. It is generally thought to be safe in pregnancy, but should not be undertaken without careful consideration. The main MR safety problems relate to the effect of powerful magnets upon ferromagnetic objects, both extraneous and within the patient.

- Ferromagnetic objects are excluded from the scanning room because the powerful magnetic field can propel them with such great speed that they become missiles, liable to cause physical injury.
- The magnetic field acts upon implanted metal including embedded foreign bodies and surgical clips. Metallic foreign bodies in the eye can become displaced and result in blindness. Similarly, clips on cerebral aneurysms can become dislodged. Most modern aneurysm clips are nonferromagnetic and unaffected by MRI but should still be fully documented in the patient's notes.
- The nature of any implanted medical devices must be known. Cardiac pacemakers and external defibrillators may malfunction when exposed to the magnetic field so alternative imaging should be used. Implanted metal may also become heated by induced electrical currents.
- Firmly implanted prosthesis, such as hip replacements made of 'MRI friendly' materials generally safe.

General Principles of Radiology

The following factors are involved in producing a useful radiographic image:

- **X-ray power and exposure time**—chosen to give a diagnostically useful exposure without excess dosage. High quality images have a range of densities appropriate to the anatomical area. For example, thoracic spine views require a larger dose than lungs.

- **Different projections (views)** produce different views of the same subject. The x-ray tube is effectively a point source giving a diverging beam (Fig. 5.2), so the subject is magnified. The distortion least affects the body part closest to the film, which is thus shown most clearly. The beam **direction** should be recorded on the film as it has consequences for interpretation, for example, a frontal chest film might be posteroanterior (PA) or anteroposterior (AP). With lateral exposures, the side nearest the film is indicated, for example, a 'Rt' lateral chest x-ray (CXR) has the right side nearest the film.
- **Patient position** during exposure (i.e., supine, prone, oblique or erect) affects the image because of gravity affecting organs, gas or fluid. Most abdominal radiographs are taken with the patient lying supine with the x-ray beam aimed vertically downwards. A horizontal beam (erect or lateral decubitus) can demonstrate fluid levels in a cavity or bowel, or free gas under the diaphragm.

Image Storage and Transfer

Virtually all images are now stored electronically in digital format and are viewed and interpreted from screens attached to computers. Images no longer need to be kept in bulky packets and space has been saved. The time and effort for staff retrieving and filing packets is now no longer needed. Of course, the systems to store the data need to be maintained and kept free from viruses and malware intrusion and so IT input is required to maintain hardware and software to keep abreast of technological changes.

Images can be viewed from multiple sites in the same institution at the same time. They can also be transferred with ease over networks to other institutions, the clinician's home or even to other parts of the world for interpretation. Adherence to strict data security principles is mandatory. In the European Union, this is defined by the General Data Protection Regulations (GDPR).

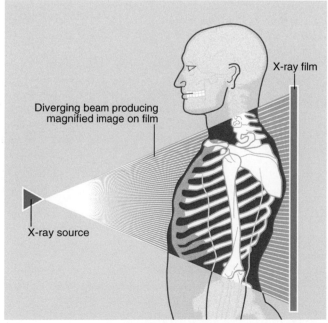

• **Fig. 5.2** Radiological Projection.

Plain Radiology

Plain radiographs of the chest and abdomen are now used much less in surgical practice. Their limitations are better recognised and there is increased availability of CT. Studies have shown that CT is far more accurate in diagnosing a wide range of acute abdominal conditions, so it is used more often and earlier in the diagnostic pathway than previously. In cases of suspected perforation or bowel obstruction, plain radiographs of chest and abdomen are often still used as the first imaging test. Plain abdominal radiographs are also useful to monitor colonic dilatation in patients with colitis. In the nonemergency state, they are also useful to follow up renal tract calculi for size, number and position.

Chest Radiograph

Interpreting plain CXRs requires a methodical approach. Several informative documents are available on the subject (see for example https://geekymedics.com/chest-x-ray-interpretation-a-methodical-approach/). Sites like these are useful guides, but can be modified to suit individual preferred methods and sequence of analysis.

Abdominal Radiograph

Interpretation of abdominal radiographs demands a systematic approach. It is helpful to consider the organs in and around the abdominal cavity methodically, both intraperitoneal and retroperitoneal, the lung bases, bones and the hernial orifices. The following site should be informative as a starter: https://geekymedics.com/abdominal-x-ray-interpretation/.

When examining an abdominal x-ray, important features to look for are:

- calcification in areas prone to stone formation (e.g., kidney, ureters, bladder or biliary tree);
- dilated bowel (stomach, small or large bowel);
- free intraperitoneal gas indicating bowel perforation;
- gas in abnormal places (e.g., biliary tree or urinary tract) suggesting a fistula with bowel);
- nonbiological objects (e.g., foreign bodies, surgical tubes or pieces of metal);
- pathological calcification (e.g., aortic aneurysm, pancreas, adrenals or uterine fibroids).

Most abdominal films are taken with the patient supine. Bowel is visible when it contains gas (Figs 5.3 and 5.4); normal **small bowel** is less than 3 cm wide and tends to occupy the centre of the abdomen. When dilated, it shows transverse folds (**plicae circulares**) which completely cross the lumen. The colon usually lies peripherally and has **haustrations**; these folds only partly traverse the lumen (see Fig. 5.3). Normal colon is less than 6 cm wide and often contains faecal lumps with a mottled appearance.

The limitations of plain abdominal radiography are summarised in Box 5.1

Free Intraperitoneal Gas

Free gas is diagnostic of **bowel perforation** except after recent laparotomy. Free air usually persists for 3 to 6 days after laparotomy, although can remain for longer. This can cause difficulty in diagnosing a possible anastomotic leak. Carbon dioxide gas used in laparoscopic surgery is usually absorbed more quickly than air.

An erect chest radiograph is the best technique for demonstrating free air from a perforation (see Fig. 19.8, p. 302). Perforation can also be diagnosed when both the inside and outside of bowel wall are outlined by radiolucent shadows. This is known as *Rigler's sign*, Fig. 32.7, p. 437). CT should be requested where the clinical diagnosis is not obvious or the plain x-ray result is doubtful or the patient too ill to sit or stand, or if perforation is clinically suspected but plain radiography does not show free air (see Fig. 5.4).

Bone Radiographs

Conventional radiographs of bones still have an important role in diagnosis of bone disease: fractures, infection, neoplasia and degenerative conditions. Other investigations including bone scintigraphy, CT, MRI and ultrasound are used when either

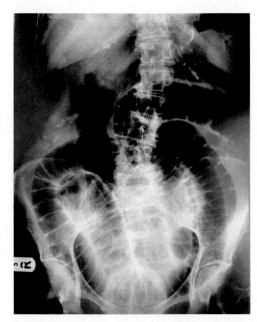

• **Fig. 5.3** Abdominal X-Ray. Supine plain abdominal film showing gross small bowel dilatation. At laparotomy, the cause proved to be an obstructing carcinoma of the caecum.

radiographs are normal, or for further evaluation of radiographically demonstrated abnormalities. If in doubt, discuss with a radiologist.

Contrast Radiology

Many previously used contrast studies have been replaced by other, better, tests:

- Intravenous urogram (IVU) → CT urogram, CT KUB (kidneys, ureters, bladder). Occasionally MR urogram
- Barium enema → CT colonography
- Barium follow through → MR or CT enterography
- Catheter angiography → MR angiography (MRA), CT angiography (CTA) or Doppler ultrasound
- Venography → Doppler ultrasound, CT or MR venography

Contrast studies remain useful in the following situations:

- Oesophagus—allowing the swallowing mechanism and oesophageal peristalsis to be observed in real time.
- Enterocutaneous fistulae—to evaluate deep connections of potential fistulae by using direct contrast injection via the cutaneous orifice.
- Assessing integrity of an anastomosis—for example, after rectal cancer surgery before reversing a defunctioning ileostomy or colostomy.
- When the alternative CT or MR investigation is contraindicated or not available.

Contrast Materials

Barium sulphate is very dense and useful for outlining the gastrointestinal (GI) tract directly, unless a leak or perforation is suspected or there is a risk of aspirating into the lungs. In these cases, a water soluble iodinated compound should be used (see Box 5.2).

Iodinated benzoic acid derivatives are water soluble compounds that can be injected into arteries or veins to opacify them. Contrast enhancement of CT scans is a development

CASE HISTORY

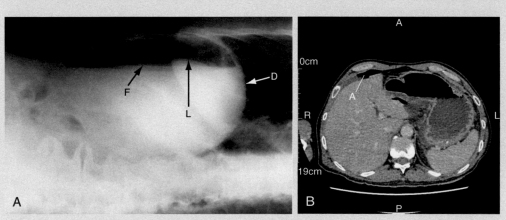

• **Fig. 5.4** Abdominal X-Ray. This 78-year-old woman presented with a sudden onset of severe abdominal pain. Erect chest x-ray **(A)** failed to show free abdominal gas but a perforation was clinically suspected so this lateral decubitus x-ray was performed. The right side is raised and the head is to the right of the picture; the x-ray beam was horizontal. Free intraperitoneal gas is seen above a fluid level *(F)* beneath the diaphragm *(D)* and 'floating' over the liver *(L)*. At laparotomy, the cause proved to be a perforated duodenal ulcer. Transaxial CT **(B)** showing free extraluminal air from perforated duodenal ulcer *(A)*.

that can provide useful extra information. For example, imaging arterial stenoses or venous thromboses effectively using lower doses of contrast, and thus replacing direct studies. Enhanced CT can increase the visibility of liver metastases compared to unenhanced CT.

Gadolinium chelates—are ferromagnetic compounds injected to enhance tissues during MRI examinations. They are analogous to the iodinated contrast agents used with CT and can increase the visibility of lesions and provide information about arteries and veins.

Ultrasound contrast agents —consist of a micro air bubble within a shell. The air bubble reflects sound waves and so the contrast agent shows up brightly in the examination. Contrast enhanced ultrasound is mainly used in evaluating liver lesions, differentiating benign from malignant lesions by virtue of their differing vascular characteristics. Secondly, these agents are useful for increasing the clarity of a vessel or cardiac chambers and determining the presence or absence of clots or occlusions.

• BOX 5.1   Limitations of Plain Abdominal Radiography

- Intraperitoneal structures are not visualised unless they contain gas themselves, displace gas-filled bowel or indent structural fat.
- Stones that are not calcified (90% of gallstones, 10% of urinary tract stones) are not visible.
- Bowel gas and faeces easily obscure stones.
- Phleboliths, calcified abdominal lymph nodes and costal cartilages readily mimic stones.
- Liver and spleen size cannot be estimated accurately.
- Free intraperitoneal gas is not usually visible on a supine film (a horizontal beam film is needed).

Examples of Contrast Radiology

Large Bowel

With improved technology, CT has almost completely replaced the barium enema. It can be performed without laxative preparation in cases where it would be acceptable to miss small polyps. CT can be particularly useful in the frail elderly when a right-sided colonic cancer is suspected because of anaemia or a palpable mass.

In cases where it is important to detect polyps as well as larger cancers, **CT colonography (CTC)** is requested. This test involves bowel cleansing to eliminate particulate matter. During the procedure, air or carbon dioxide is insufflated into the colon and the technique is sensitive enough to detect lesions of 1 cm or even smaller. With good technique, the accuracy of CTC is equivalent to optical colonoscopy in detecting polyps and cancers (Fig. 5.5).

Small Bowel

The use of barium studies to examine small bowel is declining and being replaced by CT or MR enterography. These techniques also enable the attached mesentery to be examined for complications, such as abscesses or fistulae. **Capsule endoscopy** can be used to look for small lesions that remain undetected by other tests (see later).

• BOX 5.2   Limitations of Barium Contrast Studies

- It is often impossible to distinguish between different types of pathological lesion, for example, between malignant and inflammatory colonic stenosis, or between malignant and peptic ulcer of the stomach.
- Fine mucosal detail is not shown, for example, gastric lesions, such as inflammation, shallow ulceration or early cancer, or angiodysplasias of the colon. In acute gastrointestinal bleeding, barium meal may miss the bleeding lesion.
- Small bowel is difficult to examine in detail because of contrast dilution by bowel contents and loops of bowel overlying each other.
- Major abnormalities may be concealed because of tissue overlap. Multiple projections, double contrast techniques and tube angulation reduce this deficiency.

Biliary Radiology

Magnetic Resonance Cholangio-Pancreatography (Fig. 5.6C and D)

Magnetic resonance cholangio-pancreatography (MRCP) now produces images that rival the quality of endoscopic retrograde cholangio-pancreatography (ERCP). MRI differentiates tissues and organs by their varying water content. Since bile and pancreatic juice are mostly water, hence MRCP gives clear images of bile in the gall bladder and ducts and outlines the pancreatic duct. It reveals filling defects caused by stones or tumours. MRCP can identify bile leaks, gallstones in bile ducts, and duct obstruction from any cause. There are no known hazards. MRCP is increasingly used ahead of ERCP for pancreatico-biliary investigation to reduce the number of more invasive (and potentially risky) investigations.

Indications for MRCP include:
- Suspected stones in the biliary tree.
- Bile duct strictures: benign—postsurgical or sclerosing cholangitis; malignant—cholangiocarcinoma.
- Congenital ductal anomalies: pancreas divisum causing acute pancreatitis of unknown aetiology. Choledochal cysts.
- Biliary-type pain with abnormal liver function tests in patients without stones on ultrasound.
- Patients unsuitable for ERCP because of intolerance or have had previous gastrectomy.

Endoscopic Retrograde Cholangio-Pancreatography

This is described subsequently (see *Diagnostic and therapeutic duodenoscopy*); its use in obstructive jaundice is described in detail in Chapter 18. The basic technique is illustrated in Fig. 5.6A and B.

Operative Cholangiography and Choledochoscopy

It is usual to perform operative cholangiography during open cholecystectomy. For laparoscopic cholecystectomy, some surgeons perform operative cholangiography routinely whilst others prefer no imaging at all for selected cases or else preoperative assessment using MRCP for those deemed likely to have duct stones.

Operative cholangiography allows the (highly variable) biliary anatomy to be displayed, it demonstrates stones in the bile ducts and shows whether contrast flows freely into the duodenum. A fine plastic cannula is introduced into a small cystic duct incision and passed into the common bile duct. Water-soluble contrast

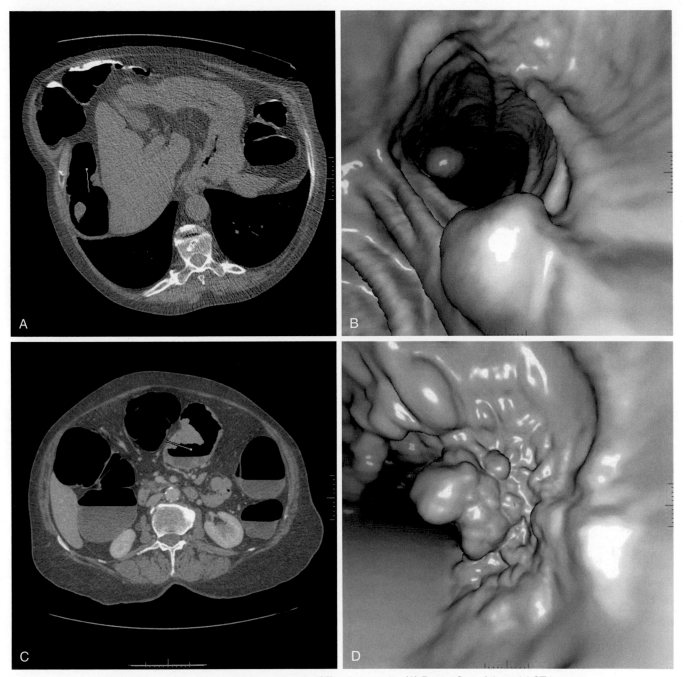

• **Fig. 5.5** Examples of computed tomography (CT) colonography. **(A)** Prone. One of the axial CT images used to reconstruct the three-dimensional (3D) image showing an adenomatous polyp in **(B)**. **(C)** One of the axial CT images used to reconstruct the 3D image showing a transverse colon carcinoma in **(D)**.

material is injected to outline the duct system and fluoroscopic images or x-ray films are taken. If duct stones are demonstrated, they are often retrieved surgically at the same operation. At open cholecystectomy, this is via a longitudinal incision in the common bile duct (**exploration of the common bile duct**). At laparoscopic surgery, a similar technique is used via the transcystic route or via a small transverse or longitudinal choledochotomy, depending on the duct size and size of the stone to be retrieved. A flexible 5 mm or 3 mm endoscope called a *choledochoscope* can be passed into the bile duct and stones can be retrieved using a range of techniques including snares, baskets, balloons, or they can even be shattered with lithotripsy probes. The choledochoscope enables the bile and

intrahepatic ducts to be inspected afterwards to confirm that all stones have been removed. A further cholangiogram is often also done afterwards to ensure the duct is clear. Duct stone removal may be deferred and performed later at ERCP, although this carries risk of complications, including biliary leakage and acute pancreatitis and death.

T-Tube Cholangiography

Following exploration of bile ducts for stones, a T-tube was often left in situ to drain the duct. The short transverse limb lay within the duct and the long limb drained to the surface. This allowed contrast to be injected postoperatively to outline the biliary

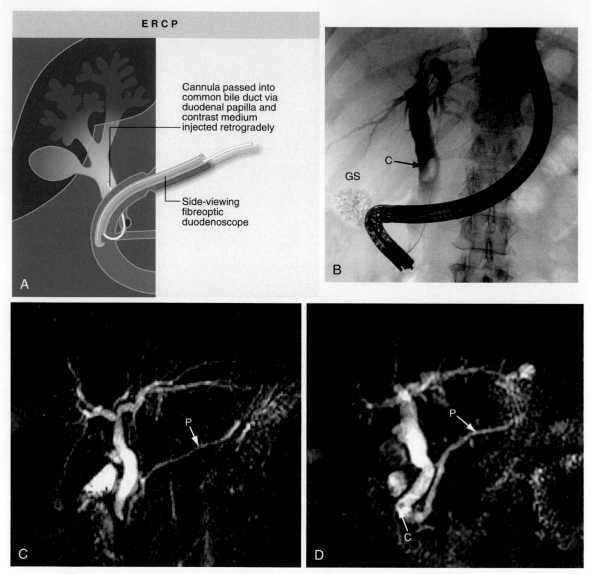

ERCP

Cannula passed into common bile duct via duodenal papilla and contrast medium injected retrogradely

Side-viewing fibreoptic duodenoscope

• **Fig. 5.6** Some Techniques for Demonstrating the Biliary System. **(A** and **B)** Endoscopic retrograde cholangiography. The patient is sedated and a side-viewing gastroscope passed down so the tip reaches the second part of the duodenum. The ampulla of Vater is cannulated under direct vision and contrast medium injected to outline the bile ducts. **(B)** A large gallstone *(C)* is seen within the dilated common bile duct and a collection of radiopaque gallstones *(GS)* is seen in the gall bladder. **(C** and **D)** Magnetic resonance cholangio-pancreatography (MRCP). The technique produces images of static fluid, thus the images are of native biliary and pancreatic secretions. Each image was obtained in one second using a thick slab 'projection' method that generates images very similar to ERCP. The pancreatic duct in each image is labelled *(P)*. (C) An example of normal biliary and pancreatic duct systems. (D) A small calculus, *(C)*, in the distal common bile duct. There is also mild dilatation of the pancreatic duct with some side branches visible.

tree and show residual stones, bile leakage or duct stenosis, as well as confirming free drainage of bile into the duodenum. If residual stones were present they could be retrieved at ERCP or sometimes by the radiologist via the T-tube. The regular use of T-tubes is now reducing, with most laparoscopic duct explorations not requiring one owing to greater certainty of duct clearance, better cross-sectional imaging and the availability of ERCP to access the duct later.

Vascular and Interventional Radiology

General Principles and Hazards of Arteriography and Venography

Further detail about applications of vascular radiology is given in Chapter 41.

The veins or arteries of an anatomical region can be opacified by intravenous or intraarterial injection of contrast medium.

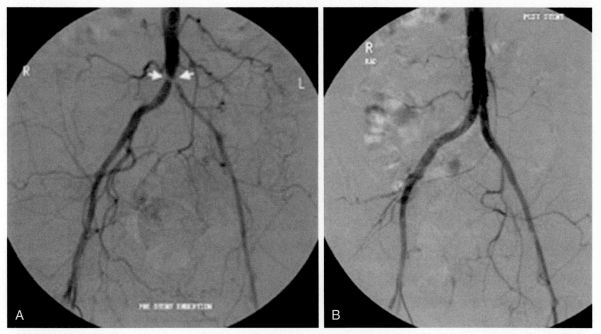

• **Fig. 5.7** Percutaneous Transluminal Angioplasty. This man of 55 years presented with bilateral calf and thigh claudication. **(A)** A localised severe stenosis of the distal abdominal aorta. **(B)** The 'kissing balloon' technique used to dilate the stenosis. Two balloons, shown inflated, are used to prevent asymmetrical dilatation which might compromise the opposite common iliac artery, kissing stents were then deployed to maintain patency due to significant recoil following angioplasty.

This is **angiography** and includes arteriography and venography. In **arteriography**, needle puncture of the access artery is followed by guide-wire insertion, needle removal and catheter insertion over the guide-wire. Shaped catheters and wires are used to advance the catheter tip to an appropriate position for arteriography. Favoured access sites are the femoral artery in the groin, the brachial artery at the level of the elbow and, more recently, the radial artery at the wrist, using smaller diameter sheaths.

Clotting studies should be performed beforehand to anticipate potential haemorrhagic complications from the vessel puncture site, particularly if the patient is on anticoagulants or if there is a suspicion of an underlying clotting disorder.

The contrast medium is the same as that used for CT and carries similar hazards, that is, allergic reaction and nephrotoxicity (see earlier).

Complications from the vascular access site include bleeding or thrombosis in veins and dissection, arteriovenous fistula or pseudoaneurysm formation in arteries.

Arteriography

Digital subtraction angiography (DSA) is the gold standard for direct contrast vascular studies. The unchanging opacities of a plain radiographic image (particularly bone and bowel gas) are **subtracted** from the image after injection of contrast medium so lower doses produce better images. However, due to advances in cross-sectional imaging (CT and MRI), satisfactory diagnostic images can be produced to help demonstrate the pattern of disease and aid treatment planning. Furthermore, CT and MRI are less invasive than DSA.

Direct diagnostic angiography better evaluates stenoses or occlusions, particularly in heavily calcified vessels. This is because CT often overestimates the severity of calcified stenoses.

Endovascular Techniques

Percutaneous Transluminal Angioplasty or Balloon Angioplasty

Angioplasty under local anaesthesia is a less invasive alternative to surgery for treating many peripheral and coronary arterial stenoses. In general, short stenoses in large vessels are most suitable. The method is particularly useful for atherosclerotic disease involving the lower limbs, coronaries and abdominal visceral arteries (coeliac, SMA and renal arteries). Carotid artery disease is also suitable for angioplasty in some cases; filters or embolic protection devices are usually placed above the stenotic segment before dilatation to reduce the risk of distal embolisation to the brain.

Major complications of angioplasty are rare in experienced hands but there is a small risk of precipitating acute ischaemia because of distal embolisation or dissection. Thus surgical salvage should be readily available should complications develop. Unfortunately, 25% to 40% of angioplastied lesions undergo restenosis or occlusion within 1 year, but the process can usually be repeated. Where stenoses fail to remain open at plain balloon angioplasty, **stents** can be placed across the treated lesion to provide a sustained outward radial force, thereby keeping the vessel patent. Advances incorporate certain drugs (with antiproliferative properties) into balloons and stents to reduce rates of restenosis and improve long-term patency. These stents are mounted on an angioplasty balloon before deployment or are self-expanding once deployed in the vessel. Stents are increasingly used in iliac, superficial femoral artery and popliteal stenoses and occlusions. Overall, angioplasty causes minimal interventional and anaesthetic stress to the patient and is often performed on a day-case basis.

Techniques of Percutaneous Angioplasty

Angioplasty is usually performed under local anaesthesia (Fig. 5.7). A needle is first inserted into an accessible artery and a short flexible guide-wire passed through it into the artery and the needle removed. A working sheath with a valved side-arm is passed over the guide-wire and advanced into the artery. A catheter is inserted and a long guide-wire is then substituted for the first and manipulated up to and through the stenosis guided by contrast injections and fluoroscopic control. An **angioplasty catheter** with a plastic inflatable balloon at its end is then passed over the guide-wire and manipulated across the stenosis. Angioplasty balloons are now no wider than the catheter before inflation, and designed to inflate to a fixed diameter at a given pressure. It is possible to measure the arterial pressure above and below the stenosis to determine the pressure gradient before and after angioplasty, and although not performed routinely, it can provide an objective measure of the physiological response to treatment. The balloon is inflated to a typical pressure of between 6 and 15 atmospheres depending on the balloon type, to dilate the stenosis, then further contrast is injected to check the result. Angioplasty techniques and equipment have progressively improved and many patients now return to near-normal life after minimal intervention. Many patients with ischaemic legs or coronary heart disease who might not have been suitable for reconstructive surgery can now have angioplasty because of its minimally invasive nature and low complication rates.

Local Arterial Thrombolytic Therapy

An artery freshly occluded by thrombus and causing ischaemia can be recanalised by local intraarterial infusion of thrombolytic agents. High local concentrations with limited systemic spill-over were intended to avoid the serious bleeding and allergic complications of systemic thrombolysis. However, experience has shown that the risk of major haemorrhage still exists, with some episodes having been fatal. Examples of serious complications include intracerebral haemorrhagic strokes, bleeding from recent surgical wounds, from the GI tract or intraocular bleeding in patients with untreated proliferative diabetic retinopathy. For this reason, the treatment has strictly limited indications, that is, recently occluded native arteries or bypass grafts. The thrombolytic agent usually used is **recombinant tissue plasminogen activator** (R-tPa). R-tPa acts more quickly and does not have the frequent allergic effects of older agents, for example, streptokinase.

For recent acute embolic ischaemia, surgical embolectomy remains the best treatment.

Therapeutic Embolisation

Highly vascular lesions or vessels that are actively bleeding that would be difficult or impossible to treat by surgery alone can have their arterial supply reduced or obliterated by embolisation. The main supplying artery is identified by selective arteriography and a catheter manoeuvred into it, close to the lesion. The materials chosen for embolisation depend on the nature of the lesion but include **gelatine foam**, **polyvinyl alcohol particles**, **minute steel coils**, **plugs**, **cyanoacrylate glue** or **liquid polymers**. The process can be repeated for all the feeding vessels.

Embolisation is particularly useful in the treatment of GI haemorrhage, some pseudoaneurysms, uterine fibroids and internal iliac arteries before endovascular aneurysm repair (EVAR). The technique is also used to treat hepatic tumours (primary and secondary) and some bone metastases before surgery.

Minimal Access Graft Placement

EVAR is now widely used to treat both abdominal and thoracic aortic aneurysms. There are several different types of device available, all composed of metal stents and graft material, and technical improvements are continuing. The device is introduced via a femoral artery and accurately positioned in the aorta, and then deployment consists of unsheathing the device under fluoroscopic guidance. Graft limbs are added to extend the device into the iliac arteries. There are now stent grafts capable of treating more complex aneurysms with side branches/grafts into renal, mesenteric, internal iliac or aortic arch arteries. These techniques create a better seal for the aortic stent graft without compromising flow to the visceral arteries. One disadvantage of EVAR includes **endoleakage**, that is, continued slow bleeding into the aneurysm sac because of an inadequate seal or, more commonly, from lumbar arteries or the inferior mesenteric artery. Other complications include graft migration, limb occlusion or limb dislocation. Although reintervention rates are higher than with open aneurysm repair, these techniques have allowed many patients to be treated who would never be fit for open surgery. There is now an increasing application of EVAR to leaking or ruptured aneurysms. This avoids the massive physiological insult associated with open surgery. The late complication rate of EVAR is about 10% per year, considerably greater than for open aneurysm grafting, but rates are falling with improving techniques.

Venous Techniques

Venography

Colour duplex Doppler ultrasound scanning has replaced contrast venography for diagnosing **deep vein thrombosis** (DVT), as well as for demonstrating reflux from deep to superficial vessels in varicose veins. A skilled operator can demonstrate the patency or otherwise of all the lower limb veins and the presence of fresh or old thrombus. Valve competence can be demonstrated in deep and superficial veins and perforating veins. Vein wall irregularity caused by previous DVT can also be displayed. Contrast venography can sometimes be helpful in defining the anatomy of complex superficial varicose veins and very occasionally to diagnose or exclude calf vein DVT where duplex is inconclusive.

Placement of Vena Caval Filters

After venous thromboembolism, a few patients experience **recurrent pulmonary embolism** despite adequate anticoagulation. In others, anticoagulation therapy is contraindicated and other methods of preventing pulmonary embolism must be found, for example, in pregnancy, after a haemorrhagic stroke, in patients with a high risk of falling or those with certain bleeding disorders. In these groups, the risk of large pulmonary embolism can be markedly reduced by placing a filter in the inferior vena cava, usually below the renal veins. This still allows venous blood to return to the heart but traps substantial embolic material in the flowing blood. Since the mid-1960s, a range of filtration devices have been developed that can be inserted relatively simply using a catheter via the femoral or jugular vein. Typical examples are the Celect or Optease filter. Most filters can be retrieved later by percutaneous techniques if necessary, within a limited period. Complications are uncommon and include caval occlusion, migration and strut fracture.

Minimally Invasive Treatment of Varicose Veins

Several methods of ablating the long or short saphenous vein have appeared in recent years including foam sclerotherapy and laser or radiofrequency ablation (RFA). These are described in Chapter 43.

Biliary Intervention

Percutaneous Transhepatic Cholangiography

This technique involves percutaneous puncture of bile ducts, usually under ultrasound and fluoroscopic guidance. The cholangiogram can demonstrate the site of a biliary obstruction or bile leak.

Percutaneous transhepatic cholangiography (PTC) is often performed with a view to biliary drainage (external or internal) and biliary stent insertion. The main indications are to decompress an obstructed biliary tree, dilate biliary strictures and divert bile from bile duct defects and stent them.

Percutaneous biliary drainage and stenting are especially indicated when ERCP has been unsuccessful, for example in patients who have had previous gastric surgery.

Other Percutaneous Hepatobiliary Interventions

Patients with coagulopathy or ascites requiring nontargeted liver biopsy can have a transjugular liver biopsy in which the biopsy is performed via jugular venous access. It is possible to treat liver tumours using embolisation - **transarterial chemoembolisation** and **radio-embolisation**. RFA is a thermoablative technique that can be used to treat hepatic tumours. RFA can be applied percutaneously or laparoscopically. Portal vein embolisation can be used before hepatic resection to increase the size of liver segments that will remain after surgery. This can reduce the postoperative morbidity and increase the number of patients suitable for curative intent resection.

Upper Urinary Tract Imaging

Acute Ureteric Colic

An unenhanced, low radiation dose CT examination usually referred to as **CT KUB**, has almost completely replaced the IVU to diagnose ureteric colic. CT KUB is more sensitive for detecting stones than the IVU and is quicker to perform.

Haematuria

Macroscopic or persistent microscopic haematuria are evaluated initially with cystoscopy for bladder causes and ultrasound (initially) for upper or lower urinary tract causes. In the upper tracts, the investigation must be able to accurately identify renal tract calculi, and renal parenchymal and urothelial lesions. CT is often needed for this because of the low sensitivity of ultrasound for calculi and urothelial tumours. CT series taken before and after administration of intravenous contrast are required. This is called a **CT urogram**.

Evaluation of Renal Masses

When a renal mass is discovered on non-CT imaging (usually ultrasound), serial noncontrast and contrast-enhanced CT images are needed to characterise the mass more precisely and determine definitively whether it is cystic or solid. Images are taken at intervals after intravenous contrast to provide information about the renal parenchyma and the arterial supply and assess for venous invasion. CT is also used for staging cancer by assessing local, regional or distant spread.

Percutaneous Therapeutic Techniques

These techniques can be used to remove stones from the renal pelvis and to relieve upper tract obstruction causing hydronephrosis. Guided by ultrasound or CT scanning, the renal pelvis can be punctured percutaneously with a needle. The tract is then dilated to allow tubes of various types and sizes to be inserted. Gaining access to the kidney in this way is known as **percutaneous nephrostomy**.

Imaging Techniques

Ultrasound

Medical ultrasound grew out of sonar used for submarine detection in the Second World War. The technology remained an official secret until the 1960s but since then, the principle has found numerous applications, from identifying shoals of fish to noninvasive imaging of body organs.

Medical ultrasound was pioneered in obstetrics where it has long been an important part of prenatal assessment. Its use in the body is now protean and there is hardly an organ or system where diagnostic ultrasound does not have a role. It is important to recognise that interpreting ultrasound depends on the skill of the operator and the dynamic picture seen during the examination; the film record provides a few representative images of part of the study.

General Principles of Medical Ultrasound

Ultrasound is noninvasive, painless and safe. An ultrasound probe containing the transducer is applied to the skin over the area of interest and an image of deeper structures displayed on a screen. The probe must be 'coupled' to the skin with jelly to exclude an air interface and is moved in different directions and angles to best display the organs of interest and any abnormalities.

The piezo-electric transducer both transmits and receives ultrasound, and reflections show as bright spots on a dark screen in real time. This is known as **B-mode** (brightness mode) with the intensity of each spot proportional to the reflectivity of tissue interfaces.

The length and breadth of organs or lesions can be accurately determined by electronically measuring the image, and the volume of some structures, such as the urinary bladder or left ventricle can be estimated. This can provide functional information, such as the volume of residual urine in chronic retention, or the completeness of left ventricular emptying in cardiac failure.

Bone, stones and other calcified tissues cause an abrupt and marked change in acoustic impedance, giving complete reflection of ultrasound. Thus the surface of hard tissue, such as gallstones is revealed by the **acoustic shadow** it casts (see Fig. 20.4, p. 310). A smaller change in acoustic impedance occurs at gas/soft tissue interfaces, such as bowel wall and its gas-filled lumen.

Minimal patient preparation is needed. For biliary examinations, the patient should be fasted to minimise bowel gas shadows and enable the gall bladder to fill with fluid. For pelvic examination, the bladder should ideally be full of urine. This provides a fluid-filled, nonreflective 'window' for ultrasound to reach the pelvic organs.

Duplex scanning combines the images from two-dimensional (2D) imaging and Doppler ultrasound. A further refinement is **colour duplex** in which the image has false colour added to show the direction and approximate volume of flow, with red indicating one direction and blue the opposite.

Special Transducers

Probes have been developed for use via different body orifices, and for body cavities via endoscopic instruments, percutaneous cannulae and laparoscopes. These devices can be placed closer to the structures being examined than surface probes so that higher-frequency sound can be used. This has lower penetration but greater spatial resolution and gives a more detailed display. These transducers are often combined with biopsy devices to enable tissue sampling.

Rectal probes are used for examining the rectal wall and prostate gland in detail and **vaginal probes** for investigating the pelvic organs. **Endoscopic probes** (e.g., transoesophageal) can examine and monitor the heart, upper GI organs and adjacent tissues. Oesophageal Doppler Monitoring measures blood flow velocity in the descending thoracic aorta and can provide a continuous estimate of cardiac output during operations and hence guide fluid replacement.

Laparoscopic probes can be applied directly to viscera to seek the extent of tumour spread or metastases, for example, pancreas, kidney, liver. They provide a more reliable diagnosis of liver metastases than percutaneous ultrasound or cross-sectional imaging.

Applications of Ultrasound in General Surgery

Ultrasound is frequently used as a first imaging test for investigating symptoms related to the upper abdomen, urinary tract and pelvis. Ultrasound is preferred to other tests in children and in women of child-bearing age (where it is appropriate) because it avoids potentially damaging ionising radiation. Bedside ultrasound examinations on wards, the Emergency Department and the intensive treatment unit are frequently used to aid interventional procedures or to make a diagnosis quickly for example, Focused Assessment with Sonography for Trauma (FAST) in abdominal injuries.

Ultrasound is useful for:

- Reliably distinguishing **solid** from **cystic** lesions (e.g., a thyroid cyst from solid nodule, renal or pancreatic cyst from solid tumour).
- Assessing palpable **abdominal masses** in the abdomen or pelvis.
- Detecting **abnormal tissues** in a homogeneous organ (e.g., liver metastases or renal adenocarcinoma).
- Detecting **damage to solid organs after trauma** (e.g., splenic or liver rupture). Bleeding into the peritoneum can provide indirect evidence of liver or spleen injury in the patient with abdominal trauma, but an immediate ultrasound examination in the Emergency Department can gain this information very soon after the patient arrives. This is referred to as **FAST** scanning.
- Detecting **abnormal fluid collections** (e.g., pseudocyst of pancreas, ascites, pleural effusions, abscesses).
- Assessing the nature of lesions from the way the **echo texture** contrasts with the normal, for example, distinguishing liver secondaries from benign lesions or normal liver.
- Detecting **movement**, such as pulsation of an aneurysm, contraction of the heart (echo shows valve morphology and movement, ventricular wall movement and cavity volumes), and foetal anatomy and movement.
- Detecting upper urinary tract **dilatation** (hydronephrosis).
- **Measuring physical dimensions** (e.g., the diameter of an abdominal aortic aneurysm or a dilated bile duct, or the volume of residual urine in the bladder after micturition).
- Investigating the **biliary system** for gallstones, thickened gall bladder wall, dilated ducts, masses in the head of the pancreas or porta hepatis.
- **Guiding percutaneous procedures**: aspiration of ascites, biopsy of liver lesions, insertion of drains for fluid collections into the chest or abdomen or insertion of vascular lines (central venous catheterisation).
- Investigating **breast lumps** (e.g., distinguishing cystic from solid lesions, suspected malignant lesions, guided cyst drainage, guiding fine-needle aspiration [FNA] for cytology, or core biopsy).

The limitations of diagnostic ultrasound are summarised in Box 5.3.

Doppler-Shifted Ultrasound

Ultrasound can detect and study blood flow by applying the Doppler principle. Simple hand-held equipment is cheap and portable, and is invaluable in the vascular clinic (Fig. 5.8). Using a probe coupled to the skin with conduction gel, a beam of ultrasound is directed at an artery or vein. Ultrasound reflects from moving red cells and causes a shift in sound frequency related to blood velocity. Reflected ultrasound is used to generate an audible signal (for detecting blood flow) or is processed to reveal information about the nature of flow. The audio pitch is related to blood **velocity** and provides some qualitative assessment of whether flow is normal or abnormal.

Main Applications of Hand-Held Doppler Ultrasound

- Measuring systolic blood pressure when it is low. This includes brachial pressure in shocked patients or in infants, and ankle systolic pressures in lower limb ischaemia. For this, a sphygmomanometer cuff is placed around the arm or ankle and a flow detector is applied to an artery beyond the cuff (see Fig. 5.8).
- Detecting foetal heart rate.
- Simple detection of venous blood reflux at the sapheno-femoral or sapheno-popliteal junction in varicose veins, particularly if recurrent.

Duplex Doppler Ultrasound Scanning

Duplex Doppler scanning adds frequency spectral analysis of blood flow using Doppler ultrasound to 2D B mode imaging of the vessel. **Colour flow Doppler** adds false colour to show the direction of blood flow and gives qualitative information about flow volume.

Duplex equipment is still expensive, and the diagnostic process is time-consuming and requires special training. However, it has largely superseded established methods in some areas, replacing venography for deep venous insufficiency and arteriography for carotid artery disease. Blood vessels can be imaged in longitudinal or transverse section to reveal the direction of flow, its velocity (which rises as blood passes through a stenosis), and the presence of abnormal vessel walls or mature thrombus in the lumen.

Cardiac echo investigation (transthoracic echocardiography) uses similar instruments and provides comprehensive information about cardiac structure and function. As with ultrasound generally, images are best viewed and interpreted as moving pictures. Echocardiography allows the study of pathological anatomy, patterns of blood flow, cardiac wall movement, cardiac output and valve movements. The most common reason for requesting an echo is to study **left ventricular function**, particularly when symptoms suggest heart failure. Echo can determine the severity and underlying cause of heart failure, for example, ischaemic left ventricular dysfunction, dilated cardiomyopathy, valve dysfunction or right ventricular dysfunction. In addition, ischaemic regional wall

---

• BOX 5.3   Limitations of Diagnostic Ultrasound

- Bone almost completely reflects ultrasound and, as a result, obscures any tissues beyond it. Ultrasound is therefore of little use for examining the brain and spinal cord, although it is valuable in examining the heart (echocardiography) and for fluid collections in the chest; special **transcranial** Doppler probes are used for monitoring during neurosurgery and carotid artery surgery.
- Bowel gas partly reflects ultrasound, which may prejudice the examination. Starving the patient and giving laxatives may help.
- A thick layer of fat degrades the ultrasound image. Thus ultrasound is less accurate (but still the first choice) for investigating suspected gall bladder disease in obese patients.
- Ultrasound is unreliable for showing stones at the lower end of the common bile duct.

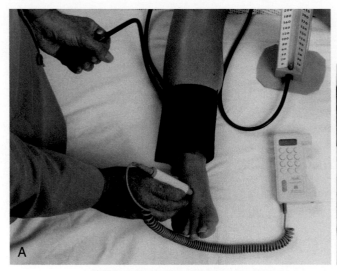
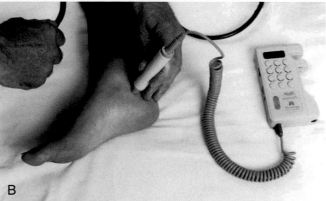

• **Fig. 5.8** Measuring Ankle Systolic Pressure Using a Hand-Held Doppler Flowmeter. **(A)** A standard sphygmomanometer cuff is placed around the ankle just above the malleoli. Ultrasound conducting gel is applied to the tip of the probe and the probe placed lightly over the likely position of the dorsalis pedis (DP) pulse, between the first two metatarsals. The probe is moved a tiny amount at a time so as to obtain the strongest signal, then the cuff is inflated until the pulse disappears. The cuff is then released gradually and the systolic pressure recorded at the point of return of signal. **(B)** The same process is repeated at the posterior tibial pulse (PT), using the midpoint of a line between the heel and the medial malleolus to find the pulse. Note that accurate measurements require considerable experience, especially when the pressure is low. Headphones are recommended to reduce interference.

movement abnormalities can be identified. These include **hypo-kinesis** (diminished movement), **akinesis** (absent movement) and **dyskinesis** (passive outward bulging in systole suggesting ventricular aneurysm). The **ejection fraction** (ratio between stroke volume and end-diastolic volume) can easily be assessed.

Echo is the investigation of choice for **valve abnormalities**. It can define the cause of a heart murmur, assess the severity of valvular stenosis or reflux and guide the need for antibiotic prophylaxis in patients with a murmur. In patients with **atrial fibrillation**, echo can detect underlying structural defects and inform the need for anticoagulation or cardioversion. In patients with **systemic embolism**, echo rarely shows intracardiac thrombus but is likely to show an underlying cardiac defect that is the source of embolism, such as mitral valve disease or vegetations, left ventricular aneurysm or a patent foramen ovale.

Applications of Duplex Doppler.
•   **Deep vein thrombosis**—this is the method of choice for detecting postoperative DVT. Thrombus more than 24 hours old can be seen and venous flow changes detected. However, the profunda vein and small calf veins are often poorly seen.
•   **Chronic lower limb deep venous insufficiency**—patency and valvular competence in deep veins (e.g., femoral and popliteal) can be determined dynamically; perforator incompetence is detectable.
•   **Varicose veins**—duplex ultrasound is useful for detecting and guiding marking of the short saphenous/popliteal junction before operation and for detecting communications between superficial veins and the sapheno-femoral junction in 'recurrent' long saphenous varicose veins. There are advantages to performing ultrasound in all varicose vein patients before treatment to clarify the diagnosis.
•   **Carotid artery disease**—duplex has now become the standard test for investigating extracranial vascular disease in preference to carotid angiography (which carries distinct risks). Duplex

shows the morphology of diseased arteries and the velocity of flow, allowing the percentage of stenosis to be calculated. The severity (percentage) of stenosis helps determine whether operation is required. Duplex is useful for evaluating asymptomatic bruits and following up patients after carotid endarterectomy, including in the early postoperative period.
•   **Femoro-popliteal bypass grafts**—duplex is used for marking out the saphenous vein graft before surgery and for graft surveillance after surgery to detect remediable vein graft stenoses.
•   **Aorto-iliac and femoro-popliteal occlusive disease**—duplex is proving valuable for estimating the sites and severity of stenoses and occlusions and replaces arteriography in some circumstances.
•   **Deeper blood vessels**—these can be imaged for blood flow and obstruction, for example, superior mesenteric and renal arteries, and renal veins for spread from renal cell carcinoma.
•   **Cardiac disease**—echocardiography is used for detecting abnormal anatomy and function including heart failure, ventricular dysfunction, valvular abnormalities including stenoses, congenital cardiac defects including septal defects, and intracardiac abnormalities predisposing to embolism.

Computerised Tomography (CT scanning)

General Principles of CT Scanning

Computerised tomography involves x-raying a series of thin transverse 'slices' of the patient's head, body or limbs. A precise fan-shaped beam of x-rays is repeatedly pulsed from successive angles around the circumference of each slice and the transmitted radiation is electronically recorded on the opposite side (Fig. 5.9).

Since CT was first introduced in the 1970s, the pace of development has been rapid. Modern machines capture images in a continuous spiral around the patient (**spiral CT**), usually as

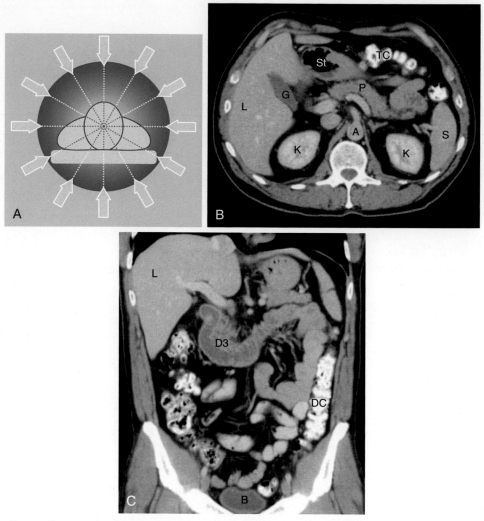

• **Fig. 5.9** Computerised Tomography (CT). **(A)** Principle of CT scanning. All images are fed into a computer and a single image of each slice produced. **(B)** Normal transverse CT scan. Liver *(L)*, gall bladder *(G)*, stomach *(St)*, kidneys *(K)*, aorta *(A)*, pancreas *(P)*, spleen *(S)*. **(C)** Normal CT scan reconstructed in the coronal plane. Liver *(L)*, bladder *(B)*, 3rd part of duodenum, descending colon *(DC)*.

multislice CT which captures several slices simultaneously with each revolution of the x-ray tube. Modern machines now generate up to 128 slices for each turn with an individual slice thickness of less than 1 mm. The result is rapid image capture of thin slices at high resolution. Spiral multislice CT machines can now produce images of chest plus abdomen in less than 1 minute. The data quality also allows images to be accurately reconstructed in three dimensions or in any chosen plane, for example, sagittal, coronal or oblique, to improve the detection and evaluation of abnormalities.

Note that the best CT images are obtained in well-nourished patients with some fat lying between the organs, enabling them to be differentiated more precisely than in very thin patients.

Further information can often be gained by performing CT after or during intravenously injected or orally ingested contrast media. Intravenous contrast can show blood vessels, and increase the visibility of tumours, for example, liver metastases. In some cases, such as liver haemangioma, the specific enhancement pattern can enable the diagnosis of a benign lesion to be made. In acute pancreatitis, areas of absent blood flow in the pancreas can indicate necrosis in acute pancreatitis. Oral contrast can be used to outline the bowel, but is not always required and in fact opacification with water can be useful when evaluating the upper GI tract.

CT, MRI and ultrasound are complementary techniques, each having advantages and disadvantages. The decision to use one or other depends on patient factors and availability of equipment, as well as the suspected disease. Very often, more than one imaging modality is required to completely evaluate a patient's illness.

Applications of CT Scanning

Pathological anatomy can be studied in great detail and a huge array of information can be obtained noninvasively to assist surgical diagnosis. Often the information is more accurate than could be obtained by exploratory operation. The technique enables timely and appropriate surgical intervention and avoids unnecessary exploratory operations.

CT is now being used earlier in the diagnostic process, particularly in emergency cases, and for an increasing range of clinical conditions, but clinical method and clinical common sense must be used before requesting such tests. Complete and accurate clinical information must be given on the request form to help in interpretation.

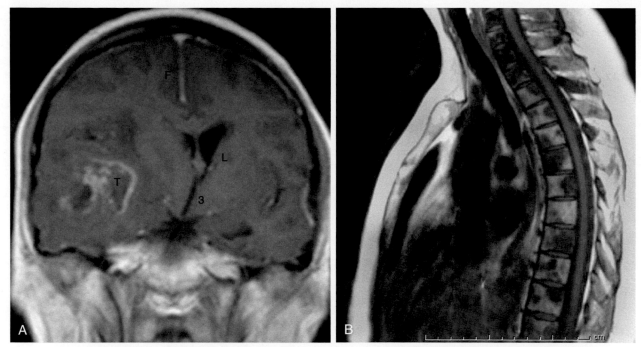

• **Fig. 5.10** Magnetic Resonance Images (MRIs). **(A)** Gadolinium enhanced T1-weighted coronal MRI of the brain. Note enhancement of a tumour *(T)*, midline shift with compression of the right lateral ventricle *(L)*. The falx *(F)* and third ventricle *(3)* are also labelled. **(B)** T1-weighted sequence sagittal MRI of the thoracic spine in a patient with known prostate cancer, back pain and an elevated prostate specific antigen. The image demonstrates bony metastases as dark areas in the vertebral bodies and spines; the white areas are normal fat in the marrow.

Some indications for CT scanning are:
• Investigating areas difficult to examine by standard radiology or ultrasound. Examples include the retroperitoneal area and pancreas (deep inside the body), the lungs and mediastinum, and the brain and spinal cord (encased in bone).
• Investigating acute abdominal pain—early CT misses fewer serious diagnoses and may reduce mortality and shorten hospital stay.
• Investigating abdominal pathology when ultrasound has proved unsatisfactory.
• Replacing more intrusive or invasive investigations used in the past, such as barium enema or diagnostic angiography.
• Pretreatment planning and follow-up of malignant tumours being treated with radiotherapy and/or chemotherapy, for example, for staging lymphomas, where historically, laparotomy was necessary.
• Planning surgery (e.g., establishing the extent of local invasion of oesophageal, pancreatic or rectal carcinoma, identifying the upper level of an aortic aneurysm, preoperative assessment of intrathoracic tumours including retrosternal thyroid enlargement).
• Assessing solid organ damage in abdominal or thoracic trauma. CT is increasingly used here and is performed earlier after admission. It can be performed rapidly and has the ability to image the solid organs, and also the lungs and pleura, hollow abdominal organs, blood vessels and bones in a single examination.
• Guiding needles during biopsy of masses, drainage of fluid collections or obtaining aspiration cytology specimens.

• Diagnosis of pulmonary embolism, renal tract calculi and arterial disease. Multislice CT has now also developed to a stage where it can often replace diagnostic coronary arteriography.
• CT is used occasionally in conducting noninvasive autopsies.

Magnetic Resonance Imaging

Principles of Magnetic Resonance Imaging

MRI was introduced into clinical practice in the early 1980s. MRI involves applying a powerful magnetic field to the body which causes the protons of hydrogen nuclei to become aligned. The protons are then excited by pulses of radio waves transmitted at a frequency that causes them to resonate and emit radio signals; these are recorded electronically. Sophisticated computation then produces images which can be viewed in any plane, transversely, longitudinally or at any obliquity (Fig. 5.10).

Lipids have particularly high hydrogen content and are clearly seen on MRI. For this reason, the initial applications of MRI were in examining the brain and spinal cord. The technique has also proved to be good for investigating joints and in some cases, replaces the need for arthroscopy. Examination times have reduced and good-quality images of chest, abdomen and pelvis can now be obtained rapidly. MRI is not generally useful for imaging gas-filled organs.

Disadvantages of Magnetic Resonance Imaging

See also section on Magnetic Resonance Imaging Safety, earlier.

Scanning times are still longer than for CT (though falling) and so MRI is less suitable for young children, those with claustrophobia, the elderly or confused, patients in pain, ventilated patients and emergency patients with active bleeding. The diagnostic applications of MRI continue to expand in parallel with the technical improvements.

Applications of Magnetic Resonance Imaging

General Surgical Diagnosis

MRI is especially useful for assessing musculoskeletal tumours, liver tumours, biliary anatomy and pelvic disease. For soft tissue tumours of the extremities, MRI is valuable in planning surgery. It can demonstrate the true extent of the tumour and its relationship to vital structures, so excision margins can be accurately decided before operation.

MRI is useful for imaging the biliary tree by MRCP as previously discussed. Pelvic MRI is invaluable for assessing the sites and anatomical complexity of **anorectal fistulae,** as well as the extent of **rectal**, **prostatic** and **female pelvic organ malignancies**. MRI is now used to image prostate cancer and show abnormal areas that can be targeted by biopsy. In many cases, a normal MRI would mean that invasive biopsy is not necessary.

There is also a role for MRI in **breast cancer**: contrast enhanced MRI may prove to be better than mammography in distinguishing benign from malignant disease and in assessing multifocal disease. In young women with a strong family history or genetic predisposition to breast cancer, screening needs to begin at an age at which mammography would be unlikely to have sufficient discrimination. MRI may accomplish this role without using irradiation.

Blood Flow

MRI is able to demonstrate **blood flow** in the heart and blood vessels, that is, **MRA**. Blood vessels can be visualised without need for contrast injection and abnormalities detected as in conventional angiography. In addition, flow volume can be calculated in particular vessels. Spatial resolution can be improved by injecting paramagnetic materials, such as compounds containing **gadolinium**. MRI is playing a growing role in diagnosing cardiac and arterial disease and may in time replace conventional and even CT coronary angiography.

Interventional Radiology

Many of the conventional x-ray, ultrasound and CT techniques already described have been adapted to guide needles for biopsy, to place drains, to dilate diseased arteries, for example, enabling less invasive therapeutic manoeuvres than formerly. Some techniques have revolutionised treatment and established the interventional radiologist as a front-line clinician, and the field is still growing. Important surgical applications are described in this chapter or in relevant sections elsewhere.

Tissue Sampling

Fine-Needle Aspiration Cytology and Core Biopsy

A fine needle (22 gauge) can be safely passed through most organs or small bowel to aspirate fragments of tissue from a suspicious lesion. Special larger-diameter needles can be used for direct core biopsy of masses. The depth and direction of the needle can be accurately guided by ultrasound or CT to ensure a representative sample is taken. For example, pancreatic masses can be reached by transfixing bowel lying in front of the pancreas; this causes remarkably few side-effects. Where practicable, many surgeons and pathologists prefer the larger specimens obtainable with **core biopsy** techniques using special needles, such as the **Trucut**, available in various configurations and dimensions.

Minimally invasive applications in breast disease include ultrasound- or mammographically-guided FNA or core biopsy of asymptomatic abnormalities detected on mammography, including those found on screening. **Stereotactic apparatus** can be used to make this process more accurate. Mammographic guidance is also sometimes used to place a hooked wire close to an impalpable abnormality immediately before operation to locate it before surgical excision (**mammographic localisation**).

Guided core biopsy or FNA techniques are also important in the diagnosis of thyroid lumps, for sampling liver nodules and for taking renal biopsies in diffuse renal disease.

Drainage of Abscesses and Fluid Collections

Ultrasound and CT are often used to guide percutaneous drainage of well-defined fluid collections in the abdomen or chest (e.g., pancreatic pseudocysts) or abscesses (e.g., paracolic or subphrenic). Ultrasound or CT can demonstrate the site and the dimensions of the fluid collection and show the least harmful route for drainage. Fluid can be drained via a needle on a once-only basis or else a self-retaining 'pigtail' drain can be placed and drainage allowed to continue. In the first category, a subphrenic or other localised abscess can be drained; in the second, a drain can be placed into a pancreatic pseudocyst or locally to drain a biliary leak after surgery or a gaseous/purulent diverticular perforation. In this way, many major surgical interventions can be avoided.

Radionuclide Scanning

Principles of Radionuclide Scanning

Radionuclide or isotope scanning uses nuclear medicine (also called *molecular imaging*) for diagnosis, by identifying sites of abnormal physiology or metabolism. These include detecting the presence of pus, abnormal phagocytic activity within infective/inflammatory foci, areas of excessive bone turnover, such as in bone metastasis, renal function, the presence of clinical or subclinical bleeding or blood clots, biochemical changes related to myocardial ischaemia and hypermetabolic changes in tumours and metastases.

A different tracer substance is administered for each type of scan, with the choice depending on the physiological, metabolic or cellular mechanism to be imaging and assessed. The tracer is nothing more than a metabolically active substrate (carbohydrate, lipid, protein, enzyme, antibody or cells) involved in the pathophysiological process to be analysed. The substrate is administered in pico- and nano mol doses as it is intended to be visualised but not interfere with the pathophysiological process. To visualise the metabolically active substrate from outside the body, it is labelled with a radioactive substance (radionuclide/isotope) emitting low energy photons that can be depicted by scan camera, also called *scintigraphic scanners*. The substrate injected is usually called a **radiopharmaceutical**. The most often used low energetic radioactive substances in imaging are either gamma emitters such as technetium-99m (^{99m}Tc) or iodine-133 (^{133}I), or positron emitters such as fluorine-18 (^{18}F), carbon-11 (^{11}C) or nitrogen-13 (^{13}N).

The radiopharmaceutical tracer is concentrated in a particular type of tissue (such as iodine in the thyroid) or else in tissues with similar physiological or pathological activity, such as reticuloendothelial cells, areas of infection/inflammation or tumour. The radionuclide scanning can be **dynamic**, that is, during a certain time span, with continuous recording of changes in uptake in specific parts of the body, or as **static** imaging at specific time points.

The scintigraphic scanners, either a gamma **camera** or a positron emission tomography (PET) camera, consist of multiple

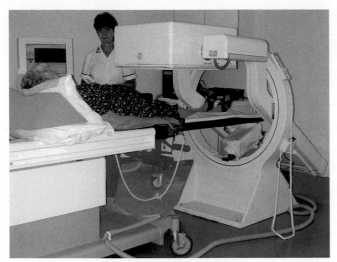

• **Fig. 5.11** Isotope Scanning Using a Gamma Camera. The patient has received an intravenous injection of radiolabelled tracer. The pattern of uptake is imaged by the detector array and transmitted electronically to be displayed on a monitor.

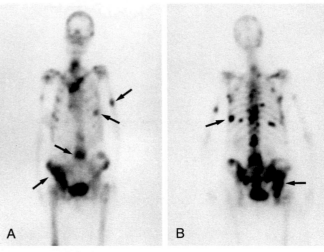

• **Fig. 5.12** Isotope Bone Scans. (A) Anterior view of bone scan in a patient with multiple bony metastases *(arrowed)* from breast cancer. (B) Posterior view of bone scan in the same patient.

detector units which collect and count the level of radioactivity across the area of interest. This produces a complete image in one exposure (Fig. 5.11). Several views are taken from different directions (usually anterior, posterior and oblique). However, newer scanners offer three-dimensional (3D) imaging, known as single photon emission tomography (SPECT) or PET. Radionuclide scanning is a very sensitive imaging tool for pathological metabolic processes, but has lower specificity as it lacks anatomical detail. To overcome this, newer scanners have been coupled with CT or MRI, forming hybrid scanners which greatly increase the effectiveness of identifying lesions and functionally abnormal tissues.

Applications of Radionuclide Scanning

Lung Scanning

Lung scanning was widely used in the diagnosis of pulmonary embolism but is used much less since multislice CT became widely available. However, the scan is still advised where radiation dose plays an important role, such as pregnant women, and also in patients with suspected chronic pulmonary embolism.

Bone Scanning

Phosphate-based agents (phosphates or bisphosphonates) labelled with technetium are usually used. The tracer is taken up in areas of increased bone deposition and resorption, indicating sites of bone growth and repair (Fig. 5.12). These include growth plates, some primary tumours, secondary tumours, foci of bone infection, healing fracture sites, active arthritis and Paget disease (Fig. 5.13).

Bone scanning is highly sensitive but interpretation requires caution because it lacks specificity. Scans are usually interpreted alongside plain radiographs to improve specificity. However, this drawback is overcome by hybrid SPECT-CT which can accurately diagnose active osteoblastic bony lesions.

The tracer agent is injected intravenously and becomes distributed throughout all body fluids. The highest concentration collects at sites of osteogenesis about 6 hours later and the patient is then scanned. The tracer is also taken up in areas of **dystrophic calcification** and may sometimes reveal an unsuspected carcinoma of breast, an old myocardial infarction scar or a uterine fibroid.

The main indications for bone scanning are:
1. Suspected bone metastases (e.g., staging prostate carcinoma) or investigation of bone pain
2. Biochemical abnormalities suggesting bone disease (e.g., hypercalcaemia or raised plasma alkaline phosphatase)
3. Suspected occult (stress) fractures of bone
4. Suspected osteomyelitis
5. Localising abnormalities in unexplained skeletal pain

Renal Scans

Renal scanning is an important method of investigating the urinary tract. It can obtain information not available from any other source, is quick and simple and allows the function of each kidney to be assessed separately.

Three main varieties of scan use different isotopes. **Dynamic** renal scintigraphy provides functional information and uses two isotopes:
- DTPA (diethylene tetramine penta-acetic acid) is excreted in urine like urographic contrast and provides a measure of glomerular filtration rate.
- Technetium-99-MAG3 (mercaptoacetyltriglycine) provides information on split renal function and drainage.
- DMSA (dimercapto-succinic acid) is a static scan where the isotope remains in cortical tissue, and so provides information on the renal parenchyma anatomy and function. (*Aide-mémoire*: DT 'Pee' A, excreted in urine; D 'Meat' SA, retained in cortical tissue.) Examples are shown in Fig. 5.14.

DTPA scanning is used to follow up children with reflux nephropathy. The isotope is instilled into the bladder; the child then voids urine while being scanned and any vesicoureteric reflux is demonstrated. Equally, a MAG3 renogram can provide an indirect micturating cystogram by imaging the patient as they void to assess for reflux. DTPA is also used to diagnose ureteric obstruction and to distinguish obstructed from merely capacious nonobstructed renal tracts.

When unilateral renal parenchymal disease is being investigated, DMSA and DTPA can both give an estimate of excretory activity. The two agents can be used to estimate differential renal function when investigating renal artery stenosis or the function of a transplanted kidney. DMSA is used specifically to image the renal parenchyma to demonstrate renal scars or tumours.

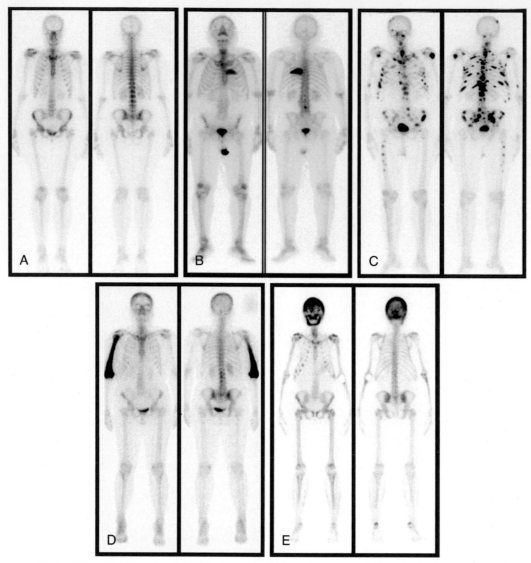

• **Fig. 5.13** Bone Scintigraphy in Adults. **(A)** Normal scan with symmetrical uptake in the skeleton. **(B)** Single bone metastasis on a left rib. **(C)** Widespread bone metastases with multiple focal uptake on skull, spine, pelvis and right femur. **(D)** Monostotic Paget disease on right humerus. **(E)** Hyperparathyroidism with intense osteoblastic activity on skull and focal uptake in ribs.

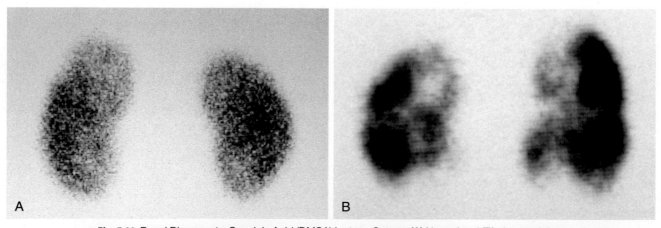

• **Fig. 5.14** Renal Dimercapto-Succinic Acid (DMSA) Isotope Scans. **(A)** Normal and **(B)** abnormal showing patchy scarring caused by episodes of pyelonephritis. In this case, there had been bilateral reflux of urine in childhood.

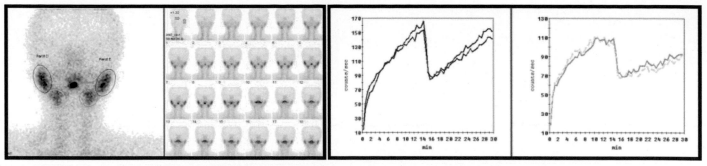

• **Fig. 5.15** Normal Salivary Gland Imaging. Dynamic images are performed over 30 minutes and citric stimulus is given after 15 minutes. Regions of interest include right and left parotid *(red and dark blue)* and submandibular glands *(yellow and light blue)*. Time–activity curves show quantitative uptake and excretion analyses.

After a renal transplant, renal dynamic studies are commonly used to evaluate its most common complications, such as tubular necrosis or rejection. The scintigraphic pattern of acute tubular necrosis shows reduced flow and glomerular filtration that improves in time. In contrast, transplant rejection shows reduced glomerular filtration rate that deteriorates progressively.

Scanning for Gastrointestinal Bleeding

Scanning using the patient's own isotopically labelled red cells may be used to locate a source of continuing or intermittent GI bleeding. This is useful where the rate of bleeding is relatively slow or in a patient with recurrent haemorrhage, particularly where a source cannot be identified by endoscopy or arteriography.

The patient's blood is labelled with radioactive technetium and reinjected, then the abdomen is scanned at intervals over the next 24 hours or so for 'hot spots' indicating accumulating GI haemorrhage. If the rate of bleeding is more than about 0.1 mL per minute, the scan usually reveals activity concentrated in one part of the bowel. This indicates the general area of haemorrhage and enables the surgical search to be focused, for example, on the distal stomach or right side of the colon. Radionuclide scanning can detect blood accumulating over a period, whereas **selective angiography** requires a higher rate of bleeding at the moment of injection; however, it can reveal the site more precisely.

In children, rectal bleeding may be caused by bleeding from a Meckel diverticulum caused by ulceration of ectopic gastric mucosa. A radionuclide compound of ^{99m}Tc concentrated in gastric mucosa may reveal the source.

Leucocyte Scanning for Inflammation and Infection

When an abscess or other infected focus is suspected but cannot be localised, the patient's white blood cells can be labelled with indium-111 or ^{99m}Tc, then reinjected and scanned. Typical indications are patients with a high swinging fever after operation, or with sepsis of unknown origin. The process is expensive but has a high degree of specificity and sensitivity; however, there is a small proportion of false negatives where an occult abscess is not revealed.

Leucocyte scanning can determine the extent of bowel involvement in inflammatory bowel disease, both ulcerative colitis and Crohn disease. Tc-hexamethylpropyleneamine oxime-labelled leucocytes migrate towards areas of inflamed bowel which are then revealed on imaging.

Thyroid Scans

Thyroid scanning is described in Chapter 49. Its use is declining in favour of FNA and cytology except in specific disorders of thyroid function.

Cardiovascular Imaging

A multiple-gated acquisition scan can provide information about ventricular function. This can be useful following myocardial infarction or for patients receiving doxorubicin (Adriamycin) chemotherapy which can damage heart muscle. Radionuclide lymphangiography in chronic lymphoedema can demonstrate the patency and capacity of lower limb lymphatics.

Myocardial perfusion imaging (MPI) has high sensitivity for evaluating left ventricular wall perfusion and thus indirectly assessing coronary flow. Impaired left ventricular wall perfusion is the first detectable change in the ischaemic cascade (see http://www.pharmstresstech.com/stresstesting/ischemic.aspx) and diagnosing it is the main justification for nuclear imaging in evaluating and risk stratifying coronary artery disease.

Salivary Gland Imaging

This assesses the function and excretion of the salivary glands, in the initial diagnosis and in posttreatment follow-up. The main indications include: tumours, cysts, inflammatory or infectious diseases, calculous disease and Sjögren syndrome.

The radiopharmaceutical is concentrated and secreted by the epithelial cells of the salivary glands in the same way as the anions that make up saliva. Thus the tracer reflects the production and physiological secretion of the saliva. The radiopharmaceutical is administered intravenously and sequential images of the head are acquired over time. Over the first 10 minutes, increasing concentration of the tracer is observed in salivary glands, representing their function. After giving citric stimulus, generally lemon, the excretion phase begins. The uptake peak usually occurs 5 to 10 minutes after starting to administer the tracer and complete excretion begins immediately after the stimulation with lemon (Fig. 5.15).

Oesophageal and Gastric Imaging

Investigation of Gastro-Oesophageal Reflux

Scintigraphy is the most sensitive noninvasive method for detecting gastro-oesophageal reflux, especially in children. Colloids with low absorption rates by the oesophageal and gastric mucosa are used to reflect the kinetics of the tracer in the digestive system.

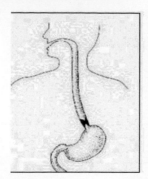
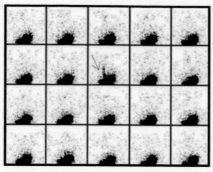
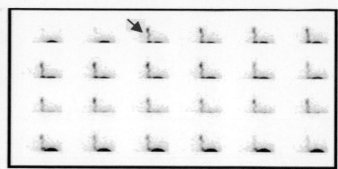

• **Fig. 5.16** Gastrooesophageal Reflux Scintigraphy. A single, short episode of reflux *(black arrow)* and a long, persistent episode of reflux *(red arrow)* during the dynamic scanning.

After oral administration of ^{99m}Tc colloid, episodes of gastro-oesophageal reflux are identified and information on the quantity and duration of the reflux and the level it reaches can be obtained (Fig. 5.16).

Gastric Emptying

This is a noninvasive examination performed after intake of solid foods, liquids or a mixture into which a small amount of radioactive ^{99m}Tc was incorporated. The emptying time and kinetics of the radiopharmaceutical in the stomach depend on the type of food ingested. Computer analysis of the dynamic images determines the half-emptying time and/or percentage emptying and generates gastric emptying time–activity curves. The main indications include diabetic gastroparesis, anorexia nervosa, gastro-oesophageal reflux, gastritis, gastric ulcer, connective tissue disorders, along with postsurgical evaluations, vagotomy and gastrectomy.

Liver and Spleen Scans

Hepatobiliary Imaging (HIDA Scanning)

Technetium-labelled imido-diacetic acid (IDA) derivatives are concentrated by hepatocytes and excreted into bile even in the presence of jaundice. This provides a means of testing the patency of the biliary tree and cystic duct in jaundice.

Hepatobiliary imaging can be used for:

- Demonstrating cystic duct obstruction in suspected acute cholecystitis.
- Demonstrating whether bile ducts are obstructed in jaundiced patients. This is often used in neonates. The patency of the extrahepatic biliary system is confirmed if there is unequivocal evidence of intestinal excretion of the radiolabel.

Sentinel Node Imaging for Various Malignancies

The sentinel node is the first lymph node to be involved by malignancy during the metastatic process. When a sentinel node is removed and found not to contain metastases, other nodes in the area are unlikely to be involved and extensive lymph node surgery can thus be avoided.

The radiopharmaceutical, a ^{99m}Tc-labelled nanocolloid, is injected around the primary tumour. Dynamic scanning over a few minutes shows the radiopharmaceutical migrate via lymphatic vessels and accumulate in the first lymph node draining the tumour site (Fig. 5.17). This procedure identifies the sentinel node on a scan and also assists the surgeon to quickly locate the node during surgery using a small radiation detector.

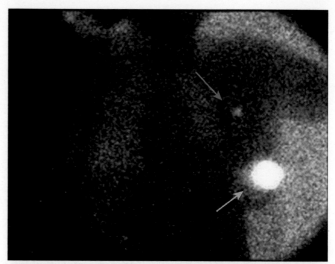
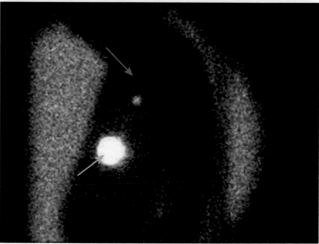

• **Fig. 5.17** Breast Cancer Sentinel Node Imaging. Anterior and left lateral images of patient's chest. After injection of radiopharmaceutical into the left breast *(yellow arrow)*, the sentinel node was identified in the left axillary lymphatic chain *(blue arrow)*.

Positron Emission Tomography Imaging for Tumours

PET measures physiological function by looking at blood flow, metabolic rates of tissues and the distribution of neurotransmitters and radiolabelled drugs. PET is usually combined with CT (PET-CT) or with MRI (PET-MRI) to enable accurate 3D location of abnormalities.

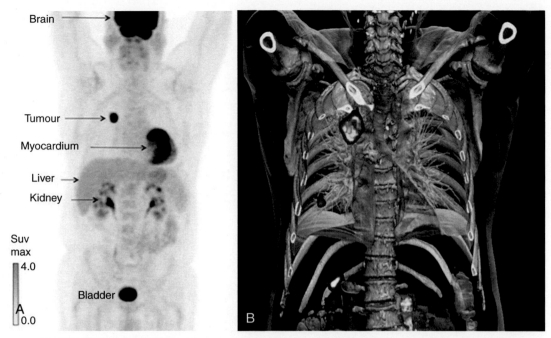

• **Fig. 5.18 (A)** Fluorine-18 labelled fluorodeoxyglucose positron emission tomography computed tomography (18F-FDG PET-CT) Scan. Maximum intensity projection image of a patient with suspected lung cancer. There is a normal high uptake of the glucose-like 18F-FDG radiopharmaceutical in the brain, myocardium, liver, kidneys and bladder. There is also an intense focal uptake in the right lung. **(B)** The metabolic PET images are fused with the anatomical CT images producing a hybrid image.

Fluorine-18 labelled fluorodeoxyglucose (18F-FDG), a glucose analogue, is a commonly used radiopharmaceutical for PET imaging in tumours; it is taken up in sites with intense glucose consumption and is thus a measure of the rate of **glucose consumption** in different parts of the body. Cancer cells are metabolically very active and usually use glucose as an energy substrate, so 18F-FDG is greatly taken up in tumour sites. Thus in many cases, 18F-**FDG-PET** imaging can detect malignancy and differentiate between malignant and benign tissue. 18F-FDG PET can be more sensitive than CT or MRI for detecting cancer. Whole body PET-CT or PET-MRI scanning is used to stage some cancers before attempting curative surgery, for example, oesophagus and lung, or to distinguish recurrent tumours from radiation necrosis or scar tissue, for example, following treatment of lymphoma (Fig. 5.18).

Radiolabelled tracers designed for different macrophage, B-or T-cell receptors are used for identifying lymphomas and active inflammatory sites. Specific radiolabelled tracers can identify specific tumour types, such as neuroendocrine tumours or prostate cancer. Newer radiolabelled tracers are increasingly used to detect specific tumour characteristics, such as neoangiogenesis (18F-endothelin) or hypoxia (18F-pimonidazole). All this information can be crucial in choosing the right anticancer therapeutic approach and in following up cancer patients.

Radiolabelled amino acids, such as 18F-labeled tyrosine, are highly sensitive for detecting brain tumours (Fig. 5.19). Moreover, blood flow and oxygen consumption in the brain can be examined using PET to help understand strokes and dementias. Tracking chemical neurotransmitters in Parkinson disease is also possible using 18F-labeled dopamine, whilst 18F-radiolabelled antiamyloid plaques are used for Alzheimer diagnosis.

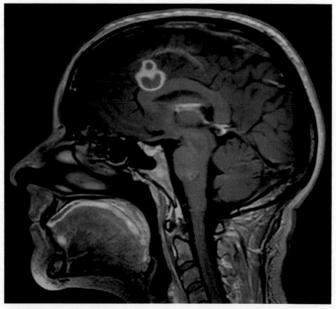

• **Fig. 5.19** 18F-Tyrosine Amino Acid Positron Emission Tomography Magnetic Resonance Imaging (PET-MRI). Hybrid PET-MRI image shows a high radiopharmaceutical uptake in the frontal lobe indicating the presence of a brain tumour.

Flexible Endoscopy

Principles of Flexible Endoscopy

Strictly speaking, endoscopy applies to any method of looking into the body through an instrument via an orifice, such as nose or mouth, or via an artificially created opening (e.g., laparoscopy, thoracoscopy or arthroscopy). Endoscopy using simple tubular instruments was

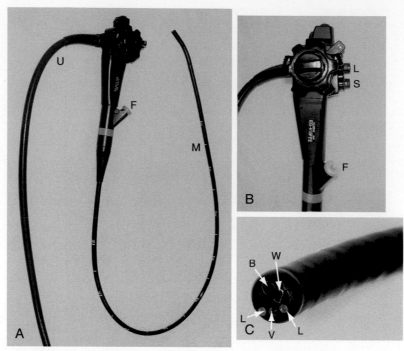

• **Fig. 5.20** Flexible Fibreoptic Gastroscope. **(A)** This end-viewing gastroscope is composed of a flexible main shaft *(M)* which is 1-m long and marked at 10 cm intervals; the distal 10 cm can be flexed in four directions to steer the instrument to advance it and to obtain the best view. There is also an 'umbilical cord' *(U)* which is plugged into the control box. This carries air to inflate the viscus, water to wash the viewing lens and suction to aspirate fluid from the lumen. There is a flush tube *(F)*, through which fluid can be injected to wash the stomach wall. The steering controls are better seen in **(B)**. **(B)** The steering controls consist of two concentric wheels with direction indicators *(D)* and *(U)* (down and up) and *(L)* and *(R)* (left and right, respectively). The channel *(F)* is also used to pass instruments; buttons control suction *(S)* and air inflation and lens washing *(L)*. **(C)** Shows the tip of the instrument in detail. The two light guides are marked *(L)*, *(V)* is the lens for the imaging chip, *(W)* is the exit for the inflation air and lens washing water and *(B)* is the channel for passing instruments and for suction. Note that the video image is transmitted up the 'scope and along the umbilical cord to the processor unit, from where it is displayed on a video monitor.

undertaken for many years and some methods are still in use, for example, rigid sigmoidoscopy. Developments in fibreoptics first led to improved illumination for rigid endoscopes and later to flexible image guides leading to construction of flexible instruments. These greatly extended the range and sophistication of endoscopic diagnosis and therapy. The unqualified term **endoscopy** is now generally applied to GI and urology endoscopy using flexible instruments with fibreoptic illumination and video image transmission.

Practical advances in endoscopy include the introduction of **chromoendoscopy** where dyes are sprayed onto tissues during endoscopy to highlight abnormal tissues. The stains are often the same as those used in histological examinations and have three mechanisms of actions: absorptive stains, such as methylene blue, contrast stains, such as indigo carmine and reactive stains, such as Congo red. Chromoendoscopy applications include identifying Barrett epithelium and sessile (flat) colonic polyps.

Endoscopy units are increasingly governed by strict quality assurance guidelines involving staffing and staff training, physical infrastructure and unit processes and governance.

Fibreoptic Illumination

Rigid endoscopes and early flexible instruments were illuminated by tiny incandescent bulbs prone to failure. These were superseded by **fibreoptic light guides** in both rigid and flexible endoscopes. Fibreoptic light guides channel light from a powerful, remote fan-cooled light source to the distal end of an endoscope. They are made up of thousands of glass fibres, each with total internal reflection, so very little light is lost and no heat is transmitted. A powerful, cool light beam emerges from the distal end of even the longest endoscope.

Image Transmission

The next development crucial to the design of early flexible endoscopes was the invention of **coherent viewing bundles** where the orientation of fibres at the distal end exactly matched the proximal viewing end. Each fibre transmitted a tiny part of the distal scene to the viewing end. The distal end of most endoscopes allowed a viewing angle of over 100 degrees, and lenses gave a remarkable depth of focus. Accurate diagnosis could often be made on inspection alone.

A later development was the charge-coupled device **video camera**, a light- and colour-sensitive microchip positioned at the distal end. The image is transmitted via wires to a colour monitor. This system has now replaced the older direct viewing method.

Structure of Flexible Endoscopes

Most flexible endoscopes include a mechanism to steer the distal end in four directions (except for specialised ultraslender scopes), a distal imaging chip for video endoscopy, one or two fibreoptic light guides, a suction channel and a channel for inflating the hollow viscus under inspection with air, doubling as a lens washing channel (Fig. 5.20). The suction channel is also used to pass slender flexible operating tools, such as tiny forceps for biopsies, grasping forceps for retrieving foreign bodies, laser guides for therapy (haemostasis or tumour destruction), snares for excision of polyps, diathermy wires, scissors for cutting sutures and needles for injecting haemostatic agents.

Applications of Flexible Endoscopy

Flexible endoscopes were first used to inspect the stomach in the late 1960s and the range of instruments has progressively expanded since then. There are now instruments available to inspect and cannulate the duodenal papilla, to examine all or part of the large bowel, to inspect the interior of the bile ducts at operation, to examine bronchi and to examine the bladder interior using only local anaesthesia.

Choledochoscopes are rigid or flexible instruments to inspect the interior of the bile ducts at open or laparoscopic operation to ensure stones are cleared. Their use has improved the rate of clearance during exploration of the common bile duct.

Narrow fibreoptic **bronchoscopes** can be passed under topical (surface) anaesthesia. They are used to inspect bronchi for disease and take biopsies and can aspirate mucus plugs responsible for postoperative lobar collapse.

Diagnostic Upper Gastrointestinal Endoscopy

Oesophago-gastro-duodenoscopy, also known as *OGD* or *gastroscopy*, involves inspecting the upper GI mucosa using a steerable, flexible endoscope. It is usually carried out under intravenous sedation and local anaesthetic spray on a day-case basis. Among other applications, gastroscopy enables the whole area prone to peptic ulcer disease and cancer to be directly and comprehensively examined.

Flexible endoscopy has the following advantages over GI contrast radiology:

- Structural abnormalities, such as chronic ulcers can be inspected directly whereas radiology provides only a 2D image with little information about surface characteristics.
- Benign ulcers and early malignancies are often indistinguishable on radiology whereas at endoscopy, suspicious lesions, such as ulcers can be inspected and biopsied.
- Shallow mucosal abnormalities invisible on radiology, such as superficial ulceration or vascular malformations can be inspected at endoscopy.
- Bile reflux through the pylorus may be visible.
- Fibrosis and anatomical distortions from previous disease or surgery interfere much less with recognition of what is abnormal on endoscopy than on radiology.
- In acute upper GI haemorrhage, endoscopy can often identify the exact site of the lesion causing it and give an indication of the rate of haemorrhage and the likelihood of rebleeding. Tracing the source is often impossible using radiology.
- During endoscopy, therapy may be applied during the same procedure, for example, injection of the source of acute bleeding, retrieving swallowed foreign body, placement of feeding gastrostomy tube.

Therapeutic Upper Gastrointestinal Endoscopy

Treatment of Upper Gastrointestinal Haemorrhage

First-line therapy for upper GI haemorrhage caused by bleeding ulcers typically involves injection of the ulcer base with adrenaline solution alone or in combination with sclerosants. Other treatments, such as laser or direct heat coagulation have proved less effective, but are sometimes used. With these techniques, the need for

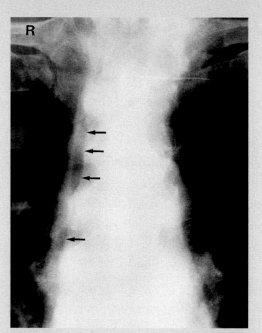

CASE HISTORY

• **Fig. 5.21** Pneumomediastinum Following Perforation of an Oesophageal Tumour During Endoscopy. This 56-year-old man who was being investigated for difficulty in swallowing complained of chest pain after the examination. Crepitus was found in the neck because of surgical emphysema resulting from oesophageal air leaking out of the perforation and tracking up the mediastinum into the neck.

urgent surgery for bleeding has been substantially reduced. Patients successfully treated for acute haemorrhage from benign lesions can often be managed in the long term without surgery; this subject is discussed in detail in Chapter 19. Haemorrhage caused by oesophageal varices is now best treated in most cases by endoscopic band ligation or injection sclerotherapy rather than surgery.

Treatment of Oesophageal Strictures

Endoscopic methods are often used for dilating benign strictures. The endoscope is passed until the stricture is visible and then a flexible wire is passed through into the stomach. The endoscope is removed, leaving the wire in situ. Plastic or metal dilators of increasing size are then passed over the wire which guides them safely through the stricture until sufficient dilatation is achieved. The technique is relatively safe, can easily be repeated and avoids the need for general anaesthesia. There is a small risk of oesophageal perforation (Fig. 5.21).

Large balloon catheters similar to angioplasty catheters can also be used to dilate benign oesophageal strictures caused by oesophagitis. For **achalasia**, balloon dilatation is now a standard technique. Balloon dilatation is sometimes used for benign rectal strictures, such as may occur at an anastomosis site, provided they are not caused by recurrent tumour.

Cloth-lined expanding metal stents are now successfully deployed, usually after dilatation, for palliation of oesophageal, gastric outlet and colonic strictures caused by malignancy. They are usually placed endoscopically, often after contrast radiology. Stenting is not indicated as a permanent solution for benign conditions as it is far from trouble free.

Dysphagia caused by an inoperable malignant stricture can be improved by creating a pathway through the tumour with endoscopically guided **laser fulguration**. Unfortunately, the tumour inevitably recurs and multiple treatments are likely to be necessary, but swallowing can be maintained and the patient's quality of life improved without major surgery. In other cases, a **stent** can be placed endoscopically to keep the oesophagus open. This involves first dilating the stricture, then pushing a collapsed metal expanding stent covered with cloth down until it lies across the stricture. The cover is removed from the stent to deploy it and it expands outwards. This avoids a risky operation and may provide worthwhile palliation for an obstructing tumour.

Diagnostic and Therapeutic Duodenoscopy

A side-viewing duodenoscope can be used to inspect the duodenal papilla and guide insertion of a cannula or therapeutic tools. Cannulation allows injection of contrast material into the common bile duct and separately into the pancreatic duct. The technique is known as **ERCP** (Fig. 5.22 and see Ch. 11) and is an important part of gastroenterological investigation.

ERCP can be both diagnostic and therapeutic. Indications for diagnostic ERCP may be decreasing as newer and safer techniques, such as **MRCP** become available. Therapeutic ERCP allows many bile duct disorders that would previously have required difficult, time-consuming and dangerous operations to be managed by minimal access techniques, with short hospital stays. For example, bile duct stones can often be removed endoscopically by slitting the sphincter at the lower end (**sphincterotomy**) and retrieving them with a balloon catheter or a Dormia

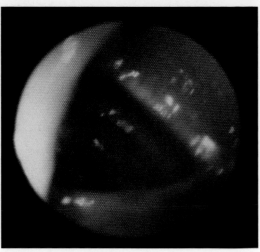

• **Fig. 5.23** Colonoscopic View of Normal Transverse Colon. When seen colonoscopically, the transverse colon is typically triangular in cross-section; the taenia coli form the apices.

basket. Other therapeutic measures include inserting bile duct stents for palliating malignant biliary obstruction (cancer of pancreatic head, bile duct or duodenum) and for managing postoperative bile leaks.

Enteroscopy

Barium follow-through, CT and MRI have low rates of positive diagnosis in small bowel disorders. Direct small bowel visualisation used to be achieved by 'push' enteroscopy (with a 2-m endoscope that could examine up to a metre beyond the duodeno-jejunal flexure) or by operative enteroscopy via a laparotomy. Later, a technique of double-balloon enteroscopy appeared, with an endoscope passed via the mouth and then coaxed along the small bowel using attached balloons as countertraction. None of these methods was convenient or reliable.

A later development for small bowel investigation is **capsule endoscopy**, introduced in 1999. This enables the entire 3 to 5 M of small bowel to be visualised with relative ease. The patient swallows a capsule which is propelled through the GI tract by peristalsis. An imaging device continually transmits images to sensors on the abdominal wall and the capsule-camera then passes in the stool.

One device, the PillCam SB capsule endoscope, is only 26×11 mm, weighs under 4 g. It contains a battery, light-emitting diodes, an imaging chip camera that captures images at two frames a second and a radiotransmitter that passes images to a sensor array for up to 8 hours. The camera has an image field of 140 degrees. If obstruction is suspected, a different model with a body made of lactose can be used. This disintegrates in less than 48 hours if arrested.

Capsule endoscopy has a positive diagnosis rate of around 65% compared with around 20% for other methods. In obscure GI bleeding, there is a positive diagnostic yield of 45% to 75% in patients who have already had negative upper and lower GI endoscopy. Typical findings include angiodysplasia, tumours, varices and ulcers. Other indications include suspected small bowel Crohn disease, particularly in children, assessment of coeliac disease, screening in familial polyposis syndromes and diagnosis of Barrett oesophagus (by attaching a string). Biopsies cannot yet be taken.

Large Bowel Endoscopy (Colonoscopy)

Flexible endoscopes of different lengths are available for large bowel examination (Fig. 5.23). The shortest, the **fibreoptic**

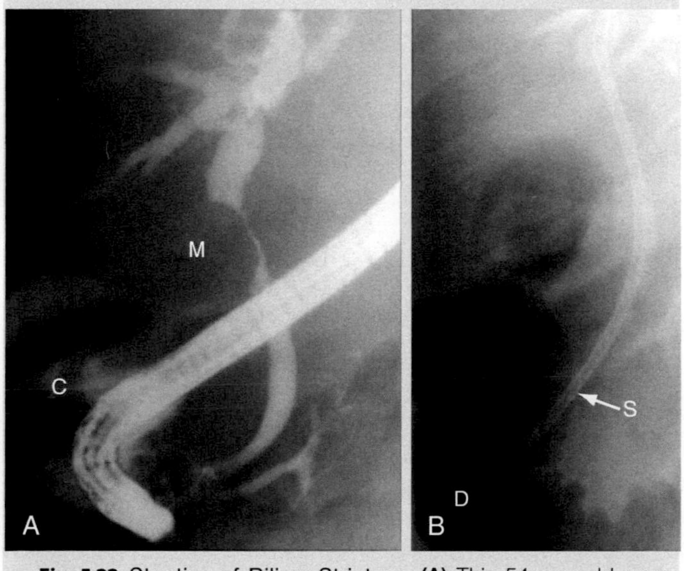

• **Fig. 5.22** Stenting of Biliary Stricture. **(A)** This 54-year-old man developed painless, unremitting obstructive jaundice. This endoscopic retrograde cholangio-pancreatography (ERCP) shows a malignant stricture of the common bile duct *(M)* because of cholangiocarcinoma. Contrast has been injected to outline the bile ducts and has leaked back into the duodenum *(C)*. **(B)** A stent *(S)* was placed endoscopically across the stricture for palliation. The second part of the duodenum is outlined by gas *(D)*.

sigmoidoscope, is about 60 cm long. It is simple to use and allows examination of the rectum, sigmoid colon and descending colon with minimal bowel preparation. Longer colonoscopes enable the entire large bowel to be inspected, and vary in stiffness to assist intubation to the caecum. Other techniques also help reach the caecum, including insufflation with carbon dioxide rather than air, and releasing seed oil from the tip to lubricate the instrument.

Colonoscopy allows inspection of pathological lesions, biopsy of suspicious lesions and resection of lesions, such as polyps. Colonoscopy is also used for surveillance and follow-up of patients treated for colorectal cancer or polyps. New tumours or polyps (metachronous lesions) are looked for and the original site of surgery can be examined. Similar examinations are also used for surveillance of patients with longstanding ulcerative colitis; multiple biopsies are taken to examine for dysplasia, and the entire large bowel is inspected for adenomas or carcinomas. Acutely bleeding angiodysplastic lesions in the large bowel can be treated with diathermy.

Colonoscopy is the most reliable method of screening asymptomatic people for colorectal carcinoma. However, its application is limited by the lack of trained endoscopists, by cost and by lack of patient compliance.

Urological Endoscopy

Endoscopic urology is a progressively larger part of urological surgery with flexible instruments used for diagnostic cystoscopy and ureteroscopy.

Cystourethroscopy (cystoscopy) using a rigid instrument is the main diagnostic and therapeutic tool for disease of the urethra, prostate and bladder, allowing biopsy and diathermy of tissues. An irrigating resectoscope is used for removal of prostate in bladder outlet surgery (transurethral resection of the prostate and holmium laser enucleation of the prostate), which have virtually eliminated the need for open retropubic prostatectomy. Most early bladder tumours can be treated endoscopically with transurethral resection of bladder tumour. An instrument similar to the cystoscope (but longer), the rigid **ureteroscope**, can be used to guide laser treatment of stones or tumours in the ureter, whilst a longer, finer flexible ureteroscope can access the upper ureter and pelvicalyceal system of the kidney for treatment (see Ch. 27, Fig. 37.6).

Endoscopic methods of percutaneous stone removal from the renal pelvis have become widely available (**percutaneous nephrolithotomy**). These involve creating a channel from the skin into the renal pelvis and dilating it until an endoscope can be passed. When the stone is seen, various instruments can be used to fragment it and achieve its removal (see Ch. 37, Fig. 37.7B).

Image-Guided Surgery

Image guidance techniques are in their infancy, but the ability to enhance the surgeon's view and awareness of the operative field is an exciting development. Currently, indocyanine green (ICG)-guided surgery has regained popularity. This was first used in the 1950s but the technique has now been adapted for laparoscopy. The fluorescent ligand ICG is injected intravenously and excited by a special light source at 850 nm. Specially adapted laparoscopes can detect the fluorescence, which can identify and quantify tissue perfusion (e.g., before colorectal anastomosis) as well as assess biliary anatomy and bile leaks. This is an important area of imaging that is expected to enhance surgical performance in real time.

Diagnostic and Therapeutic Laparoscopy

This is covered in Chapter 10.

6

Screening for Adult Disease

CHAPTER OUTLINE

Principles of Screening

Introduction

Medical screening is a public health activity that involves examining or testing asymptomatic, apparently healthy people to detect disease at an early stage. Measures can then be taken to prevent the disease (if there is a precursor stage), treat it early (hoping for improved cure rates), or at least offer treatment to delay advanced disease. For example, colonic screening can detect adenomas and carcinomas; removing adenomas prevents the well-recognised adenoma–carcinoma sequence, and actual cancers detected are often earlier and at a more curable stage. Unfortunately, for other cancers without an easily detected early precursor stage, such as breast or prostate, beneficial outcomes are elusive.

Screening can detect disorders that predispose to other diseases, for example, hypertension or elevated cholesterol levels, to ascertain people at increased risk of atherosclerotic heart disease and stroke. Screening is also useful for infection control, for example, preoperative screening of patients for methicillin-resistant *Staphylococcus aureus* (MRSA) carrier status to enable elimination therapy before operation.

An entire population can be screened (**mass screening**) but more usually, it is **targeted** at at-risk groups. Selection might be by age, gender or cardiovascular risk factors, for example (Box 6.1).

Opportunistic screening involves a more random approach, such as screening patients who happen to attend a particular clinic.

Assessing the Potential Benefits of Screening

Many lay people subscribe to the simplistic view that screening must be 'a good thing'. These include the public, people associated with distressing diseases, populist politicians and people with vested financial interests. Poorly conceived screening, however, may consume massive resources to identify just a few new cases with little clinical benefit, for example, computed tomography (CT) scanning for lung cancer in low risk populations. Worse still, early diagnosis of a condition where early intervention brings no advantage may cause suffering. These people can be prematurely placed into an anxiety-provoking sick role and given unrealistic expectations. They may also be subjected to unnecessary treatments with potentially severe side-effects, for example, some breast or prostate cancers that might never progress to metastatic disease.

As with any public health measure, medical and social benefits accruing from any screening programme need to be rigorously evaluated and the process separated entirely from the incentive to screen for profit. Whole-body scanning by CT or magnetic resonance imaging (MRI) is currently strongly marketed on the basis that a scan will show unsuspected abnormalities and allow early treatment. Abnormalities are bound to be discovered by such extensive screening, but it is difficult to reliably determine which signify serious disease and which (if any) should be treated. Doctors should not perform unvalidated screening tests any more than they should use unproven drugs, and should resist patient pressure for inappropriate screening.

Premature Introduction of Screening

Politicians can play a part in initiating inappropriate screening programmes. UK prime minister, Margaret Thatcher sanctioned nationwide breast screening in 1988, 2 weeks before a general election; some believe this was to gain the women's vote. The decision was premature and based on insufficiently validated evidence from the Swedish two-county study and the UK Forrest report. In the 1970s screening for cancer of the uterine cervix was widely introduced, also before its efficacy had been fully evaluated. Fortunately, it has proved successful despite the difficulty of engaging women at high risk. Sadly, the natural history of untreated dysplastic cervical cellular abnormalities was not properly established before the impact of widespread screening made this ethically impossible. This severely hampered scientific study of the disease, its early diagnosis and best treatment. More recently, the human

Infections
- Tuberculosis
- Methicillin-resistant *Staphylococcus aureus* (MRSA)

Malignancy and Premalignancy
- Cervix; colorectal (current programmes show benefit)
- Breast (reduces deaths but overdiagnosis)
- Prostate; bronchus (no proven benefit)
- Oesophagus (beneficial in parts of China with a high incidence)
- Stomach (beneficial in Japan with a high incidence)

Cardiovascular Disease
- Hypertension (beneficial in preventing future cardiovascular events)
- Cholesterol (beneficial in preventing future cardiovascular events)
- Abdominal aortic aneurysm (proven benefit)
- Ischaemic heart disease; carotid atherosclerosis; peripheral arterial disease (no proven benefit but lifestyle changes likely to bring benefit in subjects with disease detected)

Metabolic Disease
- Diabetes (beneficial in population screening and opportunistic screening)
- Retinopathy in diabetes (screening programmes now show evidence of benefit)
- Thalassaemia—successful national premarital screening programme for 3 million couples has reduced the expected birth rate of affected infants by 70%

[a]This list is not exhaustive and does not include genetic screening or conditions with special risk factors.

• BOX 6.2 World Health Organization Guidelines for Assessing When Screening Is Appropriate (Wilson and Jungner 1968[a])

1. The condition being screened for should be an important health problem.
2. The natural history should be well understood.
3. There should be a detectable early stage.
4. Treatment at an early stage should be of greater benefit than at a later stage.
5. There should be a suitable test for the early stage.
6. The test should be acceptable.
7. Intervals for repeating the test should be determined.
8. There should be adequate health service provision for the extra clinical workload resulting from the screening.
9. The risks should be less than the benefits.
10. The costs should be balanced against the benefits.

[a]Wilson JMG, Jungner G. Principles and practice of screening for disease. Geneva: WHO; 1968.

• BOX 6.3 Summary of Attributes of a Good Screening Programme

The Disease
- Important health problem
- Detectable truly early stage
- Predictable biological behaviour
- Long period between first detectable stages and overt disease

The Diagnostic Test
- Valid (sensitive and specific)
- Simple and cheap
- Safe and acceptable
- Reliable and reproducible

Diagnosis and Treatment
- Effective, acceptable and safe treatment available
- Evidence of better outcomes if treated early
- Benefits of screening must outweigh risks
- Treatment facilities must be adequate
- Screening overall must be cost effective
- Screening must be sustainable

papilloma virus (HPV) has become recognised as the cause of cervical cancer and is tested for in screening. This recognition has led to widespread and successful campaigns of HPV vaccination and proven major reductions in cervical cancer.

Criteria for Assessing a Screening Programme

Many years ago, the World Health Organization (WHO) realised that even beneficial screening could be expensive, unpleasant, inaccurate and unproductive, and could adversely affect psychological or physical well-being. In 1968 they published a list of criteria for effective screening programmes (Box 6.2) including attributes of the disease, the test and the treatment. These principles are still relevant today and have been added to by the UK National Screening Committee and other groups. Box 6.3 shows a summary of these modified criteria.

Evolution of Screening Programmes

Once begun, any screening programme must remain under constant evaluation and modified or discontinued when criteria are no longer being met. For example, in the 1950s and 1960s, screening for pulmonary tuberculosis (TB) by mass miniature chest x-ray was highly successful, but it was disbanded in the 1970s when new cases fell below a level at which the unit cost per new case could be justified; interestingly, by then, the yield of new cases of lung cancer from screening began to exceed that of TB, but there was virtually no effective treatment for lung cancer at the time.

Criteria for an Effective Screening Programme

To initiate a new national screening programme, certain criteria must be fulfilled. There must be a perceived need in the medical community or in the wider public. Pilot studies are then carried out. If outcomes are promising, large scale **prospective randomised controlled trials (RCTs)** need to be performed, seeking robust evidence for implementation. This is critical because it is politically difficult to stop a screening programme, even when evidence shows little benefit, for example, some early breast screening programmes (Nordic Cochrane Collaboration 2001 and 2006).

The Disease

The screened condition should be an **important health problem** either because it is common (such as lung or prostate cancer) or has serious but preventable consequences, such as carotid artery disease or abdominal aortic aneurysm (AAA). The **prevalence** (proportion of cases already in a defined population) and the **incidence** (number of new cases in a defined population within a specified period of time) of the disease in the population at risk are discovered from pilot studies. There should be a truly early stage where treatment outcomes are better than at a late stage. Colorectal adenomas and early cancers are good examples.

The biological behaviour or natural history of the disease should be well understood, including how latent disease progresses to clinical disease, and the disease course should be reasonably predictable. For example, AAAs are known to expand smoothly for the most part and rarely rupture until they are large. The risks of untreated disease also need to be understood, and there should be a long period between the first detectable stages and overt disease.

The Diagnostic Test

The test must be valid, that is, reliable in detecting the disease. This is defined by **sensitivity** and **specificity**. Sensitivity is the capability of the test to identify affected individuals in the screened population, that is, the proportion of people who have the disease and are detected. A test with many false negative results is unreliable. A UK appeal court ruled that sensitivity is paramount in (cervical) screening and awarded damages to women with missed diagnoses at screening. Specificity is the degree to which a positive test can be relied upon to prove the disease is present; in other words, the higher the false positive rate, the lower the specificity.

The test should ideally be simple and cheap and it must identify the disease by a reliable, validated and reproducible method. The distribution of test values should be understood well enough to define normality or relative risk (RR) associated with particular stages, for example, for an AAA, the diameter that carries a high risk of rupture. Intervals for repeating the test should be worked out for normal subjects and for those with positive results near the threshold.

The complete screening programme must be clinically safe and acceptable socially and ethically to health professionals and the public. This includes the test and any diagnostic procedures, treatments or interventions screening initiates. For example, if a test is perceived as unpleasant, for example, colonoscopy, uptake is low and the benefits are proportionately smaller.

The overall benefits should be greater than the risks; this includes any physical and psychological harm caused by the test, diagnostic procedures and treatment.

Diagnosis and Treatment

Cases identified by the test must be amenable to effective, acceptable and safe diagnostic procedures and the potential benefits of medical or surgical intervention prompted by earlier diagnosis need to be understood.

There should be clear evidence from high-quality studies that early treatment produces better outcomes than treatment at later stages, that is, 'cure' should be more likely, survival longer, or earlier treatment easier. Treatment should have minimal side effects. There also needs to be agreement in advance about who should be offered treatment and its nature; this evidence may emerge from RCTs.

The overall benefits of screening must outweigh the risks. This includes any physical and psychological harm caused by the test, the diagnostic procedures and the treatment. Treatment facilities must be adequate with the capacity to deal with the extra workload from screening.

Screening overall must be cost effective compared with other healthcare interventions and needs. Costs include the testing, further diagnostics and treatment, administration, staff training and quality assurance. For example, because of its high unit cost, CT screening is unlikely to be implemented unless proved extremely effective in early diagnosis of a common, highly remediable life-threatening condition. In a world of competing public health measures, debate continues about what is an acceptable cost per life year saved: £100—£5000—£35,000?

Any screening programme must be sustainable in terms of management, monitoring and quality standards. High-quality, realistic, unbiased information needs to be offered to potential participants about the consequences of testing, investigation and treatment to help them decide whether to go ahead. This is currently a subject of debate regarding breast screening in the United Kingdom.

Ideally, any primary prevention interventions for the disease should be implemented before or in parallel with the screening programme.

Limitations of Screening

Screening is conceptually and ethically different from usual clinical practice as the process is aimed at an entire population, and achieved by dealing with apparently healthy individuals. Participants expect the diagnosis of the presence or absence of disease will be accurate, and that if disease is found, the outcome will be favourable. However, there is no guarantee of this because there will always be false positive and negative results, however good the test. Also, the disease may appear or progress unexpectedly rapidly between screenings. This emphasises the importance of good population education and properly informed consent for individuals engaging in the programme. Participating in screening must be a free choice and it may or may not have health benefits and significant adverse effects.

Bias

A number of phenomena can lead to mistaken claims for efficacy of a screening programme:

Lead time bias—screening relies on the principle that a serious or fatal disease can be diagnosed at an early stage, and that doing so will definitively improve morbidity and mortality. However, if it does not alter the disease course, earlier diagnosis gives the statistical illusion of prolonged survival. It also makes affected patients acutely aware of the presence of their disease for longer.

Selection bias occurs if more health-conscious people, often at lower risk of the disease, undergo screening.

Length bias occurs when screening detects less aggressive variants than those the screening programme was set up to discover. Length bias is frequently cited in the context of breast cancer screening.

Participation Rates

Universal participation is not usually necessary to achieve measurable community benefit and cost effectiveness. This is because community benefit is the sum of individual benefits (except for infectious diseases, such as TB). If a validated screening programme has low set-up costs, benefits are usually proportional to costs. For colorectal cancer screening, for example, cost effectiveness falls off only at extremely low levels of participation.

Other Aspects of Screening

Cost Effectiveness

Imponderables, such as the economic value of saving a life or extending survival need to be considered. All screening studies cost money in detecting and treating cases. The cost effectiveness of a screening programme is usually reported as **cost per life-year saved** or the cost of increasing 'quality adjusted life years'.

The acceptable cost per life-year saved is a matter for debate; in developed countries, somewhere between £12,000 and £30,000 is often quoted as acceptable.

Research Benefits

Screening a population can teach the clinical community and the public much about the natural history and progression of a disease, its aetiology and its various associations, for example the link between coronary heart disease and smoking. Different investigations and treatments can be trialled in large groups of affected individuals, to the ultimate benefit of the population at large.

Consent

Organisers are obliged to provide participants with reliable and unbiased information about the benefits and risks of any screening process and its consequences. There must not be any form of coercion to participate. Much current information tends to overemphasise the benefits of screening and minimises the risks, often not indicating that participation is voluntary. Breast cancer screening in the United Kingdom has been criticised in this respect.

Screening for Cancer

Early Detection of Cancer

As a principle, the earlier in its natural history that malignancy is diagnosed and treated, the better the prognosis. The ideal would be to detect cancer before invasion or metastasis had occurred, that is, during the preinvasive stage. However, many cancers invade and spread before they reach a detectable size or produce tumour markers. Where true early detection is possible, health education can alert the public to early symptoms and warning signs. In skin and testicular tumours, this should include regular self-examination. Self-examination is still promoted for breast cancer but large trials have shown it to be ineffective and that it causes harm by leading to more biopsies.

The common cancer killers are shown in Table 6.1, with breast, prostate and bronchus still leading the field.

In women, breast cancer is a huge public health problem, followed by carcinoma of the cervix and ovary. In men, prostate cancer is a large and growing problem. Colorectal cancer is common and evenly matched in frequency in both sexes in the United Kingdom; 30,000 new cases are detected each year and 16,000 die of it. Gastric and pancreatic cancers are also big killers but screening is of little value except in areas of exceptionally high incidence. In China, high-risk areas for oesophageal cancer have been identified and brush cytology without gastroscopy has proved beneficial.

Several genetic predispositions to cancer have been identified, for example, polyposis coli for colorectal cancer and *BRCA1* and *BRCA2* for breast and other cancers. Genetic screening is not covered in this chapter but individual disorders are described in other chapters.

Cervical Cancer

Poorly organised screening trials using cervical smears and Papanicolaou staining began in the United Kingdom in the mid-1960s and national screening started in 1988. Nearly all reports show early detection and treatment prevents 80% to 90% of invasive cervical cancers and has greatly reduced cervical cancer mortality. The International Agency for Research on Cancer

TABLE 6.1	Most Frequent Deaths From Cancer, United Kingdom 2016[a]	
Cancer Site	Female	Male
Lung	16,306	19,314
Genital (ovary + uterus in female; prostate + urinary tract in male)	8344	21,764
Breast	11,482	81
Colorectal (inc. anus)	7515	8869
Oesophagus	2504	5500
Pancreas	4725	4538
Stomach	1597	2860
Leukaemia and non-Hodgkin lymphoma	4157	5475
Other sites[a]	19,639	23,678

[a]Note that in males, three cancers—lung, prostate and bowel—account for just under half of all cancer deaths; in females, three cancers—lung, breast and bowel—also account for nearly half of all cancer deaths. Note also a large proportion of deaths occur where the primary has not been identified.

indicated that yearly screening between the ages of 25 and 64 years reduces invasive cancer by 94%, 3-yearly screening reduces it by 91%, 5-yearly by 84%, and 10-yearly by 64%. These figures are the basis for the present UK policy—that yearly screening is unnecessarily frequent and 3-yearly screening is recommended for women aged 25 to 49 years and 5-yearly screening for women aged 50 to 64 years. Over 65 years screening is only recommended for women who have not been screened since age 50 years or with recent abnormal tests. Screening now includes cytology for abnormal cells and a test for HPV. If the latter is positive, colposcopy is advised.

In the United Kingdom, 4 million women are screened annually and 78% of the 14 million eligible women have been screened over the 5 years up to 2014. The programme costs £150 million a year, amounting to £37.50 per screen. Both the number of invasive cancer cases and deaths from it halved between 1988 and 2005, taking the disease from sixth most common cancer in women to 13th.

British data show that about a quarter of all cervical cancers occur in each of the four age groups: 25 to 39, 40 to 54, 55 to 69 and 70+ years, but there are problems with recruiting young women and women from lower socio-economic strata. Both groups have been shown to be at higher risk. In a study from Hawaii in 2003, only one in 12 eligible women had not been screened in the preceding 5 years, but this small group accounted for two-thirds of the invasive cancers in the community. Thus there are real concerns that those at greatest risk are not being tested. In addition, those with positive results may not be treated effectively.

A cost effectiveness study from Peru, India, Kenya, Thailand and South Africa indicates that a single screen (and treatment if necessary), using testing for HPV in cervical cells or visual inspection of the cervix after swabbing with acetic acid rather than a cervical smear is a cheap and effective way to reduce a woman's lifetime risk by 25% to 36%. Types 16 and 18 HPV cause most cervical cancer worldwide and effective vaccines are now available. Two rounds of screening at 35 and 40 years could reduce lifetime risk by a further 40%. If screening were introduced across the developing world, then the global incidence of cervical cancer could fall by about 50%. Ideally, all young women should be vaccinated against HPV with modern effective quadrivalent vaccines; this would virtually eliminate cervical cancer and the need for screening.

Ovarian Cancer

Ovarian cancer screening is not yet reliable enough for general use, but a study has reported on 200,000 women aged 50 to 74 years who were screened with transvaginal ultrasound (US) alone or with blood testing for the tumour marker CA125. Sensitivity for US + CA125 was 89% and specificity was 99.8%; both tests proved better than US alone. Only 84 cancers were detected overall in preliminary screening and 13 interval cancers were detected in the ensuing year.

Breast Cancer

Mammographic screening for breast cancer was introduced nationally in the United Kingdom in the late 1980s following the Forrest report of 1986. Most developed countries followed suit after results from the Health Insurance Plan (HIP) study of New York, the Swedish two-county study and the Canadian National Breast Screening Study. These appeared to demonstrate a 30% reduction in mortality from breast cancer in screened women. In the Swedish study, there was also a significant 13% reduction in all-cause mortality.

Mammographic screening detects breast cancers of smaller size than those presenting clinically, with around 30% being either carcinoma in situ or invasive cancers less than 0.5 cm in diameter. A high proportion are node negative—only about 20% have axillary spread compared with 40% for symptomatic cancer. By detecting small lesions, screening substantially increases the reported incidence of invasive breast cancer. This might be expected to mean fewer new cases in later years, as prevalent cases would disappear from the population. In Norway and Sweden, this has proved untrue, suggesting that screening is not detecting most of the clinically important cases that progress to become invasive or metastasise.

In any population of women with breast cancer, lesions will be at different stages of development and pathological potential. These may be grouped as follows:
- **Biologically early cancers**—these include lesions too small to be detectable but with metastatic potential.
- **Small cancers and carcinoma in situ**—these predominantly nonaggressive lesions may never metastasise.
- **Large or advanced tumours**—these are usually symptomatic and quickly fatal.

Large trials have concluded that as many as one-third of cancers detected by screening would never have presented clinically.

The sensitivity of screening for clinically significant cancers is poor; in particular, lobular or mucinous cancers and some rapidly proliferating, high-grade tumours may not be detectable. This is illustrated by the high proportion of **interval cancers** presenting clinically between screening visits. In one representative series, 38% of all breast cancers presented as interval cancers. These tended to occur in younger patients with dense breasts and with a higher usage of hormone replacement therapy or the oral contraceptive pill. A study in New South Wales estimated that screening overdiagnosed invasive cancer by 30% to 42% in women aged 50 to 69 years and other studies have confirmed this. A Dutch study

showed that false positives adversely affect quality of life for at least a year.

On the basis of tumour doubling times, breast cancers detected clinically have been present for an average of 8 years, whereas mammographically detected lesions have been present for about 6 years—a long period in which to metastasise. This may explain the failure of screening to increase the cure rate for clinically significant cancers, and also calls into question the political pressure for patients with suspected breast cancers to be evaluated in clinic within a very short time.

Effectiveness of Mammographic Screening

Mammographic screening every 2 years has been estimated to avert only two deaths in 1000 women aged between 50 and 59 years over a period of 10 years. To achieve this requires 5000 screens and 242 recalls, and for 64 women to have at least one biopsy. Five women will have ductal carcinoma in situ detected, some of which may never progress to invasive cancer. Less than 1% of women invited for screening will benefit; a much larger percentage have to endure false alarms, unnecessary surgery and inappropriate labels of cancer.

In the United States, the independent Health Services/Technology Assessment Texts reviewed published clinical trials and concluded that 'in absolute terms, the mortality benefit shown with mammography screening was small enough that biases in the trials could erase or create the observed mortality reduction'.

The Cochrane View of Breast Screening

The Cochrane Collaboration is an international nonprofit organisation that rigorously and dispassionately reviews published research evidence and provides up-to-date information about the effects of health care. Over 11,000 articles have been published in 20 years on breast screening. The Nordic Cochrane Centre reviewed all RCTs in 2001 and found that astonishingly few were of sufficient rigour to reliably determine whether screening reduced morbidity and mortality. Only seven RCTs were identified, of which only two were of sufficiently high quality. Evidence from the adequately randomised Canadian and Malmö trials showed screening had no significant effect. The other five trials in which randomisation was inadequate, found that screening decreased the risk of death by about 25% but showed a slight **increase** in risk for screened women for death from any cause. A further Cochrane review was published in 2006, which reanalysed data from published trials. Both reviews found little benefit from breast screening and in 2006 they stated that the absolute risk reduction for breast cancer from screening was only 0.05%. They also found that screening led to substantial overdiagnosis and overtreatment. They concluded: 'the currently available reliable evidence does not show a survival benefit of mass screening for breast cancer, and the evidence is inconclusive for breast cancer mortality.' These controversial conclusions imply that breast screening does no good, causes actual harm and probably should be abandoned. This, however, is unlikely to happen. An updated review in 2012 again concluded that screening is ineffective at preventing deaths.

Why Breast Screening Is Claimed to Improve Survival

Several factors could explain how screening could appear to reduce mortality, as follows:
- Lead time bias and overdetection of clinically insignificant lesions
- Mortality from breast cancer can occur over a very long period. Even 35 years after treatment, the commonest cause of death in

a Cambridge UK series was still breast cancer. Thus screening studies need to be prolonged.

- Improvements in breast cancer treatment were introduced over the period of the main trials. Tamoxifen and perhaps improved chemotherapy undoubtedly extended absolute survival between the early and late 1980s. Over a similar period, other cancer rates fell for largely unknown reasons: thyroid cancer fell by 12%, testis by 17% and melanoma by 23%.
- Subjectivity, unrealistic optimism and perhaps vested interests may lead to misleading presentation of statistics and unsustainable claims for the industry of breast screening.

Other Benefits From Breast Screening

Experience gained from breast screening and managing patients detected has brought rapid improvements in mammographic equipment, techniques and interpretation, as well as a more sensitive approach to patients. It has generated much scientific study of the management of early breast cancer. All of this will bring benefits for women with breast cancer and for people with other types of cancer.

For the future, there is interest in using MRI for screening, particularly among high-risk women, as MRI detects more cancers than mammography and is better able to discriminate between cancer and a scar.

Colorectal Cancer

Colorectal cancer is a major health hazard that kills 16,000 people a year in the United Kingdom; only about 10% are diagnosed early. Early cancers have survival rates of better than 90% but the all-stage 5-year survival rate of 35% has hardly improved despite treatment advances, because most cases present late. Nine out of 10 cases occur in people over 50 years.

Screening for colonic cancer has a good chance of being effective. It fulfils many criteria required for a screening programme. In particular, there is a clear sequence of adenomas progressing to adenocarcinoma. Also early cancers are detectable and progress steadily to advanced cancers. About 75% arise sporadically, most likely in preexisting adenomas. Thus a window of opportunity exists for detecting adenomatous polyps at a premalignant stage or cancers at an early invasive stage (i.e., pathologically less advanced than those with symptoms), where they are potentially curable. The transition phase from benign to malignant is long, shown by the cumulative risk of cancer in polyps 10 mm or larger being only 8% at 10 years.

However, detection methods are the stumbling block. Screening by symptoms alone is very unreliable. The **sensitivity** of guaiac faecal occult blood (FOB) testing is no better than 50% and the **specificity** is also low. A newer quantitative FOB test, faecal immunological testing is much more sensitive and specific and is replacing the guaiac test. With 2-yearly FOB testing alone, there are many **interval cancers**: 30% to 60% of cancers and as many as 80% of polyps are missed after three rounds of testing. Sensitivity and interval cancer rates can be improved by adding flexible sigmoidoscopy. A randomised multicentre once-only trial of flexible sigmoidoscopy in 100,000 people found it reduced the rate of colorectal cancer by 33% and deaths from it by 43%. Rectosigmoid cancers were reduced by 50% (Lancet 2010; 375; 1624–1633) but right-sided cancers are not detected. Unfortunately, both FOB testing and flexible endoscopy are distasteful and patient participation is low. Better forms of screening would undoubtedly improve participation.

Despite the drawbacks of FOB testing, meta-analysis of four RCTs has shown that FOB screening can reduce mortality from colorectal cancer by 16% for those allocated to screening and by 23% of those actually screened. On this basis, a 2-yearly FOB screen offered to 10,000 people aged over 40 years, with two-thirds attending for at least one test, would prevent 8.5 deaths (confidence interval [CI], 3.6–13.5) from colorectal cancer over 10 years, a mortality reduction of 23% (RR, 0.77; CI, 0.57–0.89); 2800 participants would have a colonoscopy and there would be 3.4 major complications from this, that is, perforation or haemorrhage (Cochrane). The cost of screening was £5290 per cancer detected and an estimated £1584 per life year gained, well within acceptable norms.

Reports of pilot screening studies suggest screening could improve mortality by 33%, and national screening with FOB testing every 2 years has been approved for implementation in the United Kingdom. This started in April 2006 for men and women in England and now targets those aged 60-74 years. In addition, large-scale pilots of endoscopic colorectal screening (by flexible sigmoidoscopy) are being trialled in patients in their mid-50s but have yet to show real benefit.

Prostate Cancer

Prostate cancer is the most common cause of cancer deaths in older men and 84% of deaths are in men over 70 years. Unfortunately, the prospects for prevention remain poor. The problem is not so much in detecting the disease but in avoiding false positives, detecting it early enough and predicting its clinical course. Many cancers remain forever dormant, as shown by postmortem studies in men who have died of something else: foci of prostate cancer occur in 70% of 70-year-olds, 60% of 60-year-olds and 50% of 50-year-olds. These patients died *with* the disease rather than from it and offering radical treatment for them is clearly inappropriate. Serum prostate specific antigen (PSA) levels increase with the volume of tumour, so high levels indicate extensive disease. In one study, the age-specific median concentration was 40 µg/L in men who died within 3 years, 6 µg/L in men who died between 3 and 6 years and 4 µg/L in those who died between 6 and 10 years. In another study, using a cut-off level of 10 µg/L, the false positive rate was 4% (similar to breast screening) but 15/16 men with prostate cancer had extraprostatic disease. Using the common cut-off of 4 µg/L, false positive rate was 18% and 22/33 had extraprostatic disease. Thus PSA is a good test only for cancers that cause death within 3 years; after that the common cut-off of 4 µg/L detects only half of those that would cause death or serious morbidity. Unfortunately, histological grade only partly predicts clinical outcome.

In the United States, uncontrolled screening using PSA spawned an apparent epidemic of prostate cancer. The chairman of the UK National Screening Committee stated that 'the scientific evidence is that screening for prostate cancer does not reduce mortality, and causes actual harm by exposing people to a procedure which has side effects of incontinence and impotence and where there is no evidence that they will benefit'. In 2012 the US Preventive Services Task Force recommended against PSA screening, although this was revised in 2018 to recommend screening only to those aged 55-69 years who wish it.

The UK government sponsored a Health Technology Assessment on prostate screening in 1997, which stated that the criteria for a population screening programme had not been met. Their findings were that:

- The epidemiology and natural history of the disease were ill understood.
- Screening tests were inaccurate and staging was unreliable.
- There was poor evidence of the effectiveness of treatment.
- Little research had been conducted into the complications and quality of life after radical treatment.
- On present evidence, there was no justification for PSA testing in primary care and there was insufficient evidence to support national screening.
- PSA testing should be limited to symptomatic men, to monitoring prostate cancer treatment and to randomised trials investigating screening.

Overall, PSA screening causes harm. Some men receive unnecessary treatment because the cancer is incurable or because it would never have presented clinically, and those treated risk infection (from biopsies), incontinence and impotence.

Lung Cancer

A Cochrane review of all RCTs showed that no screening test had an impact on the treatment or deaths from lung cancer, despite early stage cancers being detected and resected (most likely because these would not have progressed). Tests examined include chest x-ray, sputum tests and CT scanning. Low-dose CT scans are still being looked into as a screening test in high risk cases, such as smokers, but these tests have risks: lungs are very sensitive to radiation and frequent scans might cause damage, and scans can find changes that look like cancer and need to be biopsied, which has its own risks. Lung screening might also cause overdiagnosis in that some cancers found might never become life threatening. Researchers need to carefully balance the risks and benefits of a possible screening programme, but evidence is now emerging for low dose CT screening in high risk populations.

Screening for Cardiovascular Disease

Hypertension

Hypertension is an important cause of myocardial infarction and stroke. Lowering elevated blood pressure substantially lowers the risk. However, blood pressure on its own has proved a poor screening tool; in one large study, the 10% with the highest blood pressures suffered only 21% of the ischaemic cardiac events and only 28% of the ischaemic strokes. Even after adding other risk factors, including low-density lipoprotein cholesterol, diabetes and smoking history, the top 5% had only 28% of the deaths from myocardial infarction. Advancing age or a previous cardiovascular event are probably the best predictors of future cardiovascular events, thus all patients with risk factors should receive best advice and appropriate treatment. Several web-based risk calculators are available for individuals and recommendations produced may help reduce risk by appropriate intervention.

Abdominal Aortic Aneurysm

Introduction

Before screening, ruptured AAA caused at least 6000 deaths each year in the United Kingdom and 1.4% of all deaths in men over 65 years. The peak mortality is between 65 and 85 years and the risk of rupture is roughly proportional to the diameter; when this reaches 6 cm, the risk rises sharply. A ruptured aortic aneurysm is nearly always an acute emergency and carries a very high mortality. About half the cases never reach hospital and die at home or in transit to hospital. Half of the remainder (25%) die without an operation and half undergoing operation die. Thus the true mortality rate is 85% to 90%. An emergency operation requires a trained vascular surgeon, ties up an emergency team for 3 or more hours, requires an intensive care bed for 3 or more days, uses large quantities of bank blood, and costs 25% more than an elective procedure, whether or not the patient survives. The growing ability to treat ruptures by endovascular procedures has reduced these figures somewhat, but is still costly in terms of manpower and equipment. Detecting aneurysms before rupture means that less risky elective interventions, with a mortality of 5% or less, can be used.

Appropriateness of Screening for Abdominal Aortic Aneurysm

By WHO criteria, AAA is a near ideal candidate for screening. It is an important health problem, the natural history regarding expansion and rupture is fairly well understood, there is an easily detectable early stage, and treatment at an early stage is more beneficial than at a later stage (i.e., ruptured). Ultrasound is a suitable and highly reliable test for the early stage and it is acceptable, with an average of 80% of those invited attending. Appropriate intervals for retesting have been determined by randomised trials. There is adequate health service provision for the extra workload: a screening programme generates approximately six extra aneurysm repairs per year per surgeon.

Several trials have shown that the risks are less than the benefits, with up to 75% reduction in rupture rate, a low elective operative mortality, no excess psychological morbidity in those screened, and survival after operation being little different from an unaffected population. Costs appear to be balanced against benefits, with trials estimating the cost per life year saved at between zero (Huntingdon and Danish studies) and £12,500 (2006 figures from the UK Multicentre Aneurysm Screening Study).

Trials of Abdominal Aortic Aneurysm Screening

Several large studies have published data, with a remarkable concordance between results. The prevalence of AAA, the age distribution, attendance rates, reduction in AAA mortality and the cost effectiveness calculations from studies in Chichester, Gloucester, Huntingdon, Denmark, Western Australia and the large UK Multicentre Aneurysm Screening Study all concur.

Only one study, from Chichester, has randomised women into screening. The prevalence of AAA was six times lower (1.3%) than in men (7.6%). Over 5- and 10-year follow-up intervals, the incidence of rupture was the same in the screened and the control groups. Screening women for AAA was considered to be neither clinically indicated nor economically viable.

The Danish Study

A Danish study randomised 12,500 men of 65 years and over to AAA screen or nothing. Of these, 75% attended and 4% had aneurysms. Screening reduced the rate of emergency surgery by 75% (CI, 51%–91%); 59 were operated on electively with a 5.1% mortality. As regards to cost effectiveness, 352 needed to be screened to save one life, 4 years after screening. The screened population was rescreened after 5 years: 30% of those with aortas 25 to 29 mm developed an aneurysm but none of those originally less than 25 mm did so. People with aortas of 25 mm or greater diameter therefore need periodic rescreening.

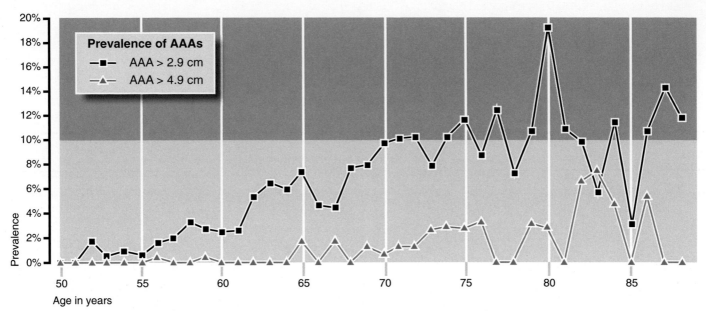

• **Fig. 6.1** Prevalence of Abdominal Aortic Aneurism (AAA) in Men Over 50 Years in the Huntingdon Screening Programme. The graphs show the percentage of those screened found to have small aneurysms *(black line)* and large aneurysms *(green line)*. Note that the lines are approximately parallel, suggesting that small AAAs become large AAAs some years later.

The Huntingdon Study

In the Huntingdon study, 15,000 men of 50 years and over were screened over 7 years: 540 were found to have an AAA larger than 2.9 cm, and 69 an AAA larger than 4.9 cm (Fig. 6.1). Very few small and no large aneurysms were found under the age of 60 years, an important factor when planning screening. Over the age of 70 years, there was virtually a 10% incidence of small AAAs. In this study, AAA mortality also fell by 75% and the number needed to be invited to save one life was 600.

The UK MASS Study

Screening was undertaken in four centres and 68,000 people were randomised to screening or not, beginning in 1997. Some 98% of people in both groups were matched with national mortality statistics. After 7 years, 21% of men had died. There was a 76% attendance among those invited (27,147 were screened) and 4.9% had an aortic diameter of 3 cm or greater. All-cause mortality fell by 4% in those invited and there was a 47% risk reduction for AAA deaths in this group. The cost of screening and treating detected aneurysms was £12,500 per life year saved and no adverse effects

were found on quality of life. The 30-day mortality for elective cases was 6%; for emergency cases operated upon, mortality was 37%. It was calculated that if screening were offered to a population, only 6% of AAA workload would eventually be on ruptures compared with around 30%. After 10 years, the RR-reduction of aneurysm-related deaths was still 49% (CI, 37%–57%), the cost per man invited was £100 and the cost per life year gained was £7600. Thus the benefit of a single screen lasted at least 10 years, though the incidence of rupture rose after 8 years.

The Consequences of Screening for Abdominal Aortic Aneurysm in an Area

There is a rise in elective AAA surgery during the first 5 to 7 years, as the existing but undiagnosed cases are progressively detected. This is gradually offset by a fall in rupture rates and a reduction in surgical referrals of symptomatic and incidentally discovered aneurysms. This becomes apparent 4 years after screening starts and continues rising until the entire population has been screened. The cost per life year saved compares favourably with colonic and cervical cancer.

SECTION B

Perioperative Care

7

Preoperative Assessment and Management of Postoperative Problems

Preoperative Assessment

Introduction

Patients with medical comorbidity and advanced age are increasingly being considered for surgery. Timely and considered preoperative assessment is crucial for ensuring any patient is safe and in the best possible condition before the operation and that healthcare resources are not wasted. This process needs both surgical and anaesthetic input.

For **elective surgery**, patients are seen first by the surgeon who evaluates the patient and discusses the procedure. Once the decision to proceed has been taken, the patient usually attends an anaesthetic preoperative assessment clinic. This evaluation is to detect and anticipate medical and social needs and, if necessary, optimise the patient for surgery. The initial assessment is usually performed by specialist nurses and the more complex patients (see Table 7.1 for examples) referred on for review, ideally by a consultant anaesthetist.

For **emergency admissions**, initial assessment is by emergency department doctors or junior surgical staff followed by senior medical staff review to formulate a management plan. The urgency of operation may limit the time to assess and optimise the patient, but major comorbidity must be sought (e.g., angina, chronic obstructive airways disease, chronic kidney impairment), not least to inform discussions about the options for the patient and the risks. For **major trauma**, senior staff are mobilised by phone before the ambulance reaches hospital.

Principles of Preoperative Assessment

The essence of preoperative assessment is a structured approach to questioning, a targeted clinical examination and careful consideration of which investigations are needed to plan for best perioperative care and to discuss risks. An accurate history of current medication must be taken and a plan for perioperative medication made. Most surgical cases are uncomplicated but avoidable complications occur unless the approach has been systematic. The combined preoperative assessment by surgeons and anaesthetists aims to answer the questions in Box 7.1. Review informs the need for further investigation and optimisation of patients with medical comorbidity to reduce the risk of perioperative problems. Investigations can provide baseline information against which later changes can be measured, for example, echocardiography in heart failure. Common problems of high-risk groups are summarised in Table 7.1.

Essentials of Preoperative Assessment

Standard preoperative preparation procedures vary in different hospitals but basic steps ensure the greatest patient safety (Box 7.2). The nature and urgency of the operation and the state of the patient ultimately determine precisely what is needed.

• BOX 7.1   Preoperative Assessment and Planning

1. Diagnosis
- (Provisional) diagnosis; how confident is it?
- Are any further investigations needed to confirm the primary diagnosis?
- Important aspects of the history?
- Findings on examination?
- Results of investigations already performed?
- If appropriate, have tissue diagnoses been obtained before admission to hospital?

2. Operation
- What operation or procedure is planned?
- Have any circumstances changed relating to the planned operation?
- Has the patient got better or worse?
- Has any new diagnostic information appeared (e.g., pulmonary metastases on a chest x-ray)?
- Is the planned operation still appropriate?
- Any special risks attending this particular operation, intraoperative or postoperative (e.g., risk of deep vein thrombosis [DVT] after pelvic surgery)?
- Any standard procedures needing to be performed for this operation (e.g., ordering blood if heavy blood loss anticipated)?
- Any operation-specific actions needing to be performed (e.g., examining vocal cord movement before thyroid surgery, arranging perioperative radiology)?

3. Anaesthesia
- What type of anaesthesia is to be used?
- Can any anaesthetic complications be anticipated (e.g., risk of postoperative chest infection after thoracotomy or upper abdominal surgery, risk of a patient with bowel obstruction inhaling vomitus during anaesthetic induction)?

4. Fitness for Operation
- Any intercurrent diseases and are they being appropriately treated (e.g., insulin-dependent diabetes) or any that might pose special problems (e.g., rheumatoid arthritis with cervical spine involvement)?
- Are any preoperative investigations or treatments needed for intercurrent disease (e.g., lung function tests and physiotherapy for chronic bronchitis, cervical spine radiology for rheumatoid arthritis)?
- Does the surgical condition pose special problems (e.g., fluid or electrolyte disturbances from vomiting)?
- Is the patient taking any drugs which might cause problems with anaesthesia or operation (e.g., monoamine oxidase inhibitors or corticosteroids)?
- Is the patient fit for the planned anaesthetic and operation?

5. High Risk
- Is this patient particularly predisposed to anaesthetic or surgical complications (Table 7.1)?

6. After the Operation
- Can any special problems be anticipated during the postoperative period and after discharge (e.g., elderly patients living alone)?
- Any problems specific to this anaesthetic or operation regarding recovery and rehabilitation, and is any special planning required (e.g., prostheses after mastectomy, stoma care, limb fitting and rehabilitation following amputation)?

TABLE 7.1   High-Risk Groups for Perioperative Complications

Group	Particular Risks	Management
Premature or tiny babies, neonates and infants	Fluid and electrolyte loss Heat loss in operating theatre	Careful measurement and replacement of fluids and electrolytes Warming blanket, temperature monitoring
Patients over 60 years	Increased risk of comorbidity	Investigations guided by comorbidity and risk of surgery (National Institute of Health and Care Excellence Guidance on preoperative testing)
Very elderly patients	Delirium Hyponatraemia Deconditioning	Multifactorial—see Chapter 8 Early postoperative detection, investigation for cause ± fluid restriction. Serial electrolyte tests until back to normal Perioperative care targeting early mobilisation
Smokers	Postoperative chest infection and atelectasis Increased risk of myocardial infarction	Stop smoking before operation—ideally at least 4 weeks beforehand Early postoperative physiotherapy Preoperative ECG; avoid hypoxia during and after operation; postoperative oxygen therapy
Obese patients	Increased risk of DVT Increased risk of wound infection Reduced mobility	DVT prophylaxis—see Chapter 12 Preoperative counselling during consent process Early mobilisation with assistance Encourage patients to lose weight before surgery
Patients with intercurrent medical disease	Depends on medical condition	Early referral to anaesthetist and/or medical specialist

DVT, Deep vein thrombosis; *ECG*, electrocardiogram.

• BOX 7.2 Essential Steps in Preoperative Assessment and Preparation

- History taking
- Physical examination
- Collating preadmission information about diagnosis, medical history, allergies and medication
- Arranging any further diagnostic investigations
- Making special preparations for the particular operation
- Optimising medical comorbidity
- Investigating any intercurrent or occult illness revealed during assessment by enlisting appropriate specialist help
- Explaining the operation and recovery and the risks and benefits with the patient, and obtaining signed consent
- Marking the operation site
- Making arrangements with operating theatre staff
- Arranging and informing the anaesthetist
- Prescribing medication, prophylactic antibiotics and thromboembolism prophylaxis, as appropriate
- Planning rehabilitation and convalescence

Explanations to the Patient, Informed Consent and Shared Decision Making

See Ch. 1 for the legal framework and further detail.

To make informed choices, patients need to understand their condition as far as possible, and the range of treatments available with their attendant risks and benefits. Patients often absorb little of what is said initially. They are often anxious and overwhelmed by the surgical clinic visit and so cannot take in the full implications of what has been said, so discussions often need to be repeated.

For **elective operations**, consent should be in two stages: first an initial explanation, with the range of options and pros and cons of each procedure discussed well in advance, and without pressure of an imminent operation. Patient information leaflets and guidance about accurate internet sites should also be given. Second, before surgery, the patient's understanding is checked and consent confirmed. In general, complications should be discussed if there is a 1% or greater risk, or if there are rarer but serious procedure-specific risks, such as recurrent laryngeal nerve injury in thyroid surgery. In addition, the Montgomery court ruling of 2015 (https://www.bmj.com/content/357/bmj.j2224) demands that patients are informed of all material risks of all the treatment options that might adversely impact on them as an individual, such as the inability to perform a certain task or outcomes which might compromise their ability to continue to work. Important questions the patient should consider during the surgical consent process are:
- What are my options?
- What are the risks and benefits of those options to me?
- How do I get further information that will help me make a decision?

For some diagnoses, the UK National Health Service has developed decision support tools to help patients. For most settings and conditions, however, it is up to the perioperative care team—surgeons, anaesthetists and specialist nurses—to support the patient with the best available information and individual risk assessment.

Methods of Evaluating Patient Risk

These fall into three broad categories
- Clinical judgment
- Risk scores or models
- Evaluation of functional capacity

In practice, a combination is likely to provide the best estimate of a patient's risk of complications, death or other poor outcomes. However, no risk prediction tool can be entirely accurate because of the complexity of patients and procedures, and the risk of unexpected events occurring (e.g., anaphylaxis to a drug in the perioperative period).

There are numerous individual **risk scores** and models designed to help predict risk. In general, the most accurate risk estimates come from using a **procedure specific tool** (e.g., the Nottingham Hip Fracture Score, or the National Emergency Laparotomy Audit model for emergency laparotomy) or one which has been tested and validated in the **same type of healthcare system** (e.g., the Surgical Outcome Risk Tool for the United Kingdom, www.sortsurgery.com, or the American College of Surgeons National Surgical Quality Improvement Program risk calculator for the United States, www.riskcalculator.facs.org).

There is a direct and clear link between reduced functional capacity (cardiorespiratory fitness) and adverse perioperative outcomes, and sedentary lifestyles are a risk factor for this. **Functional capacity** can be undertaken using a self-assessment tool, such as the Duke Activity Status Index, or through face-to-face evaluation of exercise capacity (such as, a 6-minute shuttle walk test or a cardiopulmonary exercise test on a bicycle ergometer). For older patients, **frailty** evaluation (e.g., by Frailty-VIG Index, https://bmcgeriatr.biomedcentral.com/articles/10.1186/s12877-018-0718-2) can provide a holistic assessment of a patient's health and function. The purpose of preoperative risk assessment is for clinical teams to use it to tailor a perioperative plan so as to obtain the best possible result from the operation and to reduce the risk of adverse outcomes.

For **emergency surgery**, there may not be time for a two-stage consent process but the risks are often substantially higher than for elective surgery. Quality improvement programmes have shown that senior input into risk assessment and decision-making can improve outcomes, for example, the UK's National Emergency Laparotomy Audit, https://www.nela.org.uk.

Planning the Perioperative Period

For elective surgery, it may be in the patient's best interest to defer operation until any detected comorbidities can be optimised, although the option to delay does depend on the underlying diagnosis. A good example of this might be chronic iron deficiency anaemia in a patient awaiting elective orthopaedic surgery. Correction of haemoglobin preoperatively using iron supplements may reduce the need for blood transfusion perioperatively, and thus the risks of transfusion—increased length of stay and poorer oncological outcomes, for example. Similarly, there is increasing interest in the concept of **prehabilitation**, where a patient might be placed on a structured exercise programme to improve their functional capacity (general fitness) before undergoing a major procedure. Innovative approaches, such as 'surgery schools' are also being evaluated, where patients are brought together with each other and surgeons, anaesthetists, physiotherapists and specialist nurses to have explained in detail what to expect during their recovery period and how they can help themselves prepare for operation and recovery more quickly.

Enhanced recovery pathways (see Ch. 2) encourage a protocol-driven but individualised approach to patient care, guided by the principle of trying to return patients to their optimal physiological state as quickly as possible. Enhanced recovery means using minimally invasive surgical approaches, precise fluid management using oesophageal Doppler, avoiding tubes and drains where possible, encouraging drinking, eating and mobilising as soon as possible after surgery and supporting all of this with multimodal analgesia.

Planned admission to a critical care unit after surgery is an intervention recommended for high-risk patients. For some types of elective surgery (e.g., open cardiac) this is a normal standard of care, and patients should be counselled on this as part of the consent process. Patients admitted to normal wards after surgery can be closely monitored with help from critical care outreach teams, or through continued monitoring via acute pain teams, intensivists and anaesthetists.

Plans for rehabilitation and convalescence should be discussed with the patient and relatives, including the likely rate of recovery and levels of activity likely to be possible on discharge, allowing social, business and domestic arrangements to be made early. If necessary, domestic or home nursing help can be arranged. Uncertainty about these matters often causes anxiety and may prolong hospital stay.

Marking the Operation Site

When obtaining final consent, the surgeon should **mark the operation site** on the patient's skin with an indelible pen. This is particularly important if the operation could be performed on either side, for example, an inguinal hernia repair or limb amputation. It is even more important if the patient is likely to be turned prone (face down) in theatre as this can cause confusion. Failure to mark the site represents a **never event** in-waiting (and there is no legal defence). Checking processes for identity, type of operation, side and marking must be in place at several stages during the patient's journey to the operating theatre. The World Health Organization checklist (see Ch. 1, Box 1.8) is now used in most environments where surgical procedures are undertaken and has been shown to reduce morbidity and mortality.

Immediate Preoperative Starvation and Fluid Restriction

General anaesthesia depresses the protective airway reflexes of gag and cough. To minimise the risk of aspiration of gastric contents into the lungs at induction of anaesthesia or in the early recovery period, the patient must be adequately fasted. Patients can usually eat until 6 hours before surgery and drink clear fluids up to 2 hours before. They must be allowed to have a small amount of water to take their regular medication. As part of an Enhanced Recovery After Surgery programme, clear nonparticulate carbohydrate drinks have been shown to reduce postoperative insulin resistance and inflammatory responses, thereby contributing to improving surgical outcome after major surgery. These drinks are specially formulated complex carbohydrates with low osmolality facilitating a fast transit time through the stomach. They are given up to 2 hours before surgery (provided gastric emptying is not impaired).

For patients at higher risk of aspiration, for example, gastro-oesophageal reflux, intestinal obstruction and pregnancy, the anaesthetist may prescribe antacid medication. In all patients for operation, starvation and hydration need to be checked carefully.

Liaison With Anaesthetist

For elective cases, the anaesthetist will know in advance of the proposed operation or list of operations. For emergency cases, the anaesthetist needs to know which patient is having which operation, how urgent the procedure is and the condition of the patient. The anaesthetist visits to evaluate the patient, advise on patient preoperative management and discuss the anaesthetic. The anaesthetist is responsible for ensuring that the patient is fit for surgery and often assists in resuscitation if needed.

Operating Theatre Arrangements

For any operation, the junior surgeon (intern) is usually responsible for informing the operating department about the operation(s) and any special arrangements needed. A formal **operating list** should be prepared, giving name, age, sex, ward and proposed operation for each patient. The side of the body to be operated on should be clearly noted. Any special instruments, intraoperative radiography or patient positioning must be listed. The presence of transmissible infections for example, methicillin-resistant *Staphylococcus aureus* (MRSA) or hepatitis C, should be recorded, as well as any allergies, for example, to latex or iodine. In some hospitals, the amount of bank blood ordered for a patient is also noted. If changes are made, a completely new list must replace the old to avoid error and harm.

Planning the Order of an Operating List

For elective cases, the following order can normally be recommended:
1. **Latex allergy**—remove all latex containing products from theatre and pressure ventilate for several hours beforehand.
2. **Paediatric cases**—to minimise the period of starvation and reduce anxiety.
3. **Diabetic patients**—to make perioperative diabetes management as smooth as possible, minimise the period of starvation and return rapidly to normal diet and treatment.
4. **Adult day cases**—to maximise the amount of available recovery time before discharge.
5. **Inpatients** with no special theatre requirements.
6. **Contaminated, infected cases, colorectal cases, gangrenous limbs**—so as not to infect later cases.
7. **Patients with transmissible infections**, for example, MRSA, hepatitis C. Preparation includes all nonessential equipment and personnel being removed from theatre; disposable items replace recyclable items of linen, and theatre must be cleaned before next list.

Preparation for Major Operation

The following example illustrates the way a patient might be prepared for a major operation and the considerations in preoperative management.

History

James Brown, a 70-year-old retired farmer, with a proven carcinoma at the rectosigmoid junction admitted electively for anterior resection of the rectum.

Presenting Complaint

Seen urgently in outpatient clinic, 3 weeks ago, with a 5-week history of loose stools three to five times a day, without blood or mucus. GP reported three stool specimens positive for occult blood. Lost about 4 kg over the last 3 months, but has been trying to lose weight anyway.

Results of Outpatient Investigations

- Flexible sigmoidoscopy—obvious fungating tumour of upper rectum. Scope could not be passed beyond it. Biopsies confirmed adenocarcinoma.
- Contrast enhanced computed tomography scan of chest, abdomen and pelvis—no other synchronous colonic cancers seen; liver and lungs free of metastases.

- MRI Rectum for local staging—no spread outside bowel wall.
- Blood tests: full blood count—haemoglobin 11.6 g/L, otherwise normal. Urea and electrolytes, liver function tests—normal.

Systems Enquiry

Generally well, but recent onset of shortness of breath after walking 200 metres on flat ground; occasional fast palpitations. No other cardiorespiratory symptoms. Poor stream on micturition. Nil else on systems enquiry.

Past Medical History

Appendicectomy aged 14 years; no anaesthetic complications. Serious farming injury to left elbow aged 20 years. Jaundiced during the Second World War in Asia, nil since. Hypertensive for 10 years and on drug treatment for 5 years. Diabetes discovered 3 years ago on routine urine testing, controlled by diet alone.

Family History

Mother was obese; died age 55 years from complications of diabetes (gangrene). Older brother had major stroke at 64 years but partially recovered. No family history of bowel cancer.

Social History

Widowed for 2 years, wife died of breast cancer. Has one son and one daughter, both married with young children but living far away. Lives in own house with an upstairs lavatory, on a smallholding with a few stock animals. Lives independently, and uses car for shopping. Smoker—20 cigarettes a day since age 15 years; alcohol intake averages 4 units a day.

Drug History

Takes atenolol 50 mg (a beta-blocker) and bendroflumethiazide 2.5 mg (a diuretic) once a day in the morning for hypertension. Takes aspirin 75 mg daily 'for his heart'. Told in the past not to have penicillin, but cannot recall why; does not remember when he last had penicillin. Not allergic to iodine.

Examination

General. Fit-looking man of 70 years, not obviously anxious. Tanned; not evidently anaemic; no cyanosis, jaundice, lymphadenopathy or clubbing; no thyroid enlargement. Fingers tobacco stained. Not febrile.

Cardiovascular and respiratory system. Pulse 68 beats per minute, regular. Blood pressure (BP) 150/110 mmHg. Soft systolic murmur at the left sternal edge. No ankle swelling and jugular venous pressure (JVP) not elevated. Extensive bilateral varicose veins. Chest examination unremarkable apart from a few crepitations which do not clear with coughing.

Abdomen. Moderately obese. Appendicectomy scar. Soft to palpation. No organomegaly. Possible mass in left iliac fossa—not indentable (i.e., not faeces). No groin hernias. External genitalia normal. Rectal examination—moderately enlarged smooth prostate and normal-coloured stool.

Central nervous system and locomotor system. Fixed flexion deformity of left elbow at 90 degrees, otherwise normal.

Summary

A 70-year-old man with proven rectosigmoid carcinoma without obvious dissemination, admitted for anterior resection of the rectosigmoid.

A problem list was constructed from this information, which led to further investigations and a management plan. The reasoning is shown in Table 7.2.

Postoperative Management

Introduction

Despite good preoperative assessment, surgical and anaesthetic technique and perioperative management, unexpected symptoms or signs can arise after an operation that may herald a complication. Detecting these early by regular monitoring and clinical review means early treatment can often forestall major deterioration. This chapter uses a problem-orientated approach to help junior (and more senior) doctors deal with such problems (see Box 7.4).

Managing problems such as pain, fever or collapse requires correct diagnosis then early treatment. Determining the cause can be challenging, particularly if the patient is anxious, in pain or not fully recovered from anaesthesia. It is vital to see and assess the patient clinically and if necessary, arrange investigations, whatever the hour, when deterioration suggests potentially serious but often remediable complications. Consider also whether and when to call for senior help.

Postoperative Pain

Some types of wounds are more painful than others, for example, vertical abdominal incisions and skin graft donor sites. It is better to prevent pain preemptively than react to established pain.

Methods of Management

Postoperative pain can be minimised by preoperative counselling, perioperative measures and postoperative analgesia. Counselling lets the patient know the probable extent of pain, the plans for pain relief and the likely degree of mobility after operation. During the operation, **preemptive analgesia** ensures that pain does not become established.

This may involve:
- Long-acting analgesic drugs given intravenously.
- Local anaesthetic infiltration into the wound edges at the end of the operation with a long-acting agent, such as bupivacaine.
- Regional nerve blocks (e.g., intercostal nerves for upper abdominal surgery using a transversus abdominis plane block).
- Epidural analgesia using local anaesthetic and often morphine, during and after abdominal and pelvic surgery.
- Nonsteroidal analgesics given before the patient wakens by suppository or intravenous injection. These must not be given to patients with known allergy to aspirin or other nonsteroidal anti-inflammatory drugs, a history of severe asthma or angiooedema, bleeding disorders, renal impairment, hypovolaemia or pregnancy. Mild asthma is not a contraindication. It is also unwise to use these in operations with a high risk of haemorrhage.

Analgesia for Minor and Intermediate Surgery

Patients vary greatly in their pain tolerance and need for analgesics. For minor and intermediate surgery, preemptive analgesia with simple analgesic tablets is often sufficient. However, anxiety, exhaustion and sleep deprivation may reduce pain tolerance and the amount of analgesia must be adapted to individual need.

Problem	Surgical Significance	Plan of Action for Each Problem
1. 'Mild' diabetes mellitus	No such thing as mild diabetes! Is it under good control? Are any other organs affected (kidneys, heart)?	All urine samples to be tested for glucose Fasting blood glucose estimation and HbA1c May need variable rate insulin infusion (VRII) perioperatively
2. Obesity	Multiple potential problems Lifting and handling on the ward and in the operating theatre May make intravenous and surgical access difficult at operation Predisposes to wound infection Increased risk of deep vein thrombosis or pulmonary embolism	Early referral to anaesthetist Is special bed or operating table required? Availability of hoist postoperatively Ensure adequate theatre time available plus at least two assistants Consider delayed primary closure of wound if contaminated Prophylaxis, for example, low dose heparin plus graduated compression stockings
3. Hypertension	How well is hypertension controlled on present medication? Is elevated BP on admission just because of anxiety? Are there other complications of hypertension, such as ventricular hypertrophy?	Acquire recent BP measurements from preassessment clinic and GP Check pulse rate and BP at intervals over several hours Perform (and check) ECG. Defer elective surgery if BP>180/110 mmHg
4. Recent shortness of breath on exertion and palpitations	Are these merely symptoms of anxiety or significant cardiac or respiratory disease?	Consult cardiologist re palpitations if patient feels unwell with them ECG Possibly echocardiography, exercise testing or lung function tests Recheck Hb—has anaemia worsened?
5. Poor urinary stream and enlarged prostate	Possible carcinoma of prostate Possible difficulty with catheterisation required at operation Risk of postoperative urinary retention when catheter removed	Measure plasma PSA Transrectal ultrasound; biopsy if necessary Anticipate—may need suprapubic catheterisation kit in theatre Anticipate
6. Jaundice in the past	History suggestive of hepatitis	Serological tests needed if hepatitis B or C is likely
7. Smoker	Possible occult lung cancer Possible impaired lung function Increased risk of postoperative chest infections Increased risk of myocardial infarction	CT chest if suspicious Respiratory function tests Preoperative breathing exercises, early postoperative physiotherapy Postoperative oxygen therapy
8. Left elbow injury	May cause inconvenience during operation	Inform theatre staff about need for careful positioning on the operating table
9. Diuretic therapy	Are electrolytes and renal function normal?	Plasma urea, electrolytes and creatinine estimations
10. Aspirin therapy	Could gastric irritation partly account for mild anaemia? May cause excess bleeding at operation	Use nongastric irritant analgesics Consider cardiovascular risk factors before stopping aspirin—may increase risk of MI
11. Possible penicillin allergy	Penicillin often used for prophylaxis or treatment of infections	Ask GP for allergy history. Record possible penicillin allergy; alternative drugs can be used
12. Cardiac murmur	Is this clinically significant? Is cardiac antibiotic prophylaxis necessary?	Consult anaesthetist or cardiologist; ECG, consider echocardiogram Consult guidelines (e.g., British National Formulary (BNF))
13. Lives alone, looks after animals	Who will look after him when he returns home? Who will look after animals while he is in hospital?	Discuss domestic arrangements and convalescence plans with medical social worker
14. Low haemoglobin	Transfused patients respond less well to chemo and radiotherapy Potentially extensive operation—may have large blood loss	Iron studies to identify if iron-deficient anaemia Consider IV iron infusion preoperatively to normalise Hb (can be of benefit up to 5 days before surgery) Order at least two units of blood to cover operation Order extra blood (i.e., at least four units in all)
15. May need temporary or even permanent colostomy	Does he understand about stomas? Will he be able to cope?	Refer to stoma nurse for counselling and possible preoperative 'trial' of colostomy appliance (see Ch. 27)
16. Bowel will be opened during operation	Potential for faecal contamination of abdominal cavity and wound	May need bowel preparation and will need perioperative prophylactic antibiotics
17. Lesion at pelvic brim	Does it involve the ureter?	Consider ultrasonography of kidneys to exclude hydronephrosis
18. Varicose veins	Increases risk of DVT (already high because of major pelvic operation and age 70 years)	Give prophylaxis—low dose heparin, antiembolism stockings Early mobilisation

BNF, British National Formulary; *BP,* blood pressure; *CT,* computed tomography; *DVT,* deep vein thrombosis; *ECG,* electrocardiogram; *Hb,* haemoglobin; *IV,* intravenous; *MI,* myocardial infarction; *PSA,* prostate specific antigen.

• BOX 7.3 **Postoperative Analgesics and Their Indications (Approximate Ascending Order of Analgesic Strength)**

Mild-to-Moderate Pain

- Paracetamol
- Compounds of paracetamol and low-dose codeine, for example, co-codamol
- Milder nonsteroidal anti-inflammatory drugs (NSAIDs), for example, ibuprofen

Moderate Pain

- Paracetamol
- Codeine or dihydrocodeine 30–60 mg
- Stronger NSAIDs, as tablets or suppositories, for example, diclofenac

Moderate-to-Severe Pain

- Other opiate analgesics stronger than codeine, for example, oxycodone, tramadol
- NSAIDs by intravenous injection, for example, diclofenac
- Morphine slow-release tablets
- Morphine or diamorphine—patient-controlled intravenous injection

• BOX 7.4 **Important Causes of Postoperative Collapse or Rapid Deterioration**

Cardiovascular

- Myocardial infarction
- Other cause of rapid deterioration of cardiac function, for example, sudden arrhythmia or fluid overload
- Pulmonary embolism
- Stroke (may be without obvious limb paralysis)

Respiratory

- Failure to reverse anaesthesia adequately (early)
- Drug-induced respiratory depression
- Hypoxia caused by a respiratory disorder or respiratory depressant drugs

'Surgical' and Infective

- Hypovolaemic shock from acute blood loss, or sudden decompensation in unrecognised hypovolaemia
- Bowel strangulation or obstruction
- Systemic sepsis (often caused by anastomotic leakage)
- Severe localised infection, for example, chest or operation site

Metabolic

- Electrolyte disturbances, for example, hyponatraemia
- Hypoglycaemia or hyperglycaemia associated with diabetes
- Adrenal insufficiency, for example, adrenal suppression by preoperative or earlier corticosteroid treatment; causes hypotension

Drug Effects

- Drug reactions, for example, anaphylaxis

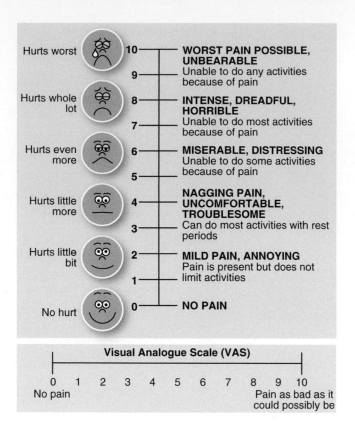

• **Fig. 7.1** Pain Measurement Scales.

Following major abdominal and perineal operations **epidural analgesia** using local anaesthetic drugs and morphine can be valuable. A single dose can provide anaesthesia for the operation, for example, transurethral prostatectomy, plus several hours of complete postoperative analgesia. For more extensive surgery, an epidural cannula can be left in situ to allow 'topping-up' to extend postoperative analgesia. These patients need careful observation for signs of toxicity, severe hypotension or respiratory depression. Note that moderate hypotension is merely an indication of satisfactory sympathetic blockade.

For major surgery and trauma where epidural analgesia is inappropriate, the analgesic dose needs to be enough to eliminate the pain without causing dangerous side-effects, and to be given often enough for continuous pain relief. Effective pain control can be achieved by allowing patients to give themselves small intravenous increments of opiates using a **patient-controlled analgesia** device (Fig. 7.2). This allows presetting of the incremental dose (often 1 mg of morphine), with a 5-minute lockout to prevent it being given too frequently, as well as control of the total dose. Continuous effective pain relief is thus easily achieved and the total dose used is often less than with intermittent injections. This technique causes minimal sedation and respiratory depression whilst maintaining excellent continuous analgesia, although it can cause opiate-induced nausea.

Excessive Postoperative Pain

If the pain is not controlled by an apparently adequate dose and frequency of analgesia, complications should be suspected. The dose should first be reviewed in relation to the expected severity of pain and the weight of the patient.

- **Local postoperative complications** should be considered. Wound pain may be caused by pressure from a **haematoma.** In limb trauma, bleeding into or inflammatory oedema within

Analgesia for Major Surgery and Trauma (Box 7.3)

Many hospitals now provide an **acute pain service**, run by anaesthetists and specialist nurses. This team can plan individual analgesic strategies and help deal with pain problems as they arise. Truly objective rating of pain is difficult but some form of **visual analogue scale** chart can be helpful (Fig. 7.1).

a fascial compartment must be diagnosed before ischaemia ensues ('compartment syndrome'). Wound pain increasing after the first 48 hours may be caused by **infection.** The wound is unusually tender even before redness and induration develop and there is usually a pyrexia. Other complications with lower limb pain include deep vein thrombosis and acute ischaemia. Lastly, major comorbid conditions may be the cause of pain, for example, myocardial ischaemia, or a fractured neck of femur may follow falling out of bed.

- **Major complications** in the operation area. After an abdominal operation, excessive pain can be caused by intraabdominal complications. These include haemorrhage, anastomotic leakage, biliary leakage, abscess formation, gaseous distension caused by ileus or air swallowing, intestinal obstruction, urinary retention and bowel ischaemia, any of which is likely to require reoperation. Constipation may also cause late postoperative pain.

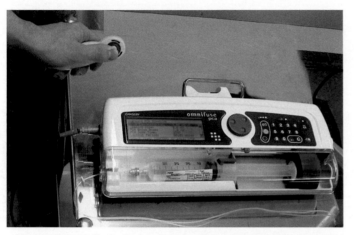

• **Fig. 7.2** Patient-Controlled Analgesia. This microprocessor-controlled device prevents overdosage by 'locking out' if used too frequently. The patient's control handset is seen on the left.

As a rule, serious complications cause deterioration in the patient's general condition, whereas with less serious complications, such as urinary retention or constipation, the patient remains well.

Pyrexia (Fig. 7.3)

Fever is a common postoperative observation not always caused by infection. Pyrexia within 48 hours is usually caused by basal lung atelectasis and should be treated with physiotherapy and mobilisation. After this period, a search should be made for a focus of infection. The common ones are **superficial** or **deep wound infection, chest infection** (pneumonia), **urinary tract infection** and infection of an **intravenous cannula site**. If there is a central venous line, infection should always be suspected in unexplained pyrexia. Unfortunately, this can only be diagnosed by removing the line and culturing the tip for organisms. Blood cultures alone are often positive but do not reveal the source of infection. Patients usually recover spontaneously once the central line is removed.

Common noninfective causes of pyrexia include **transfusion reactions, wound haematomas, deep venous thrombosis** and **pulmonary embolism**. Pyrexia is sometimes the only sign of an idiosyncratic or allergic **drug reaction**. A rare cause is **malignant hyperpyrexia** following general anaesthesia.

Tachycardia

Tachycardia (rapid heart rate) may simply indicate **pain** or **anxiety** but it is also a feature of **infection, circulatory disturbances** and **thyrotoxicosis**. Mild tachycardia may be a sign of incipient **hypovolaemic shock** as a result of haemorrhage or dehydration. It may also herald **cardiac failure**. Tachycardia may be a sign of recent onset **atrial fibrillation or flutter**; this is confirmed by electrocardiography, and may indicate the patient has suffered a myocardial infarction. In bowel surgery patients, this is often a sign of **anastomotic leakage**, presumably mediated by cytokines released as a result of the leakage.

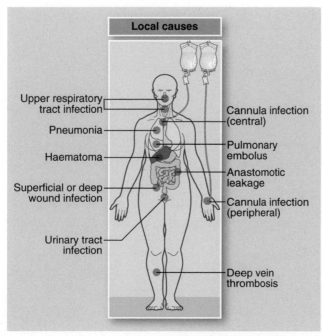
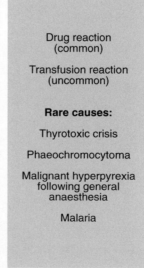

Local causes	Systemic causes

Upper respiratory tract infection
Pneumonia
Haematoma
Superficial or deep wound infection
Urinary tract infection
Cannula infection (central)
Pulmonary embolus
Anastomotic leakage
Cannula infection (peripheral)
Deep vein thrombosis

Drug reaction (common)
Transfusion reaction (uncommon)

Rare causes:
Thyrotoxic crisis
Phaeochromocytoma
Malignant hyperpyrexia following general anaesthesia
Malaria

• **Fig. 7.3** Causes of Pyrexia.

Cough, Shortness of Breath and Tachypnoea

These symptoms are often associated with an overt respiratory problem, such as **acute bronchopneumonia, aspiration of gastric contents, lobar collapse, pneumothorax** or an exacerbation of a **preexisting chronic lung disorder**. Clinical examination and chest x-ray will rapidly diagnose most of them.

Shortness of breath and rapid shallow breathing are a feature of alveolar collapse (**atelectasis**), which may not be detected by clinical examination or chest x-ray. Atelectasis usually responds to chest physiotherapy. **Abdominal distension** may also cause rapid shallow breathing by inhibiting diaphragmatic movement. Shortness of breath and tachypnoea may be early features of **cardiac failure** or **fluid overload** but there are usually other clues, such as tachycardia and basal crepitations.

A sudden onset of shortness of breath and tachypnoea, often with general collapse, may indicate **pulmonary embolism**. This must be recognised, investigated and treated vigorously. **Acute respiratory distress syndrome** may occur in chest trauma, acute pancreatitis or systemic sepsis and should be anticipated in these patients. Finally, respiratory symptoms may be caused by **hyperventilation** induced by pain, anxiety or hysteria.

Collapse or Rapid General Deterioration

The doctor on call is commonly asked to deal with a patient who has 'collapsed' or 'gone off' in a nonspecific way. To make matters more difficult, the patient is often under the care of another surgical team. The more serious possibilities are summarised in Box 7.4.

In practice, the problem is tackled in the following order, which usually leads to a logical diagnosis:
- Brief history of the collapse and postoperative course to date
- Rapid clinical appraisal—check **A**irway, **B**reathing and **C**irculation, then changes in conscious state and neurology
- Chart review reveals changes in temperature, pulse, BP, and respiratory rate
- Check urinary output and fluid balance
- Review of:
  - reason for admission and preoperative state
  - preexisting comorbid conditions
  - nature and extent of surgical operation, including any operative problems
  - likely extent of perioperative blood and other fluid losses (including sequestration in bowel)
  - adequacy of fluid replacement
- Drug therapy—prescribed drugs? Have important drugs been given or omitted?
- Detailed physical examination
- Check blood glucose using reagent strips
- Special tests as suggested by clinical findings, for example, electrocardiogram (ECG), chest x-ray, serum electrolyte estimation, arterial blood gas analysis, full blood count, urinalysis

Nausea and Vomiting

Drugs as a Cause

Nausea and vomiting are common postoperative problems. The usual causes are side-effects from drugs used for general anaesthesia or postoperative analgesia, particularly opiates. Antiemetics are usually given with opiates 'as required' for the early postoperative period but may have been missed. Nausea and sometimes vomiting later in the postoperative period may be caused by drugs. The worst offenders are erythromycin and metronidazole given orally, and **digoxin** overdosage (particularly in the elderly and in chronic renal failure).

Causes in the Immediate Postoperative Period

- Vigorous handling of the patient in the operating department and in recovery may stimulate vestibular input causing motion sickness
- Oropharyngeal stimulation—caused by a nasogastric tube or aspiration of secretions
- Hypoxia
- Hypotension
- Pain
- Anxiety

Bowel Obstruction Causing Nausea and Vomiting

Sustained vomiting 48 hours or more after operation is usually caused by **mechanical obstruction** or by **adynamic bowel** (see Ch. 12, p. 180). Adynamic small bowel (**ileus**) is common after bowel operations and is difficult to differentiate from adhesional obstruction, but if it persists beyond 5 days after surgery, obstruction is more likely than ileus.

Mechanical obstruction, usually of small bowel, can follow any abdominal operation. Early obstruction because of fibrinous adhesions occurs within 4 days of operation and may respond to conservative treatment but often requires a further operation.

Finally, **faecal impaction** is a common problem in the elderly or immobile patient and may cause vomiting.

Systemic Disorders Causing Nausea and Vomiting

Electrolyte disturbances, uraemia, hypercalcaemia and other systemic disorders may cause vomiting via central effects. Centrally-mediated vomiting also occurs with raised intracranial pressure. This must be considered following head injuries, neurosurgical operations or in patients with cerebral metastases.

Haematemesis

Elderly postoperative patients sometimes produce a small quantity of so-called **coffee ground vomitus** positive for blood on 'stick' testing. This usually results from trivial bleeding from mild, stress-related gastritis or reflux oesophagitis and rarely indicates major haematemesis. The patient should be closely observed for signs of internal bleeding, and antacid preparations, such as a proton-pump inhibitor given.

Occasionally, a major upper GI haemorrhage occurs in the postoperative patient. If there has been forceful vomiting, a Mallory–Weiss tear at the oesophagogastric junction may be the cause. Major bleeding may also arise from exacerbation of a peptic ulcer or even oesophageal varices. Seriously ill patients and the victims of burns and head injuries are susceptible to **acute stress ulceration**, which may cause catastrophic GI haemorrhage (see Ch. 21, p. 325).

Other Disorders of Bowel Function

Diarrhoea

Transient diarrhoea frequently follows abdominal operations, and should be regarded as normal in the recovery phase following bowel resections or operations to relieve intestinal obstruction, once any ileus has resolved.

Diarrhoea may also complicate **antibiotic therapy**. Several days after starting treatment, loose, frequent stools are passed for a short period, probably as a result of bacterial or fungal overgrowth. Less commonly, **antibiotic-associated diarrhoea** may develop, often caused by overgrowth of *Clostridium difficile*, which can be highly infective. If it progresses to **pseudomembranous colitis** or **toxic megacolon**, it can become life threatening. This is characterised by severe and persistent diarrhoea, sometimes containing blood (see Chs 3 and 12, pp. 46, 180).

After surgery of the abdominal aorta, blood-stained diarrhoea may occur a few days postoperatively. This may indicate **large-bowel ischaemia** caused by ligation of the inferior mesenteric artery. This is a dangerous complication and requires urgent investigation and surgical exploration.

Constipation

Constipation is common after surgery. The causes include restriction of oral fluids and fibre, difficulty or reluctance in using a bed pan, slow recovery of normal peristalsis, the use of opiate analgesia and general lack of mobility. **Anal pain** is a powerful disincentive to defaecation following anal surgery. Constipation causes great distress, especially in the elderly. It should be anticipated and prevented if practicable by prescribing **bulk-forming agents** (e.g., methylcellulose or ispaghula husk preparations), **stool softeners** (e.g., docusate), **osmotic laxatives** (e.g., lactulose) or gentle **stimulant laxatives** (e.g., Senokot). Rectal preparations, such as glycerine suppositories or enemas, can be used if there is still no progress.

Impacted faeces in any patient may result in **overflow incontinence**; thus any patient with abnormal bowel function must undergo digital rectal examination to exclude faecal impaction.

Poor Urine Output

Retention of Urine

Low urinary output or complete failure to pass urine is a frequent postoperative problem. The most common cause is urinary retention, usually occurring in males. It is readily diagnosed if there is a palpable suprapubic mass which is dull to percussion. A portable bladder scanner readily provides confirmation.

Acute retention needs to be distinguished from true oliguria resulting from poor renal perfusion or acute renal failure; retention can readily be confirmed by ultrasound examination or by passing a urinary catheter.

Pathophysiology

Postoperative retention is much more common in men, particularly when there is prostatic hypertrophy. Patients with bladder outflow obstruction symptoms ('prostatism') are at risk of developing acute retention, although young males can also be affected.

Acute postoperative urinary retention seems to result from a combination of the following factors:

- preexisting bladder outlet obstruction;
- difficulty in passing urine in the supine position;
- embarrassment at passing urine without sufficient privacy;
- accumulation of a large volume of urine during the operation and recovery, causing overfilling of the bladder;
- transient disturbance of the neurological control of voiding by general or spinal anaesthesia
- pain from an abdominal or inguinal wound inhibiting normal contraction of the abdominal musculature and relaxation of the bladder neck;
- problems after certain operations which predispose to acute retention, for example, abdomino-perineal resection of rectum or (bilateral) inguinal hernia repair;

- constipation—gross faecal loading is common in the elderly in hospital and is probably the most frequent cause of acute retention (and faecal incontinence).

Management of Postoperative Urinary Retention

Conservative Measures. The first step is to ensure there is adequate **analgesia** and this may be sufficient to enable the patient to pass urine. The next step is to help the patient out of bed to use a commode at the bedside or a urine bottle.

If these measures fail, the patient should be wheeled into a bathroom for privacy and left alone for a while, if fit enough. The familiar sound of a tap left running often encourages micturition. If the patient still does not pass urine and there is a history of constipation, encourage a bowel movement by means of a glycerine suppository. Defaecation is usually accompanied by bladder neck relaxation and micturition.

Catheterisation. If conservative measures fail or if the patient has suprapubic pain from the overdistended bladder, catheterisation is necessary. In females, bladder drainage and immediate removal of the catheter can be done. In males, the catheter is usually left in situ until the following morning or until the patient is well. If there is an untreated underlying cause, this should be corrected before the catheter is removed (i.e., tamsulosin treatment if evidence of bladder outlet obstruction, treat any urinary tract infection, treat any constipation).

Blocked Catheter. If the patient is already catheterised, the catheter may have become blocked. The catheter can be checked for patency and flushed using a bladder syringe or replaced as necessary.

Diminished Urine Production

A degree of reduced urine output after operation is normal and results from increased release of antidiuretic hormone and aldosterone caused by surgical stress. **Oliguria** requiring attention in an adult is defined as less than 0.5 mL per kg per hour.

Low urine output is most often caused by **reduced renal perfusion**, resulting from relative hypovolaemia or low cardiac output. This leads to diminished glomerular filtration and enhanced tubular reabsorption. The usual reason is inadequate replacement of perioperative fluid deficit. Potentially more serious causes of reduced renal perfusion include cardiac failure and acute myocardial infarction. Acute renal insufficiency should only be diagnosed if poor renal perfusion (prerenal failure) can be excluded.

A urinary catheter should be inserted to ensure the bladder is emptying and to enable hourly measurement of output. When retention has been excluded and true oliguria or **anuria** is diagnosed, the problem is to differentiate between acute tubular necrosis and reduced renal perfusion. Poor renal perfusion may be caused by **hypotension** during the operation or **hypovolaemia**. If untreated, this may progress to acute kidney injury and in advanced cases, acute cortical necrosis. Renal insufficiency from other causes, in particular systemic sepsis or drug toxicity, should also be considered.

If **hypovolaemia** is suspected, an intravenous **fluid challenge** of 250 mL of crystalloid solution should be given over 15 minutes or so, while monitoring JVP and urine output (Fig. 7.4). This can be repeated after 30 minutes. If this restores output, underhydration is confirmed and fluid balance corrected to prevent acute tubular necrosis.

If the patient is **hypotensive**, the cause (cardiac failure or hypovolaemia, for example) must be identified and treated. A bladder ultrasound scan will show urine is being produced; a urinary catheter may be needed. If urine output is still poor, an oesophageal

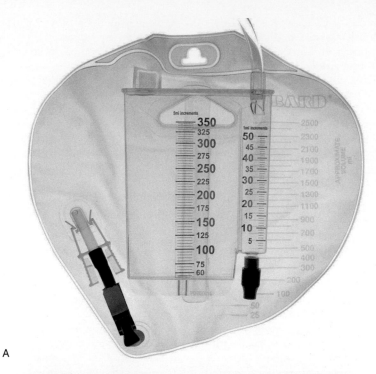

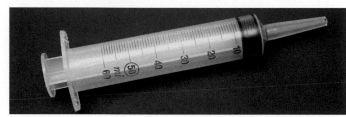

• **Fig. 7.4** Urine Burette and Bladder Syringe. **(A)** Urine burette for precise measurement of urine output. Urine first enters the narrow compartment on the right to enable small quantities to be measured. It is then tipped into the main container to measure running totals. **(B)** Bladder syringe to flush urinary catheters suspected of blockage with debris. The nozzle is shaped to fit the end of a Foley urinary catheter. Note that full sterile precautions must be used to reduce the risk of urinary infection.

Doppler should be placed for monitoring stroke volume to allow goal-directed fluid therapy. Failing this, a central venous line can be used to monitor central venous pressure. If simple measures fail, acute kidney damage must be suspected and investigated.

Lastly, bilateral ureteric obstruction should be considered (or unilateral if only one kidney is present). This is rare as a cause of postoperative low urine output. It can be diagnosed by renal ultrasound which will reveal bilateral hydronephrosis and an empty bladder.

Changes in Mental State

Marked mental changes may occur early after operation and are most common in older patients. These changes are loosely called confusion or delirium. Elderly patients are vulnerable to dementia and cerebrovascular insufficiency so may have a low tolerance of systemic insults that interfere with cerebral equilibrium. Common phenomena include clouding of consciousness, perceptual disturbances, incoherent speech and agitation or destructive behaviour, such as pulling out cannulas or catheters. Other features are loss of orientation, apathy and stupor, and stereotypical movements, such as plucking at the bedclothes.

Factors which predispose to postoperative mental changes in the elderly include:
• disorientation brought about by rapid changes of environment (from ward to operating theatre or ward to ward for example, or moving wards)
• dehydration
• hyponatraemia
• hypoxia (e.g., from pneumonia or cardiac failure)
• infection (especially of the urinary tract)
• drugs (particularly opiates and hypnotics)
• uraemia
• hypoglycaemia
In addition, pain, anxiety and sleep deprivation may precipitate confusion.

Other Causes

Pronounced alterations in behaviour, particularly in younger patients, may indicate alcohol withdrawal or craving for drugs, such as cocaine or heroin, with a history concealed at admission. Patients with a recent history of head injury may behave abnormally if hypoxic, or if intracerebral bleeding develops.

Jaundice

General Causes

Jaundice may develop several days after operation in a patient with no history of biliary disease. In these patients, the cause is usually a prehepatic or hepatic disorder. Causes of **prehepatic jaundice** include large blood transfusions, absorption of large haematomas or emergence of a haemolytic disorder, such as thalassaemia or sickle-cell trait (exacerbated by postoperative hypoxia, dehydration or hypothermia).

Hepatic causes are less common. They include cholestasis (caused by infection near the liver or drug idiosyncrasy), hepatitis and liver cell toxicity from drug idiosyncrasy and visceral ischaemia caused by shock.

Causes Related to Biliary or Liver Surgery

Patients having biliary tract or liver surgery may become jaundiced after operation. The most likely cause is **obstruction** of the extrahepatic bile ducts caused by retained stone, unrecognised surgical trauma or inadvertent duct ligation. Other causes include **infection**, such as ascending cholangitis, and systemic absorption of an intraabdominal collection of bile (biliary peritonitis).

8

Medical Problems

CHAPTER OUTLINE

Introduction

General surgical operations are now performed on patients who are older, more frail and with significant and often multiple (medical) comorbidities, so it becomes even more important to appreciate and consider these 'medical' conditions. Detailed reports of emergency abdominal surgery outcome audits have been published by the UK National Emergency Laparotomy Audit (see: http://www.nela.org.uk/reports). A high-risk patient is usually defined as one whose estimated risk of mortality is greater than 5%, and includes any patient over the age of 65 years undergoing major gastrointestinal or vascular surgery, and any patient over 50 years with diabetes mellitus or renal impairment. Recommendations include preoperative risk assessment with a tailored management plan. This was traditionally directed by consultant surgeons and anaesthetists, but increasingly for older patients, a specialist geriatrician is involved. This was pioneered with orthogeriatricians working with anaesthetists and orthopaedic surgeons in management of hip fracture. In many centres, geriatricians with expertise in perioperative management of general surgical problems are being appointed. A major role for the team is rapid identification and treatment of postoperative infection and potential sepsis.

Medical disorders appear in surgical practice in four main ways:
- A preexisting medical condition may precipitate a surgical admission because of exacerbation, progression or complications of the condition: for example, foot problems in diabetes.
- A preexisting medical condition may be made worse by operation. In chronic obstructive pulmonary disease (COPD), for example, general anaesthesia and postoperative sputum retention may precipitate life-threatening pneumonia.
- A surgical condition may be complicated by an unrelated medical disorder. For example, a patient with rheumatoid arthritis on steroid therapy is vulnerable to impaired healing and recurrent infection.
- An occult condition can become manifest under the stress of anaesthesia and operation. For example, perioperative or postoperative myocardial infarction can be caused by occult ischaemic heart disease.

A new medical problem may be precipitated by a surgical complication. For example, new onset rapid atrial fibrillation (AF) occurring after anastomotic leakage.

Cardiac and Cerebrovascular Disease

Emergency surgery in patients with cardiac disease is about four times more likely to result in death than the same operation done electively. Thus preoperative assessment is vitally important in emergency patients, so any cardiac condition can be recognised and stabilised, electrolyte imbalances corrected and appropriate anaesthesia, surgical technique, monitoring and aftercare used to minimise risk.

Ischaemic Heart Disease

The clinical manifestations of ischaemic heart disease are:
- chronic stable exertional angina; previous myocardial infarction
- acute coronary syndrome (ACS)
- cardiac failure
- arrhythmias (e.g., AF)
- conduction system disturbances (e.g., complete heart block)
- asymptomatic atherosclerotic coronary artery disease

Asymptomatic coronary artery disease may progress to infarction under anaesthetic and surgical stresses, including laryngoscopy and endotracheal intubation, pain, hypoxia, rapid blood loss, anaemia, hypotension, hypocarbia and fluid overload. For major operations, general anaesthesia and spinal anaesthesia carry similar risks. Local anaesthesia, when practicable, is much safer.

Clinical Problems

Stable Angina and Myocardial Infarction More Than 3 Months Previously

There is usually little increased risk during operation and exercise tolerance is by far the most important indicator of the patient's ability to tolerate anaesthesia and surgery. This can be assessed in the history (remembering that exercise tolerance may be limited by mobility problems rather than cardiorespiratory problems). A convenient measure is the MET (metabolic equivalent of a task). A patient with 4 METs can climb a flight of 18 stairs, walk at 4 mph on level ground, run short distances, use a vacuum cleaner, lift heavy furniture, play golf or doubles tennis. Such patients have a low risk of cardiac events. Formal assessment on a treadmill may be helpful; if patients are immobile, pharmacological cardiac perfusion imaging may be helpful. Occasionally coronary angiography is required to fully assess cardiac risk. The indications are the same for nonsurgical patients, that is, unstable angina, limiting stable angina or adverse noninvasive test results.

In general, all cardiac medication should be continued perioperatively. Nitrates, which dilate the coronary arteries and reduce preload and left ventricular (LV) work, may reduce cardiac ischaemia during general anaesthesia and should not be stopped in the perioperative period. A transdermal nitrate patch is a useful alternative to tablets or sprays. Beta-adrenergic blockers, which reduce cardiac work and oxygen demand, should be continued unless non ischaemic cardiac failure develops. Most patients will be taking aspirin (and some clopidogrel in addition, see bleeding disorders, later). Angiotensin-converting enzyme (ACE) inhibitors may be continued, though hyperkalaemia can be a risk especially if co-prescribed with nonsteroidal anti-inflammatory medications. ACE inhibitors should be stopped if acute kidney failure occurs. Statin medications can be discontinued for a few days perioperatively without detriment.

Acute Coronary Syndrome

This is a term applied to a spectrum of conditions from unstable angina to non-ST-elevation myocardial infarction to ST-elevation myocardial infarction (STEMI). ACS associated with surgery usually occurs during the first few days after operation, particularly on the second to fourth postoperative nights, rather than during the operation. Typical chest pain is not always a feature and postoperative ACS may present 'silently' (i.e., painlessly) with otherwise unexplained hypotension, cardiac failure, arrhythmias or cardiac arrest, particularly in patients with diabetes. Diagnosis is made on the basis of at least two of the following: appropriate symptoms (particularly typical cardiac ischaemic pain); a significant rise in a cardiac biomarker, usually troponin; and electrocardiogram (ECG) changes consistent with ischaemia (dynamic changes including ST depression, T-wave flattening or inversion) or infarction (ST elevation). It is always helpful to have a preoperative ECG for comparison, which should be performed on all patients over 50 years of age and any with cardiac symptoms or signs.

Troponin is a very specific marker of myocardial damage, but be aware that this damage may result from conditions other than ischaemia or infarction caused by coronary artery disease, for example, sepsis, hypotension or heart failure, and therefore the management may differ from that of ACS.

The medical treatment of ACS includes aspirin, clopidogrel (for antiplatelet activity) and fractionated heparin given subcutaneously. These drugs adversely affect clotting in the perioperative period and are discussed under bleeding disorders later. Other treatments, such as nitrate and beta-adrenergic receptor blockade are less likely to have adverse 'surgical' effects. STEMI is ideally treated by emergency primary angioplasty but this depends on the surgical stability of the patient, and on how close the nearest coronary intervention centre is. Thrombolysis is obsolete except where there are no facilities for primary angioplasty. In these circumstances, it remains an option, but the potential salvage of myocardium has to be weighed against the serious risk of major haemorrhage.

Chronic Heart Failure

This is a complex clinical syndrome with symptoms and signs resulting from impairment of the heart as a pump owing to structural or functional abnormalities. The severity of heart failure correlates poorly with objective measurements of heart function (such as ejection fraction), such that up to 50% of patients presenting with symptoms and signs of heart failure will have 'preserved ejection fraction' (previously called *diastolic heart failure*). This is especially common in older patients. Assessment of severity is based on clinical features, particularly when exercise tolerance is limited (New York Heart Association classification: http://www.heart.org/HEARTORG/Conditions/HeartFailure/AboutHeart-Failure/Classes-of-Heart-Failure_UCM_306328_Article.jsp). Patients with renal impairment or electrolyte abnormalities have a poorer prognosis and tend to decompensate more readily with operative stress.

Most patients will be taking diuretics, an ACE inhibitor and a beta-blocker as first-line treatment, and nitrates and digoxin if the condition is more severe, and these treatments should be continued if possible.

Patients with chronic heart failure (CHF) should be optimised before major surgery, but there is still an increased mortality of up to 5%. The causes, symptoms and signs of cardiac failure are shown in Fig. 8.1.

Clinical Problems

Chronic Heart Failure Before Operation

Surgery should be postponed until treatment has been optimised and the clinical condition stabilised. Hasty preoperative diuretic

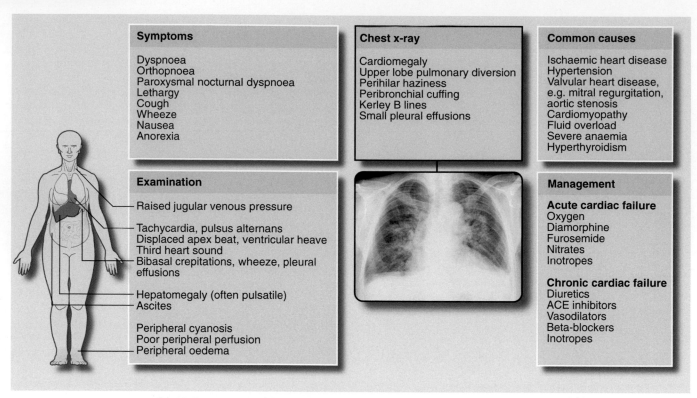

Symptoms

Dyspnoea
Orthopnoea
Paroxysmal nocturnal dyspnoea
Lethargy
Cough
Wheeze
Nausea
Anorexia

Examination

Raised jugular venous pressure

Tachycardia, pulsus alternans
Displaced apex beat, ventricular heave
Third heart sound
Bibasal crepitations, wheeze, pleural effusions

Hepatomegaly (often pulsatile)
Ascites

Peripheral cyanosis
Poor peripheral perfusion
Peripheral oedema

Chest x-ray

Cardiomegaly
Upper lobe pulmonary diversion
Perihilar haziness
Peribronchial cuffing
Kerley B lines
Small pleural effusions

Common causes

Ischaemic heart disease
Hypertension
Valvular heart disease,
e.g. mitral regurgitation,
aortic stenosis
Cardiomyopathy
Fluid overload
Severe anaemia
Hyperthyroidism

Management

Acute cardiac failure
Oxygen
Diamorphine
Furosemide
Nitrates
Inotropes

Chronic cardiac failure
Diuretics
ACE inhibitors
Vasodilators
Beta-blockers
Inotropes

• **Fig. 8.1** The Causes, Symptoms and Signs of Cardiac Failure. The chest x-ray is of a 60-year-old woman with a history of ischaemic heart disease. The signs indicate congestive heart failure. Note: some of these changes are subtle and do not reproduce well in illustrations. *ACE,* Angiotensin-converting enzyme.

therapy is dangerous because it may provoke intravascular volume depletion, hypotension and electrolyte abnormalities. Patients taking diuretics (and often ACE inhibitors or angiotensin-receptor antagonists in addition) may have abnormalities such as:

• Hypokalaemia (usually caused by potassium-losing diuretics prescribed without potassium supplements).
• Hyponatraemia.
• Raised plasma urea and creatinine with hyperkalaemia (particularly if taking an ACE inhibitor and spironolactone)—the urea is often raised to a greater extent than creatinine, indicating intravascular volume depletion. However, in severe cardiac failure, the glomerular filtration rate falls causing urea and creatinine to rise. Clinical assessment by an experienced physician may be needed to differentiate dehydration from overload in patients with cardiac failure and a raised urea and creatinine.
• Postural hypotension.

Decompensated Heart Failure Developing During or After Operation

This problem results from poor tolerance of intravenous fluids, unaccustomed supine posture, myocardial infarction or ischaemia in the perioperative period, or arrhythmias (particularly AF) induced by the stresses of surgery and anaesthesia. Prompt and vigorous diuretic therapy with intravenous furosemide and nitrate is required to prevent worsening cardiac failure, hypoxia, renal failure or other potentially lethal complications. In addition, treatment of any precipitating factors should be instituted, such as reducing cardiac stress by giving good pain relief. Postoperative cardiac failure is best managed in an intensive care unit, using a central venous pressure line to guide fluid replacement.

Preoperative Assessment of Cardiac Failure

Chest x-ray may demonstrate cardiomegaly and there may be signs of pulmonary oedema including upper lobe diversion, hilar congestion, septal Kerley B lines and pleural effusions (see Fig. 8.1). ECG may show an arrhythmia, myocardial ischaemia, ventricular hypertrophy, left bundle branch block or loss of R waves.

LV function can be assessed by echocardiography and documented more precisely by radionuclide studies using multiple-gated acquisition, but the best assessment is a clinical one based on exercise tolerance. Measurement of blood urea and electrolytes is important as baseline and also indication of severity of the condition. A preoperative body weight is crucial but is sadly often omitted.

If there is any doubt about the fitness of a patient for operation, a cardiological opinion should be sought ideally well before planned surgery.

Cardiac Arrhythmias

Clinical Problems

Atrial Fibrillation (Fig. 8.2)

Preexisting (preoperative) AF is very common and affects 2% of the population overall, rising to 10% to 17% among over 80s. In many patients, the heart is structurally normal, but AF may indicate underlying cardiomyopathy, ischaemic heart disease, thyrotoxicosis or (in the developing world) mitral stenosis. It is often associated with hypertension. Acute onset AF postoperatively may be caused by a major surgical complication (e.g., anastomotic leakage after bowel resection) or medical complication (e.g., pneumonia) (see Fig. 8.2). If the onset

Common causes in surgical patients	Diagnosis	Management

Acute causes
  Anastomotic leakage after bowel
  resection
  Myocardial infarction
  Pneumonia
  Pulmonary embolism
 	
Chronic causes
  Ischaemic heart disease
  Heart failure
  Hypertension
  Mitral valve disease
  Hyperthyroidism
  Alcohol abuse
	Examination
	Pulse irregularly irregular
	Apex rate is greater than radial pulse rate
	
	ECG
	Absent P waves
	Irregular QRS complexes
	Atrial fibrillation
		1 Treat any reversible precipitating
		   factors
		2 Control ventricular rate.
		   Drugs commonly used include:
		     Digoxin
		     Beta-blockers
		     Verapamil
		     Amiodarone
		3 Consider cardioversion to sinus
		   rhythm (if acute onset)
		4 Anticoagulation to prevent emboli

• **Fig. 8.2** Atrial Fibrillation—Causes, Diagnosis and Management. *ECG,* Electrocardiogram.

of atrial arrhythmia (particularly AF) is associated with right bundle branch block on the ECG, this suggests a diagnosis of pulmonary embolism.

AF with a controlled ventricular rate (i.e., a pulse rate of less than 90 beats per minute at rest) causes minimal extra risk. An uncontrolled ventricular rate may cause perioperative heart failure. Adequate control of ventricular rate should be achieved before operation with beta-blocker and digoxin, occasionally supplemented with verapamil or amiodarone. Digoxin can be given intravenously if rapid control is necessary but potassium levels need to be monitored closely as digoxin given in the presence of hypokalaemia can lead to further arrhythmias. AF (even with a controlled ventricular response) increases the risk of **arterial embolism** from any thrombus present in the left atrium. For this reason, all patients with intermittent or permanent AF should be considered for anticoagulation.

The Surgical Patient on Anticoagulants. The aim here is to maintain necessary anticoagulation but to reduce the risk of surgical bleeding. Warfarin should be stopped for 5 days before major elective surgery and the international normalised ratio (INR) checked on the day of surgery. Patients with recent venous thromboembolism (VTE) or recurrent VTE on anticoagulation should have 'bridging' therapeutic low-molecular-weight (LMW) heparin, with the last dose 24 h before operation. Bridging is also recommended for patients with most mechanical heart valves and for patients with AF who have had a stroke or transient ischemic attack (TIA) in the previous 3 months; also for patients with a previous stroke and three or more of these risk factors: congestive cardiac failure, hypertension (>140/90 mmHg or on medication), age over 75 years or diabetes. Prophylactic LMW heparin is used for other situations, that is, VTE over 3 months before, patients with AF that are not high risk and those with bi-leaflet aortic valves. For emergency surgery, 5 mg of phytomenadione intravenously reverses warfarin within 6 to 8 h. If surgery cannot wait that long, four-factor prothrombin complex concentrate should be given in consultation with the on call consultant haematologist. Warfarin can be restarted on the evening of surgery owing to its slow onset of action.

Increasingly direct oral anticoagulants (DOACs) are replacing warfarin; they do not require monitoring blood tests, have fewer interactions and are less likely to cause intracranial bleeding than warfarin. They are also rapidly acting and do not need 'bridging' heparin. However, patients on a DOAC may not be aware they are

on anticoagulants because of the variety of trade and generic names without the familiarity of warfarin. Reversing DOACs is more problematic than warfarin. If renal function is normal, DOACs should not be taken for 24 h before elective procedures and 48 h if the procedure is high risk. If renal function is abnormal, this interval is calculated according to the individual DOAC and the creatinine clearance. Anticoagulation can normally be restarted 6 to 12 h postprocedure but not until 48 h if the patient is at risk of bleeding. In patients with higher thrombosis risk, prophylactic doses of DOAC can be given earlier. Clotting studies are unpredictable in assessing DOAC effect, but a normal thrombin time indicates minimal circulating dabigatran. For emergency surgery with a significant bleeding risk, **andexanet alfa** can be used for urgent reversal. Tranexamic acid can also reduce bleeding in those with residual anticoagulant effect. Drugs, such as nonsteroidal anti-inflammatory drugs (NSAIDs) and colloids that impair haemostatic mechanisms, should be avoided in patients on DOACs.

Bradycardia
Bradycardia is common in young fit athletic patients and is not a problem. In patients taking beta-blockers or digoxin, if the apex rate is below 60 beats per minute, that day's dose should be omitted and the regular dose reviewed.

Bradycardia may be caused by **complete heart block**, which should be easily diagnosed on the ECG. This may require urgent temporary **transvenous pacing**, particularly when there is significant haemodynamic compromise or syncope ('Stokes Adams attacks').

If a patient has a **cardiac pacemaker**, it is important to know the reason for its insertion: is the patient pacemaker-dependent, has the pacemaker been checked recently, what type of pacemaker has been inserted? Surgical diathermy, particularly monopolar diathermy, can interfere with the pacemaker if the current flows close to the heart. Ideally, bipolar diathermy should be used if diathermy is required. In addition, a strong magnet should be available; if placed over the pacemaker this will return the rate to 100 beats/min In certain cases within the abdomen ultrasonic shears can be an alternative energy source for dissection and haemostasis.

Other Arrhythmias
Bifascicular block, in which conduction is impaired down two of the three main fascicles (right bundle plus anterior or posterior divisions of the left bundle, manifest by right bundle branch block

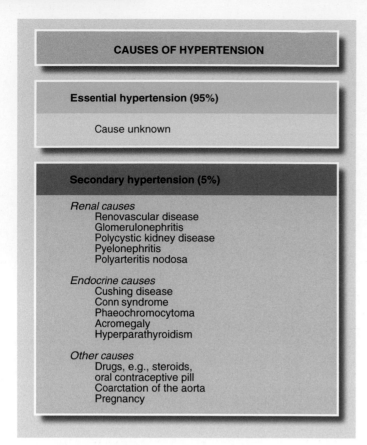

CAUSES OF HYPERTENSION

Essential hypertension (95%)

Cause unknown

Secondary hypertension (5%)

Renal causes
    Renovascular disease
    Glomerulonephritis
    Polycystic kidney disease
    Pyelonephritis
    Polyarteritis nodosa

Endocrine causes
    Cushing disease
    Conn syndrome
    Phaeochromocytoma
    Acromegaly
    Hyperparathyroidism

Other causes
    Drugs, e.g., steroids,
    oral contraceptive pill
    Coarctation of the aorta
    Pregnancy

• **Fig. 8.3** Causes of Hypertension.

and left axis deviation on the ECG), may progress to complete heart block (and low cardiac output) under anaesthesia. For these patients, a prophylactic temporary transvenous pacemaker should be considered before operation.

Hypertension

About one in four patients coming to surgery is either hypertensive or is receiving antihypertensive therapy. Most have **'essential' hypertension**, but causes, such as renal artery stenosis and phaeochromocytoma must be considered in patients presenting with raised blood pressure (BP) which has not been appropriately investigated. (For other causes see Fig. 8.3.) Undiagnosed renal artery stenosis puts the patient at risk of severe acute kidney injury if there is an episode of hypotension, and phaeochromocytoma of potentially fatal hypertensive crisis.

Clinical Problems

Mild-to-Moderate Essential Hypertension

Patients with a systolic pressure of less than 180 mm Hg and a diastolic pressureless than 110 mmHg are at minimal risk of cardiac complications, unless there is some other cardiovascular disease. Sometimes, anxiety about the operation contributes to the hypertension. A labile BP or systolic hypertension at any time may, however, indicate widespread atherosclerosis.

Treated Hypertension

Most common antihypertensive drugs are 'cardioprotective' and should not be stopped before general anaesthesia. Despite the patient being 'nil by mouth' in the immediate preoperative period,

the normal dose of oral antihypertensive drugs should usually be given with a small amount of water. Sudden withdrawal of antihypertensive drugs may cause rebound hypertension. Withdrawal of beta-blockers may trigger autonomic hyperactivity and lability of BP. Postural hypotension may occur after operation, especially if there is dehydration.

Severe or Poorly Controlled Hypertension

If the BP is greater than 180/110 mmHg, then treatment needs to be instituted and any non urgent operative procedure delayed. During anaesthesia the untreated hypertensive patient has a very labile BP and is at high risk of perioperative myocardial infarction, cardiac failure or stroke.

Preoperative Assessment of Hypertensive Patients

Chest x-ray may identify cardiomegaly or cardiac failure, both of which increase the perioperative morbidity and mortality. An ECG may reveal signs of ventricular hypertrophy and ischaemia. Plasma urea and electrolytes should be measured in all patients taking diuretics or ACE inhibitors and in any patient with suspected chronic renal impairment.

Cerebrovascular Disease

A patient has cerebrovascular disease if there is a **history of stroke or TIAs**. Cerebral atherosclerosis may render the blood flow to the brain precarious, with an increased risk of perioperative stroke from hypoxia, hypotension or increased blood viscosity resulting from dehydration.

After a **stroke**, operation should be avoided for at least 2 months if practicable. This is because autoregulation of cerebral BP becomes disrupted, so that cerebral arterial pressure becomes directly related to systemic arterial pressure. Brain perfusion thus loses the buffering effect of autoregulation on peaks and troughs of BP that tend to occur during anaesthesia and surgery. If operation cannot be delayed, it is important to prevent hypertension and hypotension in the perioperative period.

Patients with cerebrovascular disease will usually be on platelet inhibitors (see bleeding disorders, later).

Valvular Heart Disease

The common valvular abnormalities are mitral regurgitation, aortic stenosis and aortic regurgitation. Any of these may dangerously alter cardiovascular dynamics, but stenotic lesions are more serious than regurgitant ones, as the cardiac output tends to be fixed.

Under perioperative stress, valvular disease may precipitate acute myocardial ischaemia, hypotension, cardiac failure, arrhythmias or thromboembolism. Valvular heart disease also predisposes to infective endocarditis (IE).

Aortic Stenosis

Aortic stenosis is potentially the most serious valvular disorder in a surgical patient because it limits the cardiac output and reduces blood flow to the coronary arteries. Indeed, the patient may already be functioning close to the limit with almost no reserve. Perioperative hypotension and tachycardia can be life threatening in such cases. **Aortic 'sclerosis'** produces a similar ejection systolic murmur and is caused by fixed, rigid valve leaflets, usually with systolic hypertension but does not have a significant transvalvar gradient. The perioperative risk is that of the hypertension and arterial disease.

In a patient with an ejection systolic murmur, any associated **cardiac symptoms** may help identify the murmur as pathological, for example, a history of syncope, angina or shortness of breath on exertion. Note, however, that any systolic murmur is difficult to categorise clinically, particularly in the elderly, and an **echocardiogram** including colour Doppler must be performed to identify the valvular cause and offer an assessment of severity. A specialist cardiology assessment may also be required.

Clinical signs of aortic stenosis are:
- Slow rising upstroke of the carotid pulse.
- A harsh ejection systolic murmur radiating into the neck.
- Hyperdynamic apex beat indicating LV hypertrophy. (Note: the apex beat is only displaced laterally if aortic stenosis coexists with aortic regurgitation or is complicated by cardiac failure.)
- LV hypertrophy on ECG.

If aortic stenosis is suspected, an echocardiogram and Doppler will confirm the diagnosis and aid assessment of severity by measuring the aortic valve area, the gradient across the valve and an estimate of LV systolic function. A mean pressure gradient of >40 mmHg, a valve area of <1.0 cm^2 and impaired LV function all imply severe aortic valve disease.

Nonurgent surgery may be best delayed until after operative intervention to the aortic valve. This may now be carried out percutaneously in frail or elderly patients (transcatheter aortic valve implantation [TAVI]) in whom previously the risk of valve replacement was prohibitive.

Symptomatic valvular disease is potentially dangerous and requires full preoperative assessment and treatment. Major valvular heart disease may be discovered in recent immigrants from developing countries where **rheumatic heart disease** is prevalent. Patients with valvular heart disease require cardiac monitoring during operation and usually intensive care afterwards. For management of anticoagulation for patients with artificial heart valves, see the surgical patient on anticoagulants, earlier.

In all cases, it is advisable to involve the haematologist in discussion for advice on management, and in anticipation of specific treatment.

Infective Endocarditis and Indications for Antibiotic Prophylaxis

Valvular disease, and in particular prosthetic replacement valves, carry a risk of **IE**. When blood is forced under pressure through a narrow orifice, laminar flow is disrupted and eddy currents predispose to local thrombus formation and deposition of circulating bacteria. The vegetations of IE thus form on the low-pressure side of the jet of blood passing through a damaged valve or a ventricular septal defect. The left side of the heart is more susceptible than the right because of the higher pressures and greater potential for turbulence.

Streptococcus viridans is the most common causative organism of IE. Other bacteria, such as coliforms or fungi, for example, *Candida*, may also be responsible. Many types of operation and some invasive investigations cause transient bacteraemia. Although the incidence of IE following such procedures is small, the consequences can be catastrophic. In recent years, recommendations for prophylaxis against IE have radically changed and the current consensus is that antibiotic prophylaxis should be confined to those at highest risk. These are patients with prosthetic heart valves or prosthetically repaired valves; those with previous IE; and those with untreated cyanotic congenital heart disease or congenital heart disease with palliative shunts, conduits or other prostheses. Other valvular heart disease patients need no prophylaxis but should have good dental and cutaneous hygiene. These downgraded recommendations result from the following considerations: overuse of antibiotics encourages resistance and there are no randomised controlled trials of antibiotic effectiveness. The risk following dental procedures is now known to be low with low-grade bacteraemia being common after tooth brushing (and even chewing), especially in those with poor dental health, and does not seem to cause IE. For patients at high risk, prophylaxis is indicated for dental scaling, root canal treatment and manipulation of gingival or periapical regions of the teeth or perforation of the oral mucosa. For all other procedures on respiratory, gastrointestinal, urogenital tract (including foetal delivery), skin or musculoskeletal system prophylaxis is not recommended. Since the main target for prophylaxis is oral streptococci, oral amoxicillin or clindamycin in case of penicillin allergy is recommended.

Respiratory Diseases

Respiratory complications (mainly atelectasis and pneumonia) occur in as many as 15% of surgical patients and are the leading cause of postoperative mortality in the elderly. The risk of a respiratory complication increases with the increasing duration of anaesthetic and is amplified by preexisting respiratory disease, such as COPD, asthma or bronchiectasis. Other important factors include smoking, cardiac failure, obesity, old age and general debility. Good postoperative pain relief allows the patient to breathe deeply and cough, which, along with effective physiotherapy, helps reduce the risk of respiratory complications.

Clinical Problems

Chronic Obstructive Pulmonary Disease

COPD (smoking-related lung disease—chronic bronchitis and emphysema) is common and strongly predisposes to postoperative respiratory complications, particularly bronchopneumonia, lobar collapse and pneumothorax. There is often a degree of reversible **bronchoconstriction**, and this can be assessed before operation by measuring peak expiratory flow before and after bronchodilator treatment, if necessary using a low-reading instrument. Many patients will already have had spirometry and vitalography in family practice or in specialist hospital COPD services and their treatment optimised. Otherwise preoperative assessment by the hospital 'chest team' will help bring the patient into optimum health. The forced expiratory volume in 1 second (FEV_1) is perhaps the single most useful assessment of severity of chronic lung disease.

Other chronic lung diseases include bronchiectasis, pneumoconiosis, pulmonary fibrosis, sarcoidosis and pulmonary tuberculosis.

Cigarette Smoking

Smokers of cigarettes have a fivefold greater risk of postoperative respiratory problems than nonsmokers. This is partly caused by preexisting smoking-related respiratory disease but also because smokers have a highly reactive airway. This increases the intraoperative risk of laryngeal spasm and bronchospasm.

Smoking should be stopped at least 4 weeks before operation and ideally 8 weeks before if any early benefit is to be achieved. This gives time for recovery of physiological respiratory functions, such as bronchial ciliary activity. Stopping smoking just before surgery may actually be detrimental because it causes an increase in bronchial mucus production.

Current Respiratory Infections

Acute upper respiratory tract infections (usually viral) are common and these patients have reduced resistance to surgical trauma and infection. This alone may be grounds for postponing an elective operation.

Conditions associated with chronic infection, such as bronchiectasis and cystic fibrosis are more difficult. Elective operations should be carried out during remissions where possible, with intensive physiotherapy and perioperative prophylactic antibiotics.

Asthma

Asthma is common in children and adolescents but may occur later in life, particularly as a component of COPD. The main elements of asthma are airway hyperreactivity (with constriction), bronchial wall oedema, excessive mucus production and airway plugging. All these factors predispose to atelectasis, infection and hypoxia.

Asthmatic problems can be exacerbated by the following factors associated with general anaesthesia and surgery:
- Endotracheal intubation—increases airway sensitivity.
- Increased airways secretions—caused by intubation or the autonomic side-effects of anaesthetic drugs, such as muscle relaxants.
- Dehydration—increases mucus viscosity.
- Limitation of movement and posture because of pain—inhibits coughing to clear secretions
- The direct effects of other drugs, for example, bronchoconstriction caused by beta-blockers or morphine-associated respiratory depression.

In patients with asthma, the usual medication should be continued in the perioperative period, given via a nebuliser if necessary. Operations should be postponed during acute exacerbations.

Previous Pulmonary Embolism or Deep Venous Thrombosis

These patients have a greatly increased risk of recurrent thromboembolism. Prophylactic measures are mandatory for all but the most minor procedures.

Preoperative Investigation of Respiratory Disease

A chest x-ray should be performed on any patient with symptoms or signs of chest disease. There is no need for 'routine' chest x-rays on all preoperative patients as undirected screening of asymptomatic patients has a low yield of abnormalities likely to influence surgical outcome.

Appropriate **lung function tests** should be performed in patients with chronic lung disease. Spirometry (± bronchodilators), arterial blood gases and pulse oximetry should be requested. Peak flows help evaluate airflow limitation. The reversible element of bronchospasm can be assessed using peak flow measurements before and after bronchodilators. Blood gas measurements are indicated if hypoxaemia or carbon dioxide retention is likely.

Always record the inspired oxygen concentration and flow rate when blood gases are measured.

Perioperative Management of Respiratory Disease and High-Risk Patients

The following measures will maximise respiratory function and reduce the risk of postoperative complications:
- **Preoperative physiotherapy**—helps prevent postoperative chest complications. Physiotherapy should include teaching the patient breathing exercises and correct posture.
- **Drug therapy**—adjust to achieve optimum respiratory function. Theophyllines may be added in patients with asthma but regular blood levels are needed for optimum dosing. Nebulised bronchodilator drugs (such as salbutamol) may improve the reversible component of COPD and help to prevent a perioperative exacerbation of asthma. Adequate hydration reduces the risk of retained secretions which might cause airway obstruction. Prophylactic antibiotics are not recommended for COPD.
- **Encouragement of smokers to quit**—should be started at the time of booking for elective surgery.
- **Alternative methods of anaesthesia—local, regional or spinal**—should be considered for patients with chronic respiratory disorders, but are not necessarily the best solution. With the use of newer anaesthetic drugs and techniques, patients may be better off with endotracheal intubation and ventilation using short-acting muscle relaxants. These techniques allow good bronchial toilet at the end of operation. Certain abdominal operations are technically more difficult under spinal anaesthesia, for example if a patient with chest trouble coughs persistently during the procedure; general anaesthesia avoids this.
- **Early postoperative physiotherapy**—aims to enhance deep breathing, coughing and general mobility, reducing the incidence of respiratory complications.
- Noninvasive ventilation (NIV) avoids endotracheal intubation and can be used to manage episodes of acute respiratory failure postoperatively. Bi-level positive pressure ventilation and continuous positive pressure ventilation are the usual modalities, though high-flow nasal oxygen is increasingly popular and can deliver heated and humidified oxygen comfortably at up to 60 L/min.

Gastrointestinal Disorders

The main gastrointestinal conditions giving rise to complications in surgical patients are malnutrition, dental problems, peptic ulcer disease, gastro-oesophageal reflux (GORD) and inflammatory bowel disease. Previous abdominal surgery may also complicate inpatient treatment.

Malnutrition

Many surgical patients are malnourished because of reduced food intake, malabsorption and changes in metabolism (in trauma, burns and sepsis). Studies have shown that 50% of patients undergoing gastrointestinal surgery are mildly malnourished and 30% are moderately or severely malnourished. Malnutrition is particularly prevalent in older patients, those living alone and in patients with dementia. The severity of malnourishment proportionately increases postoperative morbidity and mortality. For example, severely malnourished patients experience eight times the rate of complications and three times the expected mortality following gastrointestinal surgery. Wound healing is delayed, immune resistance is impaired and muscles are weakened.

Nutritional Assessment

There is no universal tool for assessing malnutrition but the combination of a body mass index of less than 18.5 kg/m^2 with weight loss exceeding 5% of usual body weight over the preceding 1 to 2 months and a serum albumin level below 35 g/L (in the absence of renal or hepatic disease) indicates significant malnutrition. Other tools include measuring mid–upper arm circumference, skin fold thickness and grip strength.

Indications for Nutritional Support

If enteral support (i.e., supplemental nutrition into the gastrointestinal tract) is practicable before operation, certain patients benefit from it by reduced mortality and morbidity. Indications published by the British Society of Gastroenterology include patients with severe anorexia, with moderate or severe malnutrition unable to eat or swallow sufficient by mouth, with recent weight loss of 10% or more, or with intestinal failure, and patients not expected to resume oral intake for 10 or more days after operation. Nutritional support is best given as supplements by mouth if possible or else via a fine-bore nasogastric tube.

Dental Problems

Teeth and artificial fixed crowns and bridges are vulnerable to damage during intubation. This causes not only cosmetic and medicolegal problems, but also exposes the patient to the risk of aspirating foreign bodies into the bronchial tree. Similarly, infected material from carious (decayed) teeth or inflamed gums may be aspirated. This causes particularly grave aspiration pneumonia. Dentures must be removed before operation and labelled so the patient can retrieve them afterwards. In unconscious trauma victims, the possibility of aspiration, swallowing or pharyngeal obstruction by a dental prosthesis should always be considered.

Peptic Ulcer Disease

Peptic ulcer disease may be a surgical problem in its own right, but patients admitted for other reasons may have an active peptic ulcer exacerbated by hospital stresses. These include serious illness and trauma, operations, and drugs, such as aspirin, NSAIDs and corticosteroids. The result may be a sudden catastrophic **haemorrhage** (presenting as haematemesis or melaena), or occasionally **perforation**. Bleeding may also result from **acute stress ulceration** in the seriously ill patient. Note that stress ulceration is distinct from chronic peptic ulcer disease.

Patients with known peptic ulcer disease or strongly suggestive symptoms should receive perioperative prophylaxis with proton-pump inhibitors. NSAIDs and irritant oral drugs should be avoided.

Previous gastrectomy may have a number of long-term side effects. These include anaemia (deficiency of iron, vitamin B$_{12}$ and occasionally folate) and, rarely, osteomalacia. A full blood count should be included in the preoperative assessment of these patients.

Gastro-Oesophageal Reflux Disease

Patients with GORD are at risk of aspirating acidic gastric contents during induction of anaesthesia and should receive preoperative treatment with proton-pump inhibitors. Aspiration may cause interstitial lung damage which, in its severe form, is known as **Mendelson syndrome** (chemical pneumonitis).

Inflammatory Bowel Disease

Patients with chronic inflammatory bowel disease may be anaemic or malnourished if the disease is active. Patients may also be **steroid dependent** because of adrenal suppression from long-term steroid therapy, requiring perioperative hydrocortisone. Immunosuppressive drugs, such as azathioprine, methotrexate, cyclosporine and antitumour necrosis factor agents could be being taken and may increase the predisposition to infection.

Hepatic Disorders

Preexisting liver disease may have important consequences in the surgical patient and generally increases postoperative morbidity and mortality. A history of jaundice must be evaluated as it may be a clue to serious risks for both patient and medical staff.

Clinical Problems

History of Jaundice

A past history of jaundice raises the possibility that the patient may be a carrier of hepatitis B or C and this can readily be transmitted to healthcare staff. The main danger is from needle-stick injuries.

Most previously jaundiced patients will have suffered acute infective hepatitis (hepatitis A) and this poses no risk to staff because the infective agent does not cause a chronic carrier state. In contrast, lifetime **chronic hepatitis** develops in 5% to 10% of those infected with hepatitis B virus and in 80% of those infected with hepatitis C virus. These diseases should be suspected if the illness associated with the previous jaundice was prolonged or serious. Jaundice contracted in developing countries should be regarded with suspicion because hepatitis B and C are often endemic. Hepatitis C causes a high long-term rate of cirrhosis, although it often develops slowly over many years. Hepatitis B and C are also common among men who have sex with men and intravenous drug abusers who share syringes. Blood product transfusion is also a risk factor though the risk is very low in the developed world. The history should include questions to determine whether the patient falls into a high-risk group. Clinical examination should include a search for intravenous injection sites characteristic of drug abuse. In high-risk patients, screening for hepatitis B surface antigen and hepatitis C antibody should be performed (see Ch. 3).

Presence of Obstructive Jaundice

Surgery in this situation is usually performed to relieve an obstruction in patients where endoscopic stenting of the bile ducts is inappropriate, has failed or is unavailable. This surgery carries a number of special risks and management problems which are described in Chapter 18. These include ascending cholangitis, clotting disorders, deep vein thrombosis and acute renal failure.

The Patient With Known Hepatitis

Patients with any form of hepatitis, whether viral or alcoholic, tolerate general anaesthesia and surgery badly and there is a definite

- Have you ever felt you ought to **Cut down** on your drinking?
- Have people **Annoyed** you by criticising your drinking?
- Have you ever felt bad or **Guilty** about your drinking?
- Have you ever had a drink first thing in the morning to steady your nerves or get rid of a hangover (**Eye-opener**)?

mortality risk. Surgery should be avoided unless essential. If alcoholism is suspected, a CAGE questionnaire (Box 8.1) should be completed. Positive answers to two or more of the four questions suggest a drinking problem.

An elevated serum gamma glutaryl transpeptidase level and mean corpuscular red cell volume are fairly good indicators of excessive alcohol intake.

The Patient With Known Cirrhosis

Patients with cirrhosis have a high risk of perioperative morbidity and mortality. The main factors are:

- anaemia
- portal hypertension
- defective synthesis of clotting factors and thrombocytopenia
- malnutrition
- electrolyte disturbances (particularly hyponatraemia)
- defective energy metabolism (gluconeogenesis and glycogenolysis)
- abnormal drug metabolism and distribution (because of hypoalbuminaemia)
- ascites

The main postoperative complications of cirrhosis are excessive bleeding, defective wound healing, hepatocellular decompensation leading to encephalopathy, and susceptibility to infection.

Excessive bleeding results from several factors:

- Defective synthesis of clotting factors (all but factor VIII are synthesised in the liver).
- Thrombocytopenia (because of hypersplenism and depressed platelet production).
- Abnormal polymerisation of fibrin.
- Portal hypertension (greatly expanded intraabdominal venous network under high pressure). This, together with numerous vascular adhesions, makes dissection in the abdominal cavity tedious, difficult and bloody.

Portal hypertension may initially be discovered because of ascites or splenomegaly or an acute upper gastrointestinal haemorrhage from oesophageal varices, gastroduodenal ulcers, Mallory–Weiss tears or gastric erosions. If a patient with known oesophageal varices requires an operation, preoperative endoscopic assessment is important and sclerotherapy or banding may be appropriate.

Preoperative Assessment and Management

Preoperative blood tests for patients with liver disease are listed in Box 8.2. If the prothrombin ratio is prolonged, intravenous vitamin K injections are given for several days before operation. If this fails to correct the abnormal clotting (as in severe hepatocellular impairment), it is important to liaise with a haematologist who may recommend perioperative administration of **fresh-frozen plasma or prothrombin complex concentrate** (e.g., Octaplex or Beriplex), containing factors II, VII, IX, X, protein C and protein

Initial Tests

- Serological testing for hepatitis B and C
- Consider HIV testing

Further Tests

- Full blood count
- Clotting screen
- Consider blood group and cross-match if excess bleeding anticipated
- Plasma urea and electrolytes
- Bilirubin
- Transaminases
- Gamma glutaryl transpeptidase
- Albumin
- Calcium
- Phosphate

HIV, Human immunodeficiency virus.

S. If the patient is thrombocytopenic, platelet transfusion may also be required.

Renal Disorders

Renal impairment is commonly encountered in general surgical patients. There is impaired homeostasis of fluid and electrolytes and reduced excretion of nitrogenous compounds. The risk of perioperative complications increases with the degree of renal impairment. Conversely complications, such as sepsis, increase the risk of acute kidney failure. Drugs, such as NSAIDs, loop diuretics, ACE inhibitors, intravenous radiological contrast and gentamicin are also nephrotoxic. Patients fall into two groups: mild and severe chronic kidney failure (CRF). Acute kidney injury is usually a postoperative complication, often with several contributory causes including hypovolaemia, and is described in Chapter 12. Patients with preexisting renal disease are particularly vulnerable to progress to acute renal failure ('acute-on-chronic renal failure').

Clinical Problems

Mild/Moderate Chronic Renal Failure (Chronic Kidney Disease [CKD] Stage 1–3, Estimated Glomerular Filtration Rate [eGFR] >30 mL/min)

This is common in the elderly and often associated with hypertension and diabetes. The main management problems in surgical patients are:

- **Impaired excretion of drugs**—drugs handled by the kidney must be given in smaller doses or less frequently, as documented in official drug formularies. In practice, digoxin, gentamicin, vancomycin and intravenous radiological contrast pose the main problems.
- **Fluid and electrolyte homeostasis**—only becomes a problem if fluid balance is not monitored carefully in the perioperative period. Monitoring should include regular checks of plasma urea, electrolytes and creatinine, especially if the patient is receiving diuretic therapy.
- **Reduction in renal reserve**—even a small increase in plasma creatinine implies a significant reduction in renal reserve. For example, major reconstructive surgery to the abdominal aorta in a patient with mild renal impairment may interfere with renal function because of aortic cross-clamping near the renal

arteries. This is exacerbated by transient hypotension caused by blood loss. The lack of renal reserve in these patients may then progress to acute renal failure.

Severe Chronic Renal Failure (CKD Stage 4–5, eGFR <30 mL/min)

These patients are usually under the care of specialist physicians who should be involved in perioperative management. Patients may be receiving regular haemodialysis or ambulatory peritoneal dialysis; in such patients, surgery may be for renal transplantation (Fig. 8.4).

CASE HISTORY

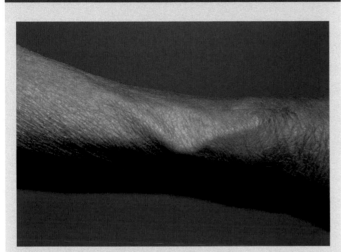

• **Fig. 8.4** Cimino–Brescia Arteriovenous Fistula. This recently constructed fistula was performed for chronic renal failure in a diabetic woman of 56 years. It involved dividing the cephalic vein and suturing its proximal end to the side of the radial artery. It was performed under local anaesthesia via the visible incision. The wrist veins are already dilating and will soon be usable for renal dialysis.

The main perioperative problems of severe CRF are:
- **Fluid overload**—caused by impaired glomerular filtration and may require correction with large doses of diuretics, fluid restriction and haemofiltration if necessary.
- **Regulation of plasma osmolality**—this is disordered in patients with severe CRF who are particularly vulnerable to hypo- and hypernatraemia. Care must be taken that the sodium content of intravenous fluids is appropriate.
- **Hyperkalaemia**—this is a particular risk in advanced CRF. Patients with lesser degrees of CRF are vulnerable to an increase in potassium load (because of transfusion, tissue damage or hypoxia) or changes in GFR (caused by cardiac failure or hypotension). Hyperkalaemia may cause cardiac arrest and susceptibility to this may be assessed by monitoring the ECG. To minimise this risk, the preoperative plasma potassium level should be stabilised below 5.0 mmol/L, but in chronic hyperkalaemia a plasma potassium up to 6.5 mmol/L rarely causes problems.
- **Metabolic acidosis**—this tends to develop in chronic renal failure but it is usually compensated by respiratory alkalosis. This compensation is disrupted by general anaesthesia and also by additional metabolic acidosis resulting from tissue ischaemia or hypoxia.

• BOX 8.3	Specific Perioperative Problems in Patients With Diabetes

Predisposition to Ischaemic Heart Disease
- Greater risk of perioperative myocardial infarction, and has a substantially higher mortality, particularly females
- Infarction may be painless or 'silent' (possibly caused by autonomic neuropathy)

Increased Danger of Cardiac Arrest
- Because of autonomic neuropathy

Renal Problems
- Predisposition to diabetic nephropathy
- Tendency to chronic renal failure

Predisposition to peripheral vascular disease
- Greater risk of perioperative strokes and lower limb ischaemia

Predisposition to Heel Pressure Sores
- Especially if there is peripheral neuropathy and/or ischaemia

Increased Incidence of Postoperative Infection
- In the wound, chest or urinary tract

Obesity
- Particularly common in type 2 diabetes
- Associated with increased operative morbidity

- **Chronic normochromic normocytic anaemia**—this results from decreased erythropoietin (EPO) production by the kidney. Cardiovascular function is usually well adapted to this anaemia and preoperative transfusion is unnecessary. If the haemoglobin concentration is substantially below 10 g/dL, the patient is usually treated with **EPO.**

Preoperative Assessment

Patients with severe renal failure should be asked about their daily urine volume, as those who are oliguric are at risk of overhydration. The state of hydration should be assessed clinically, looking for dehydration or fluid overload (particularly jugular venous pressure). Plasma urea, electrolytes, creatinine and bicarbonate, calcium and phosphate should be checked, and also haemoglobin.

Diabetes Mellitus

Severe hypoglycaemia and hyperglycaemia are life-threatening conditions. The blood glucose levels of a surgical patient with diabetes need to be closely monitored and treated.

Patients with diabetes are at special risk from general anaesthesia and surgery for the following reasons:
- Some complications of diabetes are associated with a higher perioperative risk. These are summarised in Box 8.3.
- Stress (including surgery, trauma and infections) causes increased production of catabolic hormones which oppose the action of insulin (see Ch. 2), making diabetic control more difficult.
- General anaesthesia, surgery, deprivation of oral intake and postoperative vomiting disrupt the delicate balance between dietary intake, exercise (energy utilisation) and diabetic therapy.

- Diabetic ketoacidosis is a cause of elevated leucocyte count and raised amylase level, which may be confusing in the diagnosis of patients presenting with an acute abdomen. Indeed, ketoacidosis may sometimes present with abdominal pain.
- There is a greater risk of hospital-acquired infection, which may be elusive as a cause of deterioration.
- Episodes of cardiac ischaemia and infarction may be painless.
- There may be reduced renal reserve or more overt evidence of renal impairment.

Clinical Problems

Preoperative assessment in patients undergoing major surgery should include evaluation of current diabetic control by serial blood glucose and **glycosylated haemoglobin** measurements. Potential cardiovascular and renal complications should be assessed by performing an ECG (with Valsalva manoeuvre to look for autonomic neuropathy) and measuring plasma urea and electrolytes.

Perioperative management aims to maintain blood glucose between 4 and 10 mmol/L, and hypoglycaemia must be avoided. Above 13 mmol/L, the risk of ketoacidosis or a hyperosmolar nonketotic state is unacceptable unless surgery is critically urgent. Surgery in the presence of ketoacidosis has a high mortality and should be avoided if possible until the acidosis is under control, that is, until bicarbonate is greater than 20 or pH >7.3.

For the purposes of perioperative management, patients with diabetes fall into three groups: those who are **insulin dependent**, those taking **oral hypoglycaemic** medication and those who are **diet controlled**. These are general guidelines—there are usually local guidelines and readily available clinical advice (often led by specialist nurse teams).

Insulin-Dependent Diabetes

Insulin-dependent diabetics depend for their metabolism on administered insulin. If the blood glucose level is low, insulin is not withheld but glucose infusion is increased. The general principles of perioperative management are:

- establish good diabetic control before operation;
- put the patient early on the list;
- give rapidly acting insulin (Humalog or Novorapid) as a continuous intravenous infusion during the operative period;
- give an infusion of dextrose (glucose) throughout the operative period to balance the insulin given and to make up for lack of dietary intake;
- add potassium to the dextrose infusion;
- monitor blood glucose and electrolytes frequently throughout the operative and early postoperative period.

A typical management protocol is given in Box 8.4 and a recommended insulin infusion regimen (a 'sliding scale') in Box 8.5. The key is to adjust the insulin dose hourly according to blood glucose results.

Diabetics Controlled on Oral Hypoglycaemic Drugs

Many patients are receiving short-acting sulphonylureas, such as glipizide. Metformin should be discontinued because of the risk of lactic acidosis. If glycaemic control is difficult then an insulin regimen should be used as mentioned earlier.

On the morning of the operation, the patient is starved in the usual manner and the short-acting sulphonylurea omitted, to be reintroduced when oral intake is resumed. Blood glucose should

---

> ### • BOX 8.4 Perioperative Management of Insulin-Dependent Diabetes
>
> **Before Operation**
> 1. Arrange preoperative outpatient stabilisation of diabetes with diabetes physician and specialist nurse in advance.
> 2. If outpatient preparation is unavailable or unsatisfactory, admit patient at least 1 day before operation.
> 3. Establish optimal preoperative control—may need advice from diabetic management team.
> 4. Monitor capillary blood glucose by fingerprick throughout the day, for example, before and after meals and at bedtime.
> 5. Check capillary blood glucose by fingerprick and electrolytes before operating list commences—postpone if glucose level greater than 13 mmol/L or electrolyte abnormalities found.
> 6. Arrange for the operation as early as possible in the day.
>
> **Operation Day**
> 1. Starve from midnight and omit first dose of insulin.
> 2. Commence intravenous dextrose and rapidly acting insulin infusions.
> 3. Check capillary blood glucose by fingerprick and electrolytes at conclusion of operation (or at 1–2-hour intervals in a long operation).
> 4. Adjust concentration of infusions and rate of administration as required.
>
> **After Operation**
> 1. Check glucose hourly initially and electrolytes 6–12-hourly and adjust infusion as indicated.
> 2. Continue infusion until full oral diet is established, then reintroduce subcutaneous rapidly acting insulin, using the preoperative regimen.

> ### • BOX 8.5 Perioperative Management of Diabetics Using Insulin Infusion
>
> 1. Intravenous 5% or 10% dextrose infusion at 125 mL per hour.
> 2. Constant pump-controlled intravenous rapidly acting insulin infusion. This is adjusted according to 2–4-hourly blood glucose estimations.
> 3. If there is a need to limit fluids—use 20% dextrose solution and infuse at 50 mL per hour.

---

be monitored regularly (at least 4-hourly). If glucose rises above 13 mmol/L, it can be controlled by small subcutaneous doses of short-acting insulin, for example, 6 units of rapidly acting (Humalog or Novorapid) insulin. If a major operation is planned or if postoperative 'nil by mouth' is likely to be prolonged, it is best to use rapidly acting insulin and glucose infusions as for insulin-dependent diabetes.

Diabetics Controlled by Diet Alone

If preoperative control is adequate, these patients require no special perioperative measures; they do not become hypoglycaemic and blood glucose rarely drifts above acceptable levels. Fingerprick blood glucose measurement may be used if there is any doubt.

Poorly Controlled Diabetes on Emergency Admission

Any diabetic patient may present with uncontrolled diabetes, particularly if admitted as an emergency. This may be caused by infection or vomiting. The diabetes must first be brought under control with rehydration and infusions of rapidly acting insulin, glucose and potassium.

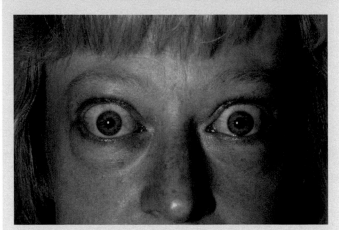

• **Fig. 8.5 Thyrotoxic Eye Signs.** This woman of 36 years presented with a typical history of primary thyrotoxicosis (Graves disease), with weight loss, irritability and menstrual irregularity. In addition, her eyesight had become blurred. She had florid exophthalmos with protruding eyeballs (proptosis) and lid lag. She was barely able to close her eyelids and would soon be at risk of corneal drying.

Thyroid Disease

Thyrotoxicosis

Thyroid or non thyroid surgery for a patient with uncontrolled thyrotoxicosis carries a risk of thyrotoxic crisis and this carries a high mortality. Thus any patient with features of thyrotoxicosis should have thyroid function tests (free thyroxine [fT4] and thyroid stimulating hormone [TSH]) included in the preoperative assessment.

In surgery for hyperthyroidism, the patient should be rendered euthyroid before operation using antithyroid drugs (propylthiouracil can be useful as it blocks peripheral conversion of T4 to the active T3) and nonselective beta-blocking drugs.

Hypothyroidism

Patients with untreated hypothyroidism are at moderately increased risk when undergoing surgery. They are more sensitive to central nervous system depressants, have a decreased cardiovascular reserve, and are also susceptible to electrolyte disorders (particularly water retention). Severe infection, especially accompanied by trauma, a cold environment or depressant drugs, may precipitate myxoedema coma which, though very rare, is often fatal.

If there is clinical suspicion of hypothyroidism, operation should be postponed and thyroid function checked by measuring fT4 and TSH levels. If hypothyroidism is diagnosed, oral replacement therapy is commenced, but it may take several weeks to achieve the euthyroid state. If surgery must be performed urgently, it is usually best to proceed with the operation and begin oral treatment later.

Disorders of Adrenal Function

Adrenal Insufficiency

The most common cause of adrenal insufficiency is hypothalamo–pituitary–adrenal suppression by long-term corticosteroid therapy. It is occasionally caused by primary adrenal failure (**Addison disease**) or secondary to pituitary dysfunction (because of tumour or surgery). Very rarely, it results from previous adrenalectomy for treatment for a hypersecretion syndrome or bilateral primary adrenal tumours.

In primary or secondary adrenal failure, the patient is usually already taking oral steroid replacement therapy, but the lack of additional adrenal response to the stresses of trauma, surgery or infection may cause acute postoperative cardiovascular collapse with hypotension and shock (**Addisonian crisis**).

The 'typical' abnormal biochemical profile which should raise concern of the possibility of adrenal insufficiency is hyponatraemia, hyperkalaemia and raised blood urea (intravascular volume depletion). However, these abnormalities are neither sensitive nor specific and a short Synacthen test will be diagnostic. If the patient is sick and an Addisonian crisis is strongly suspected then take blood for random cortisol and commence hydrocortisone treatment.

Perioperative 'Steroid Cover'

Patients with potential adrenal insufficiency must be given steroid cover during the perioperative period. This is usually in the form of intravenous hydrocortisone, for example, 25 to 50 mg before the operation and 50 mg daily until recovery. It is better to give prophylactic hydrocortisone in doubtful cases than risk acute hypoadrenalism. For any steroid-dependent patient, a doctor should write clearly in the notes '*Treat any unexplained collapse with hydrocortisone.*'

Cushing Syndrome

Cushing syndrome results from excess secretion of cortisol. This may be in response to excess adrenocorticotropic hormone (ACTH) secretion by a pituitary tumour, ectopic ACTH secretion (usually by a malignant tumour) or, rarely, caused by a primary tumour of an adrenal gland. The most common cause of Cushingoid features is long-term steroid therapy for conditions, such as polymyalgia rheumatica or asthma. Clinically, the patient may be plethoric, 'moon-faced', hypertensive, hirsute and obese with abdominal striae and have a characteristic 'buffalo hump'. The main surgical problems in Cushingoid patients are hypertension, hyperglycaemia, poor wound healing, infection and peptic ulceration. If the condition is caused by steroid therapy, there is an additional risk of secondary adrenal insufficiency.

Musculoskeletal and Neurological Disorders

Musculoskeletal and neurological disorders influence the outcome of surgery in two main ways. First, any condition which hinders mobility predisposes to chest infection, deep venous thrombosis and pulmonary embolism, aspiration pneumonitis and pressure sores. The last is even more likely if there is also sensory impairment because of stroke or diabetic peripheral neuropathy. Second, specific aspects of these disorders must be considered in relation to general anaesthesia, positioning of the patient on the operating table and the use of drugs. Finally, it is essential that patients with epilepsy and Parkinson disease get their treatment throughout the perioperative period.

Rheumatoid Arthritis

Rheumatoid arthritis poses special problems related to chronic anaemia, drug therapy and spinal complications. (Note that some of these problems are shared by other collagen disorders.)

- **Normochromic normocytic anaemia**—common in chronic inflammatory disorders, including rheumatoid arthritis, although less common now that active inflammation is better controlled with modern drug therapy. The anaemia is refractory to iron therapy and there is no benefit from preoperative transfusion unless haemoglobin concentration is <8 g/dL, or the patient is symptomatic.
- **Gastrointestinal disorders**—most will be taking NSAIDs, which together with long-term steroid therapy, predispose to peptic ulceration and perforation. Chronic low-grade bleeding from the upper gastrointestinal tract may exacerbate the existing anaemia in these patients. Operative stress may also precipitate acute gastrointestinal haemorrhage. NSAIDs may contribute to kidney injury.
- **Long-term steroid therapy**—may result in adrenal insufficiency under stress.
- **Other medications**—powerful drugs now used include chloroquine, methotrexate, sulfasalazine and cytokine inhibitors. Perioperative renal elimination of methotrexate may be reduced and fatalities have occurred when the usual dose has been continued. It is essential to involve rheumatologists and it may be safer to discontinue immunosuppressants until convalescence.

CASE HISTORY

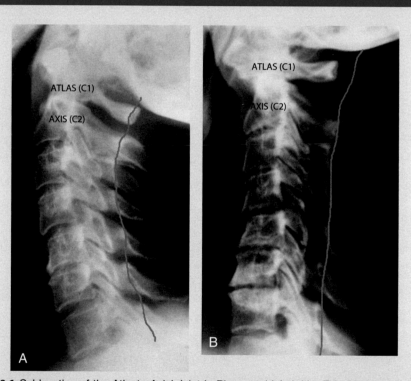

ATLAS (C1)

AXIS (C2)

ATLAS (C1)

AXIS (C2)

A

B

• **Fig. 8.6** Subluxation of the Atlanto-Axial Joint in Rheumatoid Arthritis. This 62-year-old woman with longstanding severe rheumatoid arthritis required a major abdominal operation. Cervical radiographs were taken before operation to anticipate problems during anaesthesia. **(A)** Cervical spine in extension. **(B)** The same patient in flexion. On each x-ray, a line is drawn along the posterior limit of the spinal canal. Anterior subluxation (i.e., partial dislocation) is most obvious if the most posterior part of the spine of the atlas is compared with the line and with that of the axis in the two pictures. This mobility is caused by destruction of the transverse axial ligament of the odontoid by pannus (excessive granulation tissue) from the synovial joint. Under general anaesthesia, muscle relaxation may allow exaggeration of the subluxation, causing damage to the cervical cord.

- **Odontoid subluxation** (see Fig. 8.6)—if rheumatoid arthritis involves the atlanto-axial joint, the transverse ligament may be destroyed, allowing the odontoid process to sublux. During general anaesthesia, the protective reflexes are lost. If the neck is hyperextended during intubation, there is a serious risk of injury to the spinal cord by the unrestrained odontoid.

Preoperative Assessment of a Patient With Rheumatoid Arthritis

Full blood count is essential to check for nonspecific anaemia or iron deficiency anaemia; and plasma urea, electrolytes and creatinine are measured to identify chronic or drug-induced disturbance of renal function; inflammatory markers (erythrocyte sedimentation rate and C-reactive protein) indicate the activity of the disease. Preoperative assessment must include clinical examination of neck movements and cervical spine x-rays.

Haematological Disorders

Anaemias

Severe anaemia leads to increased perioperative morbidity and mortality. General anaesthesia poses the greatest risk. Whilst this should be assessed on an individual case and patient basis, for elective surgery, the haemoglobin concentration should ideally be above 8 g/dL before operation but long-standing chronic anaemia probably poses little increased risk.

Management depends on the cause of the anaemia. Whether to transfuse before operation depends on the level of anaemia (trigger levels have come down in recent years as a response to the shortage of blood for transfusion and absence of clear benefit; see local guidelines), whether the anaemia is acute, and the expected operative blood loss. Transmission of human immunodeficiency virus (HIV) and other infective agents by transfusion is a very small risk in developed countries where sophisticated screening of donors is usual, but remains a serious risk in countries without such precautions. Transfusion for anaemia can usually be avoided in young, fit patients but elderly or very ill patients with less cardiorespiratory reserve are more likely to need transfusion. Transfusions should be given at least 24 hours before operation to allow fluid balance to stabilise and ensure optimal red cell function. For diagnosed deficiency anaemias, treatment as appropriate with iron, vitamin B_{12} or folate may be all that is necessary before operation. Treatment with EPO for patients with chronic renal failure is expensive but effective.

Haemoglobinopathies

Patients with sickle-cell disease and beta thalassaemia have a high operative mortality and morbidity, particularly if the condition is unrecognised (e.g., in emergencies). They require intensive perioperative management, avoiding hypoxia, infection, acidosis, dehydration and hypothermia. Patients with sickle-cell trait are at much lower risk and develop complications only if they become severely hypoxic. Sickle-cell trait and disease occur amongst black and mixed race people, who should always be asked specifically about a history of sickle-cell disease. A sickle-cell test must be performed before operation on any patient at risk so that the anaesthetist can be prepared.

Polycythaemia

Polycythaemia may be caused by a primary myeloproliferative disorder, such as **polycythaemia vera** or be secondary to chronic cardiac or pulmonary disease or heavy cigarette smoking. There is an increased red cell mass in primary and secondary polycythaemia producing a high haematocrit and increased blood viscosity. In primary polycythaemia, the platelet count may be increased which, paradoxically, is associated with defective haemostasis as well as the risk of thrombosis.

The main complications of polycythaemia vera are **haemorrhage** and **arterial or venous thrombosis**. The risk increases once the haematocrit rises above 50%. In general, operation should be postponed to allow treatment by venesection or myelosuppression. If possible, the cardiovascular system should be allowed to stabilise for about a month after treatment. In an emergency, the haematocrit may be reduced by preoperative venesection, restoring the volume by colloid infusion.

Leukaemia, Leucopenia and Thrombocytopenia

Patients with these haematological disorders may need surgery for unrelated conditions. Prophylactic antibiotics may be required in neutropenia, and haematologists give specific advice in patients on chemotherapy. In thrombocytopenia, haemorrhage can be minimised by transfusing platelet concentrates.

Bleeding Disorders

Bleeding diatheses, such as thrombocytopenia, von Willebrand disease (abnormal platelet function and factor VIII deficiency) and haemophilia are occasionally encountered in surgical practice. Most surgical haematological bleeding problems, however, are caused by poorly controlled anticoagulant therapy, liver disease, aspirin therapy and sometimes vitamin K malabsorption. The last occurs in obstructive jaundice and malabsorption syndromes.

A history of abnormal bleeding or factors which may predispose to abnormal bleeding should be sought from every surgical patient as follows:
- Excessive bleeding from simple cuts, previous surgery, dental extractions or childbirth.
- Current use of anticoagulant drugs or antiplatelet drugs (aspirin and clopidogrel).
- A family history of bleeding disorders.
- Intercurrent haematological or liver disease, cystic fibrosis or other malabsorption syndromes.
- Recent jaundice.
- Previous intestinal resection or bypass surgery.

Recognising and treating a clotting problem before operation is vital because runaway haemorrhage can easily occur, causing clotting factor depletion. At this point, bleeding may be impossible to control even with transfusion of clotting factors.

If a bleeding disorder is suspected, a **platelet count** and **clotting screen** must be performed. The latter includes prothrombin time or ratio and activated partial thromboplastin time. If an abnormality is found, assays of individual clotting factors may be needed. Operation should be deferred if possible until the problem is overcome.

Clinical Problems of Bleeding Disorders
Inherited Clotting Disorders
Haemophilia occurs in males. The disorder is an X-linked deficiency of factor VIII or, less commonly, factor IX. Specific antihaemophilic factors are administered before operation and for up to 2 weeks afterwards until the danger of secondary haemorrhage is past. **Von Willebrand disease** is an autosomal dominant

condition with abnormalities of both factor VIII and platelet function. It is managed with replacement of the specific factors.

Anticoagulant Therapy

The management of patients on warfarin and other anticoagulants is described earlier in this chapter and in Chapter 12.

Liver Disease

Bleeding disorders in cirrhosis are described earlier in this chapter, and disorders in the jaundiced patient are described in detail in Chapter 18.

Aspirin and Clopidogrel Therapy

Aspirin has an irreversible inhibitory effect on platelet aggregation which persists clinically for at least 10 days. The effect is reversed only when the affected platelets have been replaced. Most NSAIDs act on platelets in a similar but less profound way. High doses of intravenous penicillin cause a similar but short-lived effect. Antiplatelet therapy is important for secondary prevention of cardiovascular disease. Aspirin can be continued throughout most surgical procedures but if the risk of bleeding is high, it can be stopped 3 days before and restarted a week after. For urgent surgery on patients on antiplatelet agents, perioperative intravenous **tranexamic acid** may be beneficial. With excessive peri- or postoperative bleeding, two pools of donor platelets may be infused. In patients with recent ACS or coronary artery stents, it is especially important to continue dual antiplatelet therapy, for example, aspirin plus clopidogrel and these should be continued for low risk procedures. Procedures with a high bleeding risk should be deferred; if not possible, aspirin should be continued and clopidogrel or ticagrelor stopped 5 days preoperatively.

Malabsorption of Fat-Soluble Vitamins

Vitamin K absorption may be impaired in pancreatic dysfunction, after resection of the proximal ileum or in malabsorption syndromes. The problem is readily overcome by preoperative injections of vitamin K.

Psychiatric Disorders

Mental Illness and Learning Disability

Antidepressant drugs (tricyclic antidepressants) and antipsychotic (neuroleptic) drugs (such as phenothiazines) have a wide range of interactions (see *British National Formulary*). Plasma lithium (do not take samples in a lithium heparin bottle!), urea, electrolytes and thyroid function should be checked in patients taking **lithium** (usually for bipolar disorder), which may cause renal parenchymal damage and disturbed thyroid function.

Alcoholism and Drug Addiction

Alcoholics are prone to delirium tremens, cirrhosis, malnutrition and peripheral neuropathies. Drug addicts are at risk of hepatitis, HIV/acquired immunodeficiency syndrome (AIDS) and other infections. Alcohol acutely potentiates general anaesthetic agents, and an inebriated patient needs smaller doses. In contrast, chronic alcohol abuse induces liver enzymes which break down anaesthetic agents. This also increases tolerance to central nervous system depressants and higher doses of anaesthetics are needed. Similarly, larger doses of sedatives are required for gastrointestinal endoscopy. Opiate addiction leads to similar dosage problems.

Problems of Drug Withdrawal

Withdrawal symptoms may develop unexpectedly after operation if drug or alcohol addiction has been concealed. Alcohol withdrawal is characterised initially by irritability and tremors. Convulsions may develop after 24 to 48 hours. Full-scale **delirium tremens** may appear as long as 10 days after alcohol withdrawal. It is characterised by confusion and visual hallucinations accompanied by fever, tachycardia, pallor, vomiting and sweats. Similar symptoms and signs also occur in a range of other postoperative complications and alcohol withdrawal can be overlooked.

Alcoholic cirrhosis may cause episodic hypoglycaemia, the symptoms of which may be confused with those of delirium tremens. Hypoglycaemia should be excluded by measuring blood glucose.

Mild alcohol withdrawal states may be managed with regular reducing oral doses of chlordiazepoxide. Parenteral B vitamins are usually given daily. Opiate withdrawal symptoms are broadly similar to those of alcohol. Treatment is usually with a substitute drug, such as methadone.

Even patients with mild dementia become more confused when subject to the strange and ever-changing environment of the surgical ward. They poorly tolerate the stresses of general anaesthesia and operation and so the benefit of elective procedures should be carefully weighed against possible adverse effects. Where operation is necessary, mental capacity should be assessed and if lacking, consent obtained from two doctors.

Delirium ('acute confusional state') is common, characterised by acute onset of disturbed consciousness, cognitive function or perception. It has a fluctuating course. It is serious and associated with several adverse outcomes including death, increased length of stay, complications, such as pressure sores and falls and admission to long-term care. Patients at risk are older, have underlying cognitive impairment and severe illness, particularly hip fracture. Suspect delirium on admission if there is confusion, restlessness, hallucinations and/or lack of cooperation. **Hypoactive delirium** is often missed and is suggested by worsening concentration, slow responses, reduced mobility and altered appetite. Preventing delirium is best achieved by lack of change—a single care team familiar with the patient and not moving the patient between wards or rooms. If delirium is suspected, prompt action is needed: a short Confusion Assessment Method score should be administered:

1. Acute onset or fluctuating state
2. Inattention (easily distractible)
3. Disorganised thinking (rambling conversation)
4. Altered level of consciousness (hyperactive to stuporose)

1 plus 2 and 3 or 1 plus 4 indicates delirium. Management should be to identify and treat the cause, reassurance, reorientation and involvement of family and carers. 'Specialing' by a member of staff trained in managing delirium may be needed. Appropriate lighting, signage, an accurate clock and calendar should be present. Ensure adequate fluid intake, address constipation, correct hypoxia, glucose and electrolytes, treat infection, avoid catheterisation except for acute retention, address pain, mobilise, review medication with a ward pharmacist and address nutrition. Ensure that patient's glasses, hearing aids and dentures are available and fit. Promote a good sleep pattern by avoiding procedures (including medication rounds) at night. If these measures fail and the person is distressed or a risk to themselves or others, cautious short-term (less than 1 week) haloperidol or olanzapine may be tried under liaison psychiatrist guidance. Antipsychotic drugs must be avoided in patients with Parkinson disease or Lewy Body dementia. Delirium in Parkinson should be managed by a specialist team: reducing L-dopa (madopar or sinemet)

TABLE 8.1 Surgical Complications of Obesity

Complication	Factors
Cardiopulmonary complications, such as cardiac failure and chest infections	Predisposing factors are atherosclerosis, increased demands on the cardiovascular system, decreased chest wall compliance, inefficient respiratory muscles and shallow breathing
Wound complications, such as infection, dehiscence	Poor-quality abdominal wall musculature with fat infiltration. Large 'dead space' in which fat predisposes to haematoma formation
Venous thromboembolism—increased risk of deep venous thrombosis and pulmonary embolism	Poor peripheral venous return; delayed return to normal mobility
General anaesthesia complications	Anatomic problems, for example, intravenous cannulae difficult to insert and intubation more difficult. Clinical signs of dehydration and hypovolaemia are more difficult to elicit. Physiological problems: metabolic, for example, altered distribution of drugs
Predisposition to various **medical disorders**	Hypertension, ischaemic heart disease, type 2 diabetes, gallstones, gout
Operative difficulties	Operations take longer because of difficult access and obscuring of vital structures by fat. Leads to a higher incidence of anaesthetic and surgical complications, particularly of the wound
Problems of manual handling	Weight and size limitations of standard equipment including computed tomography scanners, operating tables, beds. Need for hoists, powered beds. Risks to staff involved in lifting and handling

BOX 8.6 Potentially Dangerous Drugs in the Surgical Patient

- Glucocorticoids
  —Predispose to peptic ulceration, delayed wound healing and infection.
  —Adrenal atrophy caused by long-term steroid therapy may lead to acute adrenal insufficiency causing cardiovascular collapse.
- Antihypertensive and antianginal drugs
  —Should not be stopped. Hazardous if abruptly stopped, which may cause rebound hypertension or angina.
- Antidepressants
  —Monoamine oxidase inhibitors are rarely used but should be stopped 2 weeks before surgery. Tricyclic antidepressants need not be stopped but carry risks of arrhythmias, hypotension and interaction with vasopressor drugs. Selective serotonin reuptake inhibitors should be continued. Stop lithium 24 hours before major surgery but not minor surgery.
- Oral contraceptives (OCP) and hormone replacement therapy (HRT)
  —Mildly increased risk of deep venous thrombosis and pulmonary embolism. HRT should be stopped 2 weeks before major surgery. Stopping OCP risks pregnancy but is advised 4 weeks before surgery.
- Anticoagulants and antiplatelet drugs
  —Predispose to haemorrhage and need careful management since omission may lead to cardiac and cerebrovascular events.
- Diuretics
  —May cause electrolyte abnormalities and dehydration. Potassium-sparing diuretics should be stopped on the morning of surgery.
- Nonsteroidal anti-inflammatory drugs may predispose to electrolyte disturbance and peptic ulceration

worsens mobility but improves hallucinations, whereas increasing L-dopa achieves the opposite. Relatives become extremely anxious about delirium particularly where it appears suddenly in someone who is cognitively intact. They will be reassured by knowing it is usually temporary.

Obesity

Gross obesity carries two to three times the risk of perioperative death or morbidity, as outlined in Table 8.1. Whenever possible, weight should be reduced before operation, particularly if it is not urgent. Referral to a dietician may be helpful although self-help groups often provide stronger motivation. Preoperative investigations for obese patients include blood glucose measurement, respiratory function tests and ECG, even if the patient is asymptomatic.

Chronic Drug Therapy

Many drugs prescribed for long-term treatment of medical conditions can complicate management of the surgical patient. Note that the risk of stopping long-term medication before surgery is often greater than the risk of continuing it throughout. Drugs that should not normally be stopped include anticonvulsants, anticoagulants (recent or recurrent VTE and certain mechanical heart valves), antiplatelet agents (recent ACS or coronary stent), antiparkinsonian drugs, antipsychotics, anxiolytics, bronchodilators, cardiovascular drugs, glaucoma drugs, immunosuppressants, drugs of dependence and thyroid or antithyroid drugs. The most important of these commonly encountered in practice are summarised in Box 8.6.

9

Blood Transfusion

Principles of Blood Transfusion

The ability to safely transfuse blood and blood products has revolutionised outcomes from major trauma and from complex surgery involving heavy blood loss, such as arterial reconstruction, open-heart surgery and organ transplantation. For replacing blood loss, stored blood restores the circulation, increases oxygen carrying capacity and helps prevents hypoxia. Modern blood transfusion is very safe but deaths and major morbidity still occur. Potential hazards include clerical errors leading to incompatible transfusion, transfusion reactions and transmission of infection.

Over the last two decades, indications for blood transfusion have been carefully scrutinised. As a result, **restrictive blood transfusion strategies** have been adopted and used in conjunction with clinical assessment. Patients requiring blood transfusion must be informed about the indications, risks, benefits and any alternatives and given the option to refuse (see the National Institute for Health and Care Excellence [NICE] Blood Transfusion guidance: https://www.nice.org.uk/guidance/ng24). Before transfusion, **valid consent** should be obtained and documented in the patient's notes (see: https://www.gov.uk/government/publications/patient-consent-for-blood-transfusion). Details about any blood transfusion given should be included in a patient's discharge summary to their GP.

Reducing the Need for Bank Blood Transfusion

Surgical blood use in the United Kingdom has fallen by more than 20% since 2000 in line with the increasing evidence for the benefits of restrictive transfusion policies. However, deaths and serious reactions still occur from incompatible transfusions, particularly when blood products are administered under general anaesthesia. Serious infections, such as hepatitis, malaria, human immunodeficiency virus (HIV) and variant Creutzfeldt–Jakob disease (vCJD) can be transmitted despite careful screening of donors and donations. The risk increases proportionately to the number of units transfused and can be reduced by critical scrutiny of the indications for transfusion.

Recognition and Treatment of Preoperative Anaemia

Anaemia is an independent factor predicting adverse outcomes from surgery. Patients who are anaemic preoperatively (haemoglobin [Hb] <130 g/L in adult males and Hb <120 g/L in adult females) are more likely to be transfused, and anaemic patients are at increased risk of mortality and major morbidity in proportion to the severity of the anaemia.

Iron deficiency is the most common type of anaemia found in preoperative screening. For men and postmenopausal women, potential gastrointestinal (GI) causes of bleeding must be investigated. Once identified, iron deficiency should generally be treated with oral iron (https://www.nice.org.uk/guidance/ng24). If time does not permit or if patients are unable to tolerate oral iron, parenteral iron should be offered. Other causes of anaemia (vitamin B_{12} and/or folate deficiency, renal anaemia or an underlying haematological condition) should be identified and addressed.

Erythropoietin-stimulating agent is not recommended before surgery except for patients with renal anaemia on dialysis or where avoiding transfusion is highly desirable (e.g., in patients refusing blood or those with complex antibodies and complex cross-match requirements).

Patients at Risk of Bleeding

Patients at risk of bleeding include those with thrombocytopenia, coagulopathies and those on anticoagulation and antiplatelet therapy. A management plan should be agreed in advance of surgery, including timely discontinuation of medications. In surgical emergencies, anticoagulation may need urgent reversal. Intravenous vitamin K reverses the anticoagulant effects of warfarin in 6 to 8 hours; prothrombin complex concentrate acts immediately. Heparin is reversed with protamine sulphate. Antiplatelet agents and newer anticoagulants (direct oral thrombin and anti-Xa inhibitors) can be reversed in some cases (i.e., idarucizumab is an antidote for dabigatran) and requires haematology guidance.

Minimising Blood Loss During Surgery

In addition to scrupulous haemostasis with diathermy, clips, ties or the use of other products, such as tissue sealants during surgical procedures, additional measures such as intraoperative cell salvage (IOCS) can be used where appropriate.

Intraoperative Cell Salvage

IOCS involves collecting blood spilled at operation by suction, then washing it in physiological solution and concentrating it. This blood, with a packed cell volume of 50%, can then be reinfused. It is recommended for patients with anticipated blood loss >20% of blood volume, those with risk factors for bleeding, in major haemorrhage, and for patients with rare blood groups. Some patients who do not accept donor blood are prepared to accept and consent to IOCS (including some Jehovah's Witnesses). The technique remains controversial in malignant disease.

Antifibrinolytic Agents

Tranexamic acid is recommended by NICE for operations with an expected blood loss of >500 mL. It is also recommended in major haemorrhage because of trauma or GI haemorrhage.

Avoiding Unnecessary Transfusion After Surgery

Postsurgery blood transfusion can be minimised by accepting restrictive transfusion triggers and by adhering to the single unit transfusion policy described later. Prescription of oral or parenteral iron can minimise use of bank blood and contribute to the patient's recovery.

Postoperative cell savers enable blood lost in the postoperative period to be collected via a filtered wound drain and transfused via another filter. This is suitable for procedures with an anticipated substantial 'clean' postoperative blood loss, such as total knee replacement.

Laboratory Aspects of Blood Transfusion

When transfusion is deemed appropriate, **the correct component(s)** must be selected according to clinical indications. The types of transfusion components and the general indications for their use are summarised in Table 9.1.

The patient's history, including current/previous diseases and treatment, can give important information to help select suitable blood and blood components (e.g., irradiated platelets must be used for patients at risk of graft-versus-host disease).

Blood Grouping and Compatibility Testing

Transfusion of ABO incompatible blood is characterised as a **'never event'** and may be fatal. Transfusion practice aims to minimise this risk and involves two steps: determining the patient's ABO and Rhesus (Rh) groups and then screening the patient's plasma for clinically significant antibodies. **Pretransfusion blood samples** must be scrupulously labelled with four points of identification, in the presence of the patient and during one continuous event. In many hospitals, confirming the patient's ABO group via a second sample is required before blood transfusion. For patients who have received blood or were pregnant during the previous 3 months, pretransfusion samples are only valid for 3 days.

Traditionally, each unit of group-compatible donor blood was directly **cross-matched** against the patient's serum to ensure compatibility. Nowadays, most hospitals issue most of their blood using computer or 'electronic' cross-matching. In some centres, electronic blood selection and matching can be performed at designated computer-supported blood fridges located in the clinical area and linked with the laboratory. This process is known as *remote issuing*.

For patients with detectable or historical clinically significant antibodies, manual cross-match is required, enabling blood to be selected that is negative for the detected antibodies. For patients in the throes of massive haemorrhage, antibodies become so depleted that ABO group-compatible blood can safely be given.

Storage and Useful Life of Blood (See Table 9.1)

Blood and blood components have specific requirements for preserving their quality and ensuring patient safety, and compliance is a legislative requirement (BSQR 2005). Blood and blood components should be retained in the designated conditions until just before use. Blood removed for more than 30 minutes and not transfused should be returned to the laboratory for disposal.

Blood Transfusion in Clinical Practice

Blood Transfusion and Elective Surgery

Surgical patients fall into one of three categories: transfusion not anticipated (e.g., hernia repair), transfusion possible but unlikely (e.g., cholecystectomy), and transfusion probable (e.g., major arterial reconstruction). For patients in the second category, blood should be sent for ABO and Rh grouping and antibody screening, and serum retained for compatibility testing in case blood should be required later ('group and save'). For patients in the third category, an appropriate number of units are requested for the operation as per the hospital Maximum Blood Ordering Schedule. If the antibody screen is negative and the criteria for electronic cross-match are met, group-specific blood can be immediately issued.

Thresholds and Targets of Transfusion for Surgical Patients

For haemodynamically stable hospitalised adult patients, **a restrictive red cell transfusion threshold** is recommended. This means that transfusion is not generally indicated until the Hb level reaches 70 g/L, but symptoms must be taken into account. A restrictive transfusion threshold of 80 g/L is recommended for cardiac surgery and those with preexisting cardiovascular disease. Hb level must be tested during the 24 hours before blood transfusion. If transfusion is needed, the target posttransfusion Hb is usually 80 to 90 g/L. The **dose** of red cell transfusion for non bleeding adult patients is a single unit followed by clinical and laboratory reassessment. The rate of administration depends on the patient's age, weight, fluid balance, cardiovascular stability, liver and renal function.

TABLE 9.1   Types of Blood Component Transfusions and Indications for Their Use[a]

Component	Indication	Volume	Adult Dose	Storage Temperature	Shelf Life	Comments
Red cells	Substantial haemorrhage and severe anaemia	220–240 mL	One unit (which increases Hb concentration by 10 g/L)	2°C–6°C	35 days from donation	Whole blood is centrifuged to separate red cells, platelets and plasma. Red cells can be washed or irradiated and suspended in preservative solution.
Fresh frozen plasma (FFP)	Replacing clotting factors during major haemorrhage	274 mL	10–15 mL/kg (four units)	< −25°C	Frozen: 36 months; thawed at 4°C: 24 hours to 5 days; room temperature: 4 hours	Prepared from fresh whole blood or donations by apheresis[b] and then frozen. FFP contains near normal amounts of clotting factors. Also used to treat TTP and acute DIC
Platelet concentrate	Treatment or prevention of bleeding for patients with thrombocytopenia or platelet dysfunction defects	200–300 mL	One unit (which increases platelet counts by 10×10^9/L per unit transfused)	20°C–24°C	2–7 days (if bacterially screened)	Mean platelet count is 165–500 $\times 10^9$/L. Platelet counts should be >50 $\times 10^9$/L for most surgical procedure and >100 $\times 10^9$/L for neurosurgery, back or eye surgery and multiple trauma. Platelets are prepared from pooled buffy coats (four donors per pack) or from apheresis donations
Cryoprecipitate	Source of fibrinogen in major haemorrhage and DIC	43 mL	Available as pools of 5 units (total volume: 189 mL). Adult dose is 2 pools	< −25°C	Frozen: 36 months. Use within 4 hours of thawing	Cryoprecipitate is made by thawing FFP at 4°C, producing a cryoglobulin rich in fibrinogen, Factor VIII and von Willebrand factor

[a]National and hospital-based guidelines are produced giving indications for red cell, platelet and fresh frozen plasma transfusion. For regular updates and for information about granulocytes and other plasma derivatives, such as human albumin solution, clotting factor concentrates and immunoglobulin solutions, please visit https://www.transfusionguidelines.org/red-book.

[b]Apheresis = process which involves removal of whole blood from the donor; blood components are separated by centrifuge, the desired constituent (i.e., plasma) is withdrawn and the remaining components retransfused into the donor.

DIC, Disseminating intravascular coagulation; *TTP,* thrombotic thrombocytopenic purpura.

For bleeding patients, the rate of administration of blood is guided by the rate of blood loss, Hb results and physiological observations (blood pressure, heart rate, respiratory rate). Managing patients with major haemorrhage is discussed separately.

Blood must be **prescribed** by a doctor or 'authorised' health professional with appropriate training according to hospital policy. The prescription must include the type of blood component, the volume, rate of transfusion and any additional instructions. Blood must only be administered by a trained and competence-assessed registered practitioner. Before **administration,** patient identification by wrist band together with verbal confirmation must be checked against the prescription, patient's blood group, special requirements and information on the unit of blood and compatibility label including expiry time. If any discrepancy is identified, the process must be stopped. In some hospitals, patient identification wrist bands are checked electronically against the unit of blood as an additional safety step. Legislation in the United Kingdom demands that retrievable records of transfusion and the fate of each unit of blood must be kept for 30 years.

During blood transfusion, patients must be observed at regular intervals (0, 15 min, and then hourly with monitoring of blood pressure, pulse, temperature and respiratory rate) to ensure transfusion reactions can be identified early.

Transfusion Management of Major Haemorrhage (Fig. 9.1)

Major haemorrhage is defined as haemorrhage of 2 litres blood in 3 hours, 4 litres in 24 hours or >150 mL blood per minute. Loss of less than 1500 mL (30% of blood volume) normally requires only crystalloids or colloids except in cases of preexisting anaemia. Loss of 30% to 40% of blood volume requires red cell transfusion; more than 40% loss, equivalent to 2 litres in an adult, can be immediately life threatening and requires urgent blood and blood component transfusion according to the local **Major Haemorrhage protocol** (see Fig. 9.1). Laboratory results and estimates of blood volume loss can be misleading and therefore the initial diagnosis of *major haemorrhage requiring transfusion* should be based on clinical criteria and observations. A pragmatic clinically-based definition is: bleeding which lowers systolic blood pressure to less than 90 mmHg or causes a heart rate of more than 110 beats per minute. In an emergency (e.g., major traumatic haemorrhage) where group-compatible blood

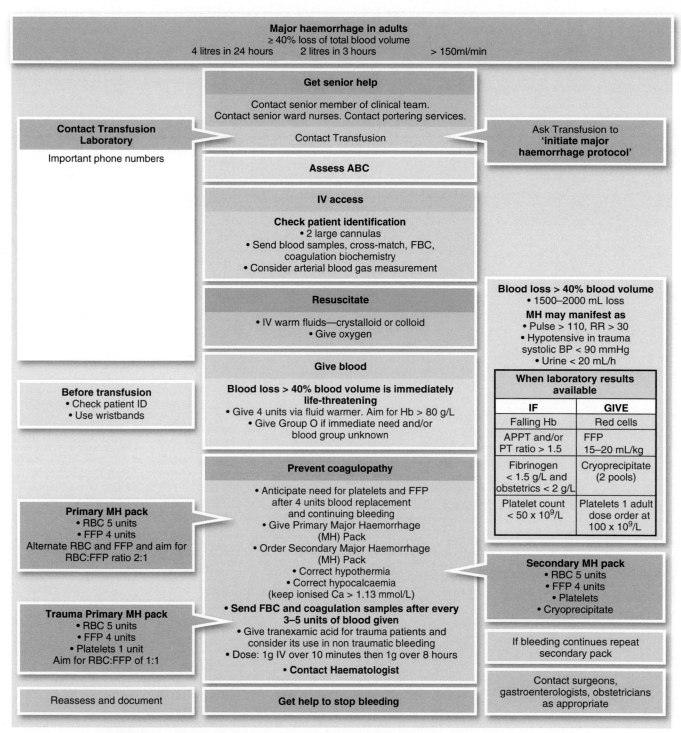

Major haemorrhage in adults
≥ 40% loss of total blood volume
4 litres in 24 hours   2 litres in 3 hours   > 150ml/min

Get senior help

Contact senior member of clinical team.
Contact senior ward nurses. Contact portering services.

Contact Transfusion

Contact Transfusion Laboratory

Important phone numbers

Ask Transfusion to 'initiate major haemorrhage protocol'

Assess ABC

IV access

Check patient identification
• 2 large cannulas
• Send blood samples, cross-match, FBC, coagulation biochemistry
• Consider arterial blood gas measurement

Resuscitate
• IV warm fluids—crystalloid or colloid
• Give oxygen

Blood loss > 40% blood volume
• 1500–2000 mL loss

MH may manifest as
• Pulse > 110, RR > 30
• Hypotensive in trauma systolic BP < 90 mmHg
• Urine < 20 mL/h

Give blood

Blood loss > 40% blood volume is immediately life-threatening
• Give 4 units via fluid warmer. Aim for Hb > 80 g/L
• Give Group O if immediate need and/or blood group unknown

Before transfusion
• Check patient ID
• Use wristbands

When laboratory results available	
IF	**GIVE**
Falling Hb	Red cells
APPT and/or PT ratio > 1.5	FFP 15–20 mL/kg
Fibrinogen < 1.5 g/L and obstetrics < 2 g/L	Cryoprecipitate (2 pools)
Platelet count < 50 x 10^9/L	Platelets 1 adult dose order at 100 x 10^9/L

Prevent coagulopathy
• Anticipate need for platelets and FFP after 4 units blood replacement and continuing bleeding
• Give Primary Major Haemorrhage (MH) Pack
• Order Secondary Major Haemorrhage (MH) Pack
• Correct hypothermia
• Correct hypocalcaemia (keep ionised Ca > 1.13 mmol/L)
• **Send FBC and coagulation samples after every 3–5 units of blood given**
• Give tranexamic acid for trauma patients and consider its use in non traumatic bleeding
• Dose: 1g IV over 10 minutes then 1g over 8 hours
• **Contact Haematologist**

Primary MH pack
• RBC 5 units
• FFP 4 units
Alternate RBC and FFP and aim for RBC:FFP ratio 2:1

Secondary MH pack
• RBC 5 units
• FFP 4 units
• Platelets
• Cryoprecipitate

Trauma Primary MH pack
• RBC 5 units
• FFP 4 units
• Platelets 1 unit
Aim for RBC:FFP of 1:1

If bleeding continues repeat secondary pack

Contact surgeons, gastroenterologists, obstetricians as appropriate

Reassess and document

Get help to stop bleeding

• **Fig. 9.1** Example of Major Haemorrhage Protocol in Adults. *APPT*, Activated partial thromboplastin time; *BP*, blood pressure; *FBC*, full blood count; *FFP*, fresh frozen plasma; *Hb*, haemoglobin; *PT*, pro-thrombin time; *RBC*, red blood cells. (Reproduced with permission from East of England Regional Blood Transfusion Committee.)

is unavailable, group O RhD negative blood can be given with comparative safety. Group O red cells must continue until the ABO group has been reported and confirmed on a second sample according to local policy. ABO group-specific and fully cross-matched blood should then follow.

Transfusion of large volumes of red cells and administration of other fluids that contain no coagulation factors or platelets causes **dilutional coagulopathy.** Major traumatic haemorrhage is often associated with coagulopathy owing to activation of coagulation

and fibrinolytic systems. Coagulation is also impaired by hypo-thermia, acidosis and reduced ionising calcium.

Blood Component Transfusion in Major Haemorrhage

Fresh frozen plasma (FFP) should be transfused in a dose 10 to 15 mL/kg to maintain prothrombin time at less than 1.5; at least four units should be given to the average adult. Fibrinogen levels need to be maintained above 1.5 g/L, and the platelet count needs to be greater than 50×10^9 /L (ideally the aim is for 75×10^9 /L). For patients with multiple trauma, traumatic brain injury or ophthalmic injury, platelets should be above 100×10^9 /L.

If bleeding continues and blood results are unavailable, haematological support should be initiated and continue empirically, aiming to transfuse in a ratio of red cells to FFP of 2:1. For trauma patients, this ratio should be close to 1:1, and consideration should be given to early administration of platelets (after the first four units of blood). It is common for any primary Major Haemorrhage pack to contain four to six unit of red cells and four units of FFP. If patients need more than more than five units of red cells, additional component requirements must be anticipated with further red cells, FFP, platelets and a source of fibrinogen in the form of cryoprecipitate. Blood should be administered through blood warming devices and acidosis and hypocalcaemia must be corrected. See: *A practical guideline for the haematological management of major haemorrhage:* https://onlinelibrary.wiley.com/doi/full/10.1111/bjh.13580.

After every five red cell units transfused, repeat blood tests should be ordered to determine the need for additional blood components. **Point of care testing**, that is, in the relevant clinical area, has an increasing role in providing 'real time' laboratory data to guide blood component replacement.

Early administration of the antifibrinolytic drug, **tranexamic acid**, improves survival of patients with major traumatic haemorrhage or at risk of significant bleeding after trauma (CRASH-2 trial 2010, https://www.thelancet.com/journals/lancet/article/PIIS0140-6736(10)60835-5/abstract). Tranexamic acid should be given as soon as possible after the injury in a loading dose of 1 g IV over 10 minutes followed by a maintenance infusion of 1 g over 8 hours.

Adverse Effects of Blood Transfusion

Modern blood transfusion is very safe provided established protocols are followed, but preventable problems still occur. Identification errors are the usual cause for wrong transfusions, including ABO incompatibility. In the United Kingdom, data about adverse effects are regularly collected by the Serious Hazards of Blood Transfusion, see: https://www.shotuk.org. Adverse effects of transfusion are commonly classified into acute or delayed, infective and noninfective, and those caused by errors or pathological reactions. Classification is also by severity—mild, moderate or severe.

Acute Transfusion Reactions

Severe acute reactions (occurring <24 hours from transfusion) are the most common cause of major morbidity and occur in one in 7000 units transfused.

Acute Haemolytic Transfusion Reactions

The most serious reactions are caused by transfusion of ABO incompatible red cells; these react with the patient's anti-A or anti-B antibodies. There is a rapid complement-mediated destruction of the circulating transfused red cells and a release of inflammatory cytokines. The patient very quickly becomes shocked and develops acute kidney failure and disseminated intravascular coagulation. Massive haemolysis, haemoglobinaemia and haemoglobinuria may also occur. The diagnosis of incompatible transfusion is confirmed by blood tests—finding hyperbilirubinaemia and a positive Coombs test. Major morbidity occurs in up to 30% of patients and 5% to 10% of episodes contribute to the death of the patient.

Acute Nonhaemolytic Transfusion Reactions

Other acute immunological reactions include allergic or anaphylactic and transfusion related acute lung injury. This presents with symptoms of hypoxia and x-ray changes suggestive of acute respiratory distress syndrome during transfusion and for up to 6 hours afterwards. The injury is caused by donor antibodies reacting with the patient's leucocytes.

Acute nonimmunological transfusion reactions also include **Transfusion Associated Circulatory Overload (TACO), febrile nonhaemolytic transfusion reactions (FNHTR)** and **bacterial contamination** of blood components.

TACO can present with a range of severity and is currently considered to be the major cause of transfusion morbidity and mortality. Patients with low body weight, positive fluid balance, cardiovascular instability, low albumin, liver or kidney failure are at higher risk.

FNHTR is an acute, normally nonsevere reaction, usually initiated by leucocytes from the transfused component, and is rare since universal leucodepletion of blood products. A temperature rise of greater than 1°C and shivering during or after transfusion indicates a likely FNHTR. Symptoms usually subside after stopping the transfusion for 15 to 30 minutes and administering antipyretics and antihistamines. The reactions are rarely life-threatening, but fever with or without rigors may herald a serious reaction.

Bacterial contamination of blood components is very rare. Platelets kept at room temperature are the most susceptible component.

If any severe reaction is suspected, transfusion must be stopped. Patient identification must be rechecked against details on the blood unit. Urgent medical review is undertaken. The suspect unit must be returned to the blood bank and haematological advice sought. Additional support may include adrenalin if anaphylaxis is suspected, or diuretics for fluid overload. If bacterial contamination is likely (temperature above 39°C or >2°C above baseline/or other symptoms of sepsis), this is treated with intravenous antibiotics on a 'best guess' basis initially. For patients with severe haemolytic reactions, symptomatic support should be given and care escalated; similarly if TACO is suspected.

Delayed Transfusion Reactions

Delayed haemolytic transfusion reactions can occur more than 24 hours posttransfusion in patients who have been 'alloimmunised' to red cell antigens by previous transfusion or pregnancy. The antibody may have fallen to an undetectable level and the patient is then inadvertently reexposed to red cells of the immunising group. These patients present with jaundice and failing Hb up to 14 days posttransfusion; treatment is supportive. Information about the type of antibody must be kept on the hospital laboratory system and antigen-negative cross-matched blood must be offered for all later transfusions. It is good practice for patients to carry cards containing this relevant information.

Transfusion Associated Graft-Versus-Host Disease

This is an exceptionally rare complication of blood transfusion with mortality of almost 100%. It presents when viable lymphocytes in the donated blood escape recognition by the recipient's immune system, start to proliferate and then mount an immune response against the recipient. The disease is characterised by pancytopenia together with skin, liver and GI manifestations. The most important risk factors are common human leucocyte antigen haplotypes between donor and recipient, transfusion of fresh, nonleucocyte depleted blood and recipient susceptibility as a result of underlying disease (e.g., Hodgkin lymphoma, T-cell dysfunction) or treatment (bone marrow transplantation, chemotherapy or other immunosuppressive agents). Since leucodepletion became universal, the number of reported cases has declined rapidly. Susceptible patients must be recognised and receive **irradiated cellular blood components.** Patients at risk must carry warning cards.

Post Transfusion Purpura

This is a rare delayed complication of blood transfusion (at between 5 and 12 days). Affected individuals present with thrombocytopenia and bleeding caused by restimulation of platelet-specific alloantibodies able to damage the patient's own platelets. This severe and potentially fatal complication of blood transfusion has become rare since universal leucodepletion. If suspected, expert advice must be sought. Patients may benefit from administration of intravenous immunoglobulin.

Infective Hazards of Transfusion

Transmission of infections by blood products is now rare in developed countries. Donated blood can now be screened for most significant transmissible infective agents using serological and polymerase chain reaction-based technique. In the United Kingdom, blood donations are routinely tested for hepatitis B, hepatitis E, HIV, human T-lymphotropic virus I & II and syphilis.

Cytomegalovirus

The virus can remain latent in leucocytes and potentially be transmitted during blood transfusion. Leucodepletion can significantly reduce the viral load and hence transmission. Cytomegalovirus-negative blood components are only recommended for intrauterine transfusions, transfusions in neonates and planned transfusions in pregnancy.

Variant Creutzfeldt–Jakob Disease

vCJD is a rare disorder believed to be caused by misfolded prion proteins and is the human version of bovine spongiform encephalitis which predominantly affected the United Kingdom. It is considered to be transmissible through blood transfusion, with four presumed cases reported up to 2018, all of which were in the United Kingdom. As there is no method of screening donors, UK

• BOX 9.1   Blood Transfusion—Summary

General
- Education, training and compliance with regulatory requirements underpin safe transfusion practice.
- Failure to check patient's identification can be fatal. Patient must wear an ID band (or equivalent) with first name, surname, date of birth and unique ID number. Confirm identity at every stage of transfusion process including pretransfusion sample labelling. If there is any discrepancy, DO NOT TRANSFUSE.
- Blood transfusion is generally safe but major morbidity and mortality still occurs. Patients must be monitored during transfusion to identify a transfusion reaction early.

For Individual Patients
- Are there alternatives to blood transfusion for this patient?
- Is transfusion really necessary for this patient? (Transfusion should only be offered when benefits outweigh risks and there are no suitable alternatives; clinical assessment plus laboratory results guide transfusion practice.)
- Before transfusion, discuss the risks, benefits and alternatives with the patient and gain their consent if possible.
- If transfusion is needed, ensure the right blood is given at the right time. Early recognition of major haemorrhage and rapid provision of blood and blood components improves outcomes.

Blood Services have introduced the following measures to minimise possible transmission:
- Importing plasma from overseas for acquiring fractionated blood products (such as immunoglobulins, albumin and clotting factors for which no recombinant product is available).
- Leucodepleting all cellular blood components (since 1999).
- Importing FFP (and applying treatments to minimise pathogen transmission) for all patients born after 1 January 1996 (when dietary transmission of vCJD was considered to have ceased).
- Excluding donors later found to have vCJD.
- Excluding individuals from donating blood, tissues or stem cells who have received donor blood, as well as those at elevated risk of iatrogenic or familial CJD.

The risks and recommendations are under regular review and further updates are expected from The Advisory Committee on the Safety of Blood Tissues and Organs (SaBTO). See: https://www.gov.uk/government/groups/advisory-committee-on-the-safety-of-blood-tissues-and-organs).

10

Principles and Techniques of Operative Surgery Including Neurosurgery

CHAPTER OUTLINE

Introduction

This chapter describes the operating environment and outlines the principles of operative surgery including those used in 'minor' surgical techniques. All of these should be understood by all doctors, not just surgeons, to help them appreciate the scope of surgery, to enable them to give meaningful explanations to patients before and after surgery and to help them assist intelligently at the operating table. Furthermore, most doctors are required to perform minor operations, emergency department procedures or invasive investigations at one time or another and these require knowledge of techniques.

Various suffixes derived from Greek and Latin are used in describing particular surgical techniques; these are summarised in Box 10.1.

Principles of Asepsis

Introduction

The main bacteria and viruses involved in surgical infections have been described in Chapter 3. The chief sources of infection are the patients themselves (particularly bowel flora), less commonly the hospital environment, food or cross-infection from other patients, and occasionally bacteria and viruses carried by ward staff or theatre personnel. Rare sources of infection are contaminated surgical instruments or equipment, dressings or parenteral drugs and fluids. The viruses causing hepatitis B and C and particularly human immunodeficiency virus (HIV) pose sinister risks of transmitting infection from patient to operating staff and vice versa. These risks

> **• BOX 10.1 Surgical Terminology**
>
> - *oscopy* = examination of a hollow viscus, body cavity or deep structure using an instrument specifically designed for the purpose, for example, gastroscopy, colonoscopy, laparoscopy, arthroscopy, bronchoscopy. The general term is **endoscopy**
> - *ectomy* = removal of an organ, for example, gastrectomy, orchidectomy (i.e., removal of testis), colectomy
> - *orrhaphy* = repair of tissues, for example, herniorrhaphy
> - *ostomy* = fashioning an artificial communication between a hollow viscus and the skin, for example, tracheostomy, colostomy, ileostomy. The term may also apply to artificial openings between different viscera intraabdominally, for example, gastrojejunostomy, choledochoduodenostomy (i.e., anastomosis of duodenum to common bile duct)
> - *otomy* = cutting open, for example, laparotomy, arteriotomy, fasciotomy, thoracotomy
> - *plasty* = reconstruction, for example, pyloroplasty, mammoplasty, arthroplasty
> - *pexy* = relocation and securing in position, for example, orchidopexy (for undescended testis), rectopexy (for rectal prolapse)

make it mandatory to observe **universal blood and body fluid precautions** described in Chapter 3.

Postoperative Infection

The risk of postoperative bacterial infection depends on the extent of contamination of the wound or body cavity at operation or, in the case of intestinal perforation, before operation. Bacteria enter a surgical site by five possible routes:

- Direct inoculation from instruments and operating personnel
- Airborne bacteria-laden particles
- From the patient's skin
- From the flora of the patient's internal viscera, especially large bowel
- Via the bloodstream

Modern operating theatre design and correctly observed aseptic procedures minimise wound contamination but when infections occur, results can be devastating, especially in relation to artificial prostheses, skin grafts, bone and the eye. Furthermore, some patients are particularly vulnerable to infection, notably neonates, the immunosuppressed, the debilitated and the malnourished. Note that treatment of established infection is no substitute for prevention.

The use of preoperative prophylactic antibiotics began in the 1970s and has revolutionised the outcome of certain types of operative surgery in a manner comparable to the changes heralded by Lister's introduction of antisepsis in the late 19th century.

It is also important to consider **Creutzfeldt–Jakob disease (CJD)**, a rare disorder caused by accumulation of an abnormal prion protein in the brain and lymphoreticular tissues resulting in fatal neurodegeneration. The variant form (vCJD) is potentially transmissible through certain (usually neurosurgical) procedures. It is common practice to assess a patient's risk of CJD before surgery as prions are resistant to standard chemical and physical decontamination regimens. Surgical instruments that come into contact with tissues at particularly high risk of infection (i.e., brain, spinal cord, eyes) need stringent chemical and autoclave sterilisation. Instruments used on 'high-risk' tissues in patients with confirmed or suspected CJD require quarantining or destruction if single-use disposable instruments cannot be used.

The Operating Environment

Modern **operating theatre design** plays a key role in control of airborne wound contamination. This is important mainly for staphylococci carried on airborne skin scales.

The main factors influencing airborne operating theatre infection rates are:

- the concentration of organisms in the air;
- the size of bacteria-laden particles;
- the duration of exposure of the open wound.

The first two are influenced mainly by theatre design and air supply, and the last can be minimised by avoiding unnecessarily long procedures. Operating theatre complexes are laid out so as to minimise introduction of infection from outside via air, personnel or patients. Air is drawn from the relatively clean external environment, filtered and then supplied to the theatres at a slightly higher pressure than outside to ensure a constant outward flow. **Air turnover** is the most important factor; the aim is to ensure 3 to 15 air changes per hour which 'scrubs out' the theatre air by dilution. Standard air delivery systems aim to achieve a constant flow of clean air towards the operating table, which is then exhausted from the theatre. Despite this, convection currents allow some recirculation of air, which may be contaminated, into the operation site.

The crucial importance of preventing infection in joint replacement surgery led to the development of sophisticated **ultra-clean air delivery systems**. These reduce postoperative infection two- to fourfold in joint replacement surgery, but the cost is very high. Enclosure of the patient in a sterile tent in which the surgeons wear space-type suits can reduce infection rates by a further 5% to 7.5%. However, correct use of prophylactic antibiotics gives better reduction in infection rates than any clean air system.

Minimising Infection From Operating Theatre Personnel

Only a modest proportion of wound infections derive from theatre personnel. Bacteria reach the wound via the air or by direct inoculation, often from viscera within the wound. About 30% of healthy people carry *Staphylococcus aureus* in the nose but pathogenic organisms may also be present in axillae and the perineal area, the last probably being the most important source of wound infections from theatre personnel. In addition, skin abrasions are usually infected, as are skin pustules and boils; thus personnel with these lesions must ensure that they are effectively covered with occlusive dressings or else should not enter the operating area.

Airborne, personnel-derived infection is reduced by changing from potentially contaminated day clothes to clean theatre clothes and shoes which should not be worn outside the theatre complex. Trouser cuffs should be elasticated or tucked into boots. **Face masks** are worn to deflect bacteria-containing droplets in expired air, but most types become ineffective after a very short period, especially when wet. With the exception of nasal *Staph. aureus* (particularly important in prostheses infection), bacteria derived from the head do not generally cause wound infection. The effectiveness of wearing masks and hair coverings to reduce infection is unknown.

Method	Equipment to Be Sterilised	Temperature	Time
Steam autoclave	Unwrapped instruments and bowls Instrument sets, dressings and rubber	123°C 126°C	10 min 3 min
Ethylene oxide gas	Selected heat-sensitive materials; plastics, electrical equipment	55°C	2–24 h
Manual cleaning then endoscope washer disinfector (EWD)	Flexible endoscopes	Low temperature (guided by type of disinfectant and detergent used for decontamination)	Guided by EWD manufacturer (around 30 min)

TABLE 10.1   Time and Temperature Requirements for Sterilisation by Different Methods

Sterile gloves and gowns are worn by surgeons and staff directly involved in the operation to prevent inoculation of bacteria. Gloves are impermeable to bacteria but hands and forearms need washing before gloving and gowning with antiseptics that persist on the skin. This minimises bacterial contamination if a glove is punctured (as often happens) or the sleeve of the gown becomes wet. The traditional ritual of scrubbing with a brush for 3 minutes is actually less effective than washing the hands thoroughly because scrubbing causes microtrauma and brings bacteria to the surface.

Despite the protection given by wearing gloves and gown, the less a wound is handled, the better. This principle applies particularly when aseptic conditions are less than ideal. On the ward, lesser procedures, such as bladder catheterisation or chest drain insertion should be performed using sterile precautions and a **no-touch technique**.

Minimising Infection From the Patient's Skin
The patient's skin, especially the perineal area, is the source of up to half of all wound infections.

These may be minimised by the following measures:
- **Removing body hair**—body hair was thought to be a source of wound contamination but this is no longer believed. Hair is removed only to allow the incision site to be seen and the wound to be closed without including hair. Shaving produces abrasions which rapidly become colonised with skin commensals. Most surgeons now restrict hair removal to clipping away just enough to provide skin access, which should be performed just before making the incision.
- **Cleaning the skin with antiseptic solutions**—chlorhexidine in alcoholic solution (or aqueous solution for mucous membranes) has been shown superior to povidone-iodine when applied to a wide area around the proposed operation site ('skin prep'). This should be allowed to dry before the incision to be effective. Alcohol-containing antiseptic solutions should be used with caution, especially if diathermy is used, owing to the risk of fire. In abdominal surgery, these solutions can pool, particularly in the umbilicus and around the flanks.
- **Draping the patient**—the operating area is isolated by placing sterile, (ideally self-adhesive) drapes made of impermeable paper or coated waterproof material over all but the immediate field of operation.

Reducing Infection From Internal Viscera
The large bowel teems with potentially pathogenic bacteria and the peritoneal cavity inevitably becomes contaminated in any operation where large bowel is opened. Pathogenic bacteria are also found in obstructed small bowel. The same applies to the stomach and small bowel of patients on proton-pump inhibitors where the normal bactericidal effect of gastric acid is lost. Great care should be taken at operation to minimise this contamination. Mechanical bowel preparation of the colon along with selective antibiotic decontamination before operation have been shown to help this process. Patients having bowel operations should be given prophylactic antibiotics before operation according to local microbiology guidelines.

Sterilisation of Instruments and Other Supplies (Table 10.1)
In modern surgical practice, infection from instruments, swabs, equipment and intravenous (IV) fluids has been virtually eliminated if sterile packs are available from a central sterile supply department (CSSD). Reusable instruments and drapes are sterilised by high-pressure steam autoclaving according to strict protocols. Most disposable items are purchased in presterilised, sealed packs. Sterilisation in small autoclaves near the operating theatre should only be performed if instruments in short supply are required for successive operations and is not recommended. Sterilisation by any method is ineffective unless all organic material is first removed by thorough cleaning. It is also important to transport soiled instruments promptly to CSSD as proteinaceous material becomes fixed to metal and resistant to removal. This is especially true for small and microsurgical instruments (e.g., in ophthalmology), where channels easily become blocked by organic matter and prevent effective sterilisation.

Instruments which would be damaged by heat, including plastics and electrical equipment, can be sterilised using a range of chemical methods. Ethylene oxide gas is selectively used for items that are moisture and heat sensitive and cannot withstand high temperature or steam sterilisation, however its toxicity and potential hazard to staff (and patients) limits its use.

In processing flexible endoscopes, there should be a one-way flow of used instruments from the procedure room to the clean dispatch area to prevent cross-contamination. Instruments are manually cleaned with detergent, with brushing and flushing before automated endoscope disinfection in an endoscope washer disinfector. Aldehyde- and alcohol-based disinfectants are no longer recommended.

Worldwide, many surgical instruments are prepared by boiling water 'sterilisers'. Boiling water is markedly inferior to other methods but is included here as it may be the only practical method in developing countries because of cost and technical difficulties. Boiling water kills most vegetative organisms within 15 minutes but spores are not killed. All organic debris should, as always, be scrupulously removed first, then the instruments immersed in visibly boiling water, returned to the boil and boiled continuously for at least 30 minutes to ensure hepatitis and HIV are destroyed.

Most bacteria infecting wounds during an operation do so by landing on the laid-out instruments in theatre rather than directly inoculating the wound itself.

Preoperative Preparation

For many elective operations, preoperative screening for methicillin-resistant *Staph. aureus* (MRSA) is commonly used. This involves taking bacterial swabs from the nose, groin and other places. If positive, local antibacterial cream and other measures reduce the risk of MRSA infection for the patient and the risk of cross-infection of other patients.

Surgical Technique

Surgical technique plays an important part in minimising the risk of operative infection. Non-vital tissue and collections of fluid and blood are vulnerable to colonisation by infecting organisms, which may then enter via the bloodstream even if direct contamination has been avoided by aseptic technique. Tissue damage should be kept to a minimum by careful handling and retraction and by avoiding unnecessary diathermy coagulation. Haematoma formation is minimised by careful haemostasis and placing drains into potential sites of fluid collection; **closed-drainage** or **suction-drainage** systems reduce the risk of organisms tracking back into the wound from the ward environment.

During extensive resections of bowel, early ligation of its blood supply allows bacteria to permeate the wall (**translocation**) and this may contaminate the peritoneal cavity. Prolonged operations are a recognised risk factor for postoperative surgical infections.

Faecal contamination is associated with a high risk of infection and great care needs to be taken in operations where the bowel is opened. In emergency operations for large bowel perforation, free faecal matter is meticulously removed. A planned 'second-look' laparotomy after 48 hours can be considered to deal with remaining contamination and new abscesses even if the patient appears well.

Prevention of Cross-Infection (Nosocomial Infection)

Cross-infection is the transfer of harmful bacteria from one person (or object) to another, or from one part of the body to another part. Strict policies on hand-washing, staff dress code being 'bare below the elbow', and universal access to alcoholic hand gel and education of staff and patients has reduced infection rates in hospitals. Cross-infection can still occur and is spread via staff, medical equipment, ward furnishings or rarely food. Doctors and nurses are still offenders as regards to transfer of infection—by removing dressings to inspect wounds in the open ward, by failing to wash hands between patients and by careless aseptic technique when performing ward procedures, such as bladder catheterisation or inserting IV catheters. Minimising patient movements between wards and hospital units also decreases cross-infection rates.

A patient with an infection that is potentially dangerous to other patients, such as MRSA, *Clostridium difficile* or extended spectrum beta-lactamase (ESBL) bacterial infections, should be isolated and barrier-nursed in a single room.

Prophylactic Antibiotics

Despite using the best aseptic techniques, some operations carry a high risk of wound infection as well as other infective complications; these can be reduced by using appropriate prophylactic antibiotics for selected procedures. The chosen antibiotics should be matched to the organisms likely to occur in the area of the operation and should be bactericidal rather than bacteriostatic (Table 10.2). The relative risk of postoperative infection in different types of operation is summarised in Box 10.2.

TABLE 10.2	Examples of Antimicrobial Prophylaxis for Clinical Conditions and Surgical Procedures[a]	
	Likely Organisms	**Antibiotic**
Abdominal Surgery		
Severe acute pancreatitis	Enterobacteriaceae Anaerobes	Co-amoxiclav OR Ciprofloxacin 400 mg IV + metronidazole 500 mg IV
Colonic and other bowel surgery	Enterobacteriaceae Anaerobes *Staphylococcus aureus* *Streptococcus pyogenes* (Group A *Strep.*)	Co-amoxiclav 1.2 g IV
Appendicectomy	Anaerobes	Metronidazole OR co-amoxiclav
Endoscopic gastrostomy Gastroduodenal surgery Oesophageal surgery	Anaerobes *Staph. aureus* *Strep. pyogenes* (Group A *Strep.*) Enterobacteriaceae *Candida* spp.	Co-amoxiclav 1.2 g IV + fluconazole 400 mg IV
Inguinal or other hernia repair with mesh	*Staph. aureus* *Staphylococcus epidermidis* (coagulase-negative) *Strep. pyogenes* (Group A *Strep.*) Enterobacteriaceae	Co-amoxiclav 1.2 g IV
Hernia repair without mesh		Not recommended
Laparoscopic cholecystectomy		Co-amoxiclav (but little clinical evidence of efficacy)

Continued

TABLE 10.2   Examples of Antimicrobial Prophylaxis for Clinical Conditions and Surgical Procedures[a]—cont'd

	Likely Organisms	Antibiotic
Orthopaedic Surgery		
Total hip replacement or prosthetic knee joint	Staph. aureus Staph. epidermidis (coagulase-negative) Strep. pyogenes (Group A Strep.) Enterobacteriaceae	Flucloxacillin three doses plus gentamicin If MRSA risk factors or known MRSA: vancomycin or teicoplanin for two doses
Trauma with contaminated wounds	Staph. aureus Strep. pyogenes (Group A Strep.)	Co-amoxiclav If heavily contaminated or dead tissue, co-amoxiclav 1.2 g IV for 7 days
Elective orthopaedic surgery without prosthetic device		Not recommended
Vascular Surgery		
Lower limb amputation or vascular surgery, abdominal and lower limb	Staph. aureus Staph. epidermidis (coagulase-negative) Strep. pyogenes (Group A Strep.) Enterobacteriaceae	Co-amoxiclav 1.2 g IV If MRSA, **add** vancomycin 1 g or teicoplanin IV
ENT Surgery		
Head and neck surgery	Staph. aureus Strep. pyogenes (Group A Strep.) Enterobacteriaceae Anaerobes	Co-amoxiclav 1.2 g IV If MRSA, **add** vancomycin 1 g IV
Ear, nose, sinus Tonsillectomy		Not recommended
Urology		
Transrectal prostate biopsy Transurethral resection of prostate (TURP) or laser enucleation	Enterobacteriaceae Enterococcus	Ciprofloxacin 500 mg Co-amoxiclav 1.2 g IV + gentamicin 120 mg IV

[a]Please also refer to local microbiology and national guidelines. Note that the antibiotic doses provided are a guide and refer to a normal weight adult with normal renal function. The European Medicines Agency advices restricting use of ciprofloxacin (and other quinolone antibiotics) due to tendon and joint risks.

ENT, Ear, nose and throat; IV, intravenous; MRSA, methicillin-resistant Staphylococcus aureus.

• **BOX 10.2   Relative Risk of Infection in Surgical Wounds**

Risk 2%–5%

Clean operations with no preoperative infection and no opening of gastrointestinal, respiratory or urinary tracts (e.g., inguinal herniorrhaphy, breast lump excision, ligation of varicose veins).

Risk Less Than 10%

Clean operations with gastrointestinal, respiratory or urinary tracts opened but with minimal contamination (e.g., elective cholecystectomy, transurethral prostatectomy excision of un-inflamed appendix).

Risk About 20%

Operations where tissues inevitably become contaminated but without preexisting infection (e.g., elective large bowel operations, appendicectomy where the appendix is perforated or gangrenous, fresh traumatic skin wounds [except on the face]).

Risk Greater Than 30%

Operations in the presence of infection (e.g., abscesses within body cavities, small bowel perforation, delayed operations on traumatic wounds).

Risk Greater Than 50%

Emergency colonic surgery (bowel unprepared) for perforation or obstruction.

As a general principle, pre- or perioperative prophylactic antibiotics are indicated if the anticipated risk of infection exceeds 10%, for example, all emergency abdominal surgery and all elective colonic operations. Prophylactic antibiotics are also used by many surgeons for operations in the 5% to 10% risk category, for example, cholecystectomy. Prophylactic antibiotics are also indicated for inherently low-risk cases where the consequences of infection would be catastrophic, for example, operations using prosthetic implants. Prophylactic antibiotics can reduce postoperative infection rates in high-risk cases by 75%, and may almost entirely eliminate infection where the risk is lower.

In most wound-related infections, the organisms are introduced during the operation and become established during the next 24 hours. Thus for prophylactic antibiotics to be effective, high blood levels must be achieved during the operation when contamination occurs. To achieve this, the first dose should be given within the hour before operation (for IV antibiotics) or within 2 hours for most oral options; prophylactic antibiotics should not be given earlier as this can encourage resistant organisms to proliferate (Box 10.3). A single preoperative dose of antibiotic is generally sufficient, if it is rapidly bactericidal and the inoculum of bacteria is small; long operations with heavy blood loss, for example, ruptured abdominal aortic aneurysm, merit a second perioperative dose of antibiotics later in the operation. Longer courses of prophylactic antibiotics are of no advantage.

In general, IV antibiotics give the most predictable blood levels and peak tissue levels are achieved within 1 hour of injection. However, for prophylaxis against anaerobes, metronidazole administered rectally gives blood and tissue levels equivalent to IV administration but later, 2 to 4 hours after administration.

Operations Involving Bowel and Biliary System. Patients having these operations are at risk mainly from a mixture of gram-negative bacilli (Enterobacteriaceae family), anaerobes (*Bacteroides fragilis*) and *Staph. aureus*. Less commonly, enterococci cause surgical infection, notably *Enterococcus faecalis* and *Enterococcus faecium*.

The most commonly used prophylactic antibiotic regimens are shown below. A more comprehensive list is given in Table 10.2:

- For biliary surgery—co-amoxiclav.
- For colonic and other bowel surgery—either co-amoxiclav or a combination of gentamicin, benzylpenicillin and metronidazole.
- For appendicectomy—rectal metronidazole alone can be given 2 hours before operation; this has proved as effective as any other regimen.

The choice of antibiotics for prophylaxis must be kept under review because organisms change their sensitivities. Aminoglycosides such as gentamicin have the important advantage that they do not alter the bowel flora because their concentration in the lumen is low; this is in contrast to the cephalosporins and amoxicillin, which have caused a rising tide of beta-lactam–resistant bowel organisms insensitive to cephalosporins and ampicillin but susceptible to aminoglycosides. If MRSA is a problem, vancomycin or teicoplanin may become necessary for prophylaxis.

Operations Involving Implantation of Prostheses. Vascular grafts and joint replacements are at particular risk from *Staph. aureus* infection. Coagulase-negative slime-forming staphylococci (e.g., *Staphylococcus epidermidis*) are a common source of chronic infection. Enterobacteriaceae are a very rare cause. Flucloxacillin is the agent of first choice for prophylaxis but gentamicin is usually added for extra protection. MRSA is becoming a common cause of prosthetic infection. In areas where the risk is substantial, prophylaxis with a glycopeptide (e.g., vancomycin or teicoplanin) is appropriate. Some implants such as Dacron grafts are impregnated with anti-bacterial agents.

Operations Where Ischaemic or Necrotic Muscle May Remain. Lower limb amputations for arterial insufficiency and major traumatic injuries involving muscle are susceptible to gas gangrene and tetanus. **Clostridia** are highly susceptible to benzylpenicillin and metronidazole, one of which should be given in high dose as early as possible after major trauma, and before major amputations for ischaemia. Co-amoxiclav is an alternative.

Basic Surgical Techniques

Anaesthesia

General Principles

Some form of anaesthesia is needed for almost every surgical procedure, with the aim of preventing pain in all cases, minimising stress for the patient in most, and providing special conditions for some operations, for example, muscular relaxation in abdominal surgery. The choice of anaesthetic techniques includes **topical (surface) anaesthesia, local anaesthetic infiltration** or **peripheral nerve block, spinal** or **epidural anaesthesia** and **general anaesthesia**. Methods other than general anaesthesia may be supplemented with IV sedation if the patient is anxious or agitated (e.g., with benzodiazepines). IV sedation with these drugs produces relaxation, anxiolysis and amnesia, whilst retaining protective reflexes. However, these drugs can also cause unconsciousness and they must be carefully titrated to produce just the desired effects. IV sedation of this type does not provide pain relief; if needed, this is achieved with local anaesthesia or IV analgesics.

Choice of Anaesthetic Technique

Combining local or regional anaesthesia (for pain relief) with general anaesthesia can minimise postoperative respiratory and cardiovascular depression compared with general anaesthesia alone, reducing morbidity. An example is the use of caudal anaesthesia in perineal operations. Local or regional anaesthesia with bupivacaine or levobupivacaine can also be administered during an operation to provide postoperative pain relief; for example, intercostal nerve blocks during an abdominal operation allow more comfortable breathing and coughing, reducing respiratory complications. Another common example is wound infiltration with the same long-acting local anaesthetics. The main factors influencing choice of anaesthesia are summarised in Box 10.4.

Incision Technique

Choice of Incision

The purpose of most skin incisions is to gain access to underlying tissues or body cavities. When planning an incision, the first concern is to achieve good access and to allow it to be extended if necessary. It must also be sited in such a way that it can be effectively closed to give the best chance of primary healing and the lowest chance of an incisional hernia later. Despite patients' impressions, the length of an incision (and the number of sutures) has little bearing on the rate of healing, and the success of an operation should not be put at risk by inadequate access.

Secondary considerations in the choice of incision are as follows:

- **Orientation of skin tension lines (based on Langer lines) and skin creases**—where possible, incisions should be made parallel to the lines of skin tension determined by the orientation of dermal collagen (e.g., a 'collar' incision for thyroid operations) as the wound is less likely to break down, there is minimal distortion, and healing occurs with little scar tissue to give the best cosmetic result
- **Strength and healing potential of the tissues**—the nature and distribution of muscle and fascia influences the strength of the repair, particularly in different parts of the abdominal wall. For example, a vertical lower midline incision along the linea alba, a strong layer of fascia, is less prone to incisional herniation than a paramedian incision, lateral to the midline
- **The anatomy of underlying structures, particularly nerves**—the incision line should run parallel to, but some distance away from the expected course of underlying structures, reducing the risk of damage. For example, to gain access to the submandibular gland, the incision is made 2 cm below the lower border of the mandible, to avoid the mandibular branch of the facial nerve

• BOX 10.4   Choice of Anaesthetic Technique

1. Local Anaesthesia

In general, this safest form of anaesthesia is used for calm and rational patients when no autonomic discomfort is anticipated:

- Minor operations, for example, excision of small skin lesions or dental operations.
- Minor but painful procedures, for example, insertion of chest drain, siting of peripheral venous cannulae.
- Unavailability of general anaesthetic expertise, for example, in developing countries.
- Patients unfit for general anaesthesia, for example, cardiac and respiratory cripples.
- Ambulatory ('day case') surgery especially if comorbidity.
- Patients unwilling to undergo general anaesthesia.
- Use of combined local anaesthetic and vasoconstrictor to provide a relatively bloodless operative field. (Note: this must never be used in the extreme peripheries, i.e., digits, penis, nose.)

2. Regional Nerve Block

- Minor surgery requiring wide field of anaesthesia, for example, femoral nerve block for varicose vein surgery, pudendal block for forceps delivery.
- When it is undesirable to inject local anaesthetic into the operation site, for example, drainage of an abscess (local anaesthesia works less well in inflamed tissue).
- To avoid tissue distortion from local infiltration in delicate surgery.
- Short-lived, wide-field ambulatory anaesthesia for reduction of forearm fractures or hand surgery (Bier intravenous regional anaesthesia).

3. Epidural and Spinal Anaesthesia

- Lower limb surgery, for example, amputations.
- Lower abdominal, groin, pelvic and perineal surgery, for example, Caesarean sections, inguinal hernia repair, transurethral prostatectomy, bladder and urethral surgery.

4. Intravenous sedation or intravenous analgesia alone

- Short-lived uncomfortable procedures where local anaesthesia is impractical, for example, gastrointestinal endoscopy, musculoskeletal manipulation.

5. Intravenous Sedation Combined With Local Anaesthesia

- Potentially unpleasant procedures despite adequate local anaesthesia, for example, wisdom tooth extraction, toenail operations, siting of central venous lines.

6. Regional Analgesia With Light General Anaesthesia

- Caudal epidural plus general anaesthesia for operations in the perineal area, for example, transurethral prostatectomy or resection of bladder tumours, haemorrhoidectomy, circumcision. This provides perioperative and postoperative analgesia.

7. General Anaesthesia

- Where all aforementioned are unsuitable or difficult to achieve.
- Severe patient apprehension or patient preference for general anaesthesia.
- Major or prolonged operations.
- Abdominal or thoracic operations requiring muscle relaxation.
- Where it is necessary to secure the airway by intubation.
- Special indications, for example, neurosurgery.

- **Cosmetic considerations**—wherever possible, incisions should be placed in the least conspicuous position, such as in a skin crease or a site that will later be concealed by clothing or hair, for example, a transverse suprapubic (**Pfannenstiel** or bucket-handle) incision below the 'bikini' line for operations on the bladder, uterus or ovary, or a periareolar incision for breast biopsy

Dissection and Handling of Deeper Tissues

The skin consists of thin **epidermis** and dense, somewhat thicker **dermis,** as well as the underlying fatty **hypodermis,** which may be 10 or more cm thick in an obese individual.

Once the skin incision has been made, the scalpel is reserved mainly for incising fascia and other fibrous structures, such as breast tissue, and for very fine dissection. Anatomic detail is exposed and displayed by a combination of blunt and sharp dissection. **Blunt dissection** involves teasing or stripping tissues apart using fingers, swabs or blunt instruments, following natural tissue planes. **Sharp dissection** with scissors and forceps or scalpel is used where tissues have to be cut and also to display small structures. Some surgeons prefer sharp to blunt dissection in general, believing it causes less tissue trauma. Most dissection, however, involves a combination of both.

Principles of Haemostasis

Bleeding is an unavoidable part of surgery. Blood loss should be minimised because bleeding obscures the operative field and hampers operative technique (the finer the surgery, the more bleeding affects visibility and quality of outcome), and because the loss has to be made up later. Excessive bleeding can be averted by judicious dissection with control of bleeding as the operation proceeds, and by minimising the area of raw tissue exposed at the operation site by accurately siting the incision and by avoiding opening unnecessary tissue planes.

Clipping, Ligation and Underrunning

Ligation or specialised bipolar diathermy is obligatory when large vessels are divided and is desirable for vessels larger than about 1 mm calibre (Fig. 10.1). If the end of a bleeding vessel cannot be grasped by haemostat forceps, a suture can be used to encircle the vessel and its surrounding tissues, a technique often described as **underrunning**. It is particularly useful for a bleeding artery in the fibrous base of a peptic ulcer.

Diathermy

Diathermy achieves haemostasis by local intravascular coagulation and contraction of the vessel wall caused by heating (-*thermy*), generated by particular electrical waveforms. However, enough heat is also produced to burn the tissues and these may be needlessly damaged by careless use, particularly near the skin, nerves or bowel. Ordinary diathermy is ineffective for large vessels, which should be ligated. There are three main variants of diathermy, illustrated in Fig. 10.2, and all three modes are available on modern diathermy machines.

Monopolar diathermy is the most widely used for operative haemostasis but there is wide dispersion of coagulating and heating effects, making it unsuitable for use near nerves and other delicate structures. Since the current passes through the patient's body, there is a risk of coagulating vessels *en passant* (e.g., monopolar diathermy used in circumcision may cause penile thrombosis and therefore it is essential that only bipolar diathermy is used on the penis), as well as provoking arrhythmias in patients with cardiac pacemakers. Monopolar diathermy may also result in skin burns at the **indifferent electrode plate** if skin contact is poor or if the plate becomes wet during operation. To improve contact, hair should be shaved from the skin where the plate is placed.

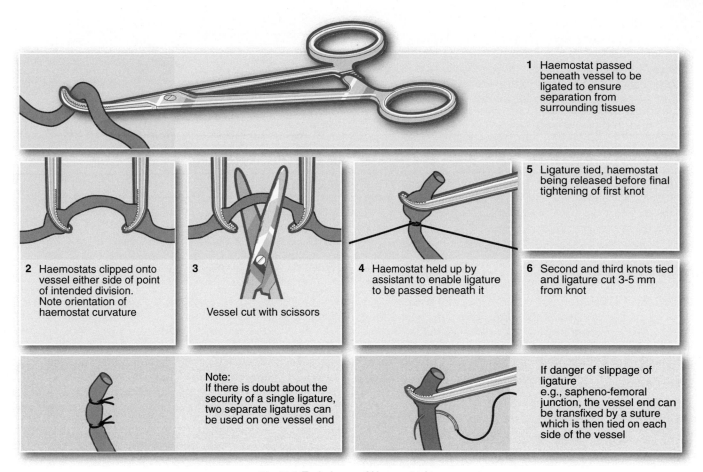

1 Haemostat passed beneath vessel to be ligated to ensure separation from surrounding tissues

2 Haemostats clipped onto vessel either side of point of intended division. Note orientation of haemostat curvature

3 Vessel cut with scissors

4 Haemostat held up by assistant to enable ligature to be passed beneath it

5 Ligature tied, haemostat being released before final tightening of first knot

6 Second and third knots tied and ligature cut 3-5 mm from knot

Note:
If there is doubt about the security of a single ligature, two separate ligatures can be used on one vessel end

If danger of slippage of ligature e.g., sapheno-femoral junction, the vessel end can be transfixed by a suture which is then tied on each side of the vessel

• **Fig. 10.1** Techniques of Haemostasis.

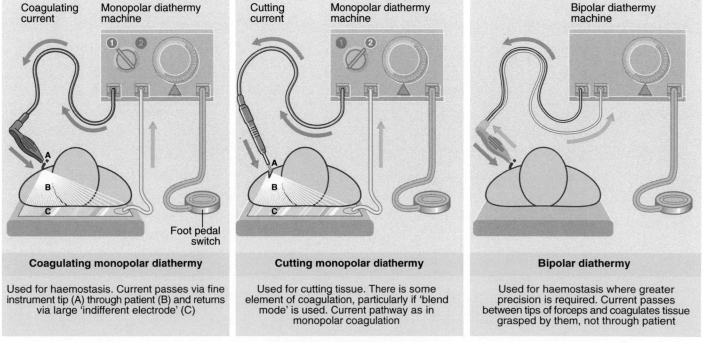

Coagulating current   Monopolar diathermy machine

Cutting current   Monopolar diathermy machine

Bipolar diathermy machine

Foot pedal switch

Coagulating monopolar diathermy

Used for haemostasis. Current passes via fine instrument tip (A) through patient (B) and returns via large 'indifferent electrode' (C)

Cutting monopolar diathermy

Used for cutting tissue. There is some element of coagulation, particularly if 'blend mode' is used. Current pathway as in monopolar coagulation

Bipolar diathermy

Used for haemostasis where greater precision is required. Current passes between tips of forceps and coagulates tissue grasped by them, not through patient

• **Fig. 10.2** Three Modes of Diathermy.

Bipolar diathermy is used mainly for finer surgery, digits and the penis. The current passes only between the blades of the forceps and it requires fairly accurate grasping of the bleeding vessel. It uses low levels of electrical power, there is almost no electrical dispersion from the tip of the forceps and much less heat is generated. The main advantages are minimal tissue damage around the point of coagulation and safety in relation to nearby nerves, blood vessels and cardiac pacemakers. Specialised computer-controlled bipolar diathermy is often used for larger vessels during laparoscopic surgery.

Cutting diathermy is mainly used for dividing large masses of muscle (e.g., during thoracotomy or access to the hip joint) and cutting vascular tissues (e.g., breast). The intention is a form of sharp dissection, at the same time coagulating the numerous small blood vessels as the tissue is cut; unfortunately, this is not always wholly effective. A blend of cutting and coagulation is sometimes used.

Tourniquet and Exsanguination

This technique is used in surgery of the limbs and hands where a bloodless field is desirable. For the whole limb, a pneumatic tourniquet is placed proximally. The limb is exsanguinated by elevation and spiral application of a rubber bandage (Esmark) or a ring exsanguinator from the periphery; the tourniquet is then inflated. Upper limb tourniquets must not be left inflated for more than 30 minutes and lower limb tourniquets for more than about 1 hour to avoid the risk of necrosis.

Pressure

Pressure is a useful means of controlling bleeding until platelet aggregation, reactive vasoconstriction and blood coagulation take over. It can be used for emergency temporary control of severe arterial or venous bleeding, but is equally useful for controlling diffuse small-vessel bleeding from a raw area, for example, liver bed after cholecystectomy. Pressure is usually applied with gauze swabs which must be kept in position for at least 10 minutes by the clock. Even if bleeding is not arrested completely, this process usually allows a clearer view and facilitates haemostasis by standard means.

For intractable bleeding which is not amenable to ligature, diathermy or suture, various resorbable packing materials, for example, oxidised cellulose, can be left in position until haemostasis occurs, allowing the wound to be closed. If bleeding simply cannot be controlled—for example, after liver injury—the bleeding cavity can be packed with gauze swabs which are left in situ and removed 48 to 72 hours later at a further operation. Bleeding, once controlled by this method, rarely recurs.

When a raw cavity has been created beneath the skin, external pressure dressings are sometimes a useful method of controlling potential superficial postoperative oozing and minimising haematoma formation.

Suturing and Surgical Repair

Types of Suture Material and Needles

Numerous types of suture are available (Box 10.5), with the most important distinction being between **absorbable** and **non absorbable** materials. The groups can be subdivided into **natural** and **synthetic** materials (although natural materials are being phased out) and further subdivided into **monofilament** and **polyfilament** (braided) materials. The choice of suture material depends upon the task at hand, the handling qualities and personal preference.

• BOX 10.5 Suture Materials and Their Characteristics

Typical brand names are given in parentheses

Absorbable
- Plain catgut—natural monofilament (no longer used)
- Chromic catgut—natural monofilament (no longer used)
- Polyglycolic acid-synthetic braided (Dexon)
- Polyglactin—synthetic braided (Vicryl)
- Polydioxanone—synthetic monofilament (PDS, Maxon)

Nonabsorbable
- Silk—natural braided
- Linen—natural braided (no longer used)
- Stainless steel wire—monofilament or braided
- Nylon—synthetic, usually monofilament (Ethilon)
- Polyester—synthetic braided (Ti-cron, and others)
- Polypropylene—synthetic monofilament (Prolene)
- Polytetrafluoroethylene (PTFE)—synthetic 'expanded' monofilament (Goretex)

Absorbable Versus Nonabsorbable Materials

The strength of absorbable sutures declines at a predictable rate for each type of material, although the suture material remains in the wound long after it has any useful ability to hold tissues together.

In increasing duration of useful strength, the main absorbable materials are:
- Plain catgut and chromic catgut—useful strength 3 and 5 days, respectively (no longer available in many countries).
- Modified polyglactin (e.g., Vicryl Rapide)—useful strength about 6 days.
- Polyglycolic acid (Dexon) and polyglactin (Vicryl)—useful strength about 10 days.
- Poliglecaprone 25 (Monocryl)—useful strength about 20 days.
- Polydioxanone (PDS)—retains its strength for at least 28 days.

The eventual elimination of absorbable materials from the body overcomes the problem of a permanent foreign body which can harbour infection. Absorbable sutures are often used in skin to avoid the need for removal. Polyglycolic acid/polyglactin (undyed) gives good results as the sutures are removed by hydrolysis without inflammation. The modified short-lived polyglactin has ideal properties for skin closure where short suture life is required, for example, inguinal hernia repair, and the monofilament poliglecaprone 25 (Monocryl) is ideal for situations when longer wound support is required.

Non absorbable sutures retain most of their strength indefinitely. They are used where the repaired tissues take a long time to reach full strength (e.g., abdominal wall closure) or will be inherently weak (e.g., inguinal and incisional hernia repairs, arterial anastomoses). Nonabsorbable sutures are also used for skin closure; synthetic monofilament sutures give reasonable cosmetic results and are easily and painlessly removed. Subcuticular sutures, which do not penetrate the epidermis, give excellent cosmetic results.

Natural Versus Synthetic Materials

Catgut has been used as a suture and ligature material since before Roman times, derived from the material used for musical instrument strings. It consists mainly of collagen and is actually made from the dried small bowel submucosa of sheep or cattle. Whilst popular in the recent past, this is no longer in clinical use. Silk and linen also have a long and distinguished history. Many surgeons believe that silk has the best handling and knotting properties of any material, but it provokes a strong inflammatory response exceeded only by linen. Silk is still used for skin sutures to secure drains (in the form of Mersilk braided silk suture), but sutures should be removed after 1 to 2 weeks to avoid skin irritation. Increasingly, nylon is used to secure drains to avoid irritation. Linen suture is not in clinical use. In general, natural materials are cheaper than synthetics, a factor of importance in developing countries.

The main advantages of synthetic absorbable suture materials are that they are stronger and provoke little or no inflammatory reaction. There is no risk of biological contamination with prions or viruses and they can be designed to meet specific requirements of absorbability, period of strength retention and handling properties.

Non absorbable synthetic materials, similarly, do not provoke inflammatory reactions. Polyesters, nylon and polypropylene all retain virtually all of their strength over long periods in the tissues; this is particularly important when they are used to suture arterial prostheses where healing alone would not retain the prosthesis, and for rectus sheath closure after laparotomy.

Monofilament Versus Polyfilament Sutures

Monofilament materials have a smooth surface and can be pulled through the tissues with minimal friction; this makes them easier to insert and remove than polyfilament braided materials. On the other hand, monofilament materials are stiff, springy and more difficult to knot. Braided materials have the best handling qualities, but their interstices are a haven for bacteria. When used at a surface (e.g., skin or bowel wall) they tend to act as a 'wick', drawing infected material in. This problem is partly overcome by the manufacturers' application of surface coatings.

Wire Sutures

Metal wire sutures have largely been displaced by nonabsorbable synthetics. Stainless steel wire is, however, extensively used in orthopaedic surgery for bone fixation and sometimes for closure of sternotomy wounds in cardiac surgery. It is virtually inert but its main disadvantages are high rates of glove penetration and late breakage because of metal fatigue.

Gauge of Suture Material

The gauge of suture chosen for a particular task depends largely on practical experience. This takes into account the following factors:
- strength of repair required;
- number of sutures to be placed—the greater the number, the finer can be the gauge;
- type of suture material used—for a given gauge, the various materials have different strengths;
- cosmetic requirements—multiple fine sutures give a better cosmetic result than fewer heavier sutures.

The traditional method of describing suture gauge (US Pharmacopoeia) is confusing for the newcomer and derives from the time when sutures were much thicker than those used today. The finest suture then was designated gauge 1, with gauge 2 and upwards applying to heavier sutures. As finer and finer sutures came into use, the scale had to be taken progressively backwards from 1, that is, gauges 0, 00 (i.e., 2/0), 000 (3/0) and so on. Nowadays, the finest suture is 11/0, used for extremely delicate surgery, such as in the eye. A more rational metric gauge, based on suture diameter, is in use but the traditional gauge is still widely used. A simple guide to the use of different gauges is outlined in Box 10.6.

> **● BOX 10.6** **Guide to Suture Gauges for Common Procedures**

Skin
- Face 5/0 or 6/0
- Hands and limbs 3/0 or 4/0
- Elsewhere 2/0 or 3/0

Abdominal Wall
- Two strands of gauge 0 ('loop nylon'), gauge 1 or gauge 2

Gut anastomoses
- 2/0 or 3/0

Arterial Anastomoses
- 2/0 down to 7/0 according to size of vessel

Microsurgery (e.g., eyes, microvascular, nerve repair)
- 7/0 down to as fine as 11/0

> **● BOX 10.7** **Types of Suture Needle**

1. Method of Use
- Hand-held needles—routine for skin suturing; sometimes used for abdominal wall closure. Less common nowadays because of needle-stick risks
- Instrument-held needles—necessary for deeper access and fine control

2. Shape of Needle
- Straight—skin suturing
- Curved—half-circle used for most purposes, quarter-circle for microvascular anastomoses, three-quarter-circle for hand closure of abdominal wall

3. Length of Needle
- Range from 2 to 60 mm—according to depth of penetration and delicacy of surgery

4. Tissue Penetration Characteristics
- Round-bodied with smooth pointed tip—most soft tissues, for example, gut, fat, muscle
- Trocar point (semi-cutting)—moderately tough tissues, for example, atherosclerotic arteries, fascia
- Cutting point—tough tissues, for example, skin, breast tissue

5. Means of Attachment of Suture to Needle
- Needles with an eye requiring suture material to be threaded by hand—mainly used in developing countries so that needles can be reused
- 'Atraumatic' needles with suture material already attached (swaged into the end)—this avoids a double thickness of suture material to cause extra drag and trauma as it is pulled through the tissues, and the suture material does not detach from the needle during use

---

Types of Suture Needle

Vast ranges of needles have been designed to accommodate the breadth of different demands of general and specialist surgery and the stringent requirements of microsurgery. Characteristics of needles and broad indications for their use are summarised in Box 10.7 and illustrated in Fig. 10.3.

Methods of Skin Suturing

The objective of skin suturing is to approximate the cut edges so they will heal rapidly, leaving a minimal scar. Edges to be apposed

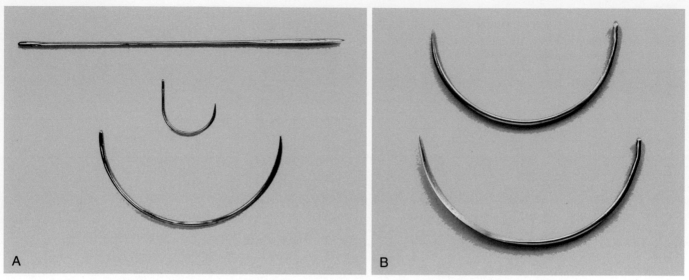

• **Fig. 10.3** Various Types of Surgical Needles. (A) Three shapes of needle. The straight needle has a cutting point and is used for skin suturing. The J-shaped needle is used mainly for femoral hernia repairs, and the large half-circle needle is for abdominal wall closure. (B) Two large needles showing the difference between 'round-bodied' (above) and 'cutting' ends (below).

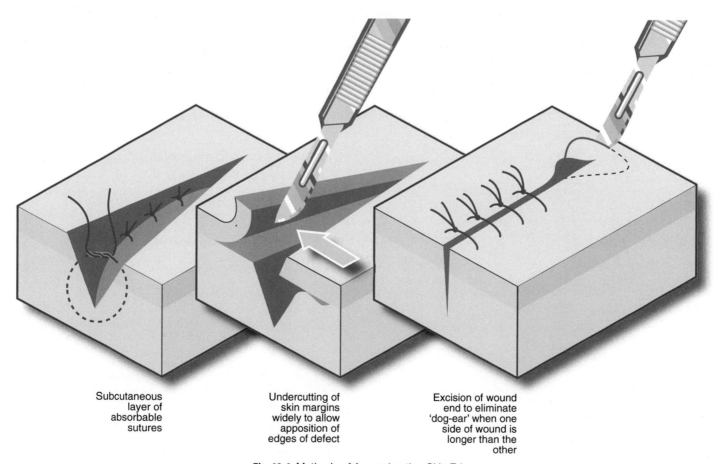

Subcutaneous layer of absorbable sutures

Undercutting of skin margins widely to allow apposition of edges of defect

Excision of wound end to eliminate 'dog-ear' when one side of wound is longer than the other

• **Fig. 10.4** Methods of Approximating Skin Edges.

should have been cut in a clean line and perpendicular to the skin surface; ragged or angled edges should be trimmed. The cut edges should be capable of being brought together neatly and without tension; otherwise the wound may break down or the scar slowly stretch, giving an ugly result. To achieve this, it may be necessary to insert a layer of subcutaneous sutures or even mobilise the skin by undercutting in the fatty layer (Fig. 10.4). Undue laxity should also be avoided by trimming excess skin.

There are many techniques of skin closure, the choice being governed by the nature and site of the operation and by the surgeon's

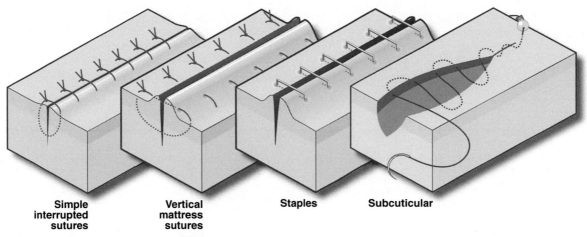

Simple
interrupted
sutures

Vertical
mattress
sutures

Staples

Subcuticular

• **Fig. 10.5** Commonly Used Skin Closure Techniques.

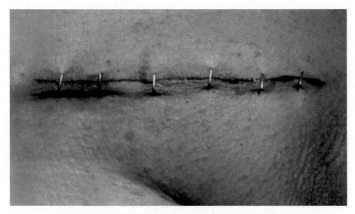

• **Fig. 10.6** Inguinal Hernia Wound Closed With Staples.

preference. In general, facial wounds are closed with multiple fine sutures removed after 4 or 5 days. Abdominal and chest wound sutures are generally removed after 7 days, while sutures for wounds on the back are best left for 14 days to minimise wound stretching.

Subcuticular sutures, either nonabsorbable or absorbable, are often used for longer wounds in cosmetically sensitive areas, provided the risk of infection is low. Elsewhere, the choice is between interrupted and continuous suture techniques. Interrupted sutures are indicated if there is a risk of infection; if infection develops, some sutures can be removed early to facilitate drainage. If the risk of infection is high, for example, large bowel perforation, skin wounds are better left open and closed 48 to 72 hours later by **delayed primary closure.** The commonly used methods of skin suturing are illustrated in Fig. 10.5.

Staples and Other Wound Closure Techniques

Staples are used for both skin closure and bowel surgery. The skin closure devices are similar in concept to ordinary paper staplers, with staples stored in a magazine and applied singly instead of sutures (Fig. 10.6). More complex devices, which apply multiple staples simultaneously, either in a linear or circular fashion, are available for bowel anastomoses and closure of tubular viscera. Some devices have revolutionised surgical practice, for example, reanastomosis of colon to rectum after Hartmann's resection or bronchial stump closure. When used for internal viscera, the staples remain in place indefinitely.

Skin glue (e.g., Dermabond) is a suitable alternative for shallow wounds without tension, particularly in children. Steristrips

('paper stitches') can be used in a similar way, but may not adhere in moist or mobile wounds, such as in the palm or around the mouth.

Postoperative Wound Management

Once a wound has been closed, the doctor has three main responsibilities: choosing the dressing, monitoring the progress of healing and deciding when to remove the sutures.

The purposes of dressings for surgical wounds are as follows:
- To maintain the wound in a warm and moist state most conducive to healing.
- To absorb or contain any superficial bleeding or inflammatory exudate.
- To protect the delicate healing tissue from trauma, bacterial contamination and interference.
- To prevent sutures catching on clothing or other objects.
- To conceal the wound from view.
- To apply pressure to the wound if haematoma formation is likely.

Types of Wound Dressing

For small surgical wounds, particularly on the face, a dressing is often unnecessary as the linear crust of inflammatory exudate performs this task very well. For other simple wounds, plastic spray dressing is suitable, for example, Opsite. In most other cases, **prepacked adhesive dressings** are used, incorporating an absorbent pad with nonstick film in contact with the wound surface. While convenient, these dressings may conceal accumulations of blood, inflammatory exudate or infected discharge. Wound inspection then requires painful removal of the dressing which can be an opportunity for infection to enter. Transparent **semipermeable plastic film dressings** neatly overcome this problem but are unsuitable for discharging wounds.

A flexible polyamide net coated with soft silicone (e.g., Mepitel) is useful for covering raw areas. This has very low wound adherence and is usually easy to remove. Other dressings include **calcium alginate** (seaweed origin), **hydrocolloids** and **hydrogels**. These dressings offer a better wound environment with increased hydration, fewer dressing changes, easier dressing removal and greater comfort.

Gamgee is a thick cotton wool dressing material enveloped in a thin layer of gauze; this is variously used for padding sites vulnerable to trauma (e.g., amputation stumps) or as pads beneath pressure bandages or as absorbent dressings for leaking wounds. **Dry dressings** are wads of dressing material (e.g., cotton gauze), usually taped or bandaged in place. Dry dressings need regular replacement and may be prevented from sticking by placing a piece of nonadherent dressing (e.g., Melolin, N/A dressing) against the wound.

Removal of Dressings and Sutures

Provided the dressing remains clean and dry and the patient afebrile and generally well, there is no need to inspect clean surgical wounds until the time of suture removal. If wound complications are suspected, the dressing should be removed and the wound checked and redressed. If infection is evident, a wound swab should be taken for culture and sensitivity. Localised abscess formation requires suture removal and probing to effect drainage, whilst spreading cellulitis requires systemic antibiotic therapy in addition.

Skin sutures (nonabsorbable) should be removed as soon as the wound is strong enough to remain intact without support. On the back and around joints, this can take 14 days; on the abdomen, it takes about 7 days (longer in the case of steroid therapy or infection). On the face and neck, healing is rapid and less influenced by functional stresses. Here, sutures can be safely removed after 3 to 5 days, giving a better cosmetic result.

Management of Drains in the Postoperative Period

Abdominal drains provide a potential route for infection to enter, even though the intraabdominal pressure nearly always exceeds external pressure. The risk can be minimised by ensuring the drain opens into a sterile environment, such as a drainage bag (**closed drainage**) and by removing the drain as soon as its task is completed. Decisions about removal of drains should rest with the operating surgeon who will undoubtedly have personal preferences.

The general principles of drain management are as follows:
- Suction drains help to collapse spaces left in the tissues at operation as well as to drain blood and inflammatory exudate. These are mainly used after extensive surgery where a large covered raw surface remains, for example, after mastectomy, thyroidectomy or large incisional hernia repair. Suction drains should not be used near bowel for fear of suction perforation. A suction drain is usually retained for only 24 hours unless substantial drainage persists (e.g., >30 mL/24 h).
- Non suction drains (e.g., large-bore silicone or rubber tubes or corrugated drains) are mainly used for bowel and biliary anastomoses and for abscess drainage. In this case, the drain is left in place for about 5 days. Some surgeons prefer to withdraw the drain in stages so that the deep part of the drainage tract can collapse progressively, reducing the risk of leaving a deep pool of fluid

Soft Tissue Surgery

Methods of Obtaining Tissue for Diagnosis

Open or Endoscopic Biopsy

If major surgery or other therapy is being considered for a suspected malignant lesion, an accurate **tissue diagnosis** should be made.

Skin lesions can be **biopsied** by incision under local anaesthesia. Rectal lesions can be biopsied without anaesthesia using forceps through a rigid or flexible sigmoidoscope or colonoscope, while gastric and colonic lesions can be biopsied via a flexible endoscope. Breast lumps or suspicious mammographic lesions can be sampled using percutaneous core needle biopsy or by fine needle aspiration cytology (see later). Gastroscopy allows biopsy of upper gastrointestinal (GI) mucosal lesions, as well as lesions of the pancreatic head transmurally.

Enlarged lymph nodes can often be diagnosed by **incision biopsy** or by removing one or more completely for histological examination (**excision biopsy**), although many units can now obtain satisfactory results by needle biopsy. Lymphadenectomy often requires general anaesthesia, particularly for lumps in the neck.

Biopsy Guided by Ultrasound or Computed Tomography Scanning

Abdominal masses, such as liver metastases, or pancreatic and renal lesions can be biopsied percutaneously with the aid of ultrasound or computed tomography (CT) scanning. The suspicious lesion is first located as an image and then a biopsy needle is guided into it with the help of further imaging. The technique can be used to sample abdominal masses or suspicious paraaortic lymph nodes in staging lymphomas or following treatment for testicular germ cell tumours.

Cytology

Special staining techniques for malignant cells can be applied to material obtained by fine needle aspiration. Cytological diagnosis requires particular laboratory skills but often permits accurate diagnosis (e.g., of malignancy), which renders more invasive investigations unnecessary. A negative cytological result, however, must be interpreted with great caution because it may be caused by sampling error.

Cytological diagnosis can be useful for the following:
- Examining cells aspirated from solid masses. This is particularly useful for thyroid nodules (see Ch. 5, p. 66 and Ch. 49), breast lumps, mammographically detected lesions and pancreatic masses.
- Examining ascitic fluid obtained from the abdomen by **paracentesis**, or pleural effusions aspirated from the chest. Fluid may also be sent for microbiological analysis.
- Examining cellular material scraped from surfaces, for example, uterine cervical smears, or fluid obtained from within hollow viscera, for example, urine, pancreatic secretions, sputum.

Microbiology

Infective causes of lesions should be considered before biopsy or aspiration is attempted so an appropriate sample can be sent (i.e., not fixed in formalin). Tuberculosis, for example, mimics many 'tumours' and culture (with sensitivity testing) can be very helpful for clinical and public health reasons.

'Minor' Operative Procedures

Many skin lesions are amenable to simple excision or biopsy, often under local anaesthesia. These may be performed in general practice or in dermatological or surgical clinics. Aseptic technique must be used.

Local Anaesthesia for Skin Lesions

The usual method of administration is by infiltration (injection) of local anaesthetic agents (e.g., lidocaine 0.5% or 1%) into the skin surrounding the lesion. Between 1 and 10 mL of solution is usually required, but care must be taken to remain within maximum safe dosages (Table 10.3). A vasoconstrictor (e.g., adrenaline [epinephrine] 1 in 200,000) may be incorporated to reduce vascularity in the operative field, but this must **never** be used on the extreme peripheries, that is, fingers, toes, penis or nose, because of the risk of ischaemic necrosis. The injecting needle should be as fine as possible and inserted into the skin as few times as possible to avoid causing unnecessary pain. Before each injection, aspiration is attempted to ensure that the solution is not injected directly into a blood vessel as intravascular injection may cause systemic toxicity. Methods of infiltration of local anaesthetic are illustrated in Fig. 10.7.

Biopsy Techniques

Excision Biopsy

The technique of excision skin or mucosal biopsy illustrated in Fig. 10.8 is appropriate for most small lesions not thought to be malignant. The lesion is removed with a fusiform piece of normal skin, with the long axis orientated along skin creases and tension lines. The specimen should include a millimetre or two of normal skin on either side of the lesion and should include the full depth of the dermis down to the subcutaneous fat. For small round lesions, a circular biopsy punch aids neat excision.

Incision Biopsy

Incision biopsy is a technique of obtaining a tissue sample from a lesion that is too large or anatomically unsuitable for excision biopsy, for example, a skin rash or a suspected malignant tumour.

TABLE 10.3	Maximum Safe Doses of Local Anaesthetic Agents for Infiltration in Fit Patients	
Lidocaine	**Bupivacaine (Marcain) or Levobupivacaine (Chirocaine)**	
2% lidocaine is probably no more effective for achieving anaesthesia than 1% or even 0.5%, so use lowest concentration needed; 10 mL of 1% lidocaine contains 100 mg	0.5% bupivacaine is probably no more effective than 0.25%; 10 mL of 0.5% bupivacaine contains 50 mg	
The maximum safe dose of **plain lidocaine** is 4 mg/kg body weight	The maximum safe dose of **plain bupivacaine** is 2 mg/kg body weight	
For a fit 60 kg adult, the maximum safe dose of 1% plain lidocaine is 16–24 mL	For a fit 60 kg adult, the maximum safe dose of 0.5% bupivacaine is 24 mL	
With adrenaline (epinephrine), this dose can be increased to 7 mg/kg body weight	Addition of adrenaline (epinephrine) does **not** increase the safe dose of bupivacaine and there is little point in using it for infiltration except to provide vasoconstriction	
For a fit 60 kg adult, the maximum safe dose of 1% lidocaine with *adrenaline (epinephrine)* is 30–40 mL	No increase	

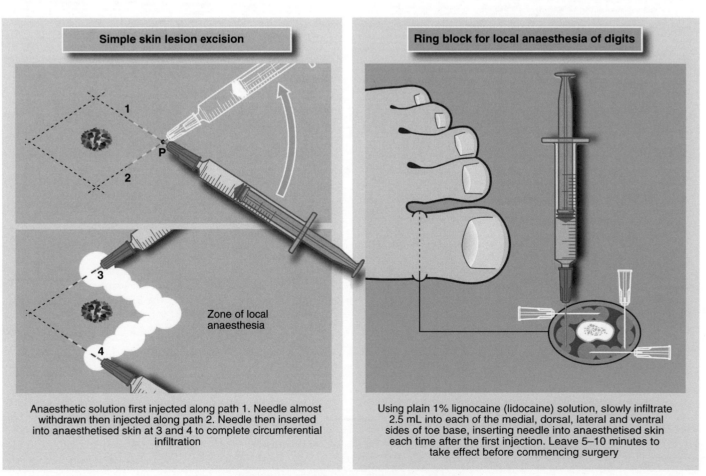

Simple skin lesion excision

Anaesthetic solution first injected along path 1. Needle almost withdrawn then injected along path 2. Needle then inserted into anaesthetised skin at 3 and 4 to complete circumferential infiltration

Zone of local anaesthesia

Ring block for local anaesthesia of digits

Using plain 1% lignocaine (lidocaine) solution, slowly infiltrate 2.5 mL into each of the medial, dorsal, lateral and ventral sides of toe base, inserting needle into anaesthetised skin each time after the first injection. Leave 5–10 minutes to take effect before commencing surgery

• **Fig. 10.7** Local Anaesthetic Infiltration Techniques.

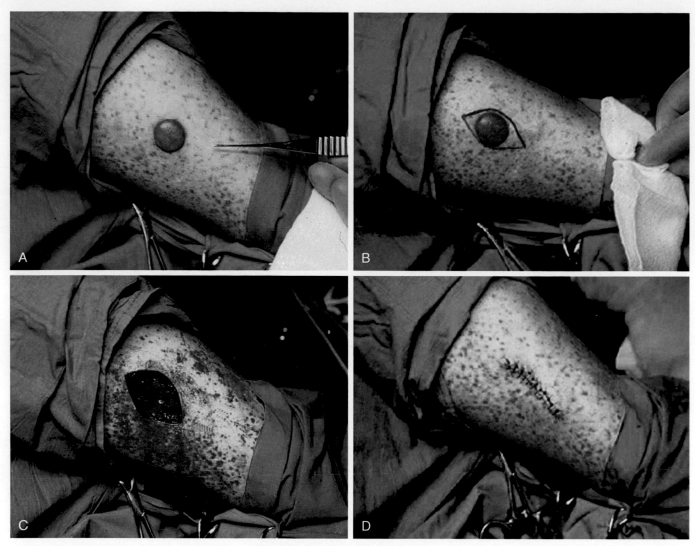

• **Fig. 10.8** Excision Biopsy Technique.

For the latter, major surgery or radiotherapy should not be performed without histological confirmation of the diagnosis. The biopsy objective is to obtain a representative sample of the full depth of the lesion, including an area of the margin and adjoining normal tissue (Fig. 10.9).

Destruction of Lesions by Diathermy, Electrocautery, Cryocautery or Curettage

These techniques are used for small lesions where there is no clinical suspicion of malignancy or for small basal cell carcinomas where a histological diagnosis is not required; the lesion is destroyed in the process of removal. Local anaesthesia is needed except for cryocautery, which is relatively painless.

Removal of Cysts

A cyst is a fluid-filled lesion, lined by epithelium and usually encapsulated by a condensation of fibrous tissue. The aim of treatment is to remove the whole epithelial lining because any remnant leads to recurrence. The technique of removal is outlined in Fig. 10.10. Ideally, the cyst is dissected out intact without puncturing the cavity. If a puncture occurs, the cyst collapses, making it difficult to identify and remove the epithelial lining.

Inflamed cysts are best simply drained and excised later when the inflammation has settled.

Marsupialisation

This is usually used for cysts or other fluid-filled lesions that are too large, inaccessible or technically difficult to remove. It is rarely appropriate for skin lesions but is often used for large salivary retention cysts in the floor of the mouth, cysts in the jaw and pancreatic pseudocysts. The surgeon usually removes a disc from the wall of the cavity and sutures the lining to the overlying epithelium around the cut edge. This leaves a pouch, which slowly fills in from below once the pressure of the cyst contents has been removed.

Surgery Involving Infected Tissues

Management of Abscesses

The first principle of managing an abscess is to establish drainage of the pus. When an abscess is 'pointing' to the surface, surgical drainage involves a skin incision at the site of maximum fluctuance followed by blunt probing with sinus forceps or a

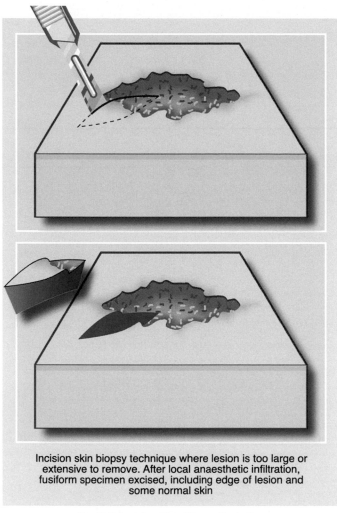

Incision skin biopsy technique where lesion is too large or extensive to remove. After local anaesthetic infiltration, fusiform specimen excised, including edge of lesion and some normal skin

• **Fig. 10.9** Incision Skin Biopsy Technique.

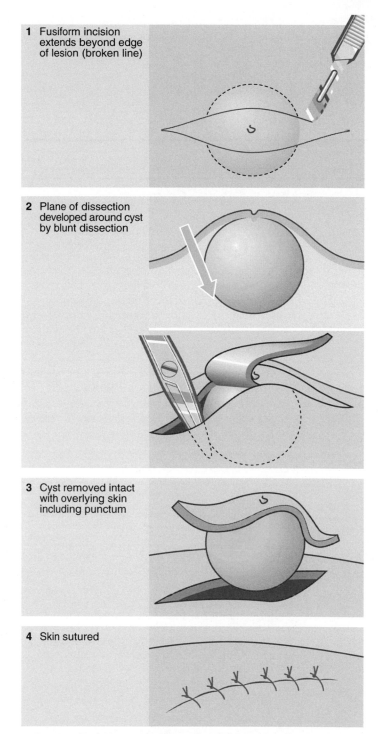

1 Fusiform incision extends beyond edge of lesion (broken line)

2 Plane of dissection developed around cyst by blunt dissection

3 Cyst removed intact with overlying skin including punctum

4 Skin sutured

• **Fig. 10.10** Technique of Excision of an Epidermal (Sebaceous) Cyst.

finger (usually under general anaesthesia) to ensure that all loculi are drained; necrotic material is removed at the same time by curettage.

After drainage, small abscesses need only a dry dressing, the cavity filling in rapidly from beneath. Larger and deeper abscesses need a method of keeping the skin opening patent until the cavity has filled with granulation tissue. A corrugated drain, which is gradually withdrawn ('shortened') over a few days, will achieve this or else the cavity may be packed with ribbon gauze soaked in antiseptic solution, or one of the newer absorbent dressings, such as an alginate (e.g., Kaltostat); these packs are usually changed daily or every other day. Good analgesia is required in the early stages.

Management of Infected Surgical Wounds

Grossly infected surgical wounds must be opened up to ensure free drainage, and cleaned. All necrotic tissue is excised leaving only healthy tissue, and the wound packed daily afterwards with antiseptic-soaked gauze or an alginate or hydrocolloid dressing. Wounds with large amounts of necrotic tissue may need more than one operation. Wounds are usually allowed to heal by secondary intention, although a large wound can be sutured later when infection is no longer a problem ('**delayed primary closure**').

Management of Dirty or Contaminated Wounds

Major soft tissue injuries result in crushing and tearing of tissues, leaving devascularised areas and deep impregnation with soil, road grit or fragments of clothing. If such a wound is merely sutured, pyogenic infection is certain, and there is a serious risk of gas gangrene or tetanus.

The principles of managing these wounds were first established during the First World War, as follows:
• Thorough removal of all foreign material from the wound (**debridement**).

- Excision of all non viable tissue (**necrosectomy**).
- Loose open packing of the wound with gauze without suturing.
- Inspection of the wound under anaesthesia 2 to 4 days later, plus drainage of any new abscesses and removal of any newly apparent nonviable tissue.
- If appropriate, suturing of the wound when it looks clean and granulating, but avoiding tension, that is, **delayed primary closure.** Alternatively, split skin grafting may be used without wound closure.

Principles of Plastic Surgery

History

Modern plastic surgery evolved during the First and Second World Wars, where pioneer Harold Gillies and later, his cousin Archibald McIndoe, invented and conducted various reconstructive operations for injured soldiers, including limb and facial reconstructions. Their techniques involved skin grafting and pedicled soft tissue flaps. The early flaps were **random pattern** in terms of vasculature, not usually based on named blood vessels. These flaps were hinged on one edge, so their dimensions and range of movement was limited, and patients often required multiple operations.

Reconstructive techniques improved with greater understanding of the vascular anatomy. The introduction of microvascular free tissue transfers eliminated the need for multistage reconstruction, allowing complex defects to be reconstructed in a single procedure. The scope of modern plastic surgery is outlined in Box 10.8.

The Reconstructive Ladder (Box 10.9)

If wounds cannot be closed directly or are not suitable to be allowed to heal secondarily, then more complex reconstructive solutions are needed using grafts or flaps. The **reconstructive ladder** is a step-wise configuration describing possible options available for any given defect.

Definitions (Fig. 10.11)

A **graft** is defined as a block of tissue completely disconnected from the body and transferred to another site where it is wholly reliant on the recipient site for survival. In contrast, a **flap** is a block of tissue moved from one site to another but always connected by its blood supply (the vascular pedicle). As one progresses up the reconstructive ladder, flaps become increasingly complex and are further classified into local, regional, distant and free (microvascular) flaps.

Skin Grafts

Whether following trauma or cancer resection, successful reconstruction of soft tissue defects relies on a satisfactory wound bed. Ideally also, the replacement tissue should result in a like-for-like reconstruction.

Skin grafts are the simplest reconstructive option but can be used only if the wound bed can provide enough nutrition to sustain the graft, allowing it to 'take'. This demands a vascularised wound bed such as viable fat or muscle, and is impossible where the bed is bare bone, tendon or cartilage. If such structures are covered by viable periosteum, paratenon or perichondrium, however, a skin graft should be possible.

• BOX 10.8   The Scope of Plastic Surgery

Congenital Problems
- Correction of congenital defects, for example, cleft lip and palate, syndactyly and polydactyly, prominent ears, hypospadias, vascular malformations, craniofacial deformities, congenital skin conditions (e.g., 'port-wine stains')

Trauma
- Reconstruction after mutilating surgery or trauma, for example, skin cover for compound lower limb fractures, vascularised bone transfer
- Management of facial soft tissue trauma
- Management of burns—grafting, management of scars and deformities
- Hand trauma—tendon repairs, microsurgical nerve and artery repairs, replantation surgery, for example, digits and limbs

Elective Hand Surgery
- Dupuytren contracture, nerve decompressions, joint replacements in rheumatoid disease

Cancer
- Cutaneous malignancies—excision and reconstruction with grafts or local flaps
- Major cancer surgery of the head and neck—excision and reconstruction with free tissue transfer
- Breast reconstruction after mastectomy

Aesthetic (Cosmetic) Surgery
- Scar removal, breast reduction and augmentation, 'face-lifts', eyelid skin reduction, nasal adjustment including after trauma
- Surgery for obesity, for example, abdominal skin reduction, liposuction, apronectomy (for pendulous abdomen)

Miscellaneous, Including Reconstruction of Large Defects
- Reconstruction for facial palsy, decubitus (pressure) sores, soft tissue sarcoma excision, leg ulcers, reconstruction of skin after radiotherapy, destructive infections (e.g., necrotising fasciitis, compartment syndromes)

• BOX 10.9   The Reconstructive Ladder

Heal by second intention
Primary closure
Split skin graft
Full thickness skin graft
Local flap
Regional pedicled flap
Distant pedicled flap
Free flap

A **full-thickness (Wolfe)** skin graft contains the entire thickness of skin (i.e., epidermis and dermis), whereas a **split-thickness** graft consists of epidermis and a variable amount of dermis, according to its chosen thickness.

Split-thickness (Thiersch) skin grafts are often harvested as sheets from the thigh (or other donor sites), using devices that may be manual (e.g., Watson or Humby knife) or air- or electrically-powered **dermatomes**. Dermatomes are often used for large grafts, such as following debridement of burns. The donor site is left raw under special dressings (alginates, such as Kaltostat are often used) and allowed to heal by second intention from residual epithelial elements. This process takes about 2 weeks.

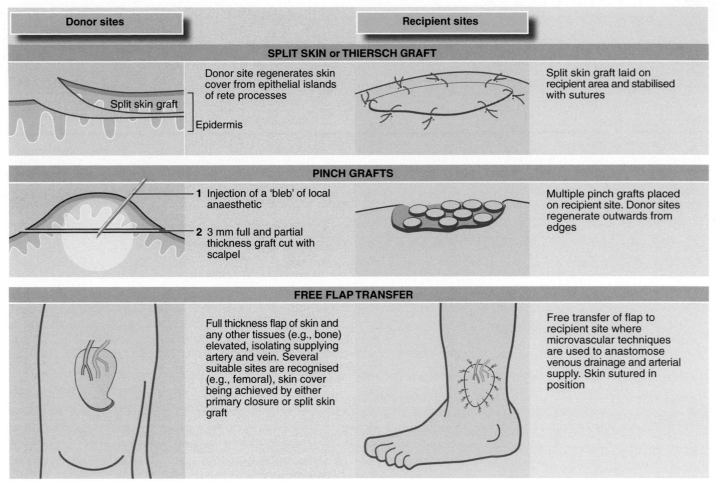

Donor sites		Recipient sites

SPLIT SKIN or THIERSCH GRAFT

Split skin graft

Donor site regenerates skin cover from epithelial islands of rete processes

Epidermis

Split skin graft laid on recipient area and stabilised with sutures

PINCH GRAFTS

1 Injection of a 'bleb' of local anaesthetic

2 3 mm full and partial thickness graft cut with scalpel

Multiple pinch grafts placed on recipient site. Donor sites regenerate outwards from edges

FREE FLAP TRANSFER

Full thickness flap of skin and any other tissues (e.g., bone) elevated, isolating supplying artery and vein. Several suitable sites are recognised (e.g., femoral), skin cover being achieved by either primary closure or split skin graft

Free transfer of flap to recipient site where microvascular techniques are used to anastomose venous drainage and arterial supply. Skin sutured in position

• **Fig. 10.11** Examples of Skin Grafting Techniques.

Split-thickness skin grafts are often **meshed** manually by making many small fenestrations with a blade, or more often by using a meshing tool. Meshing a graft allows it to expand over a wider area which is useful in large wounds. The fenestrations allow fluid to escape that might otherwise remain beneath the graft and compromise its 'take'. Meshing also allows the skin graft to be contoured better over uneven surfaces than sheet grafts.

Full-thickness skin grafts can be used for smaller grafts, as the donor site is closed primarily. Donor areas are thus limited to sites with enough excess skin to both harvest a graft and close the defect. These include parts of the neck and behind the ear (when required for facial reconstruction) and the groin. Full-thickness skin grafts tend to give a better cosmetic appearance, and they contract less over time.

Skin grafts undergo a unique healing process, with sequential but overlapping phases. Within the first few minutes, there is a period of **fibrin deposition** that causes the skin graft to adhere to the recipient site. Over the first couple of days, **plasma imbibition** occurs, where nutrients pass directly from the recipient bed into the graft. Next there is a phase of **inosculation**. This means that blood vessels in a full thickness graft connect with those in the bed, and split thickness grafts become neovascularised, that is, new blood vessels also grow into the graft. Thereafter, **graft maturation** occurs and this phase can last weeks to months.

Graft Failure

If conditions are right, most skin grafts will take. Graft failure is often caused by shearing and graft displacement, or infection, or if a physical barrier, such as a haematoma develops between graft and bed. Special dressings are used to anchor the skin graft to the recipient for the first week or so to minimise shearing. When the recipient bed is unsuitable for a skin graft, reconstruction must usually be carried out with a flap.

Local Flaps

Small defects, such as after skin cancer excision, can be reconstructed using a local skin flap, that is, a flap of tissue taken from immediately next to the defect. These local flaps are random-pattern, relying on the subdermal plexus for blood supply. They are classified according to the way they are moved into the defect—by **transposition, advancement or rotation**.

Pedicled Flaps

Larger flaps can be classified according to their constituents. They can include **skin** (e.g., a groin flap), **fascia** (e.g., temporo-parietal fascial flap), **muscle** (e.g., latissimus dorsi [LD], pectoralis and gracilis muscle flaps), **bone** (e.g., fibula and iliac crest flaps), or combinations of these.

Pedicled flaps are based on named blood vessels and can potentially be larger. Those taken from the wound region are called **regional flaps** and those from other parts of the body are **distant flaps**. Examples include LD myocutaneous flap from the back (often used in breast reconstruction) and the pectoralis major flap from the anterior chest wall used in head and neck reconstruction.

Microvascular Free Flaps

Pedicled flaps are inevitably limited in their reach so an important advance in reconstructive surgery was the appearance of microsurgery. This enabled harvesting **microvascular free flaps**, in which the flap and its vascular pedicle are dissected out and the artery and vein transected. Using microsurgery, these blood vessels are then anastomosed to matching vessels at the recipient site, reestablishing blood flow through the flap. This technique has allowed flaps from distant sites with appropriate texture, thickness and pliability to be used and causes less donor site morbidity.

Although elegant reconstructions can be achieved with free flaps, the surgery is more risky than pedicled flaps as the blood supply is divided and then reanastomosed and there is a risk that the flap can fail. Harvesting the flap is also more time-consuming, adding to overall operation time.

Non-autologous Reconstruction

Reconstructive surgeons have used a range of non-autologous materials over the years with varying success. Popular options include **alloplastic** materials, such as silicone implants for breast reconstruction and **biosynthetic** (often animal-derived) products, such as acellular dermal matrices used in breast and abdominal reconstruction, as well as dermal regeneration templates for burn wound reconstruction.

In recent years, advances in transplant immunology and microsurgical techniques have allowed reconstructive surgeons to push boundaries further. Successful **face** and **hand transplants** have been carried out around the world for defects that might otherwise have been unreconstructable.

Laparoscopic Surgery

Introduction to Minimal Access Surgery (Table 10.4)

The last few decades have seen an explosion of interest and rapid development of techniques to achieve accurate diagnosis and treatment with the least possible tissue injury and trauma. Laparoscopic surgery was among the first to catch surgeons' imagination but other techniques, such as lithotripsy, percutaneous stone removal and angioplasty advanced earlier or more or less in parallel. Initially called **minimally invasive surgery**, the principle is that if less tissue is damaged by minimising surgical incisions, then less pain is likely afterwards and the physiological responses to injury which slow recovery will be reduced. The intention is to reduce pain and allow more rapid return to normal life. Patients still need to be informed that even with short-stay laparoscopic surgery, there will still be a period of physiological recovery.

Gynaecologists led the way with laparoscopic diagnosis and procedures, particularly tubal ligation, but little development in instrumentation occurred until laparoscopic cholecystectomy emerged as a viable and popular option. Early laparoscopic cholecystectomy was hampered by poor equipment, poor imaging and lack of experience. Now that equipment is first class, training and experience have disseminated and audit is in place, the indications, contraindications and risks have become clear; as a result, laparoscopic cholecystectomy has become the standard procedure for removing gall bladder.

Interest in minimal access techniques has spread through the surgical specialties, prompting surgeons to seek new ways of performing operations that cause less trauma to their patients. Thus orthopaedic surgeons perform many operations **arthroscopically** and joint replacements are being performed through smaller incisions, allowing rapid mobilisation. **Thoracoscopy** uses similar instruments to laparoscopy for diagnostic and therapeutic applications in the thorax (see details in Ch. 31, p. 422). Endocrine surgeons now sometimes perform parathyroidectomy through very small incisions using special microscopes and retractors. Breast surgeons perform **sentinel lymph node biopsy** for diagnostic purposes using dye or radioactive marker techniques instead of axillary clearance. Urological procedures, such as nephrectomy, prostatectomy and cystectomy are undertaken endoscopically or laparoscopically, and vascular surgeons even have performed aortic aneurysm operations laparoscopically (though this difficult technique has been superceded by endovascular techniques). In fact, there is probably no abdominal operation that has not been attempted laparoscopically, although the difficulties of many larger procedures make them impractical for standard use. Laparoscopic techniques have proved most useful in areas of the body with limited access, such as the gastro-oesophageal junction, the adrenal gland and the pelvis, allowing delicate instruments to be used in confined spaces with excellent views unhampered by the surgeon's hands.

Laparoscopy

Laparoscopy or peritoneoscopy was in wide use clinically by gynaecologists from the early 1970s for diagnosing pelvic disorders and for sterilisation by tubal ligation. The first therapeutic GI procedure was probably an appendicectomy performed by Semm in 1983. In 1987 Mouret first removed a diseased gall bladder laparoscopically in France. Since then, the techniques have been adopted on an increasing scale by general and thoracic surgeons for performing abdominal and thoracic operations via a series of small punctures rather than through large incisions.

Advantages of Laparoscopic Surgery

The advantages of laparoscopic surgery, beyond simply avoiding large painful wounds to give better cosmesis and less postoperative pain include:

Surgical Advantages
* Improved access and vision in difficult areas, for example, adrenal, pelvic organs and gastro-oesophageal junction.
* Avoids handling, exposure, desiccation and cooling of abdominal tissues, which may reduce adhesion formation.
* Reduced contact with patient's blood and body fluids for healthcare professionals.
* Fewer wound infections, dehiscences and incisional hernias.

Postoperative Advantages
* Fewer postoperative chest complications.
* Lower analgesia requirements and sometimes shorter hospital stays.

TABLE 10.4	Summary of Minimally Invasive/Minimal Access Approaches to Diagnosis and Treatment[a]	
Specialty Area (In Alphabetical Order)	**Diagnostic Applications**	**Therapeutic Applications**
Abdomen CT or ultrasonography	• Diagnosis of fluid collections, for example, ascites, pancreatic pseudocyst, abscess • Percutaneous guided biopsy of enlarged lymph nodes, liver or pancreatic masses, other masses • Diagnosis of acute or chronic abdominal symptoms including detection of colorectal cancer	• Guiding drainage of fluid collections by aspiration or drain insertion • Guiding sampling of suspected pancreatic necrosis for infection in acute pancreatitis • Stent placement for obstructing colonic lesions
Anal canal	• Proctoscopy to inspect the anal canal and, if necessary, biopsy lesions	• Injection or banding of haemorrhoids • Perineal operations for rectal prolapse • Transanal endoscopic microsurgery (TEMS) • Transanal total mesorectal excision (TaTME) of the rectum
Arterial	• Conventional arteriography or magnetic resonance angiography—demonstrating the sites, severity and morphology of arterial obstruction or aneurysms—selective or highly selective angiography for detecting the source of acute intestinal bleeding or bleeding after pelvic fracture, or determining the blood supply of an organ • Ultrasound or CT diagnosis of aortic and other aneurysms • Duplex Doppler ultrasound scanning—for carotid artery disease, peripheral arterial disease, femoro-popliteal and other graft surveillance	• Angioplasty of arterial stenoses (percutaneous transluminal angioplasty—PCTA) • Stenting of obliterative arterial disease • Intraluminal stent grafting for aneurysms • Percutaneous thrombolysis • Embolisation for bleeding/tumours/arteriovenous malformations/ preoperative treatment of vascular lesions to reduce vascularity
Biliary (see also Pancreas)	• Distal duodenoscopy for ampullary tumours • Diagnostic ERCP for suspected bile duct stones or strictures, or for suspected duct damage after surgery	• Endoscopic sphincterotomy to retrieve bile duct stones, for example, in obstructive jaundice • Stent placement across bile duct strictures, traumatic leaks or tumours
Breast	• Detection and fine needle aspiration cytology or needle biopsy of solid lumps • Stereotactic fine needle aspiration or biopsy of mammographically detected lesions suspected of malignancy	• Ultrasound guided aspiration of cysts
Cardiac	• Endomyocardial biopsy for detecting rejection in heart transplants	• Angioplasty and stenting of obstructed coronary arteries • Off-pump coronary artery bypass (OPCAB) • Small incision or thoracoscopic approaches to standard cardiac operations using cardiopulmonary bypass or without, for example, via partial sternotomy • Transcatheter aortic valve implantation (TAVI)
Chest	• Ultrasound diagnosis of fluid collections • Thoracoscopic pleural or lung biopsy • Mediastinoscopic node biopsy	• Thoracoscopic cervicodorsal sympathectomy for hyperhidrosis of the hands • Pleurectomy or lobectomy for benign disease
Gynaecology	• Laparoscopic diagnosis for infertility or chronic pelvic pain caused by endometriosis or adhesions • Diagnosis of cause of acute abdomen in suspected pelvic inflammatory disease, tubal pregnancy, ovarian problems	• Laparoscopic sterilisation (tubal clipping) • Laparoscopic assisted hysterectomy (but carries 2.5 times the risk of urinary tract injuries compared with abdominal or vaginal) • Laparoscopic oophorectomy for palliation of breast carcinoma • Laparoscopic obtaining of eggs for in vitro and other forms of assisted fertilisation • Laparoscopic pelvic lymphadenectomy for radical cancer surgery • Laparoscopic operations for urinary stress incontinence
Oesophagus	• Diagnostic oesophagoscopy and biopsy—flexible instruments usually used	• Dilatation of benign oesophageal strictures • Pulsion (pushing) placement of luminal tubes and cloth-covered stents for obstructing carcinoma • Palliative laser ablation of obstructing tumours—'reboring' • Injection of bleeding ulcers • Balloon compression and endoscopic sclerotherapy injection of varices • Balloon dilatation of narrow cardia in achalasia • Thoracoscopic myotomy for achalasia (Heller operation) • Laparoscopic antireflux surgery

Continued

TABLE 10.4   Summary of Minimally Invasive/Minimal Access Approaches to Diagnosis and Treatment[a]—cont'd

Specialty Area (In Alphabetical Order)	Diagnostic Applications	Therapeutic Applications
Orthopaedics	• Diagnostic arthroscopy—hip, knee, ankle, shoulder, elbow and wrist	Therapeutic arthroscopy: • Knee—removal of loose bodies; articular cartilage and meniscal surgery; cruciate reconstruction; irrigation for infection • Shoulder—impingement decompression; shoulder stabilisation; rotator cuff repair • Hip, elbow and ankle—removal of loose bodies; articular cartilage surgery • Wrist—percutaneous screw for scaphoid fracture
Pancreas	• Endoscopic pancreatography for suspected duct abnormalities • Endoscopic collection of exocrine secretions for cytology? Malignancy	• Early sphincterotomy and trawling of biliary and pancreatic ducts to relieve stone-induced pancreatitis • Transgastric cystgastrostomy for pseudocyst
Rectum and colon	• Diagnostic flexible sigmoidoscopy or colonoscopy (including biopsy) for bleeding, suspected tumour, inflammatory bowel disease and surveillance after polyp or cancer removal, tumours for palliation, or benign rectal strictures • Endoluminal ultrasound imaging for staging rectal cancer and determining sphincter damage • Magnetic resonance imaging for detailing the anatomy of complex fistulae	• Snare excision of polyps and adenomas • Diathermy to bleeding angiodysplasias • Diathermy loop resection of inoperable rectal cancer • Argon beam laser ablation of rectal cancer (palliative)
Stomach and duodenum	• Diagnostic inspection for ulcers and cancer • Biopsy of ulcers and tumours • Biopsy to diagnose *Helicobacter* infection as a cause of ulceration	• Injection treatment of acutely bleeding ulcers • Endoscopic retrieval of foreign bodies • Combined percutaneous and endoscopic placement of feeding gastrostomy tubes ('PEG')
Urology Endoscopic— rigid and flexible	• Haematuria (diagnosis, treatment and follow-up of bladder tumours) • Poor urinary stream (assessment of bladder neck and prostatic obstruction) • Ureteric obstruction (ureteroscopy or retrograde pyelography)	• Resection of bladder tumours • Resection of bladder neck or prostate (TURP) • Holmium laser enucleation of prostate (HoLEP) • Stenting of ureter to relieve stone obstruction, strictures or external compression • Balloon dilatation of stenosed pelvi-ureteric junction via trans-urethral route (not commonly performed) • Stones—laser fragmentation of ureter and pelvicalyceal system calculi
Percutaneous, laparoscopic and robotic-assisted		• Direct endoscopic stone destruction and removal; indirect stone destruction using lithotripsy • Placement of suprapubic catheters • Nephrostomy inserted for obstructed kidney • Laparoscopic and robot-assisted nephrectomy, cystectomy, prostatectomy and lymph node dissection
Venous system	• Duplex Doppler ultrasound scanning—for diagnosing deep and superficial venous insufficiency	• Percutaneous ablation of long or short saphenous vein in varicose veins using foam sclerotherapy, radiofrequency or laser ablation • Subfascial endoscopic perforator surgery (SEPS) for treating venous ulceration

[a]Note: laparoscopic and robotic-assisted techniques are also covered in the adjoining text and Boxes 10.9 and 10.10.

CT, Computed tomography; *ERCP,* endoscopic retrograde cholangiopancreatography; *TURP,* transurethral resection of the prostate.

Risks and Complications

Certain complications are common to open and laparoscopic surgery, but laparoscopic operations carry their own particular risks. Specific problems include:

• Induction of the pneumoperitoneum (inflating the abdomen with gas) may cause subcutaneous emphysema or injury to bowel or major blood vessels and must be performed with care, preferably using an open technique rather than a blind Veress needle.

• Trocar insertion may injure the abdominal wall (including the diaphragm), intraabdominal organs and blood vessels. It must be performed under direct vision, being alert to structures that could be damaged.

- The raised intraabdominal pressure and head-down position mean that patients have to be ventilated at higher inflation pressures. This reduces venous return and cardiac output and may cause circulatory compromise in patients with cardiac ischaemia. To mitigate this, intraabdominal pressures should be kept to the minimum necessary for the procedure to be performed safely, that is, 8 to 12 mmHg; patients should not be placed in extreme head-up or head-down positions for prolonged periods. IV infusion should be stopped whilst head-down.
- The diaphragm is 'splinted' by the pneumoperitoneum and this can precipitate cardiorespiratory complications in patients with respiratory problems. Again, minimising inflation pressures reduces this effect.
- The pneumoperitoneum compresses intraabdominal veins and reduces venous return. This predisposes to thromboembolic complications, such as deep venous thrombosis. Patients should receive appropriate prophylaxis at all times.
- Inadvertent injury can occur to a range of structures during dissection, diathermy or laser instrumentation, often through excess heating. The damage may go unrecognised if the damage occurs out of the sight of the laparoscope, leading to late complications including haemorrhage and bowel perforation.
- Postoperatively, bowel may strangulate through peritoneal defects, and incisional hernias can occur through port sites. The latter should be carefully closed under direct vision to minimise this risk.

Technique of Laparoscopy

Laparoscopy is usually performed under general anaesthesia, most often with muscle relaxation to allow full and safe insufflation of the abdominal cavity. A **pneumoperitoneum** is first created by introducing carbon dioxide under controlled pressure to lift the abdominal wall away from the viscera, allowing inspection of the peritoneal cavity.

Gas is most safely introduced via a blunt cannula placed by an open technique to enable direct visualisation of the peritoneal contents. The technique has largely replaced 'blind' insufflation via a Veress needle, which has a significant risk of vascular injury. The gas pressure should be kept as low as possible while maintaining a satisfactory view, to minimise cardiac and respiratory risks. A 5- or 10-mm diameter laparoscope with video camera is then introduced into the abdominal cavity, displaying the image on monitors.

Most laparoscopic procedures need additional cannulae (trocars) through which to pass diathermy hooks, graspers, needle holders, clip appliers and linear staplers. These secondary trocars are inserted through new access points under direct vision from within the abdomen to prevent injury to bowel and other viscera. Different operations each require different port placements. Preferences vary from surgeon to surgeon and port siting also depends on the particular conditions of the operation; for example, cholecystectomy in an obese patient necessitates different port sites from those used in a slim patient.

The laparoscopic operation is performed by an operator and one or more assistants, all observing progress on monitors. Sharp or blunt dissection may be used as in open surgery. Sharp dissection uses laparoscopic scissors whilst blunt dissection is carried out using fine dissecting forceps ('Petelins' or 'Marylands'), laparoscopic gauze pledgets or the tip of a suction probe. Blunt dissection tears rather than cuts small vessels, deliberately causing minor tissue damage that rapidly activates the coagulation cascade and causes spontaneous cessation of bleeding. This is safer than sharp dissection which may require (potentially excessive) use of diathermy. Haemostasis still requires diathermy and this must be cautiously used to prevent arcing to adjacent organs. Increasingly, safer alternatives are being used, such as **bipolar** diathermy forceps or the **harmonic scalpel**, which uses ultrasound to coagulate and cut vessels and tissue.

In laparoscopic-assisted surgery, for example colectomy, a large part of the dissection is performed laparoscopically and then a small abdominal incision is made to deliver the bowel for anastomosis outside the abdomen or to remove the resected specimen. There are techniques available to extract viscera through natural orifices, such as the anal canal or vagina, to minimise wound complications, however, this has not become mainstream treatment and requires substantial training, skill and support.

After operation, patients experience abdominal discomfort at trocar insertion sites and shoulder discomfort from retained gas in the peritoneal cavity. Few restrictions are placed on the patient after discharge; he or she can return to work as soon as comfortable, often after a few days.

Robotic-Assisted Surgery

Robotically assisted surgical systems are increasingly being used for certain technically challenging operations, such as laparoscopic prostatectomy, nephrectomy and cystectomy, pharyngeal operations for cancer via the mouth and cardiothoracic operations. These robots are not autonomous, but aid the surgeon who sits at a remote console (which may be close to the patient or far away). The surgeon very precisely controls the robotic manipulation of laparoscopic instruments, previously inserted into the anaesthetised patient, via the surgical arm unit. The imaging system provides three-dimensional vision. The da Vinci system allows manipulation of all instruments whilst other simpler systems control just the camera.

Potential benefits include increased precision of movement, greater ranges of movement, 'smoothing' of tremor, reduction of fatigue in long operations and perhaps eventually the need for fewer assistants in the theatre. In the longer term, a surgeon could, at least theoretically, operate on a patient many kilometres away by **tele-surgery**. Disadvantages of robotic surgery include the high capital cost (currently around $2–3 million), lack of tactile feedback for the surgeon and long set-up times for individual patients. The place of robotic surgery remains to be defined.

Applications of Laparoscopy

Laparoscopy in general surgery has **diagnostic** and **therapeutic applications**. The diagnostic applications are well recognised and are increasingly used as first-line investigative procedures.

Diagnostic Laparoscopy

Diagnostic laparoscopy has long been used by surgeons for assessing chronic liver disease and ascites of unknown origin. Advances in instrumentation and imaging now allow surgeons to perform abdominal exploration almost as thoroughly as is possible via a long laparotomy incision. A key application is in assessing abdominal trauma and is wholly appropriate for use in the developing world. It is also invaluable for staging gastric or pancreatic cancer to assess operability. This is achieved by inspection, by obtaining peritoneal washings for cytology and by performing biopsies. By this method, patients with incurable disease can be spared the trauma of exploratory open surgery (Box 10.10). Diagnostic

Potential Indications for Diagnostic Laparoscopy

- Evaluation of acute or chronic abdominal pain, for example, suspected appendicitis, gynaecological pain
- Diagnosis and staging of intraabdominal malignancies (sometimes with direct ultrasound) (including evaluating the results of chemotherapy or radiotherapy on intraabdominal malignancies)
- Assessing blunt or penetrating abdominal trauma in stable patients with proven free intraabdominal fluid
- Evaluation of acute or chronic liver disease
- Diagnosis of ascites of unknown cause
- As a 'second-look' procedure in patients operated on for mesenteric ischaemia
- Exclusion of acute acalculous cholecystitis after major trauma or surgery in intensive care patients

• **BOX 10.11** **Current Therapeutic Applications of Laparoscopy**

- Cholecystectomy (described in Ch. 20) and common bile duct exploration
- Appendicectomy
- Colonic resections and colostomy formation—benign and malignant disease (although evidence of benefit is scarce)
- Abdominal operations for rectal prolapse
- Division of symptomatic adhesions
- Inguinal, femoral, Spigelian and incisional hernia repairs
- Small bowel surgery—including resection and enteral access procedures
- Peptic ulcer disease (plugging of duodenal perforations)
- Symptomatic hiatus hernias and oesophageal reflux (Nissen fundoplication and other antireflux operations)
- Nephrectomy, pyeloplasty, prostatectomy, cystectomy and other ureteric procedures
- Splenectomy and adrenalectomy
- Laparoscopic liver biopsy and deroofing of liver cysts
- Distal pancreatectomy
- Laparoscopically assisted oesophagectomy and gastrectomy
- Laparoscopic drainage of pancreatic pseudocysts and pancreatic necrosectomy
- Laparoscopic bypass or banding surgery for obesity
- Laparoscopically assisted total hysterectomy and all tube and ovarian procedures including marsupialisation of ectopic pregnancy

laparoscopy is valuable for assessing right iliac fossa pain, particularly in women of menstruating age. The procedure allows more accurate assessment of the gynaecological organs, improves diagnostic accuracy, allows appendicectomy if appropriate and minimises negative appendicectomy rates.

Therapeutic Laparoscopy

Laparoscopic cholecystectomy is already the standard operation for removal of the gallbladder, in both the elective and the emergency situation (described in Ch. 20). Other procedures described later and listed in Box 10.11 are becoming standard operations in the armoury of laparoscopic surgeons.

Laparoscopic Appendicectomy

Open appendicectomy for acute appendicitis has largely been replaced by laparoscopic appendicectomy, which can offer improved diagnostic accuracy with the ability to examine the entire abdomen if the appendix is normal, a lower rate of wound complications, reduced postoperative pain and hospital stay, and more rapid return to normal activities. Laparoscopic appendicectomy may offer a lower rate of pelvic adhesions because of reduced trauma; this is an advantage in young women.

Laparoscopic Inguinal Hernia Repair

Inguinal hernias can be repaired laparoscopically using a transperitoneal or an extraperitoneal approach. Both techniques involve less dissection than the open approach and are believed to reduce the likelihood of damage to testicular vessels and the ilioinguinal nerve (particularly for recurrent hernias), resulting in a lower incidence of long-term chronic groin pain.

Learning laparoscopic inguinal hernia repair requires a great deal of supervised experience, but the procedure is now widely performed, and controlled trials show that it can have results comparable with open hernia repair techniques, including term recurrence rates. Laparoscopic repair is of particular value for recurrent hernias, allowing surgery to be performed in tissue planes free from scarring. It is also recommended for bilateral hernias, when both sides can be repaired through three small incisions. Nevertheless, the Lichtenstein open mesh hernia repair remains a standard operation alongside laparoscopic operations.

Laparoscopic Fundoplication

Laparoscopic fundoplication can be used for patients suffering from large hiatus hernias or gastro-oesophageal reflux disease resistant to medical management. The technique involves dissecting the gastro-oesophageal junction at the hiatus, repairing the crura and wrapping the gastric fundus around the lower oesophagus (Nissen-type wrap). Clinical trials show that it offers rapid return to normal activity and results are as durable as open fundoplication.

Laparoscopic Management of Duodenal Ulcer Perforation

Duodenal ulcers usually perforate anteriorly and the perforation can readily be seen with the laparoscope. Under laparoscopic visualisation, the ulcer is closed in the same way as at open operation, with part of the greater omentum secured over the duodenum to seal the perforation with laparoscopically placed sutures. The peritoneal cavity is irrigated with a suction irrigator and the fluid aspirated.

Laparoscopic Placement of Enterocutaneous Jejunostomy Tube

In patients requiring long-term enteral feeding in whom a gastrostomy is unsuitable, a fine-bore feeding tube can be placed into the jejunum using laparoscopy, avoiding the need for laparotomy.

Laparoscopic Splenectomy

Laparoscopic splenectomy has become the gold standard for elective splenectomy, particularly in haematological conditions. Substantially enlarged spleens can be removed laparoscopically but the risk of conversion to open operation rises steeply once the spleen weighs over 1 kg (such spleens usually reach the costal margin). At operation, the patient lies on the right side for best access and vision, and the hilar vessels are divided between clips or with vascular staplers. The spleen is placed in a laparoscopic retrieval bag and broken up or liquidised to enable removal via one of the small port incisions.

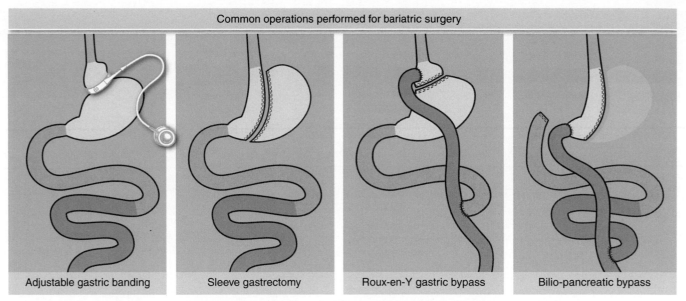

• Fig. 10.12 Common Operations Performed for Bariatric Surgery.

Laparoscopic Adrenalectomy

Laparoscopic adrenalectomy has proved a highly beneficial procedure, allowing adrenal tumours of all sizes to be removed safely and with much less trauma than the muscle-cutting flank incisions previously used. It is particularly useful in **phaeochromocytoma** where very delicate handling of the tumour is needed. This includes precise delineation and clipping of the vessels in the appropriate order to avoid catecholamine surges.

Laparoscopically Assisted Colectomy

Laparoscopic techniques were first used to perform uncomplicated colorectal procedures, such as rectopexy and formation of colostomies. Early experience with colorectal cancer showed port site metastases appearing more commonly than wound metastases at open surgery. This led to concern that the cancer was being disseminated by the pneumoperitoneum. However, further research and refinement of 'no touch' techniques have laid these fears to rest. Laparoscopically assisted resection of benign and malignant colonic lesions is becoming more commonplace, and all elective colonic resections can now be undertaken laparoscopically. Short-term benefits have been demonstrated along with reduced wound-related long-term complications for both rectal and colonic surgery. There are still controversies as to the oncologically best approaches to the pelvis for rectal cancer.

Laparoscopic Surgery for Obesity (Fig. 10.12)

In recent years, there has been a major expansion in laparoscopic surgery for obesity (**bariatric surgery**). The most common technique involves placing an adjustable restrictive silicone band around the upper part of the stomach to create a small proximal pouch that causes early satiety. Results are excellent in carefully selected, well-motivated patients who have good support and follow up. More radical bariatric operations, such as gastric bypass and biliary-pancreatic diversion operations are also being performed laparoscopically. These operations achieve greater weight loss and more rapid regression of diabetes but may carry higher rates of morbidity and mortality, largely operator dependent.

Principles of Neurosurgery

Introduction

Neurosurgery is a broad speciality concerned with diagnosis and treatment of disorders affecting the nervous system—the brain, spinal cord, peripheral nerves and cerebrovascular system. Neurosurgery is performed only in specialised centres with subspecialists in head trauma, vascular problems, paediatrics, spinal disorders, oncology, functional (e.g., movement disorders, chronic pain and epilepsy) and skull base problems. Neurosurgical conditions present complex challenges to the multidisciplinary team, which includes neuroanaesthesia, neuroradiology, neurooncology, neurointensive care and neurorehabilitation, as well as specialist nurses and physiotherapists.

Cerebral Perfusion Pressure

Cerebral perfusion pressure (CPP) is the difference between the intracranial pressure (ICP) and mean arterial pressure and is the net pressure gradient driving cerebral blood flow (CBF). **Cerebral autoregulation** maintains stable CBF over a range of CPPs and is the key to maintaining a healthy perfused brain. The mechanism involves the body varying the cerebrovascular resistance, that is, a vasoconstriction response to increased systemic (and mean) blood pressure (BP) or vasodilation if systemic BP falls.

Variations in partial pressure of carbon dioxide in arterial blood ($PaCO_2$) also alter CBF. Raised $PaCO_2$ causes vasodilatation and increased blood flow and lowered $PaCO_2$ causes vasoconstriction and reduced blood flow. Many patients with head injuries are electively hyperventilated to lower the $PaCO_2$ and lower the raised ICP, however this is a fine balance as reducing the blood flow can reduce perfusion too much and cause hypoxia.

Maintaining a constant CPP is important in managing neurosurgical patients because once beyond the limits of cerebral autoregulation, increased ICP can result in a sudden fall in CPP and blood flow, risking brain hypoxia. Prolonged reductions in CBF following head injuries cause hypoxia and a worse outcome.

• BOX 10.12 **Causes of Raised Intracranial Pressure**

Central nervous system infections
- Meningitis
- Encephalitis

Space occupying lesion
- Abscess
- Tumour

Head injury
Cerebral infarct
Intracranial haemorrhage
Cerebral oedema
Hydrocephalus
Benign idiopathic intracranial hypertension

• BOX 10.13 **Important Factors to Remember in Managing Raised ICP**

A: Maintain patent airway (requires intubation if GCS<8)
B: Maintain saturations >95%
C: Maintain normotension (caution treating hypertension too aggressively—it may be required for brain perfusion)
D: Avoid hypoglycaemia
E: 15–30 degrees of head elevation maximises venous return and can help reduce ICP

ICP, Intracranial pressure; *GCS*, Glasgow Coma Scale.

Raised Intracranial Pressure

Three components contribute to ICP within the rigid skull: brain tissue, blood and cerebrospinal fluid (CSF). ICP is normally between 5 to 15 mmHg when supine. In addition to autoregulation, the body has other mechanisms to maintain stable ICP: when the volume of one component increases (e.g., brain volume), it causes a shift of venous blood and/or CSF out of the cranium. This buffers the rise in ICP for a given volume increase in skull contents but only up to a tipping point. Beyond this, there is a massive increase in ICP which may result in catastrophic brain herniation. Causes of raised ICP are shown in Box 10.12.

Clinical Features of Raised Intracranial Pressure

Reduced consciousness, lethargy, irritability
Headache: characteristically worse in the morning, on coughing, moving head or lying down (all increase ICP)
Vomiting: worse in the morning and on lying down
Papilloedema
Focal neurological signs, including but not limited to the following:
- Hemiparesis or hemiplegia
- Cranial nerve (CN) palsies: CNIII and CNVI are most vulnerable and the first to become compressed with expanding brain tissue/herniation secondary to raised ICP
  - CNIII palsy: eye will sit down and out, ptosis, mydriasis. An enlarging and unresponsive pupil is a late sign associated with coning
  - CNVI palsy: diplopia, inability of eye to turn outwards—esotropia/convergent strabismus

Cushing reflex (very late sign): raised BP, bradycardia, irregular breathing
Rising ICP manifests initially with deteriorating conscious level. Untreated, raised ICP may cause **coning** in which one or both temporal lobes herniate down through the tentorium cerebelli, compressing the third nerve and midbrain, whilst herniation of the cerebellar tonsils through the foramen magnum compresses the medulla, causing neurological deterioration and often death. Late clinical signs are: an enlarging and unresponsive pupil, central respiratory depression, falling heart rate and rising BP (Cushing reflex).

Investigations

- Bedside
  - Observations: BP, heart rate, respiratory rate, oxygen saturations, temperature
  - Capillary glucose: hypoglycaemia can present in the same way
- Bloods:
  - Full blood count, urea and electrolytes, liver function tests, C-reactive protein, coagulation studies, bone studies
  - Arterial blood gases: indicates $PaCO_2$ to aid future management
- Imaging:
  - CT or magnetic resonance imaging (MRI)
- Special tests
  - ICP monitoring—this is invasive monitoring involving placing an ICP bolt. It is appropriate in patients with:
    1) Severe head injury and abnormal CT
    2) Severe head injury, normal CT and >40 years OR motor posturing OR systolic BP <90 mmHg

ICP monitoring is also used in subarachnoid haemorrhage, brain tumours, hydrocephalus and idiopathic intracranial hypertension (Box 10.13).

Managing Raised Intracranial Pressure

- Avoid and treat situations likely to increase ICP: maintain normotension, avoid pyrexia and hypoglycaemia, treat seizures aggressively, give appropriate analgesia and sedation (e.g., IV propofol).
- Hyperventilation—reduces $PaCO_2$ causing cerebral arteriolar vasoconstriction.
- Hyperosmolar therapy—IV hypertonic saline or mannitol is often used. These osmotic agents shift excess fluid from brain to the intravascular space.
- Neuromuscular blockade—muscle activity can raise ICP by increasing intrathoracic pressure and obstructing cerebral venous outflow. Drugs prevent transmission at the neuromuscular junction causing paralysis of skeletal muscle and prevent this from occurring.
- CSF drainage—via an external ventricular drain or ventriculoperitoneal shunt.

Benign Idiopathic Intracranial Hypertension

This is raised ICP without a mass lesion or hydrocephalus and appears to be caused by impaired CSF absorption from the subarachnoid space. It is more common in obese premenopausal females and prompt treatment is needed to prevent permanent visual impairment. It is often associated with adrenal insufficiency, Cushing syndrome, thyroid dysfunction and various medications (steroids, levothyroxine, nitrofurantoin).

Typical symptoms include throbbing headache worse in the morning and relieved on standing, gradual onset of visual field defects or transient reduction of vision on bending/stooping, blurring or haloing of vision, nausea and vomiting. Investigations should include visual field charting. Medical management includes weight reduction, smoking cessation, diuretic therapy, stopping causative medication, and serial lumbar punctures to remove CSF to control raised ICP. Surgical management is possible, including optic nerve sheath fenestration (decompression) and CSF diversion (shunting).

Hydrocephalus

Hydrocephalus results from a mismatch between CSF production and reabsorption, increasing CSF volume and raising ICP. It is classified into **communicating** and **non communicating** types, depending on whether the obstruction lies within ventricles or the subarachnoid space.

- Communicating hydrocephalus—caused by impaired CSF reabsorption. Meningitis, intraventricular haemorrhage and congenital absence of arachnoid villi.
- Noncommunicating hydrocephalus—caused by obstruction to the flow of CSF. This can occur at a number of anatomic points. Normal flow is from lateral ventricles to third ventricle via the Foramen of Monro, then to fourth ventricle via the cerebral aqueduct of Sylvius, then to the subarachnoid space via median or lateral apertures. CSF is normally then reabsorbed by arachnoid villi and drains into the superior sagittal sinus. Narrowing at any of these points results in a build-up of CSF and hydrocephalus.

Common causes of hydrocephalus include:
- congenital—spina bifida and neural tube defects, aqueduct stenosis
- trauma—blood clot, brain swelling, venous sinus injury
- infection—meningitis
- vascular—subarachnoid or intracerebral haemorrhage
- tumour

Clinical Presentations of Raised Intracranial Pressure

Hydrocephalus in infants may manifest with gradually enlarging head circumference or, in the elderly, with the triad of ataxia, dementia and incontinence ('normal pressure hydrocephalus'). An urgent CT scan can help identify a cause.

Normal pressure hydrocephalus involves an increase in CSF volume causing ventricular expansion. ICP is often normal and patients do not have symptoms of raised ICP. However, a typical triad of symptoms occurs: dementia, urinary incontinence and gait disturbance caused by pressure effects of enlarged ventricles on surrounding brain tissue. It can often be misdiagnosed as Parkinson disease or Alzheimer dementia.

Treatment of Hydrocephalus

This depends on the cause. Communicating hydrocephalus can be relieved temporarily via lumbar puncture (but never in noncommunicating hydrocephalus). Long-term management requires CSF diversion via a shunt.

Non communicating hydrocephalus secondary to a tumour may respond to dexamethasone to temporise before tumour removal. Otherwise the obstruction needs to be bypassed by endoscopic third ventriculostomy, insertion of an external ventricular drain, or creation of a permanent CSF diversion with a shunt. Shunting is usually via a catheter between lateral ventricle and peritoneum incorporating a pressure regulating valve.

Brain Tumours

Brain tumours can be primary or secondary in origin.

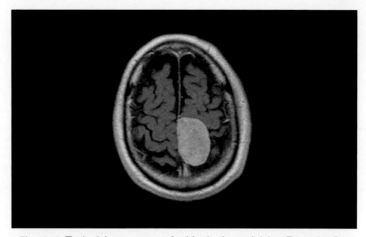

• **Fig. 10.13** Typical Appearance of a Meningioma Arising From the Dura Adjacent to the Superior Sagittal Sinus.

Primary Tumours

These are tumours originating in brain tissue and are categorised by histological type, location and histological grade. The terms benign or malignant are not normally used because these tumours rarely metastasise outside the craniospinal axis, and long-term survival depends on whether tumour growth can be controlled. **Glioma** is the most common primary tumour, whilst **meningioma** is the most common extraaxial tumour (Fig. 10.13). The World Health Organization classification is more precise, embracing the tissue of origin and its behavioural characteristics. Potential modes of tumour presentation are shown in Table 10.5.

Secondary Brain Tumours

These are metastatic tumours that have originated elsewhere in the body and have spread to the brain. Secondary tumours are most likely from lung, breast, bowel and kidney, as well as melanoma. Presentation is similar to that of primary brain tumours, together with symptoms from the causative tumour.

Principles of Craniotomy

Craniotomy is the standard method of accessing the cranial cavity. A bone flap is fashioned and lifted and is replaced at the end of the operation. Bevelling the bone edges and using titanium plates and/or screws facilitates closure. If bone is not replaced, this is termed **craniectomy** and the bone is used as a template for a titanium or acrylic plate, or is stored for later reimplantation. Indications for craniectomy include raised ICP refractory to medication, bone infection or osteomyelitis, or infiltration of bone by tumour.

Preparation for operation begins with optimal patient and head positioning. Planning the incision and craniotomy takes the following factors into account:
- Cosmesis (e.g., avoiding forehead incisions and excessive hair shaving).
- Scalp blood supply: occipital and superficial temporal arteries should be preserved.
- Avoiding placing implants or foreign material (e.g., screws/plates) directly under wounds.
- Location of scalp nerves: damage to temporalis and frontalis branches can cause unsightly muscle asymmetry of the forehead.

TABLE 10.5	Presentation of Brain Tumours According to Site	
Mode of Presentation	**Significance**	
Incidental finding	Intracranial pathology identified during imaging for another purpose (e.g., sinusitis). A period of active observation may be appropriate	
Seizures	**Generalised tonic-clonic seizures**—usually only in supratentorial tumours **Partial sensory or motor seizures**—particularly in tumours around the sensory or motor strip **Complex partial seizures**—particularly in temporal lobe tumours	
Raised intracranial pressure	Reduced conscious level, confusion, headache, vomiting, papilloedema, unilateral or bilateral pupillary dilatation	
Altered brain function	**Frontal**—altered personality, contralateral face, arm or leg weakness, expressive dysphasia (dominant side), incontinence **Temporal**—upper homonymous quadrantanopia, receptive dysphasia (dominant hemisphere) **Parietal**—lower homonymous quadrantanopia **Occipital**—homonymous hemianopia **Cerebellar**—nystagmus, ataxia, speech disturbance including dysarthria and staccato speech and intention tremor **Brainstem**—vomiting, lower cranial nerve palsies, long tract signs, reduced consciousness, pupil changes, altered eye movements **Hypothalamic/pituitary**—visual deficit (bitemporal hemianopia), endocrine disturbance	

- Position of cranial landmarks and underlying structures in relation to the pathology, including major dural venous sinuses, cranial arteries and areas of special importance, such as motor and visual pathways. Modern planning includes CT- or MRI-guided navigation, but it cannot replace knowledge of anatomy.

In elective surgery, craniotomy flaps are 'tailored' to best access the operative area, but when an intracranial haematoma after trauma needs rapid and safe evacuation, a standard fronto-temporo-parietal craniotomy is used. Meticulous haemostasis before wound closure is vital in all operative neurosurgery.

Special Postoperative Considerations

Patients are recovered in a monitored environment with regular neurological observations. The surgeon should be informed of any neurological deterioration. Depressed consciousness is usually an early sign of rising ICP but pupillary dilatation and autonomic changes occur late (e.g., Cushing reflex).

Postoperative seizures, reduced conscious level or altered neurology may herald intracranial complications, such as oedema or bleeding. Urgent repeat CT is needed after stabilising BP and oxygenation. Sedating analgesics should generally be avoided—paracetamol and codeine phosphate or small doses of morphine may be appropriate. Nonsteroidal anti-inflammatory drugs (NSAIDs) impair platelet function and should be avoided early on in high-risk patients.

IV fluids need care: dextrose may increase cerebral oedema so 0.9% saline or Hartmann's solution is usually ordered. Plasma sodium abnormalities are relatively common in neurosurgical patients. These include the syndrome of inappropriate antidiuretic hormone hypersecretion which causes hyponatraemia and sometimes fluid overload, and diabetes insipidus which causes polyuria and polydipsia by diminishing the ability to concentrate urine.

Spinal Lesions

Spinal Cord Anatomy

The spinal cord extends from the foramen magnum to L1 or L2. It lies in the vertebral canal and transmits nervous impulses from the periphery to the cortex.

Sciatica

Sciatica is pain caused by compression of a spinal nerve root (usually L4/5) that affects the lower back, hip, buttock and outer side of leg in the myotome and dermatome supplied by that nerve root. It is most often a result of prolapse of a degenerated intervertebral disc but there are many other causes, such as malignancy (primary or secondary), inflammatory disease (arthritis, ankylosing spondylitis), bone disorders (Paget, osteoporosis) and infections (tuberculosis).

Red flag symptoms include: recent trauma, constitutional symptoms (fever, night sweats, unexplained weight loss), saddle anaesthesia and changes in bladder or bowel habit; these suggest a more worrying cause. Sciatica pain is worsened by a straight leg raising as this stretches the nerve root. Knee flexion then relieves the pain.

Imaging includes x-ray of lumbar spine. MRI would be considered if symptoms were suspicious of malignancy, cauda equina compression (see later), fracture or infection.

Management options include:
- physiotherapy and encouraging physical activity
- analgesics including NSAIDs
- referral for surgical spinal decompression

Spinal Cord Compression

Spinal cord compression is a neurosurgical emergency. The spinal cord has poor regenerative ability, unlike other neurons, so neurological deficits are likely to remain after intervention.

Causes include:
- trauma or spinal haematoma
- tumours
- prolapsed intervertebral disc (usually L4/5 or L5/S1)
- infection
- cervical spondylitic myelopathy—narrowing of spinal canal in old age
- hemisection of spinal cord known as Brown-Sequard syndrome—usually caused by penetrating trauma

Clinical features include:
- vertebral pain
- motor disturbance depending on level of compression: abnormal gait, weakness, paralysis; above C3,4,5 may cause respiratory failure; thoracic lesions may cause paraplegia
- sensory loss and paraesthesia
- abnormal reflexes: typically normal above level of injury, absent at level of injury and increased below

- sphincter disturbance with incontinence of bladder or bowel—a late sign. Rectal examination will confirm saddle sensation and anal tone
- loss of autonomic activity below level of compression: anhydrosis, hypotension, loss of thermoregulation
- hypertonia

If cord compression is suspected, the patient should be laid flat with the spine in neutral alignment and given analgesia. Dexamethasone can reduce inflammation and oedema around the spinal cord. MRI is the gold-standard investigation and should be obtained within 24 hours of presentation. Rapid intervention gives better outcomes and may include surgical decompression or discectomy.

Cauda Equina Syndrome

Cauda equina syndrome is caused by compression of the bundle of nerve roots below L2 level in the lumbar spine. It is a neurosurgical emergency and requires early decompression for a favourable outcome. It presents with lower back pain, saddle anaesthesia, absence of anal tone, voiding difficulty or urinary retention, bowel dysfunction, lower limb weakness, reduced or absent reflexes and lower motor neuron signs and gait disturbance. It most frequently results from lumbar disc herniation but also spinal tumours, infections, lumbar spinal stenosis, trauma, haemorrhage or an adverse result of spinal surgery/anaesthesia.

Brown-Sequard Syndrome

This is a syndrome caused by hemi-section of the spinal cord. It is rare but most often results from spinal cord trauma by gunshot or puncture wounds. It can also be caused by spinal tumours or tuberculosis although this is rare. The syndrome presents with paralysis and loss of proprioception on the same (ipsilateral) side as the injury or lesion and is caused by injury to the corticospinal tract and posterior/dorsal column. Patients will also have loss of pain and temperature sensation on the opposite (or contralateral) side caused by injury to the spinothalamic tract. MRI is the standard investigation.

Infections in Neurosurgery

Infections of the nervous system include meningitis, brain abscess and vertebral osteomyelitis/discitis. Meningitis can be caused by community onset infections (e.g., *Streptococcus pneumoniae*, *Neisseria meningitidis*) but can also complicate shunt surgery, when coagulase negative staphylococci are the principle pathogens. These organisms cause biofilms, so removal of the shunt system, with IV and sometimes intrathecal therapy are often required.

Brain abscesses can result from haematogenous spread (e.g., from an infection elsewhere in the body such as abdomen/chest) or can spread from a local source (e.g., dental abscess or middle ear infection). Treatment is by surgical drainage plus systemic antibiotics.

Vertebral osteomyelitis/discitis can also result from haematogenous or local spread. A wide variety of organisms are capable of causing this but *Staph. aureus* is the most common pathogen identified.

Tuberculosis should also be suspected as a cause of any infection in high risk groups and appropriate samples should be sent.

11

Elective Orthopaedics

Introduction

Anatomy Of The Skeleton

Basic musculoskeletal anatomy needs to be understood when managing orthopaedic care. The normal locomotor system relies on a stable skeleton to provide attachment for muscles and a base for positioning the hands and feet in space.

The **axial** skeleton consists of the skull, spine and rib cage (Fig. 11.1A). The **appendicular** skeleton evolved from fins in early fish to form the limbs (arms, shoulder girdle, legs and pelvis, Fig. 11.1B). The skeleton is the foundation for musculotendinous attachment allowing locomotion, support, protection, haematopoiesis, mineral storage and endocrine regulation.

Bone

Bone consists of an inorganic component (60% dry weight) and an organic matrix (40% dry weight). The **inorganic** calcium hydroxyapatite provides compressive strength and rigidity whilst the **organic** component, which is 90% collagen (primarily type 1), provides the tensile strength through its triple helix structure.

Structure of Long Bone

Bones can be classified by their shape (**long vs. flat**), macroscopic structure (**cortical vs. cancellous**) and microscopic structure (**lamellar vs. woven**). **Long bones** (e.g., femur, humerus, forearm, metacarpal and metatarsal bones) have three regions: epiphysis, metaphysis and diaphysis (Fig. 11.2). **Flat bones** (e.g., cranium, pelvis, scapula) are composed of cortical bone enclosing a minimal trabecular region.

Periosteum consists of fibrous (fibroblastic) and inner cambium (osteogenic) layers and is tightly bonded to bone by Sharpey fibres. It covers the outer surface of all bones, except at the joints of long bones. **Cortical bone** has a slow turnover (formation and removal) and consists of packed Haversian systems (osteons, neurovascular canals and interstitial lamellae) which give bone its strength. **Cancellous** bone is softer, porous, more elastic and has a higher turnover, undergoing 'stress-dependant' remodelling. **Woven bone** is immature or pathological bone. It is typically weaker, more flexible, has a high turnover rate and greater osteocyte density than lamellar bone.

Managing the Orthopaedic Patient

General Considerations

A good clinical history and thorough examination is essential. Decision making in orthopaedics and fracture management never rests purely on x-ray or magnetic resonance imaging (MRI) scan findings. Factors to be considered before imaging include:

- Age: many fractures and orthopaedic conditions are very age specific.
- Occupation: some occupations are more likely to produce orthopaedic problems but, in addition, knowing a patient's occupation (and hobbies) gives insight into their financial responsibilities and aspirations. Retired people too have

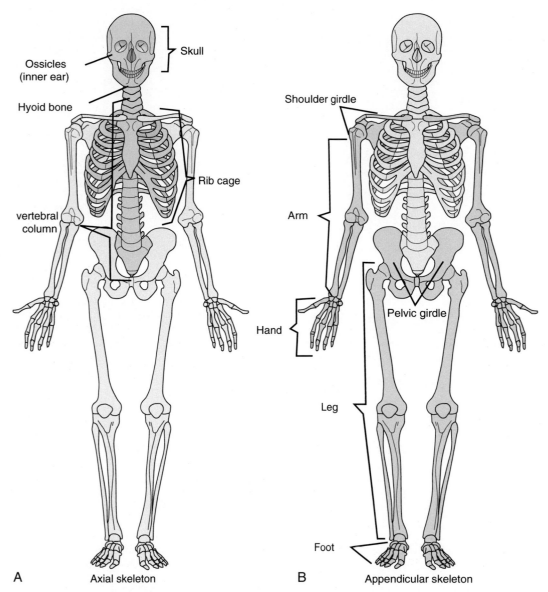

- **Fig. 11.1** The adult human skeleton consists of 206 bones; the axial skeleton comprises 80 bones **(A)** and the appendicular skeleton 126 bones **(B)**. Unlike the axial skeleton, the appendicular skeleton is unfused, thus allowing for a greater range of movement.

aspirations. Being interested in your patient as a whole helps them help you with their management.

- **History of the main complaint:**
  - Pain: most orthopaedic problems cause pain. History includes direct questions to ascertain the following characteristic of the pain: how long has it been present; where is it felt; does it radiate; the quality of the pain; is there associated numbness, paraesthesia or weakness; when does it occur; is there associated stiffness?
  - Deformity: indicates the alignment of a body part is abnormal.
  - Are there other bone or joint problems?
  - How does the problem affect the patient's activities and life generally?
- Family history—enquire about possible inherited diseases but tread carefully: there may be issues of perceived guilt when speaking to a child's parents.

- **Examination:** simply 'Look, feel and move' was advocated years ago but is not enough; you must take account of the whole patient and not just the part in question:
  - **Look** with the patient appropriately undressed; look for deformity by comparing the sides. Look at the skin. Look at the hands—thick skin indicates a heavy physical activity and usually means the patient has recently been able to lift heavy items.
  - **Feel** for tenderness but be gentle. Feel for lumps. Do not forget to palpate pulses.
  - **Passively move** the part to check the range of movement, but be sure not to hurt the patient—watch their face. Estimate the range of movement in degrees from the 'anatomical position'. It is often easiest to estimate range starting from a right angle.
  - **Active movement:** is estimated when detecting weakness and is essential in patients with neuromuscular disease.

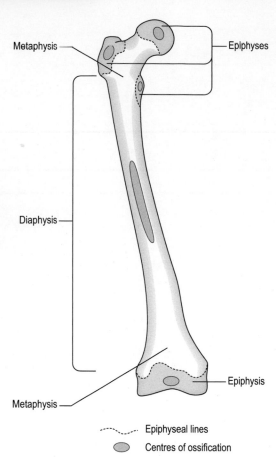

Metaphysis

Epiphyses

Diaphysis

Metaphysis

Epiphysis

- - - - Epiphyseal lines

⬮ Centres of ossification

• **Fig. 11.2** Structure of a Long Bone. The **epiphysis** lies beyond the growth plate and incorporates the articular surface, a subchondral region and a **physis** at its base. The **metaphysis** is the wider section of a long bone between the epiphysis and the **diaphysis** or shaft. Periosteum covers the whole bone except the articular surface.

The Medical Research Council grading of weakness is frequently used:

0 = No discernible muscle contraction
1 = A flicker of muscle contraction, but insufficient to move joint
2 = Muscle contaction can move joint, but only if gravity is eliminated (and limb weight is counterbalanced)
3 = Muscle contraction is sufficient to move against gravity
4 = Functional but not normal power
5 = Normal

- Investigations:
  - **Bloods tests:** full blood count; C-reactive protein (CRP) and erythrocyte sedimentation rate if systemic illness seems possible. In possible polyarthritis, a full rheumatological screen including estimation of the serum urate should be performed.
  - **Imaging**
    - **X-rays** are usually still the first-line imaging. They are cheap and readily accessible, and patients like to know about their x-rays. The usual model is two x-rays at right angles including nearby joints. Radiology of the skeleton in its loaded state can give more information, a "standing" radiograph of a joint will often give more information especially in an arthritic knee or deformed foot. This too applies in spinal fractures, where "stability" can be assessed by comparison of vertebral height/alignment to non-standing radiographs.
    - **Ultrasound** gives a dynamic view of soft tissues but bones are not imaged in useful detail. Swellings (including

cysts and ganglions), ligaments, muscles and tendons are well evaluated. A dynamic picture of a joint can help in motion disorders or impingement syndromes. Ultrasound guided injections are popular.

- **Computed tomography** (CT) scanning was the first effective three-dimensional (3D) imaging technique and revolutionised spinal imaging, replacing imprecise contrast studies. The speed of data acquisition has increased markedly and the radiation dose has reduced since its inception. CT scans can give detail of bones down to millimetre level. Images can be reformatted into 3D models, for example, for fractures or to plan complex anatomical reconstructions of acetabulum or spine
- Magnetic Resonance Imaging (**MRI**) is increasingly used to give detail of soft tissues, bones and joints. MRI is now the gold standard where x-rays and ultrasound are inadequate. MRI is particularly useful for menisci and ligaments in the knee the spine and nerve roots exiting the spinal cord; tumours; infections; some fractures and to assess synovial thickening (for contraindications, see Ch. 5).
- **Isotope scanning** is safe (see Ch. 5). Whole body bone scans can show multiple lesions, such as disseminated malignancy. Labelled white cell scanning can pinpoint suspected bone infection.
- Positron Emission Tomography (**PET**) scans are being increasingly used for investigating tumours, both locally and for systemic spread.
- **Arthroscopy.** Accurate diagnosis of a joint injury often requires internal inspection. Arthroscopy is often used shoulder, elbow, wrist and ankle pathology. It is less often in the hip. It is usually performed as a day case under anaesthesia., The arthroscope is connected to a camera so that a magnified view of the joint can be seen on a screen. **Therapeutic arthroscopy** enables abnormalities to be repaired or material removed. Most procedures take 30 to 45 minutes and recovery is usually rapid, however in more complex surgery such as hip arthroscopy this can take even longer. Arthroscopic techniques have been gradually extended to include ligament reconstruction, rotator cuff repair and cartilage repair. Similar minimal invasive technology is being employed in spinal deformity surgery, as "thoracoscopy".

Useful Jargon Words and Phrases in Orthopaedics

Osteotomy: cutting a bone, such as when it needs to be realigned.

Arthrodesis or fusion means that a joint is excised and then the two bone ends are encouraged to heal together as in a fracture healing response.

Arthroplasty is where a joint is removed and replaced with an artificial joint. This may be a total joint replacement or part of a joint (hemi-arthroplasty).

An excision arthroplasty is where a joint is entirely removed and the bone ends left without articulating surfaces (e.g., Girdlestone's excision arthroplasty of the hip). Some stability is achieved by scar tissue in the longer term but these operations are rarely performed as nowadays some form of reconstruction is usually possible.

Valgus and varus: *valgus* means the distal part points away from the midline and *varus* is the opposite. In hallux valgus, the big toe points laterally and in a bowed knee (genu varus), the lower leg angles towards the midline.

Dynamic Hip Screw (**DHS**) for extracapsular femur neck fractures but can be used for nondisplaced intracapsular fractures (see page 235).

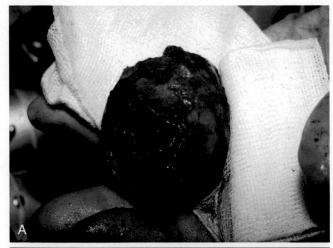

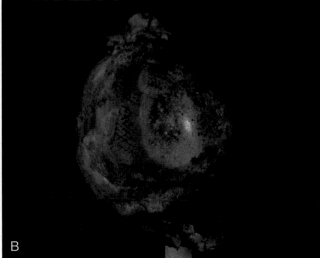

• **Fig. 11.3** Femoral Heads Removed at Operation. **(A)** Rapidly progressive erosive arthritis with femoral head collapse. **(B)** Specimen from a man with >8 years of slowly progressive disease.

Intamedullary Nail **(IMN)**. Fixation for stabilising long bone fractures.

Open reduction internal fixation **(ORIF)**, typically with plate and/or screw devices but also tension band wire (TBW) or suture techniques.

Arthritis

Rheumatologists diagnose and treat arthritis nonoperatively while surgeons are trained in surgery as well. Any condition that causes a joint to become imperfect leads to changes recognised as arthritis, but the reason a particular joint becomes arthritic is often ill understood. Malalignment or any condition that produces irregular joint surfaces are potent factors. The rate of joint deterioration is important. Fig. 11.3 shows femoral heads removed at operation. Fig. 11.3A shows a rapidly progressive erosive arthritis with femoral head collapse and Fig. 11.3B, a specimen from a man with more than 8 years of slowly progressive disease; they are quite different.

Pitfalls in Orthopaedic Diagnosis

Orthopaedic patients usually present with pain or loss of function. It is possible that patients can misdiagnose the problem as originating from a different area, such as their back, shoulder or knee, for example, but this may be incorrect. The examining doctor may miss serious pathologies affecting other areas unless a careful general health history is taken and lateral thinking sometimes used. The list of potential errors is long so beware!

Important examples include:

- a retroperitoneal, reticuloendothelial, gynaecological or prostatic problem presenting as backache;
- lung cancer or cardiac disease masquerading as arm pain;
- knee pain arising from the hip;
- diabetes presenting for the first time as numbness, foot pain and paraesthesia.

Litigation

In many parts of the world, orthopaedic and trauma surgeons have become the most likely specialists to be sued. To guard against future trouble, comprehensive contemporary notes must always be kept and it is good practice to copy any correspondence to the patient which should include a full explanation of what the problem is (as far as is known), what the management plan is and what (if any) alternative treatments are available, particularly if surgery is advocated. The risks of surgery must be fully explained and also the risk of not undergoing treatment.

Children's Orthopaedic Surgery

Always, in the back of anyone's mind who has undertaken paediatric orthopaedics, is the child's physical development. The skeleton starts forming between the 6–8th week of intra-uterine life and reaches a stable state, usually, between 15 and 18 years. Obviously, the child's development goes hand in hand with the rest of their physical and mental development. Normal development is put at risk by many diseases and injuries, both congenital and acquired. Inadequate treatment of paediatric orthopaedic problems can lead to a lifetime of disability.

The key to successful management is to understand the natural history of paediatric orthopaedic disorders; there are many conditions that appear very abnormal but turn out to grow normally if left alone; these are 'normal variants'. These need to be distinguished from serious conditions. Paediatric orthopaedic surgeons work closely with paediatricians (particularly paediatric rheumatologists), geneticists and physiotherapists which allows them a better overview of the child, the disorder, the family setting and any inherited problem.

History taking includes the birth and delivery history, family history and developmental history including milestones. Fully examining the child may include watching them walk, run and play. Only by checking every aspect of the musculoskeletal system can one reassure a parent their *child* is normal.

Normal variants include conditions such as the majority of flat feet, metatarsus adductus, genu varum or valgus, persistent femoral anteversion or retroversion. Most ligamentous laxity is a normal variation or it can occur in specific conditions such as hip dysplasia and Marfan's syndrome.

Specific Conditions and Their Treatment

Developmental Dysplasia of the Hip (Figs 11.4 and 11.5)

All children in developed countries are screened at birth for unstable hips using Barlow tests and seeking the Ortolani sign, and screened again at 6 to 8 weeks. Where there is doubt, or there is a family history of childhood hip problems, a breech birth, twin

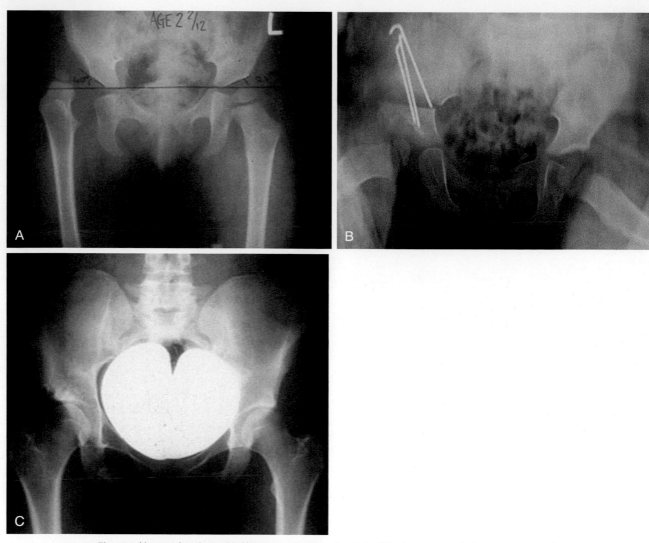

• **Fig. 11.4** X-rays of patient with late presenting hip dysplasia **(A)**, who went on to have an open reduction and pelvic (Salter) osteotomy **(B)**, and 25 years later **(C)**. The wing of the ilium supplied a bone graft.

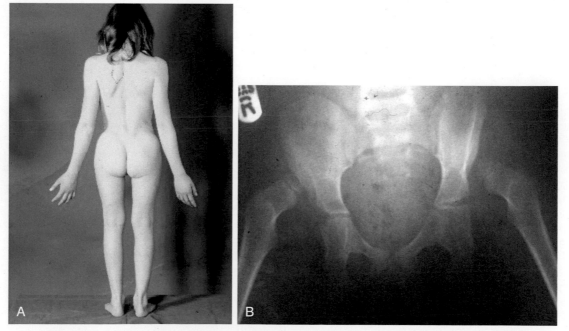

• **Fig. 11.5** A 7-year-old who had just presented with bilateral development dysplasia of the hip (DDH). **(A)** Note that the photograph was taken from behind and shows a lumbar lordosis. **(B)** The x-ray shows bilateral high DDH with bilateral dysplastic acetabulae.

birth or premature delivery, ultrasound scanning should be performed. Girls are 10 times more frequently affected than boys. At this age, treatment is conservative, with a dynamic Pavlik Harness or similar device being worn for about 3 months.

Despite screening being in use for over 50 years, some children still present with a dislocated hip later than the newborn period. Under 1 year, treatment requires surgical adductor release or formal release of medial adductors, psoas and medial capsule and about 3 months in plaster. Later presentation still occurs when the child starts walking (and sometimes into the mid and late teens). The child presents with a painless Trendelenburg short leg limp, and markedly reduced hip abduction in flexion. The incidence remains stubbornly at 1:1000 births. The femoral head is found to be dislocated, with a dysplastic acetabulum, usually with a 'false acetabulum' on the ilium. Surgery involves stabilising the hip joint without damaging its blood supply and hence growth potential. A plaster cast (hip spica) is applied for about 8 weeks.

Perthes Disease

Boys are much more likely to develop Perthes disease and girls more often have dysplastic hips. Perthes usually manifests between 3 and 12 years. The cause is unclear but the pathology involves avascular necrosis of the femoral head (Fig. 11.6). Spontaneous recovery occurs over 2 to 3 years but the final shape of the femoral head is critical in terms of later function. The outcome can be predicted from the radiological appearance. A poor outcome leads to premature hip arthritis; hip replacement is needed in 10% to 20%. Those that present before 5 to 6 years have the best outcomes.

Restricting activity (often difficult) is the mainstay of treatment if the predicted outcome is good. If predicted to be poor, containment surgery involving realigning the proximal femur can be beneficial. Valgus osteotomy and a *shelf procedure* for the acetabulum is indicated in children who develop coxa plana and adduction deformity.

Slipped Upper Femoral Epiphysis

In this, the femoral head slips off the neck metaphysis at the epiphyseal plate (Fig. 11.7); it can occur without significant trauma but can only occur if the growth plate is unfused. The presentation may be acute, acute-on-chronic or chronic. Traumatic slips are different and occur after extreme violence.

Slipped epiphysis presents with limping and pain, often in the knee. Many cases are missed because the hip is not examined. Signs include fixed flexion, markedly limited abduction and internal rotation, and the leg is often short. Typically, these children are overweight boys and short in stature.

Upon presentation, urgent diagnosis and treatment is crucial. Loder classified cases into those who can weight bear and those who cannot. The second group are surgical emergencies. Treatment always involves surgery. The slip is stabilised by passing a pin or specialised screw across the epiphysis. One screw is usually enough but accurate placement is technically demanding and should be undertaken only by experts. In severe slips, open reduction may be

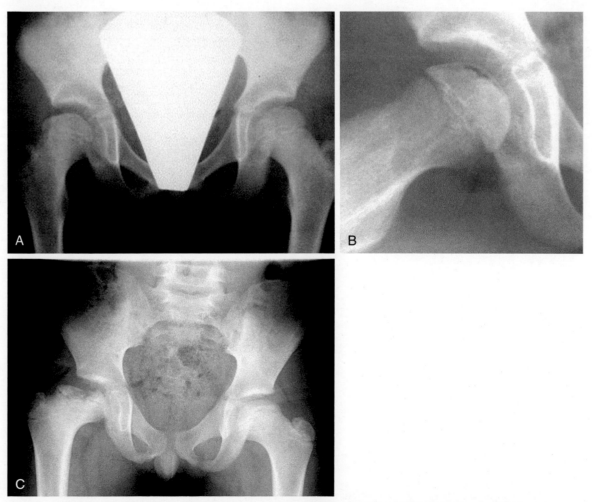

• **Fig. 11.6** Perthes Disease. **(A)** Anteroposterior pelvis showing early right sided Perthes disease. **(B)** 'Frog lateral' view x-ray showing 'head within a head' sign. **(C)** Severe right Perthes with a severely deformed 'mushroom head' deformity. The left Perthes has healed without serious deformity.

needed to avoid damaging the blood supply. Consideration should be given to prophylactic pinning of the contralateral hip. There is debate over this but the authors' view is that it should be done if the parents do not understand the potential risks, or in a premenarche girl, or in a boy whose voice has not broken.

The long-term prognosis must always be guarded as there is a marked incidence of osteoarthritis in early or mid-adulthood. Occasionally, very mild symptoms have been assumed to be growing pains and the diagnosis made only when the patient presents with an arthritic hip.

Knee Problems in Children

Pain experienced in the knee is often referred from the hip; failure to assess the hip has often led to delay in recognising a serious hip problem.

Anterior knee pain is common in children between 11 and 16 years. Full assessment needs to be made but most eventually become asymptomatic without treatment.

Osgood–Schlatter and **Larsen diseases** both affect the tibial insertion and origin of the patellar ligament. The natural history is towards spontaneous resolution but can take 18 to 24 months.

Both diseases cause activity related pain but usually resolve spontaneously. Placing the limb in a plaster cast for a month or so often speeds recovery. Osgood-Schlatter's disease often leaves a permanently prominent tubercle.

Osteochondritis dissecans is where a section of articular cartilage dissects from its femoral condyle, usually affecting the lateral side of the medial condyle. Pain and instability are typical symptoms; an intercondylar x-ray demonstrates the lesion well and MRI can be helpful in determining treatment. Many spontaneously improve but unstable lesions need to be pinned and sometimes bone grafted.

Discoid lateral meniscus—rather than being semilunar, the lateral meniscus is solid and devoid of its central recess. The condition presents as pain in the outer side of the knee, instability and clicking or clunking. Conservative management should be followed where possible. The surgical option is to 're-sculpture' it to resemble a normal lateral meniscus.

Club Foot (Talipes Equino-Varus)

About 1:1000 children is born with club foot (Fig. 11.8). For many years, early radical surgery was standard treatment. In this, all the ligaments around the joints of the hind-foot were incised,

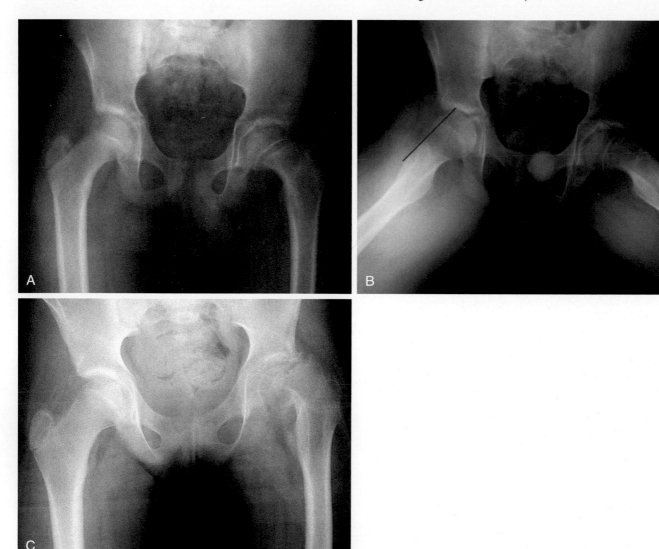

• **Fig. 11.7** Examples of Slipped Upper Femoral Epiphysis. **(A)** Anteroposterior x-ray of a moderate slip. **(B)** Frog lateral x-rays showing that Trethowan lines fail to cut the epiphysis on the affected (left) side. **(C)** Severe slip presenting with limping and a painful knee.

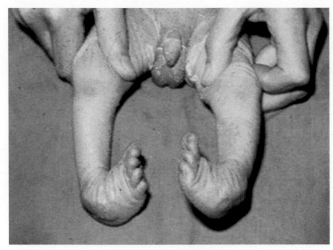

• **Fig. 11.8** Neonatal Club Feet.

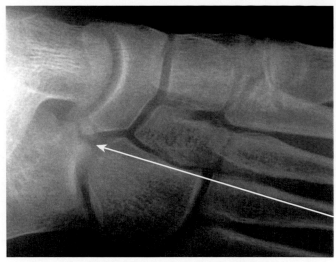

• **Fig. 11.9** X-Ray Showing Tarsal Coalition.

and the Achilles tendon and the flexor tendons lengthened. Nowadays Ponsetti's nonoperative method of manipulating and splinting the foot is usually successful. Occasionally percutaneous division of the Achilles tendon is needed and can be done in the neonatal period under local anaesthesia. The results are excellent and these patients go on to live a normal life. The condition is often picked up during a prenatal maternal ultrasound scan and the parents can be reassured about the outcome, provided more serious conditions, such as spina bifida are absent.

Pes Cavus is where the metatarsal heads lie below the heel in a neutral foot position. There is a high arch, a varus heel and usually wasting of small foot muscles. Colman's block test helps to distinguish whether the hind foot is fixed or mobile. Pes cavus can be associated with polio, hereditary sensory and motor neuropathy (Charcot–Marie–Tooth disease), spina bifida and other spinal conditions, such as diastomatomyelia. Treatment involves orthoses or reconstructive surgery.

Limb bud failures are relatively common and account for a large number of congenital deformities, such as tibial or fibular dysplasia, proximal focal deficiency and radial club hand, among others.

Tarsal coalition is an example of failure of separation (Fig. 11.9). The common types are talocalcaneal and calcaneonavicular. These coalitions can be fibrous, cartilaginous and most usually bony. They cause the child to complain of a painful foot. Examination confirms absence of hindfoot movement often with normal ankle movement. The treatment is either excision of the bar (if it is small) or surgical fusion of the subtalar and midfoot joint.

Various **eponymous syndromes** are common in a children's orthopaedic clinic. It is worth remembering that learning difficulties plus two skeletal abnormalities strongly suggests a chromosomal problem.

Primary bone tumours in children are rare although Ewing sarcoma and osteosarcoma must be considered during teenage years. Reticuloses including leukaemia can present with skeletal pain. Bone cysts and remnants of ossification errors, such as cortical fibromas are often seen incidentally on x-ray. They are usually asymptomatic and need no treatment.

Infection in Orthopaedics

Orthopaedic infections can involve soft tissues or bone or both. Soft tissue infections include those of bursae adjoining joints, tendon sheaths of hands and feet and cellulitis. Diagnosis is relatively easy but treatment is difficult without leaving a residual functional deficit or stiffness. The outcome often depends on the pathogen. Fibrosis of upper limb tendons and sheaths develops quickly even after infection has been eradicated and can severely limit hand function.

Pyogenic Joint Infections—'Septic Arthritis'

These may result from traumatic penetration of a joint, therapeutic joint injections (iatrogenic), local spread from metaphyseal osteomyelitis (particularly with intracapsular metaphyses, i.e., hip, shoulder, knee, elbow), or by haematogenous spread from a remote infection. When a synovial joint fills with pus, articular cartilage is easily damaged and can break down within hours. The blood supply can become disrupted, so treatment is urgent.

Children, including neonates, can develop primary joint infections and these must be treated urgently. *Staphylococcus aureus*, *Streptococcus pyogenes* and gram-negative cocci are the most common pathogens, but many others have been recorded. A hip full of pus can dislocate.

On examination, the child is in pain, febrile and toxic. All movements are painful so in the very young, the condition may present as apparent paralysis (pseudo-paralysis). Investigations include a full blood count, ESR and CRP. Ultrasound and MRI are useful but may be difficult, and the child may require a general anaesthetic in order to perform the imaging.

Adults: primary joint infections are uncommon and most joints affected are already abnormal, often arthritic. The usual infecting organism in septic arthritis (and in primary osteomyelitis) is *Staph. aureus*, although *Staph. pyogenes*, *Salmonella*, *Pseudomonas* and other organisms, such as Neisseria can occur, more commonly in immunocompromised patients.

Diagnosis maybe delayed because it is thought that the increased pain is caused by progression of arthritis. Delay means severe pain and rapidly progressive joint damage which will increasingly compromise potential joint. Management involves emergency investigation and arthroscopic or open washing out and debridement of the joint, followed by antibiotic treatment tailored according to culture sensitvity results (from the joint aspirate).

Crystal arthropathy: Pseudogout (calcium pyrophosphate arthropathy) can mimic infection, as can gout (monosodium urate arthropathy). Joint aspiration followed by microscopy (looking for crystals with are positively or negatively birefringent, respectively)

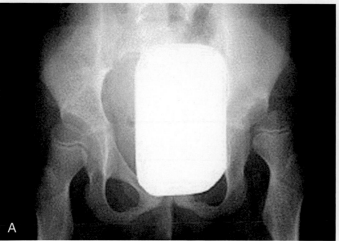
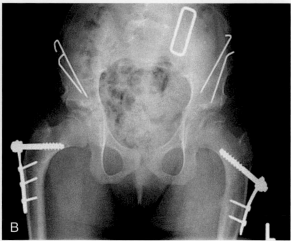

• **Fig. 11.10** Bilateral subluxing hips in a patient with severe total body cerebral palsy **(A)** treated with realignment osteotomies of upper femurs and both acetabula **(B)**.

will confirm the diagnosis. Septic arthritis can coexist with gout and pseudogout, so joint aspirations should always be sent for cultures.

Joint Replacements can become infected at the time of operation or later by metastatic infection, even years after initial surgery.

Tuberculosis (TB) can affect any joint, as well as the spine. Nowadays, it is rare in the "developed" world but common where human immunodeficiency virus (HIV) is endemic. Infection slowly destroys the affected joint. Spinal TB can lead to paraplegia (Potts paraplegia) and large ('cold') abscesses may occur. Abscesses originating from the spine can present anywhere in the lower limb but most commonly in the groin. Typically, the patient suffers from the systemic symptoms of TB, which include night sweats, weight loss and general malaise. Nowadays, treatment is usually medical (i.e. with antibiotic therapy) even in the presence of large abscesses. Immobilisation and joint arthrodesis is used much less often than in the past.

Bone Infection—Osteomyelitis

Osteomyelitis is common in "developing countries" and often presents at an advanced stage. The organisms are essentially the same as those which occur in primary joint infections.

Until antibiotics became available, the mortality in the West from acute osteomyelitis in children was >80%, because of sepsis.

Acute osteomyelitis manly affects, but is not confined to, children. It is a very painful and it causes all the symptoms of septicaemia. In patients who have sickle cell disease, the important differential diagnosis to exclude is a sickle cell "crisis". In acute osteomyelitis, the organism is usually identified from a blood culture and immediate treatment with antibiotics is usually effective. Surgical drainage is reserved for patients who fail to respond, or in abscess formation. It will progress to **chronic osteomyelitis** in neglected cases. Bone death (*sequestrum formation*), the production of a shell of new bone (*involucrum*) and the development of pus-draining sinuses may cause significant disability for the patient for the rest of their lives. The treatment of chronic osteomyelitis is often limited. Fucidic acid is often helpful during acute exacerbation and where appropriate, removal of sequestra is sometimes effective. Very occasionally massive resections of infected bone and total joint and bone replacement is indicated.

Brodie is a manifestation of chronic bone infection that has become walled off by healthy bone. It presents with chronic pain. Differential diagnosis includes osteoid osteoma. Treatment is by surgical curettage.

Diabetes and Orthopaedics

Diabetic foot problems of neuropathy and peripheral arterial disease are dealt with in Chapter 41. Diabetic medical clinics ideally work closely with orthopaedic surgeons, vascular surgeons, podiatric services and orthotic departments to ensure optimal management and supply of appropriate footwear.

Diabetes can present as a peripheral neuropathy and can intensify the symptoms of carpal tunnel syndrome and spinal stenosis. Diabetes can be responsible for neuropathic or Charcot joints, particularly in the foot and ankle. Whenever a joint has 'fallen to pieces', remember diabetes, tertiary syphilis or syringomyelia (which most commonly occurs in the upper limb), particularly when there is marked sensory loss.

Infection after total knee replacement occurs about 10 times more frequently in patients with diabetes. Patients with long standing infection of a knee replacement run a substantial risk of amputation.

Orthopaedic Surgery and Neurological Problems Outside the Spine

Central Nervous System Diseases

Cerebral Palsy (CP) is usually caused by an injury to the brain before, during, or shortly after birth, such as lack of oxygen or systemic illness. It is nonprogressive and affects upper motor neurones. The skeleton is initially normal but with growth, there is unbalanced paralysis around joints causing deformity, dislocations and contractures (Fig. 11.10). Children with total body CP may have major learning difficulties, deafness, blindness or incontinence and are unlikely ever to walk. The pain and rigidity of dislocated hips or scoliosis can prevent them sitting upright in a wheelchair but surgery can often improve the situation: children with dislocated hips can have them reduced, scoliosis can be corrected and stabilised, and hemiplegia can benefit from lengthening of a contracted Achilles tendon.

In adults, following a stroke, surgery for deformities and contractures is less successful but there are sometimes indications for tendon releases, particularly in patients who have not had suitable rehabilitation. Managing these patients is a team effort, often led by a physiotherapist.

Poliomyelitis is a viral disease affecting the anterior horn cells of the spinal cord. It can cause paralysis and this may be extensive or localised to one muscle group. It can cause death through respiratory muscle paralysis. Paralysis is often unbalanced, eventually leading to deformity and contractures. Spinal scoliosis is a common complication and can make respiration difficult. Splints and rehabilitative physiotherapy are vital and surgery can include arthrodesis of unstable joints and tendon transfers such as a tibialis posterior tendon transfer. Tibialis anterior is commonly affected whereas tibialis posterior is often spared. In these cases, tibialis posterior can be transferred through the interosseous membrane to the dorsum of the foot, so that the patient no longer needs to wear a foot drop splint.

Other peripheral neuropathies include Charcot–Marie–Tooth disease (which can cause peroneal muscular dystrophy) and other hereditary muscular dystrophies. These can lead to foot and ankle problems, such as pes cavus and foot drop. If splintage is not enough, surgery can be beneficial, until the unrelenting progress of the disease renders the patient immobile.

Peripheral Neurological Conditions

Brachial plexus trauma can be caused by penetrating injuries or by closed (avulsion) trauma. Injuries can be pre- or postganglionic. Testing for a 'triple response' (Lewis) was the traditional method of distinguishing between groups but MRI now gives a more reliable picture. Avulsion of a root as it exits the dura inevitably means a poor prognosis, with no chance of recovery.

Birth injuries to the brachial plexus include Erb palsy, caused by damage to the upper plexus, notably C5 and C6, whilst Klumpke paralysis mainly involves the lower roots.

Open injuries include penetrating stab wounds but have included iatrogenic injury by a surgeon attempting to biopsy a cervical lymph node.

Closed brachial plexus injuries in adults usually occur in motorcyclists who have landed concurrently on the side of the head and the point of the shoulder. Tell-tale signs include damage to the side of the crash helmet and a graze on the shoulder. Sadly, avulsions often involve the entire plexus, with an associated Horner syndrome, but occasionally only the C5 and C6 roots are avulsed.

Treatment for these injuries is limited. Specialist units repair some of the damaged nerves, and muscle transfers are sometimes rewarding. Rehabilitation and retraining need to start early.

Entrapment of peripheral nerves by various structures are common and surgical decompression is often indicated.

Carpal tunnel syndrome (see later).

Ulnar nerve compression at the elbow causes pain and paraesthesia in the ulnar nerve distribution in the hand. Left untreated, it may slowly lead to a weak hand with marked reduction in function of the interossei and ulnar lumbrical muscles as well as loss of sensation. The history, as with carpal tunnel syndrome, is the most important part of the diagnosis. Electrophysiological assessment can be helpful. There is usually no obvious underlying cause but cubitus valgus (sometimes following lateral condylar fracture) and osteoarthritis predispose to the condition. It can develop in patients in hospital recovering from major surgery, possibly because of long periods of elbow flexion. Surgery for uncomplicated cases involves decompressing the nerve by dividing the arch formed by the two heads of flexor carpi ulnaris. If there is an elbow flexion contracture or cubitus valgus, the nerve is transposed anteriorly to the medial epicondyle, however there is an incidence of nerve infarction after this.

Lower limb entrapments. Other notable neural entrapments include: meralgia paraesthetica, tarsal tunnel syndrome, common peroneal nerve compression and Morton neuroma.

Note that lumbar spine nerve root entrapment is dealt with in the Spine section (see page 152).

Somatisation

"It must be psychological" … how many times has this suggestion been made when there later proved to be serious disease? As a clinician's knowledge and experience of diseases increases, the idea that a patient has a 'functional disorder' or is 'making it up', somatising, being hysterical and so on, is contemplated far less often. Very few patients 'make it up' and it is always best to assume they have not done so.

Occasionally, a positive diagnosis of 'nonorganic disease' can be made by an experienced doctor, but this can only be entertained after rigorous clinical assessment and a series of negative investigations.

Examples of misdiagnosis include the patient with progressive dementia cured by removing an intracranial meningioma; or the limping adolescent whose knee is normal sent to a child psychiatrist but proves later to have a slipped upper femoral epiphysis.

Occasionally patients claim financial benefit blaming disability from musculoskeletal symptoms but are found to have thick skin on their hands and detritus under their nails. It would be reasonable to ask how this is possible if they are unable to undertake manual work.

Bone Tumours

These may be benign or malignant but some do not fall into this binary classification. More complex and serious tumours are generally dealt with in specialised centres.

Benign Bone 'Tumours'

Bone may be replaced by fluid (simple cysts), fibrous tissue or cartilage. Benign cartilage tumours may occur inside the bone (enchondroma) or outside it (ecchondroma). Some originally benign cartilaginous tumours, can undergo late onset malignant change.

Osteoid osteomas are very small benign tumours that cause severe pain and can escape diagnosis for a long time. Spinal osteomas cause marked stiffness. The pain is usually responsive to aspirin and nonsteroidal anti-inflammatory drugs (NSAIDs) and this may help diagnosis. Lesions have a soft central nidus which may be only 2 to 3 mm across, surrounded by layers of sclerotic bone. In the early stages, these are difficult to detect on plain x-rays but isotope scans and MRI show them well. Treatment is excision but as they can be difficult to locate, preoperative CT and localisation by transfixing with a sharp instrument can help. In the spine radiofrequency ablation (by interventional radiologists) has good results. The differential diagnosis is Brodie abscess (see under *Infection*) so the specimen should be assessed bacteriologically.

Giant cell tumours originate near old epiphyseal lines and grow slowly up to but not across joints. About 2% are malignant, but even benign ones can grow rapidly, weakening bone and disrupting soft tissue. They are usually surgically resectable, and the residual cavity is bone grafted.

Multiple exostoses and multiple osteochondromas (and the similar *diaphyseal achlasia*) are autosomal dominant conditions. Affected patients sometimes have tens of tumours in many bones. They enlarge with growth and can become tender. Those on flat bones, such as ribs, scapula and pelvis are susceptible to malignant change. They may expand inwards into the chest or pelvic cavity and not be evident until it is too late. Surgical treatment involves removing any tumours causing symptoms. Affected patients are favoured by examiners for 'short cases' in examinations.

Malignant Bone Tumours

Secondary Malignancy

Bony metastases are much more common than primary malignancies. They can arise from most primary cancers but bronchus, breast and prostate metastases are common. Kidney and thyroid are others that examiners expect candidates to remember. Renal bone metastases can be highly vascular, which is important when deciding whether surgical excision is appropriate. The usual presentation of bony metastases is localised pain, often followed by pathological fracture. The fractured abnormal bone is unlikely to heal and often requires surgical stabilisation.

Primary Malignant Tumours

These are rare and include osteosarcoma, chrondosarcoma and fibrosarcoma as well as diffuse malignancies like lymphomas and malignant myeloma.

Osteosarcoma is a tumour that still causes grave concern, particularly as it affects fit young people between 15 and 30 years. There are about 2000 cases a year in the United Kingdom and until recently, 12-month survival was less than 50%. Osteosarcoma typically occurs around the knee but it has been reported in most bones. Like all cancers, it invades locally (the 'sunray spicules' on an x-ray) and metastasises distantly, particularly to the lungs. It also develops 'skip' lesions further along the medullary cavity of the bone. Nowadays with team care, accurate diagnosis, surgery (including massive replacement of long bones) and oncological treatment, the prognosis has improved dramatically.

There is a second peak of osteosarcoma later in life when it manifests in preexisting Paget disease. Here it is usually multifocal and very difficult to treat.

Chondrosarcoma occurs in middle age, usually situated near the ends of long bones. It can arise in benign cartilage tumours and it tends to be resistant to oncological treatment. Surgery is the mainstay, even for secondary deposits.

Regional Orthopaedics

Upper Limb

Common Orthopaedic Conditions Around the Elbow

Tennis elbow is a condition suffered by many and talked about by more. It typically affects people between 20 and 50 years and presents with activity-related pain around the lateral side of the elbow and in the extensor muscles. Symptoms range from being severe and disabling to being an intermittent nuisance. The natural history favours spontaneous resolution. The key to diagnosis is finding intense tenderness at the extensor muscle/lateral ligament origin or over the lateral epicondyle (*lateral epicondylitis*). Wearing a tennis elbow orthosis or strap just below the elbow often helps; corticosteroid plus local anaesthetic injections are the mainstay of treatment. In recalcitrant cases, surgical release of the extensors and sometimes shaving of the lateral epicondyle is effective in most cases.

Golfer elbow. This is similar to tennis elbow except it affects the common flexor origin and the medial epicondyle. Treatment is similar.

Ulnar nerve neuritis—please see Neurology and Orthopaedics (page 160).

Olecranon bursitis (student's elbow). Inflammation of the bursa between skin and olecranon causes swelling and discomfort. An olecranon spur may be present. The condition often resolves over several months, although the bursa can become infected. Surgical excision should be reserved for patients with chronic disabling pain or where it is not resolving.

Arthritis of the elbow joint is much less likely to cause major disability than osteoarthritic hip or knee. It presents with pain and increasing stiffness. Most can be managed conservatively, with joint replacement reserved for severe cases, particularly in patients with inflammatory arthritis.

Orthopaedic Problems Around the Shoulder

Most shoulder problems present with pain and sometimes stiffness and limited mobility. Note that shoulder pain may be referred from an origin in the cervical spine, neck, heart or lung.

Subacromial Joint Disease

The subacromial space (SAS) lies between the acromion and the head of humerus. It contains the rotator cuff into which the rotator muscles are inserted. The cuff stabilizes the humeral head in the gleno-humeral joint throughout its very wide range of shoulder joint movement. The rotator cuff complex is the origin of more than 90% of shoulder pain. The rotator cuff can become:

- degenerate and partially or completely ruptured
- calcified in various parts
- inflamed, to produce a 'frozen shoulder'

The natural history of all these is unpredictable.

Calcification syndromes usually resolve spontaneously over 2 years. Those with severe pain can be helped by ultrasound guided corticosteroid and local anaesthetic injections. In extreme cases, urgent decompression and excision of the calcification may be indicated.

Tears of the rotator cuff become increasingly common in people over 50 years; they can be asymptomatic. **Major tears** require surgical repair, wherever possible.

Impingement in the sub-acromial space presents as a painful arc syndrome. Surgery can be indicated for impingement alone and this can be undertaken arthroscopically. Pain in the SAS without definite degeneration often responds to steroid and local anaesthetic injections.

Ruptured Long Head of Biceps

This is probably caused by avascular necrosis caused by trauma to its nutrient vessels in the bicipital groove. The patient, usually a middle-aged male, experiences a snap and the biceps immediately takes on a 'Popeye' shape. After the initial bruising, function steadily returns and after a few months, the odd appearance is the only legacy of the injury. Treatment is not indicated.

The uncommon injury of distal biceps tendon rupture, sometimes seen in gymnasts, needs urgent repair.

Gleno-Humeral Joint Problems

Instability. Acute dislocation may be anterior (most commonly) or posterior (usually associated with epilepsy, electroconvulsive therapy, or electrocution). Acute dislocation can lead to recurrent subluxation or dislocation. The diagnosis of recurrent dislocation is made from the history and the 'apprehension sign' on the patient's face when the shoulder is moved to where it often dislocates. The natural history is for dislocation to occur with ever increasing ease.

Treatment is surgical, with the aim of repairing any capsular detachment, adding a bone buttress to the glenoid and restricting external rotation of the shoulder by plicating the capsule.

Habitual Subluxation typically occurs in young adults who can sublux their gleno-humeral joint to order. Rehabilitation, rather than surgery, is indicated.

Arthritis. Gleno-humeral arthritis, particularly primary osteo-arthritis, is uncommon compared with hip arthritis. It presents with pain and stiffness and steadily deteriorating shoulder function. However, the disorder is common in generalised arthritides, such as rheumatoid, or conditions such as avascular necrosis. The diagnosis is confirmed on x-ray and/or MRI.

Where surgery is indicated, total shoulder replacement has largely superseded arthrodesis, although there are still indications for arthrodesis in countries where replacement is not an option. If the rotator cuff has failed, a 'reversed' shoulder replacement could be indicated to replace and stabilise the joint. Long-term results beyond 15 years are not yet available.

Hand and Wrist

A lot can be learned about a patient from their hands …
(ANON)

Students and trainees will be expected to diagnose the common conditions affecting the hand and wrist:

Carpal tunnel syndrome is the most common. The median nerve becomes compressed in the carpal tunnel causing pain, paraesthesia and numbness in the distribution of the median nerve besides weakness thenar muscles, particularly abductor pollicis brevis. Fifteen times as many females (usually over 35 years old) are affected as males. Nocturnal pain is common and debilitating, and the patient often shakes the hand to ease their symptoms. Carpal tunnel syndrome can be associated with pregnancy, hypothyroidism and acromegaly. Electromyography (EMG) will usually confirm the diagnosis in all except the milder cases. Fisrt-line treatments include splints and steroid injections into the tunnel. If these fail to provide lasting benefit, surgically dividing the transverse carpal ligament (usually under local anaesthetic) is straightforward and usually curative, relieving unpleasant chronic symptoms of pain very quickly. However, patients are unlikely to recover from the permanent the effects of chronic nerve damage, such as weakness and permanent paraesthesia.

Trigger finger is where the long flexor tendon to one (or more) fingers cannot pass easily through the A1 pulley proximally in the flexor sheath in the palm. Patients flex their fingers and then cannot straighten them without passive stretching, which is when they 'trigger'. The condition can be so painful that patients present with a flexed finger without a history of triggering. Many respond well to steroid plus local anaesthetic injections into the flexor tunnel. Surgical division of the A1 pulley is straightforward but is reserved for patients who do not respond to injections.

Dupuytren disease occurs most commonly in elderly men although an aggressive type can affect much younger people. The aetiology is unknown. The palmar fascia becomes thickened and shortened and causes fixed finger flexion to various degrees. The ulnar side of the palmar fascia is usually worst affected, together with the little and ring fingers. Thenar bands indicate radial involvement, and dorsal swellings over the knuckles (Garrod pads) often indicate more aggressive disease.

The condition usually progresses slowly but can cause major disability, particularly where hands are important for work. Surgery is the mainstay of treatment and should be performed before the deformity becomes severe when the result of operation would inevitably be poor. Even after successful operation, the condition can return. Dupuytren disease can also affect the plantar fascia (Ledderhose's disease) and the penile fascia (Peyronie's disease).

Dorsal and palmar 'ganglia' are common in younger people. A ganglion is a sac of gelatinous fluid arising in association with the wrist joint, a carpal joint or a tendon. Most disappear with time but they can be painful and disfiguring, particularly to a teenage female. Dorsal ganglia can be large—up to 3 cm across—whereas those near the flexor tendon sheath in the distal palm are the size of a grain of rice but are more likely to be painful.

Many ganglia have been excised in the past but the recurrence rate is high and the natural history is resolution so they should be left alone wherever possible.

Acquired hand deformities are common. With increasing age, many people develop nodules around finger joints (Herbeden nodes) and these do not respond to surgery. The 'swan neck' and Boutonniere deformities so common in patients with rheumatoid disease, before modern medical treatment, responded poorly to surgery.

Arthritis of the Trapezio-metacarpal joint at the thumb base is common and presents with pain and joint prominence. The condition can burn itself out after many months, leaving only moderate stiffness. In persistent cases, most surgeons offer trapezietomy, though artificial joints or fusion have met with some success.

Mallet finger describes a flexion deformity at the distal interphalangeal joint (DIPJ) of a finger. Mild trauma is usually responsible. Splintage for 6 weeks helps reduce the deformity. Surgery can help if there is an avulsion fracture at the base of the distal phalanx. Most people eventually cope with the deformity with little disability.

De Quervain tenovaginitis at the wrist is caused by inflammation and thickening of the sheath around abductor pollicis longus and extensor pollicis brevis. Opposing the thumb across the palm reproduces the symptoms, and pinpoint tenderness over the thickened sheath is diagnostic. The condition is often self-limiting. Steroid injections into the sheath often help and surgical release is usually curative in severe cases.

Lower Limb

Hip

A range of pathologies can affect the hip joint. A malfunctioning hip is more disabling than disease of almost any other joint. Body weight normally passes down through the spine, symmetrically across both sacroiliac joints and through the centres of rotation of the hips to the knees and beyond. The femoral head acts as a fulcrum around which the femur and pelvis rotate. Any pathology that interferes with this alignment or congruity of the joint leads to problems in the long term, particularly degenerative arthritis ('osteoarthritis').

Common childhood diseases that lead eventually to hip arthritis include:
- Developmental dysplasia of the hip;
- Perthes disease;
- Slipped upper femoral epiphysis (SUFE);
- Some syndromic conditions, such as spondyloepiphyseal dysplasia (SED).

Femoral/acetabular impingement (FAI) syndromes including protrusio acetabulae are also potent causes of degenerative change.

Adult pathologies that lead to similar end results include conditions that disrupt the femoral head blood supply and lead to avascular necrosis include:
- Subcapital fractures of the femoral neck or head;
- Traumatic hip dislocation;
- Sickle-cell disease and caisson disease (hyperbaric disease in divers) cause blockage of the nutrient vessels;
- Corticosteroids and excess alcohol;

- Miscellaneous conditions, such as inflammatory arthritides including rheumatoid, psoriasis and ankylosing spondylitis. The inflammation cascade leads to what is essentially a ruined joint.

Hip Arthritis

'Hip arthritis' affects millions of people worldwide, but the term represents a catch-all of different diagnoses and pathologies. The average age at presentation is about 60 years but when the condition is secondary to an earlier hip problem, age of onset is much younger.

Symptoms include pain, stiffness and instability. Treatment depends on the severity of symptoms in relation to the patient's expectations, lifestyle and personal relationships. **Pain** can cause loss of mobility and loss of sleep. **Restricted range of movement** particularly of adduction and flexion interfere with mobility. **Walking distance** should be assessed—from barely able to cross a room, barely able to cross a road to being able to walk a kilometre or more. Pain is classically felt in the groin, but often in the front or outer thigh, buttock, knee and low back or a combination of these. Occasionally it radiates below the knee. Note that knee pain alone can be a symptom of hip problems.

Examination proceeds with the patient as flat as they will allow, and the passive range of movements is measured. Active movements are of little value. There is usually stiffness and often a degree of fixed flexion, **add**uction (occasionally **abd**uction) and external rotation. Comparison with the contralateral hip is useful although that may be arthritic too. Fixed flexion deformity (FFD) is diagnosed with the Thomas test as follows: since a mobile lumbar spine can mask an FFD, the other hip is flexed until the lumbar lordosis is flattened against the examiner's hand. The affected hip may then be seen to be in fixed flexion. A 30-degree FFD can be recorded as 'minus 30 degrees of extension'. A proportion of osteoarthritic hip patients complain of leg shortness. This is usually caused by an adduction deformity rather than true shortening which is often minimal unless caused by another cause, such as hip dislocation. **Apparent shortening** is tested by measuring from the umbilicus to the ankle and comparing one leg length against the other. **True shortening** is measured from the anterior superior iliac spine to the ankle. Prescribing a shoe raise for apparent shortening is clearly contraindicated.

Conservative treatment includes the use of a stick (usually best in the opposite hand), analgesia and sometimes NSAIDs.

Operations for Hip Arthritis. Older operations, such as osteotomy and arthrodesis, have become historical curiosities. Conservative surgery for Femoro-Acetabular impingement (FAI) can be undertaken arthroscopically and some reconstructive operations are performed on top-flight sports people to better align the acetabulum with the head of the femur.

Total Hip Replacement

About 100,000 total hip replacements (THRs) are performed annually in the United Kingdom and perhaps 2 million around the world. It is a major operation and has been described as the most important new operation of the (last) century. The operation carries a moderate risk and the best THR designs often last 20 years or more without revision. There are many different designs of implant and not all are equally good. The UK National Joint Registry records the detailed attributes of each design and the outcomes of every operation, allowing problems to be analysed in depth and faulty designs to be detected early.

Other Painful Conditions Around the Hip

These include **trochanteric bursitis**, an ill-defined condition where pain and tenderness are centred around the greater trochanter, and **meralgia paraesthetica** where the lateral cutaneous nerve of the thigh becomes compressed under the inguinal ligament. Both can respond to steroid injections and the latter improves after surgical decompression

The Knee

Sports players in particular know how vulnerable the knee can be. Older people often have knees that ache and some become increasingly arthritic.

Symptoms of knee pathology include pain, instability, 'locking' and noise. **Pain** may be generalised, anterior or one-sided and is usually associated with local tenderness. **Instability** is a feeling that the knee is about to give way (and it may do so, although falls are rare). **Locking** is where the knee becomes stuck in one position and is caused by a displaced meniscus or a bony 'loose body' jammed in the joint. **Noise** is usually crepitus from one irregular surface articulating with another under load. Severely arthritic joints can 'crack' but noise is often a relatively innocent symptom.

Knee Problems in Younger People

Meniscal Problems: The medial meniscus tears 10 times more often than the lateral meniscus. Tears typically occur when the joint is loaded in moderate flexion whilst the thigh is rotated. Tears may present acutely with a 'locked knee' which is sore, swollen and cannot fully extend. MRI scanning settles the diagnosis and arthroscopic surgery is indicated when the diagnosis is confirmed. The standard treatment is to resect the torn fragment, but major peripheral or 'bucket handle' tears, particularly in young people, are more often repaired than removed.

Anterior Cruciate Ligament Tears: The anterior cruciate ligament (ACL) runs from anterior to the tibial spine to its insertion on the medial side of the lateral femoral condyle. The typical tear results from rapid deceleration, such as occurs in skiing, football and other sports. The patient often feels a 'pop' in the knee which can no longer take weight and feels unstable. A painful haemarthrosis often develops. This injury may be associated with other ligamentous, meniscal or articular damage. Intensive rehabilitation with exercises and wearing a splint during sport is enough for many patients, but others go for reconstruction using one of their own tendons or an artificial material. Most of these operations are successful.

Posterior Cruciate Ruptures: These generally occur as a result of severe direct violence to the anterior upper tibia, such as when a car hits the leg of a motorcyclist travelling in the opposite direction. The distal end of the ligament is often avulsed with a plug of bone. The upper tibia may also be fractured. Examination from the side reveals 'hang back' of the upper tibia. Surgical reattachment of the bone plug is usually effective.

Patella Problems: Recurrent dislocation or subluxation of the patella occurs most often in females from teens onwards. Pain, swelling and 'a very odd shape' of the front of the knee follow what is often a trivial event. Rarely, but importantly it may be part of a syndrome, such as *nail-patella syndrome*.

Rehabilitation by strengthening the quadriceps is often effective; otherwise surgical realignment of the patella tendon or restructuring of the deficient lateral femoral condyle is indicated.

Prepatellar Bursitis: The bursa between skin and anterior patella can become chronically swollen and inflamed and is fondly known as *housemaid's knee*. Bursitis can occur in the bursa anterior to the patella ligament; this is *clergyman's knee*. Aspirating the bursa gives a period of symptomatic relief and can be used to exclude infection. The natural history is for gradual resolution but surgical excision is occasionally indicated.

The Acutely Swollen Painful Knee

Acute Pyogenic Infection (see also section "Pyogenic Joint Infections—'Septic Arthritis'" page 159) occurs most often in already arthritic knees. Infection is often metastatic from an infection elsewhere. There is a risk that the condition is passed off as just a 'flare up' of arthritis. If infection is suspected, the knee needs to be washed out arthroscopically and specimens sent for microscopy and culture.

Sometimes microscopy reveals crystals and a negative culture. The diagnosis then becomes *crystal arthropathy* (either gout or pseudogout). This condition can mimic infection and washouts are effective treatment.

An acute *haemarthrosis* can occur in patients with bleeding disorders or on anticoagulants.

Knee Arthritis

There is often no obvious cause for a knee to become arthritic besides increasing age. However, any malalignment, any damage to the articular surface (or menisci) or ligamentous instability will predispose to osteoarthritic knee. The knee is often involved in patients with generalised inflammatory arthritis.

As the articular surface erodes, the patient complains of increasing pain and stiffness. Patients seek medical help as their activities of daily living become increasingly impaired. Conservative management with analgesia and exercises is usually tried first. If surgery, particularily where there is a varus deformity, becomes necessary, a high tibial osteotomy is to realign the knee otherwise a knee replacement is likely to be the treatment of choice.

Knee replacements can be uni-compartmental (partial) or total (TKR). Uni-compartmental replacement involves less surgery, less risk and more rapid rehabilitation but is only appropriate when the arthritis is confined to the affected compartment.

Over 100,000 TKRs are undertaken annually in the United Kingdom (2018) and the number increases each year. This major operation carries a small mortality risk and involves resurfacing the lower femur and upper tibia with combined metal and polythene implants. Nearly all patients can expect a well-performing knee for 15 years or more.

Other Conditions Around the Knee

It must be remembered that the knee is the most common site for **primary bone tumours** in young people.

Popliteal cysts occur in juveniles (and resolve spontaneously). In adults, they are associated with arthritis and are called Baker cysts. Removal is unnecessary but the arthritic joint may need treating.

Ankle, Hindfoot and Forefoot

The ankle can be affected by degenerative change and by the ravages of arthritis but fortunately, severe disability is less common than with other major weight-bearing joints. Simplistically, treatment is to provide an orthosis (a moulded foot bed for shoes) or to operate so the patient can mobilise in normal shoes. This requires detailed discussion with the patient and may include a 'do nothing' option.

Ankle arthritis can also be caused by chronic instability resulting from lateral ligament damage fracture of the ankle mortice or talus, particularly if there has been avascular necrosis. The natural history is of slow deterioration, with increasing pain and stiffness and sometimes instability. The diagnosis is clear on x-ray. Surgical options include fusion (arthroscopic or open) or ankle replacement. The long-term results of ankle replacement are as yet uncertain. A fused ankle substantial disability and at present, in most people it will be the procedure of choice.

Chronic ankle instability is usually caused by rupture of the lateral ligament complex. It is disabling and with time, becomes more painful and causes patients to fall over. Investigation should include stress x-rays, anteroposterior and lateral (*anterior draw sign*). Rehabilitation physiotherapy and splinting or taping should be tried before operation. Operations include direct repair and ligament substitution.

Tibialis posterior insufficiency is relatively common with increasing age. It causes pain and tenderness along the course of the tendon. The natural history is slowly progressive and may lead to rupture. This produces a painful, very flat hindfoot. When viewed from behind, the forefoot is splayed laterally and the patient appears to have 'too many toes'. Orthoses are often helpful in the early stages and complex tendon substitutions or os calcis osteotomy operations are possible in severe cases.

The subtalar and midtarsal joints are more often troublesome than the ankle joint. Congenital tarsal coalition (see children's section), inflammatory arthritis, posttraumatic arthritic and diabetic Charcot joints can all affect these joints. The surgical treatment is usually fusion. **Triple fusion** involves arthrodesis of the talocalcaneal, talonavicular and calcaneocuboid joints. This reliably allows a pain free and almost fully mobile existence in normal shoes.

Forefoot

In **hallux valgus**, the first metatarsal angles towards the midline (primus varus) and the big toe or hallux angles laterally, that is, valgus. It is common, particularly in women, often becoming apparent in the teens. Obtaining suitable shoes is difficult, and the condition often worsens with increasing age and splaying of the forefoot. Patients can have shoes made to fit (but not usually stylish oncs) or corrective surgery. Surgical options include various osteotomies of the first metatarsal and realignment of the big toe; outcomes are usually satisfactory but complete recovery takes several months.

Hallux rigidus occurs when arthritis of the first metatarsophalangeal joint (MTJP) causes the big toe to become stiff and painful. Alignment is usually maintained but large osteophytes can develop. Pain sometimes settles as stiffness increases, and treatment then becomes unnecessary. In others, difficulty in walking, night pain and problems obtaining footwear leads them to having the joint fused. The differential diagnosis includes gout.

Metatarsalgia is the term given to pain across the metatarsal heads of the lesser toes. It can be secondary to hallux valgus. Other specific causes include:

- **March fracture**—typically affecting the fourth metatarsal neck and first noted in army recruits unused to marching. Initial x-rays usually fail to show evidence of fracture but MRI, isotope scans and often ultrasound confirm the diagnosis. The natural history is for complete resolution over 3 to 6 months; immobilisation in a walking boot or plaster keeps the patient comfortable during healing.

- **Morton neuroma** is a thickening on the digital nerve, usually between third and fourth metatarsal heads. It causes sharp pain and sometimes paraesthesia along the two affected toes. Compressing the forefoot transversely often causes a click (Mulder click) which is diagnostic. Conservative treatment includes a steroid/local anaesthetic injection around the nerve and/or a metatarsal arch support. Surgical excision of the nerve is curative.
- **Frieberg disease** is a type of avascular necrosis that usually starts in the early teens and often affects the second metatarsal head. It is painful but the natural history is usually towards resolution. However, the head can end up misshapen and cause pain indefinitely. Surgical excision is an option.

The most common cause of metatarsalgia is nonspecific inflammatory arthritis where the mechanics of the MTPJs become deranged leading to collapse of the transverse arch so the metatarsal heads become prominent in the sole. There is also subluxation or dislocation of the proximal phalanx causing toe deformities, such as 'hammer toe' (see later).

Rheumatoid arthritis can cause similar problems and is best managed with arch-supporting orthoses and shoes that accommodate the deformed toes. Chiropody is often needed to control the thickened plantar skin. Surgical treatment includes excision of metatarsal heads and realignment metatarsal osteotomies with relocation of the toes.

Hammer toe occurs when the proximal interphalangeal (PIP) joint becomes fixed in hyperflexion, often secondary to extension of the MTPJ. The prominent PIP joint becomes chafed by the shoe. Protective ring padding or alteration to footwear is one option; surgical straightening is another.

The Spine

Most people experience back symptoms at some time. Many spinal complaints are self-limiting but a good many are serious and often disabling. The whole spine is a common site for bone metastases, myeloma and the lymphomas.

Pain from vital organs can be referred to the spine so examination should include abdominal and rectal or pelvic examinations where appropriate.

Patients mainly complain of:
- pain
- stiffness
- deformity

Pain may radiate and be coupled with neurological symptoms, such as weakness, numbness and paraesthesia (pins and needles). Night pain must always be taken seriously and fully investigated.

Stiffness normally increases as age-related degenerative changes progress, but inflammatory conditions, such as ankylosing spondylitis can produce a painful, stiff back in a young person.

Deformity can occur in the sagittal or coronal plane or both. **Scoliosis** is caused by a rotatory deformity between vertebrae but on spinal x-ray, this shows up only as a lateral curve. **Kyphosis** is when the spine becomes stooped forward; it is particularly common in elderly, usually osteoporotic people, particularly women (*dowager hump*), and in ankylosing spondylitis.

Lumbar Spine: The More Common Problems

Lumbar spine pathology leads to more days lost from work in the industrial world than any other complaint. Many resolve spontaneously or else the patient learns to live with the symptoms. Surgery for back pain is rarely indicated.

Lumbar Disc Prolapse

This occurs most commonly between 25 and 45 years of age. The onset is usually gradual and patients usually have difficulty recalling a causative event. The initial pain is limited to the lumbar spine. Once the 'disc' (the nucleus pulposus) prolapses into the spinal canal, it can compress a nerve root, sending pain into the leg and foot usually with associated numbness, paraesthesia and weakness.

Examination reveals a stiff back (this may be relative stiffness in a very flexible patient). There may be a 'sciatic list' over to one side, and tension signs are detectable when the sciatic nerve is stretched on straight leg raising. The patient may be unable to stand on tip-toes or their heels because of weakness. There may be weakness of foot evertors and toe extensors. When L4 or L5 root is compressed, weakness of the gluteus medius and minimus lead to a positive Trendelenberg sign. In an L5/S1 disc prolapse, the ankle jerk is diminished or absent.

Natural history—many resolve spontaneously but this may take a year or more. Provided the patient is improving, treatment is unnecessary. Bed rest (for as short a period as possible) and analgesia are the initial treatments along with early mobilisation. Physical therapy usually offers little help.

Investigations—MRI scans should be performed if treatment is being considered (Fig. 11.11). Surgery is reserved for those who fail to response to conservative measures. Epidural steroid injections are often useful.

Cauda Equina Syndrome 'Red Flag Symptoms'

If the cauda equina becomes severely compressed, this is an emergency requiring admission, immediate scanning and surgical decompression. This intervention has a good chance of saving the patient from potentially lifelong incontinence of urine and faeces, impotence, and an insensate perineum. The syndrome is typically caused by a large disc prolapse but tumours and spinal stenosis can also be responsible.

There is a spectrum of symptoms which include painless urinary and faecal incontinence, back pain, pain in one or both legs and numbness (perianal and perineal). Examination may reveal a distended bladder, perianal and/or perineal anaesthesia, weakness of some muscles and other abnormal neurology. Rectal examination reveals marked reduction in external sphincter tone.

Lumbar Spinal Stenosis (Fig. 11.12)

This is common and almost certainly underdiagnosed. Narrowing (stenosis) of the neural canal is typically caused by a combination of thickened ligamentum flavum, hypertrophy of facet joints and sometimes by forward slip of one vertebra on the one below (degenerative spondylolisthesis). Classically, the patient presents with 'spinal claudication. The symptoms are similar to vascular claudication but the spinal claudicant has palpable pulses. The buttock and leg pain is often accompanied by numbness and weakness. Typically, patients with spinal claudication prefer to walk uphill or cycle (spine flexion allows more blood through nerve root canals) and they like to push the supermarket trolley for support.

These patients can present to a urology clinic with impotence or urinary incontinence without having noticed typical leg symptoms because they cannot walk for other reasons.

The natural history is for it to get worse. When severe enough, treatment is surgical decompression, carefully widening the canal whilst being aware of the risk of neurological damage. Some cases may also require a one-level fusion.

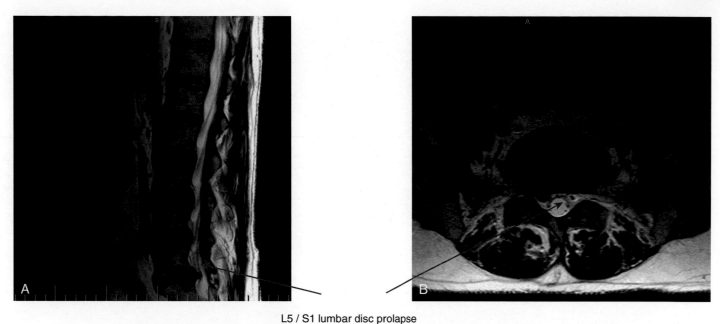

L5 / S1 lumbar disc prolapse

• **Fig. 11.11** Magnetic Resonance Imaging Scans Showing L5/S1 Disc Prolapse.

CASE HISTORY

Sagittal MRI (T2 Image)

Transverse MRI T2 at
at L 3/4 showing stenosis

Transverse MRI T2 Image
L2/3 for comparison

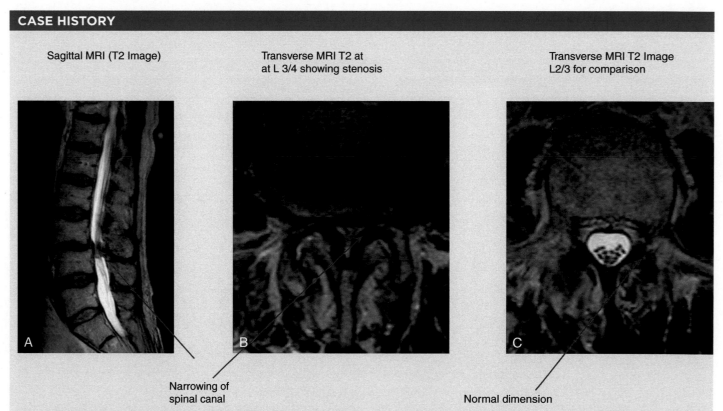

Narrowing of
spinal canal

Normal dimension

• **Fig. 11.12** Magnetic resonance imaging (MRI) images showing spinal stenosis at L3/4 in a man who complained of leg pain on walking and weakness in both feet. **(A)** Sagittal MRI (T2-weighted image where fluid is white) and **(B)** transverse image both showing L3/4 stenosis. **(C)** Transverse MRI (T2 weighted) of L2/3 for comparison. His symptoms were relieved by decompression surgery.

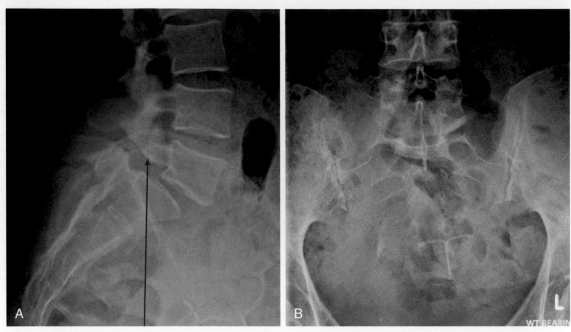

• **Fig. 11.13** Lateral and anteroposterior view x-rays showing bilateral pars defects and approximately 20% forward slip of L5 on S1. Note the patient has an intrauterine contraceptive device in situ.

Lumbar Spondylolisthesis

Forward slippage of one vertebra on another is a fairly common condition (Fig. 11.13).

- Congenital spondylolisthesis is rare and treatment of these children involves very major surgery, undertaken only in specialised spinal units.
- Degenerative spondylolisthesis results from degeneration/absorption of the disc plus erosion and bone loss at inferior facet joints.
- Isthmic spondylolisthesis occurs when there is a defect in the pars intraarticularis, the bone linking the superior and inferior facets. Some people go through life unaware that they have this condition. Treatment is conservative except in patients with disabling symptoms, in which case fusion may be indicated.
- Pathological spondylolisthesis occurs in people with conditions such as osteogenesis imperfecta.
  Neurological compromise can occur when the whole vertebra, including the posterior elements, slips forward.

Sacral Insufficiency Fractures

These have been appreciated only since MRI scanning became available. The patient is usually elderly and with osteoporosis. The pain is around the sacrum and radiates downwards and is often so severe the patient cannot walk. Treatment with intravenous pamidronate is often rapidly effective. In some vertebral (and occasional sacral) insufficiency fractures with persistent pain despite conservative measures, there is a role for vertebroplasty or baloon kyphoplasty. In these procedures bone cement is injected into the vertebra eliminating fracture micromotion.

Thoracic Spine

The thoracic spine is relatively immune from the aches and pains of the neck and lower spine, perhaps because it is stabilised by the rest of the rib cage. Thoracic disc prolapse is uncommon and generally presents with girdle pain and variable neurological symptoms. Thoracic discs can be surgically removed via an anterior approach to lessen the chances of neural damage.

In TB endemic areas, the thoracic spine is the most commonly affected and causes the classic gibbus (sharp angled kyphosis) and neurological loss (Pott paraplegia).

Cervical Spine

Cervical discs prolapse much less often than lumbar discs. Symptoms are predictable and include neck pain, radicular pain (in the distribution of the compressed nerve root), paraesthesia, numbness and weakness. Most resolve spontaneously but some require disc excision. Operation is performed via an anterior approach, with disc removal and bone grafting to achieve fusion.

Cervical Spine Stenosis

Stenosis can occur centrally or laterally and symptoms and signs are likely to be those of an upper motor neurone lesion. The patient may present with micturition difficulties, unsteadiness and radicular symptoms in one or both arms. Making this diagnosis is important as it is treatable, unlike most other conditions in the differential diagnosis. Treatment involves decompressing the theca by removing impinging bone and soft tissue There is a risk of neurological damage, which has to weighed up against the risk of leaving the condition untreated.

Scoliosis

Scoliosis spinal deformity is usually secondary to asymmetrical spinal growth. The deformity is primarily rotational, affecting the thoracic and lumbar spine (Fig. 11.14). Causes include:

- Idiopathic, the largest group in the western world. The thoracic curve is convex to the right in an otherwise normal patient with a normal spine.
- Congenital—abnormal spinal development.
- Acquired neuromuscular causes.
- Miscellaneous causes, such as neurofibromatosis and Marfan syndrome.
- Degenerative scoliosis, from the fifth decade onwards. Most of these patients have had an (often previously unrecognised) minor spinal curve.

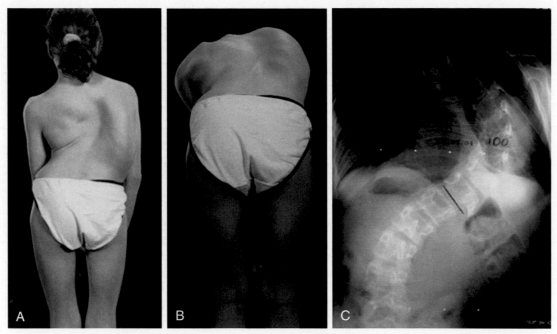

• **Fig. 11.14** Scoliosis of the Spine. **(A)** A teenager with severe adolescent idiopathic scoliosis presenting very late. **(B)** The bend down test is the hallmark of diagnosis. **(C)** The standing posteroanterior x-ray shows a Cobb angle of over 100 degrees.

The natural history is important—all curves have their own personality. Progression can only be assessed with serial consultations and x-rays. Severe scoliosis is unsightly and disabling. High thoracic curves may cause cardiopulmonary compromise. The relationship between back pain and scoliosis is less clear.

Age at presentation is important. The younger, the longer there is for the curve to progress. Most adolescent curves occur in girls and spinal growth usually stops about 18 months after periods start.

Treatment in scoliosis depends on the anticipated degree of curve at growth cessation. If a curve is predicted to remain below 40 to 45 degrees, it may stabilise and not require treatment. Many affected go through life with a substantial curve but with few problems. Physiotherapy will never alter a curve and may delay proper diagnosis and treatment. Braces were used extensively in the past and there is still a place for them in curves between 20 and 40 degrees.

Operations are very major surgery usually involving fusion but carry a potential for catastrophic neural damage. Surgery is easier and safer on smaller curves predicted to do badly. Unbalanced curves which have progressed past about 50 degrees during adolescence inevitably continue to progress through life, perhaps at one degree a year.

Complications of Surgery

Introduction

Any operation, major trauma or other surgical admission may be attended by complications, many of which are potentially preventable. Some complications are somewhat inherent to the condition being treated (e.g., deep venous thrombosis [DVT] following lower limb fractures) or arise from a comorbid (preexisting) condition, such as myocardial ischaemia, whilst others can be attributed to human or system error. **Poor communication** between hospital staff is a frequent cause of avoidable complications, including incomplete or inaccurate record keeping, failure to register allergies, and inadequate patient handover between colleagues.

A large proportion of complications can be prevented or minimised by anticipation, by taking prophylactic measures, by attention to detail and by early recognition and treatment of problems as they develop. In addition, most hospitals now have standard mechanisms designed to minimise system error, such as the World Health Organization (WHO) Surgical Safety checklists, now

completed for all operations and involving all members of the operating team.

With potentially serious complications (e.g., bowel anastomotic leak), early diagnosis and reoperation is crucial, as delay often leads to catastrophic 'snowballing' sepsis and multiorgan failure. Once two or more body systems become impaired, survival falls to only about 50%. If, for example, acute respiratory distress syndrome (ARDS) and acute kidney failure complicate an operation for obstructive jaundice in a patient with liver impairment, the odds are heavily stacked against survival.

In operative surgery, complications can be considered as those that can befall any operation or **specific** complications of individual operations. Both groups can be subdivided into **immediate** (during operation or within the next 24 hours), **early postoperative** (during the first postoperative week or so), **late postoperative** (up to 30 days after operation) and **long term**.

Surgical complications fall into the five broad categories listed in Box 12.1. 'Medical' complications are discussed in Chapter 8. Complications of specific operations are discussed in Chapters 18–51, as appropriate.

Complications of Anaesthesia

The main complications of anaesthesia are summarised in Box 12.2.

General Complications of Operations

The main complications of any operation are: inadvertent trauma to the patient in the operating department, haemorrhage, surgical damage to related structures, inadequate operation, surgical site infection and problems with wound healing.

Inadvertent Trauma in the Operating Department

Patients are at risk of injury during transport or transfer in the operating department, especially when under anaesthesia. Staff involved in handling patients are also at risk of injury, for example to the back. The WHO Surgical Safety Checklist incorporates team recognition of artificial joints, presence of devices such as pacemakers, implanted metalwork from previous operations and any other transfer concerns, to warn of the need for extra vigilance during patient positioning and during the procedure.

The most common causes of trauma in the operating theatre are:
- Injuries resulting from falls from trolleys or from the operating table during positioning.
- Injury to diseased bones and joints from manipulation or positioning. These include dislocation of rheumatoid atlantoaxial joints and dislocation of a prosthetic hip or other joint.

• BOX 12.1 Principal Categories of Surgical Complications

1. Complications predisposed to by comorbid 'medical' disorders, whether symptomatic or occult, for example, ischaemic heart disease, chronic respiratory disease or diabetes mellitus (see Ch. 8)
2. Complications of anaesthesia
3. General complications of operations, for example, haemorrhage or wound infection
4. Complications of any surgical condition, for example, pulmonary embolism, pneumonia or urinary tract infection
5. Complications of specific disorders and operations

- Ulnar, lateral popliteal and other nerve palsies resulting from pressure.
- Electrical burns from wet or poorly contacting diathermy pads or misuse of the diathermy probe.
- Excess pressure on the calves causing DVT.
- Excess or prolonged heel pressure causing pressure sores.
- Cardiac pacemaker disruption by diathermy equipment—minimised by using bipolar diathermy wherever possible. Pacemaker checks are performed pre- and postprocedure if needed but modern pacemakers are much more resistant to electrical interference.

• BOX 12.2 Complications of Anaesthesia

Local Anaesthesia

- Injection site—pain; haematoma; delayed recovery of sensation (direct nerve trauma); infection
- Vasoconstrictors—ischaemic necrosis (if used in digits or penis)
- Systemic effects of local anaesthetic agent
  - Toxicity caused by excess dosage (see Ch. 10, p. 124) or inadvertent intravenous injection. Same effect produced by premature release of a Bier's block cuff
  - Toxic effects include: dizziness, tinnitus, nausea and vomiting, fits, central nervous system depression, and cardiac dysrhythmias including bradycardia and asystole
  - Idiosyncratic or allergic reactions (very rare)

Spinal, Epidural and Caudal Anaesthesia

- Failure of anaesthetic—anatomical difficulties or technical failure
- Headache after operation—loss of cerebrospinal fluid because of dural puncture
- Epidural or intrathecal bleeding—increased risk if patient on anticoagulants
- Unintentionally wide field of anaesthesia
  - In **epidural** anaesthesia, injection into wrong tissue plane may give a spinal anaesthetic
  - In **spinal** anaesthesia, respiratory paralysis occurs if the anaesthetic agent flows too far proximally
- Permanent nerve or spinal cord damage—injection of incorrect or contaminated drug
- Paraspinal infection—introduced by the injection
- Systemic complications—autonomic block may cause severe hypotension or postural hypotension

General Anaesthesia
Postoperative Nausea and Vomiting
- Usually a response to anaesthetic or analgesic drugs. Individual sensitivity varies. Antiemetics usually administered before end of anaesthesia

Pain
- Analgesics usually administered during operation (e.g., intravenous opiates or paracetamol, diclofenac suppositories) plus local/regional anaesthetic techniques

Problems With Drugs and Fluids
- Fluid and electrolyte imbalance—too little, too much or inappropriate intravenous infusion
- Inappropriate choice of drugs or dosage in relation to age or the requirements of day surgery
- Idiosyncratic or allergic reactions to anaesthetic agents
  - Minor effects, for example, nausea and vomiting
  - Major effects, for example, cardiovascular collapse, respiratory depression, halothane jaundice
- Unexpected drug interactions—a wide range of adverse effects may occur
- Inherited disorders
  - Malignant hyperpyrexia (MH): any inhalational anaesthetic or suxamethonium may trigger MH
  - Pseudocholinesterase deficiency produces prolonged apnoea after succinylcholine
- Slow recovery from anaesthetic—many reasons including inadequate reversal
- 'Awareness' during anaesthetic—effective paralysis but ineffective anaesthesia

Cardiovascular Complications
- Myocardial ischaemia/infarction/failure, arrhythmias, hypo/hypertension, tachy/bradycardias

Respiratory Complications
- Laryngospasm/bronchospasm, atelectasis, upper or lower respiratory tract infections

Renal Complications
- Particularly in patients with comorbid renal impairment—prerenal, renal or postrenal

Hypothermia (Note: Neonates and Small Infants Are Especially Vulnerable to Hypothermia)
- Long operations with extensive fluid loss
- Large-volume transfusion of cold blood

Inadvertent Trauma
- Dental problems and prostheses
  - Teeth (particularly decayed or loose), crowns and bridges are vulnerable during intubation. Damage risks aspirating a foreign body into a bronchus and causes cosmetic and medicolegal problems.
  - Infected material from carious (decayed) teeth or inflamed gums may be aspirated and cause a particularly grave aspiration pneumonia.
  - Dentures must be removed before operation and labelled. Unconscious accident victims may aspirate or swallow a dental prosthesis or obstruct the pharynx with it.
- Corneal abrasions
- Pressure injury to nerves (especially ulnar, radial and lateral popliteal)
- Diathermy pad burns
- Initiation of pressure sores

Haemorrhage

Perioperative Haemorrhage

Haemorrhage occurring during an operation (**primary haemorrhage**) should be controlled by the surgeon before the operation is completed.

Early Postoperative Haemorrhage

Haemorrhage immediately after operation usually indicates inadequate operative haemostasis or a technical mishap, such as a slipped ligature or unrecognised blood vessel trauma. Occasionally, it is caused by a bleeding disorder.

If an operation involves major blood loss and large volume transfusion of stored blood, haemorrhage may be perpetuated by **consumption coagulopathy**, in which platelets and coagulation factors have been 'consumed' in a vain attempt at haemostasis. **Disseminated intravascular coagulopathy (DIC)** can be one facet of the systemic inflammatory response syndrome* with widespread intravascular thrombosis and exhaustion of clotting factors. Any patient giving a history of excess bleeding should have a platelet count and coagulation screen checked before operation.

Operations at particular risk of early postoperative haemorrhage include:
- major operations involving highly vascular tissues, such as the liver or spleen;
- major arterial surgery, especially ruptured aortic aneurysm (large volume blood loss may occur, and the patient may be heparinised during operation);
- operations which leave a large raw surface, such as abdominoperineal excision of rectum.

This type of postoperative haemorrhage has been traditionally described as **reactionary** in the belief that it was a 'reaction' to the recovery of normal blood pressure and cardiac output. This concept is probably misleading and should now be discarded, especially since it may hinder the decision to reoperate urgently.

Management of Early Postoperative Haemorrhage

This is really a form of primary haemorrhage and, if substantial, the patient must be surgically reexplored and the source treated. It is wise to perform a clotting screen (including platelet count) and order bank blood as a preliminary measure. Good intravenous access should be ensured. If heparin was used at the original operation, **protamine** can reverse any residual activity. If the clotting screen is abnormal, infusions containing clotting factors may be needed, as advised by a haematologist. Many patients will stop bleeding with supportive measures and blood transfusion but reexploration must be seriously considered at every stage.

Later Postoperative Haemorrhage

Haemorrhage occurring several days after operation is usually caused by infection eroding blood vessels near the operation site. This is known as *secondary haemorrhage*. Treatment involves managing the infection, but exploratory operation is often required to ligate or suture the bleeding vessels.

---

*The definitions for systemic inflammatory response syndrome (or SIRS) has recently changed. Clinicians are encouraged to use 'Sepsis-3' and the Sequential Organ Failure Assessment (SOFA) score.

Anticoagulant and Antiplatelet Therapy Considerations in Surgery

Several different anticoagulant and antiplatelet therapies exist (i.e., warfarin, clopidogrel, dabigatran, rivaroxaban, apixaban, edoxaban). These are designed to prevent intravascular thrombosis and have a lesser effect on surgically induced bleeding. All should generally be stopped preoperatively for their respective advised durations (i.e., stop warfarin 5 days before surgery; stop clopidogrel 7 to 10 days before surgery) to minimise complications with peri- and postoperative bleeding. Patients at higher risk of thromboembolism or other related complications from stopping their anticoagulant must have bridging treatment with an alternative short-acting preparation, under advice from their medical team or haematologist. An example is a subcutaneous low-molecular-weight heparin (LMWH), such as dalteparin, given once the anticoagulant is deemed to be at a subtherapeutic level (i.e., international normalised ratio [INR] falls below the target range in patients treated with warfarin), and is then stopped 24 hours before surgery. Remember to resume the patient's normal anticoagulation therapy postoperatively if there is no active bleeding, and continue bridging therapy in those needing it until their normal anticoagulation medication is therapeutic again (e.g., INR is back in range). It is no longer considered necessary to stop low-dose aspirin before surgery.

Surgical Injury

Unavoidable Tissue Damage

Anatomical structures, particularly nerves, blood vessels and lymphatics, may be **unavoidably damaged** during operation. This is particularly true in cancer surgery, illustrated by facial nerve excision during total parotidectomy. If anticipated, the probability must be discussed with the patient beforehand as part of the documented informed consent process. Sometimes, the integrity or location of vulnerable structures can be established before operation, allowing better planning of the operation. For example, indirect laryngoscopy may be done to assess vocal cord integrity before thyroid surgery.

Inadvertent Tissue Damage

Structures may be **inadvertently damaged** during operation. Examples include recurrent laryngeal nerve damage during thyroidectomy, or trauma to bile ducts during cholecystectomy. The main factors are inexperience, anatomical anomalies, attempts at arresting precipitate haemorrhage and tissue planes obscured by inflammation or malignancy. Signs of damage to structures at particular risk should be sought in the postoperative period; for example, hoarseness after thyroidectomy or jaundice after cholecystectomy.

Infection Related to the Operation Site

Minor Wound Infections

The most common infective complication is a superficial wound infection (surgical site infection) within the first postoperative week. This relatively trivial infection presents as localised pain, redness and a slight discharge. Organisms are usually staphylococci derived from skin and the infection usually settles spontaneously, or after a short course of oral antibiotics. In patients with recent prosthesis insertion, such as an arterial graft or artificial joint, any sign of infection must be treated aggressively with antibiotics to prevent infection of the prosthesis which is likely to be disastrous.

Wound Cellulitis and Abscess

More severe wound infections occur most often after bowel-related surgery, when staphylococci (methicillin-sensitive or resistant varieties) or faecal organisms are usually incriminated. Most

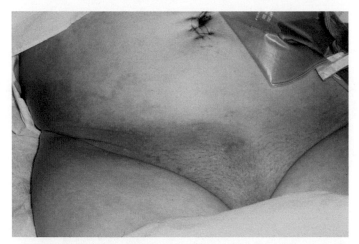

• **Fig. 12.1** Abdominal Cellulitis. This woman of 73 years presented with faecal peritonitis caused by a diverticular perforation of the sigmoid colon. She was resuscitated and underwent a laparotomy and sigmoid loop colostomy (note bag), without resection of the perforation. She remained toxic with a high fever and tachycardia, and developed spreading cellulitis in the right groin and flank. This proved to be caused by continuing leakage from the perforation. Nowadays, a Hartmann operation or resection and primary anastomosis would be performed so there is no longer a perforation leaking faecal matter into the peritoneal cavity

appear in the first postoperative week but they may occur as late as the third week, sometimes after leaving hospital. These infections commonly present with pyrexia, and wound examination reveals spreading **cellulitis** (Fig. 12.1) or localised **abscess formation**.

Cellulitis is treated with antibiotics after taking a wound swab for culture and sensitivity, whereas a wound abscess is treated by surgical drainage. This may simply involve suture removal and wound probing, but deeper abscesses may need reexploration under general anaesthesia. In either case, and for smaller defects, the wound is left open afterwards to heal by secondary intention (Fig. 12.2). Alternatively, for larger defects, the application of a vacuum dressing (**negative-pressure wound therapy**) by a tissue viability team can accelerate wound healing. This involves application of a foam pad covered by an occlusive dressing connected to a vacuum pump which continuously draws out fluid and encourages blood flow to the affected area.

Methicillin-Resistant Staphylococcus aureus Infection

Methicillin-resistant *Staphylococcus aureus* (MRSA) infection after surgery is rare but potentially serious. It can be implicated in chest, urine and wound infections and cause bacteraemia requiring patient isolation, barrier nursing and specific intravenous antibiotic therapy (e.g., vancomycin is used for severe skin and soft tissue infections). Preventative measures are widely practiced in hospitals (i.e., hand washing, dressing management and antibiotic stewardship), and all elective surgical patients ideally undergo preoperative screening with nose, throat and groin swab cultures to detect MRSA and allow eradication therapy before surgery if positive.

CASE HISTORY

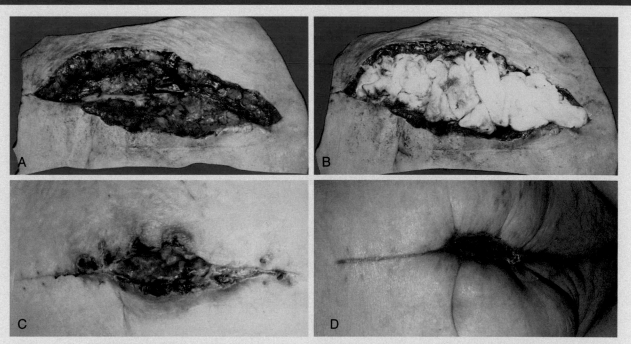

• **Fig. 12.2** Deep Wound Infection Drained and Allowed to Heal by Secondary Intention. This 80-year-old diabetic woman underwent laparotomy and the wound became infected with *Staphylococcus aureus*. This resulted in a wound abscess and necrosis of the wound edge. (A) The wound after all necrotic tissue has been excised. (B) The wound packed with gauze and allowed to heal by secondary intention. (C) and (D) The wound at 3 weeks and 8 weeks. It was completely healed after 2 further weeks. Note the degree of wound contraction, which played a major part in overcoming the tissue defect

Intraabdominal infection

Intraabdominal infection is discussed under complications of abdominal and bowel surgery later in this chapter.

Gas Gangrene

Gas gangrene is an uncommon acute, life-threatening wound infection in which the anaerobic organisms multiply in necrotic tissue, particularly muscle (see Ch. 3, p. 31).

Late Infective Complications

A late infective complication of surgery is a chronically discharging **wound sinus** emanating from a deep chronic abscess. It usually relates to foreign material, such as a nonabsorbable suture or mesh or sometimes necrotic fascia or tendon. These sinuses commonly appear following wound infections where healing is delayed and incomplete. Wound sinuses occasionally appear after apparent normal healing, particularly after insertion of a prosthesis.

Sinuses rarely heal spontaneously unless the foreign material is discharged, and the usual treatment is therefore wound reexploration and removal of the offending substance. In groin sinuses following aortofemoral bypass grafts, removal of the graft would impair the arterial supply of the lower limb and the infected graft must be replaced or bypassed. As an alternative to surgery in some noncommunicating abdominal, pelvic and retroperitoneal collections and abscesses (e.g., infected lymphocele or urinoma), ultrasound or computed tomography (CT) guidance can be used to aspirate the fluid and/or leave a drain to treat it.

Impaired Healing

Factors Retarding Wound Healing

Nearly all wounds heal without complication. It is untrue that wounds heal slowly in the elderly; this is so only when there are specific adverse factors or complications. Wound healing in general is retarded if blood supply is poor (as in lower limb arterial insufficiency) or if the wound is under excess tension. Other retarding factors are local infection, long-term corticosteroid therapy, immunosuppressive therapy, previous radiotherapy, severe rheumatoid disease, smoking, global malnutrition and specific vitamin and mineral deficiency, especially of vitamin C and possibly zinc.

Wound Dehiscence ('Burst Abdomen')

Wound dehiscence, that is, total wound breakdown, is uncommon. It affects about 1% of abdominal wounds, usually about 1 week after operation, and is preceded by profuse serosanguinous fluid discharge from the wound. The sudden bursting open of the abdomen revealing coils of bowel is alarming but is remarkably pain-free. Infection and other factors already described may play a part but the usual cause is inadequate abdominal wall repair, often in the presence of infection or malnutrition. This may be compounded by mechanical disruption caused by coughing or abdominal distension related to postoperative bowel ileus.

The wound should be covered with sterile swabs soaked in saline and the patient returned to the operating theatre within a few hours for repair. This commonly involves placement of **tension sutures** incorporating large 'bites' of the whole thickness of the abdominal wall (Fig. 12.3). In fact tension sutures should not be tight but merely snug.

CASE HISTORY

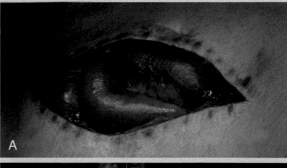
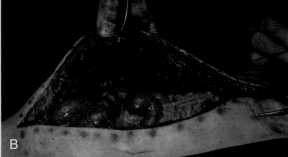
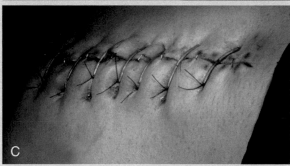

• **Fig. 12.3** Burst Abdomen and Repair With Tension Sutures. (A) Complete wound dehiscence 6 days after laparotomy for peritonitis. Note the exposed bowel spilling out of the wound. The patient had no particular risk factors so the cause was probably a poor technique of wound closure. (B) Operative photograph showing insertion of 'tension sutures' through the whole thickness of the abdominal wall. (C) The completed wound repair.

Incisional Hernia

Incisional hernia is a late complication of abdominal surgery. These usually become apparent within the first postoperative year but sometimes develop as long as 15 years later; the overall incidence is about 10% to 15% of abdominal wounds. The hernia is caused by breakdown of the abdominal wall muscle and fascial repair. Predisposing factors are abdominal obesity, diabetes, smoking, abdominal distension and poor muscle quality, poor choice of incision, inadequate closure technique, postoperative wound infection and multiple operations through the same incision.

An incisional hernia usually presents as a bulge in the abdominal wall near a previous wound. They are usually asymptomatic but occasionally a narrow-necked hernia presents with pain or strangulation. Once an incisional hernia has appeared, it tends to enlarge progressively and may become a nuisance cosmetically or for wearing clothing (Fig. 12.4). Repair is indicated for strangulation, pain or inconvenience and usually involves placing a synthetic mesh at open operation or laparoscopically.

CASE HISTORY

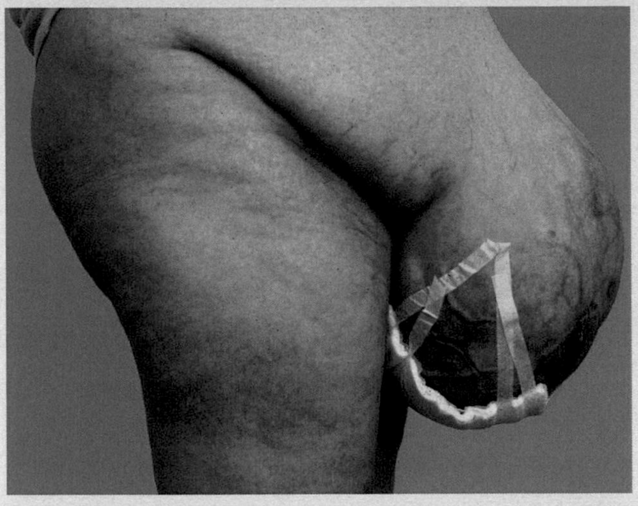

• **Fig. 12.4 Incisional Hernia.** This 55-year-old woman presented with a massive incisional hernia through an old umbilical hernia repair scar. Her only complaint was of skin breakdown at its lowermost extent. Repair presented a huge challenge but was achieved using mesh.

Complications of Any Surgical Condition

Respiratory Complications

Up to 15% of patients having major operations and general anaesthesia suffer from respiratory complications. The most common are **atelectasis** and **pneumonia**. Preexisting lung disease greatly increases the risk. Severely ill patients, including those with acute pancreatitis, and burns or trauma victims, are susceptible to **ARDS**.

Effects of Anaesthesia and Surgery on Respiratory Function

Anaesthesia and surgery predispose to postoperative complications by altering lung function and compromising normal defence mechanisms, as follows:

- **Lung tidal volume**—may be reduced by as much as 50%, depending on the incision site; thoracic, upper abdominal and lower abdominal incisions reduce lung volume in decreasing order of effect.
- **Lung expansion**—reduced by the **supine position** during and after operation, pain, abdominal distension, abdominal constriction by bandages and the effects of sedative drugs.
- **Ventilation rate**—usually increases accompanied by loss of normal periodic hyperinflation.
- **Diminished ventilation and pulmonary perfusion**—result in reduced gaseous exchange.
- **Airway defences**—compromised by loss of the cough reflex and diminished ciliary activity, which both lead to accumulation of secretions.
- **Problems associated with laparoscopic and robotic-assisted abdominal surgery**—the pneumoperitoneum and head-down position lead to diaphragmatic splinting, a reduction in functional residual capacity and changes in intrathoracic blood volume. These lead to atelectasis, pulmonary shunting and hypoxaemia. Raised ventilatory airways pressure may lead to pulmonary barotrauma.

Atelectasis

Pathophysiology and Clinical Features

Atelectasis or alveolar collapse occurs when airways become obstructed and air is absorbed from air spaces distal to the obstruction. Bronchial secretions are the main cause. Predisposing factors include preexisting lung disease and postoperative shallow ventilation, loss of periodic hyperinflation, inhibition of coughing and pooling of mucus. All of these are greater problems after thoracic and upper abdominal surgery. The resulting **ventilation/perfusion mismatch** produces a degree of right-to-left shunting of blood, which causes a fall in partial pressure of oxygen in arterial blood (PaO_2). If obstructed airways are small and cause minor segmental collapse, localising signs are minimal and x-ray appearance is unremarkable. Despite this, the overall extent of collapse may be large and cause significant hypoxaemia.

Obstruction of a major airway causes collapse and consolidation of a whole lobe, resulting in the typical signs of dullness to percussion and reduced breath sounds or **bronchial breathing**. Chest x-ray shows the lobe is contracted and opacified, with mediastinal shift and compensatory expansion of other lobes. Bronchoscopy is likely to be required to remove the obstruction.

Most cases of atelectasis are mild and pass undiagnosed, although the patient may be slow to recover from operation. The patient may be cyanosed, resulting from mild hypoxaemia, and have a mild tachypnoea, tachycardia and low-grade pyrexia, which all resolve spontaneously within a few days. Sputum culture (if sputum is produced) is usually negative but infection may complicate severe cases.

Prevention and Treatment of Atelectasis

In patients undergoing major surgery, atelectasis is best minimised by preoperative and postoperative physiotherapy. This includes deep breathing exercises, regular adjustments of posture and vigorous coughing. During physiotherapy, wounds should be supported with the patient's hand. Effective analgesia, for example, infiltration of the wound with local anaesthetic or epidural analgesia, facilitates physiotherapy and mobility. Nebulised bronchodilators, such as salbutamol may assist the patient to cough up secretions. Severe cases of diffuse atelectasis may require noninvasive positive-pressure ventilation. Lobar or whole lung collapse requires intensive physiotherapy and sometimes **flexible bronchoscopy** to aspirate occluding mucus plugs.

Hospital Acquired Pneumonias

Bronchopneumonia is often seen in surgical patients. It occurs secondarily to chronic lung disease, smoking or following atelectasis or aspiration of gastric contents. *Haemophilus* and *Streptococcus pyogenes* are the common infecting organisms but coliforms may be responsible in elderly, debilitated or seriously ill patients. *Pseudomonas* bronchopneumonia occurs in patients on ventilators or with bronchiectasis.

Infection is manifest by pyrexia, tachypnoea, tachycardia and a raised leucocyte count. The mucopurulent sputum is thick, copious and green. Antibiotics are given on a 'best-guess' (empirical) basis, guided by local microbiology protocols, until sputum culture and sensitivities are available. Physiotherapy, mobilisation and encouragement to cough are all important for recovery.

Aspiration Pneumonitis

Aspiration pneumonitis (Mendelson syndrome) is a sterile, chemical inflammation of the lungs resulting from inhalation of acidic gastric contents. There is often a clear history of vomiting or regurgitation, followed by a rapid onset of breathlessness and wheezing. This may later become complicated by infection, that is, bronchopneumonia, with typical symptoms and signs. Chest x-ray shows characteristic 'fluffy' opacities, particularly in the lower lobes, which for anatomical and postural reasons are most affected.

Aspiration occurs when protective laryngeal reflexes are suppressed or when there is intestinal obstruction and regurgitation.

Laryngeal suppression may be caused by impairment of consciousness (e.g., during recovery from general anaesthesia).

Emergency anaesthesia in the nonstarved patient poses special risks. Whenever possible, anaesthesia should be postponed for 4 to 6 hours after the last food or drink other than water. In trauma victims, it is important to note the time of last eating with respect to the incident, and to remember that stress and anxiety may greatly delay gastric emptying. Gastric emptying is also much slower in pregnancy.

A patient with **intestinal obstruction** is at risk of inhalation of gastric contents. Ideally, the stomach should be emptied by nasogastric tube. If general anaesthesia must be performed on the nonstarved or otherwise at-risk patient, a **rapid sequence induction** is used: as the patient loses consciousness, an assistant applies **cricoid pressure** to flatten the oesophagus against the cervical spine, preventing reflux. The airway is then secured with a cuffed endotracheal tube before cricoid pressure is released. Oral antacids may be given beforehand to neutralise acidity. Metoclopramide by injection may also be used to hasten gastric emptying.

Mortality from aspiration pneumonitis approaches 50% and urgent treatment must be started should it occur. This involves thorough bronchial suction via an endotracheal tube (or bronchoscope if necessary), followed by positive-pressure ventilation. Prophylactic antibiotics are commonly provided, although evidence suggests that they should be reserved for when pneumonitis fails to resolve within 48 hours, of if there is a high risk of bacterial contamination (i.e., in patients with associated small bowel obstruction). Intravenous corticosteroids are not routinely given unless there are complicating factors (i.e., sepsis, ARDS, or the patient is already on long-term corticosteroid therapy).

Aspiration Pneumonia

Aspiration pneumonia may complicate aspiration pneumonitis, but more often it develops insidiously, following chronic aspiration of infected food and oropharyngeal secretions. In the surgical context, debilitated, confused or elderly patients are the usual victims, but aspiration pneumonia is also seen in alcoholics, drug addicts and stroke patients. Achalasia of the oesophageal cardia and large hiatus hernias can lead to chronic aspiration, particularly at night. The clinical features are of infection and lobar consolidation (usually of the lower lobe) progressing to **lung abscess** formation. CT chest can helpful in providing additional detail on collections of pus (empyema) and pleural effusions that may require drainage. Organisms are usually mixed oral anaerobes sensitive to penicillin, but prognosis depends more on the patient's general condition and is usually poor.

Acute Respiratory Distress Syndrome (ARDS)

This syndrome of acute respiratory failure, formerly known as adult respiratory distress syndrome, is characterised by rapid, shallow breathing, severe hypoxaemia, stiff lungs and diffuse pulmonary opacification on x-ray. It develops in response to a variety of systemic and direct insults to the pulmonary alveoli and microvasculature. Box 12.3 lists the main conditions with which ARDS is associated.

Pathophysiology of ARDS

The lung insults causing ARDS all have the effect of increasing the pulmonary capillary permeability, leading to leakage of protein-rich fluid into the alveolar interstitium. This causes interstitial oedema which in turn **reduces lung compliance** and causes 'stiff

---

> • **BOX 12.3** **Conditions Associated With Acute Respiratory Distress Syndrome (ARDS)**
>
> **Direct Insults to the Lung**
> - Lung contusion
> - Near-drowning
> - Aspiration of gastric acid
> - Inhalation of smoke and corrosive chemicals, for example, chlorine, phosgene, nitrogen dioxide or ammonia
> - Radiation pneumonitis
>
> **Systemic Insults to the Lung**
> - Multiple trauma with shock
> - Systemic sepsis, for example, after a colonic anastomotic leak
> - Severe acute pancreatitis
> - Major head injuries ('neurogenic pulmonary oedema')
> - Fat, air and amniotic fluid embolism
> - Major blood transfusion reaction or massive blood transfusion
> - Disseminated intravascular coagulation
> - Cardiopulmonary bypass
> - Eclampsia
> - Severe allergic reactions
> - Drug overdose or sensitivity, for example, heroin, barbiturates, paraquat, bleomycin

lungs' and reduced alveolar ventilation. Release of inflammatory mediators cause these effects.

The alveolar lining cells (**type I pneumocytes**) are also damaged. This damage, combined with the increased interstitial hydrostatic pressure, causes leakage of fluid into alveolar spaces until they are filled. The result is disruption of the lung ventilation to perfusion ratio (V/Q ratio), in effect causing **right-to-left shunting** of blood. The intraalveolar fluid later condenses to form a **hyaline membrane** which lines the alveoli. This is histologically similar to the neonatal form of the disease.

The full clinical syndrome often takes 24 to 48 hours to develop after the initial insult. If the patient eventually recovers, the interstitial damage may result in diffuse **interstitial fibrosis**. It is important to note that cardiac failure is not involved in causing ARDS, but cardiac failure may later complicate it.

Clinical Features of ARDS

The main finding is rapid shallow respiration with only scattered crepitations on auscultation. There is usually no cough, chest pain or haemoptysis, but patients can rapidly deteriorate with dyspnoea at rest, tachypnoea and multiorgan failure. Blood gas analysis reveals low PaO_2; the partial pressure of carbon dioxide in arterial blood remains normal initially, although it rises in severe cases producing respiratory alkalosis, which can ultimately evolve to become a respiratory acidosis. Chest x-ray may be normal in the early stages, progressing rapidly through increased interstitial markings to complete or partial 'white-out' (Fig. 12.5). ARDS may be difficult to distinguish from cardiac failure except that cardiac diameter is normal in ARDS, and cardiac failure usually responds to diuretic therapy.

Treatment of ARDS

The objective is to maintain respiratory function and cardiovascular stability while the underlying cause (e.g., sepsis) is brought under control. This should be carried out in intensive care. The sooner treatment is begun, the greater the chance of recovery.

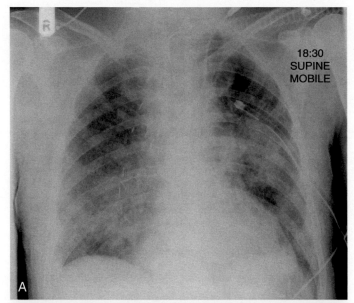

18:30
SUPINE
MOBILE

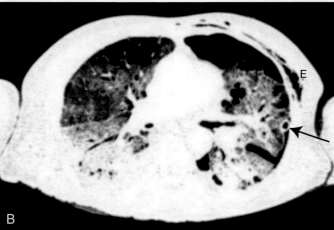

• **Fig. 12.5** Acute Respiratory Distress Syndrome (ARDS). (A) This middle-aged man underwent an oesophagectomy for carcinoma, with the proximal stomach anastomosed to the oesophageal remnant in the chest. He developed ARDS in the early postoperative period. The chest x-ray shows ill-defined alveolar opacification in the lung mid-zones. Note the metallic vascular clips on the right side, the chest drain on the left side and the endotracheal tube and central venous line. (B) The computed tomography scan shows bilateral consolidation in the dependent portion of both lungs with 'ground glass' opacification in the upper zones. There is a left pneumothorax with a chest drain in situ *(arrowed)*; subcutaneous emphysema *(E)* resulting from the thoracotomy is also visible

Most patients require mechanical **ventilation** with **positive end-expiratory pressure** at low tidal volumes to achieve adequate oxygenation and to try to reverse alveolar oedema and collapse. Fluid balance is complex and requires monitoring of **right atrial pressure** using a central venous line. Cardiac output can be measured using transoesophageal ultrasound. One of the treatment aims is to produce a negative fluid balance and thus minimise fluid accumulation in the lung and interstitial tissue. Loop diuretic infusions or continuous venovenous haemofiltration can be used to achieve this. Renal insufficiency is a common association, and can also be treated by haemofiltration. Diuretics do not control pulmonary oedema but instead aggravate the hypovolaemia and shock linked with the underlying cause. The mortality rate for complicated cases of ARDS approaches 90%.

• **BOX 12.4** **Predisposing Factors for Deep Vein Thrombosis and Pulmonary Embolism**

- Previous venous thromboembolism
- Trauma and surgery (complex systemic effects)
- Increasing age
- Direct trauma to the pelvis and lower limbs, especially fractures
- Preexisting lower limb venous disorders causing stasis
- Venous stasis during general or regional anaesthesia (loss of calf muscle pump and postural pressure on the calves)
- Malignant disease
- Immobility, for example, bed-bound patients after operation or stroke
- Cardiac failure
- High-oestrogen oral contraceptive pill, oestrogen treatment, hormone replacement therapy
- Pregnancy
- Pelvic masses causing venous obstruction
- Groin masses obstructing femoral vein, for example, femoral aneurysm, malignant lymph nodes
- Obesity
- Dehydration
- Blood disorders, for example, polycythaemia, thrombocythaemia and prothrombotic disorders

Venous Thromboembolism

Pathophysiology

Venous thromboembolism (VTE) is a major cause of complications and death after surgery or trauma and much of it is preventable. Venous blood is normally prevented from clotting within veins by a series of mechanisms that include local inhibition of the clotting cascade, prompt lysis of small clots that do form, and the flushing effect of a continuous flow of blood. In 1856 **Virchow** proposed in his '**triad**' that venous thrombosis was caused by abnormalities in the vein wall (trauma, inflammation), alterations in blood flow (stasis) and changes in the blood (hypercoagulability); this explanation largely holds good today.

The normal antithrombotic balance within veins can be upset by local and/or systemic factors, resulting in thrombus formation in venous sinuses within calf muscles and sometimes primarily in pelvic veins. About 90% of **deep vein thromboses** (DVTs) start in the calf and about a quarter propagate proximally, usually within a week of presentation, to involve femoral and pelvic veins. Calf vein thrombosis alone is rarely symptomatic early on yet it predisposes strongly to proximal propagation, and 80% of symptomatic DVTs involve proximal veins. Calf vein thrombi themselves rarely cause substantial embolism but those in larger, more proximal vessels are likely to detach and migrate proximally to impact in pulmonary arteries as **pulmonary emboli**.

The main **predisposing factors** to VTE are summarised in Box 12.4, but thromboembolism can occur in healthy individuals without evident predisposing factors. A proportion will have a **prothrombotic disorder** and investigation for these should be performed later. Note that patients may have been ill and dehydrated at home for some time before hospital admission and venous thrombosis may have begun before admission.

The risk of thromboembolism increases incrementally with the number and severity of local and systemic risk factors; this is neatly illustrated in Table 12.1. The impact of many predisposing factors can be minimised by considering **prophylactic measures against VTE** in *all* hospitalised patients.

TABLE 12.1	Factors Affecting the Risk of Deep Vein Thrombosis (DVT) After Operation		
Age (yr)	Grade of Surgery	Other Risk Factors	Risk of DVT (%)
20	Minor		1
40	Minor		3
60	Minor		10
60	Major		20
60	Major	Previous DVT	50
80	Major		40
80	Major	Previous DVT + infection or malignancy	96

CASE HISTORY

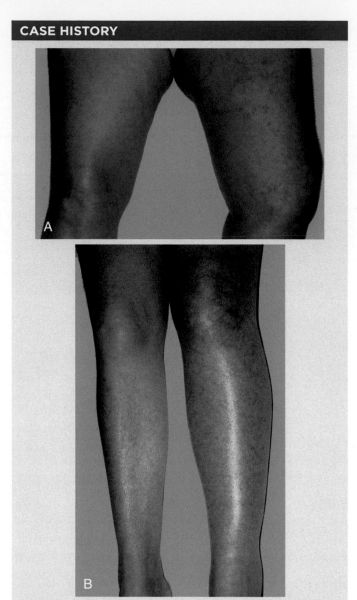

• **Fig. 12.6 Clinically Obvious Deep Vein Thrombosis.** This woman of 45 years underwent radical surgery for ovarian cancer. She suffered swelling and bursting pain in the whole of her left leg 5 days after operation. The left thigh (A) and leg (B) are both visibly swollen and blueish. On palpation, the limb felt warm. A massive iliofemoral venous thrombosis was diagnosed on venography and the patient was anticoagulated. Luckily, she did not suffer a pulmonary embolism and the limb returned to a normal diameter over 6 months. She will be at lifetime risk of postthrombotic deep venous insufficiency.

Deep Vein Thrombosis

Lower limb DVT is often silent, with classic clinical features in only a quarter of cases. These include leg swelling, calf muscle tenderness and increased leg warmth; calf pain on passive foot dorsiflexion (**Homans sign**) is unreliable.

Iliofemoral vein occlusion tends to cause diffuse and sometimes massive swelling of the whole lower limb (Fig. 12.6). In addition, there may be tenderness over the femoral vein in the groin. In severe cases (rare nowadays), the limb becomes painful and white, and boggy with oedema; this is known as **phlegmasia alba dolens** (painful white leg). In more extreme cases, the limb becomes more painful and blue, with incipient venous infarction (**phlegmasia caerulea dolens**).

Asymptomatic DVTs have the same potential as symptomatic venous thromboses for causing both pulmonary embolism (PE) and long-term chronic venous insufficiency (see Ch. 43), thus emphasising the importance of prophylaxis for all patients at increased risk. To complicate the problem, as many as half the patients who develop swelling and pain in the calf after operation do *not* have DVT.

Diagnostic Tests for Deep Vein Thrombosis

Colour duplex ultrasound is the standard technique for investigation of cases where DVT is suspected. In surgical patients, scanning is the preferred investigation as D-dimer blood tests can be misleading after operation. Colour duplex allows scanning of all the major lower limb deep veins for blood flow and contained thrombus, and when the scan is normal, can reliably exclude the diagnosis.

Pulmonary Embolism (PE)

The classic clinical picture of PE is sudden dyspnoea and cardiovascular collapse, followed by pleuritic chest pain, development of a pleural rub and haemoptysis. In hospital, this is often heralded by physical collapse whilst seated on the toilet. Ten percent of PEs are estimated to be fatal within the first hour. The electrocardiogram (ECG) may show evidence of right heart strain (S wave in lead I, Q wave and inverted T wave in leads III—'S1, Q3, T3'). This presentation, however, is uncommon and occurs only when 50% or more of the pulmonary arterial system is occluded. More extensive occlusion usually results in sudden death.

Small PEs are common and are often 'silent', presenting as nonspecific episodes of general deterioration, confusion, breathlessness or chest pain. Note that the patient suffering small embolic events is greatly predisposed to a massive or fatal embolus; it is essential to recognise the condition and to treat it seriously. The patient often has a tachycardia and low-grade fever but there are no diagnostic changes on ECG. Deterioration may be attributed to chest infection, atelectasis or cardiac failure unless PE is considered. There are sometimes more specific diagnostic symptoms of small emboli, including localised **pleuritic chest pain** and small **haemoptyses** in the form of blood-streaked sputum.

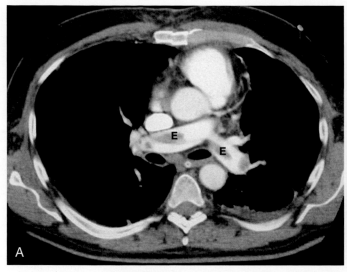
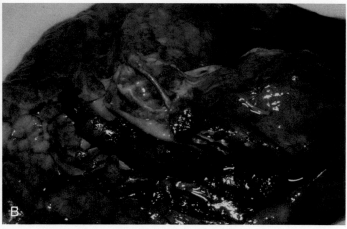

• **Fig. 12.7** Pulmonary Embolism (PE). (A) Thoracic computed tomography pulmonary artery scan (CTPA) with intravenous contrast showing large emboli *(E)* in the pulmonary arteries. This is the investigation of choice where there is a high suspicion of PE. (B) Postmortem specimen of lung from a patient who died of massive PE. Embolic material has been removed, but some remains in the pulmonary arteries *(E)*.

VTE is most common from about the fourth to the seventh day after major surgery but may present any time during the next month or so, sometimes after the patient has left hospital.

Diagnosis of Pulmonary Embolism

In suspected PE, chest x-ray and ECG changes are nonspecific and of little value. The choice of investigation depends on the level of clinical probability. Several clinical scoring schemes have been used to categorise patients to low (~10%), intermediate (~25%) or high (~80%) risk of PE. Categories are based on the sum of points allocated to **predisposing factors** (past history of VTE, immobility, malignancy) and the **presence of signs** of DVT, tachycardia or an alternative diagnosis.

Blood tests for D-dimers have a high negative predictive value for PE (D-dimers are formed when cross-linked fibrin is lysed by plasmin), although levels are elevated anyway after operation and therefore misleading. The quickest and most reliable method of confirming the diagnosis is by dynamic spiral or multislice CT pulmonary angiography using intravenous contrast (Fig. 12.7A). Where available, this has largely superseded radioisotope ventilation/perfusion scanning (V/Q scanning).

Management of Venous Thromboembolism

For most patients, removing or lysing limb thrombus or pulmonary embolus is impracticable. The usual objective in managing thromboembolism is to halt the coagulation process by systemic anticoagulation. This prevents established thrombi from propagating and new thrombi from forming. Thrombus is then gradually removed by the normal body processes of lysis.

Most lower limb thrombi eventually become organised and firmly attached to the vein wall, posing no further risk of embolisation. Thrombus is later invaded by granulation tissue and veins eventually recanalise, restoring blood flow. However, in the process, valves are often destroyed, leading to **chronic venous insufficiency** (see Ch. 43), often many years later. After PE, if the patient survives the initial episode, emboli are efficiently removed by local thrombolysis, leaving little functional deficit.

For treatment, anticoagulation is initially achieved with therapeutic subcutaneous LMWH, often started when clinical suspicion is high before the diagnosis is confirmed. Heparin anticoagulation takes effect immediately and is continued for about 5 days, by which time acute symptoms have usually subsided. Once the diagnosis is confirmed, oral anticoagulation is commenced; **warfarin therapy** (which takes several days to become fully effective) is most commonly used, and once the INR is within target range, the LMWH can be stopped. Warfarin is continued for up to 6 months, the period of highest risk of recurrent thromboembolism. Newer oral drugs that are direct inhibitors of thrombin (dabigatran) or factor Xa inhibitors (rivaroxaban, apixaban, and edoxaban) now have approval for the treatment and secondary prevention of DVT and PE and are generally easier to manage than warfarin, though are more expensive.

Untreated, about 50% of patients with proximal DVT or PE will have a further thromboembolic event within 3 months. Patients who suffer repeated thromboembolic episodes when taken off anticoagulation may need maintaining on warfarin or an alternative for life. For these patients, a **filter** may be placed in the inferior vena cava via a percutaneous route to trap emboli migrating from leg and pelvic veins towards the pulmonary arteries (see Ch. 5, p. 56).

In the rare case of submassive nonfatal PE with evidence of right ventricular dysfunction, with haemodynamic compromise and persistent hypotension, or shock despite vasopressors and optimal medical support, various options are available to try to reduce the embolic burden. **Systemic thrombolytic therapy** uses tissue plasminogen activators, such as streptokinase or urokinase to lyse clot, but this carries a high rate of serious bleeding, including intracranial haemorrhage. The technique of manipulating a pulmonary artery catheter into the embolus and instilling high doses of **local thrombolytic drugs** or performing **clot suction** is another option. Surgical **embolectomy** is considered in patients where thrombolysis is contraindicated; it is performed under cardiopulmonary bypass and is a major undertaking.

Prevention of Venous Thromboembolism

The importance of **general measures** in preventing venous thrombosis needs to be emphasised. These include preoperative encouragement to exercise, early postoperative mobilisation, adequate hydration and avoiding pressure on the calves. Women on oestrogen-containing combined oral contraceptives undergoing major surgery (lasting >45 minutes) and patients on hormone replacement therapy should consider stopping the drugs 4 weeks before surgery (ensuring an alternative contraceptive method is used during this time). This is most important for patients with preexisting risk factors for thromboembolism. In any case, low dose heparin prophylaxis should be considered for any operation.

For these and for any patients at risk (shown in Box 12.4), specific prophylactic measures should be taken to reduce the risk. Prophylactic measures include the following:

- **Low-dose subcutaneous heparin**—unfractionated heparin and LMWH both inhibit the activity of factor Xa indirectly by binding to circulating antithrombin III. Both types are as effective for preventing thromboembolism but LMWH has the advantage that it is given only once a day instead of two or three times. Low-dose heparin is currently the most effective method of reducing thromboembolism in at-risk patients. It has been shown to reduce the rate of postoperative DVT by 70% in general surgical, urological, gynaecological, orthopaedic and trauma patients. Similar reductions are achieved in PE rates. The beneficial intravascular antithrombotic effect is not caused by anticoagulation, but arises from stimulation of platelet factor antithrombin III; there should be no detectable in vitro anticoagulant effect nor any significant effect on haemostasis during or after operation, although patients on low-dose heparin probably bleed about 10% more at major surgery.
- **Factor Xa inhibitor anticoagulants**—one example, rivaroxaban, is an oxazolidinone derivative which has shown greater efficacy than enoxaparin (LMWH) in preventing thrombosis after hip and knee replacement, and with a similar safety profile, although the cost is higher. It enables predictable anticoagulation without need for dose adjustment or coagulation monitoring but is irreversible in the short term if haemorrhage occurs and clotting factors need to be given.
- **Direct thrombin inhibitor anticoagulants**—dabigatran is an alternative class of oral antithrombotic drug approved for the prevention of VTE in relation to hip and knee replacement surgery; it also has wider clinical applications.
- **Temporary vena cava filter**—placed preoperatively, this is an option for patients at very high risk of VTE, and in those whom other pharmacological and mechanical measures are contraindicated.
- **Calf compression devices**—several pneumatic and electrical devices are available for intraoperative calf compression to simulate muscle pump activity. These are noninvasive and easily applied to all patients, even those at low risk, but their effectiveness is less than low-dose heparin.
- **Graduated compression 'antiembolism' stockings**—using these stockings is simple and widely practised. Provided they are correctly fitted, stockings offer a suitable level of prophylaxis for patients at low or moderate risk. The stockings must be worn during operation, as well as during the early postoperative period.

Fluid and Electrolyte Disturbances

Fluid and electrolyte disturbances, such as **dehydration** or **fluid overload**, **hyponatraemia**, **hypokalaemia** and **hyperkalaemia** frequently develop in the postoperative period. Fluid and electrolyte abnormalities are particularly common after major bowel surgery, especially if there have been massive fluid losses through vomiting, diarrhoea or sequestration in obstructed or adynamic bowel, or surgical complications. These problems are discussed in Chapters 2 and 4.

Antibiotic-Associated Colitis

Pathophysiology and Clinical Features

Colonic inflammation and other diarrhoeal disorders may be side-effects of almost any antibiotic treatment. The conditions are largely caused by selective overgrowth of intestinal organisms which then produce toxins that cause the damage. The clinical picture ranges from a mild attack of diarrhoea to profuse, life-threatening, haemorrhagic colitis.

Antibiotic-associated colitis may develop suddenly or gradually and occasionally becomes chronic or relapsing. Surgical patients are most likely to be affected after operation. *Clostridium difficile* is responsible for many of these cases, and in severe form, the full picture of **pseudomembranous colitis** may develop. This can take a particularly virulent form. **Staphylococcal enterocolitis** is less common.

Stool specimens should be examined by microscopy and culture and by measuring levels of *C. difficile* toxin. Sigmoidoscopic inspection and biopsy of the rectum should also be performed. Treatment is based on the results of these tests. If *C. difficile* infection is diagnosed, it is treated with oral metronidazole or, in resistant cases, with oral (nonabsorbed) vancomycin and the patient must be isolated and barrier nursed (see Ch. 3).

Acute Kidney Injury

Acute kidney injury (AKI) is the abrupt decline in renal function (glomerular filtration rate), associated with rising blood urea and creatinine caused by failure to excrete nitrogenous waste products, along with a reduced urine output (oliguria or anuria). AKI may be caused by prerenal, intrinsic renal or postrenal causes. Around half of all episodes are caused by **acute tubular necrosis**, which in turn is triggered by ischaemia and nephrotoxins. Potential nephrotoxic insults include drugs, such as **aminoglycoside antibiotics** (gentamicin), antihypertensives and nonsteroidal anti-inflammatory drugs (NSAIDs); myoglobinuria (myoglobin is released in the crush syndrome), and the use of iodinated contrast in imaging. Acute renal deterioration can also be seen in fulminate liver failure (or cirrhosis) in a condition sometimes known as *hepatorenal syndrome*, and may present as a particular complication of abdominal aortic surgery, in which the renal arteries may become occluded by inadvertent damage or unrecognised embolism.

Pathophysiology

Renal tubules are acutely sensitive to a variety of metabolic insults, particularly hypoxia and certain toxins. Hypoxia readily occurs if renal perfusion falls substantially; the usual surgical cause is an episode of severe or prolonged **hypotension**. This may result from hypovolaemic shock (haemorrhage or dehydration), cardiovascular collapse (postoperative cardiac failure or myocardial infarction) or septic shock. In the last, endotoxic and cytokine-initiated renal cell damage is also an important factor. Preexisting **chronic renal disease** increases a patient's susceptibility to AKI.

If the renal tubular insult is not overwhelming, tubular cell damage is confined to disruption of cellular metabolism rather than tissue necrosis. This is potentially reversible provided the patient can be maintained in good general condition while tubular recovery takes place. The usual sequence of recovery is that poor urine output continues for a period (**oliguric phase**), followed by **spontaneous diuresis** of large volumes of unconcentrated urine consisting of unmodified glomerular filtrate (**diuretic phase**). Urinary concentrating power then slowly improves as tubules recover normal metabolic function. In contrast, when tubular damage is more extensive, the patient remains anuric or severely oliguric. Careful fluid management is required during recovery.

Prevention and Management of Acute Kidney Injury

AKI is largely preventable by careful attention to preoperative assessment, fluid balance, and prevention and prompt management of hypotension and sepsis, as well as dose monitoring of potentially nephrotoxic drugs. When AKI is mild, simple conservative measures, such as fluid restriction may sustain the patient until tubular function recovers. When complete (oliguric) renal failure occurs, plasma urea, creatinine and potassium concentrations rise inexorably and the patient usually requires **haemofiltration** or **renal dialysis**. Fortunately, many of these patients recover renal function gradually over a few weeks or months and do not require permanent renal support.

Pressure Sores

Pathophysiology

Patients with neurological or degenerative conditions, cognitive impairment, spinal cord injury, impaired mobility and those with impaired tissue perfusion are extremely susceptible to pressure sores ('bed sores'), particularly over bony prominences, such as the sacrum and heels (Figs 12.8 and 12.9). Pressure sores occur because the frequent spontaneous adjustment of position that normally occurs in bed is lost through obtunded sensation and immobility. Diminished protective pain response plays an essential part. Patients with diabetes may have a sensory neuropathy so they are unable to sense the damaging effects of prolonged pressure on a bony prominence. Tissue necrosis and any subsequent failure to heal result from a combination of factors including recurrent pressure ischaemia, poor tissue perfusion (from cardiac or peripheral vascular disease) and malnutrition. Note that patients who have experienced substantial weight loss and patients with relatively ischaemic lower limbs are at particular risk.

Prevention and Management of Pressure Sores

Once established, pressure sores are extremely difficult to eradicate so preventing them must be given high priority in patients at risk. Relatively hard surfaces, such as accident and emergency department trolleys and operating tables may initiate pressure sores in susceptible patients in less than an hour. Likewise, pressure sores can develop in a remarkably short time in a hospital bed, particularly if the patient is incontinent of urine or faeces (Figs. 12.8 and 12.9). Prevention of pressure sores on the ward is a nursing priority, and includes the following measures:

- **Special bed surfaces to spread the load**—these include (in ascending order of cost and complexity) pressure-relieving foam mattresses, electric ripple mattresses, water beds, suspended net beds and low pressure continuous airflow beds.
- **Relieving pressure on the heels**—use of ankle gel rests while on the operating table, use of heel pads, orthopaedic foam gutters and 'bean-bags' on return to the ward.
- **Regular change of posture**—for most patients, this involves encouragement to get out of bed, at least into a bedside chair, and to mobilise beyond the chair as much as possible. A bed-bound patient requires regular turning so that the same skin area is not subject to constant pressure.
- Regular checking of pressure areas.
- Management of incontinence.
- Dietician support of those with nutritional deficiency.

CASE HISTORY

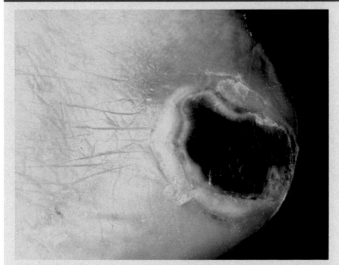

• **Fig. 12.8** Typical Heel Pressure Sore. This elderly man presented with a ruptured abdominal aortic aneurysm and had a stormy postoperative course. At some stage, this heel was allowed to remain too long in one position, resulting in deep necrosis. He had no evidence of occlusive peripheral arterial disease.

CASE HISTORY

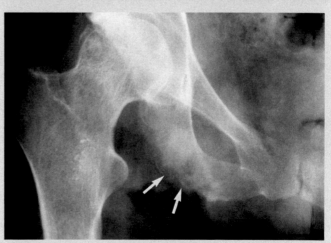

• **Fig. 12.9** Osteomyelitis of the Ischial Tuberosity Secondary to Pressure Ulceration. X-ray of the pelvis in an elderly bed-bound woman showing osteomyelitis of the ischial tuberosity (arrowed) underlying a deep, long-standing sacral pressure ulcer.

Treatment of established pressure sores is unsatisfactory unless causative factors can be eliminated. This is often impossible in the permanently disabled patient. Avoiding pressure is the mainstay of treatment, supplemented by local cleansing, barrier creams and dressings designed to remove necrotic tissue and control secondary infection. Hydrocolloid and alginate (seaweed-derived) specialist dressings both protect the affected area and speed up the healing process. For a deep sacral sore, major plastic surgery involving a rotational buttock flap is occasionally justified.

Complications of Operations Involving Bowel

These include delayed return of bowel function, mechanical bowel obstruction, anastomotic failure, intraabdominal abscesses, peritonitis, bowel fistula and acute bowel ischaemia.

Delayed Return of Bowel Function

Temporary Interruption of Peristalsis

Any abdominal operation may temporarily disrupt peristalsis. This is particularly true where the operation is for peritonitis, an abscess or intestinal obstruction, or if the operation involves extensive handling of the bowel. Operations involving the retroperitoneal area, such as aortic surgery may also upset peristalsis, probably via disturbance of parasympathetic activity. The problem mostly affects the small intestine. Patients may complain of nausea, anorexia and vomiting after oral fluids are reintroduced early in the postoperative period. This condition is described as a physiological **ileus** and is caused by reduced or absent bowel motility without obvious underlying structural abnormality, and usually resolves within 2 to 3 days. If it persists beyond 3 days, it is termed **adynamic** or **paralytic** ileus. Adynamic bowel problems may be a response to local factors (e.g., bowel handling, a bowel wall haematoma or a collection of pus in contact with bowel), sepsis, drugs such as opioids, or to systemic abnormalities, particularly hypokalaemia. Adynamic ileus requires supportive treatment with intravenous fluid support and a nasogastric tube to prevent vomiting. If the ileus becomes prolonged, another cause, such as mechanical intestinal obstruction or an intraperitoneal collection of pus should be sought.

Acute Gastric Dilatation

Occasionally, adynamic disorder involves the stomach, causing acute gastric dilatation and accumulation of large volumes of gastric and refluxed duodenal secretions. The warning feature is when the patient suddenly vomits a large volume of fluid which may, even on the first occasion, result in fatal bronchial aspiration. Preventing acute gastric dilatation is the main reason nasogastric tubes are used after upper gastrointestinal surgery or after relief of mechanical bowel obstruction. If acute gastric dilatation is suspected, the abdomen should be examined for a **succussion splash** by gently shaking the abdomen from side to side and listening for a splash. If present, immediate nasogastric intubation is necessary; two or more litres of fluid that might otherwise be vomited and inhaled may need to be aspirated. Aspiration and inhalation of gastric contents can cause mild or severe aspiration pneumonia (**Mendelson syndrome**).

'Pseudo-Obstruction'

Adynamic disorder involving the large bowel is conventionally but inaccurately described as **pseudo-obstruction**, as there is no obstruction present. It may follow any abdominal operation, especially if the retroperitoneal area has been disturbed, as in nephrectomy or aortic surgery. Pseudo-obstruction (also referred to as *acute colonic pseudo-obstruction* or *ACPO*) is also a recognised complication of nonabdominal operations, such as fractured neck of femur, especially in frail patients. It may even occur without operation as a complication of severe hypokalaemia, trauma involving the lower spine and retroperitoneal area, or anti-Parkinsonian and other drugs. The diagnosis can be made on plain abdominal x-ray or with water-soluble contrast enema by excluding mechanical causes of obstruction. CT is helpful to exclude other conditions, such as bowel perforation and mechanical obstruction. Treatment involves identification and treatment of the underlying cause, together with supportive measures, such as an indwelling flatus tube or deflation via colonoscopy, until function returns.

Mechanical Bowel Obstruction

Early Postoperative Mechanical Obstruction

This is uncommon and may be caused by a loop of bowel becoming twisted or trapped in a peritoneal defect, unwittingly created at open operation or laparoscopy. **Fibrinous adhesions** may also cause obstruction, and these usually develop about 1 week after operation. In both cases, the obstruction may be transient and settle with conservative measures (nasogastric aspiration and intravenous fluids), or may progress to full-scale intestinal obstruction. Water soluble contrast agents (such as gastrografin) can be used therapeutically in adhesive bowel obstruction; such agents act to decrease bowel wall oedema, encourage fluid movement into the lumen of small bowel and might also enhance bowel contractility to help overcome the obstruction, thus avoiding more invasive intervention. Open surgery with laparotomy is indicated for strangulated bowel, systemic signs of toxicity or in patients who have failed conservative methods. In selected uncomplicated cases, laparoscopy can also be considered. Obstruction occurring after gastrectomy or gastroenterostomy may be caused by oedema of the mucosa surrounding the anastomosis; this usually settles eventually with conservative measures, although reoperation may be required.

Late Postoperative Mechanical Obstruction

Fibrinous adhesions may organise and persist as broad **fibrous adhesions** between adjacent loops of bowel or as isolated fibrous bands traversing the peritoneal cavity. These are a common cause of an isolated episode of small bowel obstruction or even infarction. Adhesions may also cause recurrent bouts of bowel obstruction months or years after abdominal operations. Most episodes resolve spontaneously with conservative treatment, but failure of resolution or signs of strangulation (tenderness, toxaemia) necessitate laparotomy, or where clinically suitable, laparoscopy.

Patients with recurrent intestinal obstruction caused by adhesions present a serious surgical challenge. Each laparotomy becomes more difficult and hazardous for the patient. Therapeutic agents to prevent adhesions forming are also available for high risk cases.

Anastomotic Failure

Anastomotic leakage or breakdown is a major cause of postoperative morbidity after bowel surgery. Inadequate or delayed diagnosis and delayed surgical reintervention may lead to multiple and cumulative complications including fistulae, sepsis, multiorgan dysfunction and failure, and death. There should be a low index of suspicion for leaks and a readiness to undertake reoperation if leakage is suspected. This often involves exteriorising the bowel ends.

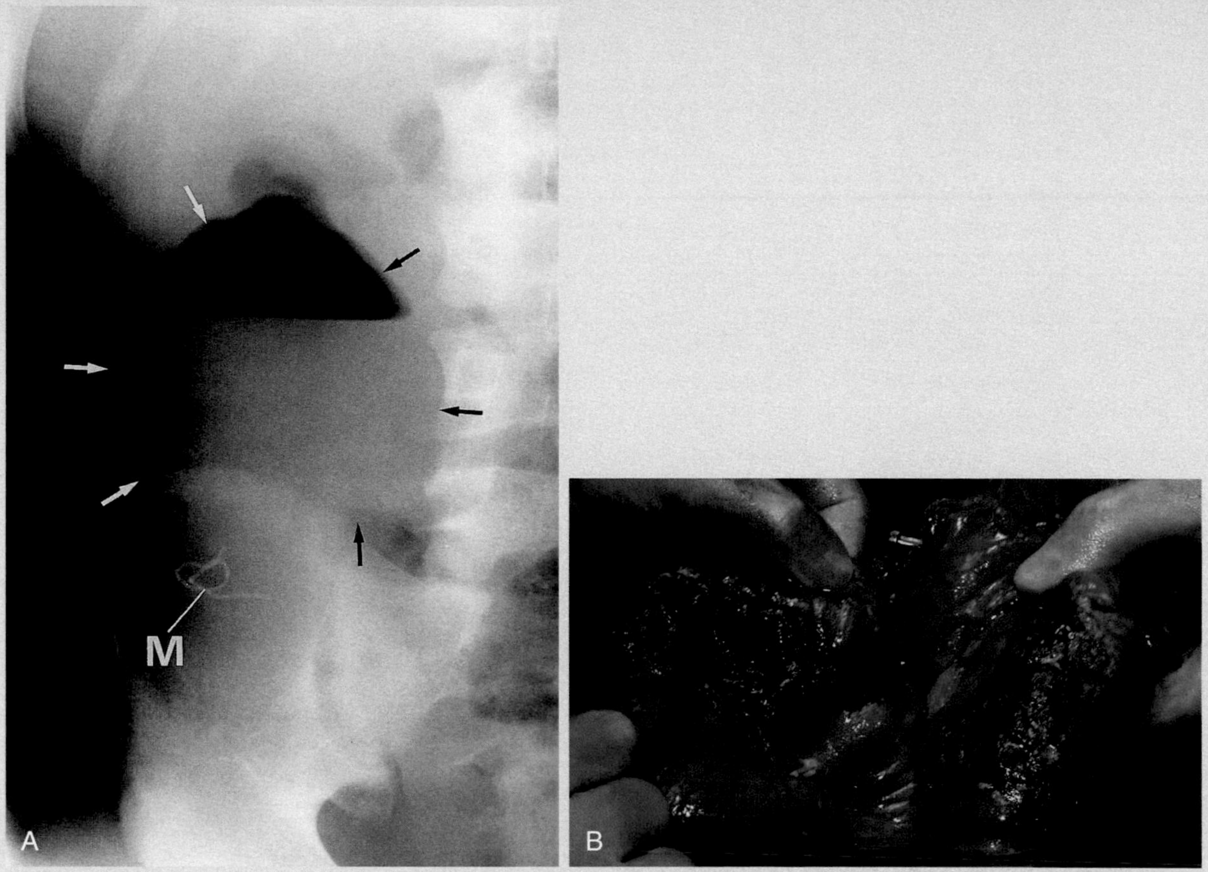

• **Fig. 12.10** Intraabdominal Abscess Following Appendicectomy. (A) This 16-year-old boy had an operation for removal of a perforated gangrenous appendix. He remained ill with anorexia and intermittent vomiting, general malaise and a swinging pyrexia. A large mass was palpable in the right side of the abdomen. Erect abdominal x-ray shows a huge abscess cavity *(outline arrowed)* with a gas bubble above a fluid (pus) level. Note the radiopaque marker *(M)* in a gauze swab packed into the open abdominal wound. (B) At operation, the abscess was surrounded by adherent small bowel, shown here. This is a *never event* and is now a rare occurrence with stringent theatre checks.

Small anastomotic leaks are relatively common and lead to small **localised abscesses** which become walled off by surrounding gut and omentum. Small leaks manifest clinically by slower than expected recovery including delayed recovery of bowel peristalsis resulting from local dysfunction. Usually, the problem eventually settles with continued intravenous fluids and delayed reintroduction of oral intake. Reoperation, however, should be repeatedly considered if recovery is slow.

Major anastomotic breakdown results in generalised peritonitis, large abdominal abscesses, progressive sepsis and fistula formation and the outcome is often fatal.

Intraabdominal Abscesses

Abscess Associated With Bowel Anastomosis

An anastomotic leak from any part of the bowel may be walled off by small bowel and omentum in a vigorous intraperitoneal response (Fig. 12.10). This results in an abscess forming near the anastomosis. The patient will either be nonspecifically unwell with delayed recovery, a swinging pyrexia and signs of local peritonitis, or more seriously ill with early signs of sepsis.

Early reoperation or radiological drainage is usually necessary to drain the abscess and prevent continued peritoneal contamination. Where the anastomosis has broken down, both ends of the bowel should be brought out to form temporary stomas, since reanastomosis will almost certainly fail. The bowel can often be rejoined once the local infection and metabolic disruption have resolved.

Other Intraabdominal Abscesses

Intraabdominal abscesses may also develop at sites remote from an anastomosis—for example, in the pelvis (**pelvic abscess**) or beneath the diaphragm (**subphrenic abscess**). These occur most often as a complication of treated peritonitis, particularly faecal peritonitis. They may also develop because of contamination of the operative site by faeces or other infected material, or by 'tracking' of an anastomotic abscess within the abdomen. Abscesses of this type usually produce a less severe illness than do those in direct communication with the bowel.

If an abscess is suspected, ultrasound or CT scanning may help to identify its location and guide needle aspiration or placement of a percutaneous drain if appropriate. Surgical exploration may, however, be necessary.

Peritonitis

Postoperative peritonitis usually results from a major anastomotic breakdown causing extensive peritoneal contamination. In other cases, the cause is perforation of **obstructed** or **ischaemic bowel** or perforation of an incidental **peptic ulcer**. The clinical picture may develop rapidly over a few hours or, if infection spreads from an intraperitoneal abscess, more gradually over a few days. The patient is systemically ill with severe, generalised abdominal pain; the abdomen is tender and rigid to palpation (see Ch. 19, p. 294 for more details). *Note*: elderly patients with peritonitis may have surprisingly little tenderness. Generalised peritonitis inevitably progresses to sepsis and multiple organ failure, unless promptly treated.

The patient is resuscitated and commenced on intravenous antibiotics and then returned to theatre for laparotomy. The abdomen is explored, the underlying cause is treated and peritoneal toilet is carried out. Early and vigorous treatment will usually save the patient's life.

Bowel Fistula

Fistula formation as a complication of surgery usually results from an anastomotic leak or infarction of a segment of bowel. A local abscess first develops then discharges to the surface via the wound or along the track of an abdominal drain. When there is obstruction of bowel beyond the anastomosis, anastomotic breakdown is more likely; the fistulous tract then provides a means of drainage for contents of the obstructed bowel. With time, the drainage tract slowly becomes lined with epithelium from the bowel and the skin surface and the fistula becomes permanent. Occasionally, a fistula develops in a patient after an operation for **bowel cancer**. In this case, the fistula may become lined with malignant cells. Fistulas, proximally in the small bowel, result in loss of large volumes of intestinal secretions containing digestive enzymes. This rapidly leads to dehydration and major electrolyte disturbances and often causes gross intraabdominal inflammation and skin destruction. The more proximal the origin of the fistula, the greater the volume of fluid and electrolyte loss and the more damaging its consequences.

The general state of the patient with a fistula depends on the extent of intraabdominal infection. If this is minimal and there is no distal obstruction, the fistula usually closes spontaneously within weeks or months, provided the patient can be sustained in the interim. Proximal small bowel fistulas require **total bowel rest** (i.e., nil by mouth and a nasogastric tube) with full **parenteral fluid replacement and nutrition.** Somatostatin analogues may be given to substantially reduce the volume of secretion into the small bowel. Distal small bowel or large bowel fistulas may be managed with **enteral feeding** using low-residue elemental or semi-elemental fluid diets. These are often given via a fine-bore nasogastric tube.

When a fistula is associated with intraabdominal infection, the patient is desperately ill, septic and hypercatabolic. These patients need management in critical care and reoperation. Laparotomy is required to bring the disrupted bowel ends to the surface as stomas and to drain the gross foci of infection; further laparotomies, even daily, may still be required before the intraabdominal infection is brought under control. Mortality from these complicated fistulas is high. A few specialist units exist to treat the most severely affected patients.

Acute Bowel Ischaemia

Acute bowel ischaemia is an uncommon postoperative complication, usually occurring after abdominal aortic surgery. Infarction of the sigmoid colon can follow inferior mesenteric artery ligation (usually a necessary part of the operation) if the collateral blood supply is compromised by obliterative atherosclerosis of the remaining mesenteric arteries. Fortunately, this is rare. The patient has usually progressed well at first then deteriorates unexpectedly several days after operation, often passing fresh blood per rectum. If untreated at this stage, the patient later collapses with peritonitis caused by colonic necrosis and perforation.

Clinical signs of acute bowel ischaemia are nonspecific, but often the degree of pain and collapse is out of proportion to the minimal abdominal signs. Plain abdominal x-ray may show 'thumb printing' of the affected bowel or the characteristic appearance of gas in the bowel wall. If acute bowel ischaemia is suspected, laparotomy and resection must usually be performed urgently as perforation will soon occur and is nearly always fatal. Even with timely surgery, the prognosis is bleak.

13

Principles of Cancer Management

CHAPTER OUTLINE

Introduction

Cancer patients make up a rising proportion of surgical cases and comprise about a third of surgical bed occupancy. Defining and ensuring optimal treatment for individual patients should be a true multidisciplinary effort involving surgeons, oncologists, pathologists, radiologists, specialist nurses, and palliative care teams. Other specialist teams often need to be involved including nutritional, psychological and social specialists. The incidence of some cancers is falling whilst others are rising, mainly owing to increased life expectancy, detection through screening programmes (see Ch. 6), and incidental findings from imaging for other reasons. Cancer has now overtaken cardiovascular disease as the most common cause of death in the United Kingdom. Cancer patients place disproportionate demands on surgical services because of their complex needs, the fact that they are usually older, recover more slowly from surgery, and are more prone to complications.

Each cancer subtype is generally treated uniquely, ideally using dynamic algorithms based on the best evidence from large-scale retrospective and prospective studies. This is designed to set the scene for the aspiring surgeon, and not as a definitive review of each area. The chapter outlines general principles of cancer management, focusing on general oncological and surgical principles, the array of systemic anticancer drugs, principles of radiotherapy and palliative care, and how these should optimally interact.

The incidences of the most common malignancies in the United Kingdom is shown in Table 13.1. Incidence rates vary markedly between countries owing to differing genetic and environmental factors and subtypes of each malignancy, and these dictate regional public health and oncological priorities. Such statistics can be misleading since a rise in incidence may reflect a true increase in the number of new cancers, or the effect of screening programmes detecting more cases (e.g., breast cancer, and pilot studies of low-dose computed tomography (CT) screening in patients at high risk of lung cancer). We focus here on **carcinomas** (epithelial malignancies), since they are the commonest and best understood, although similar principles apply to all cancers.

Cancer is diagnosed definitively by biopsy or fine-needle aspiration. Staging is the next step to determine treatment options and clarify prognosis. This helps identify patients potentially curable

TABLE 13.1	The 10 Most Commonly Diagnosed Cancers in Males and Females in the United Kingdom				
Males		Females	
Prostate	47,151	Breast	54,751
Lung	24,535	Lung	21,853
Bowel	23,082	Bowel	18,722
Head and neck	8404	Uterus	8984
Melanoma	8112	Melanoma	7794
Kidney	7919	Ovary	7270
Non-Hodgkin lymphoma	7478	Non-Hodgkin lymphoma	6204
Bladder	7310	Primary brain	5966
Oesophagus	6248	Pancreas	4960
Leukaemia	5880	Kidney	4628

From Cancer Research UK, 2015.

by surgery alone and those needing other treatments. Radical curative intent surgery can often eradicate macroscopic disease (found clinically, by imaging or during operation), but may not bring cure because of unrecognised local or disseminated micrometastatic disease. Radiotherapy alone can be curative in certain settings, with similar caveats. Additional treatments, such as chemotherapy and/or radiotherapy may therefore be appropriate to reduce the risk of recurrence—these are known as **adjuvant treatments**. Similar treatments can be given in advance to increase the operability of certain cancers (**neoadjuvant treatments**).

When a curative intent operation is not possible, or where residual macroscopic disease remains after surgery, nonsurgical **palliative** treatment may be offered, where the goal is to prolong life, preserve or improve the quality of life, or help with cancer-related symptoms rather than cure. Many newer (more) **targeted treatments** are now available, and have transformed the lives of many patients with advanced cancer. These include hormonal treatments, small molecule enzymatic inhibitors, monoclonal antibody-based drugs and immunotherapy. This is a rapidly evolving field and may transform the face of cancer treatment in the future. To increase survival in patients with inoperable cancers, massive scientific efforts are underway to identify unique susceptibilities of cancer cells to novel systemic anticancer treatments. Novel imaging techniques are also helping to identify patients where curative-intent treatment is futile.

In the fight against cancer, a range of strategies is being pursued. Lifestyle modification (e.g., programmes to reduce smoking) can reduce the true incidence of new cancers, as can prophylactic interventions in high-risk populations (e.g., bilateral mastectomy in *breast cancer [BRCA]1/2* gene mutation carriers). Early presentation is likely to increase the proportion of surgically curable cases, so education of patients and healthcare providers in cancer-related symptoms, plus appropriate screening programmes can help.

Neoplasia

It is important to distinguish between benign and malignant tumours when considering neoplastic growth. Benign tumours are only occasionally life threatening owing to their location, but are different from malignant tumours which invade surrounding tissues and metastasise. **Malignancy** results from genetic mutations of genes affecting the cell cycle which arise spontaneously or under environmental influences. Evolutionary selection of clones with favourable characteristics allows them to outcompete normal cells and other neoplastic cells. This results in some neoplastic cells progressively acquiring phenotypes categorised as the 'hallmarks of cancer'. The list of cancer-related phenotypes continues to expand and holds promise for new treatment strategies. Meanwhile, six core hallmarks are useful when considering which phenotypes cancers must evolve to progress and how they might be treated. This is alongside four enabling characteristics likely to promote malignant progression. These are shown in Table 13.2.

Malignant tumours are often highly heterogeneous in stromal cell types (e.g., fibroblasts, immune cells, endothelial and lymphatic cells) and tumour cells. The many tumour subclones make it difficult to treat all neoplastic cells alike except through surgical resection. Heterogeneity means diagnostic biopsies may show only a few dozen or hundred malignant cells which may not be representative of the cancer as a whole. Sometimes treatment decisions have to be made on cytological/biopsy specimens that only suggest malignancy (e.g., cellular atypia in pancreatic fine-needle specimen). In these cases, the whole clinical picture must be taken into account by the multidisciplinary team (MDT) to determine optimal management.

Cancer at its core is a disease of genetic change; most mutations that drive cancer are somatic (i.e., not inherited). However, inherited germline mutations (such as *BRCA1* and 2, mismatch repair proteins, or *p53*, a gene that regulates the cell cycle) can dramatically alter cancer risk and need to be understood in screening programmes and in genetic counselling for potentially affected family members.

Mutation rates are influenced by environmental carcinogens and by acquired genetic instability (e.g., by mutations in mismatch repair machinery), and both of these increase the likelihood of malignant progression. Each cancer type has a distinct constellation of mutations which can differ markedly between primary and metastatic lesions, making cancer biology and therapeutics seem infinitely complex. Much work has focused on finding common dysregulated pathways in tumours and attempting to target these.

The most commonly mutated gene in human cancers is the transcription factor *p53*, the so-called guardian of the genome, which is activated by multiple cellular stress signals to promote myriad tumour suppressor functions. The most commonly mutated oncogene (gain-of-function) is *KRAS*. Unfortunately, there are no licensed treatments yet able to directly target these common aberrations.

Benign Neoplasms

Benign neoplasms usually grow slowly, are typically well demarcated and often encapsulated, with a histological appearance closely reminiscent of the tissue of origin. Benign tumours present to the surgeon in many ways, summarised in Box 13.1. Most neoplasms can be readily categorised as benign or malignant according to histological determinants, making it possible to predict whether invasion or metastasis is likely. Sometimes this is difficult, for example, distinguishing between leiomyoma and leiomyosarcoma, or when there is insufficient tissue sampling; note that parts of benign lesions may transform into malignant lesions. Neoplasms may also be difficult to distinguish clinically

TABLE 13.2 The Hallmarks of Cancer, as Well as Enabling Characteristics, and How These Might Be Differentially Targeted

Hallmark of Cancer	Examples of How Cancers Achieve This	Examples of Therapeutic Strategies to Exploit This
Sustaining proliferative signalling	EGFR, *KRAS* and *BRAF* activating mutations	EGFR, *BRAF* inhibitors
Evading growth suppressors	TP53 and RB loss; TGF-beta pathway mutations	CDK inhibitors
Resisting cell death	TP53 loss; BCL2 overexpression, downregulation of BAX	BH3 mimetics
Enabling replicative immortality	Telomerase expression	Telomerase inhibitors
Inducing angiogenesis	Expression of VEGF/FGF	VEGF/VEGFR inhibitors
Activating invasion and metastasis	Acquisition of EMT phenotype through activation of transcription factors, such as ZEB, SLUG and TWIST1	HGF/HGFR inhibitors
Enabling Characteristic	**Examples of How Cancers Achieve This**	**Examples of Therapeutic Strategies to Exploit This**
Avoiding immune destruction	Expression of PDL1	T-cell checkpoint inhibitors
Tumour promoting inflammation	Production of proinflammatory factors; nonself proteins	Anti-inflammatory drugs
Genome instability and mutation	Loss of DNA damage repair proteins	PARP inhibitors
Deregulating cellular energetics	Promotion of aerobic glycolysis	Aerobic glycolysis enzyme inhibitors

BAX, Bcl-2–associated X protein; *BCL2*, B cell lymphoma 2; *BH3*, bcl-2 homology 3; *CDK*, cyclin-dependent kinase; *HGFR*, hepatocyte growth factor receptor; *DNA*, deoxyribonucleic acid; *EGFR*, epithelial growth factor receptor; *EMT*, epithelial-to-mesenchymal transition; *FGF*, fibroblast growth factor; *HGF*, hepatocyte growth factor; *PARP*, polyadenosine phosphate ribose polymerase; *PDL1*, programmed death ligand 1; *RB*, retinoblastoma; *SLUG*, human embryonic protein SNAI2; *TGF-beta*, transforming growth factor beta; *TP53*, tumour protein 53; *TWIST1*, TWIST-related protein 1; *VEGF*, vascular endothelial growth factor; *VEGFR*, vascular endothelial growth factor receptor; *ZEB*, zinc finger E-box-binding homeobox.
Adapted From Hanahan and Weinberg, Cell, 2011.

• BOX 13.1 Principal Modes of Presentation of Benign Tumours

- Lesion noted by the patient, often with worries about possible malignancy (e.g., breast lump)
- Overt bleeding or occult blood loss causing anaemia (e.g., bowel polyps)
- Local obstructive effects (e.g., leiomyoma of small intestine)
- Pressure causing pain or dysfunction (e.g., neurofibroma)
- Unacceptable cosmetic appearance (e.g., subcutaneous lipomas)
- Effects of the production of excessive amounts of hormone by endocrine neoplasms (e.g., parathyroid adenoma, insulinoma, phaeochromocytoma)

---

from other tumour-like disorders, such as hyperplasia (e.g., parathyroid adenoma from hyperplasia) or hamartomatous growth (a growth composed of a mixture of tissues usually found in that area of the body—these are benign but may still require removal).

Malignant Neoplasms

Malignant neoplasms are typically nonencapsulated with a poorly defined, irregular outline because of local tissue invasion. They usually grow progressively and often rapidly. Histologically, the cells range from well differentiated to **anaplastic** (i.e., little or no resemblance to parent tissue), with the aggression generally increasing with greater dedifferentiation, although well differentiated malignancies can be highly aggressive. The cells and nuclei of malignant neoplasms often vary widely in shape and size. The extent of this **pleomorphism** also tends to correlate with the degree of malignancy and the future clinical behaviour of the tumour, as can the extent of lymphovascular and perineural

invasion. These histological features are taken into account by the pathologist when classifying and **grading** the tumour. The supporting tissue **stroma** of some malignancies may undergo fibrous hyperplasia, which accounts for some of the characteristic clinical features; these include hardness to palpation (induration), intestinal obstruction caused by annular carcinomas of the large bowel, and retraction and dimpling of skin overlying breast cancers. On the other hand, in highly aggressive tumours, the supporting tissue stroma may be inadequate for metabolic support, leading to necrosis and patchy haemorrhage within the tumour. This can present with sudden onset of pain and/or a mass. Malignant tumours present in a variety of ways summarised in Box 13.2.

Carcinogenesis

Most cancers are probably caused by a complex (and chance-driven) interplay between environmental factors and patient-intrinsic factors. About two-thirds of cancers may be attributed (to some extent) to external environmental factors, such as ultraviolet light, ionising radiation, virus infections and carcinogens in air, food and water. Often the mutation pattern (e.g., guanine-cytosine>thymine-adenine transversion from carcinogens in tobacco smoke) can point to the relevant carcinogen. Given the widespread 'field' effect of preceding risk factors, patients with one carcinogen-induced cancer are at risk of developing another in that tissue, and must be kept under close surveillance after curative treatment for the first cancer—large swathes of the tissue may have inherited predisposing mutations. While this helps decide follow-up schedules after radical treatment, it can be difficult to distinguish between new primaries and recurrences. Certain tissues, particularly those of the bladder, breast, skin, head and neck, lung and large bowel, are at particular risk of new primaries.

• BOX 13.2 **Principal Modes of Presentation of Malignant Tumours**

The Primary Lesion

- Palpable or visible mass (e.g., breast or thyroid cancer)
- Obstruction or other disruption of function of a hollow viscus (e.g., bowel obstruction by colorectal carcinoma, stridor in bronchial carcinoma)
- Overt bleeding, for example, haematuria from bladder tumours, rectal bleeding from (usually left-sided) large bowel cancers, or haemoptysis from lung cancers
- Occult blood loss causing anaemia (e.g., carcinoma of stomach or caecum)
- Obstructive jaundice (e.g., carcinoma of head of pancreas or extrahepatic bile ducts)
- Skin lesion, often ulcerated (e.g., basal and squamous cell carcinomas, malignant melanoma, breast cancer)
- Abdominal distension (e.g., from primary peritoneal cancer)
- Nerve invasion (e.g., facial nerve palsy from parotid carcinoma, recurrent laryngeal palsy from anaplastic carcinoma of thyroid)
- Seizure, headache or personality change (e.g., from primary brain tumours)
  Note that pain is not a particularly common presenting feature of primary malignancy, but can be, for example, pancreatic, lung and nasopharyngeal cancers; pain is more often associated with metastases.

Metastatic Deposits

- Enlarged lymph nodes (malignant nodes tend to be hard, matted and nontender). Intrathoracic nodes may cause superior vena caval obstruction or lung collapse
- Hepatomegaly, in many cancers (e.g., stomach, large bowel and pancreatic carcinomas)
- Obstructive jaundice (usually caused by lymph node masses in the porta hepatis compressing the bile ducts, but sometimes extensive liver deposits), for example, stomach, large bowel and pancreatic carcinomas

- Abnormal masses distant from the primary lesion (e.g., abdomen, pelvis and skin)
- Bone invasion causing bone pain or pathological fractures (e.g., prostatic and breast cancers)
- Malignant effusions (e.g., pleural effusion in breast cancer, ascites with peritoneal deposits from intraabdominal or pelvic malignancies)
- Pulmonary metastases—usually asymptomatic and found on chest x-ray/computed tomography, but can present with haemoptysis, lung collapse, infection, dyspnoea or pain
- Brain metastases—behavioural or personality changes, headache, seizure, paresis, ataxia, etc.
- Neurological problems—spinal cord lesions caused by direct invasion or through associated pathological spinal fractures

Generalised Systemic Manifestations (Uncommon Except for Cachexia)

- Malignant cachexia (severe weight loss and wasting)—this can occur with any cancer, and is seen in ~50% of cases
- Fever—characteristic of lymphomas and renal cell carcinoma, also a feature of liver metastases; also occurs when there is extensive tumour necrosis
- Migrating superficial thrombophlebitis and chronic disseminated intravascular coagulation (DIC)
- Peripheral neuropathies, myopathies and rare autoimmune neuromuscular phenomena (e.g., myasthenic syndrome)
- Other rare autoimmune phenomena (e.g., haemolysis or paraneoplastic antibody production)
- Ectopic hormone production, for example, antidiuretic hormone (ADH), adrenocorticotrophic hormone (ACTH), parathyroid hormone (PTH) and gonadotrophins (all rare in malignancies seen in general surgery)

Growth and Spread of Malignant Tumours

Most malignancies probably arise from a single cell that has become capable of growing progressively. About 30 cell division cycles are probably needed to produce a clinically detectable lesion of 1 cm diameter containing 1000 million cells. Many properties must be acquired for the tumour to progress (see Table 13.2). Particular cellular properties enable a tumour to invade surrounding tissues, invade lymphatic or blood capillaries, disseminate and 'take root' in regional lymph nodes or spread to coelomic cavities or distant organs. These properties often arise through mutation and a change in cellular programming known as **epithelial-to-mesenchymal transition** (EMT), where the tumour cells lose the original tumour properties and become more migratory and stem cell-like. The precise changes that promote vascular versus lymphatic invasion, and which dictate preferred sites of distant metastases remain largely unknown, although the latter can be simply anatomical (e.g., liver metastasis from colorectal or pancreatic cancer).

These pathophysiological factors have important clinical consequences. Firstly, the earlier the primary tumour is detected and removed (i.e., the fewer cell division cycles and the fewer the number of tumour subclones), the greater the chance of complete cure. Unfortunately, changes that permit metastasis can appear very early, that is, by about 20 cell division cycles, when the primary lesion is too small to be detected (about 1 mm). The hallmarks of cancer can be acquired in any order, and additional metastasis-inducing genetic mutations may not even be required to produce the EMT phenotype as it can be promoted by other signals, such as aberrant growth factor receptor signalling.

In practice, when lymph node metastases are present and fully resectable, the probability of surgical cure depends when

the cancer develops its capacity for further spread. This can be as early as when lymph node metastases appear, so haematogenous metastases may already be multifocal and make surgical removal of detected metastases ineffective. Evidence-based guidelines dictate which groups of lymph nodes (and how many) need to be removed for optimal surgical/pathological staging. The liver, lungs, bone and brain are common organs for haematogenous spread, with each tumour type having particular propensities to metastasise most often to certain organs.

Treatment of Malignant Tumours

Principles of Cancer Management

Two broad considerations determine the approach to treatment for any cancer patient. The first is whether an attempt can and should be made to achieve a **cure** or whether **palliation** is more appropriate—note that palliation does not necessarily mean that prognosis will be short, since life can be substantially prolonged with other treatments. For example, well over 20% of metastatic oestrogen receptor-positive breast cancer patients survive beyond 5 years, and this continues to rise. The choice between curative-intent and palliative-intent management depends on the nature of the tumour, the extent of local spread and whether distant metastases are believed to be present. The next considerations are the natural history of the type of cancer (including molecular features) and the patient's age (although only if relevant and evidence based) and comorbidities determining the ability to withstand surgery.

Systems of **staging** have been devised for each tumour type, many based on the **TNM system** developed by the Union for

---

• BOX 13.3   The General Principles of Cancer Management

Note: detection of asymptomatic disease is covered in Chapter 6, including opportunistic screening, screening and surveillance of people with risk factors, and population screening.

1. Prereferral mechanisms
   - Patient education to recognise danger symptoms and signs
   - Self-examination by the patient (e.g., breast, testis)
   - Education, guidance and postreferral feedback for family practitioners in recognising danger symptoms and signs and reassuring the 'worried well'
   - Appropriate referral to specialists, helped by proformas containing indications to refer suspected skin, colorectal, breast, head and neck and upper gastrointestinal (GI) cancer
   - Ready availability of early assessment and diagnostic tests where malignancy is suspected
2. Primary diagnosis after referral
   Clinical assessment plus investigations (e.g., tumour markers, imaging, endoscopy, biopsy, fine-needle aspiration cytology, laparoscopy).
3. Staging
   Additional investigation to evaluate extent of spread:
   - Local spread
   - Lymph node spread
   - Haematogenous spread (bone, lung, liver, brain)
   - Peritoneal/pleural spread
   - Consider intracranial imaging depending on cancer type and symptoms
4. Multidisciplinary decision making
   To formulate the aims of treatment and decide optimum treatment:
   - Treatment planning and timing of treatment, based on the best available evidence and guidelines
   - Treatment may involve a single modality, or combinations of surgery, neoadjuvant or adjuvant chemotherapy and/or radiotherapy, hormonal therapy, targeted therapies
   - Patients should ideally be entered into suitable clinical trials, particularly where there is no clearly effective standard treatment
   Note that increasing specialisation and subspecialisation in the surgical treatment of rarer or more complex cancers produces better outcomes, for example, sarcoma; therefore consider carefully if the patient should be treated locally or referred to a regional/national/international specialist centre.
5. The treatment
6. Repeat staging after operation or other treatment
   With knowledge of operative findings and a review of the histology and relevant histopathological and molecular special tests. This may change the plan for postoperative adjuvant therapy and provide prognostic information to estimate the statistical likelihood of survival/cure.
7. Posttreatment surveillance
   For recurrence or appearance of new tumours in the primary field. Guidelines for different cancers are available for the desirability, frequency and duration of clinical assessment, imaging, endoscopy and measuring tumour markers
8. Audit of local outcomes to improve quality of care. Participation in national audits.

International Cancer Control, which scores characteristics of the primary **T**umour itself, the extent of regional lymph **N**ode involvement and the presence or absence of distant or other **M**etastases. Staging is used in planning treatment, as a guide to prognosis and as a standardised descriptive tool for comparing efficacies of treatments in similar populations in clinical trials, and in comparisons between different centres.

Cancer can recur at any time after the primary treatment, and treatment success is often described in terms of survival after a given number of years rather than 'cure'. **Five- or 10- year survival** are common yardsticks and can imply cure. Some tumours however, such as breast cancer, may recur in a disseminated form as long as 40 years after apparently successful treatment, probably owing to activation of long dormant micrometastases. Conversely, others, such as localised colorectal cancers, rarely recur after 10 years. Clinicians should be cautious about using the term 'cure', bearing in mind the tumour type and its likely behaviour, and the likelihood of complete elimination of tumour by therapy. The probability of cure can be discussed, but where recurrence remains possible, the term should be avoided in its absolute sense. Tumour- and risk-specific follow-up schedules are determined by prospects for treatment should recurrences be found. Most include clinical review, imaging and sometimes blood tests for tumour markers, and ideally should be able to detect recurrence early (whilst still salvageable), but balanced against the burdens and risks of active surveillance.

Tumour Markers

Proteins shed by tumour cells can be helpful in diagnosis, surveillance, and monitoring the effects of treatment. Some commonly used blood-borne tumour markers are carcinoembryonic antigen (CEA; colorectal cancer), carbohydrate antigen (CA)19-9 (pancreatic cancer), alpha-fetoprotein (AFP) and β-human chorionic gonadotropin (HCG; germ cell tumours), CA125 (ovarian cancer), prostate-specific antigen (PSA; prostate cancer), and CA15-3 (breast cancer).

Team Working in Cancer Management

There is a growing international trend towards involving a range of specialists working in cooperative teams to manage patients with complex problems. Structured MDTs are recommended for managing most cancer cases, but particularly where the diagnosis needs consideration and where treatment may involve radiotherapy, chemotherapy or targeted therapy pre- or postoperatively, meticulous planning of an operation, prostheses or reconstructive surgery, stoma care and specialist nursing or physiotherapy, as well as nutritional, social and psychological support.

The benefits of working in this way arise from the battery of experience brought by experts in different disciplines, particularly where diagnostic and therapeutic options are not clear. Cases can be discussed at any stage in the diagnostic or treatment process and an optimum treatment plan generated; the group has joint responsibility for implementing the plan. For rarer, and more difficult to manage, cancers (such as sarcoma), patients should be referred to specialist centres that deal with larger numbers to ensure optimal care.

Treatment Options

The general principles of cancer management are highlighted in Box 13.3. The treatment options for malignant disease include **surgical excision, radiotherapy, chemotherapy**, **hormonal manipulation** and other **molecularly targeted therapies (including immunotherapy)**, with two or more often used in combination. A treatment strategy usually depends on the tumour type and stage, histopathological and molecular profile (at the genetic/protein level), the patient's overall fitness and whether the aim is cure or palliation. A radical or aggressive approach may be recommended where the aim is cure, provided evidence supports this approach. Where cure is not possible, or where disease has relapsed after radical treatment, the aim is to use palliative treatments, that is, to extend or improve quality of life and/or alleviate cancer-related symptoms.

A diagnosis of cancer should never be concealed from a competent patient. Aside from the obvious ethical ramifications, suspicion and fear of the unknown often causes more distress than a frank explanation of the diagnosis and its ramifications. Likewise, prognostic information (with its associated uncertainty) should be offered, although patients should be allowed to decline this information. Time should be allowed for the patient to formulate further questions and a follow-up consultation arranged in a few days. It usually helps the patient to have a friend or relative present. Patients are also helped by well-constructed printed information, by patient groups and cancer charities, and by specially trained cancer nurses who can spend the necessary time and act as an intermediary if necessary.

All anticancer treatments can involve unpleasant and sometimes life-threatening **side-effects**, and these risks must be weighed against their intended benefits after a full and frank discussion with the patient to ensure valid informed consent. Patients need to be appropriately informed and involved in treatment decisions, though the amount of information given varies, with some patients wanting as much information as possible, and others as little as they absolutely need—nevertheless, when treatment has the potential to do harm, patients need enough information to decide if it is actually in their best interests.

Palliative Care

Palliative care focuses on quality of life when cure is not possible and involves weighing up the benefits of any treatment against its burdens and toxicities while focusing on what is important to the patient and their family. Active palliative-intent anticancer treatments (which aim to control cancer growth) should be distinguished from symptomatic palliative care (which uses supportive treatments or procedures including radiotherapy to alleviate cancer-related symptoms). In practice, these two approaches usually occur in parallel, and there is a growing trend for palliative care physicians and nurses to be involved early (alongside oncologists) in the care of patients with incurable disease, rather than when anticancer treatments have been exhausted or are not appropriate.

Specialist palliative care teams can offer invaluable outpatient support in difficult matters of symptom control, or psychological, social or spiritual problems. Some patients may need short admissions to specialist units (often called **hospices**) for symptom control and eventually for terminal care.

Surgery for Cancer

General Principles of Cancer Surgery (see Box 13.3)

The ideal result from cancer surgery is complete eradication of all malignant disease without radically interfering with organ function. Around a third of cancer patients can be cured in this way, although this varies greatly by cancer type. Decisions about whether to embark on major elective surgery depends on assessment of the nature of the disease (usually through analysis of diagnostic biopsies or cytological specimens) and its radiological stage. Modern techniques of cross-sectional imaging with CT/magnetic resonance imaging (MRI) and fluorodeoxyglucose-positron emission tomography imaging, laparoscopy, endoscopic staging (e.g., endobronchial ultrasound in lung cancer) and intra-operative ultrasound, greatly assist in accurate diagnosis, and can save patients from fruitless radical surgery. Guidelines have been produced to ensure cancer-type specific staging. Current evidence-based guidelines should be consulted to determine the best treatment approaches.

Sometimes, cancer cells can seed a biopsy tract (e.g., in soft tissue sarcoma), and these tracts need to be removed at the time of operation. For this reason, in suspected sarcoma, biopsies and surgery are performed at regional and national centres with expertise in the marking of biopsy tracts and subsequent surgery.

Metastases apparently confined to local lymph nodes are usually excised along with the primary tumour. In many cancer types, regional lymph nodes are removed and examined histologically even in the absence of evident metastases, to complete **pathological staging**. As well as a possible therapeutic benefit for removing viable cancer cells, this helps decide on optimal adjuvant treatment or surveillance.

Occasionally blood-borne metastasis appears to be a solitary event (**oligometastatic disease**) and a cure can still be achieved—for example, by partial hepatectomy for colorectal cancer or pulmonary lobectomy for renal cell carcinoma. Even in the presence of incurable metastatic disease, **palliative surgery** may be required for specific distressing symptoms from locally advanced or metastatic disease (e.g., dysphagia, pain or severe haemorrhage, spinal cord compression or bowel obstruction). Similar results can sometimes be obtained by less invasive techniques, such as radiotherapy, chemotherapy, embolisation, or other approaches to destroy cancer tissue, including radiofrequency probes or lasers. Endoscopic and interventional radiological procedures are often useful in palliation, and can prolong quality and length of life, for example, in relieving shortness of breath by stenting in superior vena caval obstruction, in relieving dysphagia by stenting a blocked oesophagus, or insertion of a biliary stent to relieve a blocked common bile duct.

Sometimes surgery is used to **debulk** a tumour, usually combined with chemotherapy to improve its efficacy (as in ovarian carcinoma), or to remove potentially viable tissue after curative-intent chemotherapy (e.g., retroperitoneal nodal masses in testicular germ cell tumours). Increasingly, chemotherapy and/or radiotherapy is used in the neoadjuvant setting to 'downsize' a malignant tumour to facilitate excisional surgery, for example, rectal cancer. This is sometimes inaccurately called 'down-staging' since the effect on metastatic disease is unclear. Sometimes, however, removal of the primary tumour by a cytoreductive procedure can result in shrinkage of metastatic disease, most notably in renal cell carcinoma.

Tissue removed at operation should always be sent for histopathological analysis. This may be to histologically confirm malignancy (e.g., after orchidectomy in presumed testicular cancer). Even after a definitive diagnostic biopsy, surgical specimens are needed for pathological staging (in curative intent treatment). They contain more tumour cells than biopsies and provide more substrate for histopathological and molecular tests to give additional diagnostic and prognostic material and better inform decisions about future treatment. This can sometimes lead to a second diagnosis, for example, lymphoma after removal of enlarged nodes thought to be secondary to gastrointestinal cancer.

Cancer patients are at high risk of venous thromboembolic events, and low-molecular-weight heparin prophylaxis should be considered in hospitalised patients but carefully balanced against the risk of bleeding (or exacerbating ongoing bleeding).

Radiotherapy

General Principles of Radiotherapy

The value of ionising radiation in treating malignant tumours was recognised soon after the discovery of x-rays in 1895, and radiotherapy is now used at some stage in about half of all patients with malignant disease. **Orthovoltage** x-rays (up to 250 kV) were the basis of radiotherapy until **megavoltage** irradiation in the late 1950s. Cobalt-60 machines provided more penetrating radiation, but have been superseded by **linear accelerators** which provide photon beams with even higher energy of 5 to 20 MeV. With increased energy, the radiation dose peaks below the skin, reducing the risk of severe skin reactions. Radiotherapy works by the target tissue absorbing radiation, which induces highly reactive free radicals that damage deoxyribonucleic acid (DNA) and cause cell death at next mitosis. Cancer cells with a high rate of proliferation are particularly sensitive but normal tissues with high rates of cell turnover (e.g., gut mucosa and bone marrow) are also vulnerable. The total dose given depends on the aims of treatment, the site and volume of the tumour and its relationship to important normal tissues. Treatment is by a variable number of sessions or **fractions**, often given as one fraction every weekday over several weeks to allow normal tissues to recover between treatments. Single palliative treatments are also used, for example, for palliation of pain from bone metastases.

The larger the volume of tumour, the greater the dosage of irradiation required. Since dosage is limited by the tolerance of normal tissues, radiotherapy is most useful for small lesions. Radiation dose is measured in **Gray** (Gy). A common daily dose is around 2 to 4 Gy, which can be sufficient to destroy about 50% of viable cells in a tumour; each subsequent dose destroys 50% of the remainder, causing a logarithmic decline in viable cell numbers as treatment proceeds. Planning radiotherapy for lesions deep in the body has improved as a result of better CT and MRI and modern immobilisation and gating techniques.

Radiation can be directed to a tumour in three ways:

1. **External beam irradiation**—the most commonly used type, but this term describes a range of different types of radiotherapy, including:
   - conformal radiotherapy
   - intensity-modulated radiotherapy
   - image-guided radiotherapy
   - stereotactic body radiotherapy/stereotactic ablative radiotherapy (including CyberKnife treatment and stereotactic radiosurgery)
   - electron beam radiotherapy
   - adaptive radiotherapy
   - proton therapy
2. **Local application of radioisotopes (brachytherapy)**—this involves placing the radiation source on or in the tissue to be irradiated. **Plaque** sources of radiation can be used for skin malignancies, and radioactive **iridium wires** or **caesium needles** can be implanted in the oral cavity, prostate, skin and sometimes breast, giving high-dose local irradiation. Implantation is usually performed under general anaesthesia. For cancers of the uterus and cervix, the radioactive source is placed in a sealed container within the uterine or vaginal cavity; it can be safely inserted without risk to staff via a flexible tube from the radiation source using computer control.
3. **Systemic radioisotope therapy**—radioactive iodine given by mouth or intravenously is a well-established treatment for thyrotoxicosis and can be used for certain thyroid cancers even if metastases are present (provided the rest of the thyroid, which would otherwise concentrate the drug, has been removed). Radium-223 is also used in prostate cancer which has metastasised to bone, where it mimics calcium and delivers radiation to the cancer cells.

Major Applications of Radiotherapy

Radiotherapy is used to some extent in most common solid tumours and in lymphomas. Radiotherapy has three major goals: (1) as a primary cure (with or without chemotherapy), (2) as an adjuvant treatment or (3) as palliation. The treatment objective must be clearly defined before treatment is begun.

Primary Curative Radiotherapy

Radiotherapy with curative intent is known as **radical**, and can be used alone or concurrently with chemotherapy (chemoradiation). Where cure rates are comparable to surgery, radiotherapy is usually used for tumours technically difficult to remove or where surgery would be particularly mutilating as in the head, neck and larynx, or debilitating (e.g., lobectomy/pneumonectomy). Radiotherapy can be directed at the primary lesion and regional lymph nodes if appropriate. Unsurprisingly, the more locally advanced the cancer, the lower the chance of cure. In general, the most radiosensitive tumours in adults are well-differentiated thyroid cancer, small cell lung cancer, germ cell tumours, lymphomas and basal cell and squamous cell carcinomas of the skin.

One advantage of surgery over radical radiotherapy for macroscopic disease or suspected microscopic disease (e.g., axillary nodes in breast cancer) is that the pathological status of the removed nodes is known, providing extra prognostic information, although this must be balanced against the risks of surgery. For example, stereotactic ablative radiotherapy is increasingly used for stage I lung cancer (instead of lobectomy), particularly in poor operative risk patients and in the elderly, especially if the tumour is peripherally located. The evidence for determining which patients should be treated with radiotherapy versus surgery is constantly changing, and up-to-date guidelines should be consulted for each case. For many, either option can be presented to patients.

Neoadjuvant/Adjuvant Radiotherapy

The principle underlying **adjuvant therapy** is targeting clinically undetectable micrometastases believed to be responsible for local, regional and systemic recurrence after macroscopic disease has been completely removed. Radiotherapy can be applied to local tissue and regional nodes before surgery (**neoadjuvant radiotherapy**), after surgery or both. Neoadjuvant therapy, comprising radiotherapy, chemotherapy or both may also be used to 'downsize' a cancer to make surgery more practicable, for example, in locally advanced rectal cancer or in oesophageal cancer. Where all three are used, this is called *triple modality treatment*.

Palliative Radiotherapy

Palliative radiotherapy is used for local control of primary or metastatic lesions to alleviate symptoms while causing minimal side-effects. It is also used to prevent impending complications, for example, spinal cord compression. Much lower total doses are used than for attempts at cure; short courses or **single high-dose fractions** are tolerable and convenient for the patient. Clearly, palliative radiotherapy is only indicated where expert assessment predicts that therapeutic benefit is likely. Radiotherapy is particularly effective in controlling metastatic deposits in bone and brain, although the radiosensitivity of cancers varies between subtypes. The pain of bone metastases can often be relieved by radiotherapy, as can some of the neurological manifestations of brain or spinal metastases.

Radiotherapy is often valuable in providing symptomatic relief in advanced disease. In ulcerating breast cancer, for example, radiotherapy can shrink the primary lesion, permitting skin healing. Similarly, the distressing symptoms of cough, haemoptysis and pleuritic pain from advanced lung cancer can often be eased. Symptoms of local recurrence can often be controlled, for example, pain or bleeding from rectal cancer. Some indications for palliative radiotherapy are summarised in Box 13.4.

Complications of Radiotherapy

Despite the precise use of high-energy radiotherapy, side-effects and complications still occur; the main early effects are outlined in Table 13.3.

Long-Term Side-Effects of Radiotherapy

Modern radiotherapy uses high-energy sources with meticulous treatment planning. Delivery causes fewer side-effects than the

---

• BOX 13.4   Some Indications for Palliative Radiotherapy

Pain control, for example in:
- Bone pain (especially breast, prostate and lung metastases)
- Nerve root and soft tissue infiltration (e.g., head and neck, brachial plexus)

Dyspnoea, for example to
- Shrink age of tumour obstructing or compressing a large airway or superior vena cava

Ulcerating and fungating lesions, for example in:
- Breast, skin, head and neck tumours

Haemorrhage, for example in:
- Haemoptysis
- Haematuria
- Rectal or cervical bleeding

Emergency complications, for example in:
- Spinal cord compression
- Superior vena caval obstruction
- Raised intracranial pressure
- Obstruction of tubular viscera (e.g., oesophagus, upper gastrointestinal tract, ureters)

Space-occupying lesions caused by symptomatic brain metastases:
- Brain metastasis causing hemiparesis

TABLE 13.3   Early Reactions and Complications of Radiotherapy

Reaction/Complication	Management
Systemic Side-Effects	
Malaise and fatigue—very common	These settle spontaneously with time and rest
Nausea, vomiting and anorexia	Antiemetics; manage contributing factors, such as mucositis/candidiasis
Effects Occurring in Irradiated Tissues	
Skin (Especially Axilla, Groin and Perineum)	
Redness, itching and mild pain Skin breakdown (in treatment of skin cancers, this heals after 3–4 weeks)	Bathe with nonperfumed toiletries Avoid friction by pat drying Aqueous cream Moisture-retaining nonadherent dressings Can consider: Silver–sulfasalazine cream Mild or moderate-strength topical steroids
Abdomen and Pelvis	
Nausea, vomiting, diarrhoea	Antiemetics, antidiarrhoeals
Frequency, dysuria, haematuria (radiation cystitis)	Urinary alkalinising agents; exclude infection
Head and Neck	
Dry mouth (xerostomia) caused by salivary gland injury	Frequent oral fluids, moist oral swabs, careful attention to oral hygiene
Painful mouth, dysphagia and altered taste. This is caused by inflammation and atrophy of oral mucosa (mucositis) and may also involve nasal mucosa	Anti-inflammatory mouthwash, topical steroids and anaesthetic gels, antifungal agents for candidiasis, artificial saliva
Chest	
Painful dysphagia (radiation oesophagitis)	Local anaesthetic solutions (e.g., low strength hydrocortisone and lidocaine) Compound antacid/alginate preparations, (e.g., Gaviscon)
Head	
Hair loss (alopecia)	Provision of wigs
Bone Marrow	
Myelosuppression	Discontinue therapy, platelet transfusion, blood transfusions, alertness for signs of infection (and prompt systemic antibiotics if so), consideration of prophylactic antibiotics (e.g., co-trimoxazole in lymphopaenia)

orthovoltage treatment used in earlier days. Side-effects such as **osteoradionecrosis** are now rare (see Fig. 13.1), but **endarteritis obliterans** may be a long-term complication affecting any tissue subjected to radiotherapy. The effect is progressive impairment of blood supply, loss of specialised tissues and replacement with fibrosis. In the chest, radiotherapy can cause pulmonary fibrosis and there is an increased risk of cardiac events in women treated for left-sided breast cancer; techniques have been modified as

a result. In the gastrointestinal tract, the effects of radiation on bowel (**radiation enteritis**) can be particularly serious, with continued bleeding (especially large bowel) and stricture formation (especially small bowel). A similar reaction probably accounts for delayed or incomplete healing after surgery with breakdown of intestinal anastomoses or formation of internal fistulae. **Radiation colitis** is most common after pelvic radiotherapy and can be difficult to manage.

CASE HISTORY

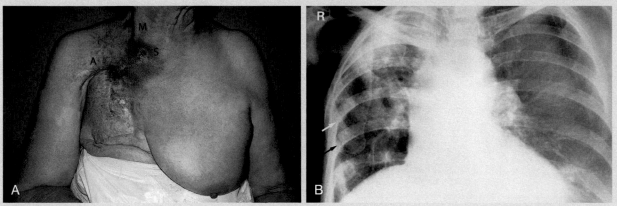

• **Fig. 13.1** Osteoradionecrosis After Early Orthovoltage Radiotherapy For Breast Cancer. This 75-year-old woman had a radical mastectomy and orthovoltage irradiation for carcinoma of the right breast in 1949, 40 years before this photograph. She presented with two discharging skin sinuses below the clavicle (S). **(A)** Gross deformity of chest wall caused by excision of pectoral muscles at radical mastectomy (axilla [A], sternomastoids [M]). Note sinus openings (S) leading down to sequestra, and widespread telangiectasia, a late result of radiotherapy. **(B)** Chest x-ray showing osteoradionecrosis of the ribs and scapula on the right side. There is typical patchy osteoporosis and osteosclerosis. Several healing pathological fractures are also evident (arrowed). Irradiation has induced lung fibrosis and pulmonary contraction resulting in a shift of the mediastinum towards the right.

Chemotherapy

General Principles of Chemotherapy

Success with cytotoxic chemotherapeutic agents, in curing many haematological and childhood malignancies, encouraged the use of similar drugs for solid tumours, previously treated only by surgery or radiotherapy. These drugs can destroy tumour cells by exploiting their increased mitotic and metabolic rates and dependencies. The main classes of chemotherapeutic agent are as follows:

- **Antimetabolites**—analogues of normal cellular nutrients, for example, antifolates (including methotrexate and pemetrexed), and fluoropyrimidines (including 5-fluorouracil [5-FU] and capecitabine).
- **Alkylating agents**—these attack negatively charged nucleophilic sites on DNA, for example nitrogen mustards (including cyclophosphamide) and triazines (including temozolomide).
- **Drugs which cross-link DNA**, for example platinum compounds, such as cisplatin, carboplatin and oxaliplatin.
- **Anthracyclines**, which promote single- and double-stranded DNA breaks, inhibit topoisomerase II and can intercalate into DNA, for example doxorubicin, epirubicin and daunorubicin.
- **Topoisomerase 1 inhibitors**, for example topetecan and irinotecan.
- **Drugs which disrupt the mitotic spindle**, for example vinca alkaloids, taxanes (including paclitaxel and docetaxel).

All of these cytotoxic mechanisms also affect normal tissues, and are responsible for most side-effects of chemotherapy. Drugs

are often used in combination, selected in terms of additive or synergistic anticancer efficacies. Ideally also, the toxic effects of each drug would impact on different organ systems so that each drug can be given in tumour-toxic doses without excessive normal tissue damage. An increasing range of new cytotoxic chemotherapeutic drugs and trials of novel combinations have led to significant improvements in survival, but at the cost of higher toxicity. Cytotoxic drugs are usually given by intravenous infusion, in a series of cycles separated by 3 to 4 weeks to allow recovery of normal tissues. Orally available cytotoxic drugs have been developed, for example capecitabine, which is metabolised in three steps to 5-FU. Chemotherapy can also be given topically (to the skin), intraperitoneally (for ovarian cancer), intrathecally (for haematological malignancies) and delivered direct to affected limbs (isolated limb perfusion for melanoma). The most sensitive cancers, and therefore the tumour types where chemotherapy alone may be curative, are shown in Box 13.5.

Major Applications of Chemotherapy

Chemotherapy can result in a substantial benefit, and even a chance of cure in some well-defined malignancies. However, clinicians treating cancer need to be clear whether their objective is cure or palliation, and base their decisions on critical review of high-quality clinical trials. Given the potential for severe side-effects and the high cost, there is no place for speculative chemotherapy especially where evidence shows no benefit.

Primary Curative Chemotherapy

This is mainly indicated for highly sensitive **germ-cell tumours**, high-grade **lymphomas** and some **solid tumours and leukaemias of childhood**. Chemotherapy may be used alone or it may follow removal of the primary tumour (e.g., testicular germ-cell tumours, Wilms tumour), or it may be used first followed by resection of any residual tumour (e.g., the causative testicle and/or abdominal paraaortic nodes in testicular germ cell tumours). Curative-intent chemotherapy with radiotherapy (**chemoradiotherapy**) often replaces the need for radical surgery, for example, with anal canal, cervical and head and neck cancers. The chemotherapy regimen can be, or can include, a radiosensitising agent. As part of a curative treatment plan, induction chemotherapy or chemoradiotherapy can be used to shrink a tumour to render it potentially operable, or to make the procedure easier or for cosmetic reasons, for example, allowing breast conserving surgery versus mastectomy.

Adjuvant Chemotherapy

This involves systemic chemotherapy added to the local treatment of the primary, with the aim to destroy already disseminated but undetectable micrometastases. Adjuvant chemotherapy regimens are used for many types of malignancies where trials have shown a proven survival benefit. For example, in colorectal cancer, adjuvant therapy has a role in extending recurrence-free survival and life expectancy. Adjuvant treatment schedules are often long and toxic—the standard adjuvant regimen (5-FU, folinic acid and oxaliplatin—FOLFOX) lasts for 6 months in colorectal cancer. Six months of gemcitabine, or gemcitabine and capecitabine, are often used adjuvantly in pancreatic cancer. Benefit from adjuvant chemotherapy is observed in many other cancer types, for example, breast, lung and ovarian cancer.

Palliative-Intent Chemotherapy

In patients with incurable disease, chemotherapy can be useful in extending life expectancy, improving quality of life and alleviating cancer-related symptoms. In clinical trials, outcomes with palliative anticancer treatments are usually expressed in terms of median progression free survivals (the time point at which ~50% of patients have progressed despite starting the treatment) and median overall survivals (the time point at which ~50% of patients have died despite starting the treatment). These are useful for comparing the efficacies of anticancer treatments, particularly when compared alongside each other in prospective, randomised controlled trials. It is less reliable to compare between trials, and it should be noted that clinical trial populations are usually fitter and younger than the general cancer population and many patients fare much better or worse than the statistics would imply.

The **Eastern Cooperative Oncology Group (ECOG) performance status** (PS) is widely used in oncology to give a reasonably objective level of an individual patient's fitness and helps interpret clinical trial findings. It is also prognostic in itself and predictive of toxicity, with ECOG PS 0 or 1 patients faring better. Cytotoxic chemotherapy in a patient with ECOG PS 2 or greater needs careful consideration (although may be appropriate in highly chemoresponsive tumours).

Side-Effects of Chemotherapy

Cytotoxic chemotherapy is especially toxic to cells with rapid turnover, for example, bone marrow and gastrointestinal epithelium. Some common toxic effects of chemotherapy are summarised in Box 13.6, but toxicity profiles vary markedly from drug to drug.

Hormonal Manipulation

The growth of certain tumours, notably carcinoma of the prostate and oestrogen receptor-positive breast cancer, is dependent on sex hormones. Removal of the gonads or use of hormone blocking drugs can have a valuable inhibitory effect on tumour growth. It can reduce the risk of recurrence in the adjuvant setting, as well as improving survival in advanced disease. Hormonal manipulation in the treatment of prostatic cancer is covered in detail in Chapter 35, and breast cancer in Chapter 45. Bone protection, for example, with bisphosphonates, should be considered in patients with bone metastatic disease and when on hormonal treatment.

Targeted Therapies

The molecular revolution in oncology has led to identification of driver mutations and pathways on which certain cancer cells are dependent for their growth or survival. These weaknesses are now being exploited in targeted ways using **predictive biomarkers**—these are changes within the cancer cell (e.g., presence of a particular mutation or overexpression of a certain protein) which predict sensitivity of a patient's tumour cells to a particular therapeutic agent. This helps avoid administering toxic drugs to those unlikely to benefit, as well as helping match individual patients to optimal therapy. Despite their targeted nature, these drugs are often very toxic, often precipitating dose reductions, treatment delays and treatment discontinuation. Even with strongly predictive biomarkers, it should never be assumed that a patient will be fit enough to tolerate treatment with a targeted agent, so expectations need to be managed when referrals are made to oncologists for consideration of treatment.

Small Molecule Enzymatic Inhibitors

These agents are bioavailable orally and can target the enzymatic activity of a single protein or multiple proteins. They can also be designed to specifically target mutant proteins, reducing adverse effects on physiological pathways. Most approved agents of this type inhibit receptor tyrosine kinases, or kinases downstream of these receptors. Sunitinib and pazopanib are multitargeted tyrosine kinase inhibitors, with targets including vascular endothelial growth factor (VEGF) receptors, platelet-derived growth factor (PDGF) receptor and c-kit, and are used in advanced renal cell carcinoma. Activating *BRAF* mutations are found in ~50% of melanomas, and this is targeted by the *BRAF* inhibitors, vemurafenib and dabrafenib. Activating epithelial growth factor

• BOX 13.6 Toxic Effects of Cytotoxic Chemotherapy

Bone Marrow Suppression

- Causes anaemia, thrombocytopenia and leucopoenia (potentially fatal, especially in the context of neutropenia—neutropenic fever is a medical emergency!). Such patients can become septic and die very rapidly if not appropriately managed); opportunistic infections (e.g., *Pneumocystis* pneumonia).

Nausea and Vomiting

- Can be early or delayed after chemotherapy (and may also be multifactorial)
- Modern antiemetics can usually control these symptoms and are usually given prophylactically, often with steroids—the nature and schedule of the antiemetic regime depends on the expected emetogenicity of the chemotherapy regime.

Disruption of Gastrointestinal Epithelial Turnover

- Causes diarrhoea and oral ulceration.

Peripheral Neuropathy

- For example, by cisplatin or taxanes.
- Can be painful and/or disabling and requires careful monitoring on treatment.

Toxicity to Hair Follicles

- For example, by etoposide, cyclophosphamide, doxorubicin, and taxanes, note that many chemotherapies can cause complete alopecia or hair thinning—this is often the most troubling feature of chemotherapy for some patients.
- Reversible, and effects can be reduced by cold capping during chemotherapy (although this is often very uncomfortable for patients).

Gonadal Injury

- Loss of libido, sterility and possible mutagenesis—have a discussion about fertility early, and consider techniques, such as gamete/zygote storage and gonadotropin-releasing hormone agonists (these reduce the risk of infertility in premenopausal women).

Long-Term Risk of Inducing Other Malignancies

- Should be discussed but this risk usually massively outweighed by benefits of chemotherapy—specific surveillance programmes may be indicated.

Rapid Tumour Destruction on a Large Scale (Tumour Lysis Syndrome)

- Leads to release of purines and pyrimidines (usually only a problem in leukaemias and lymphomas, but can complicate treatment of solid organ malignancies, particularly rapidly proliferating tumours with a high disease burden) which cause hyperuricaemia, presenting as obstructive uropathy and renal failure.
- Hyperuricaemia can usually be prevented by giving prophylactic allopurinol.

receptor (EGFR) mutations are found in lung adenocarcinomas, particularly in Asian women who were never smokers—this aberration can be effectively targeted by a range of EGFR inhibitors, including erlotinib, gefitinib and afatinib. Some kinase-targeted treatments can also be useful in the adjuvant settings. Drugs targeting the cell cycle, such as palbociclib and ribociclib (CDK4/6 inhibitors) have been approved in breast cancer alongside hormonal treatments. Certain chromosomal fusion events that turn on tyrosine kinases are particularly adept at driving malignancy, and these malignancies appear to be particularly reliant on this aberrant signalling. Imatinib is an inhibitor of the BCR-ABL tyrosine kinase, the fusion protein produced by the Philadelphia chromosome, and has transformed the treatment of chronic myelogenous leukaemia patients with this chromosomal fusion. It also inhibits the PDGF receptor and c-kit, and such properties are useful in other malignancies, such as gastrointestinal stromal tumours. Recently, larotrectenib, which targets tyrosine kinase fusion proteins, showed a response rate of 75% and a median progression-free survival of 9.9 months. Sadly, it appears that such fusion events are rare in solid malignancies. Increasing numbers of agents are targeting the DNA damage response, trying to specifically deplete DNA repair mechanisms through synthetic lethality approaches. Polyadenosine phosphate ribose polymerase inhibitors, such as olaparib, which inhibit single strand break repair, are particularly effective in cancers that have homologous repair deficiency (e.g., *BRCA* mutant breast/ovarian cancer). The number of approved agents in this class is increasing rapidly.

Monoclonal Antibody-Based Drugs

The advent of humanised monoclonal antibody technology has led to development of effective antibody-based drugs. These drugs depend on high affinity interactions between the variable domains of the antibody and a target surface or soluble antigen. Rituximab is a chimeric murine/human monoclonal immunoglobulin G_1 antibody directed against the CD20 antigen found on B-cells, and has transformed the landscape of treatment for B-cell malignancies. Bevacizumab binds to VEGF-A, thereby inhibiting angiogenesis fuelled by this soluble growth factor. Despite initial excitement that it might be a golden bullet for cancers (since all must promote angiogenesis), it has only provided modest clinical benefit in some cancers. Trastuzumab is an antihuman epidermal growth factor receptor (anti-HER)2 antibody that has transformed survival for patients with HER2-positive breast cancers, and can be used in combination with pertuzumab, which targets a distinct epitope on the HER2 extracellular region. Both are now routinely used in both neoadjuvant and metastatic settings (in combination with docetaxel). Trastuzumab is also used in the treatment of HER2-positive gastric cancer (in combination with cisplatin and a fluoropyrimidine). Cetuximab, which targets the EGFR receptor, is effective against squamous cell carcinoma of the head and neck and (*KRAS* wild-type) colorectal cancer. In head and neck cancer, it can be used in the first-line setting alongside radiation, or as a single agent after failure of previous chemotherapy. Antibody-drug conjugates use the targeting power of monoclonal antibodies to deliver payloads (usually a cytotoxic chemotherapy covalently joined to the antibody) to tumour cells expressing the target antigen. The first approved agent of this kind was ado-trastuzumab emtansine (T-DM1), which is a conjugate of trastuzumab and a microtubule inhibitor. T-DM1 has clinical utility after failure of trastuzumab in metastatic HER2-positive breast cancer. Many more antibody-based drugs are in development.

Immunotherapeutics

Cancer is a disease characterised by genetic mutations, and these mutant genes produce mutant proteins which have the potential to be recognised as nonself and be destroyed by the immune system. Recombinant interleukin-2 (IL2), which stimulates lymphocytic activity, has been approved for decades for the treatment of advanced renal cell carcinoma and melanoma, but has limited activity (despite some patients having a very long duration of response) and high toxicity. More recently, T-cell checkpoint inhibitors have been developed, which aim to overcome barriers in cytotoxic T-cell killing of cancer cells expressing mutation-induced neoantigens. The currently approved agents are monoclonal antibodies targeted at cytotoxic T-lymphocyte–associated protein 4 (CTLA4; a negatively regulating receptor on the surface of CD8$^+$ T-cells), programmed cell death protein 1 (PD1; another T-cell–associated negatively regulating receptor) and programmed death ligand 1 (PDL1; a protein upregulated by certain cancer cells to help them evade T-cell killing by ligating PD1). These have clinical activity in a growing number of cancers, for example, melanoma, lung, head and neck, and urothelial cancers. PDL1 expression and tumour mutational burden can predict response to anti-PD1 agents (although only the former is in regular clinical practice). The other factors governing response and why only a minority of patients respond overall, remain largely unknown. If patients do respond, they often do so for long periods of time, although these agents have not been in use long enough to say whether some patients are cured of advanced disease. T-cell checkpoint inhibitors have a unique constellation of common and often severe side-effects through stimulation of autoimmune organ destruction, and while activity is increased when these agents are used in combination, so are the toxicities. These include colitis, pneumonitis, and hepatitis, as well as glandular dysfunction including hypothyroidism. Some of these can be life-threatening and require very specific investigation and management with immunosuppressive and supportive medications, and as a result specialist advice from physicians competent in dealing with these toxicities must be sought for any patient where immune-related toxicity is in the differential diagnosis.

Resistance

Even in the presence of a predictive biomarker, response rates to targeted agents are often low, owing to the presence of intrinsic treatment resistance. Further, with the possible exception of a very small minority of patients treated with immunotherapy, acquired resistance is unfortunately inevitable, owing mainly to redundancy and plasticity of intracellular signalling pathways, and the presence of many subclones within the tumour with varying degrees of innate treatment sensitivity. Resistance mechanisms are often well documented, and combination approaches are being used to counteract the common pathways to prevent the outgrowth of resistant clones.

The Future

A massive academic and industrial effort is underway to find new treatments for cancer, most of this focusing on targeting particular genetic events present in small subsets of cancers, and on immunotherapeutics. Two early phase clinical trial concepts illustrate the main approaches, and rely upon in-depth genetic profiling of tumours. Umbrella trials take patients with a single disease, such as lung cancer, and give patients a particular targeted drug matched to any actionable cancer mutation found. Basket trials take patients with the same molecular cancer alterations, and give them all the same targeted drug, irrespective of the tumour type. Both approaches illustrate a shift towards treating on the basis of mutations rather than cancer type—this is truly personalised medicine, but it is unlikely to supersede cytotoxic chemotherapy any time soon.

• BOX 13.7 **Principles of Palliative Care**

1. Palliative care is not just about helping people in their last few weeks or days of life. Patients with cancer need to be helped to function as normally as they can for as long as they can. Palliative care should begin early, ideally when a patient is given a terminal diagnosis, and occur in parallel with active anticancer treatments
2. Ensure good communication by spending time with the patient and family (empathic listening, and giving information according to the patient's needs are crucial). Some patients want more information, and some want less. Find out about the patient in front of you. Explore the patient's concerns by asking open questions
3. Anticipate potential problems. Ensure the patient/family know who to call if things go wrong. At an appropriate point, find out where a patient wants to die. Many choose home, some hospital. Hospices are another option. Terminal care at home needs coordinated planning. The family often take most of the burden of care
4. Assess symptoms regularly. Medication may need to be changed frequently as the patient's condition changes. Put a plan in place so that patients and families know who will manage their care, and know who to call at any time of day for help or advice
5. Be aware of different cultural practices and religious beliefs when caring for patients and families
6. Think about cardiopulmonary resuscitation decisions early, establishing the patients' wishes about this, and answering their questions open and honestly. Review this at regular intervals to avoid circumstances in which unnecessary, futile, undignified resuscitation events occur—this can be particularly distressing for families and staff. Consult your national guidelines for information on how best to deal with this in your country, according to local law and professional regulatory guidance
7. Be aware of how looking after seriously and terminally ill patients can personally affect healthcare workers. Working as a team, being supportive of each other, and discussing patients' care regularly (e.g., in formal/informal debrief sessions) helps professionals cope both practically and emotionally.

Palliative Care

Principles of Palliative Care

The principles of palliative care are outlined in Box 13.7. The diagnosis of cancer has immense significance to the patient and the patient's family. Domains affected include:

- Psychological—for example, adjustment reaction, anxiety, depression
- Social—for example, loss of role: unable to care for family, no longer viewed as husband/wife/companion
- Financial—for example, loss of job, expense of frequent hospital visits
- Spiritual—for example, patient and family face up to mortality
- Physical—for example, pain, nausea, fatigue, dyspnoea, toxicities from treatment

For specialists, there is a danger of concentrating on the primary disease while failing to treat the patient as a whole. Palliative care is concerned with a holistic assessment of the patient, with the emphasis on the patient's priorities before, during and after treatment (particularly where complete cure is not possible or likely).

Increasingly, patients are living longer with a large tumour load. This means they often experience symptoms with multiple aetiologies, often resulting in treatment with numerous (and often too many) drugs. To reduce the burden for patients, diagnostic tests should be kept to a minimum, and used only to identify problems that can be treated. Time must be made available for clear and honest explanation of proposed treatments with patients and families. Palliative care focuses on **quality of life**, and all clinicians, including family practitioners, should do what they can to optimise this for patients, ensuring a comfortable and dignified demise. Specialist palliative care physicians and nurses can support the primary care team and the patient and family at home and in specialist palliative care units (often called hospices).

Approach to Common Symptoms Requiring Palliation Other Than Pain

Good communication is the foundation of palliative care. Giving patients and families time to talk about their thoughts and concerns often provides comfort in itself. Palliative pain relief is covered in the next section, and management of other common symptoms is detailed in Table 13.4. Effective management of the symptoms of advancing cancer requires frequent reassessment, and frequent discussion with the patient to assess his or her own priorities, which may change.

TABLE 13.4	**Common Symptoms Other Than Pain Requiring Palliation**	
Symptom	**Causes Include**	**Management**
Fatigue/asthenia (lack of energy)	Circulating factors released by tumour, chemotherapy, radiotherapy Pain, poor sleep, depression, anxiety	Open discussion with patient and family Encouraging gentle, regular exercise within limitations and a daily routine Address and treat remediable causes—check for anaemia Think of depression which often goes undiagnosed Consider a trial of corticosteroids
Loss of appetite (anorexia) and weight loss	Circulating factors released by tumour, chemotherapy, radiotherapy, chronic pain and nausea, fear, depression, anxiety, 'squashed stomach' syndrome, sore mouth, dysphagia, ascites	Explanation to patient and family of known causes Meticulous attention to oral hygiene Correct remediable factors Consider a trial of corticosteroids to stimulate appetite Drain symptomatic ascites only, but do so promptly
Dysphagia	Tumours of pharynx, oesophagus and stomach Compression of oesophagus by extrinsic tumour (e.g., mediastinal lymph nodes) Oesophageal candidiasis	Options include insertion of stents, laser ablation, cryotherapy Radiotherapy, high-dose steroids Consider stenting, radiotherapy, high dose steroids Suspect candidiasis in immunosuppressed patients or patients on steroids; diagnosis may require oesophagoscopy; may require prolonged treatment with a suitable dose of oral antifungal agent
Nausea and vomiting	Drugs: opioids, NSAIDs and others Metabolic causes, for example, hypercalcaemia, uraemia, liver failure Radiotherapy/chemotherapy Intracranial lesions causing raised intracranial pressure Gastric outlet obstruction Intestinal obstruction Constipation	Explanation to allay anxiety; review prescriptions Antiemetics (may require more than one class of antiemetic) Treat reversible metabolic causes High-dose steroids reducing to minimal maintenance dose Antiemetic drugs Radiotherapy Neurosurgical intervention sometimes indicated Antiemetic drugs, including prokinetics Consider stenting Radiotherapy may be helpful Consider nasogastric tube or venting gastrostomy If not candidate for surgery discuss with specialist. Needs honest discussion with patient—may not be able to stop patient being sick but should be able to reduce it. If incomplete (e.g., no colic and passing wind) may benefit from prokinetic agents If complete, may need antisecretory drugs (e.g., hyoscine butylbromide or octreotide) as well as antiemetics (e.g., cyclizine or levomepromazine) Consider nasogastric tube or venting gastrostomy Consider long-term parenteral nutrition Strongly consider prophylactic laxatives for all patients prescribed opioids, at least ensure they are available if required; avoid bulk laxatives in preference to softening and stimulant agents (and see later)
Breathlessness (dyspnoea), cough, choking	Pleural effusion, cardiac failure, infection, anaemia, pulmonary emboli Laryngeal tumour, pulmonary tumour or major airway obstruction	Investigate and treat all reversible causes with regard to patient's overall condition Consider thoracocentesis/pleural drain ± pleurodesis, diuretics, antibiotics, blood transfusions and therapeutic doses of low-molecular-weight heparin May require stenting or local treatment, for example, radiotherapy/laser/cryotherapy Steroids Nebulised adrenaline can be useful in stridor

Continued

TABLE 13.4	Common Symptoms Other Than Pain Requiring Palliation—cont'd	
Symptom	Causes Include	Management
	Lymphangitis carcinomatosa, multiple pulmonary metastases or infiltration	Trial of high-dose dexamethasone 16 mg daily; if beneficial slowly reduce to a maintenance dose (e.g., 2–4 mg daily)
	Multifactorial: disease and debilitation where potentially reversible causes aforementioned are not identified	Explanation to patient and family If appropriate: • Trial of intermittent oral morphine • Trial of bronchodilator therapy • Trial of oxygen (beware in CO_2 retainers) In terminal phase, continuous subcutaneous infusion of diamorphine and/or midazolam may be needed to reduce sensation of breathlessness and associated anxiety Clear explanation, appropriate reassurance
	Anxiety—common in breathlessness	Anxiolytic drugs, for example, small doses of lorazepam orally/sublingually or midazolam subcutaneously may help
Constipation	There are many factors which make patients more likely to become constipated: immobility, weakness; general debility; poor oral intake/dehydration; low dietary fibre; hypercalcaemia; hypokalaemia; serosal disease Drugs, for example, opioids, tricyclic antidepressants and 5-HT3 antagonists (e.g., ondansetron)	Discuss nutritional options; encourage increased fluid intake; prescribe antiemetic where nausea contributes to poor intake Avoid constipating drugs if possible, or limit dosage Laxatives: • Bulking agents—should generally be reserved for moderately active patients with good fluid intake who are not on opioid medication • Osmotic laxatives—lactulose (may cause flatulence and abdominal cramp); magnesium salts (sometimes unpalatable) • Stimulants—senna, bisacodyl • Lubricants—docusate (mainly a softener), liquid paraffin Often necessary to combine softening and stimulant agents Suppositories (glycerol and/or bisacodyl) Enemas are best for distal blockages (felt on PR exam) Prokinetics can be useful
Confusion	Unfamiliar stimuli Drugs, for example, opioids, anticonvulsants, tricyclics, and steroids Metabolic causes, for example, uraemia, hypercalcaemia, hyponatraemia Cerebral metastases Infection Anxiety Cerebral hypoxia	Explanation and calming reassurance to patient and family Adequate lighting; familiar objects; minimise moving of patient within hospital Investigation and treatment of any reversible causes (including withdrawal of causative medications—be careful with completely withdrawing effective analgesia; note that renally excreted drugs including opiates can rapidly build up to toxic levels in the presence of dehydration or renal failure Medication if necessary: distressed patient may respond to benzodiazepines or haloperidol—the latter is very useful for hallucinating patients
Terminal restlessness (also known as terminal agitation/terminal anguish/terminal distress)	This is a diagnosis made by exclusion and can be distressing for the family	Explanation to family Rule out treatable causes: look for urinary retention (although most such patients should already be catheterised for comfort); treat pain Sedation; often requires continuous subcutaneous infusion, for example, midazolam (benzodiazepine) ± levomepromazine
'Death rattle' (i.e., distressing sounds of retained secretions in terminal stage of illness)	Accumulation of bronchial secretions and loss of control of muscles of larynx and pharynx	Explanation to family—usually more distressing to them than to the patient Repositioning of patient often reduces sound and respiratory effort Early and continued use of antisecretory agent (e.g., glycopyrronium subcutaneously in divided doses or by continuous infusion)

CO_2, Carbon dioxide; *NSAIDs,* nonsteroidal anti-inflammatory drugs; *PR,* rectal.

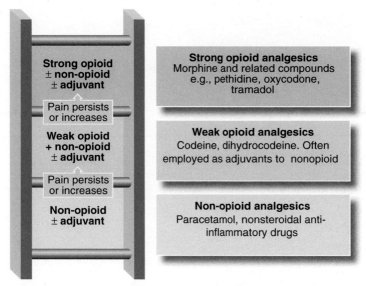

• **Fig. 13.2** Three-step analgesic ladder for cancer pain control (WHO 1986) (see Table 13.5 for adjuvants). The World Health Organization has stated that pain relief should be: (i) by the mouth—oral medication if possible; (ii) by the clock—regularly, not 'as required' (p.r.n.); (iii) by the ladder—if, after reaching top dose on one rung of the ladder, pain is not controlled, go up the ladder.

Cancer Pain

Around three-quarters of patients with advanced cancer have associated physical pain at some stage of their illness. How individuals perceive pain is influenced by what it means to them (e.g., 'my cancer is getting worse'), as well as other factors in their life, which, if deteriorating, can worsen pain. Identifying and addressing these factors is an important way of helping.

Assessment of Pain

Patients frequently have more than one source of pain and each must be assessed. Pain measurement tools (e.g., visual analogue or verbal rating scales) and charts can be helpful. It is useful to use a classification when assessing pain to help plan how to relieve it, and to monitor effects of treatment:

- **Visceral pain**—a constant 'tumour ache' caused by pressure of cancer or invasion of internal organs. Although severe, it often responds to opioids. It can acutely worsen by factors, such as intratumoural bleeding.
- **Neuropathic pain**—caused by pressure on, or destruction of nerves. Often difficult to describe, this may be a clue to their aetiology. Sometimes words like 'tingling' or 'shooting' are used and pain is in the distribution of a nerve root or peripheral nerve. Such pains are usually only partially responsive to opioids and require the use of adjuvant analgesics, such as tricyclic antidepressants (e.g., amitriptyline), antiepileptics (e.g., gabapentin) or corticosteroids to reduce oedema around tumours. Targeted radiotherapy can also be useful.
- **Bone pain**—caused by infiltration of cancer and felt in the bone itself—this can be severe and difficult to treat, although opiates, steroids and bisphosphonates can be useful. Associated clinical features depend on the location, for example, spinal lesions may cause pressure on the cord causing neuropathic pain, anaesthesia and weakness. Skull base lesions can lead to

cranial nerve palsies. Neuropathic features are treated as aforementioned. Targeted radiotherapy can often be useful for bone and/or neuropathic pain.

Bony metastases or nervous compression often lead to **incident pain** where pain is tolerable at rest but becomes much worse with movement. This is often difficult to treat. Local radiotherapy and bisphosphonate infusions (particularly in bone pain from breast and prostate cancers and myeloma), together with analgesics can be helpful. Incident pains are often not responsive to long-acting opioids but adjuvants (mentioned earlier) may help, and fast-acting opioids taken before the activity known to lead to pain can be beneficial.

Principles of Cancer Pain Management

- The aim is to control pain as well as possible, with a balance between analgesia and the side-effects of medication.
- Analgesia should be given regularly, not just 'as required' unless pain is generally infrequent and predictable.
- Analgesics should be titrated against the severity of pain using the three-step analgesic ladder developed by the World Health Organization (Fig. 13.2 and Table 13.5).

Opioid Analgesia

Morphine is generally the opioid of choice. Most patients' pain can be managed with oral morphine, the dose of long acting formulations being titrated up or down according to analgesic requirements. It is helpful to ask patients to keep a diary of how often they require breakthrough (short-acting) pain relief, and which doses they take. This can then be easily factored in when increasing their long-acting analgesia. Addiction is only very rarely a problem amongst cancer patients. If the pain is expected to abate, for example after radiotherapy or surgery, opiates should be reduced promptly—these are times when patients are particularly vulnerable to symptoms and signs of overdose. If a patient on a stable dose requires an increase for the same pain, this can reflect tolerance or disease progression.

TABLE 13.5 Adjuvant Analgesics and Other Treatments for Management of Cancer Pain

Treatment Method	Some Indications
Nonsteroidal anti-inflammatory agents	Reduce inflammatory component in pain. Have a role for bony and other musculoskeletal pains; may sometimes help neuropathic pains. Add a proton-pump inhibitor if used regularly
Tricyclic antidepressants (usually as single evening dose)	Used in treatment of neuropathic pain. Can also help insomnia. Can help mood as dose is increased
Anticonvulsants (e.g., gabapentin or pregabalin)	Valuable for neuropathic pain
Antispasmodics (e.g., hyoscine butylbromide)	Reduce visceral contractions in colicky visceral pain (intestinal, biliary, ureteric) and overt bowel obstruction—beware as can worsen subacute bowel obstruction
Muscle relaxants (e.g., diazepam)	Relieve muscle spasms (and anxiety)
Topical antibiotics (e.g., metronidazole tablets or gel)	Help treat infected superficial lesions, e.g., ulcerated skin, breast or head and neck tumours (use as per local guidelines)
Systemic antibiotics	Infections can precipitate or worsen pain, and will likely shorten life if untreated—this is not always appropriate and should be discussed with the patient and family
Corticosteroids (dexamethasone is usually preferred)	Shrink oedema associated with tumour to relieve pressure effects, for example, cerebral tumours, spinal cord and peripheral nerve compression, liver capsule stretching, tumour swelling causing obstruction of bowel, biliary or urinary tracts Balance use against side-effects, and aim to stop if ineffective (avoid abrupt withdrawal and use slow tapering)
Topical anti-inflammatory agents	For oral and nasal mucositis, ulcerated skin lesions, radiation proctitis
Local palliative radiotherapy	For painful bone metastases, compressive lesions of brain and spinal cord, large airway and superior vena caval obstruction, fungating or bleeding superficial lesions
Bisphosphonates	Predominantly used in this setting for the relief of bone pain Can be given parenterally as bolus or continuously as oral therapy
Paracetamol	Even in severe pain, this can have beneficial effects and reduce opiate requirements (and their attendant side-effects)
Chemotherapy	Can relieve pain by shrinkage of chemosensitive tumours
Nerve blocks (often under radiological/endoscopic guidance)	Very helpful in treating pain in specific areas, for example, intercostal blocks for chest wall pain, coeliac plexus blocks for pancreatic and other 'foregut' pain. Often reduces the overall requirement for systemic analgesia
Physiotherapy and associated physical modalities (e.g., massage, TENS, hot or cold packs)	Muscle spasm, inflammatory component of pain. Massage for muscle spasms and lymphoedema. TENS may help neuropathic pain
Skeletal immobilisation	Elective internal fixation of long bones for incipient or actual pathological fracture of long bones

TENS, Transcutaneous electrical nerve stimulation.

Strong opioids can be administered parenterally when patients cannot take oral medication owing to dysphagia, nausea, vomiting, poor absorption or fatigue. The intravenous route can be used in hospital, although the **subcutaneous route** is preferred. This route is suitable for single 'breakthrough' doses as well as for continuous infusion. Infusions are given via an indwelling 'butterfly' needle, usually controlled with a battery-operated syringe driver. In the United Kingdom, **diamorphine** is preferred to morphine since smaller volumes can provide equianalgesic doses.

Approaches for Establishing Opiate Treatment. The preferred method for establishing opiate requirements is by **titration**, and should be tailored to the individual, taking into account organ function and diurnal variation in pain. For those not requiring round the clock analgesia (the minority of patients with cancer-associated pain), the usual starting dose will be 2.5 to 10 mg of immediate-release morphine 4-hourly (or 2.5–5 mg for elderly patients), and depends on the severity of the pain—it is useful to give patients a range, and for them to up-titrate the dose if ineffective, or reduce the interval if analgesia does not last long. For those with renal or liver impairment or in the very elderly, 6- to 8-hourly intervals may be required. For those requiring round the clock relief, a twice daily preparation of controlled release morphine is preferred, often starting at 5 to 10 mg twice daily. In addition to the regular dose, a further dose of immediate-release morphine should be prescribed on an 'as required' basis to treat pain which 'breaks through' before the next dose is due—this is usually around one-sixth of the total daily dose of controlled-release morphine. If morphine relieves the pain, the total daily morphine requirements are added together to give the new recommended long-acting total dose.

Other opioids are often used in palliative care, and usually for specific indications. These are summarised in Table 13.6.

TABLE 13.6	Common Opioid Drugs Used in Palliative Care		
Analgesic	Equianalgesic Dose of Oral Morphine	Duration of Action	Indications
Codeine 60 mg	6 mg	4–6 h	Codeine or dihydrocodeine alone or in combination with paracetamol are used to treat mild to moderate pain. May cause nausea and is highly constipating
Tramadol 50 mg	5 mg	6 h	Limited use, but useful in certain settings. Its effect on monoamine reuptake means that it may be useful for neuropathic pain
Diamorphine injection 10 mg	20–30 mg	4 h	Where local regulations permit, it is preferred to morphine if parenteral route required as high solubility means smaller injection volume. Side-effects as morphine
Fentanyl transdermal patch Lowest dose now 12 mg/h	12 mg/h equivalent to 30–60 mg of oral morphine in 24 h	72 h	Patch works by releasing depot drug into the skin. Takes 12 h to reach analgesic levels so breakthrough treatment must be available when starting. *Contraindicated* in unstable pain. Often preferred to oral tablets by patients. Causes less constipation
Fentanyl lozenges Lowest dose 200 mg		1–4 h	Can start to have its effect after 5–10 min. May be useful for patients with incident pain who can take a lozenge before they want to move
Alfentanil	Start only under specialist guidance	Seek specialist guidance	Alfentanil is not renally excreted so is very useful in patients with renal impairment
Oxycodone 5 mg—lowest strength capsule	10 mg	4–6 h	May be better tolerated in some patients (e.g., elderly) as may cause fewer side-effects, particularly confusion or hallucinations. Can be useful in renal failure. Should be used only as second-line to morphine

Note: there is no role for meptazinol or pethidine in the long-term treatment of cancer pain as they have major limitations, for example, analgesic ceiling, short duration of action or accumulation of toxic metabolites, which render them unsuitable for regular long-term use.

14

Principles of Transplantation Surgery

CHAPTER OUTLINE

Introduction

Organ transplantation is the optimal treatment for end-stage organ failure and has the potential to both improve the quality of life and prolong life. It can now be considered for patients with kidney, liver, heart, lung and intestinal failure, as well as for patients with diabetes and bone marrow failure. While the availability and long-term outcomes of transplantation have significantly improved in recent years, this remains an area of intense research and clinical development.

The scene for clinical organ transplantation was set early in the 20th century by Alexis Carrel. He was awarded the Nobel Prize for Physiology and Medicine in 1912, for his pioneering work in vascular surgery and transplantation, with Charles Guthrie. Carrel, working with laboratory animals, found that **autografts** (organs removed and reimplanted into the same animal) could be expected to function indefinitely, whereas **allografts** (organs transplanted between animals of the same species) rarely functioned for more than a few days. Early attempts at transplantation in man used **xenografts** (transplantation between different species) to transfer renal tissue from pigs, goats, rabbits and apes; these were uniformly unsuccessful.

The first clinically useful transplant for humans involved pig heart valves. These consisted of simple avascular tissue, treated to render it nonimmunogenic to avoid rejection. Porcine cardiac valve transplants have been used regularly since the mid-1970s and have advantages over artificial valves in younger people and where anticoagulation must be avoided. The first successful 'solid organ' transplant was a kidney transplanted from a living donor to his genetically identical twin, by Joseph E Murray in 1954. The key to organ transplantation between nonidentical twins lay in the developing field of immunology, first with detection of the mechanisms involved in **graft rejection** and then the elaboration and application of techniques to minimise or prevent it.

Pharmacological immunosuppression designed to attenuate graft rejection has continued to advance, leading to improving success rates with transplantation of an expanding range of organs and tissues (Table 14.1). Human cornea, kidney, liver, pancreas, heart, heart and lung, single or double lung and bone marrow transplantation are all now standard, although not free of rejection or other complications (see http://www.ctstransplant.org/). Promising results are also achieved with small bowel transplantation, in isolation or together with other intraabdominal organs, such as stomach, duodenum, pancreas and liver in **multivisceral transplants**. Even limb, face and uterus transplants are now achieving success.

Transplant Immunology

Major Histocompatibility Complex

When transplanted from one individual to another, nucleated cells have a number of different surface **glycoproteins** known as **histocompatibility antigens** that are recognised by the recipient's immune system as foreign and elicit a response. The immune response involves cell- and antibody-mediated mechanisms, which cause destruction of the transplanted cells.

Each individual has several histocompatibility antigens, but one group is predominantly responsible for graft rejection. These **major histocompatibility antigens** are coded for by a set of genes known as the **major histocompatibility complex (MHC)**. In humans, the MHC gene is located on a segment of the short arm of chromosome 6. It was first discovered in leucocytes and, although now shown to be present in all cells, it is still known as the **human leucocyte antigen (HLA) complex**. Two major groups of HLA antigens, known as HLA class I and class II, have been described, each with different structures and specificities.

TABLE 14.1 **Summary of the Main Immunosuppressive Agents Used in Transplantation**

Class of Drug	Examples	Mechanism of Action	USES			Adverse Effects and Comments
			Induction	Maintenance	Rejection	
Biological Agents						
Non-depleting antibodies	Basiliximab	Inhibition of IL2-induced T cell activation (mAb)	√			Hypersensitivity and adverse effects are rare
Depleting antibodies	Alemtuzumab (Campath-1H)	Prolonged depletion of B and T lymphocytes (mAb)	√			Cause moderate cytokine release syndrome
	ATG (antithymocyte globulin)	Prolonged depletion of T lymphocytes (polyclonal Ab)	√		√	Cytokine release syndrome common
	Rituximab	Depletion of B lymphocytes (mAb)	√		√	Not formally licensed for use in transplantation
Nonbiological Drugs						
Calcineurin inhibitors (CNIs)	Ciclosporin	Inhibition of calcineurin phosphatase and T cell activation		√		Nephrotoxicity is a significant adverse effect
	Tacrolimus			√		
mTOR[a] inhibitors	Sirolimus (rapamycin)	Inhibits IL2-induced T cell proliferation		√		Cause impaired wound healing, pneumonitis
Antimetabolites	Mycophenolate mofetil (MMF)	Suppression of B and T cell proliferation		√		Myelotoxicity (pancytopenia) and GI disturbance common
	Azathioprine	Inhibition of DNA synthesis in lymphocytes		√		In general, well tolerated
Corticosteroids	Prednisolone (PO)	Suppression of cytokine production, T cell activation and migration		√		Cause the full spectrum of Cushing syndrome adverse effects
	Methylprednisolone (IV)		√		√	

[a]*DNA*, Deoxyribonucleic acid; *GI*, gastrointestinal; *IL2*, interleukin-2; *IV*, intravenous; *mAb*, monoclonal antibody; *mTOR*, mammalian target of rapamycin; *PO*, orally.

The principal class I loci are the **A, B** and **C antigens** and the principal class II loci are the **DP, DR and DQ antigens**.

Tissue Typing and Organ Allocation Schemes

ABO blood group compatibility is an obvious prerequisite for organ transplantation. Allocation of organs to recipients further involves determining the donor and recipient HLA haplotypes ('HLA typing'). This is done by detecting genetic variation in the expressed HLA molecules using antisera (serological typing), or now almost universally, at deoxyribonucleic acid (DNA) sequence level (DNA typing). The antigens at HLA A, B and DR loci are particularly important determinants of the immune response to transplanted organs. Since each individual receives one set of genetic information from each parent, there are six principal loci, and any two individuals can differ at any or all of these loci.

In kidney transplantation, close HLA matching gives significantly better graft survival. HLA typing of individuals is therefore used to match the donor and recipient as closely as possible in kidney (and pancreas) transplantation. HLA matching is not currently regularly performed for other organs, such as heart or liver transplants, as the number of available organs is too small to allow optimal matching. However, even a fully HLA matched transplant evokes a profound immunological response from the recipient

because of differences in other major (non-A, non-B and non-DR) and minor histocompatibility antigens. Immunosuppression is therefore a prerequisite for successful organ transplantation.

Most developed countries have a national transplant sharing mechanism so that donors and recipients can be matched as closely and fairly as possible. Systems are designed to achieve an optimal balance between **utility** (the optimum use of an organ in terms of graft survival) and **equity** of access (the chance that an individual patient will receive a graft within a reasonable period). This typically combines the important matter of tissue matching with other factors, such as age and time spent on the waiting list.

Immunosuppression

Immunosuppressive therapy needs to be continued indefinitely after transplantation, although the dosage can usually be progressively reduced to maintenance levels after high-dose **induction therapy**. This is because a partly tolerant state is established by diminution of the **alloimmune** response with time. Episodes of **rejection** are often treated with strong or high-dose immunosuppression.

Immunosuppressant drugs are broadly classified into biological (monoclonal or polyclonal antibodies) and nonbiological agents; the characteristics of the main examples are summarized in Table 14.1. Immunosuppressive drugs are almost always used in combination to allow lower doses of individual agents to minimise side-effects. These adverse effects include infections, impaired wound healing, predisposition to certain malignancies (e.g., skin and lymphoproliferative disorders) and bone marrow suppression. A widely used combination is induction with **basiliximab**, followed by maintenance on **prednisolone**, **tacrolimus** and **mycofenolate mofetil**.

Graft Rejection

Graft rejection continues to be a problem despite improved efficacy of immunosuppressive agents. It can present in several ways:

Hyperacute Rejection

Hyperacute rejection is caused by the presence of high levels of preformed antibodies (e.g., against ABO antigen) in the recipient. It occurs within minutes of reperfusion and is now exceedingly rare owing to improvements in tissue-matching techniques.

The presence of lower levels of preformed antibodies against a donor's HLA is not uncommon and may be caused by previous blood transfusions, pregnancies or transplants. While this increases the risk of rejection, it is not necessarily prohibitive and can be safe when using strong immunosuppression. In fact, it is now even possible to perform, in some cases, successful 'ABO- or HLA-incompatible' kidney transplants. This is made possible by preemptive removal of the preformed circulating antibodies in the recipient, in conjunction with pretransplant treatment with immunosuppressive drugs, in carefully-designed **desensitisation** protocols.

Acute Rejection

Acute rejection occurs in up to 30% of transplants, most commonly during the first 3 months posttransplant. It is predominantly T-cell-mediated but can be antibody-mediated in about 10%. It can usually be reversed by a temporary increase in immunosuppression, most often in the form of a short course of high-dose corticosteroids.

Chronic Rejection

Chronic rejection occurs months to years after transplantation and is probably the result of antibody-mediated rejection. It is often associated with gradual occlusion of arteries in the graft and can occur even with effective long-term immunosuppression. A gradual and chronic deterioration in graft function is a feature of many organ transplants and has a multifactorial aetiology, including chronic immune rejection, toxicity from immunosuppressive drugs and recurrence of the original disease.

Organ Donation and Preservation

Sources of Organs for Transplantation

Organs for transplantation may be procured from living or deceased donors. Approximately 60% of donors in the United Kingdom are deceased donors with around 22 donors per million population per year. However, this still lags significantly behind the rate of 28 to 43 per million achieved in comparable countries, such as United States of America, France and Spain.

Deceased donation in the United Kingdom can proceed after 'brain death' (donation after brainstem death—DBD) or after 'circulatory death' (donation after circulatory death—DCD).

> **• BOX 14.1** **Legal Criteria for Diagnosis of Brain Death (United Kingdom)**
>
> *Note:* this diagnosis is clinical and does not require special tests.
> 1. There must be a positive diagnosis of severe structural brain damage.
> 2. The condition causing brain damage must be irreversible.
> 3. There must be complete loss of brainstem function—evidenced by fixed pupils, no spontaneous eye movements or response to caloric testing, absent corneal, eyelash and blink reflexes, absent laryngeal and cough reflexes, and no response to deep painful stimuli. (*Note:* some spinal reflexes may be retained despite brain death.)
> 4. On removal of ventilatory support, there must be no spontaneous respiratory activity in the presence of a physiologically adequate increase in partial pressure of carbon dioxide (PCO_2).
> 5. Any possible effects of hypothermia and drugs (e.g., muscle relaxants, respiratory depressants, alcohol) must be excluded.

Approximately 60% of deceased donors are DCD and 40% are DBD. The number of organ transplants from DBD and DCD donors has increased steadily in the United Kingdom over recent years, while the number of living donors had remained reasonably constant. Consent for deceased organ donation can be given by the donor during his/her lifetime by registration with the Organ Donor Register, or by the donor's next of kin immediately before death (in the case of a DCD donor) or after the diagnosis of brainstem death (DBD donor).

'Brainstem Death'

In most Western countries, the legal definition of death is dependent upon the diagnosis of brainstem death following irreversible brainstem injury (e.g., from head injury or intracranial vascular catastrophe). Death can therefore be legally confirmed even in the presence of an intact circulatory system. Once the established criteria have been satisfied and appropriate consent obtained from relatives, the legally deceased patient becomes eligible for DBD donation and the organ retrieval operation can proceed with the donor ventilated and the organs perfused with oxygenated blood. If brainstem death has not occurred or cannot be confirmed, ventilatory and circulatory support is withdrawn if the patient has a hopeless prognosis and further treatment is deemed futile. Life supporting treatment is then withdrawn in an intensive care setting and organ retrieval can only proceed after circulatory arrest and death are confirmed by irreversible cessation of neurological (pupillary), cardiac and respiratory activity (DCD donation).

The legal criteria for brain death in the United Kingdom are summarised in Box 14.1; similar criteria are used in other countries. In the United Kingdom, the diagnosis of brain death is made on purely clinical criteria; electrocardiography, cerebral blood flow and other neurophysiological tests are not required. Appropriate clinical examination must be performed by two senior doctors independent of the transplant team and must be repeated at least twice.

Living Donation

UK law permits kidney transplants from living genetically or emotionally related, as well as from altruistic donors. This can only proceed after comprehensive medical and psychological assessment of the donor. Living donor nephrectomy is performed laparoscopically. The advantages of living donor transplantation include elective rather than emergency procedures, better long-term graft outcomes, lower delayed graft function rates, and potentially, preemptive (predialysis) transplantation. Living kidney donation has a mortality risk of ~1:2500, and a major and minor complication rate of approximately 2% and 20%, respectively, in the donor.

Living liver donation is also becoming more common. It was introduced to allow donation of a small portion of the left liver from parent to child, but has now expanded to include right liver donation, and allows adult to adult transplantation. The donor risks are greater than in kidney donation. In countries where the availability of deceased donor organs is limited for cultural reasons, such as Japan, these procedures are the mainstay of organ transplantation. The growing shortage of organs for transplantation has led to this being adopted even in countries where cadaveric liver transplantation is well established.

Organ Preservation and Transport

Donors are often in hospitals many miles from where the recipient operation is to be performed. There may be delay in locating the recipient, and in getting the recipient into hospital and ready for operation. As a result, the organ to be transplanted is usually removed from the donor several hours before transplantation, driving the search for reliable techniques of organ preservation. **Hypothermia** (at 0°C–4°C) is the main method of organ preservation by reducing the metabolic demands of the organ. Organs are first flushed with and then stored in preservation solutions which usually have the following components:

- an osmotic agent to provide extracellular oncotic force to prevent cellular oedema;
- a buffer to counter intracellular acidosis;
- electrolytes to maintain cellular ionic composition.

After retrieval, the bag containing the organ and preservation fluid is usually packed in ice (**static cold storage**), while awaiting transplantation. Alternatively, kidneys may be connected to a machine to continuously circulate cold preservation solution (**hypothermic machine perfusion**). Machine perfusion is more expensive and cumbersome than static cold storage; however, its potential advantages include a more physiological environment and the ability to identify and discard nonfunctioning kidneys with poor perfusion characteristics. Hypothermic machine perfusion is also being investigated for liver preservation.

The period of **warm ischaemia** is the time from circulatory arrest to effective cooling of the organ. Warm ischaemia must be minimised to prevent irreversible damage to the organ (less than 40–60 min in kidney transplantation). This warm ischaemia endured by DCD organs is thought to account for some of the inferior outcomes after DCD compared to DBD transplantation. The period of **cold ischaemia** is from perfusion with cold preservation solution to transplantation. Cold ischaemia time should also be minimised to best preserve graft function and ideally should be less than 24, 12 and 6 hours for kidney, liver and heart transplantation, respectively.

There is intense interest in developing superior methods for organ preservation. A promising approach is perfusion of organs with oxygenated blood at 37°C as a method to assess organ quality or to restore energy reserves and recondition organs, for example through delivery of therapeutic agents. Early evidence suggests that **normothermic machine perfusion** of organs may offer advantages in liver, heart, lung and kidney transplantation.

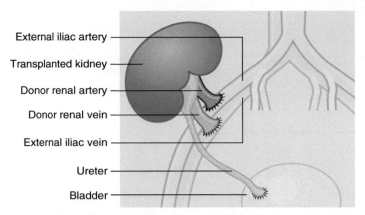

• **Fig. 14.1 Renal Transplantation.** The usual site for the transplanted kidney is in the pelvis, with anastomoses being formed between the donor renal artery and vein, and the recipient iliac artery and vein, and between donor ureter and recipient bladder.

Specific Organ Transplants

Kidney Transplants

Kidney transplantation is the longest established and most widely practised of solid organ transplants. It offers a substantial improvement in quality of life for patients with end-stage renal failure who are otherwise faced with thrice-weekly haemodialysis or a regimen of daily treatment with chronic ambulatory peritoneal dialysis. Donor organs can be obtained from any generally healthy donor up to or even beyond 80 years of age.

The kidney is transplanted into an extraperitoneal location in the iliac fossa (i.e., **heterotopic** as the graft is placed into a different anatomical position), and the renal vessels anastomosed to the iliac artery and vein (Fig. 14.1). The ureter is implanted into the bladder either directly or using an intramural tunnel to prevent reflux. A temporary ureteric stent is placed to protect the ureteric anastomosis, and removed 4 to 6 weeks later at cystoscopy under local anaesthesia. Nonfunctioning kidneys are usually left in situ unless infected or causing unmanageable hypertension.

Overall results have steadily improved owing to better tissue matching, more effective and safer immunosuppression, superior organ procurement and preservation, as well as improved surgical technique and perioperative care of recipients. The survival rate of transplanted kidneys can be as high as 90% to 95% at 1 year and falls to about 70% at 10 years.

Liver Transplants

Current indications for liver transplantation in adults are end-stage nonmalignant parenchymal liver disease (e.g., cirrhosis caused by viral hepatitis or alcohol), acute hepatic failure, certain inborn errors of hepatic metabolism and hepatocellular carcinoma (within specific criteria). In children, liver-based inborn errors of metabolism and biliary atresia are the most common indications; the operation often needs to be performed during early infancy.

Liver transplantation is a technically challenging operation, not least because most patients have advanced liver disease with disordered coagulation and often severe portal hypertension. A team approach has evolved, with close cooperation between surgeons and specialist anaesthetists. The diseased liver is removed and the new liver in placed into the same anatomical position (i.e., **orthotopic**),

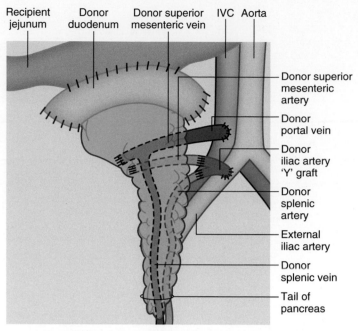

• **Fig. 14.2** Pancreas Transplantation. *IVC,* Inferior vena cava.

with vena cava, portal vein and hepatic artery being reanastomosed in turn. Biliary reconstruction can be performed using a direct duct-to-duct anastomosis or a Roux-en-Y loop. Results have improved greatly since the first successful liver transplant in 1967, and 1-, 5- and 10-year patient survival rates are respectively around 80%, 70% and 60%. Biliary complications (e.g., strictures) and disease recurrence, particularly when transplantation is for hepatitis C, are important remaining challenges, although the advent of novel therapies for hepatitis C are likely to have a significant beneficial impact in the future. For paediatric cases, the problem of an insufficient supply of donor organs has been largely addressed with reduced-size liver grafts. An adult liver can be divided into two to allow a child and an adult to receive grafts from a single organ.

Pancreas Transplants

Pancreas transplantation is a potentially curative treatment for diabetes, thus avoiding its many late complications including myocardial ischaemia, peripheral vascular disease, peripheral neuropathy, nephropathy leading to renal failure and retinopathy leading to blindness. Pancreas transplantation presents particular challenges since the gland combines endocrine and exocrine function, the latter of which can lead to serious posttransplant complications including graft pancreatitis (Fig. 14.2). The technique involves transplanting the whole pancreas with a small segment of duodenum. The arterial supply to the pancreas is reconstructed using a donor iliac artery 'Y graft' which is joined to the donor superior mesenteric artery (to supply the head of pancreas) and donor splenic artery (to supply the body and tail of pancreas). Venous drainage of the pancreas is through the portal vein. The graft is sited in the pelvis and the vessels are anastomosed to the recipient iliac vessels. Alternatively, the portal vein can be anastomosed to the inferior vena cava. In an early technique, the attached duodenal segment was anastomosed to the bladder, allowing exocrine secretions to drain into the urine. This has been largely replaced by anastomosing the pancreas directly to small bowel or

via a Roux-en-Y loop to allow enteric drainage of enzymes. Five-year graft survival rates of 70% to 80% are now being obtained and there is evidence that the procedure can arrest and sometimes partly reverse the long-term complications of diabetes. Most pancreas transplants currently performed are in diabetic patients with renal failure and advanced complications of their disease. In these, the pancreas transplant is combined with a renal transplant (simultaneous pancreas and kidney transplant—SPK).

A different approach is transplanting pancreatic endocrine tissue alone using **human islet cells** extracted from pancreases by collagenase digestion. The islets are injected into the portal venous system and lodge in liver sinusoids. The extraction yield has improved markedly, allowing a substantial proportion of islets to be recovered from each pancreas. Whilst the success rate is improving, it typically requires islet cells from more than one donor to achieve euglycaemia, so the procedure is less efficacious than whole pancreas transplantation while organ donors remain scarce.

Heart and Lung Transplants

Cardiac transplantation has become a standard treatment for patients with ischaemic heart disease not amenable to coronary artery bypass grafting, and for patients with certain cardiomyopathies. A standard operative technique uses orthotopic placement; the donor atria and vessels are sutured directly to those of the recipient. Monitoring for early rejection requires regular right-heart catheterisation and endomyocardial biopsy.

Using immunosuppressive protocols similar to kidney transplantation, results of cardiac transplantation are now excellent, with 1- and 5-year patient survival of 80% and 75%, respectively. In recent years, hearts from DCD donors have successfully been transplanted after 'reanimation' using normothermic machine perfusion, with excellent outcomes. Nonetheless, the shortage of donor organs means cardiac transplantation, in the foreseeable future, is unlikely to be an option for all those who could benefit.

Common indications for lung transplantation include cystic fibrosis, pulmonary hypertension, idiopathic pulmonary fibrosis and chronic obstructive pulmonary disease. One- and 5-year lung transplant survival rates are 80% and 55%, respectively. Transplantation can be performed as a single or double lung transplant, or in a combined heart-lung transplant where there is secondary heart disease. In other cases where the recipient's heart is healthy, it can be transplanted into another patient. This is known as the **domino heart** procedure.

Small Bowel Transplants

Small bowel transplantation is a relatively recent advance. There are a growing number of patients who have lost all or most of their small bowel from vascular problems, volvulus, necrotising enterocolitis, desmoid tumours or Crohn disease, and who are maintained on long-term parenteral nutrition. Specialist units can sustain them in good health for years but treatment is expensive, inconvenient for patients, and leaves them at constant risk of infective and thrombotic complications from feeding lines, as well as liver disease from parenteral feeding. Small bowel may be transplanted alone or combined with stomach and pancreas, as well as the liver in coexisting irreversible liver disease. Outcomes have improved significantly so that in selected cases, small bowel transplantation rivals long-term total parenteral nutrition in survival and has clear advantages in quality of life.

Principles of Trauma Surgery

15

Major Trauma

Injury Epidemiology

Injury is one of the major causes of death and disability in the world. The World Health Organization defines injury as physical damage that results when a human body is subjected to levels of energy that exceed tissue and physiological tolerances. Injury encompasses a wide range of causative energy sources, mechanisms and circumstances (Fig. 15.1). Many factors also influence a patient's exposure to, and tolerance of, energy transfer. These include physical, genetic, physiological, environmental, behavioural, cultural and social variables. In terms of consequences, there is also a spectrum of severity that ranges from simple self-limiting minor injury, through life *changing* severe injury to complex, life *threatening* major trauma (Fig. 15.2). Conceptualising and quantifying the epidemiology of injury can therefore be challenging. One useful approach is to consider injury like any other disease process with the pathophysiology being the result of interaction of a host (patient), an injurious agent (energy) and the sociocultural and physical environment. Applying the 'host/agent/environment' model and seeing injury as a disease caused by energy allows a public health approach to

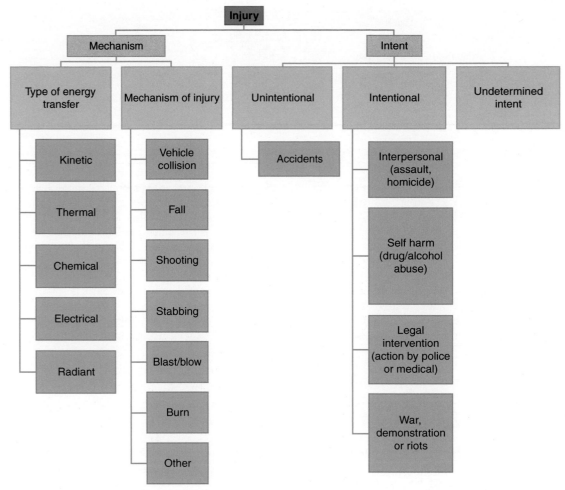

• **Fig. 15.1** A Schematic Illustration of the Classification of Injury in Terms of Range of Energy Sources, Injury Mechanisms and Circumstances.

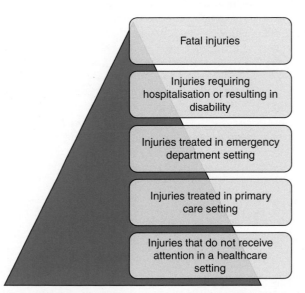

• **Fig. 15.2** The Injury Pyramid or Iceberg—illustrating the spectrum of severity of injury.

be taken to injury prevention and control. The Haddon Matrix (Box 15.1) relates the 'host/agent/environment' model to events before, during and after the injury. It illustrates how factors associated with the patient or victim, the energy transfer and the sociocultural or physical environment can be identified for any specific injury problem in the preevent, event and postevent phases.

Understanding these factors allows them to be targeted for primary (preevent) or secondary (event) prevention in much the same way as for any other disease process. In the United Kingdom, the commonest causes of severe injuries are road traffic related injuries (typically involving younger patients) and falls (typically involving older patients). The Haddon Matrix (Box 15.1) illustrates how the approach to prevention in these groups could be very different.

Injury severity is typically defined using anatomical scoring systems. The most widely used system is the Injury Severity Score (ISS). Application of the ISS methodology results in a score between 1 and 75—with the higher scores being associated with increased mortality and morbidity. By convention, severe injury is defined as an ISS score between 9 and 15, and major trauma as an ISS score of greater than 15. Using the ISS, the incidence of severe injury and major trauma in the United Kingdom is between 15 and 30 patients per 100,000 population per year. ISS is anatomically based and calculated retrospectively (when all injuries are known). The time-sensitive nature of injury and the limited knowledge about the extent of injury at first assessment means that the emergency services and trauma receiving hospitals must be able to quickly assess, triage, transport and treat a much larger number of patients (as illustrated in the injury pyramid) to ensure effective care for the most seriously injured.

Trauma Systems

A trauma system integrates injury prevention, prehospital care, emergency department (ED) care, acute hospital care, reconstruction, rehabilitation and reablement in a structured and organised

• BOX 15.1   **The Haddon Matrix Applied to Falls in Older Patients**

Phase/Factor	Host (Injured Person) Factors	Injurious Agent (Energy) Factors	Environment Factors (Physical or Socioeconomic)
Preevent phase	Bone density, flexibility, balance and strength, comorbidity	Height of fall, contact with other surfaces/objects	Optimised medication, availability of care and supervision
Event phase	Protective measures, such as hip protectors	Energy absorbing flooring and surfaces	Room lighting, trip/slip hazards, handrails and supervision
Postevent phase	Severity of anatomical injury, physiological consequences and comorbidity	Alarm systems and supervision (to reduce long lie).	Access to emergency care. Policy on falls prevention and care

way. The fundamental premise underpinning a trauma system is that patients with the most severe and complex injuries should be managed in designated Major Trauma Centres (MTCs) with access to the full range of specialist services and a significant caseload. There are two broad conceptual models for trauma system design. These 'inclusive' or 'exclusive' models differ, in the simplest terms, with respect to the extent to which all components of the emergency medical system (and wider healthcare system) are involved. In 'exclusive' systems, the focus is predominantly, or exclusively, on the MTC. The underpinning philosophy is that all patients with suspected major trauma within the area covered by the MTC are primarily transported there from the scene, bypassing all other facilities. Exclusive systems are ideally suited for urban areas with short prehospital journeys. In contrast, an 'inclusive' system is better suited to more dispersed populations where prehospital journeys may be much longer and primary transfer to the MTC is not necessarily a safe or publicly acceptable option. Arrangements must therefore be put in place to designate a range of smaller trauma receiving hospitals, often referred to as Trauma Units, who can undertake initial assessment, resuscitation and stabilisation before secondary transfer to an MTC where necessary. Regardless of system design, injured patients require rapid assessment and, in many cases, rapid interventions, to save life and reduce disability. In some case, prehospital interventions or care in a local hospital ED are essential before a patient can be moved to an MTC. In others, a patient's only chance of survival might be rapid transport to the MTC, bypassing other hospitals. There is no single solution—each trauma system must be designed and tailored to the injury epidemiology of the population and managed to maintain effective care from point of injury through to rehabilitation.

Prehospital Trauma Care

A key component of any trauma system is early access to the emergency services. In most developed countries, a single national telephone activation number (112 or 999) connects callers to an Ambulance Service call handler who uses sophisticated telephone triage systems to identify the main problem, mobilise the right resources and provide prearrival care advice. Ambulance Services can deploy a range of healthcare professionals from paramedic practitioners through to physician-paramedic critical care teams and may use a range of land and air transport platforms to deploy personnel and move patients. The clinical priority for prehospital personnel is to search for immediate threats to life, initiate resuscitation as necessary and transport patients safely to hospital. In some cases, prehospital care can be very basic and rapid (e.g., a stable and alert stabbing victim in an urban area). In others, prehospital care may be particularly complex and take considerable time (e.g., the provision of prehospital anaesthesia to an unstable and trapped driver in a rural area). Time is important but the historical characterisation

of prehospital personnel as undertaking either a 'scoop and run' or 'stay and play' approach to trauma care no longer applies. The key prehospital time is 'time to meaningful intervention related to the effect of the injury' rather than time to the nearest hospital. The challenge is to understand the nature of the meaningful intervention, provide the minimum necessary care to deliver that and then undertake safe transfer to the appropriate destination. In recognition of the challenges of prehospital care, the public are being encouraged to provide citizen aid, paramedics are becoming increasingly sophisticated healthcare practitioners and Prehospital Emergency Medicine has become a recognised medical subspecialty.

Prehospital Assessment

An overarching consideration for prehospital personnel is safety. Trauma patients are often in an uncontrolled, high-risk environment. Industrial accidents, falls from height, road traffic collisions, scenes of public disorder, fires, railway incidents and building collapses all have very specific hazards that place both the patient and the emergency services personnel at risk. Whatever the mechanism, it is essential for risks to be managed as far as possible. The priority in terms of patient care is to undertake an initial clinical assessment, often referred to as a *primary assessment* or *primary survey*, to identify and control any immediate threats to life. In contrast to the conventional medical model, where a detailed history leads to a focused clinical examination, trauma care cannot rely on a detailed history (or sometimes any history) and the rapid focused clinical examination takes priority. As with the initial approach to all critically ill or collapsed patients, this examination follows a standard structured sequence. The most widely used is the CABCDE sequence (Box 15.2). Prehospital personnel will undertake this primary assessment in a linear or stepwise approach—addressing specific life threats as they are identified. As more personnel become available, concurrent activity can take place both in terms of clinical care and in planning rescue (for those who require extrication) and the transport and destination hospital options.

Prehospital Resuscitation

Resuscitative interventions should ideally be performed concurrently with the primary assessment—as CABCDE threats to life are identified, the relevant technical and therapeutic interventions can be undertaken. This is no different from the hospital setting although it is often extremely challenging, given constraints around physical access to the patient, environmental circumstances and availability of resources. Nonetheless, emergency services are able to undertake a wide range of prehospital medical interventions and doctors qualified as subspecialists in Prehospital Emergency Medicine can often be deployed to the incident scene with additional knowledge, skills and equipment.

• BOX 15.2   **The CACBCDE Sequence for Undertaking the Primary Assessment (see also Fig. 15.5 Primary Survey and Initial Resuscitation, later)**

C   Immediate search for and control of **catastrophic external bleeding** with combinations, as necessary, of direct pressure, indirect pressure, wound packing, use of haemostatic dressings (i.e., dressings with procoagulant and/or mucoadhesive properties) and application of a tourniquet

A   Supporting the **airway** as necessary with manual positioning or manoeuvres, suction, basic airway adjuncts (nasopharyngeal and oropharyngeal airways), supraglottic airway devices and possibly direct laryngoscopy and tracheal intubation (with or without drugs) or surgical cricothyroidotomy

C   Controlling and restricting movement of the **cervical spine** until a deliberate decision regarding the risks and benefits of spinal immobilisation can be made

B   Assessment of the effectiveness of **breathing,** excluding or treating life-threatening thoracic injuries, such as tension pneumothorax, open pneumothorax, flail chest, and providing supplemental oxygen and/or noninvasive or invasive ventilatory support

C   Assessment of the **circulation** to identify physiological markers of shock, gaining access to the circulation and looking for signs of life-threatening injuries in the chest, abdomen, pelvis and limbs that could contribute to shock, controlling those that can be controlled (e.g., splinting the long bones and pelvis)

D   Assessment of neurological **disability** (Glasgow Coma Scale Score, pupil responses, limb weakness and lateralising neurological signs) to identify brain or spinal injuries and assist with decision making regarding the continued need for spinal immobilisation

E   Establishing a controlled safe **environment**, protecting the patient from extremes of heat or cold, exposing the patient to ensuring there are no missed or external injuries and establishing a brief history

Traumatic cardiac arrest is one circumstance where prehospital resuscitation may need to be very extensive. Regardless of mechanism, the reversible causes are hypoxia, hypovolaemia, tension pneumothorax and cardiac tamponade. Every effort is made to simultaneously control external bleeding, ventilate and oxygenate the patient, decompress the chest, splint the pelvis and any long bone fractures, and give appropriate fluids or blood if available. If the mechanism is penetrating trauma, then prehospital resuscitative thoracotomy may be necessary. If the mechanism is major pelvic and/or lower limb injury, then surgical control of the aorta, via thoracotomy or endovascular approaches, may be required. There is considerable complexity and risk associated with this level of resuscitation at the roadside and in-transit to hospital but it can be life saving. Most patients do not require such complex care but prehospital services must be prepared for the worst.

Prehospital Damage Control

The concept of damage control is often applied to surgical interventions in hospital rather than in prehospital resuscitation. The idea is simple—do not undertake interventions that may exacerbate the effects of the injury either physically or physiologically. In surgical terms, this means limiting surgical intervention to that which is absolutely necessary and then focusing on optimising physiology. However, there are a number of nonsurgical damage control strategies that can be applied in the prehospital phase and that can reduce the risk of secondary injury from hypoxia, hypovolaemia, metabolic derangement and patient handling. Damage control resuscitation in hospital is discussed in more detail later—prehospital damage control strategies follow the same principles. Once primary assessment and resuscitation is underway, deliberate decisions should be made about which, if any, damage control strategy could be applied. The most common strategies include: permissive hypotension (see later), haemostatic resuscitation, wound-protection, neuroprotection and lung-protection (Fig. 15.3).

Transport to Hospital

Injured patients need to be transferred rapidly to an appropriate hospital. A key principle for safe transport is that the patient's in-transit care should not be compromised. Once primary assessment, resuscitation and any damage control strategies have been completed to the point at which transfer is deemed safe, then it is important that good work at the scene is not undone by rough or careless handling, loss of inadequately secured tubes and lines or the physiological consequences of the transfer itself. A neuroprotective strategy might, for example, be compromised by allowing the patient to be conveyed in a head down posture (as often happens in helicopters) or subjecting them to rapid acceleration and deceleration forces during emergency driving. The destination hospital should be determined by preagreed trauma system and field triage criteria and the receiving hospital should be prealerted both the moment the emergency services identify that there is a seriously injured patient, who is likely to be transferred to them and when leaving the scene. The aim should be seamless transition from the scene to the receiving ED regardless of transport platform (helicopter or land ambulance).

Initial Assessment in Hospital

A key element of effective trauma care is preparation. Every ED should have an appropriate physical environment (Fig. 15.4), a well-rehearsed process and prepared staff and equipment to manage an undifferentiated trauma patient arriving with short notice. If there is more than one patient, then predefined major incident plans should be available. Whether there are one or more patients, an early and comprehensive prealert to the receiving ED is essential. A common prealert system for a single patient is the ATMISTER system:

- **A**ge
- **T**ime
- **M**echanism
- **I**njuries
- **S**igns
- **T**reatment
- **E**xpected time of arrival (ETA)
- **R**equests (such as activation of massive blood loss protocols)

A common prealert system for a multiple casualty incident is the METHANE system:

- **M**ajor incident declared
- **E**xact location
- **T**ype of incident
- **H**azards present or suspected
- **A**ccess—routes that are safe to use
- **N**umber, type, severity of casualties
- **E**mergency services present and those required

Success in managing patients with life-threatening multiple injuries depends on good preparation and organisation—as a system,

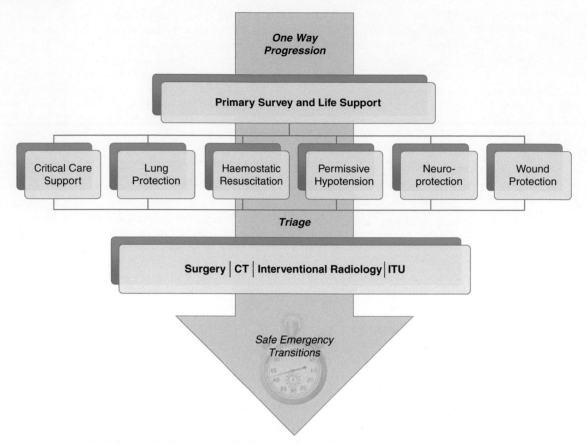

- **Fig. 15.3** A Conceptual Framework for Damage Control Resuscitation. *CT,* Computed tomography; *ITU,* intensive treatment unit.

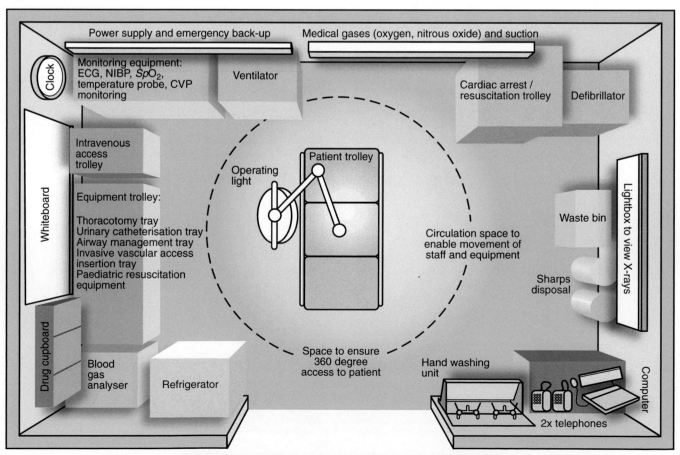

- **Fig. 15.4** 'Bird's Eye View' Drawing of an Ideal Resuscitation Room.

BOX 15.3 The Trauma Team

- Team leader (senior doctor experienced in trauma care)
- Airway manager (typically an anaesthetist)
- Airway assistant (typically a trained Operating Department Practitioner or Nurse)
- A primary assessment doctor (typically a surgeon or emergency physician)
- A procedures doctor (typically a surgeon or emergency physician)
- Two experienced ED nurses to support the team
- A scribe to record contemporaneous notes related to team members, timings, history, clinical findings and any initial care decisions
- Support staff (porters, healthcare assistants, radiographers, phlebotomists)

More comprehensive teams, especially in MTCs, include:
- An emergency general surgeon
- An orthopaedic surgeon
- Specialist surgeons, such as vascular, cardiothoracic, plastics, maxillofacial, neurosurgical and plastics according to the prealert information and injuries
- A radiologist (particularly when ultrasound may be required to help triage patients or where interventional radiology is being considered)
- A transfusion practitioner (particularly when massive blood loss protocols have been activated)
- Specialist obstetric or paediatric staff as necessary

ED, Emergency department; *MTC,* major trauma centre.

TABLE 15.1 Triage Priority Groups

Category	Definition	Colour	Treatment
P1	Life-threatening	Red	Immediate
P2	Urgent	Yellow	Urgent
P3	Minor	Green	Delayed
P4	Dead	White/Black	

department and hospital. Each ED should have protocol for managing prealert calls and mobilising the appropriate resources—both to attend the ED to receive patients and to prepare for transition of patients from the ED to imaging, operating theatres, critical care units and wards. Initial management often involves a trauma team response within the ED and concurrent activity between several disciplines throughout the initial phases of care (Box 15.3). Training for the initial management of trauma patients has been standardised through **Advanced Trauma Life Support** (ATLS) and similar courses, now widely available throughout the world. The ATLS principles are simple—a systematic approach should be followed, using a common language and terminology, and the greatest threats to life must be treated first. Following these principles, the severity of physiological derangement is often used as the basis for triage systems that are applied when there is more than one patient to assess. Most systems differentiate ambulatory from nonambulant patients and then follow the principles of the primary assessment to identify patients with the greatest threat to life. Triage categories and their associated meaning are illustrated in Table 15.1.

Special provisions are often made for obstetric and paediatric cases. Obstetric cases include all the elements of the trauma teams described in Box 15.3 with the addition of obstetric and neonatal expertise. Paediatric cases require additional medical paediatric, paediatric surgery, and paediatric anaesthetic or intensive care involvement.

Initial Assessment

As with the prehospital phase of care, the priority is to undertake an immediate CABCDE assessment to identify and control any immediate threats to life (see Box 15.2). The overarching priorities for the trauma team are:
- Rapid primary assessment combined with damage control resuscitation

- Prioritisation and initial treatment of identified injuries
- Safe emergency transfers to computed tomography (CT), critical care and/or the operating theatre
- Detailed history and secondary, head-to-toe, assessment
- Consideration of the need for early transfer to an MTC or specialist unit

A team leader, often a surgeon or emergency physician, is required to coordinate the efforts of the trauma team and maintain tempo and control—particularly if there are parallel and competing priorities for care. Trauma team leaders require additional training to help them both apply the principles of effective team leadership and maintain their knowledge and skill related to the trauma care. The trauma team initial assessment (or reassessment) is often taught in a sequential manner and may be performed in a sequential manner when resources are limited. If there has been adequate preparation and prealert, they can often be undertaken in parallel by a team coordinated by the trauma team leader. Fig. 15.5 provides an outline of the components of the primary assessment in hospital.

On completion of the primary assessment, resuscitative interventions and initiation of any damage control strategy, further information should be gathered and a secondary assessment or survey should be undertaken. A useful mnemonic for gathering further history is **AMPLE**:
- **A**llergies
- **M**edicines and drugs currently taken
- **P**ast medical and surgical history and possibility of pregnancy
- **L**ast meal (including alcohol)
- **E**vents leading to the injury event

The secondary survey is a systematic head-to-toe physical examination looking for signs of physical injury in each body system and/or region. It may not be possible to progress to the secondary assessment in very unstable patients during initial care, but it is imperative that a full secondary survey is carried out as soon as possible after admission. Some examples of clinical features to be sought are given in Fig. 15.6.

Damage Control

Early mortality following major trauma is predominantly associated with uncontrolled bleeding and three associated key pathophysiological changes termed the *lethal triad*: coagulopathy, hypothermia and acidosis. Later mortality is associated with organ failure and infection. Following primary assessment and immediate life support interventions, trauma team leaders must decide whether to use a damage control resuscitation strategy in an attempt to reduce early and late mortality and morbidity, and which particular strategy to follow to ensure ongoing organ and

PRIMARY SURVEY (CACBCDE)

C. CATASTROPHIC BLEEDING – is there life-threatening uncontrolled bleeding?
1. Apply immediate **direct pressure** to source
2. Apply **indirect pressure** to the artery proximal to the bleeding point
3. Apply a **tourniquet** above the bleeding site in limbs
4. Consider **haemostatic dressings** and agents in junctional areas (groin, axilla, neck) and trunk
5. Early aggressive **surgical intervention** for proximal control may be required

A. AIRWAY – is the patient maintaining and/or protecting their airway?
1. **Manual airway manoeuvres** (jaw thrust), removal of foreign bodies, suctioning and postural drainage
2. **Use of airway devices:** oral (Guedel) airways, nasopharyngeal airways and supraglottic airway devices
3. **Rapid transition to a definitive airway** (a cuffed tracheal tube), using drug-assisted intubation or front-of-neck access (surgical cricothyroidotomy), may be required

C. CERVICAL SPINE – re-assess the need to restrict motion of the cervical spine using validated clinical decision rules

National Emergency X-Radiography Utilization Study (NEXUS) Criteria
Trauma patients do not require immobilization or x-rays if they meet ALL low risk criteria:

1. No posterior midline cervical spine tenderness
2. No evidence of intoxication
3. A normal level of alertness
4. No focal neurological deficit
5. No painful distracting injuries

Canadian C-spine Rule (CCR) Criteria

Trauma patients under the age of 65 years old do not require immobilization or x-rays if they are alert and stable, have no neurological symptoms or signs, have only low-risk presentation features (simple rear end road traffic collision, ambulatory at any time, sitting position in the ED, delayed onset of neck pain and no midline tenderness) and can actively rotate their neck 45° left and right

B. BREATHING AND VENTILATION – only assess breathing on the airway is secure.
Is the patient breathing spontaneously and adequately ventilating?

Physical examination
Inspection, palpation, percussion and auscultation
Early log-roll in penetrating trauma to examine the back of the chest
Search for evidence of life-threatening chest injuries
Obtain early blood gas analysis
Consider chest x-ray and/or ultrasound if patient too unstable for CT

Emergency treatment
1. Open (sucking) chest wound: seal with occlusive dressing + tube thoracostomy
2. Flail segment: positive pressure ventilation (invasive or non-invasive) + tube thoracostomy
3. Cardiac tamponade: emergency thoracotomy, pericardiocentesis may be temporising measure
4. Tension pneumothorax: needle thoracocentesis + tube thoracostomy
5. Haemothorax: tube thoracostomy and monitoring of output
6. Increased oxygen requirement and ventilatory failure: positive pressure ventilation

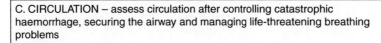

C. CIRCULATION – assess circulation after controlling catastrophic haemorrhage, securing the airway and managing life-threatening breathing problems

Physical examination
Look for physiological markers of shock (impaired perfusion). Are there sources of concealed or external heamorrhage?
Obtain all vital signs
Consider chest x-ray, pelvic x-ray and/or ultrasound, if patient too unstable for CT

Emergency treatment
1. Continue to control any external haemorrhage
2. Insert two peripheral wide-bore IV cannulae or intraosseous needles, if necessary
3. Send samples of blood for cross matching, lactate, venous blood gases, clotting and full blood count
4. Minimise coagulopathy and consider causes of shock state (obstructive, hypovolaemic/haemorrhagic, neurogenic)
5. Undertake balanced resuscitation with crystalloids and/or blood products depending on cause of shock and physiological responses to early treatment
6. Undertake definitive surgical control of bleeding as soon as possible – consider permissive hypotensive strategy as bridge to surgery or interventional radiology

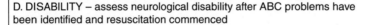

D. DISABILITY – assess neurological disability after ABC problems have been identified and resuscitation commenced

Physical examination
Assess Glasgow Coma Scale (GCS) score, pupil responses and peripheral motor and sensory function (mini-neurological examination)
Look for evidence of raised intracranial pressure

Emergency treatment
1. Asymmetric pupil responses or a unilateral dilated pupil in context of reduced GCS may indicate critically raised intracranial pressure and need for hypertonic saline, hyperventilation and rapid surgical intervention
2. Flaccid areflexia distributive shock and/or priapism may indicate spinal cord injury and early need for neuro-protective strategy and spinal injury care

E. EXPOSURE – of the whole patient and control of the environment

Patient must have full top-to-toe assessment. Environment must be controlled to prevent hypothermia and lines and tubes must be properly placed and secured prior to transfer to CT, intensive care or theatre (intravenous lines, airway circuites, orogastric tubes, chest drains, catheters and monitoring equipment)

• **Fig. 15.5** Primary Survey and Initial Resuscitation. Management priorities for the patient with multiple injuries. In practice, trauma team members from relevant specialties undertake simultaneous assessment and interventions are coordinated by the trauma team leader.

SECONDARY SURVEY

Head and neck

Look for bruising, soft tissue swelling; signs of basal skull
   fracture — Battle sign (bruising over mastoid process),
   'racoon eyes'
Lacerations
Depressed vault fractures
Facial and jaw fractures
Pupil size and responsiveness
Range of active neck movements

Chest (front and back)

Signs of respiratory distress — grunting/stridor
Bruising and skin imprinting
Penetrating injuries
Pattern and rate of respiration
Symmetry of chest movement
Gross mediastinal shift
Pattern of air entry throughout lung fields
Crepitus (subcutaneous air)

Abdomen and pelvis

External injuries as for chest (front and back)
   Note: buttock injuries may penetrate abdominal cavity
Distension by gas or fluid (including blood)
Tenderness
Presence of palpable or percussible bladder
Pelvic fractures
Bleeding from urethral meatus
PR bruising, palpable pelvic haematoma or loss of anal tone
(spinal injury)

Limbs

Neurovascular status of each limb
Lacerations
Deformities
Soft tissue swelling

Further definitive management of lesser injuries

Depends on findings from Primary and Secondary survey
May involve **further imaging** ± **surgery** or **ITU admission**
Before leaving the Emergency Department, **reassessment**
is essential to ensure that the patient is safe to be
transferred elsewhere

• **Fig. 15.6** Secondary Survey. Special points to note in systematic examination of the seriously injured patient.

system support, optimise physiology and reduce risk of further tissue injury.

The concept of damage-control resuscitation, illustrated in Fig. 15.3, acknowledges that no two trauma patients are the same and that separate injury types and physiological presentations may require very different approaches to resuscitation. A major challenge for the trauma team leader is to assimilate all the information from the primary assessment and determine whether one or more damage control strategies should be used. Some of the strategies may compete and risk further harm.

Critical care support refers to the early introduction of anaesthesia, positive pressure ventilation, invasive monitoring and use of vasoactive drugs. Almost all major trauma patients will require a period of critical care support, either in the resuscitation room, operating theatre or intensive care unit. Critical care

support may also be essential to undertake other damage control strategies but there are some patients where less may be more, particularly in the early stages of resuscitation. The most striking example of this is the concept of permissive hypotension (see earlier). This strategy is not a therapeutic goal but a deliberate decision to allow the shocked patient with exsanguinating non-compressible haemorrhage (typically intraabdominal or intrathoracic) to remain shocked to prevent further bleeding. A permissive hypotensive strategy can be dangerous and is only ever utilised as a bridge to definitive surgical control of bleeding within a limited time window. Patients who remain shocked for over an hour may, for example, succumb. These patients would typically move to the operating theatre before induction of anaesthesia (similar to abdominal aortic aneurysm patients).

Haemostatic resuscitation refers to an approach that combines minimising bleeding (through meticulous attention to haemorrhage control and wound, fracture and patient handling), optimisation of coagulation (on the assumption that all trauma patients are at risk of coagulopathy and many are already coagulopathic on arrival), and early judicious replacement of volume with blood products (red cells plasma and platelets). Coagulation is supported with tranexamic acid and clotting factors whilst coagulopathy can be minimised by careful attention to the environment, avoidance of haemodilution and correction of metabolic derangement. In an emergency, universal donor packed red cells (group O, Rh negative) can be transfused but evidence from recent conflicts has demonstrated the advantages of early administration of whole blood (or combined blood products) in reducing the risk of haemodilution and coagulopathy. EDs are increasingly using massive blood loss or massive transfusion protocols, which include several units of, packed red cells, fresh frozen plasma and platelets. These may be transfused in a 1:1:1 ratio or in a goal-directed manner, guided by clinical response, coagulation testing and thromboelastography.

A lung protective strategy recognises that injured lungs, through contusion, laceration and aspiration combined with mechanical chest wall injury need support but that all invasive ventilation is harmful. Ventilation may cause further structural injury to the alveolar–capillary unit through hyperoxia, volutrauma (overdistention) and barotrauma (overpressure). Lung protective ventilation (low tidal volume, low minute volume, lower mean airway pressures) combined with thoracic decompression (drainage of haemothorax and extraalveolar gas) may reduce ventilator associated lung injury. However, a lung protective ventilation strategy may be associated with permissive hypercapnia that may be harmful in traumatic brain injury.

A neuroprotective strategy recognises that although the primary neurological injury has already occurred, there is scope to reduce the extension of injury to surrounding neurological tissues by optimising perfusion. This is achieved by reducing cerebral metabolic demand (anaesthesia) and optimising cerebral blood flow through a combination of controlling ventilation, improving cerebral venous drainage and maintaining an optimum mean arterial pressure (see Ch. 16). Clearly, a permissive hypotensive strategy and a neuroprotective strategy are directly competing—the patient with traumatic brain injury and a ruptured spleen who is exsanguinating must receive a balanced approach. Wound protective strategies are discussed in Chapter 17.

Imaging

In major trauma, there is now consensus that adults should undergo whole body CT or 'trauma' CT a soon as possible after completion of the primary survey. In some systems, patients are now received directly into hybrid imaging suites/resuscitation room/operating theatres and undergo whole body imaging within a few minutes of arrival. Trauma CT involves CT of the head and neck without contrast, followed by CT of the chest, abdomen and pelvis with contrast. Historical characterisation of the CT scanner as the 'doughnut of death' related to incidents where CT scanners were remote from the resuscitation room, patients were not sufficiently stable or supervised and the scanning itself took a long time. Current protocols involve the whole trauma team moving with the patient to an adjacent or colocated CT suite, continuing resuscitation throughout scanning and achieving diagnostic images within a few minutes that permit prioritisation of emergency interventions.

If a patient is considered too unstable to undergo CT, then there is still a role for ultrasound and chest and pelvic x-rays in the resuscitation room. Focused Assessment with Sonography for Trauma (FAST) reliably detects free intraabdominal fluid and concentrates on five areas, the 'five Ps'—Perihepatic (hepatorenal space or Morison pouch), Perisplenic (splenorenal recess) and Pelvic (inferior portion of the peritoneal cavity and pouch of Douglas) in the abdomen, and Pleural and Pericardial in the chest. It is, of course, user-dependent. Chest x-rays, typically anteroposterior (AP) supine projections, can assist in confirmation of tube and line placement, identification of pneumothorax, pulmonary contusion, lung collapse and haemothorax. Pelvic x-rays can identify major pelvic disruption.

Abdominal Injuries

Abdominal and thoracic injuries often coexist, so it is logical to think in terms of **torso trauma**. Major torso injuries are a common cause of death at the scene, for example from avulsion of the thoracic aorta, cardiac injury or massive liver injury. Immediate diagnosis and urgent laparotomy or thoracotomy offers almost the only hope of survival, but the injury is often too extensive or time too short to intervene.

The site and signs of external injury provide clues to internal injuries. This is obvious with penetrating injuries but is also true of blunt injuries. For example, trauma to the left upper abdominal quadrant or lower ribs is often coupled with **splenic rupture**; similarly for the **liver** with right-sided injuries. Lower abdominal injuries may injure the **bladder**, and loin trauma the **kidney**. Central anterior chest trauma can damage the **heart** whilst clavicular area injury may traumatise the **brachial plexus** or **subclavian blood vessels**.

Abdominal injuries are less common than head and chest injuries and mortality can be low with prompt and appropriate management. When death occurs, it is usually from massive haemorrhage arising from bursting of liver or spleen or from penetration of major arteries or veins, particularly with gunshot wounds. Note that **unrecognised injuries** are a significant **avoidable** cause of death.

Areas of the abdomen other than the main peritoneal cavity may be wounded; **pelvic** viscera lie within a bony cage but extend low enough to be injured by buttock or perineal wounds. Similarly, **retroperitoneal** viscera may seem protected but are vulnerable to flank or back wounds, or to deep anterior stab wounds or any gunshot wounds. This area is not easily palpated and diagnosis usually requires CT.

Overall, 20% of patients with closed abdominal trauma require operation. In penetrating injuries, 30% with stab wounds require operation and close to 100% of those with gunshot wounds.

Diagnosis of Abdominal Injuries

Clinical diagnosis is unreliable in blunt injuries because overt signs of bleeding or hollow viscus perforation may not develop until hours after injury. If the patient is stable but the injury involved high-energy transfer or other significant injuries are present, early CT scanning should be performed.

Clinical Observation

If surgical intervention is not needed, regular nursing observations and serial clinical examination should be performed for signs of peritonitis or intraabdominal bleeding. Note that significant injuries almost always become manifest within 24 hours.

Penetrating Abdominal Wounds

Stab Wounds and Other Sharp Abdominal Wounds

Stab wounds may or may not penetrate the peritoneal cavity. They often cause little damage unless the blade penetrates the retroperitoneal area and injures great vessels or pancreas. It used to be thought that all abdominal stab wounds required surgical exploration but current policy in most cases is more conservative management. A large series from Baragwanath Hospital, Soweto, South Africa, demonstrated that 70% of patients or more, could safely be managed by observation in hospital for 24 hours, and operated upon only if there were signs of deterioration. However, haemodynamically unstable patients and those with extensive or potentially contaminated penetrating wounds **must** be explored surgically without delay.

For most patients, the first step is to determine whether the peritoneum has been breached, by exploring the wound under local anaesthesia. If it has, then laparoscopy, ultrasonography or CT scanning can be used to explore intraabdominal viscera. If the peritoneum is intact and/or imaging is negative (as in most cases), conservative management with careful monitoring is appropriate. However, about one third who later proved to have significant injury were initially free of signs, emphasising the need for repeated clinical and radiographic reassessment.

Bullet and Other Missile Injuries

The severity of internal injury depends on the path and mass of the missile and especially on its velocity. Low-velocity wounds (e.g., hand-gun bullets) cause damage confined to the wound track, whereas high-velocity (i.e., rifle) bullet wounds injure widely and deeply. This is because the much higher kinetic energy is dissipated in the tissues. In addition, **cavitation** is caused and debris is sucked into the wounds, causing contamination with clothing and soil. If a bullet hits bone, secondary missiles cause further injury. The size of the entry wound is often small because of elastic recoil of the skin and is no guide to the extent of injury. Given the unpredictable extent of injuries, **all** gunshot wounds must be surgically explored to check for visceral organ, intestinal and vascular damage. Buttock wounds may penetrate the pelvic cavity and should be treated in the same way.

Closed (Blunt) Abdominal Injuries

Closed abdominal injuries usually result from road traffic collisions, falls, sporting contact injuries and accidents involving horses. Following substantial blunt injury, about 20% will require laparotomy. The **spleen** is the most vulnerable organ, especially in left-sided injuries (Fig. 15.7). **Liver injury** requires greater impact force, usually from the front or right side. **Pancreatic and duodenal injuries** are uncommon and usually result from a heavy central abdominal impact, transecting the pancreas or retroperitoneal duodenum across the vertebral bodies. This most commonly occurs in children falling across the handlebars of bicycles. The **kidneys** are vulnerable to punches or kicks in the loins.

Bowel is damaged by rapid deceleration or crushing, and is particularly vulnerable at sites where freely mobile bowel becomes attached to the retroperitoneum, that is, at each end of the transverse colon, at the duodenojejunal flexure and in the ileocaecal area. A full **bladder**, common after a bout of heavy drinking, may rupture into the peritoneal cavity (or sometimes retroperitoneally) after abdominal impact. The **bladder** and **urethra** are also liable to be torn in displaced pelvic fractures. The clinical features and investigation of closed abdominal injuries are shown in Box 15.4.

Injuries to Specific Solid Organs

Spleen

The spleen is the most commonly injured organ in blunt abdominal trauma. The organ should be preserved wherever possible

---

CASE HISTORY

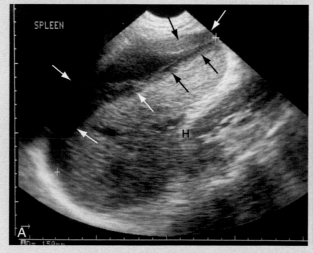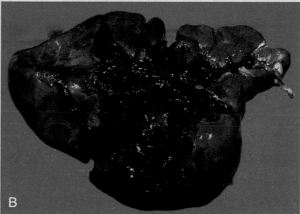

• **Fig. 15.7** Ruptured Spleen. (A) This 67-year-old woman sustained fractures of the left lower ribs in a fall. Discharged from hospital the next day but represented 6 weeks later with abdominal swelling, tenderness and anaemia. This ultrasound scan shows a large subcapsular splenic haematoma *(arrowed)*, which had developed slowly, and intrasplenic haemorrhage *(H)*. She rapidly recovered after splenectomy. (B) This operative specimen comes from a 15-year-old girl who fell off her pony, which then trod on the left chest. She was admitted with bruising over the lower ribs and tachycardia. At laparotomy, her spleen was found to be split completely in half, necessitating removal because of the dangers of postsplenectomy infection and sepsis. In one study, 2.4% of all postsplenectomy patients suffered sepsis and more than 50% of those were fatal.

CT scanning enables accurate assessment and classification of the extent of injury. Haematomas and capsular tears not extending deeply can often be managed conservatively. More severe injuries are treated by urgent laparotomy and where possible, splenic repair (splenorrhaphy) by direct suture, fibrin glue or absorbable mesh bags. Segmental resection or splenic artery ligation can be done, but 50% of splenic substance must be preserved for useful function. Whenever splenic preserving techniques are used, a period of careful observation for up to 10 days is required as catastrophic secondary haemorrhage can occur.

Liver

Isolated small liver injuries may be treated by surgical repair or local resection but paradoxically, major injuries are often best treated conservatively. This is because control of deep hepatic vessels may prove impossible, particularly bleeding from hepatic veins entering the inferior vena cava (IVC). Patients with severe liver injuries should be discussed with a regional hepatopancreaticobiliary (HPB) or liver unit. Conservative management involves large-volume blood transfusions until abdominal tamponade stops the bleeding. If operation is performed and a major liver injury is found and haemorrhage cannot be arrested, the liver should be packed with large pieces of surgical gauze, the abdomen closed and the patient stabilised. Ideally the patient should be transferred to an HPB centre, as extensive liver surgery may be necessary when the packs are removed at a 'second look' laparotomy 24 to 48 hours later.

Other Organs

Pancreatic transection is treated by surgically removing the distal part and oversewing the stump. A crushing pancreatic injury may have to be treated with drainage alone. **Renal injuries** are usually managed conservatively unless nephrectomy is required for uncontrollable bleeding.

Bowel Injuries

Injuries to small bowel are dealt with by simple suture or, if mesenteric vascular supply is impaired, by resection and anastomosis. Conventional treatment for right-sided colon injuries is resection and anastomosis of colon to ileum. Localised injuries to other parts of the colon without substantial faecal contamination can usually be resected and joined end to end. After knife or gunshot wounds, simple repair gives good results if there is minimal peritoneal contamination. Extensive injuries with contamination require **exteriorisation** of the damaged bowel ends to the abdominal wall (see Ch. 27).

High-velocity penetrating injuries wreak havoc on the gut, causing devascularisation and multiple perforations. All necrotic or ischaemic tissue must be excised. The immediate dangers are peritonitis and systemic sepsis from contamination. Exteriorisation of viable bowel ends is mandatory and planned reexploration usual.

Lower Urinary Tract Injuries

Intraperitoneal rupture of the bladder is treated by laparotomy and suturing, with a urethral catheter left in situ for 5 to 7 days. **Extraperitoneal** bladder rupture is treated conservatively, with prolonged urethral or suprapubic catheterisation. Urethral tears require specialist urological management. If the urethral wall is partly intact on urethrography, it can be treated, at least initially, by suprapubic catheterisation. Complete urethral avulsion injuries are usually treated by suprapubic catheterisation, with formal repair after inflammation has settled.

Damage Control Laparotomy

Major trauma patients sometimes have extensive and complex intraabdominal injuries. In an unstable patient, prolonged surgery to manage these definitively may exacerbate the lethal triad of coagulopathy, hypothermia and acidosis. Damage control laparotomy can be used here as a life-saving procedure that should be completed within an hour. Temporary clamping, then packing or ligating vessels controls haemorrhage. Hollow viscus injuries are stapled or resected without anastomosis. The abdomen is temporarily closed, or sometimes left open, and arrangements made for definitive surgery in 24 to 48 hours following resuscitation.

Chest Injuries

The types of chest injury, their clinical features and their treatment are summarised in Table 15.2.

• **BOX 15.4** **Clinical Features of Closed Abdominal Injury That Suggest Visceral Injury**

1. History
   • Substantial trauma to the abdomen or lower chest
   • Seatbelt not worn in road traffic collision (especially driver impacting steering wheel)
   • Abdominal pain after trauma
   • Haematuria, particularly following trauma to the back or loin
2. Physical signs
   • Skin bruising immediately after injury—suggests sufficient force to cause internal damage
   • Imprinting of cloth pattern on skin (*cloth printing*)—caused by compression of skin against vertebral bodies; implies high energy transfer impact
   • Unexplained hypotension—suggests concealed haemorrhage into abdominal cavity or elsewhere
   • Abdominal distension, that is, increasing abdominal girth—from accumulating blood, urine or gas in the peritoneal cavity
   • Increasing abdominal tenderness, guarding and rigidity (difficult to assess if abdominal wall bruising)—possible intestinal perforation or intraabdominal bleeding
   • Lateral lower rib fractures—injury to spleen, liver or kidney
   • Pelvic fractures, especially 'butterfly' fractures of all four pubic rami—often bladder or urethral injury (especially in males) and pelvic vein injury
   • Inability to pass urine and blood at urethral meatus and/or perineal bruising—imply rupture of urethra, usually at pelvic diaphragm, that is, postmembranous urethra (avoid urethral catheterisation in favour of suprapubic); rectal examination may reveal 'high-riding' prostate
   • Damage to anus or rectum may be palpable on rectal examination; presence of blood suggests anorectal injury. If anal sphincter tone low, suggests neurological damage from spinal injury
3. Investigation
   • Raised plasma amylase suggests pancreatic injury needing CT scanning
   • Chest and plain abdominal x-rays (supine and erect or lateral decubitus) for free intraperitoneal or retroperitoneal gas, rib or pelvic fractures associated with specific visceral injuries and radiopaque missiles, such as bullets, shotgun pellets and glass
   • Ultrasound and CT scanning—particularly useful for solid organs, that is, spleen (Fig. 15.7), liver, kidneys, pancreas. Intravenous contrast CT useful for large vessel injuries
   • Urethrography—for suspected urethral rupture
   • Laparoscopy—increasingly important in closed abdominal trauma in stable patients. Can be performed under local anaesthesia

CT, Computed tomography.

TABLE 15.2	Types of Chest Injury and Their Management	
Nature of the Injury	**Clinical Features**	**Treatment**
Sternal fracture	Anterior chest pain and tenderness; 'clicking' on palpation; arrhythmia and ECG changes	Consider cardiac contusion or tamponade; FAST scan; 24-h ECG; cardiac enzymes
Rib fractures	Localised pain on respiration or coughing; tenderness over fractures; usually visible on chest x-ray	Analgesia, intercostal blocks, physiotherapy, prophylactic antibiotics in chronic bronchitis
Flail chest, that is, multiple rib fractures producing a mobile segment	Respiratory embarrassment; 'paradoxical' indrawing of the flail segment on inspiration	Intercostal block analgesia; endotracheal intubation and ventilation if hypoxic
Pneumothorax, that is, air in pleural cavity causing lung collapse	Unilateral signs: loss of chest movement and breath sounds, percussion note resonant; sometimes chest wall emphysema; confirmed by chest x-ray	Intercostal drain with underwater seal
Sucking chest wound, that is, open pneumothorax with mediastinum 'flapping' from side to side with each respiration	Gross respiratory embarrassment, audible sucking of air through chest wound	Sealing of chest wound with impermeable dressing; intercostal drainage
Tension pneumothorax, that is, expanding pneumothorax causing progressive mediastinal shift to the opposite side and tracheal deviation	Signs of pneumothorax with disproportionate and increasing respiratory distress and hypoxaemia	Urgent chest drainage
Lung contusion	Deteriorating respiratory function; opacification of affected lung field on chest x-ray	Oxygenation, physiotherapy, mechanical ventilation if severe
Rupture of bronchus (uncommon)	Respiratory distress, surgical emphysema in the neck; suggested by air in mediastinum on chest x-ray (see Fig. 15.9A); confirmed by bronchoscopy	Operation by thoracic trained surgeon
Rupture of oesophagus (very rare)	May have surgical emphysema in neck and pneumomediastinum on chest x-ray but diagnosis often missed until mediastinitis or empyema develops	Surgical repair if recognised early; surgical drainage and diversion if late
Haemothorax, that is, blood in the pleural cavity. Usually arises from chest wall injury—rib fracture lung parenchyma or minor venous injury. Most are self-limiting. Arterial injuries less common and likely to need thoracotomy	Dull percussion note, breath sounds absent, tachycardia and hypotension caused by blood loss	Most have stopped bleeding by the time of examination and only tube drainage is required. Dark, venous bleeding more likely to cease spontaneously than bright arterial bleeding. Tube must be large enough to drain without clotting, ideally **32F–36F**; placed in sixth intercostal space in midaxillary line. If patient haemodynamically stable, admit and observe. If continuing drainage of 200 mL+ per hour over 4 h, should undergo thoracotomy
Cardiac tamponade, that is, bleeding into pericardial cavity (usually penetrating trauma)	Hypotension, inaudible heart sounds, distended neck veins with systolic waves; enlarged, rounded heart shadow on chest x-ray; confirmed with ultrasound	Long needle aspiration via epigastric approach; operation if tamponade recurs
Cardiac contusion	Often arrhythmia or ECG changes similar to myocardial infarction	Conservative management
Rupture of aorta (usually from deceleration injury)—fatal unless false aneurysm develops in mediastinum	Back pain, hypotension; systolic murmur or signs of tamponade in some cases; characteristic widening of mediastinum on chest x-ray; diagnosis confirmed by arteriography	Urgent thoracotomy and Dacron graft or minimal-access stent graft if available
Rupture of diaphragm, linear split usually in left diaphragm with herniation of gut into chest (penetrating or abdominal crush injury)	Respiratory distress, bowel sounds heard in the chest; diagnosis by chest x-ray and confirmed by barium meal; many cases only discovered much later; diagnosis may be made by laparoscopy or at laparotomy	Repair of diaphragm, usually via abdominal approach

ECG, Electrocardiogram; *FAST*, focused assessment with sonography for trauma.

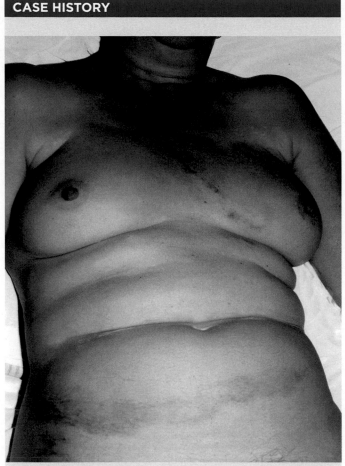

• **Fig. 15.8** Seatbelt Injury. This 60-year-old woman suffered a severe frontal impact whilst driving. The photograph shows typical seatbelt bruising. The body of the sternum had an undisplaced fracture but there were no major injuries; the seatbelt almost certainly saved the patient's life.

General Principles

Chest injuries are common in patients with multiple injuries. They are also common in road traffic collisions where, in some cases, the extent of the energy transfer to the chest can be revealed by seatbelt injury (see Fig. 15.8). Injuries that may pose an immediate life threat and which should be sought in the primary assessment include significantl tension pneumothorax, massive haemothorax, open pneumothorax, and tracheal or bronchial injuries. Signs of more subtle, but serious thoracic injuries should be sought in the secondary assessment. These include simple pneumothorax, simple haemothorax, fractured ribs, flail chest and pulmonary contusion.

Serious chest injuries may be present without external injury, particularly tearing of mediastinal contents (aorta, bronchi and oesophagus). Early imaging, typically with trauma CT, is required to exclude these injuries (see Fig. 15.9).

Mechanisms of chest injury include penetrating trauma, blunt impact and crushing injuries, deceleration injuries and rupture of the diaphragm caused by abdominal compression. Less than 10% of chest injuries require surgical intervention but early recognition of these may be life saving.

Thoracostomy (Open and Tube)

Following trauma, chest drains are usually placed in the fourth or fifth intercostal space on the midaxillary line. The technique is shown in Fig. 31.6, p. 426. Bilateral open thoracostomy is often used to decompress the chest in emergency care in ventilated patients as a precursor to formal chest drain insertion.

Vascular Trauma

Veins and arteries may be damaged by penetrating or blunt trauma. Gunshot wounds are more likely to damage vessels than stab wounds, and blunt injuries can damage arterial walls causing occlusion. Iatrogenical injuries are becoming common with the rise in radiological and minimal access procedures, and hip replacements. Damaged vessels bleed or impair distal circulation, or both.

Bleeding

Bleeding may be revealed (visible), or concealed and the rate of loss determines the presentation and risk of death. Concealed haemorrhage often occurs in the chest, abdomen or pelvis or in limb muscles with fractures; blood from facial fractures may be swallowed and unrecognised.

Ischaemia

Trauma that interrupts arterial flow to a limb or organ causes ischaemia, leading to potential limb or organ loss, stroke, bowel necrosis, and consequent multiple organ dysfunction. Skeletal muscle can survive ischaemia for 3 to 6 hours and still recover but peripheral nerves are sensitive and deficits can result from brief ischaemia.

If arterial supply is restored after delay, the release of inflammatory mediators, lactic acid and potassium into the circulation can cause **reperfusion syndrome**. In limbs, this can lead to compartment syndrome, and can also initiate a systemic inflammatory response with myocardial and other organ dysfunction.

Patterns of Vascular Injury

Laceration is the most common. Completely severed arteries contract, limiting haemorrhage, but partially transected arteries continue bleeding. Veins are unlikely to retract.

Blunt trauma causes crushing, stretching or shearing injuries to vessels. Intimal flaps can lead to thrombosis or dissection. Thrombosis may propagate down the vessel or embolise distally. Arterial 'spasm' alone does not cause limb ischaemia—the cause is thrombosis or vessel wall damage and requires urgent investigation.

False Aneurysm

An arterial puncture (e.g., femoral artery catheterisation or a stab wound) may cause bleeding that is enclosed by connective tissue, forming a pulsatile mass of clot known as a **false aneurysm.** This often presents days or weeks later. Distal flow is usually conserved and diagnosis can be confirmed by duplex Doppler ultrasound. First-line treatment is usually ultrasound-guided compression to cause thrombosis of the leak. If this fails, or for larger defects, suturing or patching may be needed.

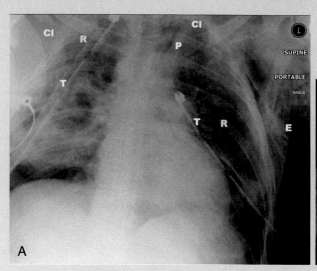
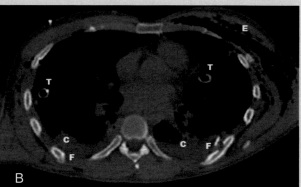

• **Fig. 15.9** Serious Chest Injuries. This 34-year-old male motorcyclist was hit by a car and then by another car whilst lying in the road. His Glasgow Coma score was 12–13 on arrival in the resuscitation room; brain, abdominal viscera and cervical spine were intact on computed tomography (CT). There were multiple fractures of ribs, scapula, clavicle, pelvis, humerus, femur and the chest injuries shown on CT (B). His thoracic injuries were successfully managed conservatively. (A) Supine portable chest radiograph taken in the resuscitation room. It is not well centred, reflecting the difficulty in radiographing sick patients being resuscitated. The film shows bilateral clavicle (CI), and rib fractures, pneumomediastinum (P), surgical emphysema (E), lung contusions and bilateral chest drains (T) inserted for pneumothorax. (B) CT on bone window settings showing surgical emphysema (E), bilateral basal atelectasis of lungs (C), chest drains (T), and bilateral rib fractures (F).

Arteriovenous Fistula

An injury to an artery and an adjacent vein can cause an arteriovenous (AV) fistula, which may eventually rupture or lead to cardiovascular compromise. These present some days or weeks after the injury. In a limb, the patient complains of a swelling with dilated superficial veins. On examination, there is a machinery-type murmur heard and diagnosis is confirmed by angiography. Treatment is by dividing the fistula and repairing the vein and artery, sometimes with a flap of fascia interposed.

Diagnosis of Vascular Injury

Clinical Signs

Visible bleeding from a traumatic wound with signs of hypovolaemia makes the diagnosis obvious. In limbs, palpable distal pulses are the most reliable sign of intact distal circulation. Hand-held Doppler probes can be misleading in detecting distal pulses and in ankle pressure measurement.

The following 'hard' signs of vascular injury indicate a need for urgent operative intervention, often without prior investigation.
• Audible bruit or palpable thrill
• Active, especially pulsatile haemorrhage
• An expanding haematoma
• Distal ischaemia (cold, pale, pulseless limb)

Patients with the following 'soft' signs of vascular injury do not require urgent investigation or exploration; they should be admitted, investigated as needed and observed over 24 hours.
• Haematoma

• History of haemorrhage at the accident scene
• Unexplained hypotension
• Peripheral nerve deficit
• Reduced but definitely palpable pulse
• Injury site near a major artery

Investigation

In expert hands, Duplex ultrasound can detect intimal tears, thrombosis, false aneurysms and AV fistulae, but **angiography** by direct puncture, CT angiography or on the operating table remains the gold standard for investigation and mapping of vascular injury. Arteriography may be needed to show the extent of injury in a stable patient with equivocal signs; to exclude injury where there are no hard signs but suspicion of vascular injury; in limb fractures with absent pulses; in injury by high-velocity missiles or multiple fragment injuries; and in blunt trauma. Angiography may be used to treat certain injuries by embolisation or stenting where expertise is available.

Management of Vascular Injury

The priorities in managing vascular injury are arrest of life-threatening haemorrhage and restoration of normal circulation. Temporary bleeding control is usually achievable by pressure over the site of injury.

Direct exploration of an actively bleeding wound is usually inadvisable because of poor visibility and the technical difficulty of achieving control. Far better to obtain proximal control, if necessary via a separate incision, isolating and clamping the artery before exploring the wound. Sometimes the artery distal to the wound needs clamping remotely too.

With proximal and distal clamps in situ, the wound is explored, debrided and the extent of arterial and venous damage assessed. In general, large veins should be repaired first to allow drainage as soon as the artery is repaired. A cut or lacerated artery may be amenable to direct repair or to patching, if direct suturing would narrow the lumen. More extensive damage may require an interposition graft, usually autologous long saphenous vein, or sometimes synthetic graft material. Before repair, proximal then distal clamps are released in turn to check for adequate blood flow. If inadequate, a Fogarty balloon catheter is passed to extract thrombus and heparinised saline instilled.

Compartment Syndrome

Delayed revascularisation of a limb risks compartment syndrome (see Ch. 17, p. 260). Prophylactic fasciotomy should be performed at the time of repair in these circumstances, particularly if the patient is ventilated or has an epidural, as these mask the symptoms of developing compartment syndrome.

Damage Control in Vascular Injury

Vessel Ligation

In extreme conditions, many arteries can be ligated. The common and external carotid, subclavian, axillary or internal iliac can be ligated with little consequence, but internal carotid ligation carries a 10% to 20% risk of stroke, and ligation of external iliac, common or superficial femoral arteries has a high risk of causing critical limb ischaemia. Coeliac axis arteries can be ligated, but not the superior mesenteric which would lead to bowel ischaemia. Almost any vein can be ligated, including the IVC (but this causes lower limb oedema).

Shunting

Where primary reconstruction cannot be performed and where ligation would risk limb loss, stroke or intestinal ischaemia, a temporary intraluminal shunt may be used to restore flow. Purpose-made shunts are available with side arms for flushing but ad hoc ones can be constructed from sterile tubing.

Primary Amputation

This is usually considered when there is severe injury, including crush injury, with a serious risk of reperfusion injury or when the limb is likely to be painful and useless.

Interventional Radiology in Vascular Injury

Interventional radiology is increasingly used in trauma as a means of controlling haemorrhage without need for a surgical procedure. In pelvic fractures, angiography and embolisation has become the gold standard for control of bleeding from iliac vessels; this remains the only firm indication for interventional radiology in unstable patients. In stable patients, embolisation can be used to control bleeding from solid organs (e.g., in splenic laceration) and covered stents can be deployed across major vessel disruptions (e.g., traumatic rupture of the thoracic aorta).

Special Patient Groups

The priorities of trauma care apply equally to all patient groups. There are, however, certain patient groups where there are important anatomical, physiological and psychological considerations.

• BOX 15.5 Important Anatomical and Physiological Differences in Children

Airway	Relatively large occiput and short neck can cause neck flexion and airway narrowing in the supine position
	Combination of small face and mandible and large tongue may impede or obstruct laryngoscopy view
	Infants less than 6 months old are primarily nasal breathers and are at risk of airway compromise
	Adenotonsillar hypertrophy in children between 3 and 8 years may contribute to obstruction and difficult laryngoscopy
	The larynx is high and anterior and the epiglottis is horseshoe-shaped and projects posteriorly at 45 degrees, making curved blade laryngoscopy more difficult
	The trachea is short and soft. Overextension of the neck as well as flexion may cause tracheal compression
	Tracheal tube displacement is more likely
B	The upper and lower airways are relatively small, and are consequently more easily obstructed
	Infants rely mainly on diaphragmatic breathing and are more prone to respiratory failure
	In the injured child, the compliant chest wall may allow serious parenchymal injuries to occur without rib fractures
	Infants and children will desaturate much more rapidly than adults
C	The child's circulating blood volume per kilogram of body weight is higher than that of an adult, but the actual volume is small—relatively small absolute amounts of blood loss can be critically important
D	Consistent assessment of neurological disability can be challenging
E	The body surface area to weight ratio decreases with increasing age. Small children, with a high ratio, lose heat more rapidly and are relatively more prone to hypothermia

Children

Injury remains the most common cause of death and disability in childhood. Almost half of child deaths are caused by road traffic collisions. Trauma care for children can seem complicated because they are a very diverse group and because of the anatomical, physiological and psychosocial differences across the ages. A basic awareness of these differences (Box 15.5), combined with the understanding that regardless of age, the primary assessment still follows ATLS principles and the CACBCDE approach, should provide reassurance that injured children can be safely managed in adult settings. Nonetheless, it is important that paediatric specialists form part of the trauma team whenever possible.

Key principles are:
- Age specific equipment must be immediately available to cover the full range of children—absolute size and relative body proportions change over time.
- A reliable means for determining or estimating weight (growth charts) must be available—drugs and fluids are typically given as the dose per kilogram of body weight.
- Aides-memoires with normal ranges of vital signs of different age groups must be available—all observations on children must be related to their age.
- Families should have information, encouragement and support to enable them to support their child and share in decisions about care. Children should also be informed about, and have active involvement in decisions related to their own ongoing care.

- Age appropriate communication and knowledge of normal child development will assist in managing fear and psychological distress.
- Safeguarding and the possibility of maltreatment should always be considered.

In relation to clinical assessment, the CACBCDE system should be followed and, with due recognition of the lower blood volume, the full range of investigations undertaken. Imaging in children takes a more selective approach than in adults and balances the need to keep radiation dose to developing tissues as low as possible, while still providing diagnostic images. Developing and maturing tissues in the growing child are more radiosensitive and the cumulative radiation risk over a lifetime alters the risks and benefits of trauma CT. Local policies and procedures for selective imaging strategies vary. In general, the criteria for CT head reflect adult criteria but there is a higher threshold for CT neck and x-rays of the neck may be more appropriate. Similarly, the threshold for CT thorax is higher and the primary investigation for blunt chest trauma is the chest x-ray. Penetrating chest injury and traumatic intraabdominal injury should undergo contrast-enhanced chest CT. Pelvic imaging is rarely necessary as pelvic fractures are rare in childhood. Again, x-ray may be more appropriate than CT in the first instance.

With respect to safeguarding, physical, emotional and sexual abuse, neglect, and fabricated or induced illness may all come to light following a presentation with injury. The following injuries should prompt specific consideration of child maltreatment and initiation of local safeguarding procedures if there is no suitable explanation.

- Bruising in the shape of a hand, ligature, stick, teeth mark, grip or an implement.
- Bruising or petechiae not caused by a medical condition and without suitable explanation, including:
  - in a child who is not independently mobile;
  - that are multiple or in clusters;
  - of similar shape and size;
  - on nonbony parts of the body, including the eyes, ears and buttocks;
  - on the neck/ankles.
- Human bite mark thought unlikely to be caused by a child.
- Lacerations, abrasions or scars on a child that are without suitable explanation, including:
  - on a child who is not independently mobile;
  - that are multiple or have a symmetrical distribution;
  - on the areas usually protected by clothing, or the eyes, ears and sides of face;
  - on the neck, ankles and wrists that look like ligature marks.
- One or more fractures in a child if there is no medical condition that predisposes to fragile bones, or if the explanation is absent or unsuitable, including:
  - fractures of different ages;
  - x-ray evidence of occult fractures.
- Burn or scald injuries on a child:
  - who is not independently mobile; or
  - on soft tissue areas not expected to accidently come into contact with a hot object (for example, backs of hands, soles of feet, buttocks, back); or
  - in the shape of an implement (for example, cigarette or iron).
- Intracranial injury in a child if there is no confirmed accidental trauma or known medical cause in one or more of the following circumstances:
  - the child is under 3 years;

- other inflicted injuries, retinal haemorrhages, or rib or long bone fractures;
- there are multiple subdural haemorrhages with or without subarachnoid haemorrhage with or without hypoxic ischaemic damage to the brain.
- Signs of spinal injury in a child if there is no confirmed accidental trauma.
- Intraabdominal or intrathoracic injury in a child if there is no confirmed accidental trauma, or with delay in presentation.

Pregnancy

There are significant physiological and anatomical changes over the course of pregnancy that can make the signs and symptoms of injury, and the response to resuscitation, harder to interpret. There are also two patients! Nonetheless, the primary assessment and structured approach is the same as for nonpregnant patients—the best treatment for the unborn child is effective resuscitation of the mother. To be effective, it is essential to know the main anatomical and physiological changes related to the gestational age.

In the respiratory system, there is increased oxygen consumption, hyperventilation and a relative hypocapnia. Upward displacement of the diaphragm leads to a decrease in functional residual capacity. In the cardiovascular system, cardiac output increases caused by increased preload (from a rise in blood volume), decreased afterload (from reducing vascular resistance) and increased resting heart rate. Plasma volume increases steadily throughout pregnancy but red blood cell volume increases to a lesser degree, resulting in haemodilution (physiological anaemia of pregnancy). Healthy pregnant patients can therefore compensate for the loss of significant volumes of blood before exhibiting signs of hypovolemia.

The principle anatomical change is the emergence of the gravid uterus from within the pelvis after the first trimester. By 20 weeks, it is at the umbilicus and at 34 to 36 weeks, it reaches the costal margin. Beyond 20 weeks, the gravid uterus can compress the IVC when in the supine position and reduce venous return to the extent that cardiac output can fall by 25% to 30%. Increased intraabdominal pressure combined with decreased lower oesophageal sphincter tone increases the risk of gastric aspiration.

Whilst all elements of the CACBCDE approach should be applied, resuscitation practice needs to be modified to take these changes into account. In particular, if the uterus is at or above the umbilicus, displacing the uterus to the left, off the IVC vessels, is critical to maximising cardiac output. This is best accomplished by placing the woman on her left side, but if this is not possible, putting a wedge or rolled towel under her right hip or adjusting her platform to achieve a 30-degrees left lateral tilt. There may need to be a lower threshold for airway protection because of the risk or regurgitation and aspiration. A careful and repeated assessment for compensated hypovolaemic shock must also be undertaken.

With regard to the foetus, the abdominal wall, uterus and amniotic fluid act to reduce energy transfer and provide a degree of protection from direct blunt injury. There is, however, a risk of injuries unique to the pregnant patient, such as uterine rupture and placental abruption—both of which may lead to the death of the foetus (see later). Physiological compensation in the mother can result in increased uterine vascular resistance, reduced foetal oxygenation and foetal distress (typically evidenced by an abnormal foetal heart rate). The foetus may be in distress and the placenta deprived of vital perfusion while the mother's condition and vital signs appear stable. Measurement of the foetal heart rate is therefore essential to determine whether the foetus is alive, and if alive, whether it is compromised.

Imaging should be undertaken early. The information obtained nearly always outweighs any radiation risk to the foetus, and concern about the possible effects of ionising radiation should not prevent medically indicated diagnostic procedures, using the best available modality for the clinical situation. Wherever possible, the risks and benefits should be discussed with the mother.

Emergency caesarean delivery is indicated in a viable foetus in the context of:
(a) A persisting abnormal foetal heart rate tracing in a critically unwell mother.
(b) Allowing surgical access for management of maternal injuries during laparotomy.
(c) Maternal cardiac arrest—optimum newborn and maternal survival are obtained when caesarean delivery is initiated within 4 minutes of maternal cardiac arrest and the foetus is delivered within 5 minutes of continuous resuscitation attempts.

Placental Abruption

Uterine distortion related to deceleration forces, even after minor injuries, can result in shear stress at the uteroplacental interface. Although a significant abruption can be asymptomatic or associated with minimal maternal symptoms, characteristic features are:
- vaginal bleeding
- abdominal pain
- contractions
- uterine rigidity and tenderness
- abnormal foetal heart rate

Ultrasound examination is of limited usefulness in diagnosing abruption. CT scanning in the context of trauma CT may identify the injury.

Uterine Rupture

Sharp or blunt abdominal trauma can lead to uterine rupture. Signs and symptoms include:
- shock
- abdominal tenderness, guarding, rigidity, or rebound tenderness
- vaginal bleeding
- uterine tenderness
- abnormal foetal lie (oblique or transverse lie)
- palpable foetal parts (because of being extrauterine)
- inability to palpate the uterine fundus
- abnormal foetal heart rate

Transplacental Haemorrhage

Transplacental or foetomaternal haemorrhage may lead to immunisation to the D antigen if the mother is D negative and the baby D positive. This can result in haemolytic disease in subsequent pregnancies. Obstetric advice should be sought regarding the necessity, timing and dosage of anti-D-immune globulin for the mother.

Elderly

As the population ages, trauma is becoming increasingly common in elderly patients. When compared to children and younger adults, patients over 65 years old have greater morbidity and mortality for virtually all injuries. This is in part caused by anatomical and physiological changes associated with ageing

• **BOX 15.6 Important Considerations in the Elderly**

- Lack of 'classic' response to hypovolaemia
- Risk for cardiac ischaemia
- Increased risk of dysrhythmias
- Elevated baseline blood pressure
- Increased risk for respiratory failure
- Increased risk for pneumonia
- Poor tolerance to rib fractures
- Interpretation of laboratory findings
- Drug dosing for renal and hepatic insufficiency
- Decreased ability to concentrate urine
- Increased risk for acute kidney injury
- Increased risk for fractures
- Decreased mobility
- Difficulty for oral intubation
- Risk of skin injury because of immobility
- Increased risk for hypothermia
- Challenges in rehabilitation

that increase risk and impair capacity to respond to the stress of injury. Another factor is the increased level of comorbidity (preexisting conditions) and medication use that may further diminish physiological reserve and response. One further factor is that older trauma patients may not be prioritised for treatment at an MTC because the injury mechanism is considered low risk and their physiology has been interpreted as normal when it is not. Yet with early, appropriate and aggressive trauma care, elderly patients can return to their baseline and continue to lead fulfilling lives.

Age-related anatomical and physiological changes can influence both the impact of the injury and the assessment by the trauma team (Box 15.6). Even apparently, benign mechanisms (e.g., fall from standing, the most common mechanism) can cause significant injury. Tissue tolerances to energy transfer are lower—reduced bone density and increased brittleness results in increased risk for all types of fractures. Changes in the compliance of the lungs and chest wall result in increased work of breathing. Combining this increased risk and reduced respiratory reserve with blunted physiological responses to hypoxia, hypercarbia, and acidosis increases the risk of delayed diagnosis of respiratory failure after, for example, sustaining multiple rib fractures. Such patients may present with a normal respiratory rate despite becoming progressively hypoxic and hypercarbic.

Older patients have less cardiovascular reserve and the cardiovascular system is less responsive to catecholamines. Tachycardia may not therefore be present despite haemorrhage, pain, or anxiety. Systemic vascular resistance is increased, often contributing to baseline hypertension, which can lead to the misinterpretation of 'normal' blood pressure readings. In other words, an older trauma patient may have a physiologically fixed heart rate and cardiac output. They will not mount a tachycardia and a 'normal' blood pressure may actually represent hypotension. Traditional physiological parameters used to identify high-risk trauma patients, such as systolic blood pressure below 90 mmHg or heart rate above 120 beats per minute, therefore do not identify older patients.

The presence of medical conditions has a major influence. In some cases, the injury event may have been precipitated by a medical condition, such as syncope, myocardial infarction, infection, and stroke. In relation to preexisting conditions, hypertension and heart disease are the most common but hepatic disease, renal insufficiency, and cancer may all be present. Dementia may also complicate assessment.

Older patients are also more likely to take multiple medications including anticoagulants, antiplatelet agents, beta-blockers, calcium-channel blockers, and glucocorticoids. These medications may play a pivotal role—not just in terms of predisposition to injury but also the consequences of, and response to, injury.

In assessment and treatment terms, older patients should be assessed in the same way as younger patients. There is a historical tendency in the older patient to withhold early aggressive airway management and positive pressure ventilation. Airway changes that are likely to complicate management include limited mouth opening, loose dentures or edentulous patients. Should drug-assisted intubation be required, doses should be reduced to limit the risk of hypotension and cardiovascular collapse. Noninvasive ventilatory support strategies should also be considered.

Interpretation of clinical and laboratory information can be complicated by preexisting disease (e.g., chronic lung disease) or normal age-related changes (e.g., renal function).

The increased risk of occult injury and lower risk associated with radiation exposure, should result in a lower threshold for trauma CT with the caveat that impaired renal function may predispose the patient to contrast induced nephropathy.

Given the limited capacity to compensate for the physiological stress of injury and the frequency by which insidious physiological deterioration occurs, the secondary survey should include assessment of trends in symptoms, physiology and investigations.

Injury patterns in older patients often include head and spinal injuries. Aging causes the dura mater to become more adherent to the skull resulting in the bridging veins becoming more vulnerable to shear stress—even after minor injury. A reduction in brain size with age increases the space in which blood from a torn bridging vein can accumulate. There may then be a delay in the development of symptoms and signs associated with subdural haemorrhage.

Older patients can sustain cervical spine fractures from seemingly minor mechanisms. In particular, high cervical fractures (e.g., odontoid) are more common. Conditions, such as cervical stenosis and degenerative rheumatoid and osteoarthritis make the spine more vulnerable to fracture and spinal cord injury. Hyperextension injury of the neck after a low fall can lead to a central spinal cord syndrome characterised by disproportionately greater motor impairment in upper compared with lower extremities, bladder dysfunction, and a variable degree of sensory loss below the level of injury.

Emergency Transfer

The safe movement of patients within a hospital is generally well structured and defined. The development of integrated trauma systems and the recognition that trauma patients have lower morbidity and mortality if managed in specialist MTCs has led to an increased recognition of the need to consider early emergency transfer of the major trauma patient between hospitals—particularly in inclusive trauma systems. Transfer should occur within a predetermined framework and each organisation, including those responsible for facilitating transfer, should be fully aware of their responsibilities. When considering emergency transfer within or between hospitals, the key principles are:

- Transfer should be initiated as soon as it becomes clear that the patient's needs exceed the capabilities of the provider.
- There should be established transfer agreements and protocols between hospitals that include the logistical elements of the transfer (standardised 'packaging', drug infusion regimes, documentation requirements, etc.).
- After recognising the need for transfer, expedite the arrangements. Do not perform diagnostic procedures that do not change the plan of care.
- Primary assessment, resuscitation and initiation of damage control strategies must have been completed before transfer. It should be anticipated that these might need to continue during transfer.
- Checklists, procedural aide memoires and standard operating procedures should be well established and used.
- Standardised documentation should be used—such that referring and receiving hospitals have a shared understanding of the patient and their needs.
- When planning transfer, the anticipated in-transit care needs and, as a consequence, the level of escort (paramedic, nurse, medical team), transport platform (ambulance or helicopter) and urgency of transfer should be considered.
- Consider the recovery of the transfer personnel and equipment. Ensure that their welfare is provided for.

Rehabilitation

Access to rehabilitation is a key component of an integrated trauma system. Rehabilitation is a process of assessment, treatment and management through which the individual (and their family/carers) are supported to achieve their maximum potential for physical, cognitive, social and psychological function, participation in society and quality of living. A large proportion of trauma patients will have an uncomplicated recovery and progress rapidly down the recovery, reenablement and rehabilitation pathway. Many have life changing injuries and require more specialist input from a range of services, including:

- Specialists in rehabilitation medicine
- Physiotherapists
- Occupational therapists
- Psychiatrists
- Clinical psychologists
- Neuropsychologists
- Nutrition and dietetics specialists
- Speech and language therapy specialists
- Prosthetic and orthotic specialists
- Pain specialists

Physical disability, cognitive impairment and psychosocial factors can all present significant challenges in providing effective rehabilitation. In some cases, patients require prolonged or permanent in-patient facilities to meet their needs. There is, however, good evidence for the effectiveness and cost benefits of rehabilitation, especially where the relevant health and social care services work together as a coordinated interdisciplinary team. The long-term results of rehabilitation are most successful where ongoing support and supervision is available for those who require it.

ORTHOPAEDIC INJURIES

Introduction to Fractures

This section covers the main points of the management of fractures, dislocations and ligament and muscle injuries, followed by detail on spinal and pelvic injuries.

General Points

- **Pain**—major orthopaedic injuries are extremely painful so good analgesia and early reduction is important, contributing to early mobilisation and reducing the risk of thromboembolism.
- **Blood loss**—internal blood loss from fractures is often substantial (Table 15.3) particularly if fractures are multiple, and blood volume needs to be replaced appropriately. External fixation may reduce blood loss in pelvic fractures.
- **Deformity**—obvious deformity should be corrected early using temporary splinting. This treats pain and may benefit vascular supply and limit blood loss.
- **Vascular and neurological integrity of limbs**—check, investigate and intervene if necessary.
- **Definitive fixation of fractures**—may be necessary early or may be deferred until life-threatening injuries have been treated.

A fracture involves a break in continuity of a bone. Bone is strong in compression but weaker in resisting torsional or bending forces. A footballer landing on one foot loads the tibia in compression and this is stable, but if a twisting force is added, it fractures. A bending force on a forearm causes fracture, with the energy applied where the bone is weakest. As velocity before impact increases, **high energy transfer** collisions can fracture the bone in multiple places (force = mass × velocity^2).

Classification

Fractures can be classified by age of the patient, outward appearance and involvement of the overlying skin, cause of fracture, and the radiological appearance.

Age—the outer layer of a willow tree shoot is tough and often remains in continuity even if the inner wood snaps. Fractures in a young person can be similar with the thick periosteum remaining intact even though the bone is broken. This is a **green stick fracture,** contrasting with adults where the periosteum is thinner and unable to resist the fracturing forces.

Outward appearance—if the skin over a fracture remains intact, it is **closed** whereas if it is broken, it is an **open** or **compound** fracture (Fig. 15.10). The skin can be broken by whatever caused the fracture (*compound from without*) or by a spike of bone bursting out from within (*compound from within*). Compound fractures are

often classified using the Gustilo-Anderson method (Box 15.7) and tibial fractures are the most common compound fracture.

Cause—The Three Main Causes of Fracture

- **Traumatic**—the bone is normal and an episode of violence causes the break. This is the usual cause in otherwise fit people.
- **Pathological fractures**—where a force not normally enough to cause a fracture has done so. These occur when the bone is inherently weak (e.g., osteoporosis, metabolic bone diseases such as osteomalacia, hyperparathyroidism, Paget disease, osteogenesis imperfecta) or where the bone has been replaced by abnormal tissue, such as a bone cyst (Fig. 15.11), chronic infection, benign tumour (e.g., chondroma) or malignant tumour. The most common 'malignant fracture' is through a metastatic deposit from a primary bronchial, breast, prostate, kidney or thyroid carcinoma besides myelomatosis.
- **Stress fractures** occur after, often relatively minor, repeated trauma. Examples include **'march fractures'** of a metatarsal neck (usually the fourth) but can occur in any lower limb

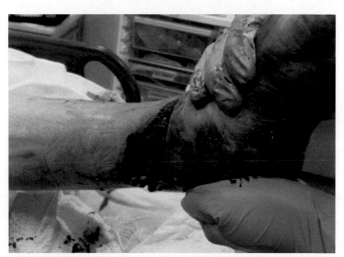

• **Fig. 15.10** Compound ankle fracture being held with manual traction. Traction being applied to a compound fracture to reduce pain, while the wound is cleaned and splinted in the emergency room.

• BOX 15.7	Classification of Open Fractures Described by Gustilo and Anderson (1976). The Grade Typically Increases as the Energy Dissipated Increases
Grade	**Description**
I	Wound >1 cm long. Usually a low energy compound 'from within' injury
II	Wound between 1 and 10 cm but without extensive soft tissue damage
IIIA	Extensive soft tissue damage but soft tissue coverage of fracture still possible. Also includes injuries where history indicates very high energy dissipation without initial overt signs of massive soft tissue damage
IIIB	Extensive soft-tissue loss including periosteal stripping and bone damage, usually associated with severe contamination. Plastic surgery reconstruction will be required to gain coverage
IIIC	An open fracture associated with an arterial injury requiring repair, irrespective of degree of soft-tissue injury

TABLE 15.3	Average Blood Loss From Fractures
Site	**Average Loss (L)**
Pelvis	1–4
Femur	1–2.5
Tibia	0.5–1.5
Humerus	0.5–1.5

bone. Tibial stress fractures form part of the differential diagnosis of anterior tibial pain in runners; femoral neck fractures can occur in weightlifters. Stress fractures of the pars intraarticularis of the lumbar spine can lead to spondylolysis. They can occur in athletes, but also in osteoporotic and elderly bones. Stress fractures may not show on x-ray until callus forms, by which time they have usually become asymptomatic. Isotope scans or magnetic resonance imaging (MRI) may be helpful in early diagnosis.

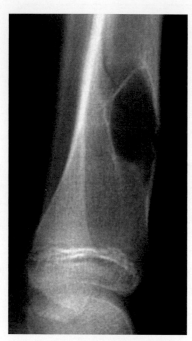

• **Fig. 15.11** A Minimally Displaced Pathological Fracture Through a Benign Bone Cyst. Note, the sclerotic white margin confirms its benign nature.

Radiological Appearance

X-rays show the fracture configuration and much evidence can be drawn from this. Traditionally, a stable fracture is one where the limb will not shorten if an axial load is applied, whilst an unstable one means that the force is likely to cause further displacement. In practice, fractures rarely displace axially more than they did at impact.

Radiological configurations:

- **Transverse**—the fracturing force impacts directly on the bone (Fig. 15.12). These fractures are stable but the area of bone in contact for healing is small, so union takes twice as long as in spiral fractures.
- **Spiral**—these are low velocity fractures (Fig. 15.13). The distal part of the limb is stationary and the heavy body twists around it. Fracture healing is more rapid because of the large areas in contact.
- **Oblique**—a combination of rotational and direct forces (Fig. 15.14). A common example is the short oblique tibial fracture in a footballer on the wrong end of a tackle. These heal quickly provided another bone in the limb does not keep the fracture ends apart. They are relatively stable, particularly if the second bone is intact.
- **Butterfly fracture**—caused by a direct blow combined with an evolving spiral fracture (Fig. 15.15). Healing is often slow.
- **Comminuted fracture**—usually the result of great force. There are more than two bony fragments to the fracture configuration (see Fig. 15.15). Blood supply is often compromised leading to delayed healing, even though there is a large contact area. These fractures are generally unstable.

Fracture Healing

The most rapid union occurs in growing children with thick periosteum and a good blood supply. In general, upper limb bones heal faster than lower limb, whilst compound (open) fractures take longer. Transverse and comminuted fractures take twice as long as spiral fractures to unite and consolidate. High energy impacts cause more damage and healing takes longer.

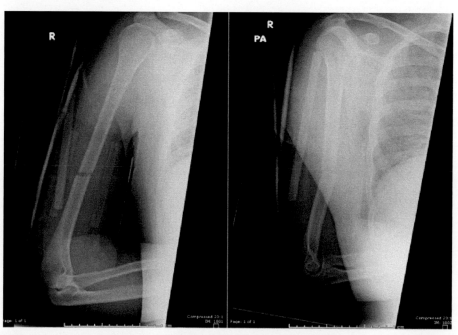

• **Fig. 15.12** Transverse fracture of a right humerus caused by direct violence, splinted in an acceptable position. *PA,* posteroanterior.

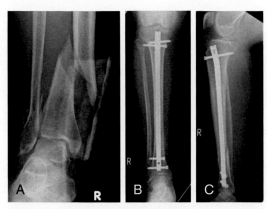

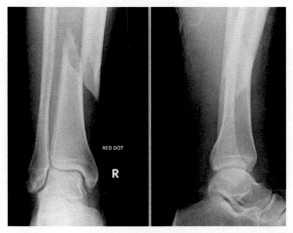

• **Fig. 15.13** (A) Spiral fracture (compound) fracture; note the visible dressing. Postoperative x-rays, anteroposterior (B) and lateral (C) views, showing the reduced fracture held by an intramedullary nail locked by screws at both ends.

• **Fig. 15.14** Anteroposterior and Lateral X-ray of a Displaced Oblique Fracture of the Tibia.

The Process of Healing

Fractures heal by restoring bone continuity. Cancellous bone heals more quickly than cortical and some movement at fracture sites stimulates healing. Healing is a cascade, like blood coagulation, and can be considered in five stages:

- Firstly, bleeding from the bone ends and the stripped periosteum produces a haematoma.
- Secondly, an acute inflammatory response occurs initiating a healing process, with fibroblasts producing a web of collagen in the haematoma.
- Thirdly, osteoblasts proliferate from the bone ends and the local periosteum and produce immature bone known as woven bone or callus. Osteoclasts gradually resorb dead bone.
- In stage four, orderly lamellar bone replaces woven bone and the fracture becomes united.
- Lastly, during stage 5, remodelling occurs. The bone recovers much of its shape and the medullary cavity is restored. Children remodel well and can often heal without a skeletal blemish by the time of skeletal maturity. Malunion is where a fracture has united but not without deformity. A classic example is a rotatory deformity at the elbow following a juvenile supracondylar fracture.

Principles of Fracture Management (Table 15.4)

The maxims of **reduce, hold and rehabilitate** were used centuries ago and still apply today.

Reduce

Displaced fractures should be reduced into an acceptable position. This can often be achieved by 'closed' manipulation. If this is not possible then open operation needs to be considered.

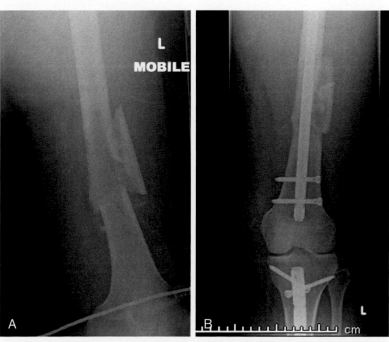

• **Fig. 15.15** Comminuted Fracture With 'Butterfly' Fragment.

Hold

Closed—if successful, external splinting is applied. This was traditionally a plaster of Paris cast but now synthetic or sometimes biodegradable casts are used.

Open—if reduction necessitates surgical opening, the aim is to achieve perfect reduction under direct vision. After this, internal fixation is used involving screws, plates, tension bands and other such devices. Internal fixation of long bones can be achieved by inserting intramedullary devices, including rods and nails, under x-ray guidance. The devices can be 'locked' to prevent rotation and shortening using locking screws (see Fig. 15.13 earlier).

Indications for Internal Fixation (Open Reduction and Internal Fixation, ORIF)

ORIF should be undertaken only when the advantages far outweigh the risks. The generally accepted indications include:
- After arterial repair or presence of nerve damage.

- Where the fracture involves a joint. Joint surfaces need to be perfectly congruent so displaced intraarticular fractures must be accurately reduced and fixed internally.
- Where conservative management is futile, such as fractured neck of femur in an elderly patient.
- Where conservative management would involve long immobilisation in bed, such as with a fractured shaft of femur.

It must be stressed that operating on fractures should be undertaken only by properly trained surgeons. Fractures usually heal in time if left alone and the long-term result after poor surgery can be far worse than after conservative treatment.

External fixation with a system of wires or screws attached to a frame is sometimes chosen, particularly with open fractures (Fig. 15.16).

Managing Compound Fractures

The most common compound (open) fracture is of the tibia. Its management is often asked in examinations. After the standard

TABLE 15.4   Types of Limb Fracture and Their Management

Site	Mechanism of Injury	Classification (Common or Important Types)	Management	Specific Potential Complications
Upper Limb				
Clavicle	Fall onto outstretched hand	Proximal one-third, middle one-third, distal one-third	Up to 98% of middle third heal with conservative management. Displaced distal may need operation	Plate fixation of middle third fractures threatens underlying neurovascular bundle
Humerus (neck)	Fall onto hand	Neer	Operate if severe displacement and incongruency	Severely broken humeral heads may need hemiarthroplasty
Olecranon	Fall onto point of elbow		Tension band wire for articular surface reconstruction	
Fracture-dislocations of forearm	Fall onto arm		Accurate reconstruction preserves full range of movement	… but neurovascular structures make operating difficult
Distal radius	Fragility fractures	Smith, Colles, Barton	Aim to restore function	Porotic bones makes perfect x-rays difficult
Base of thumb	Forced extension	Rolando, Bennett	Accurate fixation to preserve thumb movements	
Metacarpal neck	Punching/fist injuries		Many managed conservatively	
Lower Limb				
Neck of femur	Fragility fractures	Garden, intra-/extra-capsular	~100% operation rates to allow early mobilisation	High morbidity and mortality in elderly patients
Tibial plateau	High energy fractures	Schaztker	Operate to reconstruct vital articular surface	
Tibial shaft	High energy fractures		Conservative and operative methods available	High rates of nonunion compared to other bones
Ankle	Low energy fractures	Weber, AO classification	Operate to restore perfect ankle congruity if casting fails	
Calcaneum	High energy falls	Sanders class		Often lead to hind foot pain or collapse
Forefoot and toes	Low energy falls/trips		Fix and straighten bones, mobilise early	

ABC assessment of an injured patient, the compound fracture is considered. The history of injury is pivotal in choice of management: low velocity fractures compound from within are much less challenging than high velocity direct violence fractures caused by motor vehicle collisions. Such direct violence must badly damage the soft tissues. It is good practice to photograph compound fractures on admission so all specialists involved in care can plan without repeatedly disturbing the wound. The Gustilo and Anderson classification of open fractures is universally accepted and is a good discipline to use (see Box 15.7).

Initial Treatment of Compound Fractures

The wound should be covered with a sterile dressing and the limb splinted to reduce continuing blood loss and aid pain relief. An antitetanus injection (when indicated), opiates for pain and intravenous systemic antibiotics and are administered without delay. Selective peripheral nerve blocks for pain relief are useful after neurovascular assessment.

Under general anaesthesia, the wound is explored and all foreign material removed. The skin edges are excised together with all devitalised soft tissue (**debridement**). The wound is vigorously irrigated with warm isotonic saline where appropriate (*never* hydrogen peroxide). A decision is then made as to type of fixation—internal or external.

Delayed Primary Closure

This apparently simple idea was developed in the Great War of 1914 to 1918 to manage battlefield wounds that invariably became infected if closed primarily. However, the lesson often had to be learned (the hard way) in later wars, conflicts and civilian life. For a contaminated wound, debridement is the first step but the wound is left open and packed for about 3–5 days before being inspected again under general anaesthesia, and then closed or skin

grafted. Further debridement may be needed, and closure or skin grafting delayed. Failing to follow these principles is likely to lead to serious infection and possible death.

Rehabilitation

Patients often know when their fracture is healing as they begin to feel more confident using the limb. X-rays showing fracture healing help determine when casts can be removed and more activity encouraged. A physical therapist can get stiff joints moving again and help with mental rehabilitation.

Complications of Fractures (Box 15.8)

As all students know, any procedure or treatment a patient undergoes risks complications. These can be local or systemic, immediate, early or longer term. Note that sharp bone ends moving with force can cause great injury to nearby structures.

Individual Complications of Fractures

Malunion can lead later to disordered mechanics in the rest of the limb and the back, and may lead to osteoarthritis in nearby joints. Displaced intraarticular fractures with an irregular joint surface markedly increases friction, leading to posttraumatic osteoarthritis.

Delayed union leads to long periods of disuse, and the entire limb can suffer from muscle atrophy, osteoporosis and joint contractures.

Nerve damage is particularly likely in a fracture when the nerve is tethered. It can also occur if there is ischaemia from vascular damage. There is often a mixed picture, particularly with traction

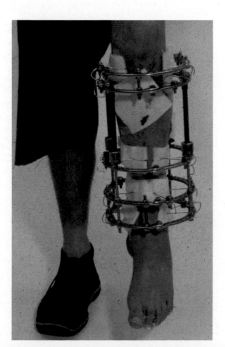

• Fig. 15.16 Patient Ambulating With External Fixation. Note that wires pass through the tibia above and below the fracture, and are secured to the rings which are locked together.

• BOX 15.8   Complications of Fractures

Local
Immediate
- Damage to skin, muscles, veins
- Damage to nerves and arteries
- Damage to joints
- Damage to viscera (lung etc.)

Early
- Fat embolus syndrome
- Infection

Late
- Nonunion
- Malunion (union in an unsatisfactory position)
- Joint damage leading later to arthritic changes
- Epiphyseal injuries, particularly Harris type 4 and 5, can lead to partial growth arrest and late deformity

Systemic (General)
Immediate
- Pain and shock
- Systemic effects of severe blood loss, such as stroke, myocardial infarction and kidney failure

Early
- As earlier plus venous thromboembolic disease
- Chest infections and confusion in the elderly
- Loss of confidence

Late
- All the problems associated with long term disability

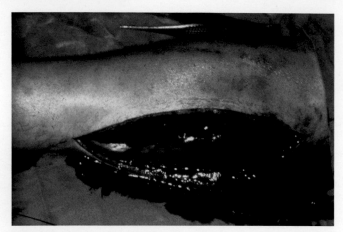

• **Fig. 15.17** Picture showing massive herniation of muscle through the lateral of three fasciotomy incisions to decompress the lower leg after delayed repair of a damaged femoral artery.

injuries. Nerve damage is evident when the part is insensate and not moving to command. Lack of sweating strongly suggests nerve damage and is useful in children who may retreat from a doctor coming at them with a pin.

Common closed injuries associated with nerve damage include shoulder dislocation (axillary nerve and brachial plexus), humeral fractures (radial nerve) and posterior hip fracture/dislocations (sciatic nerve but more often common peroneal nerve)

In children, displaced humeral supracondylar fractures are often associated with anterior interosseous nerve palsies, most of which recover spontaneously.

Vascular Damage

Damage to a major artery causes blood loss and can threaten limb survival. Arterial damage can be caused by externally penetrating injuries, such as bullets or shrapnel, or by bone ends from within.

Arteries can be severed, partially damaged (sometimes leading later to an AV fistula), or become trapped between bone ends. Sometimes only the intima/inner media is damaged causing a **lesion in continuity**; these are usually traction injuries. The inner or intima layer peels up and occlude the vessel. At operation, the vessel appears to be in spasm but still in continuity. Urgent reconstruction is required and through a longitudinal arteriotomy the damaged intima is removed and a reversed vein patch is applied to the longitudinal arteriotomy. In cases where the artery is more seriously damaged it can be excised and replaced with a (reversed) vein graft.

Arterial damage producing ischaemia causes very severe pain (unless major nerves are coincidently damaged) and progressive numbness and weakness. Examining by careful passive stretching of ischaemic muscle by joint movement, especially flexor muscles, increases the pain and is diagnostic. With severe vascular damage, it is important to consider **decompression fasciotomy** (Fig. 15.17). This is indicated:

- When it has taken more than 6 hours to restore arterial supply to the limb
- Add to this, where there is extensive distal injury including burns
- Add to this, where there is significant venous damage
- Whenever there is doubt about the aforementioned

Venous damage is much less likely to be limb threatening. Major limb veins can be ligated when blood loss is life threatening

blood loss but major trunk veins (common iliac, subclavian etc) require repair by a vascular surgeon.

Volkmann Ischaemic Contracture

Muscle death by untreated ischaemia leads later to contractures, which severely compromise limb function. Such late recognition of ischaemia may lead to litigation. The pathophysiology is that ischaemia followed by late revascularisation leads to increased pressure in the osteofascial compartment beyond the vascular injury because of fluid loss from damaged capillaries. High pressure prevents blood entering the compartment and the tissues within die. Early fasciotomy relieves the pressure and intracompartmental circulation is restored. Fasciotomy is relatively easily achieved by making longitudinal incisions in the skin and the fascial compartments. Skin grafts may be needed to close the operation, some 5 to 7 days later.

Compartment Syndrome

Limb muscles are arranged into compartments during embryological life; grouping those with similar actions limiting friction between them. The compartments have inflexible fascial walls restricting expansion beyond a limited volume, so if traumatic swelling occurs, there is a risk of **compartment syndrome** causing ischaemia (see Ch. 17, p. 260).

What Does This Mean for the Doctor on the Spot?

Any patient suffering a significant injury must have a careful neurological and vascular assessment and the results carefully noted and acted upon. The complications described happen in real life, not just in text books.

Individual Types of Fracture

Insufficiency Fractures

These are seen typically in (usually) elderly osteoporotic patients and include femoral neck and pubic ramus, lower radius (Colles type), upper humerus, vertebral body and sacral insufficiency fractures. Patients with these fractures should have a metabolic bone disease workup and, in the case of sacral insufficiency fractures, urgent medical treatment. Patients who have fallen for no obvious reason or fall repeatedly should be referred to a falls prevention clinic. Falls are responsible for many deaths in the elderly; it is often said that 'We all enter the world via the pelvis and many leave it via the neck of the femur'. Wherever possible, early treatment, mobilisation and discharge from hospital should be the aim.

Wrist Fractures

These are the most common fracture in the average adult fracture clinic. Major hospitals may see about 10 of these each day and >90% are in elderly women. The author remembers seeing 70 in one day after snow. In a Colles fracture the distal fragments are displaced/angulated dorsally (Fig. 15.18), whilst in the Smith fracture, the fragments are angulated in a palmar direction (Fig. 15.19). About 50% of Colles fractures need closed manipulation plus reduction and splintage (usually under local anaesthesia) and the others require a simple splint or plaster. Normally a 'back slab' is applied for about a week to allow for swelling and is then completed to become a full cast. The cast is usually needed for 6 weeks for a displaced fracture and 5 weeks if undisplaced.

Smith fractures (sometimes known as *Barton fractures*) usually need open reduction and a buttress plate (see Fig. 15.19).

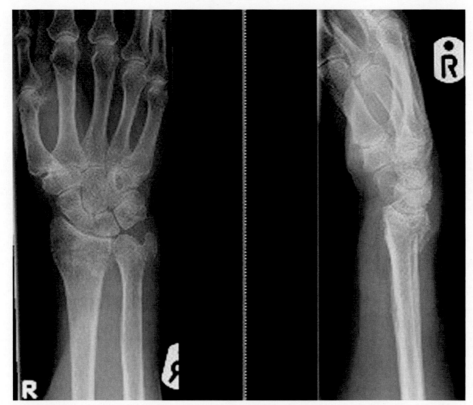

• **Fig. 15.18** Anteroposterior and lateral view x-rays of a Colles fracture of the lower radius and ulna with minimal displacement. Note the osteoporosis. It healed with a synthetic cast.

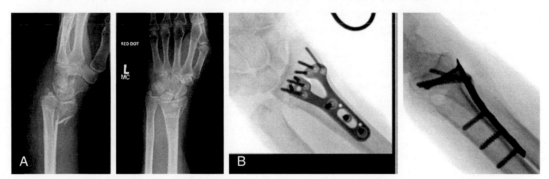

• **Fig. 15.19** Wrist Fractures. Peroperative anteroposterior and lateral x-rays of a mildly displaced Smith fracture treated with open reduction and internal fixation.

Fractured Neck of Femur (Fig. 15.20)

These fall into two groups: **Subcapital** or intraarticular femoral neck fractures, and those in the **Pertrochanteric region** (usually in an older age group) (see Fig. 15.20A). Neck-of-femur fractures are usually caused by a fall. Most patients have premorbid medical conditions that need to be addressed during treatment. Patients cared for in multidisciplinary environments with surgeons, physicians (geriatricians) and specialists in rehabilitation involved, achieve the best outcomes and lowest mortality.

Fragility fractures caused by osteoporosis far outnumber the others and affect a large number of older patients. Femoral neck fracture still carries a high mortality. Operative treatment carries risks but is still the best method of restoring mobility and preventing death from other causes. Nevertheless, death rates of 10% to 30% at 1 year are common.

Dealing with fragility hip fractures presents a challenge. Conservative treatment is rare nowadays, as spending 6 or more weeks in bed leads to high rates of venous thromboembolism, respiratory infection, pressure ulcers and death. These patients are often frail, with impaired cardiovascular and respiratory function, so surgical treatment requires anaesthetic risk assessment and optimising general health. There is a trend in the United Kingdom towards involving a dedicated care-of-the-elderly physician (geriatrician) in assessing and managing all these patients. This, together with physiotherapists, dedicated theatres to minimise delays, modern surgical stabilisation techniques and skilled anaesthesia, provides optimum care and better outcomes.

Subcapital Fractures or Intracapsular Fractures

The femoral head blood supply is principally endosteal, from one anterior and two posterior arteries and is vulnerable to fractures.

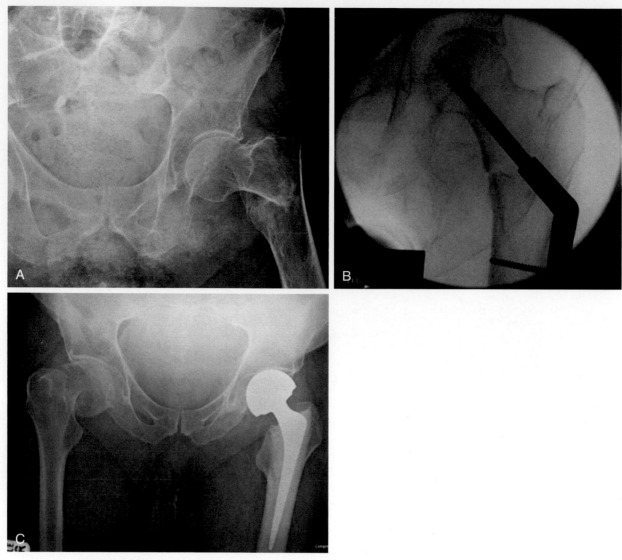

• **Fig. 15.20** (A) X-ray showing a completely displaced left pertrochanteric fracture. (B) This was treated with a 'sliding nail plate'. (C) Subcapital (intracapsular) fracture of the right femoral neck in a patient who had previously sustained a similar injury on the left side, appropriately treated with a hemiarthroplasty.

If the fracture is substantially displaced, the blood vessels are disrupted and the femoral head dies (**avascular necrosis**). In general, there is a high rate of nonunion. When x-rays show displacement is minor, the fracture can be held with accurately placed pins or partially threaded screws (see Fig. 15.20B). For displaced fractures, it is usual to replace the femoral head with a hemiarthroplasty (see Fig. 15.20C) or sometimes a total hip replacement.

Pertrochanteric or Extracapsular Fractures

These occur mainly in the very elderly, usually in women, and the comminuted fragments are often substantially displaced (see Fig. 15.20A). This group has a 3-month mortality of 15% in most series and 5-year survival is less than 25%. The principle aim of fracture treatment is early stabilisation with internal fixation to allow early mobilisation. In the developed world, nonoperative treatment is generally futile, with the patient often succumbing to pneumonia and bedsores. In some parts of the world, they are treated with traction until pain is no longer a problem when they can then mobilise but with a shortened, externally rotated leg. Patients who are small and light are less likely to suffer complications.

Other Lower Limb Fractures

To fracture a lower limb long bone in a healthy adult requires substantial force. Typical patterns of tibial and femoral shaft fractures occur in motor vehicle accidents, falls from a height, collisions and twisting injuries on the sports field and ski slopes. Femoral shaft fractures can be treated with traction for up to 12 weeks when safe operative facilities are unavailable but the preference is for an intramedullary locked nail introduced under X Ray control.

Displaced tibial fractures are treated with intramedullary nailing or an external frame. Ankle fractures occur in all age groups, caused by accidental slips, twists and falls. Undisplaced fractures can be treated with a splint or a cast, ORIF is usually indicated with displaced fractures, particularly if they involve the joint.

Spinal Fractures and Dislocations

These are dealt with in the neurosurgical section.

Fractures in Children

Children's bones are very different from adults, particularly in their ability to heal and remodel. Management of individual

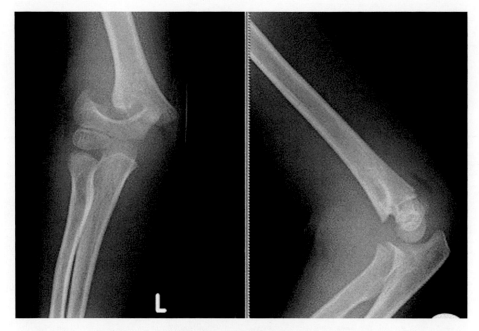

• **Fig. 15.21** X-ray of Displaced Supracondylar Humeral Fracture.

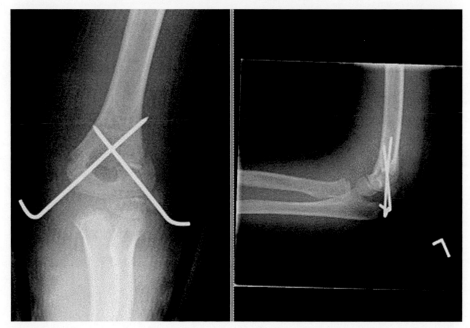

• **Fig. 15.22** Closed Reduction of Fracture Held With Two Crossed K Wires, Which Were Later Removed. The end-result was normality.

fractures depends on their natural history but some, described later, are potentially limb threatening if not treated properly.

Supracondylar fracture of humerus—usually results from a fall in a child 7 to 10 years old. It can cause neurological damage to the median, ulnar or radial nerves. Damage to the brachial artery can lead to Volkmann contracture and serious loss of hand function. Displaced fractures can be treated with reduction and fixation with K wires (Figs. 15.21 and 15.22) or traction, as originally described by Dunlop.

Epiphyseal Injuries (Fig. 15.23)

Injuries around the epiphysis cause partial or complete growth arrest if germinal cells are involved (as in types IV and V).

Complete growth arrest leads to a short limb, whilst partial arrest leads to increasing angulation, as one side grows without the other.

Some practitioners add a type VI where the periosteum is damaged as it merges with the epiphysis. This usually involves overlying skin, for example, on the inner ankle, damaged when run over by a motor vehicle. This injury is very likely to cause progressive angulation with growth.

Growth arrest is confirmed by CT scans and arrests can sometimes be resected but with variable success. Gross shortening or major angulations are managed in limb deformity clinics with osteotomies and frames (based on Ilizarov's original designs) with the deformity being slowly corrected whilst avoiding vascular damage.

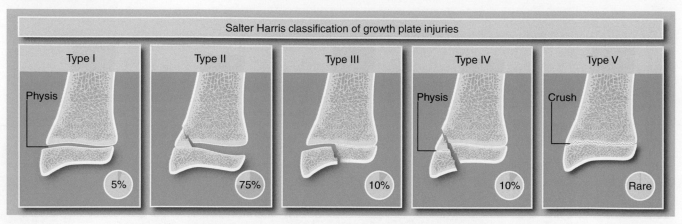

• **Fig. 15.23** Salter Harris Classification of Physis/Epiphysis in Children.

TABLE 15.5	Examples of Injuries Sustained From a Fall Onto an Outstretched Arm/Hand		
Injury	**Usual Age**	**Treatment**	**Outcome**
Fracture clavicle	All ages but mainly 9–16 years	Conservative for children Some adults benefit from plating	Excellent Satisfactory
Elbow lateral condylar	5–8 years	ORIF	Good
Elbow supracondylar	7–11 years	Closed reduction of displaced fractures and K-wires or traction	Satisfactory if well treated. Cubitus varus if poorly treated
Fracture lower radius >16 years Colles fracture Barton (Smith) fracture	10–15 years 60 years and upwards 60 years and upwards	Reduction and splintage. Occasional ORIF Reduction and splintage ORIF if displaced	Excellent Variable, usually good function Variable
Scaphoid fracture	15–30 years	Splintage if undisplaced ORIF if displaced	Good

ORIF, Open reduction and internal fixation.

Nonaccidental Injury

All doctors seeing children with fractures must be aware of possible nonaccidental injury (NAI). With the slightest suspicion of NAI, a paediatrician should become involved. Important signals suggesting NAI are repeat fractures, delays in presentation and where the history does not fit the pattern of injury. Spiral fractures in children not old enough to stand suggest that the child has been swung around by the limb. Transverse fractures of proximal limb bones suggest violent shaking. All children under the age of one with a fracture should be normally admitted to hospital for a full assessment, including a comprehensive history, careful and thorough examination, a radiologic skeletal survey, and where indicated a CT head (for old fractures and subdural haematomas) besides a welfare report from social workers.

Falls on the Outstretched Hand or Arm ('FOOSH' Injury)

Falls on the upper limb fit into distinct patterns, and certain fractures occur in certain age groups (Table 15.5).

Fractured scaphoid —note these carry a high risk of litigation.

These are typically caused by a fall on the outstretched hand in a male between 16 and 30 years old. The wrist will be mildly swollen and there is marked tenderness in the anatomical snuff box. Undisplaced

fractures are not always visible on initial 'scaphoid series' x-rays. If the diagnosis is equivocal, they should still be treated as a fracture. MRI and CT scans are often indicated to clarify the situation.

Undisplaced fractures are treated with splintage and kept under careful observation with serial x-rays. Displaced fractures are usually better treated with ORIF (Fig. 15.24).

Failure to make an early diagnosis and treat effectively can lead to avascular necrosis of the proximal pole of the scaphoid as its blood supply is entirely endosteal, and the vessels become damaged as the bone breaks. This may also lead to early onset wrist osteoarthritis.

Scaphoid fractures can be associated with other, usually major, carpal injuries, such as transscaphoid perilunar dislocation and the initial x-ray must be carefully scrutinised with these injuries in mind.

Other Specific Sites

Pelvic Fractures

Until old age, the pelvis is a very strong structure and only large forces will cause it to fracture. Most major pelvic fractures occur after high impact violence such as occurs in MVAs or when a horse rolls on its fallen rider. If the bony pelvis is disrupted, the soft organs and viscera are also threatened. High energy pelvic fractures often occur along with substantial injuries to the trunk and limbs. The

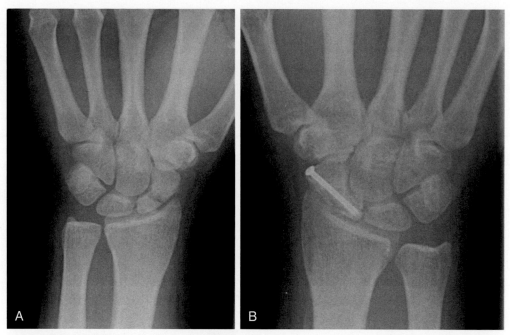

• **Fig. 15.24** (A) X-ray of fractured waist of scaphoid. (B) This was treated with percutaneous compression screw fixation.

bony pelvis is effectively a ring, and disruption depends on there being at least two fractures or joint separations with consequent instability. The pelvis can be crushed in an anteroposterior, lateral or vertical direction or a combination of all three. Life-threatening internal bleeding from arterial or, most importantly, venous injury to the iliac vessels often accompanies pelvic fractures.

Clinical indications of likely pelvic fracture include:

- Haematuria or in males, signs of urethral injury, for example, high-riding prostate on rectal examination, scrotal haematoma or blood at urethral meatus.
- Rectal bleeding, or a large haematoma or palpable fracture line on rectal examination.
- Haematomas of the proximal thigh, above the inguinal ligament, over the perineum or in the flank.
- Neurovascular deficits of lower extremities.

A plain anteroposterior pelvic x-ray reveals 90% of injuries. If a fracture is present or suspected and the patient stable, a pelvic CT scan is the best imaging for pelvic anatomy (including hip dislocation and acetabular fracture) and shows the extent of pelvic, retroperitoneal and intraperitoneal bleeding. Rapid assessment, then urgent resuscitation is often vitally important, followed by temporary stabilisation using a fabric pelvic-binder (http://www.realfirstaid.co.uk/pelvic-sling/) applied in the accident department. This may help arrest or slow the bleeding, but transfusion and angiographic embolisation are likely to be needed.

Osteoporotic fragility fractures of the pelvis are common in the elderly and usually affect either the inferior or superior rami. They do not require specific treatment other than pain relief and early mobilization.

Spinal Fractures

Spinal fractures mostly fall into two groups; acute traumatic and pathological. Numerically the most common fracture is a fragility (crush) fracture in osteoporotic bone, typically in lumbar vertebral bodies in older patients. Up to 90% of patients in their 80s have radiological evidence of a chronic vertebral fragility crush fracture. A simple fall on their backside usually results in such a fracture These cause pain and disability but do not benefit from surgical treatment and take time to

settle. Pathological fractures through metastatic deposits are a common new presentation of a known neoplasm or of an undiagnosed primary.

Nonpathological spinal fractures usually occur with high energy trauma (see Fig. 15.25), but vertebrae can be crushed in healthy adults after a vertical fall from standing height. Any patient suffering sufficient trauma should be assumed to have a spinal injury until proven otherwise. Most attention is directed to the vulnerable cervical spine (see later), but the entire spinal column should be assessed.

The cervical spine may be cleared clinically, without need for radiology, if the following conditions are met:

- patient alert and orientated
- no head injury
- no drugs or alcohol
- no neck pain
- no abnormal neurological signs
- no significant other injury that may distract the patient from complaining about the spine
- **on examination**: no bruising or deformity around the neck, no tenderness and a normal pain-free range of active movement

A cervical spine CT scan should be performed (usually with a CT head) if the criteria are not met. Thoracolumbar spine imaging is indicated if there is pain, bruising, swelling, deformity or abnormal neurological signs attributable to the region. A fracture anywhere in the spine is an indication for full spinal imaging. Unconscious patients cannot be assessed clinically and require **radiological clearance** of the whole spine (i.e., exclusion of injuries). If in doubt, spinal immobilisation devices are left in place, logrolling for movement and high frequency nursing care is continued, while seeking detail about the fracture.

The spine has a key role in structural support and fractures are classified to judge stability. Fractures occur in flexion/extension, compression and/or rotation. Understanding altered vertebral anatomy helps decide whether operation is needed. Damage to the spinal cord or peripheral nerves in the vertebral canal causes catastrophic paralysis. This can occur at the moment of trauma and may be an irretrievable neurological injury, no matter what spinal

CASE HISTORY

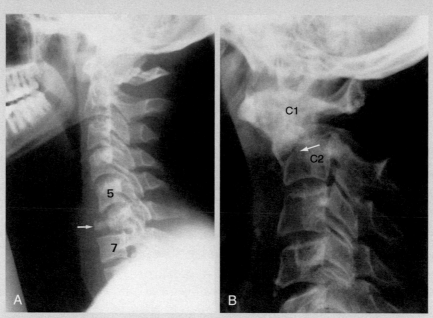

• **Fig. 15.25** Spine Fractures. (A) This 17-year-old boy was admitted semiconscious after crashing his motorcycle and landing head-first in a ditch. On examination, he was tetraplegic and unable to move his upper or lower limbs but could shrug his shoulders. This lateral cervical spine x-ray shows a burst fracture of the body of C6 (arrowed) with fragments in the spinal canal; there is also some posterior subluxation of C5. (B) Left lateral cervical spine x-ray from another unconscious young patient showing a fracture (arrowed) of the body of C2 and severe anterior subluxation of C1.

stabilisation is provided. However, the injured spinal cord can enter a period of spinal shock lasting 24 to 72 hours and sometimes recovery is seen after this. **Spinal shock** is an old term for a period of altered distal function with loss of sphincteric control and reflexes which may result from inadequate tissue perfusion secondary to the spinal injury interrupting autonomic control, leading to bradycardia and hypotension. Management of spinal shock is a period of observation, with protection against pressure ulcers and urinary retention, until the spinal cord settles to a stable state of injury, with neurological deficits at and distal to the level of injury Severe spinal cord injuries above C5 usually cause instant death.

Ankle Fractures (Fig. 15.26)

These are common in all age groups except young children. Many only involve the lateral malleolus, and if undisplaced, heal well with a splint or a "walking" plaster When there is displacement of the Talus, fracture of both malleolae ORIF is indicated. Most ankle fractures are caused by a combination of forced inversion or eversion plus rotation. If these are intraarticular fractures, there is a risk of secondary arthritis, unless they heal precisely, anatomically.

Fractured Calcaneum

This occurs with falls from a height on to a hard surface. A window cleaner falling from a ladder would be a perfect candidate for this injury. Concomitant fractures of either the spine, hips or upper tibia are common in patients with bilateral calcaneal fractures and need to be carefully excluded, bearing in mind their symptoms may be masked by the severe pain that calcaneal fractures cause. Several classifications are in use but if the fracture is extensive, displaced and involving the subtalar joint, the prognosis is poor in terms of function and wearing normal shoes. The results of surgical treatment have been generally disappointing. Elevation to reduce the enormous swelling and good analgesia are the mainstays of treatment.

Upper Limb Fractures

Upper Humerus

These fractures typically occurs in elderly females who fall on their shoulder (Fig. 15.27). They are often very painful. Many can be managed conservatively with a body bandage and a collar and cuff until they are comfortable but, with only one useful arm they will need support in their activities of daily living. A few require surgery. To regain function most will require physiotherapy.

Olecranon Fractures

These result from a fall on the elbow and are complicated by the triceps muscle causing the fracture to displace (Fig. 15.28). Most will require ORIF.

Metacarpal and Phalangeal Fractures

Vary between minimally displaced fractures of phalanges sustained in ball games (usually treated by strapping to the adjacent finger or 'buddy' strapping), to crushed hands inflicted by industrial machines. ORIF is occasionally indicated but the most important early treatment is reducing the swelling (using ice and elevation) and early mobilisation under the guidance of a therapist.

Isolated fractures of the fifth metacarpal are usually diagnosed in young men who have misguidedly thrown a punch and caught a hard object on the side of their clenched fist. Whilst they may always have a slight cosmetic deformity in the region of the fifth metacarpal neck for the rest of their lives, function will almost certainly return to normal within a few weeks without no more than a temporary splint and analgesia.

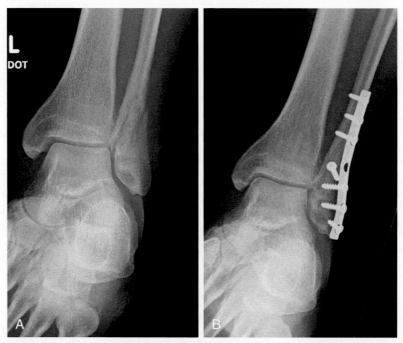

• **Fig 15.26** (A) X-ray of lateral malleolus fracture. (B) treated with open reduction and internal fixation with one interfragmentary compression screw and a contoured neutralisation plate.

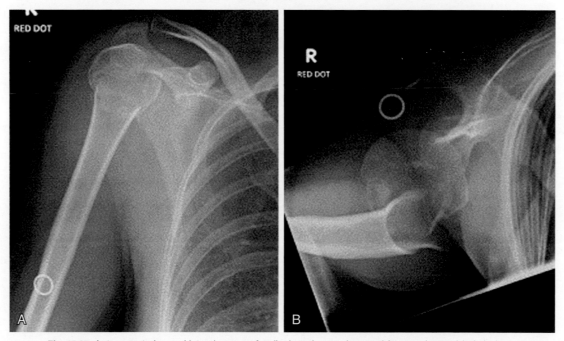

• **Fig. 15.27** Anteroposterior and lateral x-rays of a displaced upper humeral fracture in an elderly lady.

Dislocations and Subluxations

A dislocation is when the surfaces that make up a joint completely separate. A subluxation is when there is partial separation of the surfaces of the joint. Trauma is the most common cause but once the soft tissues, that normally hold the joint together, have been damaged, the joint may easily dislocate again. This is **recurrent dislocation**.

Dislocations can also be congenital, as in the hip, and can occur in neuromuscular conditions, such as cerebral palsy (see paediatric orthopaedic section). **Habitual subluxation or dislocation** is usually associated with a bony or soft tissue abnormality and occurs whenever a particular position in joint movement is reached.

Examples of Dislocation

Shoulder

Two types of dislocation occur: glenohumeral and acromioclavicular. The much commoner glenohumeral dislocation is **anterior**, whilst **posterior** dislocations are usually associated with **electricity,** such as in electrocution, electroconvulsive therapy and epileptic fits.

Anterior Glenohumeral Dislocation

Is usually caused by a fall on an abducted arm, often during contact sports (Fig. 15.29). The axillary nerve and sometimes the brachial plexus are at risk and a careful neurological assessment is essential. Closed reduction is achieved under anaesthesia by the Hippocratic or the Kocher manoeuvre.

Warnings: in older people the dislocation may be associated with upper humeral fracture which might be difficult to see and open reduction should be anticipated. Posterior dislocations are often missed in accident departments.

Acromioclavicular Subluxations and Dislocations

Occur after a fall on the point of the shoulder. One of your authors did his, landing on his shoulder on hard ground scoring a rugby try. It was painful for 6 months, but not so severe it needed surgery. Complete dislocations usually need relocating and the soft tissues repairing.

Hip Dislocations

Most traumatic dislocations of the hip are posterior (Fig. 15.30). Typically, the patient has been in a high impact motor vehicle collision, with the flexed hip forced out of the back of the acetabulum,

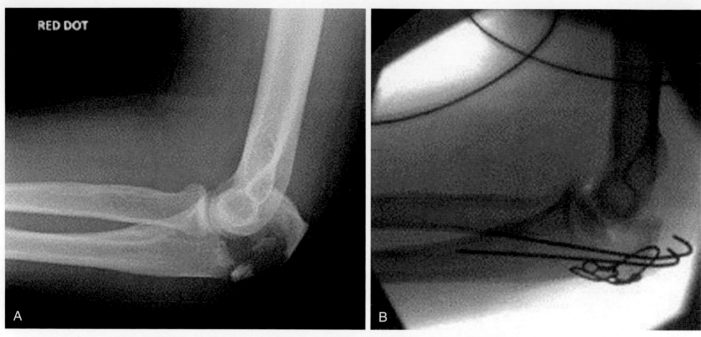

• **Fig. 15.28** X-rays of fracture olecranon treated with open reduction and internal fixation.

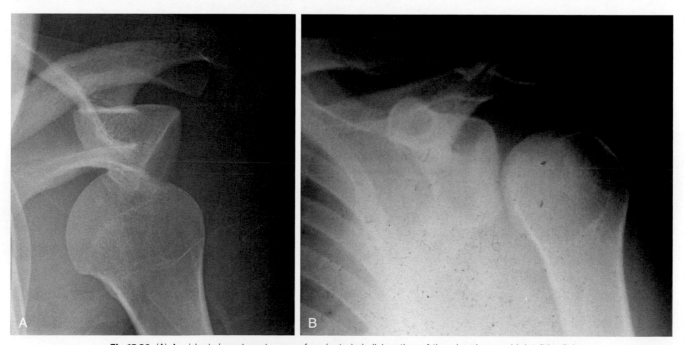

• **Fig 15.29** (A) Accident department x-ray of an (anterior) dislocation of the glenohumeral joint ('the light bulb sign'). (B) X-ray of a posterior infraglenoid dislocation of the glenohumeral joint.

often with a fracture of the posterior wall. The sciatic nerve can be permanently damaged and there is substantial risk of avascular necrosis of the femoral head, particularly if the dislocation is not reduced within a few hours.

Knee Dislocations

When you hear of someone "dislocating their knee" it is usually the patella rather than the main joint that has dislocated. In patients who suffer traumatic patella dislocation (Fig. 15.31A), there is often a minor underlying congenital abnormality. Ninety-five percent dislocate laterally and many spontaneously reduce when the knee is straightened. Conservative treatment is usually adequate but surgery will be required if dislocation becomes recurrent.

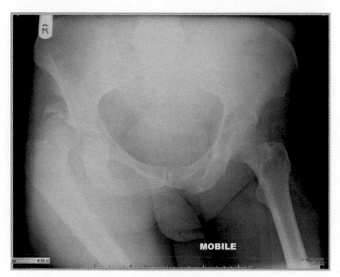

• **Fig. 15.30** X-ray showing a posterior dislocation of the right hip with an associated posterior acetabular wall fracture. This was treated with open reduction and open reduction and internal fixation.

Complete dislocations of the knee occur when there has been sufficient trauma to rupture both collateral and cruciate ligaments (Fig. 15.31B). The popliteal artery and nerves are at risk in this injury.

Initial Management of Fractures in Polytrauma Victims: Damage Control (Also See Chapter 5)

After the initial ABC regimen in a polytrauma victim has been completed, injuries other than appendicular skeleton fractures need to be prioritised.

Damage control fracture management means stabilising fractures to reduce pain and bleeding and is achieved with splints (including plaster back slabs), traction and increasingly, external fixators that can be applied under local or a short general anaesthetic.

The patient can then be managed and supported for the next 48 to 72 hours in a high dependency setting, whilst the physiological 'storm' is optimised and plans made for definitive fracture treatment by surgeons with appropriate skills. The patient needs to be regularly reassessed during this time to make sure there are no further injuries and complications overlooked initially.

Ligament Injuries

Very few people must go through life without spraining an ankle. The lateral ligament is damaged when the patient forcibly inverts or twists their hind foot on an uneven surface. Initially, patients can often weight bear but as the swelling builds up walking becomes difficult.

Other sites typically associated with 'sprains' include the medial side of the knee and wrist. Most sprains represent partial ligamentous tears and they, given time, heal without intervention.

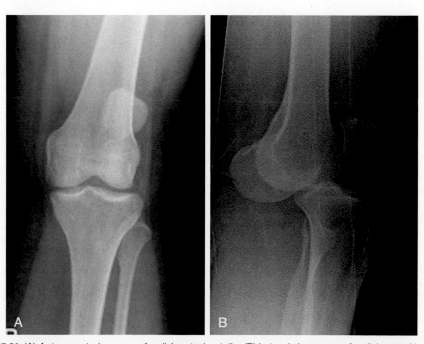

• **Fig. 15.31** (A) Anteroposterior x-ray of a dislocated patella. (B) Lateral view x-ray of a dislocated knee—a very severe injury.

More Serious Ligamentous Injuries

A simple ankle sprain usually means the anterior talofibular ligament is partially torn but if the injuring force is substantial, the whole lateral ligamentous structure can rupture. This leads to an unstable joint (see section on *ankle orthopaedics*) which needs reconstruction. At presentation, these patients cannot put any weight through the limb and there is enormous swelling and bruising. Initially they are treated along standard lines with a splint or cast. Only if a rehabilitation programme fails are they assessed for reconstruction.

Ligamentous injuries around the knee can range from minor sprains of the medial ligament to rupture of the medial, anterior cruciate and even posterior cruciate ligament they are associated with significant violence. They need to be dealt with by a specialist knee surgeon.

Ligamentous injuries around the wrist range from severe intra-carpal ligament ruptures to minor collateral ligament sprains. All too often, undisplaced fractures of the scaphoid have been misdiagnosed as a wrist sprain, with serious consequences.

Muscle Injuries

Pulled muscles are common in sports players. Even the most severe rupture is rarely treated surgically, unless there is also bony avulsion. MRI scanning makes it possible to confirm a tear and assess its magnitude which helps manage a patient's expectations.

With sports people, the commonest muscle to be torn is a hamstring, torn from the ischium. Whilst running, jumping or in some way overstretching their 'ham', the patient notices a sudden severe pain, which stops them in their tracks. They will often say they felt it go.

Partial or complete rupture of the **rectus femoris** is less common and is often sustained whilst kicking. It is painful and recovery takes a long time. There is rarely any point in surgically joining the torn ends as the patient usually ends up with a fully functioning limb with time but without any intervention. They will be left with a dent in the anterior thigh as a memento.

Calcification in a muscle can occur after a severe bruise and presents with a hard and tender lump with associated stiffness of the distal joint. The question of malignancy may arise but the history and an ultrasound or MRI scan will allay such concern.

16

Head and Maxillofacial Injuries

CHAPTER OUTLINE

Head Injuries

Introduction

Head injury with traumatic brain injury (TBI) is the most common cause of death and disability in people aged 1 to 40 years in the United Kingdom. Head injuries cause about 3500 deaths each year in the United Kingdom, amounting to about 0.6% of all deaths. Even in survivors, there may be devastating problems, which have an enormous social and economic cost. Head injuries are a common reason for patients to attend an emergency department with 431,000 attendances in the United Kingdom in 2017 (Fig. 16.1). Using the Glasgow Coma Scale (GCS, Table 16.1) as a clinical indicator, 90% are classified as minor (score of 13–15), 5% as moderate (score 9–12) and 5% as severe (score 3–8). Improving care of head-injured patients depends on prompt triage, appropriate resuscitation, ready access to computed tomography (CT) scanning, safe and rapid transfer to neurosurgery units if needed, and availability of specialist critical care. Less than half the head injury patients attending emergency departments require hospital admission or CT scanning and only a small proportion require specialist neurosurgical investigation and care. To streamline this process, various triage algorithms have been produced, notably National Institute for Health and Care Excellence (NICE) guideline CG56, https://www.nice.org.uk/guidance/CG56 (summarised in Box 16.4). The main focus is detecting clinically important brain injuries (and cervical spine injuries—Box 16.1), whilst avoiding admission of those with low risk of sequelae.

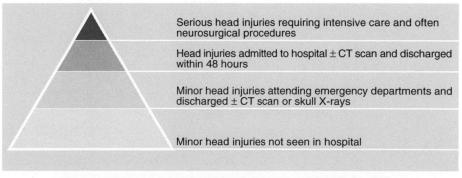

• **Fig. 16.1** Workload Caused by Head Injuries. *CT*, Computed tomography.

Pathophysiology of Traumatic Brain Injury

TBIs can be divided into **primary injury**, arising from the initial trauma, and **secondary brain injury** which evolves later. Treatment cannot reverse the primary brain injury but aims to minimise adverse sequelae. Secondary brain injury is mostly caused by raised intracranial pressure (ICP, from intracranial haematoma or brain swelling), hypoglycaemia, ischaemia or hypoxia; all are amenable to prophylactic measures and/or timely intervention.

At the cellular level, brain injury disrupts the neuronal cytoskeleton, which can lead to irreversible axonal injury in only a few hours. High levels of glutamate accumulate extracellularly, damaging neighbouring cells and causing a ripple effect of neuronal death and release of further toxic molecules. Potential neuroprotective agents, such as glutamate and calcium antagonists have so far proved ineffective.

The brain has minimal capacity to regenerate after injury but in general, the younger the patient, the better the prognosis. Young children can make remarkable functional recovery despite severe injuries because of the plasticity of the developing nervous system. However, some will suffer high-level cognitive impairment ('executive dysfunction') in their late teens from failure of frontal maturation. In adults, the primary injury consequences are likely to be more severe with advancing age. One factor here is that the brain atrophies, allowing greater mobility of the brain within the cranial vault under impact.

Primary Brain Injury

Concussion

Concussion is a brain injury associated with brief loss of consciousness, typically for only a few minutes. It causes minor cognitive disturbances, such as temporary confusion or amnesia. By definition, there are no persisting abnormal neurological signs although some patients may report long-term symptoms, such as headache, impaired concentration, poor short-term memory and altered affect (postconcussion syndrome, see later under rehabilitation).

Diffuse Axonal Injury

Diffuse axonal injury (DAI) typically follows large rotational acceleration and deceleration forces, causing widespread damage to axonal tracts. DAI involves microscopic tissue damage and so imaging may appear normal. Abnormalities are seen best on magnetic resonance imaging (MRI), which demonstrates haemosiderin deposition at the junctions of deep grey and white matter, within white matter tracts, or in the basal ganglia. This type of injury does not usually lead to raised ICP. Treatment is supportive. These injuries have a high mortality, and may later produce substantial cognitive impairment and personality change, with or without physical neurodisability.

Focal Brain Injuries

Focal injuries result from trauma to localised brain areas and are readily visible on CT scans. The site and extent of the primary injury depend on the nature of the damaging force (Fig. 16.2). The main lesions are cerebral contusion, laceration or haematoma, all of which can act as space-occupying lesions with a potential for secondary brain injury. Contusions may be small or large and occur beneath the area of impact (**coup**) or contralateral to it (**contre-coup**), caused by rebound of the brain within the skull at the time of impact (see Fig. 16.3). Serious trauma is needed to cause focal brain injury and hence usually results in a period of loss of consciousness followed by confusion.

TABLE 16.1	Glasgow Coma Scale (GCS)
Clinical Observation	**Score[a]**
Eye Opening	
Spontaneous	4
To verbal command	3
To pain	2
None	1
Motor Response	
Obeys commands	6
Localises pain	5
Flexion withdrawal to pain	4
Abnormal flexion (decorticate)	3
Extension to pain (decerebrate)	2
None	1
Verbal Response	
Orientated	5
Confused conversation	4
Inappropriate words	3
Incomprehensible words	2
None	1

[a]On this scale, a patient's Glasgow Coma score is the sum of the scores from all three sections. The worst total score is 3, the best is 15. After the initial score, the observations and scoring are repeated at intervals to assess for deterioration.

> **• BOX 16.1** **National Institute for Health and Care Excellence (NICE) Guidelines for Assessing Cervical Spine Injuries**

Indications for Immediate CT or 3-View X-Ray Imaging of Cervical Spine

- Patient unable to actively rotate neck 45 degrees to left and right
- Not possible to test range of movement in neck
- Patients with neck pain or tenderness aged 65 years or more, or who have suffered a dangerous mechanism of injury

Immediate CT Imaging of the Cervical Spine is Indicated as Follows

- GCS <13 on initial assessment
- The patient has been intubated
- The patient is being scanned for polytrauma
- Where x-ray is not possible or technically inadequate
- Where x-ray is definitely abnormal or suspicious
- If clinical suspicion remains despite a normal x-ray study

CT, Computed tomography; *GCS*, Glasgow Coma Scale.

Secondary Brain Injury

Secondary brain injury can be caused by cerebral hypoxia, intracranial bleeding or infection.

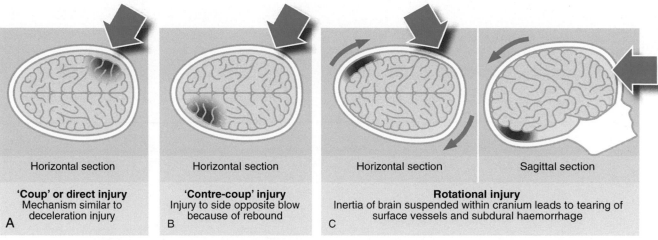

• **Fig. 16.2** Mechanisms of Brain Injury. **(A)** The mechanism of 'coup' or direct injury is similar to a deceleration injury (shown in horizontal section). **(B)** A 'contre-coup' injury affects the side opposite to the blow because of rebound (horizontal section). **(C)** In rotational injury, the inertia of the brain suspended within the cranium leads to the tearing of surface vessels and subdural haemorrhage (horizontal and sagittal sections).

CASE HISTORY

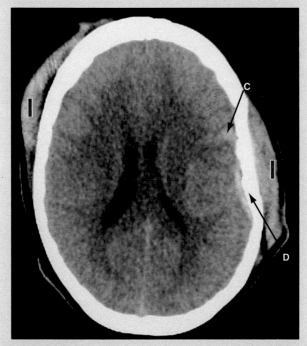

• **Fig. 16.3** Focal Brain Injury. A cyclist was knocked off his bike by a car and suffered a head injury with loss of consciousness of 45 minutes. Computed tomography scan of head shows signs of soft tissue injury *(I)*, in both left temporal ('coup') and right frontoparietal regions ('contre-coup'). There is a depressed segment of skull bone in the left temporal region *(D)* and signs of intracerebral contusion *(C)* beneath both areas of injury. He gradually recovered without need for operation, but full cerebral functional recovery took several months.

Cerebral Hypoxia

Ischaemia and hypoxia are central to most secondary mechanisms of brain injury, and lead to **cellular energy failure**. Hypoxia causes cerebral oedema, which in turn causes a secondary **rise in ICP** risking further ischaemia. Common causes of hypoxia are airway obstruction in reduced GCS, alcohol or drug overdose, chest injury, inhalational pneumonitis, acute respiratory distress syndrome or central respiratory depression. **Hypotension** caused by hypovolaemia contributes to cerebral hypoxia by reducing cerebral perfusion. Resuscitation aims to prevent or treat hypoxia and hypovolaemia.

Intracranial Haemorrhage

Posttraumatic intracranial bleeding is classified into **extradural** (epidural), **subdural**, **intracerebral** or **subarachnoid** (Fig. 16.4). Intracranial bleeding acts as a mass lesion causing a general rise in ICP, whilst local brain compression can cause focal neurological deficits.

Extradural Haemorrhage

Extradural haemorrhage occurs when blood accumulates in the space between dura and calvarium of the skull. It is most common in children and younger adults because their dura is less adherent to the skull. Most have a fracture, usually in the temporal or parietal region (Fig. 16.5). Almost 90% are caused by rupture of an artery, usually the middle meningeal or a branch running inferior to the temporal region. This normally results in a **loss of consciousness** immediately following injury. In up to half the patients, this is followed by a **lucid interval**, with no symptoms other than worsening headache. This is followed by **deteriorating conscious level**. Temporal lobe herniation then leads to compression of the third nerve and **pupillary dilatation**. Death quickly follows unless the haematoma is evacuated rapidly. Emergency CT scanning is indicated to confirm the diagnosis and show its position (typically a lentiform-shaped clot—Fig. 16.5B). Urgent transfer to a neurosurgeon for evacuation of the clot is the ideal course of action.

Subdural Haematoma

Subdural haematoma usually results from tearing of veins passing between cerebral cortex and dura, or from injury to vessels on the brain surface. Blood accumulates in the large potential space between dura mater and arachnoid mater and the haematoma tends to spread laterally over a wide area (Fig. 16.6). In contrast to extradural haemorrhage, there is usually underlying primary brain injury. Acute subdural haemorrhage is more common in older adults because the brain is more mobile within the cranial cavity.

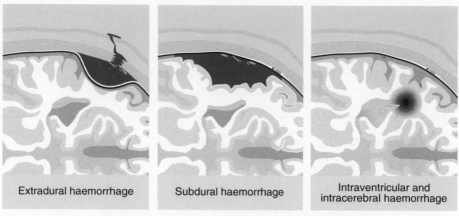

Extradural haemorrhage

Subdural haemorrhage

Intraventricular and intracerebral haemorrhage

• **Fig. 16.4** Types of Posttraumatic Intracranial Bleeding.

CASE HISTORY

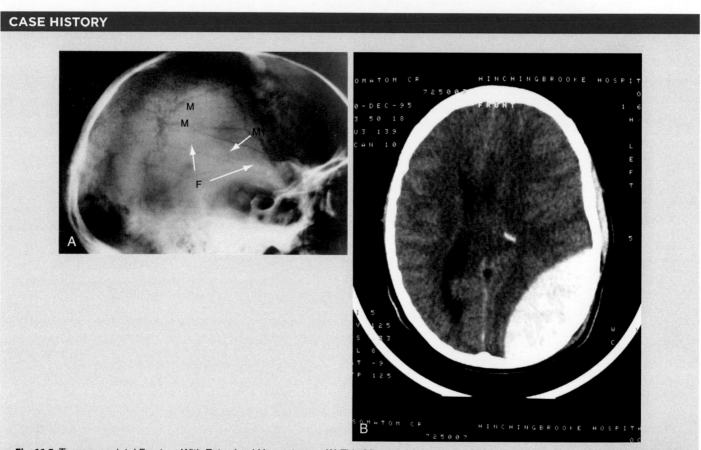

• **Fig. 16.5** Temporoparietal Fracture With Extradural Haematoma. **(A)** This 20-year-old man was admitted fully conscious after being knocked off a bicycle but deteriorated rapidly 2 hours later. Lateral skull x-ray showing a linear fracture *(arrowed 'F')* of the right temporoparietal bones crossing the course of the anterior branch of the middle meningeal artery *(M)* on the temporal bone. **(B)** Classical computed tomography appearance of extradural haematoma.

In **acute subdural** haemorrhage, there is usually clinical evidence of brain injury at the outset. A lucid interval is rare, except where the pathology is tearing of a bridging vein. Evacuation of an acute subdural haematoma cannot be achieved via burr holes because the blood is clotted. Surgical evacuation via craniotomy may halt deterioration but recovery is often incomplete because of the underlying brain injury. With increasing use of anticoagulation and antiplatelet therapy, acute subdural haematoma is now seen more after relatively inconsequential injury, particularly in the elderly.

Chronic Subdural Haematoma

In the elderly, subdural haematomas may develop gradually following trivial, often unrecalled, head trauma. This is caused by the relative ease with which atrophic brains can accommodate blood under venous pressure. The condition

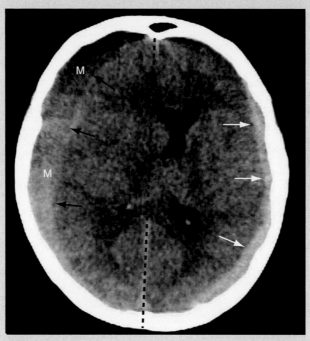

• **Fig. 16.6** Subdural Haematoma. An elderly man suffered a head injury in a road traffic collision without loss of consciousness 48 hours previously. His conscious level gradually deteriorated and so this computed tomography scan was performed. On the right side, there is a large subdural haematoma of mixed attenuation *(M)*, (*black arrows* define the edge of the brain). Such mixed attenuation suggests old liquefying thrombus and is consistent with its origin around the time of the accident. There is a smaller subdural haematoma on the left side *(white arrows)* of consistent attenuation suggesting that it arose more recently. Note the midline of the brain is shifted to the left by the mass effect of the larger haematoma and there is compression of the lateral ventricles. The patient required neurosurgical drainage.

only manifests some weeks or months later as the clot lyses and fluid is drawn into the subdural space by osmosis. Symptoms are nonspecific neurological deterioration, chronic headache or coma. At this point the liquid haematoma can be evacuated via burr holes, and the subdural space irrigated with warm saline.

Intracerebral Haemorrhage

Haemorrhage into the brain parenchyma is caused by primary brain injury. Multiple small deep lesions are often associated with DAI. Small haematomas should be managed conservatively and monitored for expansion using serial CT scans. A larger haematoma causing 'mass effect' should be evacuated early to prevent secondary brain damage.

Infection

Early debridement of compound depressed fractures is important so as to minimise the risk of infection. Prophylactic antibiotics are not indicated except in contaminated wounds. There is no evidence in favour of prophylactic antibiotics in cases of cerebrospinal fluid (CSF) leakage.

Skull Fractures

A skull fracture is a measure of impact severity. Consequently, patients with fractures are much more likely to sustain primary brain damage, and to suffer secondary brain injury by the mechanisms described earlier. Depressed fractures are often associated with injury to the underlying brain. With the advent of NICE

guidelines (Box 16.2), CT is the investigation of choice for the diagnosis of clinically significant head injury.

Linear Fractures

These involve mainly the skull vault, often with little external sign of injury, although there may be some scalp bruising or swelling. Linear fractures rarely exhibit displacement unless there are multiple fracture lines. Linear fractures appear as lucent lines on imaging.

Depressed Fractures

These are usually caused by blunt injuries (Fig. 16.7A). The overlying scalp is usually lacerated or severely bruised. Such fractures rarely produce serious primary brain injury unless they are depressed more than the full thickness of the skull vault. Elevation of closed depressed fractures is usually performed for cosmetic reasons or if there are significant focal deficits.

Open (Compound) Fractures

An open fracture indicates a communication exists between brain and the external environment. This may be overt (e.g., a penetrating injury), or result from a skull base fracture. Linear and depressed skull fractures can both be open. There is a high risk of infection in a depressed fracture if the dura is torn, so early debridement and dural closure are indicated. Prophylactic antibiotics are indicated in these cases. Compound fractures of the skull base are diagnosed clinically (Box 16.3) with or without CT. Fluid may be analysed for beta transferrin, which is present in CSF but not in plasma.

National Institute for Health and Care Excellence (NICE) Criteria for Computed Tomography Scan

General Principles

- First stabilise airways, breathing and circulation (ABC)
- Immediately clinically assess patients with a GCS below 15
- If GCS is 8 or less, involve anaesthetist for airway management and resuscitation
- Perform early CT imaging where appropriate to detect brain and cervical spine injuries (skull x-rays + inpatient observation where CT unavailable)
- Exclude brain injury before attributing depressed conscious level to intoxication
- No systemic analgesia until assessed for conscious level and neurological deficit (local anaesthesia for fractured limbs/other painful injuries)
- Record observations on a standard head injury proforma (paediatric chart for under 16s)

Indications for Head CT Within 1 Hour in Adults

- GCS less than 13 at any time since injury
- GCS <15 at 2 hours after injury
- Suspected skull fracture, open or depressed, including signs of basal skull fracture (haemotympanum, 'panda' eyes, cerebrospinal fluid otorrhoea, Battle sign—see Box 16.3)
- Posttraumatic seizure
- Focal neurological deficit
- More than one episode of vomiting
- Coagulopathy

Indications for Head CT Within 8 Hours in Adults if the 1-Hour Criteria do not Apply

- Retrograde amnesia (i.e., for events before impact) of more than 30 minutes
- Any loss of consciousness or amnesia plus:
  — Age 65 years or more
  — Dangerous mechanism of injury (e.g., pedestrian struck by motor vehicle, occupant ejected from a motor vehicle or fall from more than 1 metre or five stairs)

CT, Computed tomography; *GCS,* Glasgow Coma Scale.

Basal Skull Fractures

These usually involve the anterior skull base (frontal/ethmoidal or sphenoidal air sinuses) or the middle cranial fossa (petrous temporal bone). They should be suspected if the features in Box 16.3 are present.

Management of Head Injuries

Clinical Assessment

In a neurosurgical emergency, the aim is to treat life-threatening injuries first and all other injuries in order of priority so as to reduce further harm and prevent secondary brain injury. Assessment is divided into a primary and secondary survey but a history may be available in advance from paramedics or from the patient or relatives on arrival.

History

The most important factors indicating potential brain injury and risk of future complications are **unconsciousness,** and amnesia for events before the impact (**retrograde amnesia**).

The duration of unconsciousness and amnesia are roughly proportional to the severity of brain injury. If the patient was travelling in a motor vehicle, the extent of injuries to other passengers may give an indication of the energy transfer in the accident. Likewise, knowing the use of seatbelts and helmets can be useful.

Examination

Primary Survey Using Standard Advanced Trauma Life Support (ATLS) Protocols

A—Airway and cervical spine immobilisation

The airway should be checked for signs of obstruction and appropriate measures taken.

If cervical spine injury is suspected, this should be immobilised using a semirigid collar.

B—Breathing

Assess respiratory function and oxygen requirements.

C—Circulation

Assess haemodynamic stability—capillary refill, blood pressure and heart rate.

D—Disability

- Assess pupil size and reactivity.
- Assess responsiveness. If level of consciousness is reduced, a GCS evaluation should be made (see Table 16.1). With a GCS <8, the ability to maintain an adequate airway is impaired and intubation and ventilation should be considered.

E—Exposure

Expose the patient fully and perform a log roll (with cervical spine immobilisation if indicated) to assess for further injuries.

Specific Clinical Examination for Head Injury Patients

Observations should be recorded periodically on a standard head injury proforma (e.g., http://www.leicspart.nhs.uk/Library/NeurologicalAssessmentandObservations.pdf), and the GCS (see Table 16.1) calculated each time. If there is a deep scalp laceration or a history of penetrating injury, the scalp should be assessed carefully for the presence of a bony defect or step which may not lie directly beneath the scalp wound.

1. Level of Consciousness

This is the most important single observation in head injury patients. The GCS (see Table 16.1) is used worldwide to standardise assessment and monitoring of head injuries. Level of consciousness can be categorised simply and reproducibly by this method. Formal assessment should take place after resuscitation and before intubation if possible. Aggressive behaviour in a patient smelling of alcohol or having taken illicit drugs must **not** be assumed to result from intoxication (i.e., removal of social inhibition) because this behaviour can also be a manifestation of brain injury or hypoxia. A thorough examination should be performed to exclude significant cerebral injury. In addition to eye opening and verbal responses, the motor response is an important observation. In a patient with impaired conscious level, pressure over the supraorbital nerve at the orbital rim is usually used to elicit pain. To be scored as able to localise the pain, the patient's hand should rise above the clavicle.

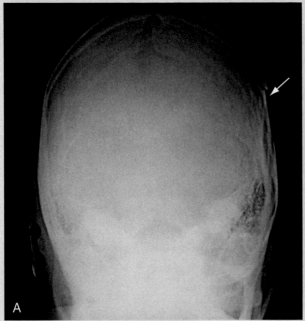

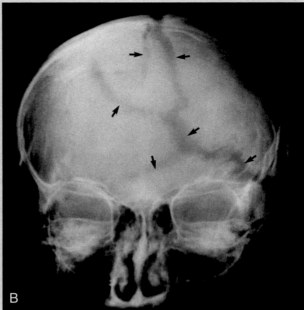

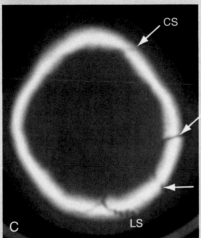

• **Fig. 16.7** Standard Skull X-Ray Views and Computed Tomography (CT) Scan Showing Skull Fractures. **(A)** Towne view from a 19-year-old woman after a blunt blow to the side of the head; she was fully conscious. This shows a depressed fracture in the left parietal bone *(arrowed)*. The segment of bone is depressed by more than the thickness of the skull and therefore needed surgically elevating. **(B)** This 24-year-old woman suffered a high-impact speed road traffic accident and was admitted to hospital deeply unconscious and with deep scalp lacerations. Her Glasgow Coma Scale was 5. This anteroposterior x-ray shows extensive fractures *(arrowed)* in the parietal, occipital and squamous temporal bones. Because of the lacerations, these fractures were considered compound. **(C)** CT scan of the upper part of the skull vault in a different patient after a road traffic collision showing a normal coronal suture *(CS)*. There are parietal fractures *(arrowed)* and diastasis *(partial separation)* of the lambdoid suture *(LS)*.

The severity of the head injury can be assessed by the elicited GCS following resuscitation. The probability of there being an intracranial haematoma likely to need surgery in different GCS groups is shown in Table 16.2.

2. Pupil Size and Reactivity

Pupillary **size** and **response to light** should be assessed, along with the full range of eye movements and, if possible, visual fields. Normal pupillary size and response to light require the integrity of both second and third cranial nerves. Pupillary changes are a late indicator of developing intracranial hypertension (Table 16.3). However, benign pupil asymmetry is relatively common in the population and it is important to consider this in conjunction with deteriorating conscious level.

3. Limb Movements and Responses

In a fully conscious patient, tone, power and coordination can be readily assessed. If a subtle abnormality is suspected, the patient should be asked to close the eyes and hold the arms outstretched with palms upwards. Pronation or downward drift on one side indicates brain injury. For the semiconscious or unconscious patient, the pattern of limb response to painful stimuli provides a useful indication of the conscious level, that is, normal is flexion whilst extension is abnormal.

• BOX 16.3   Clinical Signs of a Fracture of the Skull Base

A basal skull fracture provides a potential route for cerebral infection. Prophylactic antibiotics against meningitis are given for 7 days, or until 7 days after any cerebrospinal fluid (CSF) leak has ceased.

Anterior Fossa Fractures

- Periorbital haematomas (see Fig. 16.13)—usually bilateral 'panda eyes' and limited by the margins of the orbicularis oculi.
- Subconjunctival haemorrhage (see Fig. 16.13)—the blood tracks from behind forward and therefore no posterior limit can be seen (unlike localised subconjunctival haematomas that result from direct trauma).
- CSF rhinorrhoea—clear fluid running from the nose caused by damage to the cribriform plate. Anosmia (loss of sense of smell) is common. Dural repair likely to be required.

Middle Fossa Fractures, That Is, Involving Petrous Temporal Bone

- CSF otorrhoea—clear fluid running from the ear via a torn tympanic membrane. Repair not usually required.
- Bruising over the mastoid area behind the ear (Battle sign); may take 24–48 hours to develop.

• BOX 16.4   National Institute for Health and Care Excellence (NICE) Criteria for Admission to Hospital Following a Head Injury Where CT is Available, and Criteria Have Been Followed

- New and clinically significant abnormalities found on imaging
- GCS has not returned to 15 after imaging, regardless of imaging results
- When CT scanning is indicated but cannot be done within the appropriate period
- Continuing worrying signs, for example, persistent vomiting, severe headache
- Other sources of concern, for example, drug or alcohol intoxication, other injuries, shock, suspected nonaccidental injury, meningism or cerebrospinal fluid leak from nose or ear

CT, Computed tomography; *GCS,* Glasgow Coma Scale.

TABLE 16.2   Probability of Intracranial Haematoma Requiring Surgery According to the Severity of Head Injury as Assessed by the Glasgow Coma Scale (GCS)

GCS Score	Severity of Head Injury	Probability of Haematoma
3–8	Severe	1 in 7
9–12	Moderate	1 in 50
13–14	Mild	1 in 3500

TABLE 16.3   Significance of Pupillary Changes in Head Injury

Pupil Finding	Potential Significance
Unilateral, dilated pupil	1. Tentorial herniation caused by raised intracranial pressure (usually ipsilateral to the side of injury but may be a false localising sign) 2. Direct ocular damage—often associated with hyphaema (bleeding into anterior chamber)
Bilaterally dilated pupil, unreactive to light	Severe brainstem dysfunction
Pinpoint pupils	Primary brainstem injury or drug-induced

Secondary Survey

Once the patient has been adequately resuscitated and is haemodynamically stable, a detailed history and thorough physical examination is undertaken. In neurosurgery, symptoms to explore would be unconsciousness, amnesia, limb or facial weakness and paraesthesia. A systematic neurological examination including cranial nerves and upper and lower limbs should be performed, as well as a general head-to-toe examination.

Imaging for Suspected Head Injuries

The published NICE guidelines for head and cervical spine imaging are summarised in Box 16.2.

Practical Management of Head Injuries

Management of Moderate and Severe Head Injuries

Most trauma deaths result from head injuries or from multiple injuries involving chest, abdomen and limbs. Some head injuries are so severe as to preclude survival, whilst others require urgent recognition and surgical decompression, for example, extradural haemorrhage. The report of the Working Party on Head Injuries (Society of British Neurological Surgeons, 1998) recommended a maximum delay of 4 hours between the injury and neurosurgical intervention.

Secondary avoidable deaths from head injury relate to inadequate ventilation and resuscitation. This leads to hypoxaemia, hypercarbia and cerebral swelling, compounding the rising ICP. If patients are combative or severely agitated, there may be a need for general anaesthesia to enable control of partial pressure of carbon dioxide (PCO_2).

Initial Management

Any patient with focal neurological signs, whose conscious level is moderately depressed (GCS 14 or less) or who is unconscious, must be considered to have a significant head injury. Patients should be resuscitated along ATLS guidelines, focusing on secondary brain injury prevention, prioritisation of other injuries and the timing of CT scanning. Patients requiring urgent neurosurgery should be transferred to a specialist centre promptly, but only after adequate resuscitation.

Early Management

The most important factors that indicate potential brain injury and risk of future complications are **unconsciousness** and amnesia for events before the impact (**retrograde amnesia**). The duration of unconsciousness and amnesia are roughly proportional to the severity of brain injury.

Patients with a GCS of 15 and no risk factors requiring inpatient observation (alcohol intoxication, etc.) can be discharged safely to the care of a responsible adult with standard head injury advice. Patients with risk factors (Box 16.4) requiring admission should be observed in a ward with experience in managing head injuries. Patients with worrying presentations may require early CT scanning as per NICE guidelines.

TABLE 16.4	Essential Observations for Head Injury Patients (Findings Should Be Recorded on a Standard Head Injury Proforma)
Observation	**Sign of Neurological Deterioration**
Conscious level (GCS)	Falling score
Pupil size and light response	Dilatation, loss of light reaction or developing asymmetry
Respiratory pattern and rate	Irregularity, slowing or reduced depth of breathing
Developing neurological signs	Focal signs point to localised intracranial damage
Pulse rate	Falling pulse rate (late sign)
Blood pressure	Rising blood pressure (late sign)

GCS, Glasgow Coma Scale.

A patient with a suspected head injury should have frequent neurological observations (Table 16.4). These include GCS assessments, general observations (pulse rate, blood pressure, respiration rate) and noting of any worrying symptoms (i.e., visual disturbance, vomiting, severe headache). Together, these are sensitive enough to give early warning of developing complications. The frequency of observation depends on the state of the patient. If there is a skull fracture or any suggestion of reduced consciousness, confusion, disorientation, alcohol or drug effects, observations should be made at 30-minute intervals until a GCS of 15 is maintained, then hourly for 4 hours, then 2 hourly after that. Any deterioration noted should warrant urgent medical review. Note that transient unconsciousness or amnesia with full recovery is not necessarily an indication for admission of an adult, but may be so in a child, and patients with head injuries may have other serious internal injuries that are easily overlooked.

The care of all patients with new, surgically significant abnormalities on imaging should be discussed urgently with a neurosurgeon and, where possible, the imaging linked electronically. A report on management of head injuries by the Society of British Neurological Surgeons in 1998 recommended a maximum delay of 4 hours between injury and neurosurgical intervention. Other criteria for neurosurgical referral include:

- persisting coma (GCS less than or equal to 8) after resuscitation;
- unexplained confusion for more than 4 hours;
- deterioration in GCS after admission (most attention should be paid to deterioration of motor response);
- progressive focal neurological signs;
- a seizure without full recovery;
- definite or suspected penetrating injury;
- a CSF leak.

Continuing Care

Continuing care of the patient with a serious but stable brain injury (usually in a neurological critical care unit) involves some or all of the following procedures.

- **Intensive monitoring** of vital signs and neurological status
- **Endotracheal intubation and artificial ventilation**
- **Nasogastric aspiration** for unconscious patients to prevent inhalation of gastric contents
- **Monitoring of fluid and electrolyte balance**

- **Monitoring of ICP** using a surgically implanted ICP monitoring device
- **Measures for control of raised ICP**—escalating protocols are used for incremental rises: controlled hyperventilation (reducing PCO_2 causes cerebral vasoconstriction, reduced cerebral oedema and hence reduced ICP), CSF drainage, mannitol or hypertonic saline infusion (for its osmotic effect in reducing cerebral oedema), hypothermia, barbiturates and decompressive craniectomy
- **Measures to maintain cerebral perfusion pressure**—volume expansion and inotropic support

Rehabilitation

There is a high risk of long-term disability following severe head injury, and significant cognitive dysfunction may persist in patients even after good physical recovery. Even patients with apparently minor brain injury may be moderately or severely disabled a year after injury (**postconcussion syndrome**). Problems include headache, dizziness, mental deficits, slowness of thought, poor concentration, difficulty communicating, inability to work, poor performance at school and difficulties with self-care.

Potential or actual disability needs to be recognised early, ideally before discharge from hospital. However, no reliable mechanism has been found to exclude patients safely from the need for follow-up. Ideally, all head injury patients should be followed up at least once, and expert and prolonged follow up is mandatory following severe injuries. Long-term physical and cognitive recovery after serious brain injury is a slow process and involves a multidisciplinary approach, often led by a dedicated rehabilitation team, including physiotherapy, occupational therapy, speech therapy and neuropsychology. Patients can easily languish in the community unless the problems are recognised and supportive measures are put into place.

Maxillofacial Injuries

General Principles

Facial injuries are common and occur after falls, interpersonal violence, road traffic collisions, occupational accidents and sporting injuries. Broadly speaking they can be divided into soft tissue injuries, hard tissue injuries, and combinations of these with or without injury to other parts of the body (polytrauma). This section will deal with hard tissue facial injuries only. Frequently seen facial injuries include those of the mandible, zygoma, nasal bones and orbit. Facial fractures rarely pose urgent management problems except for major middle third fractures (in which the upper jaw becomes detached from the base of the skull) and multiple mandibular fractures, which may cause profuse bleeding and upper airway obstruction, respectively. These patients may require endotracheal intubation or a surgical airway to safeguard the airway. Facial fractures are generally managed by maxillofacial surgeons, who may not be available in smaller hospitals. In most cases, delaying treatment for a few days does not adversely affect the outcome.

Examination for Facial Fractures

Examination of the injured face uses the orthopaedic maxim of 'look, feel and move'. Table 16.5 gives examples of common findings and requires no more than a good light and a systematic approach.

TABLE 16.5	Examination for Facial Fractures		
Look	**Feel**	**Move**
• Bruising, including 'panda' or 'racoon' eyes • Swelling • Grazes and lacerations • Subconjunctival haematoma • Intraoral bruising • Floor of mouth haematoma • Gingival (gum) tears • Absent teeth	• Pain on palpation • Step deformity of the bony ridges of the face, for example, orbital rim • Crepitus (air within the soft tissues of the face) • Loss of normal facial contour, for example, flattened cheek prominence seen with zygomatic fracture	• Limitation of mandibular movement • Abnormal movement of the mandible and/or maxilla • Inability to occlude teeth correctly (altered bite) • Ophthalmoplegia (eyes not moving normally) • Diplopia (double vision)

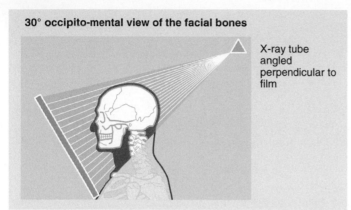

30° occipito-mental view of the facial bones

X-ray tube angled perpendicular to film

• **Fig. 16.8** Thirty-Degrees Occipitomental X-Ray for Facial Fractures.

Ideally, try and examine the face as soon as the primary survey has been completed and before oedema develops, which can obscure some findings, notably eye signs.

Radiology

If facial fractures are suspected, x-rays should be taken with views chosen according to the bones under suspicion (Fig. 16.8). Interpretation of facial radiographs can be difficult for the nonspecialist but most fractures can be identified if the main bony contours are traced and compared with the opposite side. Opacities or fluid levels in the maxillary and paranasal sinuses usually represent bleeding and are often associated with fractures of the mid and upper face. If available, CT scans typically provide definitive imaging. If CTs are being ordered for head or neck injuries, it is wise to obtain facial views at the same time, as such injuries are often encountered together. Three-dimensional images are increasingly used to appreciate the extent of injury and help with treatment planning.

Mandibular Fractures

The common sites of mandibular fractures are shown in Fig. 16.9. Because the mandible is effectively a ring of bone in continuity with the skull base, a fracture on one side is often accompanied by a fracture on the other side in a different position similar to pelvic fractures, for example, body of mandible on one side and condylar neck on the other. Fracture lines tend to occur through points of weakness, for example, mental foramina, unerupted third molar teeth or condylar necks. Many undisplaced mandibular fractures need no active intervention but displaced fractures require fixation. This is

usually achieved by open reduction and internal fixation using miniplates (see Fig. 16.10). Previously, broken jaws were wired together using the one intact jaw against which the opposing jaw can be 'set' with dental wires between the teeth of both jaws. Any fracture passing through a tooth socket defines the fracture as 'open' or 'compound' and prophylactic antibiotics should be administered.

Fractures of the Middle Third of the Face

The division of the face into thirds was first appreciated by da Vinci and can be seen in his descriptions of facial proportion. The middle third of the face runs from the frontal brow to the lip line and includes the nasal, ethmoidal, zygomatic and maxillary bones, and those of the orbit.

Fractures of the Nasal Bones

Trauma to the nose is common and often results in nasal bone fracture. Less often, fracture dislocation of the septum occurs and may interfere with the nasal airway. Diagnosis is made on clinical grounds with the main features being flattening or lateral displacement of the nasal bridge. Bleeding from the nose often indicates a nasal fracture. The fracture is usually reduced several days later by an ear, nose and throat or maxillofacial surgeon.

Fractures of the Maxilla

Fractures of the maxilla are typically complex and often known as 'Le Fort' fractures where the upper jaw is effectively separated from the skull base at different levels. Diagnosis is based on clinical and radiographic assessment. Abnormal movement of the upper jaw relative to the skull base indicates such a fracture and should be confirmed with CT imaging. Treatment may involve disimpaction followed by internal fixation. External fixation is rarely required.

Fractures of the Zygoma

There are several types of zygomatic fracture, ranging from isolated disruption of the arch itself (which can limit mandibular movements) through to complex fractures involving the orbital walls (Fig. 16.11). The fracture line often passes through the infraorbital foramen causing numbness of the cheek, upper lip, teeth and buccal mucosa and a palpable step at the inferior orbital rim. Diagnosis may be suspected by flattening of the cheek; this is best seen from above and behind the patient. Overlying oedema may

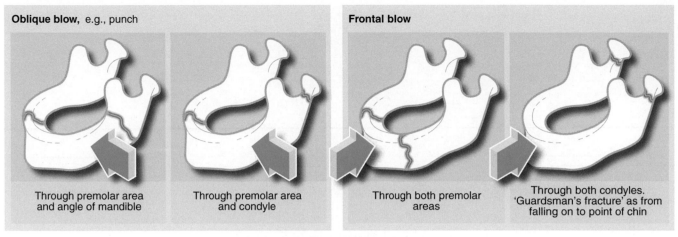

Oblique blow, e.g., punch

Through premolar area and angle of mandible

Through premolar area and condyle

Frontal blow

Through both premolar areas

Through both condyles. 'Guardsman's fracture' as from falling on to point of chin

• **Fig. 16.9** Common Sites of Mandibular Fractures.

CASE HISTORY

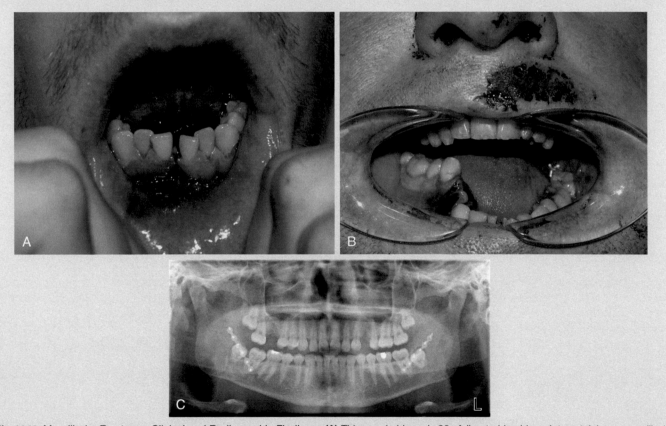

• **Fig. 16.10** Mandibular Fractures; Clinical and Radiographic Findings. **(A)** This man in his early 20s fell onto his chin point sustaining a mandibular fracture at the symphysis. This clinical image shows a gingival tear between the lower central incisors plus a space between them referred to as a *traumatic diastema*. In addition, there is a sublingual haematoma. All of these signs are pathognomonic of mandibular fractures. **(B)** This young man suffered a cycling injury. He was very aware that his teeth did not meet together properly. An altered bite should always prompt further examination to look for a bony injury of the mandible—it is very obvious in this case! **(C)** Following a single punch to the lower jaw, this patient suffered bilateral fractures at the mandibular angles. Both fractures were immobilised with direct bone plating via an intra-oral approach. Both fractures occurred via weak points in the mandible namely the third molar (wisdom tooth) sockets. However, as these teeth were firm within the sockets they could be left in situ.

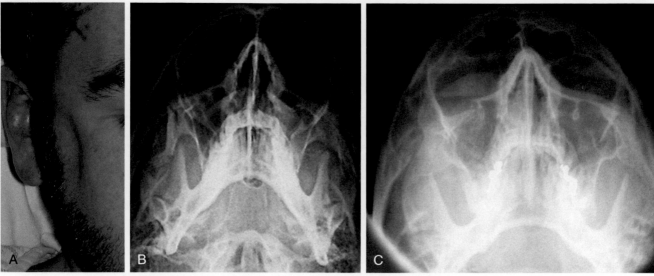

• **Fig. 16.11** Zygomatic Fractures. **(A)** This rugby player received a knee to the right face during a match resulting in a depressed fracture of the zygomatic arch. In addition to the obvious depression in his cheek, he could not open his mouth properly nor move it towards the injured side because of impingement of the arch fracture against the underlying coronoid process of the mandible. **(B)** Occipitomental view of the same patient revealing the proximity of the depressed arch to the coronoid process of the mandible. This was managed with a closed elevation via a temporal approach often referred to as a *Gillies lift*. **(C)** This patient received a blow to the right mid face resulting in a depressed fracture of the body of the zygoma. On examination, the infraorbital step deformity was readily palpable and intraorally there was a haematoma within the buccal mucosa. This patient had limited mouth opening because of impingement of the coronoid process against the depressed zygoma. There was marked soft tissue swelling on the right; these features are best appreciated by comparing each side. Interestingly, there was no mid-facial sensory change as the fracture occurred lateral to the infraorbital nerve canal. This fracture was exposed, elevated and plated via an intraoral route.

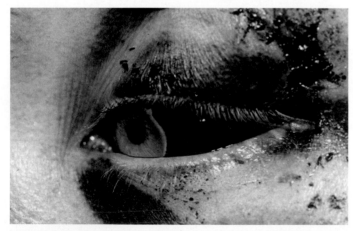

• **Fig. 16.12** Subconjunctival Haematoma Following a Head Injury. This 14-year-old boy fell off his bicycle and momentarily lost consciousness. This photograph shows a subconjunctival haematoma with no posterior limit indicating a fracture of the orbital wall, in this case the petrous temporal bone of the base of the skull.

obscure a depressed fracture, and these patients warrant radiological examination. An associated fracture of the lateral orbital wall may produce bleeding which tracks forward under the conjunctiva leading to a *subconjunctival haemorrhage* with no visible posterior limit. This is a characteristic sign of an orbital wall fracture (Fig. 16.12).

Treatment is indicated if there is inferior orbital nerve compression, deformity or functional difficulties, for example, with jaw or ocular movement. Reduction of an arch fracture is usually accomplished via a temporal or 'Gillies' approach, sliding an elevator under the root of the zygoma, deep to the temporalis fascia. Fractures of the body of the zygoma can be approached via an intraoral route and periorbital incisions, typically using fixation to ensure stability.

Blow-Out Fractures of the Orbit

An orbital 'blow-out' fracture occurs when there is disruption of one or more of the orbital walls and may be isolated or may be associated with other midfacial fractures especially zygomatic bony injuries. An isolated blow-out occurs when an object about the size of a squash ball (3–4 cm) acts like a plunger, causing compression of the orbital contents leading to the orbital walls 'bursting' open without damaging the orbital margin. This can also cause herniation of peribulbar fat into the maxillary sinus and disrupts the function of the extraocular muscles, causing diplopia and restricted upward gaze (Figs 16.13 and 16.14). Hence it is important to test eye movements in any patient with a facial injury. CT scanning of the orbit is ideal to demonstrate such fractures. Treatment involves exploring the orbital floor and may require a bone graft or repair with an alloplast of inert material.

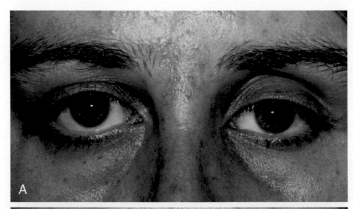

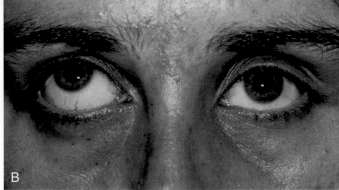

• **Fig. 16.13** Blow-Out Fracture of Orbital Floor. **(A)** This young man was punched in the left eye, causing a blow-out fracture of the orbital floor. **(B)** Note failure of upward gaze on the left caused by trapping of the extraocular muscles in the fractured orbital floor.

Injuries to the Teeth

Fractures and avulsions of the anterior teeth are common and may require immediate treatment in the emergency department. Such injuries are frequently seen in young people and are often painful. Correct first-aid treatment may preserve teeth which would otherwise be lost. Fractures involving the loss of more than one-third of the crown should be seen urgently by a dental surgeon as the dental pulp may be exposed or endangered. Partially avulsed teeth need to be pushed back into position. This can usually be done with the fingers after local anaesthetic infiltration. Urgent dental referral for tooth splinting and root canal treatment is then required.

CASE HISTORY

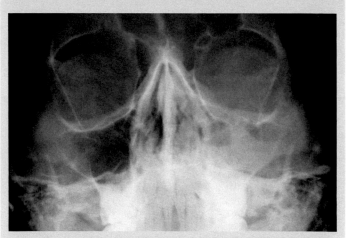

• **Fig. 16.14** Plain X-Ray Appearance of an Orbital Blow-Out Fracture. This man suffered blunt trauma to the left eye resulting in an orbital floor fracture which in turn entrapped the inferior rectus leading to vertical diplopia. The occipitomental x-ray shows a horizontal blood level within the maxillary antrum and a hanging drop sign. If this injury is suspected, an orbital computed tomography scan should be requested and an orthoptic assessment completed.

A completely avulsed tooth can be reimplanted; it should be handled by the crown only to avoid damage to the periodontal ligament and it should be cleaned and stored in saline or similar isotonic solution before reimplantation. Note that success with reimplantation diminishes proportionately to the time the tooth is out of the socket: under 30 minutes gives the best results. The discovery of missing or broken teeth in an unconscious patient should alert the examining doctor to the possibility of inhalation of tooth material into the bronchi or impaction in the lips or pharynx. Chest x-ray and examination of the perioral soft tissues should be performed in these cases.

Common Ear, Nose and Throat Emergencies

The most common ear, nose and throat emergencies are illustrated in Fig. 16.15.

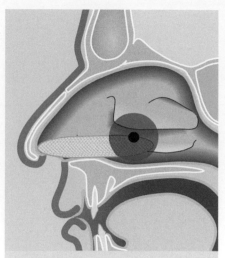

1. Epistaxis

Refer to the 2017 British Rhinological Society Consensus Guidelines. Ensure a structured resuscitative approach is taken. Gain IV access early. Apply topical local anaesthetic, e.g., co-phenylcaine. Identify a bleeding point, usually on Little area. Cauterise the blood vessel with silver nitrate or electrocautery. If the site is more posterior, the most frequent source is the sphenopalatine artery. In the event of a persistent posterior bleed, insert a nondissolvable nasal pack.

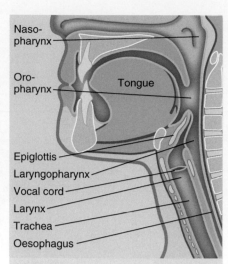

2. Stridor

This is an airway emergency. Inspiratory stridor suggests supraglottic pathology. Biphasic stridor indicates a glottic or subglottic lesion. Expiratory stridor suggests obstruction in the lower trachea. There are multiple causes but common examples include laryngeal malignancy, airway foreign body and supraglottitis/epiglottitis. Management is in conjunction with an anaesthetist. The priority is to safely secure the airway, often in theatre.

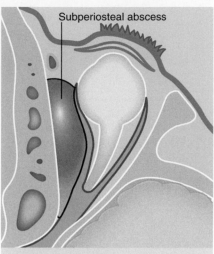

3. Periorbital cellulitis

Arises from periorbital injuries (e.g., trauma, insect bites) or sinusitis. Assess eyes, vision, nose, signs of meningism and sepsis. Grade severity according to Chandler classification (I–V). Treat with resuscitative measures, broad spectrum IV antibiotics, nasal decongestants and nasal steroids. CT may be required if there is suspicion of Chandler III (see figure). Presence of the latter will usually require surgical drainage, either endoscopically or via a Lynch Howarth incision for medial abscesses.

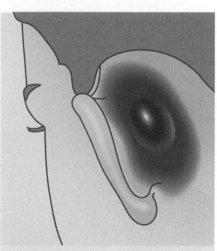

4. Acute mastoiditis +/– mastoid abscess

Complication of acute otitis media where infection spreads from middle ear to form an abscess in the mastoid air spaces. Patients present with sepsis with poor feeding and offensive otorrhoea. Examine for pinna proptosis and mastoid tenderness +/- fluctuance. CT temporal bone may be required. Treat with resuscitative measures and broad-spectrum IV antibiotics. If no improvement after 24-hours of IV antibiotics, the likely presence of an abscess may require operation. Beware meningitis or intracranial abscess.

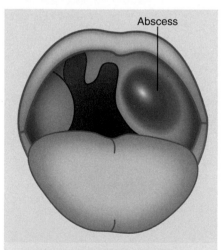

5. Quinsy or peritonsillar abscess

Complication of acute tonsillitis. An abscess collects adjacent to the tonsil (not within the tonsil). It causes trismus, uvula deviation and medialisation of the anterior pillar of the fauces. Management: 3-pass technique aspiration or incision and drainage. IV dexamethasone and IV antibiotics (1st line: benzylpenicillin and metronidazole).

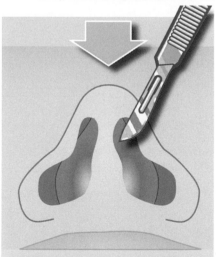

6. Septal haematoma following direct trauma

Note that the nose is blocked bilaterally. Management: incise and drain under local anaesthetic. If untreated likely to become a septal abscess leading to collapse of cartilage.

• **Fig. 16.15** Common Ear, Nose and Throat Emergencies.

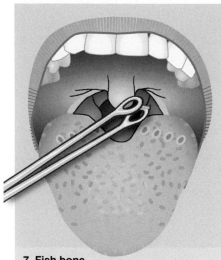

7. Fish bone

Patients can accurately indicate the position of foreign bodies above the suprasternal notch. Fish bones are often located in the tonsil or valleculae. Flexible nasendoscopy may aid diagnosis. Apply copious topical anaesthetic. Remove using Magill forceps, headlight and Lack tongue depressor (if available).

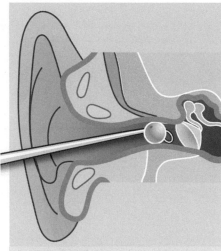

8. Aural foreign body

Most commonly a bead in a child's ear. Children will provide you with one opportunity to remove the object. Remove using Jobson-Horne probe or microsuction, dependent on the type of foreign body. Button batteries are an emergency and must be removed immediately. Organic material must be removed urgently. Failure to remove a foreign body by this means requires removal under general anaesthetic.

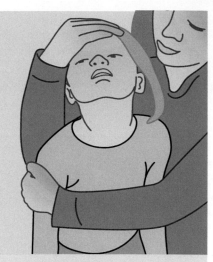

9. Nasal foreign body

Bear in mind that this is a foreign body in the airway. Try the 'Mother's kiss technique'; this is occasionally successful and minimally traumatic. Otherwise, visualise using headlight and Thudicum speculum while asking the parents and nursing staff to help hold the child still. Remove using Jobson-Horne probe – angle the instrument beyond (posterior) to the foreign body and remove swiftly. Failure to remove requires removal under general anaesthetic.

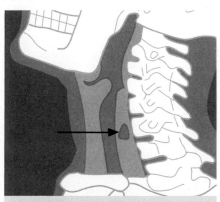

10. Oesophageal food bolus obstruction

Patients with soft food boluses (e.g., meat without bone) should be admitted to hospital and commenced upon agents to encourage passage of the bolus into the stomach (e.g., IV butyl bromide, buscopan, diazepam, nitrates, glucagon). Lateral neck radiographs are useful: look for air-fluid level and prevertebral oedema. If the bolus fails to pass within a 12-hour period, the patient should be taken to theatre for rigid oesophagoscopy. Low oesophageal foreign bodies will likely require gastroenterological input for OGD, as they are beyond the reach of a rigid scope. Patients with sharp objects (e.g., dentures, bone) should be taken to theatre immediately for surgical removal. Beware oesophageal perforation.

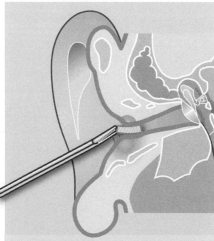

11. Otitis externa

Usually infecting agent is Pseudomonas or Staphylococcus. Presents with severe otalgia and otorrhoea. Management: microsuction of debris, insert Pope wick, if canal oedema, and topical antibiotic drops. Oral antibiotics do not play a role in uncomplicated otitis externa. Patients with secondary facial or pinna cellulitis should be admitted for IV antibiotics. Beware the diabetic patient with resistant infection – they are at risk for necrotising otitis externa.

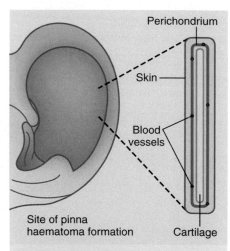

Perichondrium

Skin

Blood vessels

Cartilage

Site of pinna haematoma formation

12. Pinna haematoma

Sustained following blunt trauma to the pinna. Haematoma collects deep to the perichondrium. This is significant as the blood supply to underlying cartilage is via the perichondrium therefore delayed management can lead to avascular necrosis. Management: aspiration or incision and drainage. The authors prefer incision and drainage as there is a very high likelihood of recurrence with simple aspiration. Apply pressure dressing (secure with mattress suture through pinna) and head bandage to prevent recurrence.

Fig. 16.15, cont'd

17

Soft Tissue Injuries and Burns

Soft Tissue Injuries

Soft tissue injuries are common, and timely, up-to-date management gives the best outcomes. Traumatic soft tissue injuries include cuts, lacerations, crushing injuries, missile injuries and impalements not involving bone or body cavities. Other causes of injury include infective, oncological, surgical and vascular insults. The holistic care of soft tissue injury involves attention to the wound and to comorbid illness and patient choice. Effective care of complex injuries may require discussion with and/or transfer to a specialist plastic surgical unit for wound management and associated care.

The priority for treating soft tissue injuries depends on the outcome of the primary survey using the ABCDE system (see Ch. 15). This allows more urgent injuries to be identified and treated. Soft tissue injury is rarely imminently life-threatening, but may be distracting for the patient and healthcare providers.

Minor injuries are superficial injuries not involving 'danger areas', such as the eye or hand, without significant nerve or vascular injury and without heavy contamination. These grazes, cuts and some bites are usually self-managed. Others are treated in primary care or emergency departments. In general, such wounds need cleaning with tap water and dressing. Most heal well, but advice may be sought if the injury is outside the patient's ability to cope, or if complications develop, such as infection. **Intermediate injuries** are not life-threatening but require special attention, usually in hospital. **Major injuries** require more complex management in hospital, often with more than one specialty involved, for example, general surgery, plastic and reconstructive surgery and orthopaedic surgery. Penetrating and other major eye injuries need expert ophthalmic surgical care.

Stages of Wound Healing

Injured tissue goes through four stages on its path to healing: **haemostasis**, **inflammation**, **proliferation** and **remodelling**. There is some overlap between stages and healing may be impaired or interrupted, resulting in a poorer outcome. Several cytokines coordinate wound healing.

Haemostasis involves coagulation and vasoconstriction. **Inflammation** begins over the 4 days following injury. Early inflammation involves complement activation and neutrophil ingress by diapedesis. Later, macrophages become the predominant cell type. These perform phagocytosis and release cytokines and growth factors. **Proliferation** occurs from about day 4 to week 4. Epithelial-only injuries with an intact basement membrane restore continuity over days. Deeper injuries involve migration and proliferation of epithelial cells from the wound edge under the control of transforming growth factor (TGF-α) and epidermal growth factor (EGF). Disorganised connective tissue is initially formed in the cavity by fibroblasts migrating and proliferating in the granulation tissue, directed by platelet-derived growth factor, EGF and TGF-β. Angiogenesis occurs within this new tissue under the control of tumour necrosis factor (TNF)-α. **Remodelling** occurs over several months. The initial disorganised collagen is reorganised along lines of stress, leading to wound maturation. There is also a change from type III to type I collagen, and myofibroblasts in the wound contract its extent. The wound does not fully return to normal organisation but instead forms a scar. The wound is weak for the first 2 to 3 weeks; at around 8 months the wound reaches around 80% of its original strength.

The management of a soft tissue injury depends upon the following factors:
- the mechanism of injury (e.g., penetrating knife wounds, lacerations in road crashes, blast injuries, gunshot and missile injuries, burns, bites);

- the site of injury;
- the extent and depth of wounds;
- the types of tissue involved including nerves and blood vessels;
- the extent of tissue devitalisation;
- any contamination (e.g., with road dirt, soil or potential bacterial inoculation with animal or human bites);
- the possibility of retained foreign bodies.

Minor Soft Tissue Injuries

Most minor wounds can be cleaned and sutured immediately or closed with tissue glue. Local anaesthesia is usually required. Tetanus must be considered in any wound that is more than purely superficial, and tetanus toxoid given if immunisation is lacking or uncertain. Grazes may need cleaning of road dirt but generally just require dressing with perforated nonadherent dressings, such as Mepitel.

Intermediate Soft Tissue Injuries

Traumatic wounds are inevitably contaminated by bacteria from skin flora, but there is also potential deeper inoculation resulting from the injury. Colonisation may progress to infection that needs treatment. If there is evident nonviable tissue, debridement must be performed to permit assessment and to reduce the risk of infection. Deciding the extent of debridement requires experience.

Deep, soil-contaminated wounds (however small) in a nonimmunised patient also warrant prophylactic penicillin, effective against clostridia, and should not be closed until a few days later (delayed primary closure).

Foreign Bodies

Detailed history about the injury helps determine whether foreign bodies are likely to be retained in the wound. The main types of foreign bodies are agricultural and road dirt, wood splinters, and glass and metal fragments. Plain radiology reveals metal and usually glass (Fig. 17.1) but a negative x-ray does not exclude its presence. Remember that a foreign body unrecognised at the time may result in litigation later.

As a principle, foreign bodies should be removed, especially if organic (e.g., wood) or likely to be contaminated. Badly contaminated wounds need debridement and even scrubbing under general anaesthesia (GA). However, glass and metal fragments are often small, multiple and deeply embedded and may be difficult to locate at operation despite x-ray or ultrasound guidance. In these, it is best not to embark on exploratory surgery but to leave the fragments in situ, where they rarely cause complications. The patient must be informed about what has been left and warned that fragments often work their way to the surface and are shed, **and to return if problems occur**. This must be recorded in the patient's notes in case of future legal action.

CASE HISTORIES

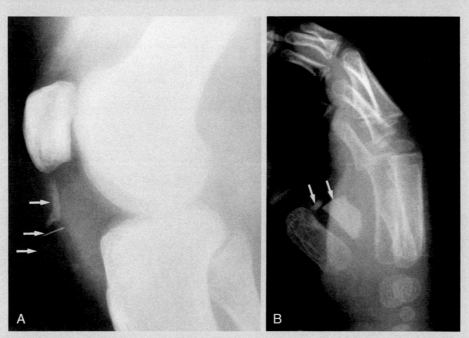

• **Fig. 17.1 Glass in Soft Tissue Wounds.** (A) A 19-year-old woman with lacerations near the knee after falling on to broken glass. Note several fragments of glass *(arrowed)* in the infrapatellar soft tissues. (B) Fragments of glass *(arrowed)* in the palm of a 12-year-old boy after he fell through a glass door. In both of these cases, the fragments were missed by casualty officers because x-rays were not requested despite a history of glass injury.

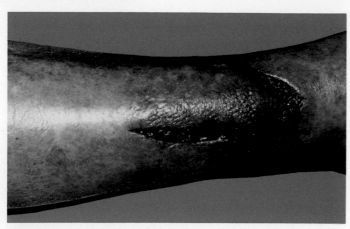

• **Fig. 17.2** Flap Laceration. This wound was caused by a fall in which the patient's shin was scraped on a stone step. It is tempting to suture such a wound, but if this is done, the flap will invariably undergo necrosis.

Wound Assessment

Factors that influence wound management include:
- site of injury
- mechanism of injury
- tissues involved
- contamination or infection
- systemic factors

Site of Injury

This influences how the wound is managed and its healing. All soft tissue injuries should be assessed early on for potential injury to deep or vital structures and certainly before using local anaesthesia. In the limbs, distal perfusion should be assessed and action taken if inadequate. When bleeding is difficult to control, focused pressure on the wound with swabs usually arrests it pending exploration. Neurological injury should be assessed in terms of sensory change and motor function. Lastly, the integrity of underlying muscles and tendons should be considered. If necessary, the wound is explored and relevant structures repaired.

Soft tissue limb injuries may be associated with an underlying fracture. Principles of wound management include early wound closure or soft tissue reconstruction, plus the need for fracture treatment. Antibiotics should be given because of the higher risk of infection. Guidelines, such as BOASTs (British Orthopaedic Association Standards for Trauma and Orthopaedics) for management of open lower limb fractures are available (see: https://www.boa.ac.uk/publications/boa-standards-trauma-boasts/).

Flap Lacerations

Relatively minor trauma to the tibia commonly produces a V-shaped **flap laceration** (Fig. 17.2), particularly in older patients or those on long-term corticosteroids. If untreated, this injury consistently fails to heal because of poor blood supply to the flap and underlying tissue. Attempting to suture or tape a flap into place increases tension, causing ischaemia, tissue loss and ulceration. The most effective management is early excision and immediate split skin grafting (see Ch. 10, p. 140). This can be performed under local anaesthesia and takes an average of 2 weeks to heal.

Facial Lacerations

Minor facial lacerations heal well and can be sutured primarily in the accident department after careful cleaning. Infection is rare because of the excellent blood supply. Even ragged skin edges do not become devitalised, so trimming is rarely necessary. The main consideration is the cosmetic outcome, so great care should be taken with technique, using GA if necessary. Complex lacerations, lacerations across the lip margin or eyelid and areas of substantial skin loss, especially on children and young people, should ideally be managed by plastic surgeons (see later).

Scalp Lacerations

With scalp lacerations, brain injury and skull fracture must be excluded, and then determine whether the aponeurotic layer (galea) has been breached. Haemostasis must be carefully achieved; it is easy to underestimate blood loss from scalp lacerations, sometimes sufficient to cause hypovolaemic shock in the elderly. Special care should be paid to haemostasis from major scalp blood vessels lying in the superficial fascia between dermis and aponeurosis. Dense collagenous bands cross the area and can prevent torn vessels contracting, hindering spontaneous arrest of bleeding. Torn vessels need to be individually ligated or sutured. Assessment and thorough exploration is made easier by shaving the wound edges; large lacerations may need exploring under GA. If the aponeurosis is breached, it should be repaired separately to prevent a subaponeurotic haematoma vulnerable to infection.

Major Soft Tissue Injuries

Major injuries of soft tissues alone requiring hospital treatment are uncommon and can be classified as in Box 17.1. A primary survey (see Ch. 15) determines the order injuries are managed, with life-threatening injuries treated first. For other injuries, the urgency depends on the potential for deterioration (e.g., blood loss, ischaemia or loss of an eye), the risk of infection and availability of appropriate specialists. Contused or contaminated wounds need early cleansing and excision of all devitalised tissue (debridement), usually under GA. If substantially contaminated, wounds are often left unsutured to prevent wound infection and are then sutured a few days later by **delayed primary closure**. Less commonly, wounds are left open and are allowed to heal by **secondary intention** (see Ch. 3, p. 34). Wounds involving skin loss may need early skin grafting (see Ch. 10, p. 140).

Injuries to a Vital Part of the Body
Eye

Injuries greater than 'sand in the eye' are best managed by ophthalmic specialists who use a slit lamp and other equipment to assess the injury. Typical injuries include abrasions to the cornea, penetrating injuries (dart or pellets) and firework injuries.

• **BOX 17.1** Classification of Major Soft Tissue Injuries

- Vital part of the body, for example, eye, hand, extensive facial lacerations
- Vascular injuries involving blood loss or ischaemia
- Nerve and tendon injuries requiring meticulous surgical repair
- Animal or human bites
- Gunshot, missile and stab wounds
- Traumatic amputation of digits or limbs
- Injuries involving substantial skin loss likely to need skin grafting, for example, degloving injuries to limbs
- Contamination with soil, road dirt—requiring debridement and/or prophylactic immune serum or antibiotics
- Crush injuries
- Chemical injuries, for example, acid, bleach, fertiliser
- Burns of more than 5% of body area or involving inhalation

CASE HISTORY

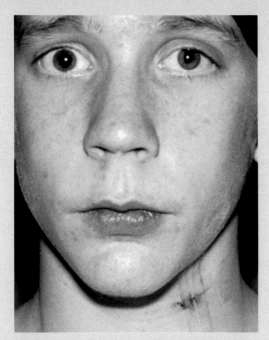

• **Fig. 17.3** Horner Syndrome Caused by Stab Wound in the Neck. This 19-year-old was stabbed in the neck: the knife missed the great vessels but succeeded in damaging the cervical sympathetic chain, causing miosis (constriction) of the pupil as a result of unopposed parasympathetic activity

Neck

Penetrating injuries to the neck must be treated with respect. Vital structures are concentrated here and may be injured. These include major arteries and veins (carotid, jugular, subclavian, vertebral), the brachial plexus, some cranial nerves, the cervical sympathetic chain (see Fig. 17.3), and lung and pleura.

Lacerations to the Limbs and Hands

(for *Traumatic amputation*, see p. 264)

Many of these are industrial injuries. The main considerations are:

- **Possible nerve, tendon or vascular injury**—assessment includes testing sensation, movement, peripheral pulses and tissue perfusion (i.e., pulses, warmth, colour, capillary refilling after blanching). Tendon and nerve injuries are covered later.
- **Tissue viability**—particularly important in crush injuries and flap lacerations. such as in the pretibial area (see earlier).
- **Risk of infection**—the fingers and hands are vulnerable to infection of pulp spaces and the deep palmar space. Wounds need antibiotic prophylaxis against *Staphylococcus* and *Streptococcus* (e.g., flucloxacillin plus amoxicillin). They also need meticulous cleansing and exploration, if possible by a specialist hand or plastic surgeon. Injuries from bites (especially by dogs, cats or humans) and bones (usually in meat workers) almost invariably become infected (see later).

Extensive Facial Lacerations

Facial injuries should be thoroughly cleaned and examined under local or GA to determine the extent of the damage before repair, ideally within 12 hours of injury. Facial wound edges need minimal trimming. Important anatomical boundaries should be aligned first; these include the vermilion border of the lip, the rim of the eyelid and the eyebrow. Tissue layers should then be approximated individually—mucosa, muscle, cartilage and skin. Parotid duct injury should be considered in deep lacerations of the cheek and the duct repaired if possible. Photographic documentation is useful to help the patient appreciate the extent of injury and to provide an accurate record of progress.

Facial nerve integrity should be determined before anaesthesia is given. Nerve branches should be repaired (usually by a plastic surgeon with microsurgical skills). Those caused by a laceration posterior to a vertical line from the lateral canthus of the eye do better than those anterior to this. Nerve repair should be performed no more than 72 hours after injury.

Vascular Injuries Involving Blood Loss or Ischaemia

Where major **blood vessels** have been damaged, haemorrhage can usually be arrested, at least temporarily, by applying pressure on gauze swabs. If there is limb ischaemia, early vascular imaging and repair is needed. Vascular grafting is required if substantial lengths of vessel have been lost. If revascularisation is delayed, **reperfusion injury** is probable and **compartment syndrome** likely (see next section). Reperfusion injury occurs when blood flow is restored after a period of severe ischaemia. Much of the damage appears to be caused by free radicals formed in the inflamed damaged tissues and is mediated by macrophages and inflammatory cytokines.

If a main artery and vein have both been severed, for example, femoral artery and vein, the vein is always repaired first to allow venous drainage before repairing the artery. If nerves have also been cut, nerve repair is required using an operating microscope (microsurgery).

Compartment Syndrome

The muscles of the leg below the knee and in the forearm lie within rigid fascial compartments. Any increase in volume results in rising intracompartmental pressure, which if sustained, compromises venous and then capillary flow resulting in compartmental ischaemia known as *compartment syndrome*. If untreated, necrosis occurs within hours.

Compartment syndrome is most common after lower leg and forearm fractures and also occurs when blood flow restoration is delayed in an acutely ischaemic lower limb. Altered distal perfusion or sensation are late and inconsistent signs; the main clinical feature is severe pain, worse on passive stretch. Untreated compartment syndrome has serious consequences, so it is reasonable to proceed to fasciotomy on clinical suspicion alone.

The treatment is to release the compartment fascia and to correct any underlying cause if possible. Fasciotomy involves a longitudinal incision in the limb to access and incise the fascia of each compartment; any necrotic muscle should be excised. The skin wound is left open initially and if the swelling does not resolve over the first few days, skin grafting may be needed.

Animal-Associated Soft Tissue Injuries

Animals can cause injury through bites, kicks, blunt trauma, goring with horns or lacerations from claws. Bite wounds in particular need prompt medical attention to reduce the risk of local infection. Tetanus is also a risk in puncture wounds or bites in a patient unprotected by immunisation.

Animal Bites

Domestic pets cause bites more often than wild animals, with dogs more likely to bite than cats; however, cat bites are more likely to become infected. In the United States, dog bites cause about 44,000 facial injuries requiring hospital treatment and 10 to 20 people are killed each year. This is about 1% of all emergency room visits. Unfortunately, most fatalities are in young children where bites to the face, neck or head are more likely caused by their small stature. *Pasteurella canis* and *Pasteurella multocida* are potential inoculated bacteria in dog and cat bites. Dogs typically cause a crushing wound because of their rounded teeth and strong jaws.

In general, the better the vascular supply and the easier the wound is to clean (i.e., laceration vs. puncture), the lower the risk of infection. Bites of the **hand** have a high risk of infection because of the relatively poor blood supply. The complex anatomical structure also makes adequate cleansing difficult.

The principles of treatment of bite wounds are inspection, debridement, irrigation and closure.

Primary closure can be considered in clean bite wounds or wounds that can be cleansed effectively. Others are best treated by **delayed primary closure**. Facial wounds are at low risk of infection, even if closed primarily. Bite wounds to the lower extremities, bites with delayed presentation, or those in immunocompromised patients should generally be left open after cleansing.

Human Bites

Human bites can be more dangerous than animal bites because of the numerous resident bacteria in the mouth. Infection risk is high, especially in 'fight-bite' injuries where a forgotten bite may have occurred during interpersonal violence. With injuries to a clenched fist, musculotendinous function should be tested across the range of movement, as tendon injury may occur distant to the skin injury. Potential contaminating bacteria include *Eikenella corrodens*, *Streptococcus* spp. and *Staphylococcus* spp. Transmission of blood-borne viruses is a rare complication.

Snakebite

Poisonous snakes are a hazard in many areas, although deaths from snakebite are rare. Snakebites are most common where dense human populations coexist with large snake populations (e.g., South-East Asia, sub-Saharan Africa, and tropical America). Highly dangerous snakes include the Australian brown snake; the black mamba, puff adder and boomslang in Africa; Russell's viper and cobras in southern Asia; carpet vipers in the Middle East; and coral snakes and rattlesnakes in the Americas. The venom of a small or immature snake can be more concentrated than that of larger ones, so all snakes should be left well alone. Less than half of all snakebite wounds actually contain venom, but travellers are advised to seek immediate medical attention whenever a bite breaks the skin. First-aid measures should include immobilising the affected limb and applying a pressure bandage that does not restrict limb perfusion (not a tourniquet), then moving the victim quickly to a medical centre. Incision of the bite is not recommended. Specific therapy varies and should be left to experienced local emergency personnel.

Arthropod Bites and Stings

The bites and stings of some arthropods (which include insects) can cause unpleasant reactions. Travellers should seek medical attention if a spider or insect bite or sting causes excessive redness, swelling, bruising or persistent pain. Patients with a history of severe allergic reactions to bites or stings should consider carrying an adrenaline (epinephrine) autoinjector (EpiPen or similar). Many insects and arthropods can transmit **communicable diseases,** for example, malaria, dengue fever or Lyme disease, even without the traveller being aware of a bite, particularly when camping or staying in rural accommodation. Travellers to many parts of the world should be advised to use insect repellents containing diethyltoluamide, protective clothing, and mosquito netting around beds at night. Stings from **scorpions** can be painful but are seldom dangerous except in infants and children. Exposure can be avoided by sleeping under mosquito nets and by shaking clothing and shoes before putting them on.

Gunshot, Missile and Stab Wounds

Gunshot wounds and missile injuries need special attention. High-energy missiles may cause a small entry wound but produce havoc within (see Ch. 15). X-rays need to be taken and wounds explored under GA.

Vascular Injury

Soft tissue trauma rarely involves arterial injury, but when it does occur, there are often other structural injuries, for example, ulnar artery, ulnar nerve and hand flexor tendons. A single arterial transection will not necessarily result in compromised distal perfusion unless it involves a single or proximal main vessel, because there is usually a collateral blood supply. Despite this, vascular repair should be performed, if possible, to control haemorrhage and to optimise distal perfusion. This is usually performed under magnification. It is unusual for venous injury to require repair, as there is normally sufficient capacity within nearby veins to compensate, so damaged veins can usually be ligated. Venous repair is required in replantation of a digit (see later) or when a large single proximal vein is divided, for example, common femoral, where ligation would lead to distal venous congestion.

Traumatic Amputation of Digits or Limbs

Replantation Surgery

Replantation of amputated anatomical parts has been performed most often for digits, but also on limbs, genitalia, ears, nose and even the face. At the place of injury, the amputated part should be cleaned, placed on damp gauze in a sealed plastic bag and then into iced water for storage.

Clean lacerations are more likely to be suitable for replantation rather than crushing or avulsing injury. The period of warm ischaemia must be short to avoid necrosis or reperfusion injury. Muscle is particularly sensitive to ischaemia. Although replantation is an emergency procedure, a short period of cold ischaemia can permit informed discussion, and assembly of an appropriate theatre team.

The patient needs to know that return of function will take several months, be incomplete, and there is likely to be pain and stiffness, and must be happy to proceed despite this. Many patients later fail to use the replanted digit; in any case, the operated limb will be out of action for purposes of employment during the recovery period. Failure rates are much higher in smokers and functional recovery in older patients is likely to be worse. A specialist microsurgical surgical team is needed to perform these procedures, which are likely to last several hours. Nursing and physiotherapy staff experienced in hand injuries are also necessary to achieve optimal results.

Indications for replantation vary between units but often include:
- children
- loss of thumb
- loss of multiple digits

- loss of upper limb or hand
- employment—relative indications are in professions, such as musicians, or where a patient will be supported in their time off work
- cultural—relative indication—in cultures where greater concern is attached to such injuries

Contaminated Injuries

Superficial wounds, such as grazes caused by motorcycle injuries and lack of protective clothing, often become widely impregnated with road debris. These need to be scrubbed clean, often under GA. In the case of large contaminated and contused wounds involving muscle, the potential for **gas gangrene** must be considered. Dead tissue must be excised, benzylpenicillin given prophylactically, and primary closure avoided in favour of a second look at 48 to 72 hours for further wound cleaning and debridement if needed, and then delayed primary closure. Note that **hydrogen peroxide** must **never** be used in any wounds other than purely superficial ones because of the dangers of oxygen embolism causing brain damage.

Crush Injuries

Rhabdomyolysis follows prolonged heavy continuous pressure on muscle and **crush syndrome** is caused by reperfusion injury when damaged muscle revascularises on removing compression. Damaged cells release potassium and potentially toxic substances, such as myoglobin, phosphate and urate, into the circulation. Water and extracellular electrolytes enter the damaged muscle. The net result is hypovolaemic shock with electrolyte disturbances leading to acute kidney injury.

Following earthquakes, the incidence of crush syndrome is 2% to 5% of those buried under rubble. About half develop acute kidney injury, and half of those need dialysis. Crush syndrome is also seen following industrial incidents, particularly in mining, and in road traffic collisions.

Diagnostic criteria for crush syndrome include:

- a crushing injury to a large mass of skeletal muscle;
- sensory and motor disturbances in the compressed limb;
- swelling and tenseness of the limb a few hours later;
- myoglobinuria and/or haematuria;
- elevated serum creatine kinase with a peak greater than 1000 U/L;
- renal insufficiency hours or days later. This may manifest with oliguria (urine output less than 400 mL in 24 hours), decreased plasma calcium concentration and elevated plasma urea, creatinine, uric acid, potassium and phosphate.

Peripheral Nerve Injuries

Anatomy

In a peripheral nerve trunk, individual axons are sheathed in **endoneurium** and groups are bundled into **fascicles**. Each fascicle is covered in tough **perineurium** composed of collagen and elastin and may contain sensory and motor axons. A **peripheral nerve trunk** consists of a number of fascicles in a matrix of **epineurium**, which also coats the nerve. Fascicles divide repeatedly along the course of a nerve, communicating with each other and intermixing rather than running neatly in parallel. This means the arrangement and type of axons and fascicles in one cross-section of the nerve may be very different from that in an adjoining one. The resulting difficulty of aligning the proximal with the distal arrangement is an important reason why functional recovery is poor if a segment of nerve is lost and has to be replaced with a nerve graft.

Types of Injury

Nerve Injuries. Nerve injuries were classified by Seddon in 1943:

- **Neuropraxia** is the mildest injury, where axonal continuity is preserved and Wallerian degeneration does not occur distal to the injury. Caused by compression, blunt impact or nearby sharp injuries, resulting in oedema and conduction delay or blockade. Demyelination may occur. Recovery normally occurs within 6 to 8 weeks.
- **Axonotmesis** occurs when there is interruption of axon and its myelin, but perineurium and epineurium are preserved. Axonotmesis results from more severe crush injury or contusion; complete denervation occurs but supporting structures remain intact. Wallerian degeneration occurs distal to the injury. Recovery takes place by axon regeneration at around 1 to 2 mm/day and is likely to be near complete unless a neuroma forms.
- **Neurotmesis** involves complete disruption of the axon and its supporting structures. It can occur with severe contusion, stretching or, most commonly, laceration. It rarely recovers without surgical intervention.

It is difficult to classify a nerve injury clinically at initial assessment. Open injuries with altered distal nerve function should be surgically explored and neurotmesis repaired to aid functional recovery and reduce the risk of neuroma formation. Repair is normally performed using a tourniquet and loupe or microscope magnification to approximate the nerve ends with epineural sutures. Tension should be avoided, and any gap can be filled using autologous (nerve or vein graft) or artificial material (such as polyglycolic acid polymer nerve conduits).

Recovery from nerve injury is influenced by which nerve is injured (for example radial better than median, which is better than ulnar), patient age, injury level (distal better than proximal), length of any defect, associated injuries, surgical technique and comorbidities, such as smoking. There is inconsistent evidence for the timing of repair; earlier exploration is generally easier and may be necessary for wound management, but risks unnecessary exploration of neuropraxic or axonotmesis injury.

Musculotendinous Injury. Substantial **muscular injury** should be treated with debridement of devascularised tissue and then gentle repair with absorbable sutures. If appropriate, the fascial compartment can then be closed. **Tendon injury** is common in hand lacerations; management involves exploration and tendon repair. There is a range of techniques for tendon repair, depending on the type and position of injury.

Physiotherapy is essential after tendon repair and as there is a balance between the risk of rerupture and reducing the risk of adhesions; protocols, such as the Belfast or Norwich regimens are used for flexor and extensor tendons respectively.

Closed tendon injury is uncommon, but may be a consequence of sudden traction or chronic injury, such as inflammatory arthritis (in which repair may not be possible).

Necrotising Soft Tissue Infections

Necrotising fasciitis (NF), and other necrotising soft tissue infections are characterised by rapidly progressive soft tissue infection often involving primary fascial necrosis and secondary necrosis of overlying soft tissue. Features include pain, skin changes moving from erythema to fixed dark staining, and blistering and crepitus from subcutaneous gas. Patients become extremely ill, resulting in a mortality rate of 25% to 50%. Around 50% of patients were previously well, with the other half immunosuppressed, as in diabetes or after organ transplantation.

NF may be categorised as follows:

- **Type 1**—Polymicrobial synergistic infection, the most common type. May occur after tissue injury because of local hypoxia.
- **Type 2**—Group A streptococcal infection. Associated with superantigen production. Rapid progression and a grave prognosis.
- **Type 3**—Clostridial infection. May follow surgery or trauma. Associated with subcutaneous emphysema.
- **Type 4**—Other infections including *Vibrio, Aeromonas, Candida*.
- **Fournier gangrene** is a subtype of NF affecting the perineum.

Treatment of Necrotising Fasciitis

If the diagnosis is uncertain, scoring systems, such as LRINEC, have been validated in stratifying risk of NF versus severe cellulitis. Broad-spectrum antibiotics should be given according to unit protocol. Debridement of NF is a surgical emergency. Exploratory incisions and radiography (for soft tissue gas) can also be used. Multiple debridements and critical care are usually required. Reconstruction later depends on the extent of tissue loss.

Principles of Wound Dressings

Wounds heal best in a moist but not saturated environment. The early stages of wound healing are fragile, and therefore the wound should be protected, and dressing choices and changes performed with care. Wounds should be clean and free of devitalised tissue. Dressings should not adhere to the wound bed. Gauze impregnated with paraffin is simplest (tulle gras, Jelonet) but tends to dry out. This gauze can contain antimicrobials, such as chlorhexidine (Bactigras). New silicone dressings, such as Mepitel maintain their nonstick character for longer. Excess fluid can be absorbed by using a layer of gauze on top of gauze dressings. Topical creams and ointments, such as paraffin and antimicrobials are also used. They may be easier to use than dressings but need to be applied several times daily.

Negative Pressure Wound Therapy

Negative pressure wound therapy (NPWT) involves a foam wound dressing covered by an occlusive dressing and connected to a suction machine. A hydrocolloid dressing protects surrounding skin from maceration. Usual negative pressure settings are between 50 and 125 mmHg; dressings are usually changed every 2 to 3 days. NPWT is beneficial in highly exudative wounds, where excess fluid is controlled and drained. In addition, the wound is kept moist but extracellular oedema is removed to reduce inflammatory mediators, and diffusion distance is reduced. The microvasculature is splinted open to improve blood flow.

Contraindications include:

- anticoagulation, ongoing bleeding or exposed vasculature risks uncontrolled blood loss;
- growth of nearby malignancy may be enhanced;
- unexplored fistulae may lead to large fluid loss;
- relative contraindications include wounds that are difficult to seal, such as the perineum, or heavily contaminated or infected wounds;
- expense—more expensive than traditional dressings but may be mitigated by improved healing.

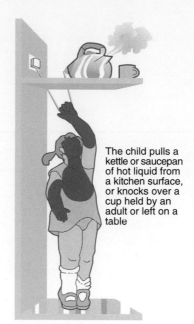

• **Fig. 17.4** Typical Pattern of Burns in a Young Child. The child pulls a teapot or cup of hot liquid from a table or when being held by a seated adult. The area shaded pink is typically burnt.

The child pulls a kettle or saucepan of hot liquid from a kitchen surface, or knocks over a cup held by an adult or left on a table

Burns

Introduction

Burns are the fourth most common trauma worldwide (after traffic collisions, falls and interpersonal violence). Most adult burns are flame injuries, whereas paediatric burns are usually scalds (i.e., caused by hot fluids). Other types of burn include flash and contact burns; chemical and electrical injuries are less common. Burns cause devastating injuries. Initially, there is severe pain and distress, but soon, there is a massive assault on both physical and psychological aspects of those affected.

Epidemiology

In the United Kingdom, about 250,000 people are burnt each year; 112,000 attend accident departments and 13,000 are admitted to hospital. About 1000 have burns severe enough to need fluid resuscitation and, sadly, half of these are children under 12 years. In an average year, burns cause 250 deaths in the United Kingdom, although the incidence has decreased owing to prophylactic measures, for example, curly cables on kettles; abandonment of open fires; and flameproof sofas and clothing. Worldwide, burns cause about 180,000 deaths a year (World Health Organization, 2018). **Most burns are preventable.** Young children and the elderly are at greatest risk and also suffer disproportionate mortality. Twenty percent of all burns occur in children under the age of 4 years; 70% are scalds caused by spilling hot liquids or by exposure to hot bath water. Toddlers frequently pull containers or cups of hot liquid over themselves from cookers and tables, which burn the outstretched arm, face, neck and front of the chest and can cover a large area (Fig. 17.4).

Overall, 60% of burns occur between the ages of 15 and 64 years, of which half are flame burns, often with inhalational injury; burns tend to be deep dermal or full thickness (Fig. 17.5). It is important to consider nonaccidental injury (NAI) in all age groups.

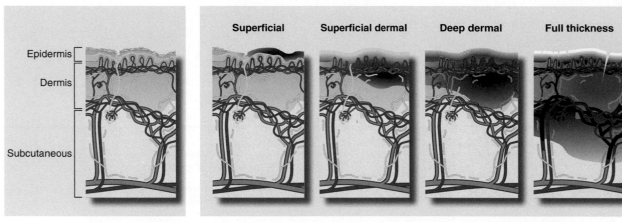

- **Fig. 17.5** Classification of Depth of Burns. Erythema—red, dry skin that easily blanches then rapidly refills (not illustrated here). Superficial—red, moist wound that blanches and rapidly refills. Superficial dermal—pale, dry, blanching wound that regains colour slowly. Deep dermal—mottled cherry red and does not blanch (fixed capillary staining). The blood is thrombosed and fixed in damaged capillaries in the deep dermal plexus. Full thickness—dry, leathery or waxy, hard wound that does not blanch. In extensive burns, full thickness burns can be mistaken for unburnt skin.

Pathophysiology of Burns

Thermal injury occurs at temperatures above 43°C owing to protein denaturation; at 45°C, permanent cell damage is inflicted. The inflammatory changes in burn injury alter intravascular Starling forces—arteries dilate and capillaries become more permeable, so fluid moves from the intravascular to the extravascular space. With larger burns, intravenous fluid replacement is needed to prevent hypovolaemic shock.

In thermal skin burns, the depth of destruction determines the local outcome. Skin burns are broadly divided into **partial** or **full thickness**. In **partial thickness burns**, epidermal elements are spared, eventually allowing spontaneous healing without grafting. In **deep partial thickness burns**, the only epithelial remnants may be hair follicles and sweat glands, extending into the hypodermis, making regeneration slower. In **full thickness burns**, all the epidermis has been destroyed. Skin grafting is needed because epithelialisation from the margins is slow and prone to complications, in particular infection, fibrotic scarring and contractures.

Three zones of a major burn were described by Jackson in 1947: a central zone of **coagulation,** where skin cells are irreversibly damaged, surrounded by a zone of **stasis,** with decreased tissue perfusion in which injured cells can survive or die according to the effectiveness of treatment. These zones extend deeply but the third, outer zone of **erythema** is superficial. Here, the cells are minimally injured and recover within 7 days. This zone should not be included in calculating the burnt area.

Systemic Effects (Box 17.2)

Extensive burns cause large fluid losses. Epidermal destruction removes the barrier that normally prevents evaporation of body water. Inflammation also causes exudation of protein-rich fluid into the extracellular space, causing oedema and blisters. The large volumes lost need to be replaced urgently (Box 17.4), with the amount lost depending on the burn area rather than its depth. Once 30% of the body surface area is burnt, particularly if there is necrotic tissue, inflammatory mediators and cytokines spill into the circulation, causing a systemic inflammatory response. This provokes a general rise in capillary permeability, escalating the volume of plasma leaving the circulation into the 'third space'. Fluid

> **• BOX 17.2   Systemic Changes Occurring With Large Area Burns (Greater Than 15% Surface Area in Adults or 10% in Children)**
>
> - Surface and third space fluid losses lead to hypovolaemia
> - Systemic inflammatory response syndrome (SIRS) occurs once burns affect 30% of body surface area
> - Myocardial contractility becomes depressed
> - In smoke inhalation, bronchoconstriction and acute respiratory distress syndrome occur
> - Basal metabolic rate (BMR) increases up to threefold
> - Function of the innate immune system becomes depressed
> - General capillary permeability is increased
> - Peripheral and splanchnic vasoconstriction occurs
> - Red cells are destroyed by the burn
> - Sepsis is likely if burns become infected, leading to organ failure and death

losses are greatest in the first few hours but continue for at least 36 hours.

Epidermal loss and necrotic tissue put the patient at high risk of infection. The main organisms are *Streptococcus pyogenes* during the first week and *Pseudomonas aeruginosa* thereafter. If burns become infected, the risk of sepsis and organ failure increases and leads to high mortality, even in this antibiotic era.

Electrocution Burns

Electrical burns are uncommon but dangerous. Electrocution is responsible for around 3% of admissions to burns units. A mix of thermal and nonthermal injury occurs; thermal because of conversion of electrical energy into heat caused by tissue impedance, and nonthermal because of depolarisation of conductive tissues, such as muscle and nerve.

Low voltage burns (under 1000 V) usually occur in the domestic setting. Entry and exit wounds are small and similar to full thickness thermal burns, but significant deep structural injury is unusual. High voltage burns (over 1000 V) can also cause substantial muscle injury, resulting in rhabdomyolysis and compartment syndrome. Blood vessels sustain intimal damage and thrombose.

Deep tissue necrosis may not become clinically apparent until some days afterwards and the extent of damage is often much greater than suspected. Together with bone necrosis and soft tissue damage, there is a risk of limb loss. If the conduction path from entry to exit wound is across the chest, there is a high risk of arrhythmia. The patient may also be thrown from the source causing additional injury. Contact with voltages greater than 70,000 V is invariably fatal.

Electrical injuries should be managed by safely removing the patient from the electrical source, performing a primary survey and delivering supportive care, which may require cardiopulmonary resuscitation. At this stage, fluid resuscitation should be titrated against urine output rather than the visible burn surface area. If there is any evidence of rhabdomyolysis, input should be such as to produce at least 1 mL/kg per h urine, and renal replacement therapy initiated if that is insufficient.

Chemical Burns

Acids, alkalis and hydrocarbons, such as petrol, can result in burn injuries. Nearly all chemical burns should be treated by removing the injuring material and then irrigating with cool water (except with reactive metals, phenol and white phosphorus). Irrigation should continue for longer than for thermal burns, and guided by relief of pain and return to neutral pH. The burns can then be treated and dressed like thermal burns.

Chemical burns usually result from industrial accidents, but sometimes from household chemicals or interpersonal violence. It is therefore important to maintain meticulous documentation for later investigation by health and safety bodies, insurance companies or the police.

Nonaccidental Injury

Between 3% and 10% of paediatric burns are caused by NAI, that is, deliberate harm to the child. Up to 30% of repeatedly abused children die. If NAI is suspected, it is vital to follow the local NAI protocol.

Assessment of the Burnt Patient

History

A history should be taken, including the nature and time of injury, other injuries, symptoms of airway injury (cough, wheeze, altered voice, facial burns, smoke inhalation), allergies, medications, past medical history and last meal. If there is a likelihood of other injuries, the patient should be examined systematically and treated as appropriate.

Calculating the Burnt Area

All of the burnt area needs to be exposed sequentially, ensuring the patient is kept warm. For adults, Wallace's rule of nines (Fig. 17.6) is fairly reliable for medium to large areas and is quick, but it is inaccurate in children. Another method is to use the patient's palm and finger area to indicate 1% of body surface area. This is useful for small burns, and in very large burns where the **unburnt area** is measured. The most accurate method is to use **Lund and Browder charts**, which compensate for variations in body shape with age; the charts are also accurate in children.

Early assessment of burn depth is difficult, but is important for management. If the burnt area is erythematous, blanches on pressure and retains pinprick sensation, it is partial thickness; charred skin or thrombosed skin vessels invariably indicate a full thickness burn. It is essential to reappraise the burn regularly until it heals.

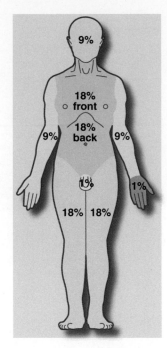

• **Fig. 17.6** Rule of Nines. Wallace rule for estimating the percentage of the skin surface area burnt. A useful alternative estimate is that the area of the patient's own palm plus fingers is approximately 1% of the total skin area.

Partial thickness burns may be classified as follows:
- **Superficial** burns—affect the epidermis but not the dermis, for example, sunburn.
- **Superficial dermal** burns—destroy the epidermis and upper dermal layers; blistering usually occurs. The burn may be covered with soot or dirt, which needs removing, and blisters should be deroofed so that the base can be checked. Capillary refill can be tested by pressure from a sterile cotton bud. A 21-gauge needle is used to test sensation and bleeding; in superficial dermal burns, pain is felt normally and bleeding is brisk. Scalds tend to cause 'superficial' to 'superficial dermal' burns.
- **Deep dermal** burns—these destroy all the epidermis and most of the dermis, leaving only the deepest skin adnexae, sweat glands and some hair follicles, all of which are scanty. Accurate depth estimation can be difficult. On needle testing, bleeding is delayed and only nonpainful sensation is experienced.
- **Full thickness** burns are insensate and do not bleed on needling.

Principles of Management of Burns

Optimal treatment reduces the morbidity of burns, as well as mortality in large burns. Effective treatment shortens the period of healing, speeds return of function and reduces the need for secondary reconstruction.

First Aid

The first priority at the scene is to stop the burning process. The heat source must be removed and any flames doused. Clothing is removed unless stuck to the burn, and **active cooling** used to remove heat and arrest progression. Cooling the burn with running tepid water within 3 hours for at least 10 minutes reduces the size and depth of burn; it may be cooled for longer for analgesia. It is important to avoid causing hypothermia, a particular risk with scald injuries to the paediatric chest.

- Associated inhalational injury
- Partial thickness > 5% in a child or > 10% in an adult
- More than 1% full thickness burns
- Partial or full thickness burns to face, perineum, external genitalia, feet, hands and across joints
- Circumferential injury
- Chemical or electrical burns
- Extremes of age
- Nonaccidental injury
- Comorbidity
- Nonhealed burn 3 weeks after injury

Analgesia

Burns are very painful, with pain being greatest in superficial burns. Pain relief is best achieved by cooling and covering burns in addition to analgesic drugs. In larger burns, opioids are given initially and nonsteroidal anti-inflammatory drugs later.

Dressings

Cling film (PVC) is ideal as an initial burn dressing. It is essentially sterile and forms a pliable, nonadherent, impermeable barrier, which is transparent to allow inspection. It should be laid on rather than wrapped around and covered with a blanket to keep the wound warm. Burnt hands are enclosed in plastic bags. Prepacked cooling hydrogels, for example, Burnshield, are available for applying at the scene of the burn.

Where Should Burns Be Managed?

Very small or erythema-only burns can be managed in primary care but all other patients should be assessed and resuscitated in an emergency unit. Initial assessment then determines whether treatment can continue as an outpatient or inpatient in a general hospital, or whether to transfer to a specialist burns unit. Patients with burns involving more than 30% of body surface should be transferred to a specialist burns unit right after initial treatment and resuscitation. Facial burns should also be referred after covering with bland paraffin ointment (repeated every 1–4 hours to minimise crust). Other referral criteria are summarised in Box 17.3.

Outpatient Management of Minor Burns

Patients appropriate for outpatient management are adults without inhalation injury or significant comorbidity, with partial thickness burns affecting less than 10% of body surface area. Children with less than 5% burns are also suitably managed in this way. Patients with full thickness burns of up to 1% can also be managed as outpatients.

Immediate care involves analgesia and reassurance. Fluid resuscitation is not needed. The main objective is to prevent local dehydration and infection of the burn site; epithelialisation progresses faster in a moist environment. The burnt area is cleaned of soot and debris with soap and water or weak chlorhexidine if necessary. Larger blisters are deroofed and covered with a nonstick impregnated gauze dressing, ideally a soft silicone-coated net, such as Mepitel. A generous layer of silver sulfadiazine cream (Flamazine) can be used instead; this antibacterial cream covers gram-negative organisms including the common infecting organism, *Pseudomonas*. Either dressing is then covered by a thick absorbent layer of gauze and wool (Gamgee). Burns on the fingers and hands are best treated with a liberal coating of silver sulfadiazine cream and enclosing the hand in a plastic bag. Burnt areas should be checked at 24 hours and the dressing changed at 48 hours, by which time the depth should be evident and the treatment plan can be reviewed. Silver sulfadiazine cream can then be applied every 24 to 48 hours and skin slough excised as it separates. Partial thickness burns reepithelialise within 14 to 21 days. If the burn has failed to heal within 3 weeks, the burn must be assumed to be full thickness and requires referral to a specialist unit.

Managing Burns of Specific Depth

Superficial burns, typically sunburn, require only supportive therapy with regular analgesia and dressings for moist areas. Healing takes place within a week by regeneration from undamaged keratinocytes.

Superficial dermal burns. Blistering is common and exposed superficial nerves make these burns painful. Healing is expected within 2 weeks. Treatment is as aforementioned, although Hypafix is a special dressing that preserves mobility and allows washing with the dressing in place. This dressing needs changing weekly by soaking in oil. Awkward facial burns are left open but liberally coated with antimicrobial creams or ointment.

Deep dermal burns. Some of these burns heal spontaneously if kept warm, moist and free of infection, but if deep dermal burns are extensive or are in functionally sensitive areas, such as limb flexures or are cosmetically sensitive, they are better treated in a burns unit by excision to a viable depth and skin grafting within 5 days. This can reduce morbidity and accelerate return to normal function.

Full thickness burns. Ideally all full thickness burns need excision and grafting unless they are sited where function would not be compromised and are less than 1 cm in diameter.

Management of Extensive Burns

Major burns are those affecting more than 20% of the body surface area. Survival depends crucially on accurate assessment, prompt and effective resuscitation, also the premorbid condition of the patient and whether there has been smoke inhalation. The main early aspects of management are fluid replacement, assessment and treatment of inhalational respiratory problems and local management of the burns.

The risk of dying is greater with increasing area, with inhalational injury, and in children under 3 years and adults over 60 years. Very high voltage electrical burns are particularly lethal. Other medical conditions also increase the risk, for example, alcoholism, epilepsy, diabetes, atherosclerosis and drug abuse.

Resuscitation and Fluid Management

Adults with 15% and children with 10% body surface burns lose sufficient fluid to be at risk of hypovolaemic shock. Fluid replacement depends on the area of the burn and the patient's weight. Hypovolaemia in the presence of myoglobinaemia readily precipitates acute renal failure. Effective resuscitation maintains tissue perfusion in the zone of stasis, inhibiting depth progression. Most fluid is lost in the first 8 to 12 hours, during which there is a general shift of fluid from intravascular to interstitial. Substantial fluid losses continue for at least another 36 hours. Rapid boluses of fluid should not be given early on as raised intravascular hydrostatic pressure drives it rapidly out of the circulation.

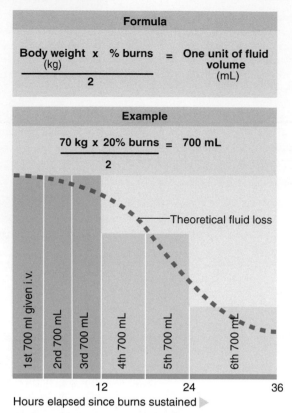

Formula
$\dfrac{\text{Body weight} \times \% \text{ burns}}{2} = \text{One unit of fluid}$
(kg) volume (mL)

Example
$\dfrac{70 \text{ kg} \times 20\% \text{ burns}}{2} = 700 \text{ mL}$

Hours elapsed since burns sustained ▶

• **Fig. 17.7** Serious Burns—A Method for Estimating Fluid Requirements Over the First 36 Hours (After Muir and Barclay). The lower panel shows an example of a fluid replacement regimen for a 70-kg man with 20% burns. Each block represents one unit of fluid volume and is calculated as follows:

$$\text{Unit fluid volume} = \frac{70 \times 20}{2} = 700 \text{ mL}$$

• **BOX 17.4** **The Parkland Formula for Fluid Resuscitation in the First 24 Hours in Major Burns**

- For adults, the total volume to be given over 24 hours is 3 to 4 mL Hartmann solution per kg body weight for each percent surface area burnt.
- For children, the calculation is the same as for adults plus normal maintenance fluids.
- For all cases, half the estimated volume is given in the first 8 hours and the rest over the next 16 hours.

Fluid requirements should be calculated from the time of injury, *not* the time of arrival in the emergency department. Colloids appear to offer no advantage over crystalloids and the volume required is estimated by referring to well-tried formulae, such as that of Muir and Barclay or the Parkland formula, Box 17.4. The Parkland formula has the advantage that it uses only crystalloids, it is easy to calculate and the rate can be adjusted by titrating against urine output.

These formulae are only a guide, however, and fluid balance must also be monitored according to pulse, blood pressure and urine output via a urinary catheter. Patients should also have 4- to 6-hourly estimations of packed cell volume, serum sodium, base excess and lactate. Note that patients with high-tension

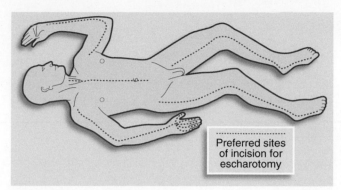

• **Fig. 17.8** Sites for Performing Escharotomy in Deep Circumferential Burns.

electrocution injuries need substantially more fluid than estimated by these formulae. In extensive full thickness burns, widespread red cell destruction occurs and blood transfusion may be needed.

Local Management of the Burns

All wounds should achieve epithelial cover within 3 weeks to minimise scarring. Partial thickness burns reepithelialise spontaneously given proper care, but full thickness burns require excision and skin grafting. Fingers, eyelids, limb flexures and genitalia nearly always require primary grafting soon after injury. For optimal care, grafting should be performed within 5 days of injury.

The best covering for excised areas is autograft split skin from unburnt areas, ideally harvested near the recipient area to ensure best colour match. Sheets rather than postage stamp grafts should be used for hands and face. Wounds to be grafted must be free of infection; large areas of deep burns need excising and grafting early to prevent infection and systemic sepsis. With extensive burns, skin grafting usually has to be performed in several stages because of a shortage of donor sites. Sites already used can be reused (**donor site rotation**) after 3 weeks or so; burnt areas can be primarily excised and covered with temporary covering until donor sites become mature. Temporary coverings include cadaveric allograft skin, xenograft skin (e.g., pigskin), specially developed synthetic products or cultured epithelial autografts (sheets can be available in 3 weeks, skin cell suspensions in 1 week).

Deep circumferential burns of the limbs and thorax begin to contract early and may restrict blood flow and respiratory movements. If excision and grafting is not done early, and if these signs develop, **escharotomy** is performed, involving incision of the eschar longitudinally down to bleeding tissue (Fig. 17.8).

Inhalational Injuries

Respiratory and systemic damage from inhalation of hot air, smoke and toxic gases (e.g., carbon monoxide or cyanides from burning upholstery) is a major cause of death and complications even if skin burns are insignificant (Box 17.5). The heat of inhaled gases is often sufficient to cause inflammatory oedema of the oral, nasal and laryngeal mucosa or even serious burns. Blackening by smoke or burnt skin around the nasal or oral cavities warns of inhalation injury. In addition, noxious gases can injure the lung parenchyma, resulting in pulmonary oedema, atelectasis and secondary pneumonias a day or two later.

Investigations include chest x-ray, blood gas and carbon monoxide estimations and upper respiratory tract examination with flexible pharyngoscopy and bronchoscopy.

• **BOX 17.5** **Clinical Indications of Likely Inhalational Injury That May Prompt Endotracheal Intubation and Ventilation**

- A history of flame burns or burns in an enclosed space
- Stridor, tachypnoea or dyspnoea
- Singed nasal hair
- Full thickness or deep dermal burns to face, neck or upper torso
- Changes in the voice with hoarseness or a harsh cough
- Carbonaceous sputum or carbon particles visible in oropharynx
- Erythema or swelling of the oropharynx on direct inspection

Initial treatment involves administration of humidified air by mask and antibiotics to prevent chest infection. More severe cases require oxygen by mask, progressing to endotracheal intubation and intermittent positive pressure ventilation if blood gases deteriorate or pulmonary oedema develops.

Follow-Up and Late Treatment of Burns

Burnt areas should be protected from sun for 6 to 12 months by avoiding the sun or using sun block. Physiotherapy may be needed if mobility is impaired, and if deformity results from the burns or the treatment, prolonged psychological support is necessary, particularly if the face is involved.

Local symptoms of severe **itching** and **dryness** can be helped by topical lanolin and specially made pressure garments. These also minimise skin contractures. If limitation of functional movement at joints or around facial orifices is not helped adequately by physiotherapy, operations to release scars and skin grafting may be needed.

Full thickness burns across joint flexures (including around the neck) may undergo fibrotic contraction even after grafting, seriously limiting movement. This difficult problem is likely to require plastic reconstructive operations. Hypertrophic and keloid scars are also common and often require custom made pressure garments worn for a year or more, and sometimes surgical management.

Symptoms, Diagnosis and Management

18

Nonacute Abdominal Pain and Other Abdominal Symptoms and Signs

Introduction

Diagnosis of nonacute abdominal complaints is an important part of the general surgical clinic workload and most patients with abdominal complaints can be managed as outpatients alone. Diagnoses made in a clinic are often quite different from those in emergency surgical admissions. Nevertheless, the surgeon in the clinic must remain alert to unfamiliar presentations that more usually present acutely, for example, an appendix mass.

The principal presenting symptoms of nonacute abdominal disorders are shown in Box 18.1. In addition, patients are often referred to a surgeon after discovery of an **abdominal mass**, **obstructive jaundice** or an **iron deficiency anaemia** caused by chronic blood loss. As ever, the history can provide 70% or more of the clues to the diagnosis, and so must be taken thoughtfully, accurately and with great care. As a general rule, history taking and clinical examination should be done first to reach a provisional diagnosis, and to direct any investigations.

Pain

Character, Timing and Site of the Pain

Key points in taking a history of abdominal pain are summarised in Box 18.2. Pain is highly subjective and the description will be coloured by the patient's perception of it and its possible significance. Patients often use vague terms such as 'indigestion' and 'dyspepsia'; these terms are imprecise, so what the patient actually means should be clarified by further questioning. Time-related

> **• BOX 18.1 Main Presenting Symptoms of Nonacute Abdominal Disorders**
>
> - Abdominal pain
> - Difficulty in swallowing (dysphagia)
> - Weight loss
> - Anorexia (loss of appetite)
> - Nausea or intermittent vomiting
> - Change in bowel habit, including rectal bleeding

Assessing Abdominal Pain From the History

1. Onset and Duration of Pain
- How long ago did it start (hours, days, weeks)?
  - Gradual or sudden onset? (sudden onset implies a mechanical cause)
  - Any previous similar episodes or attacks?

2. Periodicity
- Does pain come in bouts recurring hourly, daily, weekly, monthly?
  - Predominantly daytime or night-time?
  - Any period free from pain?
  - In females, any association with menstrual cycle? Possibility of pregnancy?

3. Location of the Pain
- Where did the pain start and where is it now, for example, central, epigastric, right or left subcostal (hypochondrial), in right or left iliac fossa, suprapubic, 'lower abdominal', or loin?
- Is pain well or poorly localised? (i.e., well localised if parietal peritoneum involved because of its somatic innervation)
- Is there any radiation of the pain? (i.e., spread to nearby areas)

4. Severity and Character of the Pain
- Discomfort only, moderate pain or severe pain?
- How much does it interfere with activities of normal living?
- What descriptive words does the patient use: 'sharp'; 'blunt'; 'burning'; 'crushing'; 'deep'; 'gnawing'; 'boring'; 'bloating'; 'knife-like'; 'stabbing'?
- Is the pain more likely to be physiological (e.g., predefaecation colic or dysmenorrhoea) or pathological?

5. Variation of Pain Severity With Time
- Does the character of the pain vary during an attack, for example, constant, intermittent or episodic, 'colicky' (i.e., coming in severe cramp-like waves), background pain with exacerbations?

6. Exacerbating and Relieving Factors
- For example, improved or made worse by food, posture, exercise or drugs?

7. Associated Symptoms
- For example, vomiting, change in bowel habit, weight loss or nausea?

features of the pain are often highly significant in formulating a differential diagnosis but will only be elicited by diligent enquiry. It is important to establish when a pain first began. Sometimes, asking when the patient was last completely well helps pinpoint the real onset. When presenting or writing a case history, say 'the pain began 6 days ago' rather than, say, 'it began last Thursday'.

Patients describe pain in many different ways, and as each entity tends to have its own pattern, recognisable patterns only come to light if all aspects of the pain history are enquired into.

The Site of Origin, Distribution and Radiation of the Pain
These, and particularly the site it first manifested, suggest likely anatomical structures involved. These are shown in Fig. 18.1.

Diseases Causing Nonacute Abdominal Pain—Typical Patterns
- **Gallstones and gall bladder dysfunction.** Biliary colic presents with irregularly recurrent bouts of severe pain which, though described as colic, characteristically last continuously for 1 to 12 hours. Severe and prolonged episodes may bring the patient into hospital. Pain is usually located in the upper abdomen—most often on the right side—and may radiate around to the back. It is often precipitated by rich or fatty foods and may be associated with vomiting.
- **Peptic ulcer disease.** Typically, there is intermittent 'boring' epigastric pain which recurs several times a year and lasts for days or weeks at a time. It is not as severe as biliary colic unless there is perforation, which presents acutely. Retrosternal 'burning' occurs in peptic oesophagitis and tends to occur after large meals and on lying down. The relationship of pain with food varies according to the site of the ulcer disease: duodenal ulcer pain is relieved by bland food and recurs 3 to 4 hours afterwards, typically in the early morning, whereas the pain of gastric ulcer and oesophagitis tends to be aggravated by food, especially if acidic or spicy. Peptic pain is generally relieved by antacids and virtually always by H_2-blocking drugs (e.g., ranitidine) or proton-pump inhibitors (e.g., omeprazole), this 'trial of treatment' providing evidence towards a diagnosis.
- **Chronic pancreatitis and carcinoma of pancreas.** Both are typically associated with severe 'gnawing', persistent and poorly localised central pain which usually radiates through to the back and is often associated with anorexia and weight loss. The pain may be relieved by leaning forwards ('the pancreatic position'). Early carcinoma of the pancreas, however, is usually painless.
- **Irritable bowel syndrome and constipation.** These may cause a chronic symptom complex mimicking partial bowel obstruction and manifested by episodes of colicky pain. This is poorly localised, often 'bloating' pain, particularly postprandially (after meals). Its intensity varies and it is often associated with transient disturbances of bowel function, particularly alternating diarrhoea and constipation. Passage of flatus or stool often temporarily relieves the symptoms
- **Diverticular disease and Crohn disease.** Partial bowel obstruction can occur with sigmoid diverticular disease or with small bowel Crohn disease. Symptoms are similar to those of complete bowel obstruction but more low key. In incomplete bowel obstruction, there is often passage of some flatus or even faeces but the patient otherwise appears obstructed.
- **Chronic renal outflow obstruction (hydronephrosis).** Causes include stones, tumour (urothelial carcinoma), ureteric stricture, extrinsic ureteric compression (i.e., retroperitoneal fibrosis) or pelviureteric junction obstruction from an aberrant crossing vessel. Patients may report a 'dull', poorly defined, fairly constant loin pain, which can radiate to the groin or genitalia. Pain is often aggravated acutely by high fluid intake. Associated urinary symptoms may include haematuria or dysuria.
- **Gynaecological conditions.** Chronic pelvic pain may be caused by pelvic inflammatory disease, endometriosis and ovarian tumours. These may reach the general surgeon because of poorly defined lower abdominal pain. A gynaecological history should be taken in female patients; pelvic examination may reveal the cause and ultrasound is usually diagnostic.
- **Nonsurgical (i.e., 'medical') disorders causing abdominal pain.** These include liver congestion in heart failure (common), splenic infarcts or diabetes (both uncommon but important), acute intermittent porphyria, sickle-cell anaemia or tertiary syphilis (very rare). Patients sometimes present with abdominal pain for which no organic cause can be found despite extensive investigation. In these, irritable bowel syndrome or sensitivity to certain foods, for example, gluten or wheat protein, need to be considered. Only as a last resort should the pain be attributed to psychological disturbances.

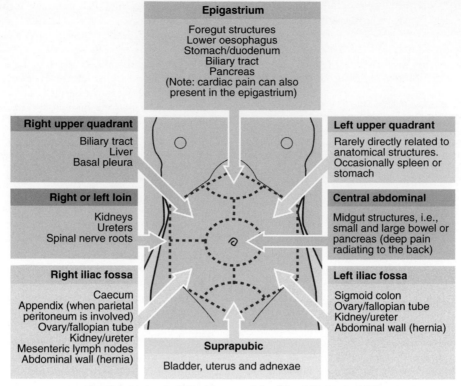

• **Fig. 18.1** Anatomical Significance of the Site of Abdominal Pain.

Nonacute Abdominal Pain in Children (Also See Ch. 51)

This is common. The main organic causes are: 'infantile colic' (sometimes caused by cow's milk allergy), irritable bowel syndrome in older children, chronic inflammatory bowel disease, recurrent streptococcal infections, and sometimes hydronephrosis caused by urinary tract obstruction. Childhood *periodic syndromes* include recurrent episodes of poorly defined and inconsistent abdominal pain and/or recurrent vomiting, sometimes sufficiently severe for the child to require admission and intravenous fluids; these are often described as a precursor to migraine. 'Abdominal migraine' describes abdominal pain with or without nausea, pallor, and photophobia which lasts for up to 3 days, is most common in the years before puberty, and is not usually associated with a headache. Psychosomatic abdominal pain may be the explanation if organic causes have been excluded and thus psychological, environmental and social factors, including the possibility of child neglect and abuse, should be explored (see Chapter 51).

Approach to Investigation of Nonacute Abdominal Pain

A differential diagnosis must first be made on clinical grounds (Box 18.3 and see Fig. 18.1). The choice (and order) of investigations should be efficient and economical, after considering how each will support or help eliminate the most probable (and common) diagnoses and how it might influence management.

Dysphagia and Odynophagia

Clinical Presentation

Dysphagia is the term for difficulty in swallowing. The most common complaint is inability to swallow solids, which the patient describes as 'becoming stuck' or 'held up' before it passes into the stomach or is regurgitated. Fibrous foods, such as chunks of meat, usually cause the most trouble. The patient can usually indicate a precise level for the perceived obstruction. The true level of obstruction is usually some distance below that point.

Dysphagia is almost always caused by disease in or near the oesophagus but occasionally the lesion is in the pharynx or stomach. Oesophageal narrowing usually causes symptoms only when the lumen is unable to expand beyond about 10 mm—the narrower the lumen, the more severe the symptoms. In many pathological conditions causing dysphagia, the lumen becomes progressively constricted and indistensible. Initially only fibrous solids cause difficulty but later this extends to all solids and eventually, even to fluids. Because narrowing is a gradual and insidious process, patients often compensate to a surprising degree (e.g., by liquidising all food) and may only present when they have difficulty swallowing fluids or even their own saliva. By this time, there is usually marked weight loss.

The common causes of dysphagia are outlined in Box 18.4. **Pain** on swallowing or **odynophagia** (usually provoked by both food and drink, particularly if hot) is a distinctive symptom highly suspicious of carcinoma.

Achalasia is an exception to the usual pattern of dysphagia, in that swallowing fluids causes more difficulty than solids. In achalasia, there is idiopathic destruction of inhibitory ganglia in Auerbach

• BOX 18.3 Abdominal Examination: 28 Points to Remember in Examining a Patient With Abdominal Symptoms

General Examination

1. Well-looking or ill (thin, emaciated, weak)?
2. Alert and responding normally or obtunded and slumped in bed?
3. Dehydrated (poor skin tone, sunken cheeks)?
4. Abnormal skin colour (pale, jaundiced, grey)
5. Signs of surgical wounds or dressings
6. End-of-bed charts—fever, tachycardia, fluid balance, trauma chart, pain chart, drug chart (e.g., strength and frequency of analgesia), modified early warning scores (MEWS)
7. 'Medical accessories'—IV infusion, urinary catheter, parenteral nutrition, monitoring equipment, oxygen mask

Peripheral Stigmata of Abdominal Disease

1. Fingernails for koilonychia (spoon-shaped nails in iron deficiency) and leuconychia (whiteness and opacity of nails, sometimes caused by hypoalbuminaemia)
2. Hands for palmar erythema and Dupuytren contracture (association with liver disease)
3. Eyes—yellow sclerae in jaundice, pale conjunctivae in anaemia
4. Mouth and tongue—for ulceration suggestive of Crohn, angular stomatitis in anaemia, dehydration, telangiectasia in hereditary haemorrhagic telangiectasia
5. Supraclavicular fossa palpation for enlarged lymph nodes, particularly medial left-sided Virchow node indicating upper GI malignancy (Troisier sign)
6. Inspect abdominal skin for jaundice and scratch marks resulting from pruritus (itching), spider naevi (indicate likely liver disease)
7. Chest in males for gynaecomastia in liver disease

Abdominal Inspection

1. Position the patient correctly (comfortable, near-flat, arms by sides) and expose the whole abdominal field ('nipples to knees', but not all at once)
2. Distended or scaphoid (sunken) abdominal shape?
3. Skin—wounds and scars, redness, purulent discharge or other signs of infection, erythema ab igne (see Fig. 18.2 in Case History)

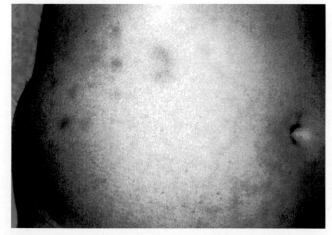

• **Fig. 18.2 Erythema Ab Igne.** This woman of 45 years suffered chronic pain in the right loin and had obtained some relief from regularly applying a hot water bottle to the area which resulted in typical skin damage. A staghorn calculus in the right kidney proved to be the cause.

4. Bruising—umbilical or flank in acute pancreatitis; cloth printing (trauma cases)
5. Herniation (including usual primary sites and incisional hernias)
6. Caput medusae—enlarged veins radiating from umbilicus indicating portal venous obstruction
7. Visible peristalsis—usually indicating long-standing small bowel obstruction

Abdominal Palpation (do not hurt the patient; watch the face for signs of discomfort)

1. Gentle overall palpation for obvious abnormalities
2. Overall firmer palpation at a deeper level provides detailed examination of abnormal masses—relationship to abdominal wall, size, shape, position, mobility, texture, hardness, fixation posteriorly or anteriorly, tenderness. Likely site or organ of origin?
3. Specific organ palpation—press in first, then ask the patient to breathe in deeply; gradually relax your pressure and seek the descending lower edge of the organ; repeat at 3 cm intervals moving upwards:
   — Liver: start as low as it might have reached, for example, right iliac fossa, and work upwards as earlier. Map out palpable lower liver edge. If large, palpate surface for irregularities, for example, metastases. The enlarging liver usually remains in contact with the anterior abdominal wall and is dull to percussion. Percuss also for upper border to gauge liver size; auscultate a large liver for vascular bruits
   — Spleen: tilt patient slightly towards right side, place left hand behind lower left ribs and gently lift. Start as low as enlargement might have reached, for example, right iliac fossa, and palpate as for liver. Seek notch in lower edge. To be palpable, spleen needs to be enlarged two to three times normal. Percuss for overlying resonance caused by gas in bowel superficial to it
   — Kidneys: as with the liver, a renal mass usually descends with inspiration since the kidneys lie just beneath the diaphragm. Bimanual palpation enables the posteriorly placed kidney to be felt by displacing it anteriorly (see Fig. 18.3). Place left hand in loin and attempt to push enlarged organ forwards on to examining hand
4. Examination for ascites (see Fig. 18.4)
5. Hernial orifices—inguinal and femoral for cough impulse; reducibility (see Ch. 32)
6. Rectal and/or vaginal examination if appropriate (see Table 18.1)
7. Percussion and auscultation if appropriate

GI, Gastrointestinal; *IV,* intravenous.

• BOX 18.4 Causes of Dysphagia

Obstruction Arising in the Oesophageal Wall

Common
- Peptic oesophagitis (often associated with hiatus hernia)—sometimes causes fibrous stricture
- Carcinoma of oesophagus or cardia (uppermost part) of the stomach

Uncommon
- Candida oesophagitis, particularly after major surgery

Extremely Rare
- Pharyngeal pouch
- Oesophageal web (Plummer–Vinson/Paterson–Kelly syndrome)
- 'Oesophageal apoplexy' caused by haematoma in the wall
- Leiomyoma of the oesophageal muscle

Disorders of Neuromuscular Function
- Achalasia—uncommon
- Bulbar or pseudobulbar palsy—rare
- Myasthenia gravis—rare

External Compression of the Oesophagus
- Subcarinal lymph node secondaries from carcinoma of the bronchus—fairly common
- Left atrial dilatation in mitral stenosis—rare
- Dysphagia lusoria (compression from abnormally placed great arteries)—very rare

---

(myenteric) plexus of the entire oesophagus, which results in functional narrowing of the lower oesophagus and peristaltic failure throughout its length. Thus the oesophagus becomes markedly distended and dilated, with solids settling towards the lower end and fluids spilling over into the airways causing **spluttering dysphagia**, particularly when the patient is lying flat. Achalasia commonly presents with chronic chest infection rather than dysphagia and the diagnosis is often reached late. Similar overspill symptoms can be caused by bulbar palsy, most commonly after a stroke.

Bolus obstruction is an acute form of dysphagia, where a lump of food sticks at a narrowed part, completely obstructing the oesophagus.

Approach to Investigation of Dysphagia

Dysphagia, particularly of recent onset, must be regarded seriously and fully investigated. A plain chest x-ray should be taken to exclude bronchial carcinoma; occasionally an oesophageal fluid level behind the heart is seen, resulting from an oesophageal stricture, hiatus hernia or achalasia. In high dysphagia, flexible pharyngoscopy followed by a barium swallow and meal is the usual sequence of investigation. In lower dysphagia, flexible endoscopy (oesophago-gastro-duodenoscopy, OGD) is usually performed, as this allows direct inspection and biopsy; however, contrast radiography can be helpful. In disorders of function, swallowing barium-soaked bread or a video record of a barium swallow may be diagnostic. Oesophageal physiology measurements using manometry and pH monitoring are helpful in reaching a diagnosis of achalasia, especially in its early stages.

Weight Loss, Anorexia and Associated Symptoms

Marked weight loss (**cachexia**) and loss of appetite (**anorexia**) are frequently manifestations of serious, insidious, often malignant abdominal disorders. There may be other symptoms, such as malaise, bloating, nausea, sporadic vomiting and regurgitation. These symptoms may have been unnoticed or dismissed as trivial by the patient and are only elicited by direct questioning.

The diseases which cause these symptoms may be grouped into four broad categories:
- **Intraabdominal malignancies**, for example, carcinoma of stomach or pancreas, metastatic disease in the liver or widespread across the peritoneal cavity (arising particularly from stomach, large bowel, ovary, breast or bronchus), bowel lymphomas.
- **'Medical' conditions**, for example, alcoholism and cirrhosis, viral diseases (e.g., hepatitis or infectious mononucleosis), uncontrolled diabetes or thyrotoxicosis, malabsorption, renal failure, cardiac cachexia.
- **Psychological disorders**, for example, anxiety, depression, anorexia nervosa, bulimia.
- **Chronic visceral ischaemia**, a very uncommon condition resulting from atherosclerotic narrowing of at least two of the three main visceral arteries—the coeliac axis and the superior mesenteric and the inferior mesenteric arteries—resulting in 'fear of food' and massive weight loss.

Approach to Investigation of Weight Loss, Anorexia and Associated Symptoms

There may be other clinical clues to the main diagnosis or to suggest a line of investigation, for example, pain, signs of anaemia or jaundice, or a palpable abdominal or rectal mass. More difficult are cases where the symptoms occur alone. In that situation, basic screening investigations (full blood count, erythrocyte sedimentation rate [ESR], C-reactive protein, urea and electrolytes, liver function tests and urinalysis) begin to differentiate 'medical' conditions from 'surgical' ones. If these screening tests fail to produce a lead, abdominal imaging using ultrasound or computed tomography (CT) scanning may be indicated to exclude liver metastases or occult intraabdominal malignancy.

If investigations still reveal no cause, positive evidence of psychiatric disturbance should be sought. In practice, by this stage, previously concealed psychiatric features often become apparent, but except for anorexia nervosa or bulimia, these are rare.

Anal and Perianal Symptoms

Anal Bleeding

This is a very common symptom. It is well tolerated by patients who usually believe that 'piles' (haemorrhoids) are responsible. Patients often present when bleeding becomes excessive or when other symptoms develop. The characteristic feature of anal bleeding is fresh blood separate from stool which may be seen only 'on the paper'. Fresh bleeding, however, can arise from malignancy in the rectum, sigmoid colon or anal canal and must be treated seriously. In addition to digital examination and proctoscopy, all patients require at least sigmoidoscopy; patients over 40 years require colonoscopy or CT pneumocolon to exclude large bowel cancer, even if a benign anal cause, such as haemorrhoids, has already been found. Barium enema is an alternative investigation that has been largely superseded by CT pneumocolon. Contrast CT of the abdomen and pelvis may be used to investigate frail and elderly patients unable to tolerate colonoscopy or CT pneumocolon, both of which require mechanical bowel preparation.

Anal Pain and Discomfort

The principal causes of chronic anal pain and discomfort is haemorrhoids. Haemorrhoids usually cause intermittent bouts of discomfort and other anal symptoms rather than severe pain. Anal carcinoma is usually painless but may present with haemorrhoid-like symptoms. The difference is obvious on digital rectal examination (DRE).

Severe perianal pain following each episode of defaecation usually indicates a fissure-in-ano. This is a longitudinal tear typically found in the posterior anal mucosa ending externally in a characteristic 'sentinel pile', a small skin tag visible at the anal margin. A fissure is often initiated by a bout of unaccustomed constipation. A perianal abscess may be responsible for anal pain even before the abscess is clinically detectable; the rare **intersphincteric abscess** may cause chronic pain and elude detection for weeks.

An acute onset of anal pain may be caused by a **perianal haematoma**, clearly visible at the anal margin, by strangulated or thrombosed haemorrhoids or by a perianal abscess.

Proctalgia fugax describes recurrent shooting pains experienced in the anal area. Investigations should be performed to exclude local causes but usually no physical cause is found.

Perianal Itching and Irritation

The most common cause of these symptoms is inadequate hygiene resulting in local skin irritation. This is exacerbated by scratching or application of topical medications. The discharge associated with haemorrhoids, fistulae or tumours tends to cause itching and keep the perianal skin moist, predisposing to low-grade fungal and bacterial infections. The longer symptoms persist, the more difficult they are to eradicate and in fastidious patients a 'fixation' can develop. In children, threadworm infestation is a common cause of perianal itching, usually worse at night.

'Something Coming Down'

Haemorrhoids, skin tags ('memorials to past haemorrhoids') and occasionally mucosal or rectal prolapse cause this symptom. It is exacerbated by defaecation. Many patients tolerate the condition for some time before seeking medical advice and may have to push the lumps back manually after defaecation, presenting medically only when this becomes impossible. A pedunculated low rectal polyp may occasionally emerge through the anus and be confused with prolapsed haemorrhoids. Perianal warts are occasionally mistaken for lumps arising from within the anal canal.

Perianal Discharge

This results from leakage of pus, inflammatory exudate or mucus from the anus or anal area. Pus may arise from a pilonidal sinus in the natal cleft or from an anal fistula. Inflammatory exudate or excess mucus may be produced by haemorrhoids, anorectal mucosal inflammation (proctitis), a villous adenoma or an ulcerating carcinoma.

Approach to Investigation of Anal and Perianal Symptoms

Inspection of the anal area, careful DRE and proctoscopy are mandatory (Table 18.1 and Fig. 18.3). Further examination follows the principles described earlier. If pain makes these examinations impossible, a young patient can usually be assumed to have a fissure. In an older person or those with specific risk factors (e.g., HIV positive), carcinoma of the anus must be excluded by examination under anaesthesia (EUA). Haemorrhoids appear as bulging

bluish masses beneath the anal mucosa. They all arise above the squamocolumnar junction or dentate line ('internal piles') but may later extend beneath the perianal skin ('external piles') or prolapse through the anus ('interoexternal piles').

A typical **anal fistula** appears as an inflammatory 'nipple' near the anal margin (see Fig. 18.4); it often exudes a discharge. In **proctitis**, the rectal mucosa is granular, erythematous and friable on proctoscopy. An anal or low rectal carcinoma is a discrete ulcerated lesion with an indurated (firm, woody) base and a thickened margin; diagnosis is confirmed by biopsy.

The lymphatic drainage of the anal canal below the dentate line is to inguinal lymph nodes and these should be examined when a suspicious anal lesion is found.

CASE HISTORY

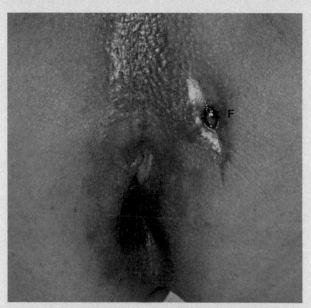

• **Fig. 18.3** Anal Fistula. This man of 39 years had presented with a perianal abscess 3 months previously that had been drained. He complained of persistent discharge which was found to be emanating from a fistulous opening *(F)*, within the drainage scar. On further examination under anaesthesia, this proved to be a low fistula.

Change in Bowel Habit, Rectal Bleeding and Related Symptoms

Normal bowel habit varies widely between individuals in frequency and consistency of stool. Transient changes in habit are usually insignificant but persistent change definitely requires investigation. The differential diagnosis of a change in bowel habit is summarised in Box 18.5.

Frequency of Defaecation and Stool Consistency

Chronic constipation or diarrhoea mark the extremes of change, although some patients develop an erratic bowel action. Any change may signify serious disease; the index of suspicion is further raised if there is rectal bleeding or tenesmus (sensation of incomplete rectal evacuation). Waking from sleep to evacuate the bowels should be treated seriously, especially if it occurs persistently.

TABLE 18.1 **Investigation of Anal and Colorectal Symptoms**

1. Digital Rectal Examination

Purpose	Inspection of the anal and perianal area for skin changes and lesions Palpation of the anal canal and lower rectum and surrounding tissues. Normally the firm walls of the anal sphincter are felt over the first 5 cm or so. Above that level, the rectal walls are soft and mobile
Preparation	Offer a chaperone 'Consent'—written or implied Patient position—left lateral with knees drawn up Equipment—good light, surgical gloves, gel lubricant, tissues
Technique • **Inspection**	Sentinel pile; excoriation; ulceration, perianal haematoma; fistulous opening; scars; abscess; prolapsed mucosa or haemorrhoids; skin tags
• **Palpation** Try not to cause pain and discomfort—if pain/spasm prevents examination, a fissure or anal carcinoma may be present *Note*: in the female, the uterine cervix is often felt anteriorly as a firm but localised mass. In the male, the normal prostate gland is felt near the tip of the finger anteriorly as a smooth, firm swelling about 3–4 cm in diameter with a midline groove between the lateral lobes	*In lumen*—faeces/blood/foreign body *In wall*—ulceration, polyp, thrombosed piles, internal opening of tract or fistula; Crohn thickening; anal carcinoma; lack of normal softness *Outside wall*—smooth prostatic enlargement (usually benign) can be palpated, as can irregularity or nodularity, which may represent carcinoma; cervix; frozen pelvis; mass in pouch of Douglas Note: glove should be checked for blood/mucus/colour of stool

2. Proctoscopy (see Fig. 18.5; see also Ch. 30)

Purpose	Direct visualisation of mucosa of anal canal Must be done even if rigid sigmoidoscopy/barium enema/MRI to be done Therapy, for example, sclerotherapy/banding of haemorrhoids
Technique	The proctoscope with obturator in situ is lubricated and gently introduced into the anal canal to its greatest extent (10 cm). The obturator is removed and the instrument slowly withdrawn, ensuring that the mucosa of the entire anal canal is inspected
Findings in mucosa	Inflammation/granular surface Superficial ulceration Haemorrhoids—bleeding, degree of prolapse Anal carcinoma Solitary 'rectal' ulcer Pus Fistula Fibrous polyps Melanoma

3. Rigid Sigmoidoscopy (for flexible sigmoidoscopy see text)

Purpose	**Visualisation** of the rectum up to rectosigmoid junction (18–20 cm) **Biopsy** of suspicious lesions or abnormal mucosa
Technique	As for proctoscopy for 10 cm or so. Obturator removed and proximal end closed with lens. Gentle inflation whilst inspecting lumen, manipulating and advancing scope with least discomfort to patient Faecal loading may prevent visualisation; pain may limit examination to lower rectum only
Examples of pathology	Inflammation/granular surface Superficial ulceration Pus Polyps and adenomas Carcinoma Melanosis coli Strictures

MRI, Magnetic resonance imaging.

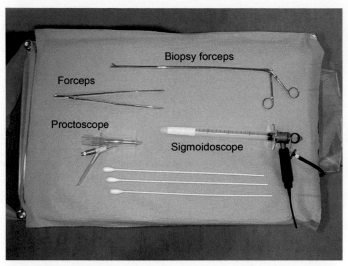

• **Fig. 18.4** Proctosigmoidoscopy Trolley. Typical layout of trolley prepared for proctoscopy and sigmoidoscopy in an outpatient clinic. Note the yellow waste bag on the left for contaminated swabs and waste and the paper bag on the right for waste wrapping from swabs, etc. Sigmoidoscopic biopsies are placed in a container of formol saline for fixation.

● BOX 18.5 Differential Diagnosis of Change in Bowel Habit

- Carcinoma of colon, rectum or anus
- Diverticular disease
- Irritable bowel syndrome
- Crohn disease of small or large bowel
- Ulcerative colitis
- Drug effects, for example, codeine phosphate, iron, laxative abuse
- Reduction or increase in fibre content of diet
- Parasitic infestations, for example, giardiasis
- Following acute bacterial or parasitic colitis
- Changes in resident bacterial flora, for example, antibiotic-associated diarrhoea
- Malabsorption syndromes
- Thyrotoxicosis

Note: in many cases, no cause is found.

Stool consistency varies according to diet but the stool is usually 'formed'. Persistently unformed stools, that is, 'looseness', is only abnormal if it represents a change from the patient's norm.

Constipation

Severe constipation arises for four main reasons:
- Incomplete bowel obstruction, for example, faecal impaction, an obstructing carcinoma or stricture in the bowel wall, or occasionally a lesion outside the bowel, such as ovarian cancer.
- Loss of peristalsis, for example, acutely caused by drugs, such as narcotics, antidepressants or iron, chronic diverticular disease, chronic laxative abuse.
- Inadequate fibre intake or poor fluid intake, which decrease faecal volume and prolong intestinal transit time.
- In bed-bound patients, multiple factors including immobility, changed diet, inadequate fluid intake, drug effects.

Diarrhoea

Chronic diarrhoea is most often caused by irritation or inflammation of small or large bowel. The inflammatory bowel diseases (ulcerative colitis and Crohn disease) are important diagnoses. Chronic parasitic infestations of large bowel with amoebae, or of small bowel with *Giardia lamblia*, are easily overlooked. In areas where these diseases are not endemic, patients may give a history of foreign travel. Chronic diarrhoea may follow an acute attack of *Salmonella* or other coliform infection. Less commonly, a blind loop of small bowel remaining after bypass surgery becomes colonised with gut flora, causing changes in intraluminal metabolism (**blind loop syndrome**). The most common diagnosis in diarrhoea after intestinal infection is irritable bowel syndrome.

Bile salts irritate the bowel. Therefore if the enterohepatic circulation is disrupted, for example, after distal small bowel resection, defective reabsorption of bile salts may cause diarrhoea. A less common cause is the increased volume of bowel contents in malabsorption syndromes. Finally, when no physical cause can be found, concealed laxative abuse or an anxiety state should be considered. Early morning diarrhoea on its own rarely indicates serious disease.

Erratic Bowel Habit

Some patients develop an erratic bowel habit with bouts of constipation interspersed with episodes of frequency and looseness of stool. The most common cause is **irritable bowel syndrome**, which can be attributed to a heightened pain response in conjunction with a possible overproduction of enteric gas. Sometimes symptoms include a marked gastrocolic reflex, that is, a call to stool immediately after eating. In **diverticular disease**, constipation and 'rabbit-pellet' faeces are the dominant characteristics (see Ch. 29). However, there may be episodic diarrhoea during periods of inflammation or following release of proximal liquefied stool past partially obstructed solid faeces (**spurious diarrhoea**). Incomplete bowel obstruction of this type may also occur in carcinoma of the left colon, Crohn disease or faecal impaction.

Patients treated with broad-spectrum antibiotics, particularly the cephalosporins, may develop **antibiotic-associated diarrhoea**. If caused by *Clostridium difficile*, this is known as **pseudomembranous colitis** in its severe form; the symptoms are caused by changes in colonic bacterial flora (see Ch. 12).

Changes in the Nature of the Stool

Stools are normally brown owing to the presence of stercobilin, a breakdown product of bile. In biliary obstruction, bilirubin fails to reach the gut and stools become pale. In obvious jaundice, stools are often described as 'putty-coloured' or 'clay-coloured'.

Stools may also be pale when they contain excess fat as in various malabsorption syndromes. In coeliac disease (gluten enteropathy) the stool is often loose and offensive. In fat malabsorption, the lipid rich stools tend to float and are difficult to flush away (**steatorrhoea**).

Undigested food in the stool indicates malabsorption or a 'short-circuit' in the bowel caused by previous bowel resection or a fistula between bowel loops. Note that this can be normal when the diet is extremely high in fibre.

Presence of Frank Blood, Altered Blood or Mucus in the Stool

Note: acute gastrointestinal (GI) haemorrhage is covered in Chapter 19.

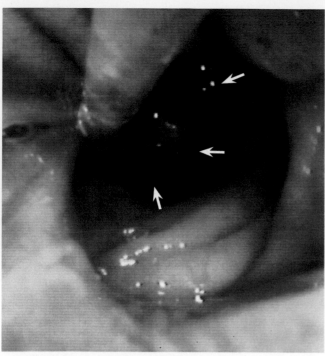

• **Fig. 18.5** Colonoscopic Appearance of a Polyp in the Sigmoid Colon. This 2-cm polyp *(arrowed)* was found to be the cause of rectal bleeding. It was easily removed with a colonoscopic snare soon after this photograph was taken.

Frank Rectal Bleeding

When a patient has seen blood in the stool, it is important to know the colour, that is, fresh or altered blood, and also the relationship of the blood to the stool. Bright red blood usually indicates a lesion in the rectum or anus. When blood is clearly separate from the stool, it suggests an anal lesion (see earlier). If blood is on the surface of the stool it suggests a lesion, such as an adenoma (Fig. 18.5) or carcinoma in the rectum or descending colon. These observations have limited diagnostic reliability and all rectal bleeding should be assumed to be caused by a tumour until proven otherwise.

When older, darker blood is mixed with the stool, it usually indicates even more proximal disease, that is, descending or transverse colon. Carcinoma or inflammatory ulceration is often the cause. When the blood originates more proximally in the GI tract, for example, peptic ulcer, it is so altered by digestion that it may not be recognised as blood by the patient. The stool is typically shiny black or plum-coloured, has a characteristic odour, and with rapid bleeding, becomes fluid or 'tarry' (**melaena**). Patients on iron therapy have greenish-black, formed stools, not to be mistaken for altered blood; faecal immunochemical test (FIT), which is used to identify blood in the stool, should be negative.

Occult Faecal Blood Loss

A persistent trickle of blood from the GI tract may not alter the appearance of the stool but can cause serious iron deficiency anaemia. This 'occult' blood may be detectable only by chemical or immunological tests; these should be repeated three times to prevent false negatives.

Rectal Passage of Mucus or Pus

Mucus ('slime') or pus may be passed alone or with the stool. The most common cause is irritable bowel syndrome. **Villous**

adenomas typically secrete copious mucus, but this may also occur with rectal carcinoma. Mucus and pus may be noted in inflammatory bowel disorders and occasionally in diverticular disease. An anal leak of mucus may be a feature of haemorrhoids and causes itching (**pruritus ani**). A patient sometimes reports passing a mass of purulent material. This usually represents spontaneous discharge of a perianal or pararectal abscess, and will often be preceded by anal or perineal pain.

Tenesmus

Tenesmus is an unpleasant sensation of incomplete evacuation of the rectum. The sensation causes the patient to attempt defaecation (often with straining) at frequent intervals. The most common causes are irritable bowel syndrome or an abnormal mass in the rectum or anal canal (e.g., polyp; carcinoma). Occasionally a prostatic carcinoma invades around the lower rectum producing tenesmus. In some cases, despite extensive investigation, no organic cause is found.

Approach to Investigation of Change in Bowel Habit

In chronic diarrhoea, stool specimens should be examined for ova and parasites and cultured for *Shigella* and *Salmonella* species. After rectal palpation and proctoscopy, the next step is sigmoidoscopy. **Rigid sigmoidoscopy** (more accurately termed *rectoscopy*) permits visual examination up to the rectosigmoid junction and mucosal biopsy for histology and microbiology. **Flexible sigmoidoscopy** allows more precise examination as far as the splenic flexure, the area in which over 50% of large bowel cancers occur and is the examination of choice when available.

Further investigation is based on the differential diagnosis assembled during clinical examination. Barium enema x-ray, contrast CT scanning or colonoscopy is indicated in most cases. Low rectal lesions cannot reliably be demonstrated on contrast studies and so preliminary sigmoidoscopy is mandatory. Note that more than one colonic adenoma or carcinoma can occur at the same time (synchronous lesions), so a full colonic examination is needed if one lesion is found. If Crohn disease is suspected, barium studies or cross-sectional imaging of the small bowel may also be required.

Iron Deficiency Anaemia

A common reason for surgical referral is persistent or severe anaemia believed to be caused by chronic intestinal blood loss. The patient may have presented with symptoms of chronic anaemia, namely lethargy, generalised weakness, breathlessness or even angina. Just as often, the anaemia has been recognised during general examination or on a blood count.

Chronic anaemia has many causes. Iron deficiency is the most common and the only one with a cause likely to need surgical treatment. In blood films, iron deficiency anaemia is characterised by **hypochromic, microcytic** red blood cells. Serum iron level is low and transferrin elevated. Iron deficiency anaemia can be caused by chronic low-grade blood loss (often occult), inadequate dietary iron intake or absorption, or a combination. The pattern of iron deficiency may be complicated by coexisting anaemia from another cause, particularly the 'anaemia of chronic illness'. For example, an elderly patient with rheumatoid arthritis may have a chronic normochromic, normocytic anaemia caused by

---

• BOX 18.6   **Conditions Causing Chronic Occult Blood Loss**

Lesions in the Gastrointestinal Tract

- Ulcerating tumours or polyps of the following (in order of frequency): caecum, stomach, the rest of the large bowel, and (rarely) stromal tumours of small bowel, for example, leiomyosarcoma (gastrointestinal stromal tumour)
- Chronic peptic ulceration, that is, hiatus hernia with reflux oesophagitis, gastric and duodenal ulcers or stromal ulceration following gastric surgery. All may be induced or aggravated by ingestion of aspirin and other nonsteroidal anti-inflammatory drugs. These drugs can also cause chronic gastric haemorrhage from superficial erosions
- Other 'ulcerating' lesions of the bowel, for example, haemorrhoids, angiodysplasias of colon or small bowel
- Chronic parasitic infestations, for example, hookworm (extremely common in some developing countries)
- Angiodysplasias—small vascular malformations, single or multiple, occurring anywhere from stomach to rectum which bleed spontaneously

Conditions Affecting the Female Genital Tract

- Heavy menstrual loss (menorrhagia is an extremely common but easily overlooked cause)
- Carcinoma of uterus or cervix (usually presents as abnormal vaginal bleeding rather than anaemia)

Lesions in the Urinary Tract (Rarely Sufficient to Cause Anaemia)

- Urothelial carcinoma of bladder, pelvicalyceal systems or ureters
- Renal cell carcinoma (may cause haematuria but rarely significant anaemia)
- Chronic parasitic infestations, for example, schistosomiasis (common in some developing countries)

---

chronic disease, as well as an iron deficiency anaemia caused by gastric bleeding provoked by nonsteroidal anti-inflammatory drugs (NSAIDs). Pernicious anaemia or folate deficiency anaemia may also underlie iron deficiency anaemia.

Approach to Investigation of Anaemia

Investigation of a patient with suspected iron deficiency anaemia has five main components:

- History—seeking sources of blood loss from the various tracts (Box 18.6) and excluding inadequate iron intake. Previous gastrectomy may cause vitamin B_{12} deficiency and also diminished acid output, which may diminish iron absorption. Drug history—aspirin, other NSAIDs and corticosteroids may be the cause of chronic gastroduodenal blood loss. A history of drug treatment for peptic ulcer or antacids for 'indigestion' may also indicate a source of blood loss.
- Physical examination—seeking an abdominal mass, an enlarged Virchow node in the left supraclavicular area (indicative of intraabdominal malignancy), a rectal lesion or signs of a 'medical' cause.
- Confirmation of iron deficiency anaemia and exclusion of common 'medical' causes of anaemia, such as rheumatoid arthritis or chronic leukaemias—examine blood film, measure ESR, serum iron and transferrin, vitamin B_{12} and folate. When there is a 'mixed' anaemia, measuring iron stores in a bone marrow biopsy is the definitive method of diagnosing iron deficiency. Small bowel biopsies may demonstrate coeliac disease in a proportion of patients with simple anaemia without bowel symptoms.

- Testing of specimens of stool for occult blood or the FIT (at least three specimens).
- Pursuing clues that suggest the origin of bleeding with special investigations, such as endoscopy and contrast radiology. When faecal occult blood is identified, colonoscopy is performed, looking for tumours, polyps, inflammatory bowel disease or angiodysplasias. If negative, this is followed by gastroscopy. Both can be performed in one session. If both are negative, it may be appropriate to proceed to small bowel contrast radiography (magnetic resonance imaging [MRI] or CT may be used), flexible small bowel enteroscopy or **capsule endoscopy** (see Ch. 5).

Obstructive Jaundice

The Normal Enterohepatic Circulation (Fig. 18.6)

The **haem** component of spent red cells is normally broken down to bilirubin (mainly in spleen and bone marrow), bound to albumin and transported to the liver. This relatively stable protein–pigment complex is insoluble in water and is not excreted in urine. In the liver, the complex is split and the bilirubin conjugated with glucuronic acid (which makes it water-soluble), before being excreted into the bile canaliculi. The normal concentration of both conjugated and unconjugated bilirubin measured in the blood is very low. Bacterial action in the bowel converts conjugated bilirubin into colourless **urobilinogen,** some of which is converted to form **pigmented stercobilin** which imparts the brown colour to normal faeces. Some urobilinogen is reabsorbed, passing to the liver in the portal blood, and is then reexcreted in the bile. The entire process is called an **enterohepatic circulation** (see Fig. 18.6). In addition, some urobilinogen is converted into **urobilin** and is excreted in the urine, colouring it yellow.

Bile acids (**salts**) are synthesised in the liver from cholesterol-based precursors. These are excreted in bile to the duodenum and facilitate lipid digestion and absorption in the small intestine. About 95% of the bile acids are reabsorbed in the distal ileum and returned to the liver via the portal vein, only to be reexcreted in the bile. Thus both bilirubin and bile acids are involved in enterohepatic circulations.

Pathophysiology of Obstructive Jaundice

If biliary outflow becomes obstructed, conjugated bilirubin is dammed back in the liver from where it enters the bloodstream and causes a gradual rise in plasma bilirubin. Once the plasma bilirubin level exceeds about 30 µmol/L, jaundice should be clinically detectable. Conjugated bilirubin, being water soluble, is excreted in the urine, turning it dark.

In obstructive jaundice, there is diminished or absent excretion of bile into the bowel, causing changes in the faeces. There is less stercobilin to darken the stool and fewer bile acids, resulting in defective fat absorption and characteristic 'putty' coloured stools.

A consequence of poor dietary fat absorption is malabsorption of fat soluble vitamins A, D, E and K. Lack of vitamin K leads to decreased hepatic synthesis of clotting factors, notably prothrombin (factor II), factors VII, IX and X, and proteins C, S and Z. Impaired blood clotting increases the risk of haemorrhage during invasive procedures, so a clotting screen must be checked beforehand. The coagulopathy is corrected with parenteral vitamin K or, in an urgent procedure, fresh frozen plasma. Biliary obstruction also dams back bile acids, which raises their blood concentration leading to deposition in the skin; this can cause intense itching.

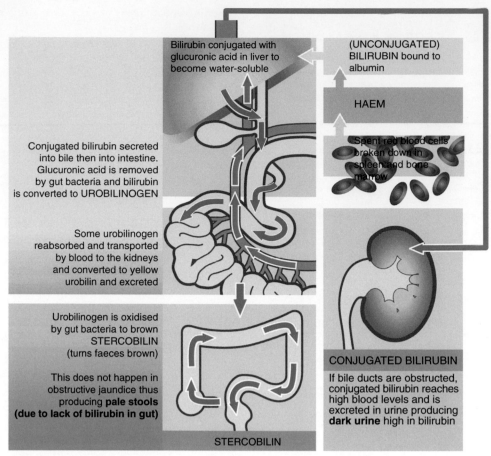

Bilirubin conjugated with glucuronic acid in liver to become water-soluble

(UNCONJUGATED) BILIRUBIN bound to albumin

HAEM

Spent red blood cells broken down in spleen and bone marrow

Conjugated bilirubin secreted into bile then into intestine. Glucuronic acid is removed by gut bacteria and bilirubin is converted to UROBILINOGEN

Some urobilinogen reabsorbed and transported by blood to the kidneys and converted to yellow urobilin and excreted

Urobilinogen is oxidised by gut bacteria to brown STERCOBILIN (turns faeces brown)

This does not happen in obstructive jaundice thus producing **pale stools** (due to lack of bilirubin in gut)

CONJUGATED BILIRUBIN

If bile ducts are obstructed, conjugated bilirubin reaches high blood levels and is excreted in urine producing **dark urine** high in bilirubin

STERCOBILIN

• **Fig. 18.6** Normal Dynamics of Bilirubin Excretion and the Effects of Obstructive Jaundice. Note that urobilinogen will appear in substantial quantities in the urine if large amounts are produced because of haemolytic anaemia, or if there is liver cell damage.

History and Examination of Patients With Obstructive Jaundice

History-Taking

This should include enquiry about episodes of pain typical of gallstone disease, previous episodes of obstructive jaundice, biliary tract surgery or attacks of acute pancreatitis. Other important aspects of the history include:

- change in colour of urine and stools, that is, dark urine and pale stools;
- drug history, for example, oral contraceptive pill—potential for intrahepatic cholestasis;
- risk factors for viral hepatitis—blood product transfusion, intravenous drug abuse, tattoos, shellfish ingestion, sexual exposure;
- alcohol intake—if excessive, predisposes to pancreatitis and cirrhosis;
- symptoms associated with malignancy—anorexia, weight loss and nonspecific upper GI disturbance is common in carcinoma of the pancreas, a disease of later life;
- a history of inflammatory bowel disease predisposes to **sclerosing cholangitis** although this is uncommon.

Examination

Early jaundice is a subtle physical sign and can be missed unless the patient is examined in a good light, preferably daylight. Jaundice is first detectable in the sclera and soon afterwards in abdominal wall skin. In some cases of obstructive jaundice, the patient develops generalised itching (pruritus) and scratch marks may be evident. The general stigmata of liver disease, such as spider naevi and liver 'flap' of the wrists are found only when jaundice is caused by primary liver disease rather than extrinsic obstruction.

The abdomen should be examined, particularly for ascites, an enlarged liver or spleen, abnormal masses or a palpable gall bladder. An enlarged liver may be caused by primary or secondary malignancy, and in the tropics, schistosomiasis or malaria. In a jaundiced patient, splenomegaly with hepatomegaly is an important sign of chronic parenchymal liver disease (usually cirrhosis) and indicates portal hypertension. Ascites in a patient with obstructive jaundice is almost always caused by disseminated intraabdominal malignancy.

Courvoisier 'law' (Fig. 18.7) was formulated in 1890 and states that obstructive jaundice in the presence of a palpable gall bladder is not caused by stone (and therefore likely to be caused by tumour). The argument is that gallstones cause chronic inflammation leading to gall bladder fibrosis or intermittent stone obstruction leading to hypertrophy of the gall bladder wall, either outcome prevents its distension. In malignancy, progressive obstruction occurs over a short period and the nonthickened gall bladder distends easily.

Particular attention is paid to the colour of stool found on rectal examination, as a pale stool is characteristic of obstructive jaundice. The urine in obstructive jaundice is usually dark yellow or orange from the presence of conjugated bilirubin, and froths when shaken owing to the detergent effect of bile acids. Conditions causing obstructive jaundice are illustrated in Fig. 18.8.

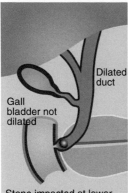
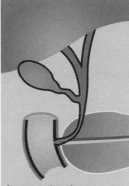
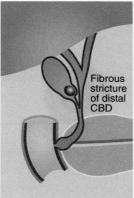
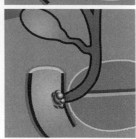
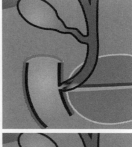

Gall bladder not dilated

Dilated duct

Stone impacted at lower end of CBD

Gall bladder may dilate and become palpable (Courvoisier's sign)

CBD compressed by carcinoma as it passes through the head of pancreas

May also invade or compress 2nd part of duodenum

Acute or chronic pancreatitis may compress CBD in a similar way to pancreatic carcinoma in 2 by inflammation or scarring

Fibrous stricture of distal CBD

1 Stones in common bile duct very common

Suggested by a history of pain typical of biliary colic. Jaundice may be progressive (If stone is firmly impacted), fluctuant without ever disappearing altogether (if a stone alternately impacts and disimpacts), or intermittent (if multiple small stones successively impact then pass through the lower end of the common bile duct)

2 Carcinoma of head of pancreas common

Typically causes painless jaundice which is persistent or progressive. The gall bladder may become palpable (Courvoisier's law, see Fig 18.9)

3 Pancreatitis uncommon

Common bile duct is obstructed by inflammatory swelling in acute pancreatitis or by scarring in chronic pancreatitis

4 Mirizzi's syndrome rare

Found in about 1% of cholecystectomy patients. Gallstones impacted in Hartmann's pouch cause inflammation of the gall bladder which then fuses with the CHD causing secondary stenosis. Large impacted stones sometimes cause pressure necrosis of the adjoining duct walls leading to chole–choledochal fistula

5 Periampullary malignant tumours uncommon

Include carcinomas of the ampulla, distal bile duct or duodenum (uncommon). Obstructive features are similar to carcinoma of head of pancreas

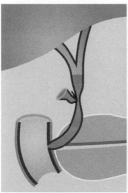
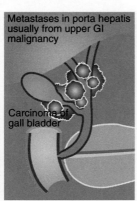
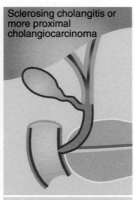
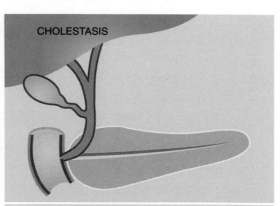

Metastases in porta hepatis usually from upper GI malignancy

Carcinoma of gall bladder

Sclerosing cholangitis or more proximal cholangiocarcinoma

CHOLESTASIS

6 Benign strictures of the common bile duct uncommon

May be due to surgical damage (fairly common) or inflammation caused by previous stone. Obstructive features are similar to carcinoma of head of pancreas in 2

7 Other malignant tumours rare

May cause bile duct obstruction above the ampulla. Examples include lymph node metastases in the porta hepatis (fairly common), primary cholangiocarcinoma (uncommon) and carcinoma of the gall bladder

8 Intrahepatic or hilar bile duct obstruction rare

Primary cholangiocarcinoma; sclerosing cholangitis (rare)

Note: hepatic metastases rarely cause obstructive jaundice

9 Intrahepatic cholestasis common

Viral hepatitis is a common cause.

Systemic sepsis often causes low grade jaundice (due to liver dysfunction).

Idiosyncrasy to certain drugs (including chlorpromazine, oral contraceptives and chlorpropamide) interferes with bile excretion from hepatocytes, presumably by affecting membrane transport.
Widespread hepatic lymphoma is a classical but rare cause

• **Fig. 18.7** Courvoisier Law. *CBD*, common bile duct; *CHD*, common hepatic duct.

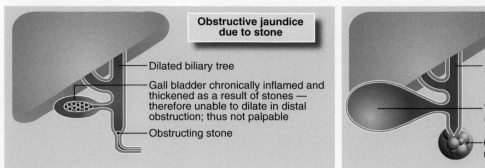
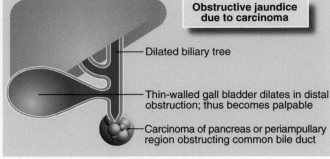

- **Fig. 18.8** Causes of Obstructive Jaundice.

Approach to Investigation of Jaundice

Urine Tests

The concentration of bilirubin in urine is easily established by dipstick tests. Substantial quantities usually mean biliary obstruction.

Blood Tests

- Infective hepatitis should be excluded by serological screening for hepatitis B and C. A history of transfusion, intravenous drug abuse or travel to developing countries may increase the likelihood of an infection.
- Confirm that the jaundice is obstructive by liver function tests, although these are not completely reliable. Obstructive jaundice is characterised by elevated plasma conjugated bilirubin and marked elevation of plasma alkaline phosphatase (liver isoenzyme). The transaminases, derived from hepatocytes, are usually only mildly elevated.
- When biliary obstruction is intrahepatic (e.g., cholangiocarcinoma obstructing one duct) there may be a mixed biochemical picture with evidence of hepatocyte damage and duct obstruction. Liver function tests are an unreliable guide here and liver ultrasonography is mandatory.
- Mild jaundice is commonly found in patients with Gilbert syndrome, caused by a mild congenital abnormality of haemoglobin metabolism without serious significance.
- Coagulation studies should be performed because of likely defects in clotting.
- Tumour markers should be tested for in patients with a previous history of GI malignancy.

Imaging

Hepatobiliary Ultrasonography

This is the simplest means of demonstrating dilated intrahepatic ducts (Fig. 18.9), liver secondaries, a dilated extrahepatic biliary system or gall bladder abnormalities including stones. Ultrasound is unreliable for demonstrating pathology in the lower part of the biliary tree, and although it may show gallstones or lesions in the head of the pancreas, it cannot be relied upon to exclude them.

Computed Tomography Scanning

This may be the next stage if ultrasound findings are equivocal. CT is particularly useful for demonstrating primary or secondary tumours but may miss a small carcinoma around the lower end of the common bile duct.

Endoscopic and Magnetic Resonance Cholangiopancreatography

If ultrasound demonstrates dilated ducts, endoscopic retrograde cholangiopancreatography (ERCP) is often the next investigation (Fig. 18.10). It is now usual practice to drain an obstructed bile duct at the same procedure if practicable, by sphincterotomy and stone removal or by placing an intraluminal **stent**. This may be the definitive treatment for duct stones or inoperable carcinomas; for patients requiring operation, stenting may be used to allow jaundice to settle and liver function to improve, but stents can interfere with endoscopic ultrasound staging of cancers. The role of diagnostic ERCP here has been largely superseded by magnetic resonance cholangiopancreatography (MRCP), described in Chapter 5.

Laparoscopy and Liver Biopsy

If bile ducts are not dilated, biopsy of liver or of demonstrated secondaries may be performed (with ultrasound or CT guidance), after correcting clotting abnormalities with vitamin K or fresh frozen plasma.

In patients unsuitable for percutaneous biopsy, or those who require visualisation of other organs, diagnostic laparoscopy can visualise the liver directly and obtain biopsy specimens from suspicious areas. Occasionally, a firm diagnosis cannot be made before a definitive operation; abdominal exploration and frozen section histology may provide the answer.

Principles of Management of Obstructive Jaundice

The primary aim of treatment is to relieve the biliary tract obstruction. Obstructed bile is often infected and a fulminant **acute cholangitis** can develop at any time. Back-pressure interferes with liver functions, such as synthesis of albumin and clotting factors. Eventually structural liver damage ensues.

Three categories of obstruction can be defined according to treatment options.
- Potentially curable obstructions
- Obstruction caused by incurable tumour
- Terminal disease

Potentially Curable Obstructions

These include bile duct stones and strictures, as well as small tumours of the lower bile ducts, duodenum or ampullary region (*periampullary tumours*) (see Fig. 18.8).

The number, size and position of **bile duct stones** may have been identified before operation by ERCP or MRCP. Stones can be removed at ERCP by dividing the ampullary sphincter using a 'bow-string' diathermy wire via a duodenal endoscope. Sometimes, if the stone is very large or impacted, obstructed bile may be drained by endoscopic placement of a stent (up to about 4 mm in diameter) alongside it within the bile duct without stone removal. Endoscopic procedures are treatments of choice for patients with common bile duct stones causing obstructive jaundice.

If cholecystectomy is the chosen treatment, bile duct stones can be identified by **perioperative cholangiography** and removed surgically using a **choledochoscope**, inserted via the divided cystic duct. Alternatively, an incision in the bile duct (choledochotomy) can be made, and closed primarily after stone extraction;

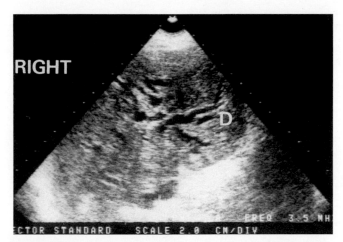

• **Fig. 18.9** Ultrasonogram Showing Dilated Intrahepatic Ducts. An ultrasound scan in an 80-year-old man with obstructive jaundice. This transverse section through the liver shows the characteristic 'double-barrel shotgun sign' *(D)*, with two parallel tubular structures representing major branches of the bile duct and portal vein. Normally, the portal vein is four times wider than the corresponding bile duct. Here they are the same diameter.

however, this carries a risk of biliary stricturing so few surgeons perform this.

Many surgeons undertaking laparoscopic cholecystectomy routinely perform operative cholangiography but only a small proportion undertake laparoscopic exploration of the common bile duct as this is a difficult and time-consuming procedure.

Benign bile duct strictures can be treated by long-term stenting or surgical reconstruction, usually by anastomosing a loop of jejunum to the bile duct proximal to the obstruction (hepaticojejunostomy). Strictures are usually caused by postsurgical fibrotic scarring (usually following iatrogenic injury) or from inflammatory scarring caused by cholecystitis (**Mirizzi syndrome**).

Small **periampullary tumours** may be amenable to complete excision, thereby relieving biliary obstruction and often achieving cure. **Adenocarcinoma of the pancreatic head** is a common cause of obstructive jaundice but the prognosis is poor even after successful radical pancreaticoduodenectomy. If an operation for potentially curable malignant disease is planned, the precautions in Table 18.2 should be used.

Obstruction Caused by Incurable Tumour

Such obstructions are caused by carcinoma of the pancreatic head (common), lymph node metastases in the porta hepatis (uncommon) and from carcinoma of the gall bladder (rare). Stenting is the palliative treatment of choice for the bile duct and, if necessary, duodenum. The alternative is palliative triple bypass surgery to bypass both biliary and duodenal obstructions (see Fig. 24.3, p. 353).

Terminal Disease

By the time obstructive jaundice has appeared, some patients have reached a terminal stage of their cancer. In these cases,

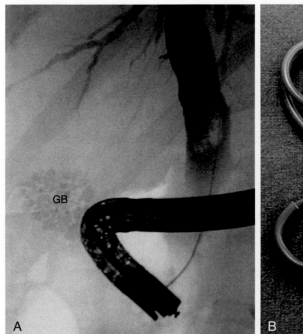
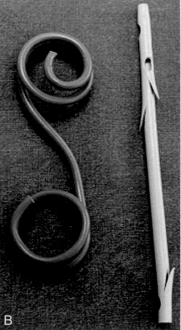
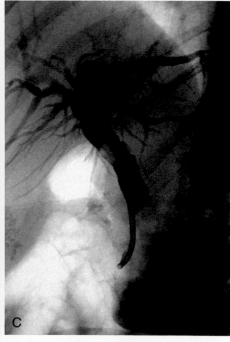

• **Fig. 18.10** Endoscopic Stenting. **(A)** Diagnostic endoscopic retrograde cholangiogram (ERC) showing an enlarged common bile duct containing a single large stone. A collection of radiopaque gallstones is seen in the gall bladder *(GB)*. **(B)** Two types of biliary stent: the pigtail type on the left and the notched variety on the right, as used in this patient. **(C)** Despite endoscopic sphincterotomy, the bile duct stone could not be retrieved so a tubular self-retaining stent has been placed to relieve the obstructive jaundice. The stone was successfully removed endoscopically on a later occasion.

TABLE 18.2	Special Precautions to Be Taken When Operating on a Patient With Obstructive Jaundice	
Potential Complication	Pathophysiology	Prophylaxis
Infection	Obstructed bile is usually infected with aerobic gut organisms, and is under pressure. Instrumentation may precipitate ascending cholangitis, leading to sepsis and multiple organ dysfunction Spillage of infected bile during operation causes peritoneal contamination and risks intraperitoneal or wound infection	Preoperative drainage of bile into the bowel by endoscopic sphincterotomy or stenting is sometimes used Prophylactic antibiotics against gut flora should be given
Endotoxaemia and kidney failure	Bacterial endotoxins appear in the systemic circulation. These predispose to multiple organ dysfunction syndrome (MODS) by activating components of the inflammatory cascade and may precipitate a systemic inflammatory response. Renal function is particularly vulnerable if renal perfusion is already impaired Postoperative 'hepatorenal syndrome' (i.e., acute renal failure) which manifests as oliguria and hyponatraemia	Prophylactic antibiotics Ensure adequate hydration during any period of restriction of oral fluid throughout—preoperative intravenous fluids and osmotic diuretics during operation Insert urinary catheter to monitor output
Hepatic impairment	Biliary back-pressure on the liver causes defective clotting factor synthesis (even if vitamin K given) and defective hepatic metabolism of certain drugs Patients with chronic parenchymal liver disease withstand the stresses of major abdominal surgery and anaesthesia poorly	Avoid drugs excreted by the liver. Give antibiotics to minimise endogenous endotoxin production
Fat malabsorption	Biliary obstruction causes diminished absorption of fats including fat-soluble vitamins, such as vitamin K (a cofactor for prothrombin synthesis). This results in defective clotting	Monitor clotting Give parenteral vitamin K to improve prothrombin ratio, 24 hours preoperatively if possible; if necessary, fresh-frozen plasma perioperatively
Thromboembolism	Paradoxically, considering the clotting deficiency, postoperative deep vein thrombosis is common	Prophylactic subcutaneous low-dose heparin injections

stenting may still be indicated but surgical interference may be difficult to justify; the aim should be to relieve distress and allow a dignified death with good palliative care. Some patients experiencing severe itching may be helped by drugs, such as antihistamines or chlorpromazine. Oral cholestyramine (used to bind bile in the GI tract to prevent reabsorption) is not indicated because it only removes bile salts which are able to reach the bowel.

Special Risks of Surgery in the Jaundiced Patient

Despite the fact that most obstructive jaundice can now be relieved preoperatively by stone removal or stenting, surgery must still sometimes be performed in a jaundiced patient. This poses a greater risk from preoperative and postoperative surgical complications, as shown in Table 18.2.

Abdominal Mass or Distension

An abdominal mass is sometimes discovered by the patient but more often by clinical examination. An older patient with a palpable mass is likely to have a malignant tumour, but benign cysts, inflammatory masses, aneurysms or atypical hernias may be responsible. Occasionally masses have a 'medical' cause, for example, hepatosplenomegaly of chronic lymphocytic leukaemia. Commonly, one of the 'five Fs'—foetus, faeces, flatus, fat or fluid—may masquerade as a 'surgical' mass or distension. Patients with an abdominal mass usually have GI symptoms, anaemia or jaundice in addition.

Clinical Assessment of an Abdominal Mass (Table 18.3)

History

A thorough history often provides clues to the organ system involved. Important features include: how long has it been there; how did the patient come to notice it; is it always present or does it sometimes disappear (e.g., a hernia may reduce); is it getting bigger or smaller? A history of intraabdominal malignancy or malignant melanoma of the eye years before should be regarded with grave suspicion: the disease may have recurred, metastasised or a related new primary developed. This is especially common in colorectal cancer but uncommon once 7 years have elapsed since treatment.

General Examination

General examination should seek systemic signs of disease (e.g., cachexia, anaemia and jaundice) or signs of malignant dissemination (e.g., supraclavicular lymphadenopathy in suspected stomach cancer). Abdominal and pelvic examination must be methodical and, if appropriate, proctoscopy and sigmoidoscopy performed.

Examination of an Abdominal Mass

The location of the mass, its relations to other structures, its mobility and its physical characteristics, such as size, shape, consistency and pulsatility give valuable information about the organ of origin and the likely pathology. **Hernias** (see Chapter 32), for example, incisional, umbilical and sometimes interstitial (Spigelian) hernias

TABLE 18.3   Causes of Hepatosplenomegaly

Hepatomegaly	Splenomegaly	Hepatosplenomegaly
Physiological		
Riedel lobe		
Malignant Tumours		
Hepatocellular carcinoma Secondary carcinoma		
Infective		
Viral		
Hepatitis, Epstein–Barr virus, cytomegalovirus	Hepatitis, Epstein–Barr virus, cytomegalovirus	Hepatitis, cytomegalovirus
Bacterial		
Tuberculosis, leptospirosis, liver abscess	Subacute bacterial endocarditis, typhoid, tuberculosis, leptospirosis	Tuberculosis, leptospirosis
Protozoal		
Malaria, schistosomiasis, amoebiasis, histoplasmosis, hydatid disease	Malaria, toxoplasmosis, brucellosis, schistosomiasis, leishmaniasis (kala-azar)	Malaria, toxoplasmosis, brucellosis, schistosomiasis, leishmaniasis (kala-azar)
Alcoholic Liver Disease		
Fatty liver Early cirrhosis		
Systemic Diseases		
Wilson disease	Sarcoidosis	Amyloidosis
Haemochromatosis Cellular infiltration, for example, amyloid, sarcoid	Amyloidosis Rheumatoid arthritis (Felty syndrome) Storage diseases (e.g., Gaucher)	Storage diseases (e.g., Gaucher)
Benign Tumours		
Hepatic Adenoma		
Congestive cardiac disease	**Congestive splenomegaly**	**Congestive hepatosplenomegaly**
Right heart failure Tricuspid regurgitation (pulsatile liver) Budd–Chiari syndrome	Hepatic vein thrombosis Portal vein thrombosis Splenic vein thrombosis Cirrhosis with portal hypertension	Hepatic vein thrombosis Portal vein thrombosis Splenic vein thrombosis Cirrhosis with portal hypertension Budd–Chiari syndrome
Haematological Disease Lymphoproliferative Disorders		
Lymphoma Leukaemias	Lymphoma Leukaemias	Lymphoma Leukaemias
Myeloproliferative Disorders		
	Chronic myeloid leukaemia Myelofibrosis Polycythaemia rubra vera Essential thrombocythaemia	Chronic myeloid leukaemia Myelofibrosis Polycythaemia rubra vera Essential thrombocythaemia
Anaemia		
	Haemolytic anaemia Megaloblastic anaemia	Megaloblastic anaemia
Miscellaneous		
Primary biliary cirrhosis Polycystic liver disease	Thyrotoxicosis	Infantile polycystic disease

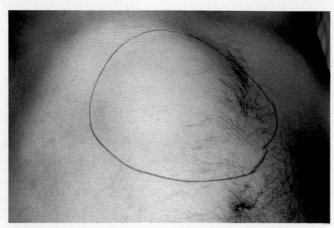

• **Fig. 18.11** Epigastric Mass. This man of 44 years presented having discovered an epigastric mass. It was asymptomatic. The margins of the mass are outlined on the skin. The mass moved downwards with respiration and proved to be a massive liver metastasis from a tiny pancreatic primary adenocarcinoma.

(see Ch. 32), may present as localised swellings but they usually shrink or reduce completely when the patient is supine or under anaesthesia, unless they are incarcerated.

Examination of Masses in Specific Regions of the Abdomen (See Fig. 18.1)

Mass in the Right Hypochondrium (Right Upper Quadrant or RUQ)

A right hypochondrial mass is usually of hepatobiliary origin. If so, it will be continuous with the main bulk of the liver to palpation and percussion. When the liver is diffusely enlarged, the inferior margin is regular and well defined and the consistency is usually normal. When infiltrated with primary or secondary cancer, it may be hard and irregular or the liver may appear diffusely enlarged. Carcinoma of the gall bladder is indistinguishable from hepatic cancer on palpation. Rarely, a Riedel lobe—a congenitally enlarged part of the right lobe—is mistaken for a pathological mass but is soft and mobile. Less commonly, a right hypochondrial mass is a diseased gall bladder. A mass continuous with the liver above and having a typical pear-shaped rounded outline is likely to be a mucocoele of the gall bladder. A more diffuse, tender mass may be an empyema of the gall bladder.

Epigastric Mass

A mass in the epigastrium is usually caused by cancer of the stomach or transverse colon or sometimes omental secondaries from ovarian carcinoma. Cancer involving the left lobe of the liver may also present like this (Fig. 18.11). These masses are usually hard and irregular, and are mobile or fixed according to the degree of invasion. Occasionally an epigastric mass consists of massive para-aortic lymph nodes caused by lymphoma or testicular secondaries. A pulsatile epigastric mass is likely to be an abdominal aortic aneurysm.

Mass in the Left Hypochondrium (Left Upper Quadrant or LUQ)

A cancer of the stomach or splenic flexure of the colon may present as a mass in the left hypochondrium. Tumour masses can usually be distinguished clinically from an enlarged spleen as the latter often has a discrete 'edge' and lies more posteriorly.

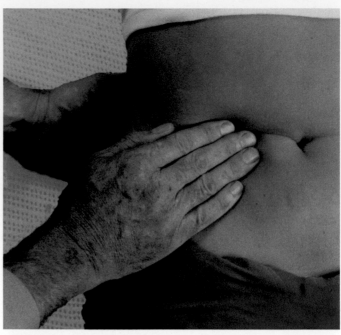

• **Fig. 18.12** Bimanual Palpation of the Abdomen. The posterior hand pushes forwards so that an enlarged viscus (usually retroperitoneal, e.g., kidney) or a mobile intraabdominal mass is pushed onto the anterior examining hand. Note that this is not ballottement, which involves short, sharp palpation anteriorly, thus displacing ascites enabling a mass to bounce onto the examining hand.

Mass in the Loin or Flank

A mass in the loin or flank is likely to be of renal origin and can best be felt on **bimanual palpation** (Fig. 18.12). Very rarely, a hernia occurs in the lumbar region; this reduces spontaneously as the patient rolls over.

Mass in the Left Iliac Fossa

Masses here usually arise from the sigmoid colon. A hard faecal mass may be mistaken for cancer but it can often be indented like putty. A solid sigmoid mass is usually caused by tumour or a complex diverticular inflammatory mass. Ovarian masses may be palpable in either iliac fossa. These lesions, however, arise out of the pelvis and can often be pushed up on to the abdominal examining hand by digital pressure in the vagina or rectum (bimanual palpation—most effectively performed under general anaesthesia). Note that rectal examination is usually regarded as mandatory in a complete abdominal examination.

Hernias in the groin are common (see Ch. 32) and may be chronically irreducible (incarcerated). Occasionally, an interstitial (Spigelian) hernia develops above the groin in either iliac fossa. This presents a somewhat confusing picture on examination by virtue of its site and because the peritoneal sac herniates between the abdominal wall layers.

Suprapubic Mass

Suprapubic masses usually arise from pelvic organs, such as bladder or uterus and its adnexae. A palpable bladder is most commonly caused by chronic urinary retention, easily confirmed on ultrasound. A distended bladder is dull to percussion and disappears on catheterisation. Bladder enlargement is usually symmetrical and may extend above the umbilicus. Only large or invasive bladder tumours tend to be palpable and these would be accompanied by urinary tract symptoms and urine abnormalities (haematuria). Sometimes large bladder stones are palpable abdominally.

A uterus may be palpable abdominally when enlarged by pregnancy or fibroids. Bimanual examination involves vaginal and lower abdominal palpation. Ovarian tumours, particularly cysts, may become enormous and extend well up into the abdomen; again, bimanual examination (under general anaesthesia if necessary) helps distinguish the origin.

Mass in the Right Iliac Fossa

The right iliac fossa is a common site for an asymptomatic mass. It may be caused by unresolved inflammation of the appendix, surrounded by omentum and small bowel, forming an 'appendix mass' (see Ch. 26, p. 279). There is usually a recent history of right iliac fossa pain and fever. Carcinoma of the caecum may become very large without causing obstruction because the caecum is large and distensible, and the faecal stream at this point is semi-liquid. Thus caecal carcinoma often presents with an asymptomatic mass, and iron deficiency anaemia. Crohn disease of the terminal ileum often presents with a tender mass, usually with typical symptoms of pain and diarrhoea.

Central Abdominal Mass

A central abdominal mass may originate in large or small bowel, be a result of malignant infiltration of the great omentum, or if they are large, from retroperitoneal structures, such as lymph nodes, pancreas, connective tissues or the aorta. A common central abdominal mass is an abdominal aorta aneurysm. Aneurysms nearly all appear over 60 years of age and usually arise just above the aortic bifurcation (at umbilical level). A characteristic feature is **expansile pulsation**; other solid masses may transmit pulsation from large vessels nearby, but those masses are not expansile.

Several different types of hernia present near the centre of the abdomen. Most common is an **incisional hernia** protruding through part or all of an abdominal wall incision. This may occur any time after operation, from days to years later. It usually results from poor closure technique or postoperative infection. **Paraumbilical** or **umbilical hernias**, common in the obese, occur centrally and diagnosis is usually straightforward. **Divarication of the recti** (rectus abdominis muscles, not a true hernia) involves the recti being splayed apart, often as a result of pregnancy or obesity, leaving the central abdominal wall devoid of muscular support. This is easily recognised because of its typical 'keel' shape and its symptomless nature and the absence of an abdominal scar; treatment is rarely necessary. Divarication and midline hernias can best be demonstrated when abdominal muscles are contracted by asking a supine patient to raise both heels from the bed.

Rectal Mass and Findings on Pelvic Examination

An abdominal or pelvic mass may be palpable solely on rectal (or vaginal) examination. The mass may be a cancer of rectum or in the loop of sigmoid colon in the pelvic cavity; the latter is unlikely to be visible on sigmoidoscopy. Sometimes, secondary deposits from an impalpable tumour in the upper abdomen may seed the pelvic cavity. This may produce a hard anterior lump or even a solid mass filling the pelvic cavity (**frozen pelvis**). Frozen pelvis can also occur with benign conditions, such as endometriosis, local spread of a carcinoma of cervix or, rarely, prostate or bladder cancer.

Interpretation of a Finding of Ascites

Ascites is defined as a chronic accumulation of fluid within the abdominal cavity and has many causes, some malignant and some nonmalignant. Ascites can usually be recognised clinically only when the volume exceeds 2 litres, but even then it is easily overlooked. Dullness to percussion in the flanks and suprapubic region with central resonance is suspicious of ascites and should be followed by an attempt to elicit a fluid thrill or 'shifting dullness' (Fig. 18.13).

Malignant Ascites

In intraabdominal cancer, the peritoneum is sometimes seeded with tumour deposits that secrete a protein-rich fluid containing malignant cells (**malignant ascites**). The peritoneum may be peppered with thousands of minute seedlings or there may be several large masses hidden by ascitic fluid. Such widespread peritoneal involvement may cause abdominal distension but can be difficult to recognise on abdominal examination. It should be suspected if a patient with a past history of GI or ovarian cancer has other symptoms suggestive of malignancy, such as anorexia or marked weight loss.

Lymphatic Obstruction

A rare cause of ascites is major obstruction of abdominal lymphatic drainage. This is usually caused by malignant involvement of paraaortic lymph nodes with lymphoma or metastatic testicular malignancy. **Chylous ascites**, in which the ascitic fluid is milky-white, is rare and is caused by proximal lymphatic obstruction and the presence of chylomicrons in the fluid originating from mesenteric lymphatics.

Tuberculosis

Abdominal tuberculosis is an uncommon cause of abdominal swelling in developed countries but is common in the developing world. Tuberculosis can occasionally present as ascites; this form is characterised by multiple tiny peritoneal tubercles, only distinguishable from tumour secondaries by biopsy.

Nonsurgical Causes

Ascites is commonly caused by gross congestive cardiac failure, constrictive pericarditis, severe hypoalbuminaemia or portal venous obstruction, the last occurring in cirrhosis and occasionally with liver metastases.

Diffuse Abdominal Distension

In diffuse distension without a palpable abdominal mass, sinister causes must be excluded. Gas within bowel is a common cause for long-standing and often intermittent abdominal pain and distension. It usually occurs in healthy young adults, particularly women, in association with irritable bowel syndrome or air swallowing during hyperventilation. Chronic gaseous abdominal distension may also be found in elderly patients with partial volvulus of the sigmoid colon. Clinical assessment usually diagnoses these problems and avoids unnecessary investigation.

Gross faecal loading may also be responsible for abdominal distension. This is often seen in children with abdominal pain and sometimes in young adults with irritable bowel syndrome. Asymptomatic chronic constipation is common in the elderly, and a faecal mass palpable through a thin abdominal wall can give the impression of a sinister mass.

Approach to Investigation of an Abdominal Mass or Distension

Laboratory Tests

Blood, urine and stool investigations are performed as suggested by the history and examination, for example, full blood count, function tests, dipstick urinalysis and faecal occult bloods or faecal immunological test (FIT).

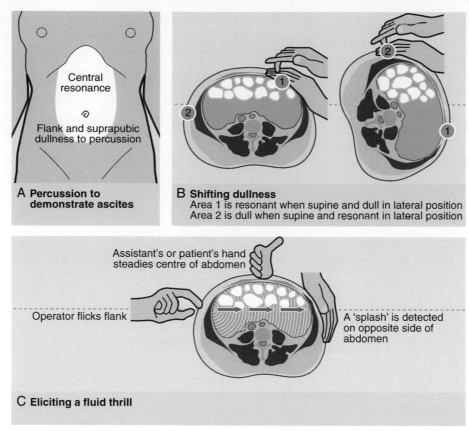

• **Fig. 18.13** Clinical Signs of Ascites.

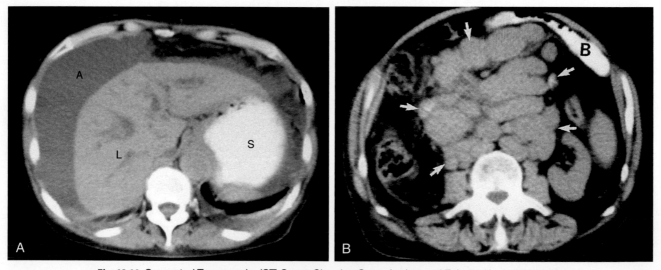

• **Fig. 18.14** Computed Tomography (CT) Scans Showing Gross Ascites and Enlarged Lymph Nodes. In **(A)** note the darker grey homogeneous shadow of fluid *(A)* around the liver *(L)* and the contrast in the stomach *(S)*. **(B)** Retroperitoneal mass of lymph nodes caused by lymphoma. This CT scan was taken to assess the stage of spread of a known lymphoma. This 40-year-old woman presented with a large rubbery lymph node mass in her neck and was also found to have a large central abdominal mass. Abdominal CT scanning showed an enormous mass of lymph nodes *(arrowed)*. Small bowel *(B)* is seen anteriorly, enhanced by orally administered contrast material.

Radiology

A chest x-ray should be performed if malignancy is suspected. Ultrasonography or CT scanning (Fig. 18.14) is useful for demonstrating the size and origin of a mass. For pelvic masses, transvaginal or transrectal ultrasound is often the investigation of first choice although MRI is often helpful. CT scanning is most valuable for defining masses in the retroperitoneal area, for example, pancreas, aorta or kidneys, but may be the preferred investigation for suspected large bowel cancer, particularly in frail patients. Ultrasound or CT scanning can be used to guide needle biopsy or aspiration cytology precisely. Contrast studies, for example, barium meal, barium enema or intravenous urography, may be indicated by the clinical findings.

Endoscopy

Flexible endoscopic techniques, such as gastroscopy, colonoscopy and ERCP enable direct examination and biopsy of many GI lesions.

Other Methods of Tissue Diagnosis

A tissue diagnosis should be obtained even if disseminated malignancy seems obvious. It can influence palliative and supportive treatment and, occasionally, an apparently hopeless case proves on histology to be treatable or even curable. Examples are tuberculosis, lymphomas or a germ cell tumour, such as teratoma. Techniques of obtaining tissue for histology include needle or excision biopsy of enlarged cervical lymph nodes, and percutaneous biopsy of liver or an intraabdominal mass. Paracentesis abdominis (i.e., needle aspiration of ascitic fluid) is a safe and simple way of obtaining a specimen for cytology and microbiology. Finally, when less invasive methods have failed to provide the necessary information, direct biopsy of tumour at diagnostic laparoscopy or open operation usually provides the definitive diagnosis.

Examination Under Anaesthesia, Laparoscopy and Exploratory Laparotomy

EUA is sometimes necessary for estimating the mobility and spread of pelvic tumours. General anaesthesia with a muscle relaxant allows thorough abdominal palpation and bimanual examination of the pelvis via rectum and/or vagina and the taking of biopsies. This may not be possible without anaesthesia because of tenderness or abdominal wall muscle tone. EUA is often combined with cystoscopy or other rigid endoscopies.

Laparoscopy is now widely used as a diagnostic tool in general surgery. It allows direct inspection and biopsy of masses and visualisation of the extent of local spread governing resectability, as well as allowing a search for intraabdominal metastases. Samples can be taken for cytology to demonstrate intraperitoneal spread. Special ultrasound probes may be applied directly to the liver and other organs where lesions are suspected.

19

The Acute Abdomen and Acute Gastrointestinal Haemorrhage

Introduction

The term *acute abdomen* is widely understood but is difficult to define precisely. Typically, the symptoms are of acute onset abdominal pain. The illness is of such severity that admission to hospital appears essential and operative surgery is a likely outcome. Many of the disorders causing an 'acute abdomen' are serious and potentially life threatening unless treated promptly. On the other hand, simple and relatively trivial conditions, such as constipation can produce acute and severe symptoms mimicking the early stages of an acute abdomen.

Major gastrointestinal (GI) haemorrhage is also a common reason for acute surgical referral, and is manifest by vomiting of blood (**haematemesis**), profuse rectal bleeding or the passage of **melaena**. Many such patients are initially referred to a general (internal) physician or gastroenterologist, especially if the presumptive diagnosis is of bleeding from a peptic ulcer or oesophageal varices.

Acute surgical emergencies constitute about 50% of all general surgical admissions. About half of these are for abdominal symptoms, predominantly pain, and half of those in this group resolve without operation.

Basic Principles of Managing the Acute Abdomen

The first goal is to resuscitate the patient with intravenous fluids and administer analgesia. The next is to make a diagnosis based on the history, examination, laboratory tests and imaging

(Box 19.1). Together these will help decide if an operation is necessary, its urgency, and clarify any nonsurgical treatment, for example, antibiotics for diverticulitis or conservative measures for acute pancreatitis. Most of the time, it will only be possible to make a differential diagnosis rather than a definitive diagnosis.

Disorders and Diseases Causing the Acute Abdomen

Intestinal Obstruction

Pathophysiology of Intestinal Obstruction

Any part of the GI tract may become obstructed and present as an acute abdomen. Gastric outlet obstruction, however, presents differently and is described in Chapter 21. The causes of intestinal obstruction are many and varied, as outlined in Fig. 19.1.

Obstruction leads to proximal dilatation of bowel and disrupts the peristalsis. The manner of presentation depends on the level of obstruction in the GI tract (i.e., stomach, proximal or distal small bowel or large bowel) and on the completeness of obstruction. The most acute presentation is upper small bowel obstruction. This manifests within hours of onset as the large volume of gastric and pancreaticobiliary secretions is prevented from progressing, and thus regurgitates into the stomach and is vomited. In contrast, distal large bowel obstruction is more insidious in onset and presentation may be delayed by as much as a week in many cases.

Symptoms of Intestinal Obstruction

Symptoms and physical signs are summarised in Box 19.2.

Vomiting

Bowel obstruction often presents as vomiting; the more proximal, the earlier it develops. Vomiting can occur even if nothing is taken by mouth because saliva and other GI secretions continue to be produced and enter the stomach. At least 10 litres of fluid are secreted into the GI tract each day. The nature of the vomitus gives clues about the level of obstruction. For example, vomiting of semidigested food eaten a day or two earlier suggests

Plain Radiology in the Acute Abdomen—What to Look for

Five Main Image Densities are Detectable on Radiographs
- White—metallic objects
- Off white—calcified structures
- Medium shades of grey—most soft tissues
- Dark grey—fat
- Black—gas

How to Review an Abdominal X-ray:
1. Check **name** is correct and **date** is current.
2. Note **type of x-ray**, that is, plain or contrast, erect or supine.
3. Is the image of adequate **diagnostic quality**, that is, appropriate density? Does it show the whole abdomen?
4. **Bowel gas and bowel wall**—note distribution and dilatation (small bowel diameter less than 3 cm, most large bowel less than 5 cm, caecum less than 9 cm). Absence of gas may indicate a displacing mass, ascites (central) or acute pancreatitis (ground glass appearance). Faeces appear mottled; 'faecal loading' may mean constipation or obstruction. Rigler sign is strongly suggestive of bowel perforation.
5. **Non-bowel gas**—free intraperitoneal gas, for example, subphrenic gas in perforation of bowel, gas within bowel wall in necrosis, gas in biliary tree after sphincterotomy or fistula of gall bladder into bowel.
6. **Calcification**—aortic wall in aneurysm; pancreatic, renal and ureteric stones; gallstones; pelvic phleboliths (calcified old venous thrombi); teratomas and foetus. Bones of spine and pelvis—osteoarthritis, metastases (lytic or sclerotic), Paget disease, fractures.
7. **Soft tissues.** Thickened bowel wall. Check outline of kidneys (are both present? Length equal to three or more vertebral bodies) and psoas muscles (obscured in retroperitoneal inflammation).
8. **Artefacts**—artificial objects placed by medical personnel—central venous line, nasogastric tube, metal vessel or Fallopian tube clips, biliary, vascular or bowel stents, inferior vena caval filter, intrauterine contraceptive device.
   - foreign bodies—embedded bullets, glass fragments, objects inserted rectally
   - projection of buttons, safety pins, rings on hand, coins, body piercing

In Patients with an Acute Abdomen, Always Review Chest X-Ray for the Following:
- hiatus hernia
- heart size
- lung fields
- pneumothorax
- diaphragms: relative height; gas under
- bony changes
- central venous pressure line position

gastric outlet obstruction. Copious vomiting of **bile-stained fluid** suggests upper small bowel obstruction. If the vomitus becomes thicker and foul-smelling (**faeculent**), more distal obstruction is likely and this change is often an indication for urgent operation. The term *faeculent* is a misnomer as the vomitus contains altered small bowel contents rather than faeces itself.

Pain
Fluid and swallowed air proximal to an obstruction in combination with continuing peristalsis cause pain. The general area of the pain gives clues to the embryological origin of the segment of affected bowel: upper, middle or lower abdominal pain originates in foregut, midgut or hindgut, respectively. In obstruction, pain may not always be the most prominent symptom. However, when it does occur, it is usually colicky, occurring in short-lived bouts as peristalsis attempts to overcome the obstruction. In small bowel, the peristaltic action often increases for 24 to 48 hours after the onset of obstruction and then fades.

Constipation
Absolute constipation, that is, no faeces or flatus passed rectally, is pathognomonic of obstruction. The longer the duration, the more noteworthy it becomes in the diagnosis of obstruction.

Effects of Competence of the Ileocaecal Valve
Symptoms develop more gradually in large bowel obstruction because of the large capacity of colon and caecum and their absorptive capability. However, if the ileocaecal valve remains competent, no retrograde flow of accumulating bowel contents occurs and the thin-walled caecum progressively distends and eventually ruptures; operation is clearly more urgent in these cases. The ileocaecal valve becomes incompetent in about half the cases of large bowel obstruction. This allows the small bowel to distend, delaying the onset of obstructive symptoms and perhaps their acuteness.

Incomplete Obstruction
If bowel is partially obstructed, clinical features are less distinct. Vomiting may be intermittent and bowel habits erratic. Chronic incomplete obstruction leads to gradual hypertrophy of bowel wall muscle proximal to the obstruction and the strong peristaltic activity causes bouts of colicky pain, often more severe than in complete obstruction. In thin patients, the pain is often accompanied by **visible peristalsis**, the hallmark of incomplete obstruction. The most common cause is a slowly growing obstructing colonic cancer. Incomplete obstruction should *not* be called *subacute obstruction* as the term is misleading.

Physical Signs of Intestinal Obstruction
General Examination
Vomiting, diminished fluid intake and sequestration of fluid into the small bowel proximal to the obstruction, lead to **dehydration**. Gas-filled loops of bowel proximal to the obstruction produce **abdominal distension**; the more distal the obstruction, the greater the distension. Examination may also reveal signs of anaemia or lymphadenopathy attributable to the primary disorder.

Groin Examination
It is essential that the groin is examined for hernias as the resulting bowel obstruction will not settle with conservative treatment. An obstructed **femoral hernia** is usually very small and rarely causes local symptoms or signs, even when strangulated. Hence it is easily missed if not specifically sought. Instead it produces the symptoms and signs of small bowel obstruction. This is an important clinical point—an obstruction caused by an irreducible hernia will not settle with the usual conservative treatment.

Abdominal Examination
On **inspection**, scars of previous operations provide a map of previous surgical disease, and raise the possibility of adhesive obstruction. On **palpation**, the most striking feature is the lack of abdominal tenderness except when strangulation has occurred. Obstruction with tenderness *must* be diagnosed as strangulation or perforation, necessitating urgent operation after fluid resuscitation. Note that a large obstructing abdominal mass may be palpable.

On **percussion**, the centre of the abdomen tends to be resonant and the periphery dull because bowel gas rises to the most non-dependant point, mimicking ascites. On **auscultation**, obstructive bowel sounds are traditionally described as loud and frequent,

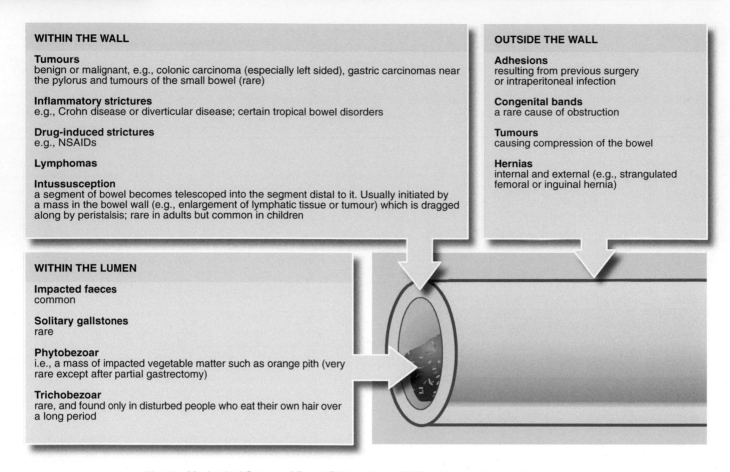

WITHIN THE WALL

Tumours
benign or malignant, e.g., colonic carcinoma (especially left sided), gastric carcinomas near the pylorus and tumours of the small bowel (rare)

Inflammatory strictures
e.g., Crohn disease or diverticular disease; certain tropical bowel disorders

Drug-induced strictures
e.g., NSAIDs

Lymphomas

Intussusception
a segment of bowel becomes telescoped into the segment distal to it. Usually initiated by a mass in the bowel wall (e.g., enlargement of lymphatic tissue or tumour) which is dragged along by peristalsis; rare in adults but common in children

OUTSIDE THE WALL

Adhesions
resulting from previous surgery or intraperitoneal infection

Congenital bands
a rare cause of obstruction

Tumours
causing compression of the bowel

Hernias
internal and external (e.g., strangulated femoral or inguinal hernia)

WITHIN THE LUMEN

Impacted faeces
common

Solitary gallstones
rare

Phytobezoar
i.e., a mass of impacted vegetable matter such as orange pith (very rare except after partial gastrectomy)

Trichobezoar
rare, and found only in disturbed people who eat their own hair over a long period

• **Fig. 19.1** Mechanical Causes of Bowel Obstruction. *NSAIDs,* Nonsteroidal anti-inflammatory drugs.

• **BOX 19.2 Clinical Features of Bowel Obstruction and Strangulation**

Symptoms
- Vomiting—time of onset and nature of the vomitus suggest the level of obstruction
- Absolute constipation (i.e., no flatus or faeces passed rectally)—pathognomonic of complete obstruction (but not present in partial obstruction)
- Abdominal pain—usually colicky in character, often mild in uncomplicated obstruction and more severe in strangulation

Physical Signs
- Dehydration—caused by vomiting, lack of fluid intake and fluid sequestration in obstructed bowel
- Abdominal distension—caused by gas-filled loops of bowel. The more distal the obstruction, the greater the distension
- Visible peristalsis—uncommon finding; usually encountered in a very thin patient with prolonged but incomplete distal small bowel obstruction
- Abdominal tenderness—important feature distinguishing bowel strangulation from uncomplicated obstruction
- Central resonance to percussion with dullness in the flanks—gas within dilated bowel loops rising to the uppermost point in the abdomen
- Abnormal bowel sounds—exaggerated, lapping, sloshing, perhaps high-pitched or tinkling. Bowel sounds are absent or normal in adynamic obstruction

high-pitched and tinkling; in practice, bowel sounds may or may not be increased but have an echoing, cavernous quality or else can sound like the lapping of water against a boat. A **succussion splash**, heard on gently shaking the patient's abdomen from side to side, may be heard in gastric outlet obstruction.

Radiological Investigation of Suspected Bowel Obstruction

The most useful initial investigation is a plain supine abdominal x-ray (Figs 19.2–19.4). The pattern and distribution of bowel gas often indicates the approximate site of obstruction. In small bowel obstruction, fluid levels may be visible on an erect or decubitus x-ray. Measuring the bowel diameter on x-ray gives the degree of distension (see Box 19.1 for norms).

In large bowel obstruction where the ileocaecal valve remains competent, profound large bowel dilatation without small bowel distension is seen on x-ray; this is a key determinant of the likely rate of deterioration of the patient. When the caecum reaches 10 cm, it is in imminent danger of rupture and an operation is needed urgently.

In large bowel obstruction of less acute onset, radiology helps demonstrate the site and nature of the obstruction (including sigmoid volvulus) and helps in distinguishing mechanical from pseudo-obstruction (see later). A contrast enema is a sensitive and reliable radiological investigation, but computed tomography (CT) scanning is increasingly used. CT scanning gives an indication of the level of obstruction and may also provide a diagnosis of the cause of obstruction. Other useful information, such as the presence of hepatic metastases may radically influence management, for example the use of a large bowel stent to relieve the obstruction rather than surgery.

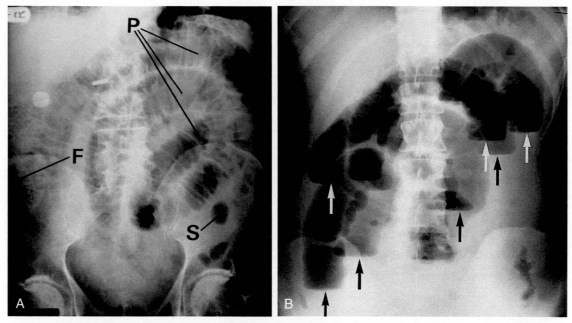

• **Fig. 19.2** Radiological Appearances of Obstructed Bowel. **(A)** Supine abdominal film of a man of 67 years presenting with vomiting and abdominal distension. The film shows mid small bowel obstruction. Dilated small bowel loops fill the upper left quadrant and centre of the abdomen, and can be identified by the valvulae conniventes (plicae circulares *[P]*) which extend across the whole width of the lumen. The small bowel distal to the obstruction is collapsed and is not visible on this film. The large bowel is also collapsed, with faecal loading of the ascending colon *(F)* and only a small amount of gas in the sigmoid colon *(S)*. Note also the metallic tip of the nasogastric tube and the incidental radiopaque gallstone. **(B)** Erect film showing multiple loops of dilated small bowel and multiple fluid levels. The obstruction was caused by a small carcinoma of the medial wall of the caecum encroaching upon the ileocaecal valve. Note: erect abdominal films are rarely taken nowadays

CASE HISTORIES

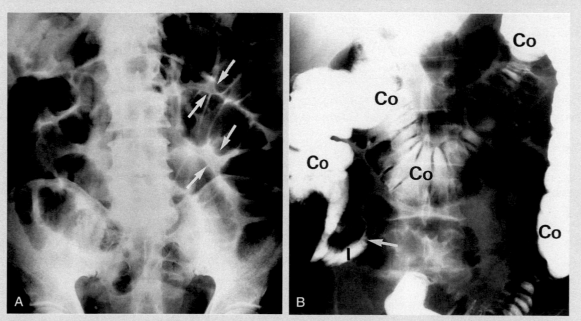

• **Fig. 19.3** Radiological Appearances of Obstructed Bowel. **(A)** Supine abdominal x-ray in a middle-aged man with several days of symptoms of small bowel obstruction. The abdomen is filled with grossly dilated small bowel loops. In addition, the small bowel wall is thickened, as shown by the apparent space between loops of bowel *(arrowed)*; this is a characteristic feature of prolonged obstruction. **(B)** 'Instant' contrast enema showing contrast filling the normal colon *(Co)* and distal ileum *(I)* which abruptly terminates at the obstruction *(arrow)*. The obstruction proved at laparotomy to be caused by a band adhesion resulting from an operation for appendicitis 25 years previously.

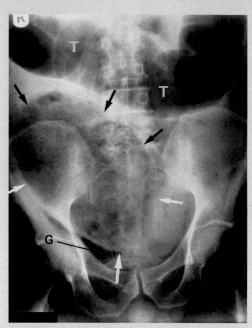

• **Fig. 19.4** Radiological Appearances of Obstructed Bowel. Supine film of an elderly man showing gross caecal dilatation with loss of haustration (surface folds). In large bowel obstruction, this typically occurs if the ileocaecal valve remains competent—a condition that carries a high risk of perforation. In this case, the transverse colon (T) is dilated with gas and there is complete absence of colonic gas on the left side of the abdomen where the descending and sigmoid colon lies. From this, it can be deduced that the colon is obstructed near the splenic flexure. In fact, this patient had an obstructing carcinoma at the splenic flexure and the caecum had perforated, as shown by the presence of gas (G) in the extraperitoneal tissues.

The Adynamic Bowel

This is covered in Chapter 12.

Pseudo-obstruction of the Colon

A form of adynamic bowel disorder peculiar to the large bowel is **pseudo-obstruction** although no mechanical obstruction is present. It can be caused by a range of apparently unrelated conditions that impair bowel peristalsis. These include retroperitoneal inflammation or haemorrhage, neurological conditions, biochemical abnormalities, certain drugs (e.g., anticholinergics), pregnancy and delivery, orthopaedic injuries or surgery (particularly in the elderly) and prolonged recumbency.

Physical signs are similar to those of mechanical obstruction except that bowel sounds are normal or inaudible. The diagnosis is based on the clinical findings and is confirmed if no mechanical obstruction is found on imaging.

Pseudo-obstruction usually resolves with conservative measures, but it is important to identify and treat any evident precipitating cause. Neostigmine is sometimes used where conservative measures fail but needs close cardiac monitoring. Surgery is sometimes indicated if the bowel perforates or if there is no recovery after prolonged conservative management.

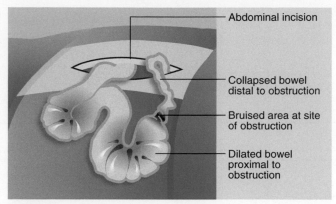

• **Fig. 19.5** Findings at Operation for Simple Band Obstruction of Small Bowel.

Principles of Management of Intestinal Obstruction

Once intestinal obstruction has been recognised and the approximate level of obstruction identified, management proceeds as follows:

- Resuscitation is an essential first step (see Ch. 4). Oral intake is discontinued and appropriate intravenous fluids are administered. After prolonged vomiting, patients may be seriously fluid and electrolyte depleted.
- If the patient is vomiting and/or has marked small bowel dilatation, a nasogastric tube is passed and gastric contents aspirated. This controls nausea and vomiting, removes swallowed air and reduces gaseous distension. Most importantly, it minimises the risk of aspiration of gastric contents, particularly during induction of anaesthesia.
- At least two-thirds of uncomplicated cases of obstruction are caused by adhesions; these usually resolve with conservative measures used for a maximum of 4 days.
- Large bowel obstruction caused by faecal impaction can be relieved by enemas or manual removal of faeces.
- Operation may be required to relieve the obstruction. Provided strangulation, obstructed hernia and caecal distension have been excluded, operation can safely be deferred for a day or two. This gives time for resuscitation and for any needed investigations. Nevertheless, few obstructions that show no evidence of settling within 48 hours will resolve without intervention.
- **Bowel stenting**—in some cases of left-sided colonic obstruction caused by cancer, the obstruction can be rapidly relieved with an endoscopically-placed self-expanding metallic stent. Surgery can then be deferred until the patient's condition has been optimised. If incurable metastatic disease has been identified, resectional surgery may be avoided altogether.
- At operation, the cause of the obstruction is confirmed and dealt with appropriately (Fig. 19.5).

Bowel Strangulation

Pathophysiology of Bowel Strangulation

Strangulation occurs when a segment of bowel becomes trapped so that its lumen becomes obstructed and its blood supply compromised. If unrelieved, this progresses to **infarction** and eventually perforation. Strangulation can occur when there is an external hernia, when loops of bowel become ensnared within the abdominal cavity or when there is mass rotation of bowel, twisting and compressing the mesentery (**volvulus**).

Strangulation begins with partial obstruction of the bowel. Venous return is occluded causing bowel wall oedema which further aggravates the obstruction. The closed loop of bowel progressively dilates with gas from fermentation. The combination of gas pressure and venous back-pressure progressively inhibits arterial inflow, causing ischaemia and then infarction.

Strangulation most commonly occurs when small bowel is caught within an **external hernia** (inguinal, femoral, umbilical or incisional). The bowel undergoes necrosis and soon perforates within the hernial sac, after which generalised peritonitis usually ensues. Clinically, the patient first develops symptoms and signs of small bowel obstruction. A newly irreducible hernia can usually be found and is likely to be tender and inflamed. However, a strangulated femoral hernia is often deceptively small and nontender and will be missed unless both groins are carefully examined.

Bowel may also become strangulated within the abdominal cavity if a loop becomes trapped by fibrous bands or adhesions (congenital or resulting from previous surgery) or passes through an omental or mesenteric defect. Similarly, strangulation occurs if a large loop of bowel becomes twisted on its mesentery, a condition known as *volvulus*. Small bowel volvulus is rare and occurs only when the mesentery has an unusually narrow base. Recognition is vital because the entire small bowel may be lost if treatment is delayed. The sigmoid colon (or occasionally the caecum) is particularly susceptible to volvulus if it becomes excessively distended; this is most commonly seen in elderly patients with chronic constipation and in countries where the staple diet is extremely high in fibre.

Symptoms and Signs of Bowel Strangulation

Intraabdominal strangulation presents with the usual symptoms and signs of bowel obstruction (see Box 19.2) but is accompanied by **abdominal tenderness,** which should be an alerting signal. When compared with uncomplicated obstruction, patients with strangulation are systemically more unwell, with a rising tachycardia and a leucocytosis.

Principles of Management of Suspected Bowel Strangulation

When strangulation is diagnosed or even suspected, an operation must be performed urgently (after rapid fluid resuscitation) to try to prevent infarction and perforation (Fig. 19.6). The patient is otherwise managed as for uncomplicated obstruction. Bowel strangulation is a clinical diagnosis best confirmed at laparoscopy or laparotomy; there are no specific investigations to confirm the diagnosis of strangulation, though a raised serum lactate level should cause concern in patients with obstruction.

Peritonitis

Pathophysiology and Clinical Features of Peritonitis

Peritonitis is defined as inflammation of the peritoneal cavity. At its onset, before becoming generalised, inflammation of an intraabdominal viscus is often **localised** and the affected viscus is contained by the wrapping of omentum, adjacent bowel and fibrinous adhesions around it. If this is insufficient to prevent spread, **generalised peritonitis** results. Sudden perforation of any viscus almost invariably leads to life-threatening generalised peritonitis.

Localised peritonitis occurs near any primary intraabdominal inflammatory process. Acute appendicitis is a typical example. At first, the pain is poorly localised and central. When the parietal

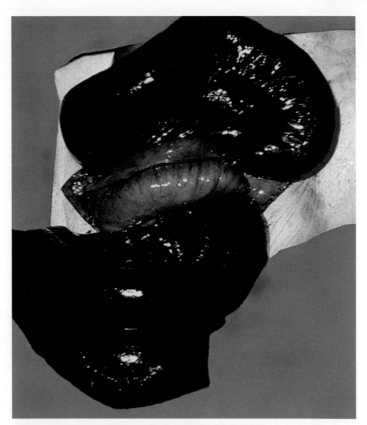

• **Fig. 19.6** Necrotic Bowel After Strangulation. This photograph, taken at operation for bowel obstruction, shows a dilated necrotic loop of small bowel, which has strangulated after passing through a congenital defect in the sigmoid mesocolon. The bowel was on the point of perforation.

peritoneum becomes involved, pain localises to the affected area and is exacerbated by abdominal muscle movement. The area is tender to palpation and overlying abdominal muscles contract when examination is attempted ('**guarding**'). If the palpating hand is quickly removed, the sudden peritoneal movement causes intense pain described as *rebound tenderness*. Rebound tenderness is better and more kindly elicited by gentle percussion. Rectal examination should be performed, as anterior peritoneal tenderness can be a sign of pelvic peritonitis. Localised peritonitis is usually accompanied by mild systemic 'toxicity', that is, low-grade fever, malaise, tachycardia and leucocytosis.

With **generalised peritonitis**, the patient becomes seriously and rapidly ill. There is massive exudation of inflammatory fluid into the peritoneal cavity (causing hypovolaemia), toxaemia from absorbed toxins, and if infection is present, sepsis. The systemic illness is most severe when there is widespread contamination by faeces, pus or infected bile. Peritonitis is less severe when infection is absent (e.g., perforated duodenal ulcer in its early stages).

On examination, the abdomen is rigid and tender (but this may not be evident in the very elderly or mentally obtunded) and bowel sounds are absent because of peristaltic paralysis. CT scans are often performed but rarely change management and may delay definitive treatment. The causes of peritonitis are summarised in Box 19.3.

Intraabdominal Haemorrhage

Blood may come into the abdominal cavity from many sources including ruptured ectopic pregnancy, leaking aortic aneurysm or blunt trauma, especially to liver or spleen. Blood causes moderate

Localised Peritonitis

- Transmural inflammation of bowel, for example, appendicitis, Crohn disease, diverticulitis
- Transmural inflammation of other viscera, for example, cholecystitis, salpingitis

Generalised Peritonitis

- Chemical peritonitis: irritation of the peritoneum by noxious materials, for example, bile, stomach or small bowel contents (caused by perforation), enzyme-containing exudates of acute pancreatitis or blood
- Bacterial peritonitis: spreading intraperitoneal infection, for example, rupture of intraabdominal abscess or faecal contamination caused by bowel perforation, trauma, surgical spillage or anastomotic leak after recent bowel surgery

peritoneal irritation and peritonitis-like symptoms, but often more muted. In an unstable patient with obvious intraperitoneal bleeding, this is best diagnosed at laparoscopy and managed at laparotomy. If less urgent, as in some cases of blunt abdominal trauma, bleeding may be confirmed by CT scan, which indicates the cause or helps the difficult decision of whether to manage conservatively or by operation.

Principles of Management of Peritonitis

Local peritonitis is treated according to the diagnosis. For example, appendicitis usually requires appendicectomy, whilst acute diverticulitis and salpingitis are usually managed with antibiotics.

With generalised peritonitis, the patient is at risk of dying from sepsis. As soon as the diagnosis is made, the patient is resuscitated and given high doses of antibiotics intravenously. With the exception of acute pancreatitis, generalised peritonitis requires urgent laparotomy to discover the cause (sometimes laparoscopy is appropriate initially), clear the contaminating material (**peritoneal toilet**) and to undertake definitive treatment.

Intraabdominal Abscess

Pathophysiology and Clinical Features of Intraabdominal Abscess

There are two common causes of intraabdominal abscess. The first occurs after bowel perforation, when omentum and adjacent bowel attempt to wall off the defect. The second is a complication of bowel surgery following an anastomotic leak or localised faecal contamination during an operation. Appendiceal perforation may cause a local abscess or one which tracks into the pelvis. Diverticular disease often causes a **pericolic abscess** or **complex inflammatory mass** in the rectosigmoid area or pelvis. Less common examples include: perforated colonic carcinoma causing a pericolic abscess, gall bladder perforation resulting in a right-sided **subphrenic abscess** and posterior gastric ulcer perforation producing a **lesser sac abscess**.

Intraabdominal abscesses tend to present with a worsening, continuous abdominal pain, diarrhoea or adynamic bowel disorder caused by local bowel irritation and a high swinging temperature. The last is an important sign of an abscess and there is usually marked leucocytosis. Patients are often relatively well, except with a postoperative abscess where a degree of systemic inflammatory response or multiorgan dysfunction is usual (see Ch. 3). There may be a palpable inflammatory mass, most commonly

originating with acute appendicitis or acute diverticular disease. Rectal examination may reveal a hot, tender mass displacing the rectum backwards (a **pelvic abscess**)—a classic finding in the febrile postappendicectomy patient. Patients usually complain of diarrhoea; a result of the abscess causing rectal inflammation .

Ultrasound or CT of the abdomen and pelvis is most useful in demonstrating the site and size of an abscess, and drainage may be possible under imaging control (see Fig. 19.7).

Principles of Management of an Intraabdominal Abscess

With a pelvic abscess in an otherwise well patient, there is usually no advantage in giving antibiotic treatment or attempting to drain the abscess because, given time, the abscess usually drains spontaneously and safely into the rectum. Discharge of the abscess is recognised when the patient passes pus and blood per rectum; this is followed by resolution of the fever and healing.

Small subphrenic abscesses may also resolve without intervention but larger ones can be drained percutaneously. Many intraabdominal abscesses can be treated using percutaneous drainage under radiological control but this deals only with the abscess and not the underlying cause. Laparotomy may be required if the underlying cause needs treatment or if the abscess is unsuitable for percutaneous drainage.

Perforation of an Abdominal Viscus

Pathophysiology and Clinical Features of Perforation

Disease of any hollow viscus may be complicated by perforation into the peritoneal cavity. The common sites are stomach and duodenum (from peptic ulcer), sigmoid colon (from diverticular disease or carcinoma) and the appendix (from acute appendicitis). The symptoms and signs of a perforated viscus depend on the nature of its contents, the volume of spillage and the effectiveness of local defences.

A small perforation may be immediately walled off by omentum and bowel but a local abscess then develops, giving symptoms of an intraabdominal abscess. A common example is appendicitis in adults. A small diverticular perforation without faecal spillage may cause local peritonitis, which may resolve spontaneously. At the opposite extreme, a large colonic perforation caused by a stercoral tear from severe constipation causes sudden overwhelming faecal peritonitis, which is often fatal. A perforated peptic ulcer causes marked abdominal signs of peritonitis, typically 'board-like' rigidity, but little initial systemic upset because the fluid spilled is usually sterile. Acute cholecystitis occasionally perforates if inflammation is severe enough to cause necrosis.

Perforation is essentially a clinical diagnosis but can be confirmed by the presence of free gas in the peritoneal cavity on plain radiography (or CT scan). This is visible as a radiolucent line beneath the hemidiaphragms on an erect chest film (see Fig. 19.8) or a lateral decubitus abdominal film. Note that CT scanning is more sensitive than plain films for detecting small quantities of free gas. Free gas is rare in perforated appendicitis or perforated gall bladder. If imaging fails to support the clinical findings, action should be based on the clinical diagnosis.

Principles of Management of Perforation

Perforation is a surgical emergency. Most cases require urgent operation to repair the defect or resect the segment of diseased bowel. Duodenal ulcer perforations can be plugged with omentum at open or laparoscopic surgery. In large bowel perforations, a Hartmann procedure, which creates a temporary colostomy (see

CASE HISTORIES

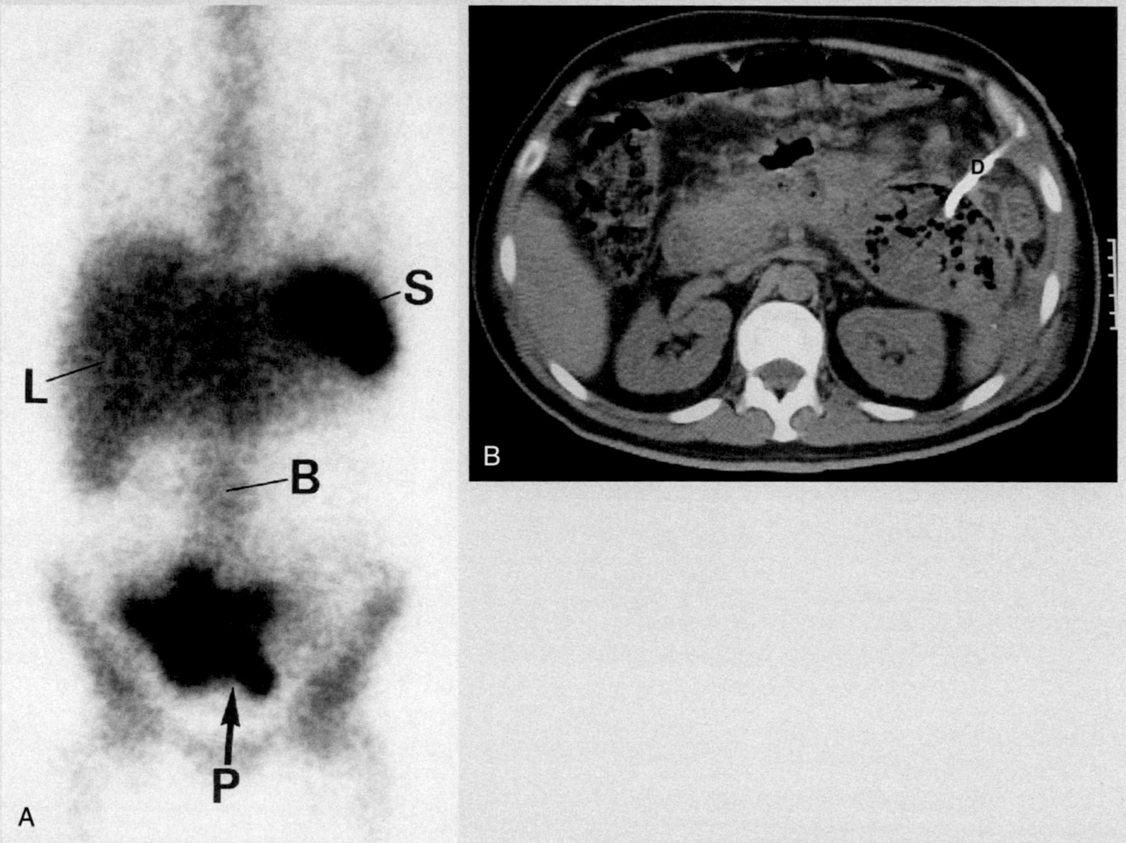

• **Fig. 19.7** Radiologically Guided Drainage of Intraabdominal Abscess. **(A)** Radionuclide scan of a 47-year-old woman who presented with lower abdominal tenderness and a swinging pyrexia. The patient's own leucocytes were labelled with a radionuclide. This image shows a large pelvic abscess *(P)*, shown later to be caused by diverticular perforation. Note also the radioisotope uptake by the spleen *(S)*, liver *(L)* and bone marrow *(B)*, which is a normal feature of such scans. **(B)** Computed tomography–guided percutaneous placement of a drain *(D)* into an abscess of the pancreatic tail following an attack of acute pancreatitis. Note: the pancreas remains generally swollen.

Ch. 27), is frequently required because healing of an anastomosis may be impaired by the gross peritoneal contamination, although there is a trend towards performing primary anastomosis even in these cases, together with a covering ileostomy. Very rarely, in perforation following colonoscopy, conservative management is appropriate if there are few clinical signs. This is because faecal contamination is minimal as the bowel is already clean. In the elderly or unfit, perforated duodenal ulcers may also be managed conservatively using restriction of oral fluids, nasogastric aspiration, acid suppression and antibiotics; however, the outcome is unpredictable and the approach should be reserved only for patients unsuitable for general anaesthesia or surgery.

Acute Bowel Ischaemia

Pathophysiology and Clinical Features of Intestinal Ischaemia

Acute occlusion of the **superior mesenteric artery** (SMA) may lead to acute ischaemia of the primitive midgut-derived structures, that is, jejunum, ileum and right colon (see Fig. 19.9). This causes massive infarction of the right side of the colon and most of the small bowel and later, fatal perforation. There are two types: **embolism** usually originates from left atrial thrombus in atrial

fibrillation or from left ventricular wall thrombus after recent myocardial infarction; and **thrombosis** of the artery, secondary to atherosclerotic stenosis. Rarely, in low output cardiac failure, occlusion may be a terminal event. The vulnerability of the SMA territory is poorly understood, as is the sparing of the coeliac and inferior mesenteric territories, but it likely depends on the quality of the collateral blood supply.

Acute bowel ischaemia can be difficult to diagnose because of the lack of specific clinical features or diagnostic tests. In the early stages, pain is often very severe and out of proportion to the clinical signs. There may be mild diffuse tenderness but the abdomen is usually soft without guarding. As the process evolves, there is a disproportionate degree of cardiovascular collapse or shock. By this stage, arterial blood gas analysis will show a metabolic acidosis and the plasma lactate may be elevated. On plain abdominal x-ray, gas may be visible within the bowel wall. By this time, surgery is unlikely to succeed. Diagnosis therefore depends on clinical suspicion and rapid action, but for most cases the outlook is grim no matter how early the diagnosis is made.

Some cases of intestinal infarction are caused by **mesenteric vein thrombosis**. The cause may be a prothrombotic disorder but is often idiopathic. In these patients, the infarction is often patchy and localised resections may allow some patients to survive.

CASE HISTORY

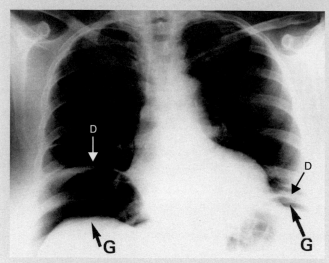

• **Fig. 19.8** Free Perforation of Abdominal Viscus Shown on Plain Chest X-Ray. Erect chest x-ray of a man of 60 years with a perforated sigmoid diverticulum who presented with a sudden onset of severe abdominal pain. The film shows large radiolucent gas shadows *(G, G)* under each hemidiaphragm *(D, D)*. Fortunately in this case, no faeces entered the peritoneum and the patient did not suffer shock or peritonitis.

CASE HISTORY

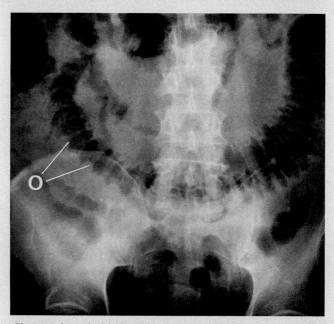

• **Fig. 19.9** Intestinal Ischaemia. This 68-year-old woman with atrial fibrillation presented with collapse but only moderate abdominal pain. The patient had embolised her superior mesenteric artery (acute SMA occlusion) which supplies the embryological midgut-derived structures. The whole of her small bowel and the right half of her colon were necrotic but the left half of the colon was intact. This film shows the typical gross thickening of small bowel folds caused by swelling from oedema and intramural haemorrhage *(O)*.

> • **BOX 19.4** Special Points to Note in Examining a Patient With an Acute Abdomen
>
> **General Examination**
> See Box 18.3
>
> **Abdominal Examination**
> • Inspection
>   — distension, visible peristalsis, previous operation scars, obvious hernias, range of abdominal movement with respiration
>   — always inspect the loins and back
> • Palpation and percussion
>   — tenderness, guarding, rigidity, rebound tenderness, pain on percussion
>   — free fluid, succussion splash
>   — groins for hernias and their reducibility, external genitalia
>   — abdominal masses (including a full bladder)
>   — abnormal pulsation (aneurysm?)
> • Auscultation
>   — bowel sounds, mesenteric arterial bruits

Principles of Management of Intestinal Ischaemia

If intestinal ischaemia is suspected, laparotomy or a laparoscopy must be performed urgently unless it is clearly going to be fruitless.

Very occasionally, it is possible to restore the mesenteric supply by embolectomy or bypass before the bowel undergoes necrosis. If the infarcted segment is limited and the rest of the bowel looks healthy, resection gives a reasonable chance of recovery and an adequate amount of bowel to sustain nutrition. Even with short segments of residual small bowel, supplementary nutrition may allow prolonged survival but in nearly half the cases, the necrosis is so extensive that the patient should be allowed to die with minimal interference. In a few patients with arterial or venous infarction, massive resection and subsequent small bowel transplantation may be appropriate.

Examination and investigation of the acute abdomen are summarised in Boxes 19.4 and 19.5.

Major Gastrointestinal Haemorrhage

Pathophysiology and Clinical Features

Major GI haemorrhage presents as vomiting of blood or passage of frank or altered blood rectally. Vomited blood (**haematemesis**) may be fresh or partly digested. In the latter case, it is dark and may have the typical appearance of 'coffee grounds'. Haematemesis usually indicates bleeding from the oesophagus, stomach or duodenum.

Blood loss beyond the duodenum is usually passed rectally. The extent to which it is altered by digestion and the degree of mixing with the stool are useful indicators of its level of origin and rate of bleeding. Upper GI bleeding is often manifest by **melaena**. This is the passage of loose, reddish-black, tarry stools with a characteristic foul smell. With upper GI bleeding proximal to the duodenojejunal flexure, haematemesis or melaena or both can occur. Haematemesis is more likely if the bleeding is rapid. The main causes of major GI haemorrhage are summarised in Fig. 19.10.

Management of Upper Gastrointestinal Haemorrhage

Initial Management and Resuscitation

Any patient with severe upper GI haemorrhage is at risk of dying from hypovolaemic shock. This may occur with the initial event

• BOX 19.5   Investigation of the Acute Abdomen

Blood Tests
Haematology
- Haemoglobin
  - may be normal immediately after an acute bleed
  - low haemoglobin concentration may represent chronic anaemia caused by occult blood loss rather than acute haemorrhage
- White blood count—leucocytosis is nonspecific and rarely of much diagnostic value unless greater than about 14×10^3/L
- Blood group and ordering of blood for transfusion—for severely anaemic patients, in major haemorrhage or when major surgery is contemplated

Biochemistry
- C-reactive protein
  - nonspecific indicator of inflammatory activation
  - confirms organic illness if substantially elevated
- Plasma amylase—whenever pancreatitis cannot be excluded
- Urea and electrolytes—indicated in vomiting and diarrhoea, dehydration, poor urine output, diuretic therapy, urinary tract disease, known or suspected renal failure, pancreatitis and sepsis
- Glucose—for diabetics or those with glycosuria (beware of hyperglycaemia caused by acute stress or steroid therapy). Low glucose often found in acute pancreatitis
- Liver function tests and calcium estimation—for pancreatitis and acute biliary disease
- Clotting studies—for acute pancreatitis and septicaemia (disseminated intravascular coagulation), severe bleeding (consumption coagulopathy) or those with a history of bleeding disorders

Urine Tests
- Ward ('stick') testing—for blood, protein, bile, glucose, nitrites and white cells
- Microscopy—for red and white blood cells, organisms
- Culture and sensitivity—in suspected urinary tract infections
- Strain urine for stones—in ureteric colic
- Pregnancy test in females if appropriate

Imaging (see Box 19.1)
Plain Radiography
- Erect chest x-ray
  - cardiovascular disease or abnormality, for example, cardiomegaly, thoracic aneurysm, aortic dissection, cardiac failure
  - respiratory disease
  - suspected visceral perforation (gas under diaphragm)
- Supine abdominal x-ray (erect or decubitus if necessary)
  - bowel (gas pattern and dilatation, fluid levels, gas in the wall, faeces and faecoliths)
  - urinary tract ('KUB' = kidneys, ureters and bladder) shows kidney size and position, calculi
  - biliary tract (gallstones, gas in biliary tree in gallstone ileus)
  - aortic calcification (aneurysm)
  - psoas shadows (obscured by retroperitoneal inflammation or haemorrhage)

Ultrasound
- Gallstones
- Pelvic abnormalities in obstetric and gynaecological practice
- 'Chronic' enlargement of the spleen
- Abdominal aortic aneurysm (AAA)
- Free abdominal fluid and gas indicating perforated bowel
- Other stones
- Dilated ducts; air in biliary tree
- Hydatid, teratomas and other cysts
- Intraabdominal abscesses and masses

Contrast Radiology
- 'Instant' barium enema in colonic obstruction or acute colitis
- Emergency intravenous urography in ureteric colic

Computed Tomography Scanning
Computed tomography (CT) can give rapid, cost-effective evaluation of acute abdominal pain but should not supplant clinical examination nor lead to unreasonable delays in surgical exploration in the deteriorating patient. Diagnostic value of CT is better if timing, contrast (intravenous and/or oral) and other variables are tailored to the working diagnosis.
- Assessment of abdominal trauma—severity and grading of solid organ injury, free intraabdominal fluid and gas; retroperitoneal injuries including pancreatic and duodenal rupture and vascular injury
- Often first choice for ureteric colic, suspected aortic aneurysm or aortic dissection
- Useful where diagnosis remains in doubt, for example, suspected bowel perforation (detects small amount of free gas), acute diverticulitis
- Investigation of postoperative complications—abscesses, fluid collections
- Severe acute pancreatitis, especially if necrosis suspected

---

or as a result of rebleeding. High-risk patients (Fig. 19.11) have about a 50% risk of rebleeding during a hospital stay; a combined medical/surgical management policy can reduce mortality for all cases of upper GI haemorrhage from 10% to about 2%. Hospitals should have clearly written and agreed protocols for this, so patients do not slip through the net and perish by default (see Fig. 19.11).

Clinical History, Examination and Investigation
In Western countries, more than two-thirds of patients with upper GI haemorrhage are over 60 years and one-third of these have taken aspirin or other nonsteroidal anti-inflammatory drugs. Alcohol consumption, previous peptic ulceration or gastric surgery, or a history of cirrhosis and variceal haemorrhage may also be important.

Abdominal examination is usually unremarkable but general examination may show signs of chronic liver disease suggesting possible gastro-oesophageal varices. Rectal examination may reveal melaena or altered blood and this can be helpful if the history of haematemesis has not been substantiated.

Estimating blood loss from the history is unreliable because a great deal of blood may remain in the bowel. It is essential to obtain good venous access early and then to perform a full blood count, urea and electrolytes and prothrombin ratio and liver function tests, to send blood for grouping and antibody screen (or cross-matching), and to order blood for transfusion in high-risk cases (see Fig. 19.11 and later). Electrocardiogram and chest x-rays are useful in patients over 65 years or with cardiorespiratory disease. *Note*: the patient should be ready to go to the operating theatre at a moment's notice if he or she suddenly deteriorates!

Stratification of Risk
Patients with acute upper GI haemorrhage should be stratified clinically into either a **low-risk group** (non–life threatening) or a **high-risk group** (where continued bleeding or likely rebleeding is potentially life threatening) (see Fig. 19.11 and next section).

COMMON CAUSES OF GASTROINTESTINAL BLEEDING

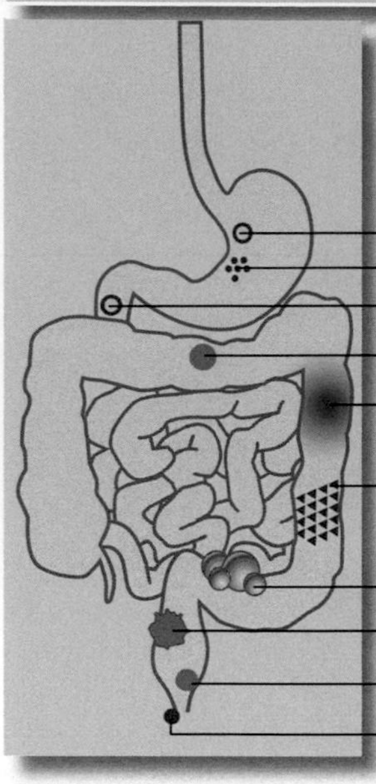

Pathology	Clinical features	Frequency
Acute and chronic gastric ulcers	Haematemesis and/or melaena	Very common
Gastric erosions		
Chronic duodenal ulcer		
Polyps or carcinoma of colon	Altered blood per rectum	Common
Ischaemic colitis	Abdominal pain then fairly fresh rectal bleeding	Fairly common
Angiodysplasias of colon	Pattern of bleeding depends on location within colon; increasingly recognised with the rise in colonoscopy	Fairly common
Diverticular disease	Fresh rectal bleeding	Common
Carcinoma of rectum	Fresh rectal bleeding but rarely in large quantities	Common
Rectal polyps		
Haemorrhoids		

UNCOMMON CAUSES OF GASTROINTESTINAL BLEEDING

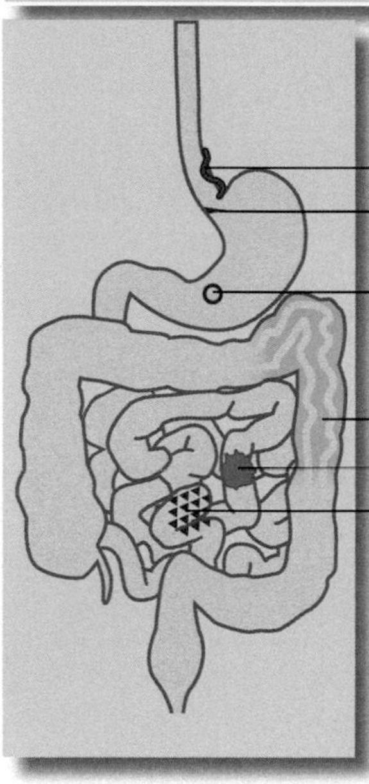

Pathology	Clinical features	Frequency
Oesophageal varices	Haematemesis and/or melaena	Uncommon
Mallory–Weiss oesophageal tears	Haematemesis or altered blood per rectum	Uncommon
Stress ulcers	Haematemesis and/or melaena	Uncommon
Acute or fulminant ulcerative colitis	Bloody diarrhoea	Uncommon
Malignant small bowel tumours	Altered blood per rectum	Rare
Angiodysplasias of small bowel	Altered blood per rectum	Rare

• **Fig. 19.10** Causes of Gastrointestinal Haemorrhage.

Patients with signs of shock must be monitored and resuscitated thoroughly; the rate and volume of intravenous fluid replacement (whether plasma expanders or blood) is adjusted against the responses of pulse rate, blood pressure, central venous pressure and hourly urine output.

Endoscopic Management of Acute Upper Gastrointestinal Haemorrhage

Patients clinically at high risk should be assessed early by a surgical team, even if admitted under the care of a gastroenterologist or (internal) physician. Effective teamwork, communication and handover are critical to the management of these patients. Patients should be closely monitored until recovery so that a prompt decision to operate can be made if conservative management fails.

Patients with upper GI haemorrhage require endoscopy to determine the site and activity of bleeding, to diagnose oesophageal varices and to determine suitability for endoscopic treatment. Endoscopy also assists in locating the source if surgery becomes necessary. Urgent endoscopy, within 12 hours of the first bleed, should be performed in high-risk patients; all others should be endoscoped on the next available list. Even in the most acute upper GI haemorrhage, gastroscopy can usually be performed on the operating table before operation. Duodenal or gastric ulceration should be easily identifiable, but its real value is the ability to diagnose unusual sources of bleeding (e.g., Mallory–Weiss tear; see Ch. 22) and to avoid operating on unsuspected variceal haemorrhage. Even in patients with known varices, endoscopy is essential, as in 50% of cases, blood loss will be from a completely different lesion, for example, peptic ulcer or gastric erosions.

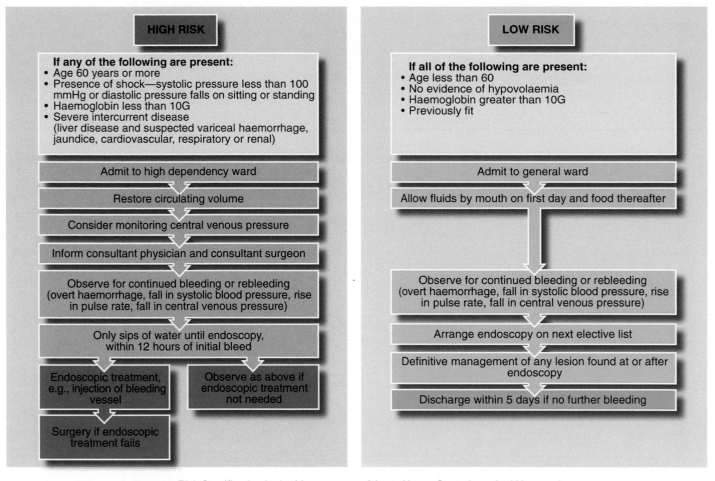

• **Fig. 19.11** Risk Stratification in the Management of Acute Upper Gastrointestinal Haemorrhage.

Certain endoscopic features may place apparently low-risk patients into a high-risk category. These are:

- **Active spurting from an artery in an ulcer bed.** Endotherapy by gastroscopic injection of adrenaline (epinephrine) or an adrenaline/sclerosant mixture should be attempted; there is a 25% to 40% rebleed rate, even in expert hands, and the patient must be closely monitored as these often need surgery.
- **A visible elevated vessel or protruding adherent clot (Dieulafoy lesion).** These lesions double the aforementioned risk of rebleeding to 50% to 80%. If the patient is hypotensive as a result of blood loss, the risk of rebleeding is 80%.
- **Bleeding gastro-oesophageal varices.** Mortality is around 30%. Immediate treatment is required with endoluminal band ligation or injection sclerotherapy. Tamponade with special balloon catheters may also be necessary before endotherapy.

High-risk patients should be commenced on a 72-hour intravenous infusion of high-dose proton-pump inhibitor. Low-risk patients usually stop bleeding with conservative management and are then unlikely to rebleed. They may be given sips of water, monitored for rebleeding, and endoscoped on the next available list.

Surgical Management

A policy of early surgery for patients over 60 years has been shown to reduce mortality. Urgent surgery is also required for patients defined clinically or endoscopically as at high risk, and who suffer one rebleed; or for any patient who suffers two rebleeds.

Immediate surgery, including unguided laparotomy, may be required for patients with exsanguinating haemorrhage or those unable to be stabilised during resuscitation.

Bleeding is arrested with underrunning sutures after gastrotomy or duodenotomy and attempts are made to preserve the pyloric ring. Gastric and duodenal ulcers should be biopsied for *Helicobacter* testing, and for malignancy in gastric ulcers. Anti-*Helicobacter* therapy is given later if perioperative or postoperative testing is *Helicobacter pylori* positive.

More Distal Gastrointestinal Haemorrhage

More distal GI bleeding is not usually investigated immediately to find the site but is managed conservatively, anticipating spontaneous cessation. If bleeding continues, it is important that the source be localised by investigation so that treatment can be accurately targeted. 'Blind' laparotomy is often unsatisfactory because the source may be difficult or impossible to find or the cause may need nonsurgical treatment.

Blood loss from diverticular disease (approximately 60% of cases) and ischaemic colitis is usually self-limiting. Several small bleeds may occur over a few days but the volume lost is usually small and hypovolaemia is rare. Typically, patients present late and the bleeding has often stopped, with blood per rectum being the only evidence.

Investigation involves **colonoscopy**, usually once the bleeding has stopped. Occasionally an unsuspected carcinoma or polyp is discovered. In ulcerative colitis, the diagnosis is evident from

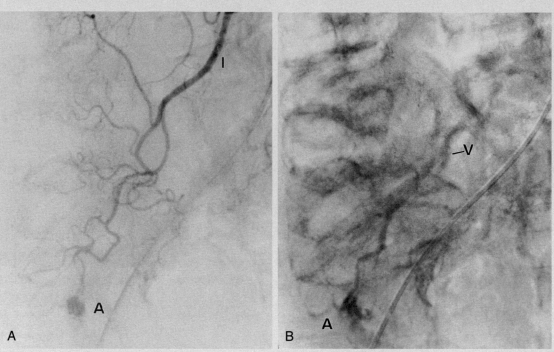

• **Fig. 19.12** Angiogram Showing Angiodysplasia of Caecum. This man of 70 years had been admitted to hospital on 12 occasions for rectal bleeding and chronic anaemia and had received 55 units of blood transfusion in all. On the last admission, this superior mesenteric arteriogram was performed, revealing the source of blood loss. **(A)** Subtraction film showing the arterial phase; the ileocolic artery *(I)* feeds a knot of abnormal blood vessels, an angiodysplasia *(A)*, at the lower pole of the caecum was responsible for the bleeding. **(B)** Subtraction film of the venous phase; the angiodysplasia *(A)* is still visible and there is early filling of a large draining vein *(V)*. These appearances are typical of angiodysplasia; the caecum is the most common site of occurrence. The lesion was resected by right hemicolectomy

the other symptoms and signs, and management depends on the success of medical treatment (see Ch. 28). Persisting large bowel haemorrhage which is less rapid but recurrent is usually caused by **angiodysplasias** (see Ch. 29). Colonoscopy can be both diagnostic and therapeutic for bleeding angiodysplasia. If colonoscopy is negative, impossible or unsatisfactory, radioisotope scanning using the patient's own labelled red cells can be used; this has the advantage of identifying bleeding at rates as low as 0.05 mL/min. Highly selective arteriography is increasingly used in diagnosis of

GI haemorrhage but relies on more rapid bleeding (greater than 0.5 mL/min) (see Fig. 19.12). At the time of arteriography, bleeding can be controlled with localised delivery of vasopressors or by embolisation with coils.

At laparotomy, the whole bowel can be examined and any suspect area resected if appropriate. However, purely mucosal lesions are undetectable at operation so, as a last resort, a colonoscope inserted through an incision in the bowel wall can be used to examine the whole colon and small bowel for bleeding sites.

20

Gallstone Diseases and Related Disorders

CHAPTER OUTLINE

Introduction

Gallstones and related disorders account for all but a small proportion of biliary tract disease in most countries. Gallstone disease is also known as *cholelithiasis* and *choledocholithiasis* is when stones are present in the bile ducts.

Most gallstone-related disease presents with pain, typically located in the epigastrium or right hypochondrium (right upper quadrant or RUQ). The character of the pain varies, but in most cases, it is acute and intermittent. Less commonly, gallstone disease presents as pain and jaundice caused by a stone passing into and obstructing the common bile duct.

Structure and Function of the Biliary System

Bile collects in canaliculi between hepatocytes and drains via collecting ducts within the portal triads into a system of ducts within the liver. These progressively increase in diameter until they become the **right** and **left hepatic ducts** which fuse to form the **common hepatic duct**. This is joined further distally by the **cystic duct** to become the **common bile duct** (Fig. 20.1). The common bile duct is 4 to 5 cm long and passes down behind the duodenum, then through the head of the pancreas to drain via the **ampulla of Vater** into the medial wall of the second part of the duodenum. In most cases, the **main pancreatic duct** joins the common bile duct at the ampulla, although it may enter the duodenum independently. The **sphincter of Oddi** within the ampulla prevents reflux of duodenal contents into the common bile duct and pancreatic duct.

The **gall bladder** is a muscular sac lined by mucosa characterised by a single, highly folded layer of tall columnar epithelial cells. The lining epithelium is supported by loose connective tissue containing numerous blood vessels and lymphatics. Mucus-secreting glands are found at the neck of the gall bladder but are absent from the body and fundus. The proximal part of the duct is disposed into a spiral arrangement called the *spiral valve*, the function of which is not well understood. The gall bladder lies in a variable depression in the undersurface of the right hepatic lobe and is covered by the peritoneal envelope of the liver. The common bile duct is a fibrous tissue tube lined by a simple, tall columnar epithelium. Normally, it is up to 0.6 cm in diameter and this can be measured on ultrasound scanning.

Bile is made continuously by the liver and passes along the biliary tract to the gall bladder where it is stored. Bile is concentrated there, by as much as 10 times, by a process of active mucosal reabsorption of water. Lipid-rich food passing from stomach to duodenum promotes secretion of the hormone **cholecystokinin-pancreozymin** by endocrine cells of the duodenal mucosa. This hormone stimulates contraction of the gall bladder, squeezing bile into the duodenum. Bile salts (acids) act as emulsifying agents and facilitate hydrolysis of dietary lipids by pancreatic lipases. If biliary tract obstruction prevents bile from reaching the duodenum, lipids are neither digested nor absorbed, resulting in passage of loose, pale, foul-smelling fatty stools (**steatorrhoea**). Furthermore, the fat-soluble vitamins (A, D, E and K) are not absorbed. The lack of vitamin K soon leads to inadequate prothrombin synthesis and hence defective clotting. If surgery is necessary in a patient with obstructive jaundice, this may pose problems of haemostasis.

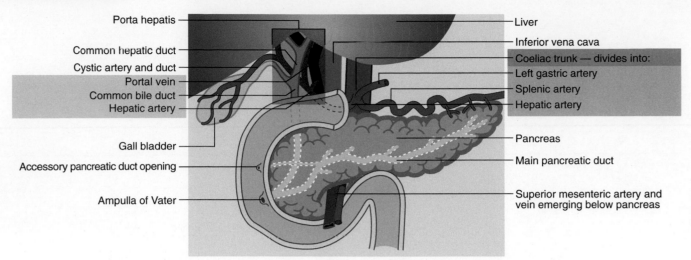

• **Fig. 20.1** Surgical Anatomy of the Gall Bladder, Biliary Tract and Pancreas. The coeliac trunk (the foregut artery) arises from the aorta and divides into the hepatic, splenic and left gastric arteries. The hepatic artery divides into right and left branches, mirrored by the extrahepatic right and left hepatic ducts. These join caudally to form the common hepatic duct; this in turn is joined by the cystic duct to form the common bile duct (CBD). The **porta hepatis** consists of the hepatic arteries, the extrahepatic bile ducts and the portal vein.

TABLE 20.1	Composition and Pathogenesis of Gallstones	
Chemical Composition	**Pathogenesis**	**Characteristics**
Mixed stones (75%–90% of all stones) Cholesterol is the predominant constituent Heterogeneous mixture of cholesterol, bile pigments and calcium salts in a laminated structure around a 'core' (see Fig. 20.2)	Combination of: • abnormalities of bile constituents • bile stasis • infection	Multiple stones with several generations of different sizes often found together Stones may be hard and faceted (where they have developed in contact) or irregular, 'mulberry'-shaped, and softer Colours range from near-white through yellow and green to black Most are radiolucent but 10% are radiopaque
Cholesterol stones (up to 10% of all stones)	As for mixed stones	Large, smooth, egg- or barrel-shaped and usually solitary ('cholesterol solitaire') Yellowish. Up to 4 cm diameter and may fill the gall bladder. Radiolucent
Pigment stones Calcium bilirubinate (uncommon in most developed countries but common in Asia)	Excess bilirubin excretion caused by haemolytic disorders, for example, haemolytic anaemias, infections, malaria, leukaemias	Multiple, jet-black, shiny 'jack' stones; 0.5–1 cm diameter. Usually of uniform size and often friable
Calcium carbonate stones (rare)	Excess calcium excretion in bile	Greyish faceted stones Radiopaque

Pathophysiology of the Biliary System

Gallstone Composition

In most developed countries, most gallstones are of **mixed** composition and contain a predominance of cholesterol; this is mixed with some **bile pigment** (calcium bilirubinate) and other **calcium salts**. A small proportion is virtually 'pure' cholesterol stones ('**cholesterol solitaire**'). In Asia, most gallstones are composed of bile pigment alone. The composition and pathogenesis of the various types of gallstone are summarised in Table 20.1 and Fig. 20.2, and some examples are illustrated in Fig. 20.3.

The physical structure of mixed gallstones gives an insight into their sequence of formation. There is usually a small core of organic material, often containing bacteria. The main body of the stone is made up of concentric layers, demonstrating that stones form in a series of discrete precipitation events. Furthermore, in the same gall bladder, there are often several 'families' of gallstones, each of a different size. This suggests each generation began at a different time, presumably because of some transient change in local conditions. All families then build up at the same rate by lamination, leading to the range of different sizes. Radioisotope dating studies have shown that the average gallstone is 11 years old when removed!

The main factors in stone formation are: (1) changes in concentration of the different constituents of bile, (2) biliary stasis and (3) infection. It is likely that several subtle abnormalities combine synergistically to bring about precipitation of bile constituents.

Bile salts and lecithin are responsible for maintaining cholesterol in a stable **micelle** formation. The normal micellar structure of bile supports a greater concentration of cholesterol than could otherwise be held in solution, and is therefore inherently unstable. An excess of cholesterol in proportion to bile salts and lecithin is probably one of the main factors in cholesterol stone formation. This is supported by the fact that patients in whom the terminal ileum has been resected or who have chronic distal ileal disease have a threefold risk of developing cholesterol-rich stones. The mechanism is likely to be as follows: the terminal ileum is the main site for reabsorption of bile salts and when it is diseased or has been removed, reabsorption declines, leading to bile salt loss via the bowel and, eventually, a decline in the bile salt pool. The remaining bile salts are then insufficient to maintain the micellar structure of cholesterol in suspension.

Precipitation from bile is enhanced by **biliary stasis**. This occurs if the gall bladder becomes obstructed or contractility becomes defective. It is not known whether obstruction of the gall bladder outlet is a primary event in formation of stones, but it probably plays a part in their continued accretion. Obstruction can be caused by dysfunction of the spiral valve in the cystic duct, by reflux of duodenal contents (which may be infected) or by small stones already formed. The muscular gall bladder wall is damaged by longstanding inflammation or infection which interferes with its ability to empty. Pregnancy is also a predisposing factor.

The Role of Inflammation and Infection

Inflammation and infection probably both play a part in gallstone formation. Abnormalities of bile composition may cause **chemical inflammation** of the gall bladder, resulting in inflammatory

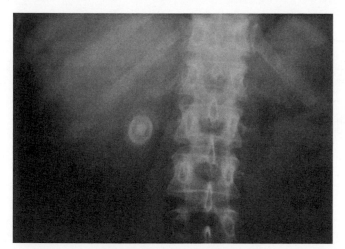

• **Fig. 20.2** X-ray of Radiopaque Gallstone. Plain abdominal x-ray showing large radiopaque gallstone in the right upper quadrant. Note that the stone is obviously laminated, having built up in layers over many years. Note also that only 10% of mixed stones are radiopaque.

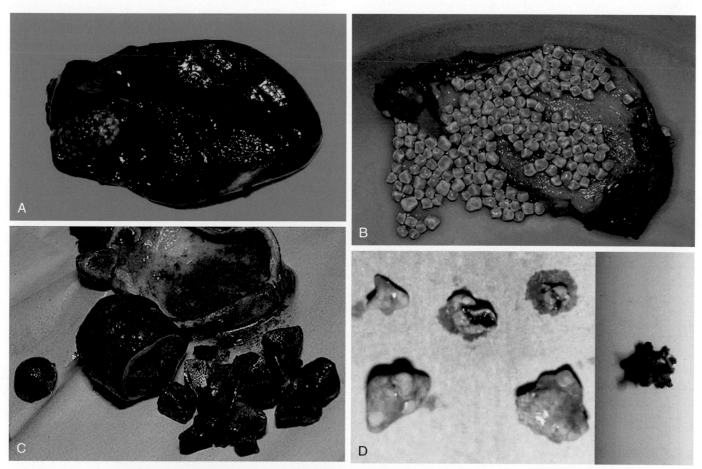

• **Fig. 20.3** Types of Gallstone. (A) Thick-walled chronically inflamed gall bladder found to be obstructed at its neck by a single stone. Note the stone is an aggregate of many smaller stones (B) Multiple small gallstones in the gall bladder, all of much the same 'generation'. (C) Gall bladder containing one huge stone and multiple smaller stones. These stones all fitted together with adjoining facets. (D) Different types of gallstones—pale irregular stones of different ages on the left and a pigment 'jack' stone on the right

exudation and accumulation of inflammatory debris. **Bacteria** usually form the organic nidus upon which gallstones are built; they enter the gall bladder intermittently by reflux from the duodenum or via the bloodstream. This process is probably normal but becomes pathological if the bacteria are not flushed out, as occurs when the gall bladder does not adequately empty. In support of this, is the fact that faecal organisms can be cultured from at least 25% of cholecystectomy specimens.

The Role of Chronic Obstruction

Most gall bladders removed for chronic pain show histological features more in keeping with a **chronic obstructive aetiology**, than an infective one. These include atrophic mucosa, submucosal and subserosal fibrosis, hypertrophy of the muscular wall, and mucosal diverticula extending into the muscular layer (known as *Rokitansky–Aschoff sinuses*). Evidence of active or previous infection is uncommon. In some cases, the gall bladder is so grossly scarred, distorted or contracted that its absorptive and contractile functions have been completely destroyed.

Other Pathological Mechanisms

In about 10% of patients with typical symptoms of gall bladder disease, no stone can be found during investigation or at operation. In some of these, a stone may have passed out of the duct system into the bowel. In others, acute or chronic inflammation occurs independently of stones, called *acalculous cholecystitis*; once again, chronic obstruction may be the cause. Finally, the terms *biliary dyskinesia* and *cystic duct syndrome* may sometimes explain the condition where patients have typical symptoms of gall bladder disease but standard investigations are essentially normal. When biliary manometry is used, some patients have an abnormally high pressure in the sphincter of Oddi. Confirming this diagnosis is difficult but a fair proportion of patients suspected of this are cured by endoscopic sphincterotomy.

Epidemiology of Gallstones

In developed countries, at least 10% of adults probably develop gallstones during their lifetime, although most remain asymptomatic. Gallstones are rare before adulthood and increase in prevalence with age. Women are affected four times more often and pregnancy appears to be an important predisposing factor; obesity and diabetes may also play a part. The typical patient is said to be a 'fair fat fertile female of forty', but many gallstone patients do not fit this description. Gallstone disease is rare in rural communities of developing countries but is increasing with urbanisation. Western-style processed foods, high in fats and refined carbohydrates but poor in fibre, may be responsible. Dietary contributions to gall bladder disease support the theory that changes in composition of bile are important in stone pathogenesis.

Investigation of Gall Bladder Pathology

When gallstone disease is suspected, investigation has the following objectives:
- Exclude haematological and liver abnormalities and other metabolic disorders.
- Establish if gallstones are present in the gall bladder and/or common duct and whether the gall bladder wall is thickened.
- Assess the integrity and patency of the bile duct system and the pancreatic duct (if there is any suggestion of obstruction).

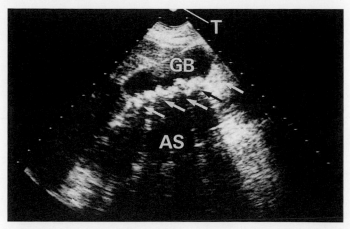

• **Fig. 20.4** Biliary Ultrasound Scans. Longitudinal scan of gall bladder in a 46-year-old woman who complained of intermittent attacks of right upper quadrant pain. The scan shows the outline of the gall bladder *(GB)* and a layer of gallstones *(arrowed)* along its posterior wall. The stones each cast a clear acoustic shadow *(AS)* beyond them. Note that these shadows can be projected back to the transducer *(T)*.

Blood Tests for Haematological and Liver Abnormalities

Haemolytic disorders, such as hereditary spherocytosis, thalassaemia and sickle-cell trait should be considered, as they may predispose to pigment stones. Liver function tests (LFTs) are indicated to look for indications of common duct stone obstruction, if there is any suggestion of jaundice, and to exclude other liver abnormalities.

Imaging in Investigating Gall Bladder Pathology

Ultrasonography (Fig. 20.4) can reliably identify stones in the gall bladder and any increase in thickness of the wall (caused by inflammation or fibrosis). Ultrasound also provides a simple and accurate means of demonstrating **dilatation of the common duct system**, often indicating distal duct obstruction. Unfortunately, it is unreliable for directly identifying bile duct stones, particularly at the lower end, because the image tends to be obscured by overlying duodenal gas. Ultrasound has the great advantage of being suitable for use in the seriously ill or jaundiced patient, as it is noninvasive and can be performed at the bedside.

Investigating the Biliary Duct System (Fig. 20.5)
The Nonjaundiced Patient

Patients with gallstones but no history of obstructive jaundice do not require preoperative investigation for duct stones, apart from an ultrasound scan and LFTs. If cholecystectomy is needed, **intraoperative** (or perioperative) **cholangiography** may be carried out. A cannula is passed through the cystic duct into the common bile duct and radiopaque contrast material injected to fill the biliary tree. X-rays or fluoroscopic imaging are then used to demonstrate the duct morphology and abnormalities, such as duct dilatation, filling defects caused by stone, or distortion of the tapering lower end of the common duct, as well as obstruction of flow into the duodenum. If cholangiography shows stones, the duct may be explored at the time or else dealt with later by endoscopic retrograde cholangiopancreatography (ERCP).

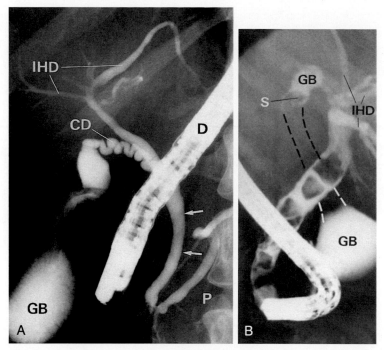

• **Fig. 20.5** Investigation of the Biliary Duct System. (A) Normal endoscopic retrograde cholangiopancreatography showing duodenoscope *(D)* in the second part of the duodenum. Contrast has been injected first into the pancreatic duct *(P)* and then into the common bile duct *(arrowed)*. Note also the cystic duct *(CD)*, gall bladder *(GB)* and intrahepatic bile ducts *(IHD)*. (B) Endoscopic retrograde cholangiogram in a woman of 77 years who presented with mild epigastric pain and obstructive jaundice. The film shows multiple large stones in the common bile duct, represented by filling defects. The common bile duct is moderately dilated, but the intrahepatic ducts *(IHD)* are not. The fundus and neck of the gall bladder *(GB)* are shown, but the body is empty of contrast *(dotted lines)*. There is a stone *(S)* near the neck of the gall bladder.

Patients with a history of **transient jaundice**, possibly attributable to stones, will have either operative cholangiography at cholecystectomy or preoperative ERCP.

The Jaundiced Patient

When obstructive jaundice has been diagnosed, it is important to distinguish between stone, benign stricture and tumour to plan appropriate management. **Ultrasonography** is usually the initial investigation. This shows the extent of dilatation of intrahepatic and extrahepatic ducts and may even show a stone lodged at the lower end of the duct. If stones are in the gall bladder, this suggests stones are blocking the duct rather than tumour, but the two can coexist. The ultrasound scan will usually demonstrate the presence of a carcinoma of the pancreatic head or enlarged lymph nodes in the porta hepatis; either may cause extrahepatic biliary obstruction.

Ultrasound may make the diagnosis, but if more information is required, biliary tract morphology can be outlined using **magnetic resonance cholangiopancreatography (MRCP)**, which produces images of the biliary tree and pancreatic ducts (see Ch. 5, p. 61; Fig. 5.6). If MRCP does not yield the necessary information, the ducts can be visualised by direct introduction of contrast. There are two methods: ERCP and, more rarely, percutaneous transhepatic cholangiography. ERCP is the more useful investigation; it also allows the ampullary region to be inspected for tumour. If stones are found in the common bile duct, it is often possible to perform immediate **endoscopic sphincterotomy** (also called papillotomy) to release the stones, thus diagnosing and relieving the jaundice in one procedure. This may be life saving for the patient with ascending cholangitis and is the treatment of choice on its own for the patient who is a poor risk for laparotomy or laparoscopy.

Percutaneous transhepatic cholangiography (Ch. 5, p. 61; Fig. 5.6) is used in exceptional circumstances, for example if ERCP is unsuccessful because of previous gastric surgery. It involves inserting a long, fine (22-gauge) needle through the skin into one of the dilated intrahepatic ducts under radiological control. Contrast medium is then injected. An obstructing stone produces a characteristic rounded filling defect, contrasting with the tapering stricture typical of tumour. Stricture dilatation and stent insertion can also be performed via this route and in difficult cases, it can be combined with ERCP in what is termed a *rendez-vous* procedure.

Endoscopic ultrasound scanning, that is, scanning via the endoscope, is a useful technique to show greater detail at the lower end of the common bile duct or to examine lesions in the ampulla or head of the pancreas with greater clarity and perform fine-needle aspiration for histological diagnosis.

Clinical Presentations of Gallstone Disease

Gallstones may cause chronic, low-grade symptoms, often labelled *chronic cholecystitis*. However, many of these symptoms may be caused by irritable bowel syndrome or chronic aerophagia (air swallowing). Transient obstruction of the gall bladder by stone may cause episodes of acute pain (**biliary colic**). If the obstruction persists, the gall bladder becomes chemically inflamed causing **acute cholecystitis**. If obstruction does not resolve by itself and the contents do not become infected, the gall bladder becomes distended with mucus; this is known as a ***mucocoele***, and is often palpable and tender. If the contents become infected, an abscess develops within the gall bladder and this is known as an ***empyema of the gall bladder***.

Rarely, free **perforation** of the gall bladder may occur. Equally rarely, large stones in the common bile duct ulcerate directly into the duodenum causing **fistula** formation. If they pass down the small bowel and impact in the terminal ileum and cause obstruction, this is called ***gallstone ileus***. Finally, gallstones probably predispose to **carcinoma** of the gall bladder in the very long term. The spectrum of clinical disorders associated with gallstones is summarised in Fig. 20.6.

Chronic Symptoms Suggestive of Gall Bladder Disease

Many patients are referred with a history of intermittent pain in the RUQ or epigastrium often accompanied by nausea or even vomiting. The pain may be brought on by large or fatty meals and may radiate around towards the back. Symptoms are often vague and ill-defined so patients often delay consulting a doctor. Examination rarely reveals more than vague upper abdominal tenderness. Many turn out not to have gallstones on ultrasonography and the pain may be caused by irritable bowel syndrome but the differential diagnosis includes peptic ulcer disease, urinary tract infection and chronic constipation. Note that even if a patient has upper abdominal symptoms and demonstrable gallstones, this does not prove the pain is caused by stones. When symptoms are less specific, a more extensive diagnostic search is needed, perhaps including upper gastrointestinal endoscopy, plasma amylase and electrocardiography as well as bowel investigations.

Biliary Colic

Clinical Features

The most common reason for symptoms from gallstones is probably intermittent cystic duct obstruction by stone. The pain is severe; it typically rises to a plateau over a few minutes then continues unrelentingly. Note that this pain does not have the strikingly intermittent brief peaks of other forms of colic (e.g., ureteric). These patients may be in agony until the pain resolves spontaneously after several hours or after opiate analgesia. Vomiting is often associated with the attack and the patient feels exhausted and sore for the next day or so. There is commonly a history of previous similar episodes. There are few positive findings on examination: the patient is afebrile but there may be some local tenderness caused by gall bladder distension. If the attack does not settle within 24 hours, acute cholecystitis is a more likely diagnosis (see later).

Management

Most cases of biliary colic can safely be managed at home if the diagnosis is recognised. Relief of pain usually requires only one injection of an opiate and the attack passes. Severe attacks of biliary colic usually prompt emergency hospital admission, since the differential diagnosis includes other conditions that may require urgent operation, for example, perforated peptic ulcer. Ultrasound examination should be performed early since early diagnosis may save several unnecessary days in hospital. In acute gallstone disease, cholecystectomy scheduled for the next available list is preferred by many surgeons and is generally safe, but others perform the operation electively, at a later date. Early operation appears to be the better option, reducing the risk of the complications of gallstones.

If a mucocoele of the gall bladder is found on ultrasonography, the attack is likely to persist and there is a high risk of an **empyema of the gall bladder** developing. In this case, cholecystectomy often becomes obligatory during the current admission.

Cholecystectomy is the definitive treatment for attacks of biliary colic. Patients are frequently put on a low-fat diet initially or whilst awaiting operation and this often relieves symptoms, presumably by removing a stimulus to gall bladder contraction. In younger patients, cholecystectomy is typically straightforward. The gall bladder is usually found to contain stones or thick dark biliary sludge and its wall is often thin, although it may sometimes be inflamed. In some patients, the gall bladder is thickened and scarred and technically more difficult to remove. Techniques of cholecystectomy are discussed on pages 315 onwards.

Acute Cholecystitis

Pathophysiology and Clinical Features

Several factors contribute to causing acute inflammation in an obstructed gall bladder. These include physical and chemical irritation and, later in the episode, bacterial infection. The clinical result is acute cholecystitis, which often presents as a surgical emergency. In contrast to biliary colic, the patient is usually systemically unwell with a fever and tachycardia. On examination, there is tenderness in the RUQ, more marked on inspiration and a tender inflammatory gall bladder mass may be palpable. The term ***Murphy sign*** is often misused in this context; it was originally used to describe tenderness at the tip of the ninth rib. Being inflammatory in origin, the clinical course of acute cholecystitis is more prolonged than biliary colic, usually lasting several days before settling or else precipitating urgent surgery.

Management

Ultrasonography is usually sufficient to support the diagnosis by revealing stones and a thickened gall bladder wall. Oral intake should be restricted to fluids, and an intravenous infusion set up if necessary. Most patients with acute cholecystitis have only a chemical inflammation and therefore do not need antibiotics. When acute cholecystitis is accompanied by gall bladder infection, symptoms and signs are more marked and antibiotics should then be given.

Acute Cholecystectomy

The patient with acute cholecystitis will need a cholecystectomy at some stage. Early cholecystectomy, performed within a few days of the onset of the attack, is becoming more popular. The procedure is as safe as elective surgery, convenient for the patient and an efficient usage of hospital beds. The alternative policy of conservative management involves discharging the patient after the acute attack resolves, with readmission for elective cholecystectomy after about 6 weeks, by which time the inflammation has usually settled. However, in the meantime, there is a risk of further acute attacks or another manifestation of gallstone disease, such as acute pancreatitis. Even if delayed cholecystectomy is preferred, the acute attack may not settle, necessitating cholecystectomy on the same admission.

When operation is performed during the acute illness, the gall bladder is found to be obstructed and tense and may be grossly inflamed, thickened and scarred. The serosal surface is oedematous and inflamed with petechial haemorrhages or even purulent

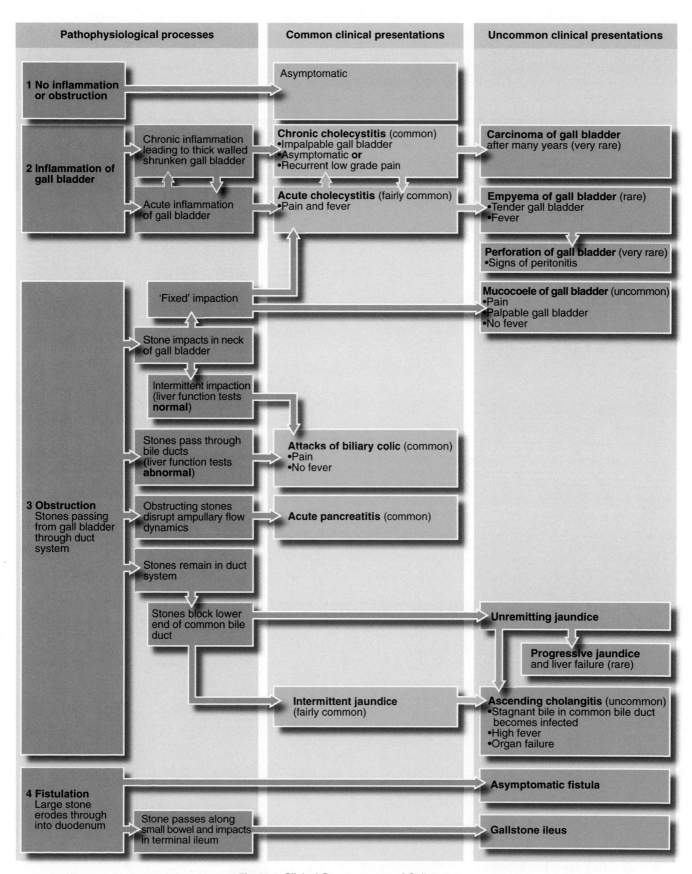

• **Fig. 20.6** Clinical Consequences of Gallstones.

exudate and there are fibrinous adhesions to nearby structures. The gall bladder neck or cystic duct is blocked by an impacted stone and the gall bladder is usually found to contain further stones or sludge mixed with inflammatory exudate. Great care must be taken to avoid damaging the bile ducts. Bowel organisms can be cultured from the contents in about 70% of cases. A bacterial culture swab should be taken from within the gall bladder at operation as any postoperative infective complications are likely to involve the same organisms.

Empyema of the Gall Bladder

In a more extreme clinical variant, the gall bladder becomes distended with pus. The condition, known as an *empyema*, represents an abscess of the gall bladder. As with abscesses elsewhere, a swinging pyrexia is often found. Sometimes part of the gall bladder wall becomes necrotic, leading to perforation, which causes a subphrenic abscess or generalised peritonitis. These patients require surgery without delay. **Gangrenous cholecystitis** and perforation are rare because the gall bladder has a rich blood supply from its hepatic bed, as well as from the cystic artery.

Cholecystoduodenal Fistula and Gallstone Ileus

These uncommon complications of gallstones occur when the inflamed gall bladder becomes adherent to the adjacent duodenum and a stone ulcerates through the wall to form a cholecystoduodenal fistula. The fistula decompresses the obstructed gall bladder and allows stones to pass into the bowel and gas to enter the biliary tree. The condition is usually painless and unsuspected, but may be diagnosed on plain abdominal x-ray by the presence of gas outlining the biliary tree (see Fig. 20.7). Sometimes a fistula is discovered at operation.

CASE HISTORY

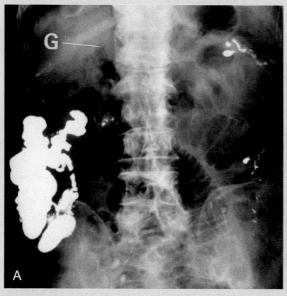
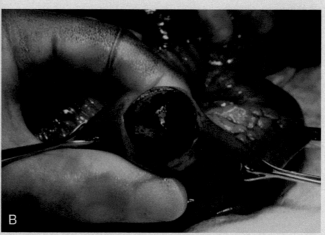

• **Fig. 20.7 Gallstone Ileus.** This 78-year-old woman presented with a gradual onset of small bowel obstruction. A large cholesterol solitaire stone had ulcerated from the gall bladder into the duodenum, travelled down the small bowel and finally impacted in the distal ileum causing complete obstruction. (A) This plain supine abdominal x-ray shows widespread small bowel dilatation. The diagnostic feature is the presence of gas *(G)* in the biliary tree (in this case, the common bile duct and cystic duct). (B) Photograph showing 'cholesterol solitaire' stone being removed from the distal ileum at operation. This had caused gallstone ileus by obstructing the terminal ileum. The gall bladder and fistula did not require surgery.

Occasionally, a solitary cholesterol stone passing into the bowel is so large that after traversing the small bowel it impacts in the narrowest part, the distal ileum, causing small bowel obstruction or **gallstone ileus** (see Fig. 20.7). This occurs in the elderly and presents as an unexplained intermittent and sometimes incomplete small bowel obstruction. Unfortunately, the diagnosis is often difficult to make as the stone is usually radiolucent, so in an elderly patient with distal small bowel obstruction, the diagnosis needs to be considered and can be confidently made if gas is recognised in the biliary tree on a plain abdominal x-ray.

Carcinoma of The Gall Bladder

Chronic irritation by stone over a long period is believed to predispose to adenocarcinoma of the gall bladder. The presenting symptoms are similar to chronic inflammatory gall bladder disease.

Jaundice may develop if the tumour obstructs the bile ducts. Carcinoma of the gall bladder is usually an unexpected finding at cholecystectomy for stones and is often incurable by the time of detection.

Bile Duct Stones

Pathophysiology

Bile duct stones nearly always originate in the gall bladder and pass through the cystic duct. Most stones are small enough to pass out of the biliary system into the duodenum but may cause biliary colic or mild jaundice during transit.

Initially, stones in the bile ducts are small but if they stay in the bile duct without passing, they may enlarge progressively in situ. This is evident from the occasional finding of multiple faceted gallstones fitting neatly together in the common duct and which could only have formed within the duct. The common bile duct is narrowest at its lower end and stones too large to pass out tend to lodge there. Such a stone becomes impacted, causing **progressive jaundice**, or acts as a ball-valve, causing **intermittent jaundice**. Obstruction results in gradual dilatation of the biliary tree; longstanding dilatation does not regress even after the obstruction is removed and may lead to stagnation of bile and further stone formation. Note that the gall bladder rarely distends in this condition even when the common bile duct is completely obstructed, because of the inflammatory fibrosis or mural hypertrophy caused by gallstones (Courvoisier law—see Ch. 18, p. 284).

Clinical Presentations of Stones in the Biliary Tract

Obstructive Jaundice
Stones in the common bile duct, as stated earlier, are a common cause of obstructive jaundice and must be considered in the differential diagnosis; details are given in Chapter 18.

Asymptomatic Duct Stones
Any patient with gallstones may have duct stones although asymptomatic duct stones are rare. Standard practice used to be to perform operative cholangiography at every operation and this continues to be adopted as best practice by many surgeons. Others perform selective cholangiography in patients with signs, symptoms or investigations suggesting passage of stones.

Acute Pancreatitis
Stones passing through or lying near the ampulla of Vater may interfere with drainage of pancreatic enzymes into the duodenum. Bile reflux into the main pancreatic duct may then cause acute pancreatitis (see Ch. 25).

Ascending Cholangitis
Bile stasis in the common duct occurs with chronic obstruction and dilatation and predisposes to bacterial infection. The condition is known as *ascending cholangitis* and is a potent cause of systemic sepsis. It is characterised by intermittent attacks of pain, swinging pyrexia and jaundice. This triad is referred to as ***Charcot intermittent hepatic fever*** and is often accompanied by marked weight loss. Ascending cholangitis is a serious condition and may culminate in life-threatening **acute suppurative cholangitis**. The bile duct must be drained urgently, either by surgical operation or preferably by endoscopic sphincterotomy.

Management of Gallstone Disease

Nonsurgical Treatment of Gallstones

Whatever the clinical manifestation of gallstone-related disease, most cases are treated surgically. A small proportion of patients are not fit for surgery and can be considered for oral drug therapy. **Chenodeoxycholic acid** (a bile acid) and related drugs increase the bile salt pool and inhibit hepatic cholesterol secretion. When administered over a long period, these drugs cause slow dissolution of cholesterol stones. Unfortunately, the drugs have several disadvantages:

- very slow action;
- only small—less than 1 cm—cholesterol-predominant stones can be dissolved;
- high rate of stone recurrence after successful treatment—up to 50% after 2 years;
- frequent drug-related side-effects, for example, severe diarrhoea and hepatic damage.

For these reasons, drug therapy has largely gone out of favour and should only be considered in patients unfit for general anaesthesia with small radiolucent stones in a gall bladder, which concentrates contrast and contracts in response to a fatty meal.

Surgical Management of Gallstones

Indications for Surgery and Preparation of the Patient
There are two main indications for cholecystectomy:
- Symptomatic gallstone disease.
- Asymptomatic gallstones, when there is a reasonable likelihood of future symptoms or complications.

In most cases, high-quality biliary ultrasound is the only imaging study required. This demonstrates gall bladder disease and gallstones and the diameter of the intrahepatic and extrahepatic bile ducts. Information from ultrasound about gall bladder wall thickness or the number and size of stones has not proved useful in predicting the feasibility of laparoscopic surgery. If there are stones in the duct system, common duct exploration is added to cholecystectomy or else stones are extracted at ERCP.

Any jaundiced patient is at particular risk during surgery because of infection, hepatic impairment, defective clotting, acute renal failure and venous thrombosis (see Table 18.2, p. 288). It is often preferable to relieve obstructive jaundice before surgery by endoscopic sphincterotomy and stone extraction or bile duct stenting to minimise some of these complications. In patients presenting with jaundice caused by operable carcinoma of the pancreas, it may be preferable to proceed to surgery without biliary stenting to avoid complications of the procedure, particularly cholangitis and pancreatitis. However, a proportion of patients require preoperative drainage to alleviate symptoms related to jaundice and improve fitness for major surgery.

Cholecystectomy—Open Versus Laparoscopic Surgery
Laparoscopic cholecystectomy is now the gold standard treatment for gallstones. All surgeons performing this operation **must** also be able to competently perform the laparoscopic operation, but also a potentially difficult open operation to cope with the occasional conversion to open operation brought about by unexpected difficulties or complications arising during a laparoscopic operation.

Laparoscopic Management of Gall Bladder Disease
Absolute contraindications to laparoscopic cholecystectomy include the late stages of pregnancy and uncorrected major bleeding disorders. Relative contraindications for less experienced surgical teams include morbid obesity, acute cholecystitis, untreated bile duct stones including obstructive jaundice, previous abdominal surgery (adhesions) and intraabdominal malignancy.

In most centres, 1% to 5% of elective patients require conversion, so patients undergoing laparoscopic surgery should be prepared for and have consented to open surgery in case conversion proves necessary. If bile duct stones are suspected, preoperative ERCP (or equivalent magnetic resonance investigation) is advisable and stone extraction may be carried out. With experience, 95%+ of stones can be successfully extracted by endotherapy. Some surgeons favour operative cholangiography in every case to give a 'road map' of the duct anatomy, to exclude bile duct stones and to provide experience for when cholangiography becomes essential. However, other surgeons practice 'selective' cholangiography in only those patients who have had abnormal LFTs at any time, have a dilated duct on ultrasound scanning, or with clinical evidence of earlier passage of stone (e.g., previous acute pancreatitis or jaundice).

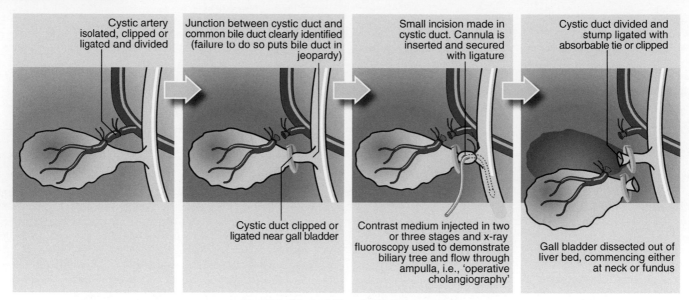

Cystic artery isolated, clipped or ligated and divided

Junction between cystic duct and common bile duct clearly identified (failure to do so puts bile duct in jeopardy)

Cystic duct clipped or ligated near gall bladder

Small incision made in cystic duct. Cannula is inserted and secured with ligature

Contrast medium injected in two or three stages and x-ray fluoroscopy used to demonstrate biliary tree and flow through ampulla, i.e., 'operative cholangiography'

Cystic duct divided and stump ligated with absorbable tie or clipped

Gall bladder dissected out of liver bed, commencing either at neck or fundus

• **Fig. 20.8** Principal Steps in Cholecystectomy.

Operative Technique

The main steps in cholecystectomy are shown in Fig. 20.8 and a common operating theatre set-up for laparoscopic cholecystectomy is shown in Fig. 20.9. The patient is anaesthetised and a pneumoperitoneum established via an open Hassan procedure using an automatic gas insufflator. The open method is very safe and has superseded the blind Veress needle technique. A 10-mm cannula is then placed into the abdomen to accommodate a video laparoscope and the abdominal cavity inspected for other pathology. Three additional abdominal punctures are usually made to introduce operating instruments. The cystic duct and artery are identified and an operative cholangiogram performed (if desired) percutaneously across the abdominal wall. It is extremely important to be certain of the ductal anatomy before cutting anything, because of the distortion introduced by retraction of the gall bladder and the limitations of two-dimensional imaging systems. If in doubt, perform a cholangiogram.

The cystic duct is doubly secured with metal or plastic clips, the gall bladder is dissected from the liver bed using diathermy or ultrasonic coagulation probes, and haemostasis is secured. The now free gall bladder is usually removed via the umbilical port, often using an extraction bag to prevent wound contamination. To achieve this, the laparoscope is moved to the upper midline port and forceps inserted through the umbilical cannula. The neck of the gall bladder is grasped and pulled into the cannula and the entire cannula and gall bladder neck withdrawn through the abdominal wall. If large stones prevent its passage, the incision is enlarged. The umbilical fascial defect should be sutured to prevent herniation, but the upper midline puncture and the lateral punctures are usually left unsutured.

Results of Laparoscopic Cholecystectomy

Most patients are able to walk and tolerate food within 6 hours of operation and up to 80% can be discharged within 24 hours. The intervals before return to work and other normal activities are significantly reduced compared with open cholecystectomy.

Bile duct injuries occur in approximately 0.5% of patients. The risk of bile duct injuries is undoubtedly related to the experience of the operating team, but has been reported to be twice as high in laparoscopic surgery as open surgery. The consequences of bile duct injury can be catastrophic; patients have died with multiorgan failure resulting from unrecognised biliary peritonitis, whilst others have required open operations to repair bile ducts and have risked the consequences of long-term bile duct strictures. Other potential complications are listed in Table 20.2.

Operations on the Common Bile Duct

Exploration of the Common Bile Duct

If stones are known to be present in the bile ducts, the common duct may be explored laparoscopically or at open surgery. The duct is opened through a longitudinal or transverse incision and stones retrieved by a combination of manipulation, irrigation, grasping with stone forceps or a Dormia basket or use of a balloon catheter. **Operative choledochoscopy** is often used to check for residual stones and to remove difficult stones. A flexible fibreoptic choledochoscope gives good visibility and manoeuvrability and can also be used in laparoscopic surgery. Intraoperative choledochoscopy can also be performed via the cystic duct, in some cases avoiding any incision of the bile duct. After exploration, a latex T-tube is usually inserted to drain bile to the exterior, with the transverse limb placed within the common bile duct, although larger ducts can be closed primarily. The purpose of a T-tube is to reduce the risk of iatrogenic biliary stricture and bile leak in addition to providing access to the biliary tree for a further cholangiogram about 1 week after operation (**T-tube cholangiography**, Fig. 20.10). This is to ensure that no stones remain and to allow any oedema at the ampulla to settle.

Endoscopic Management of Bile Duct Stones

With the widespread availability of ERCP and endoscopic sphincterotomy, stones in the common duct can often be retrieved without an operation. This technique represents a real advance in the management of duct stones over the earlier need for open surgery, but does carry its own risks. **Endoscopic sphincterotomy** may be used in the following circumstances:

- Urgent drainage of the bile duct in obstructive jaundice complicated by cholangitis. Definitive surgery can then be deferred until the risks of infection have been minimised.
- Retrieval of stones missed at operation. This avoids a difficult and hazardous operation to explore or reexplore the duct.

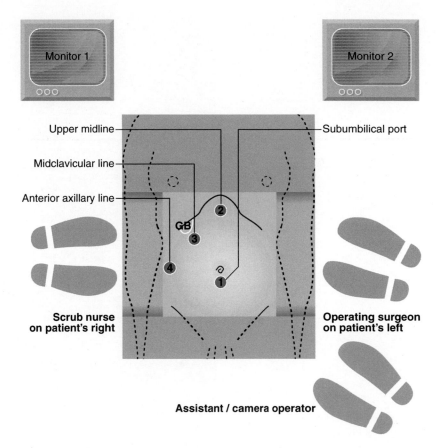

• **Fig. 20.9** Operating Theatre Arrangement for Laparoscopic Cholecystectomy. A common arrangement of the various operating ports *(numbered 1–4)* is shown. The subumbilical port *(1)* is usually placed with the Hassan open technique to take a 10-mm video laparoscope. A Veress needle is still sometimes used for initial gas insufflation. At the upper midline port *(2)*, a 10-mm trocar is placed 5 cm below the xiphoid under video vision to the right of the falciform ligament. This is used to introduce operating instruments—curved dissectors, clip applier, and suction and irrigation tubes. At the midclavicular *(3)* and anterior axillary *(4)* lines, 5-mm trocars give access for grasping forceps, which are used to retract the gall bladder, and liver retractors.

- Removal of duct stones in patients unfit for operation (gall bladder left in situ).
- Some cases of acute pancreatitis caused by gallstones.
- Preparation of a jaundiced patient for elective gall bladder surgery.

Complications of Biliary Surgery

The procedure-specific complications of laparoscopic cholecystectomy are listed in Table 20.2. General complications of cholecystectomy are described later.

The Retained Stone

Despite considerable care at exploration of the common duct, stones occasionally remain in the duct system after operation and are revealed by postoperative T-tube cholangiography. Retained stones are usually retrieved by ERCP and sphincterotomy, although it is possible to retrieve retained stones percutaneously, via a mature T-tube track using steerable grasping forceps or a Dormia basket.

Retained stones sometimes make themselves known many years later, when, having enlarged, they cause pain or obstructive jaundice. This possibility should be considered if a patient with previous biliary tract surgery develops typical pain or obstructive jaundice.

Biliary Peritonitis

Bile leaking into the peritoneal cavity is an irritant and causes a chemical peritonitis. If the bile is infected, it causes generalised peritonitis and sepsis with a high risk of fatality. Bile tends to leak through suture lines because of its detergent action. Therefore whenever the duct system has been opened, a drain should be left in the vicinity for at least 5 days. Small leaks after biliary operations usually settle spontaneously, but if biliary peritonitis develops, the area must be urgently drained percutaneously or, more often, reexplored surgically and drained, with intravenous antibiotic cover.

Bile Duct Damage

The bile ducts can easily be damaged at cholecystectomy or common duct exploration unless their anatomy, which is commonly aberrant, is carefully displayed. The most serious error is unrecognised transection or ligation of the common duct. This presents as a major biliary leak or increasing jaundice in which case, urgent reexploration and reconstruction is mandatory. Lesser degrees of bile duct damage from crushing, overuse of diathermy or a careless ligature will heal, but eventually cause a fibrotic stricture, which presents much later with obstruction. Regardless of how the bile ducts are damaged, complex reconstructive surgery is usually required, often at a tertiary centre and early referral is critical.

TABLE 20.2	**Potential Complications of Laparoscopic Cholecystectomy**

PLACEMENT OF INSUFFLATION NEEDLE, TROCAR OR OTHER INSTRUMENTS	
Stage of Procedure	**Complication**
During operation	Injuries to bowel Injuries to blood vessels, for example, iliac artery Diaphragmatic injury with tension pneumothorax
Postoperative	Bleeding from trocar insertion sites Subcutaneous emphysema
Late	Herniation through trocar entry points and bowel strangulation

TRAUMA TO BILIARY SYSTEM	
Stage of Procedure	**Complication**
During operation	Injuries to common bile ducts and hepatic ducts Bleeding from cystic or right hepatic artery Gall bladder perforation with spillage of bile and stones
Postoperative	Bleeding and bile leakage from liver bed Bile leakage from cystic duct remnant Retained bile duct stones
Other complications	Bowel damage by diathermy or laser

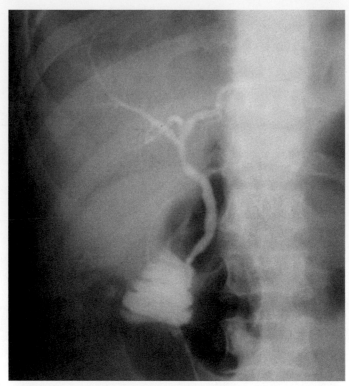

• **Fig. 20.10** Operative Cholangiograms. Normal operative cholangiogram. The bile ducts are not dilated, the hepatic ducts fill, and contrast flows easily into the duodenum. There are no filling defects in the duct and the duct tapers normally at its lower end.

Haemorrhage

The cystic and hepatic arteries and the vascular liver bed are vulnerable to operative trauma and bleed profusely. Removing a grossly inflamed or fibrotic gall bladder is particularly hazardous. Manoeuvres to control haemorrhage may damage other structures, passing unnoticed at the time; this is a common cause of bile duct trauma.

Hazards of Preexisting Jaundice

These are discussed under *Obstructive jaundice* in Chapter 18, Table 18.2 (p. 288).

Ascending Cholangitis and Other Infections

Ascending cholangitis can be a late complication of biliary surgery, where an anastomosis has been formed between bile ducts and bowel. Reflux of intestinal contents and organisms takes place continually in such cases, but active infection only occurs when bile stagnates in the duct system because of inadequate drainage. Usually the diameter of the anastomosis has shrunk to a point when it no longer drains adequately. Ascending cholangitis may also occur early after common duct exploration for jaundice, since bile in this situation is nearly always infected. Prophylactic antibiotics should always be used when operating on jaundiced patients with duct obstruction, to minimise this complication.

An early complication of biliary surgery is a **subphrenic abscess**. This must be considered if the patient develops an unexplained swinging fever a few days after operation. Diagnosis may be elusive and is best made by ultrasound. Treatment is by percutaneous needle drainage under ultrasound guidance or occasionally by open operation.

21

Peptic Ulceration and Related Disorders

CHAPTER OUTLINE

Introduction

Peptic ulcer disease affects the oesophagus, stomach and duodenum. The conditions share the symptom of epigastric pain and the common aetiology of mucosal inflammation associated with gastric acid–pepsin secretions. The most important aetiological factor in gastric and duodenal ulcer disease is chronic mucosal infection with the bacterium *Helicobacter pylori*. Peptic disorders, together with gallstone disease, are the most common causes of organic upper abdominal pain.

With highly effective pharmacological agents to block acid secretion and more reliable diagnostic, treatment and monitoring techniques, such as flexible endoscopy, surgery for peptic ulcer disease has declined by over 90% in developed countries in the last 30 years. Recent antibiotic and other treatments against *H. pylori* result in permanent cure for many peptic ulcer disorders. Most patients with suspected peptic ulcer disease are treated by family practitioners; the rest are largely managed by gastroenterologists. Only a minority present to surgeons because of failed medical treatment. Rates of emergency complications, such as perforation and haemorrhage have remained relatively static but peptic pyloric stenosis has markedly declined as chronic ulceration has become less common. Nevertheless, because of the diagnostic difficulties posed by upper abdominal symptoms, surgeons still manage many patients who turn out to have peptic disorders.

Pathophysiology and Epidemiology of Peptic Disorders

Pathophysiology of Peptic Ulceration

Inflammation, probably initiated by *H. pylori* infection and sustained by the combined effect of gastric acid and pepsin on the mucosa, is probably the cause of all peptic disorders of the upper gastrointestinal tract other than reflux oesophagitis. *H. pylori* is a gram-negative microaerophilic spiral bacterium, which has the ability to colonise the gastric mucosa over a very long period. In many cases, infection appears to have been acquired in childhood, often with poor living conditions in early life. Normally, a dynamic balance is maintained between the inherent protective characteristics of the mucosa (the mucosal barrier) and the irritant effects of acid–pepsin secretions. The delicate balance between the two may be disrupted by diminution of mucosal resistance or excessive acid–pepsin secretion or a combination of both. The mucosal surface may become eroded by direct action of an external agent, for example, alcohol. Whatever the aetiology, the range of pathological outcomes is similar and is summarised in Fig. 21.1.

Outcomes of Breaches of the Mucosal Barrier

When the protective mucosal barrier is breached, the delicate underlying connective tissue is exposed to acid–pepsin attack, exciting an acute inflammatory response. If the protective balance is restored at this early stage, inflammation resolves and epithelium regenerates. Little if any residual damage will result. If the healing balance is not restored, continued acid–pepsin attack on the unprotected submucosa leads to an **acute peptic ulcer**. This tends to become progressively larger and deeper.

Sometimes the ulcerative process continues virtually unchecked through the full thickness of the gut wall. The ulcer either erodes posterior tissues or perforates, so that intestinal contents escape into the peritoneal cavity causing peritonitis. More often, the layer of necrotic slough and acutely inflamed underlying tissue in the ulcer base temporarily resist acid–pepsin attack. This allows granulation tissue to form, which initiates the process of fibrous repair. If acid-reducing drugs are used, the ulcer may heal, leaving a small scar with normal overlying mucosa. Usually, however, a tenuous balance

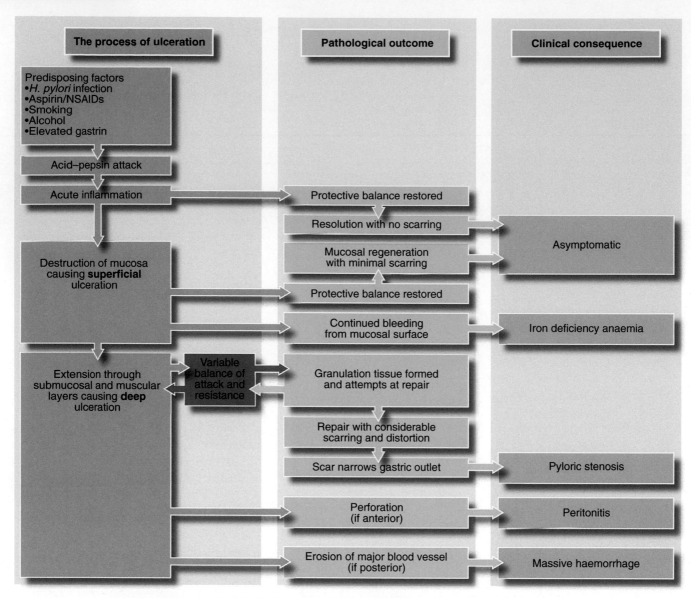

• **Fig. 21.1** Pathogenesis of Peptic Ulceration and Its Possible Outcomes. Note that pain is a common factor in any active ulceration. *NSAIDs*, Nonsteroidal anti-inflammatory drugs.

is established between resistance and attack, matched by an unstable equilibrium between the rates of repair and tissue destruction. A chronic peptic ulcer then results, which may persist for years, its size and symptoms varying as mucosal resistance and exacerbating factors fluctuate.

If local or systemic factors change and swing the balance in favour of repair, the lesion may heal completely. On the mucosal surface, the healed ulcer site is usually puckered by scar contraction in the muscular wall. If scarring occurs in a narrow part of the tract, for example, the pyloric region, the lumen may stricture, and subsequent acute mucosal inflammation and swelling may precipitate **gastric outlet obstruction**. If healing does not occur, a chronic ulcer may slowly enlarge and deepen. Continual bleeding from the ulcer may cause **chronic anaemia**. Ulceration **posteriorly** may erode into the gastroduodenal artery causing acute major haemorrhage; if the ulcer lies on the anterior wall, it may perforate into the peritoneal cavity.

Epidemiology and Aetiology of Peptic Ulcer Disease

The Size of the Problem

Chronic peptic ulcer disease is very common in developed countries, affecting around 10% of the population at some time in their lives. The incidence of **duodenal ulcer** has been falling over the last 30 years, probably because of improved living conditions, reduced smoking and good medical therapy. The incidence of **gastric ulcer** is probably constant, although increasing numbers of cases are revealed as a result of nonsteroidal anti-inflammatory drugs (NSAIDs)—provoked haemorrhage.

Peptic ulceration is somewhat less common in developing rural communities, despite a high incidence of *H. pylori* gastroduodenal infection. This implies that environmental factors associated with Western life are additional aetiological factors in the disease.

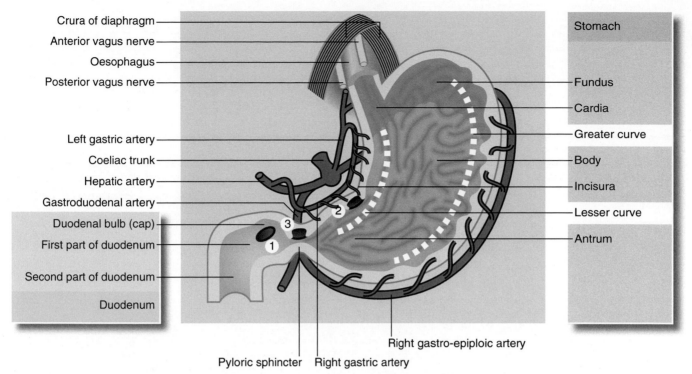

Crura of diaphragm
Anterior vagus nerve
Oesophagus
Posterior vagus nerve

Left gastric artery
Coeliac trunk
Hepatic artery
Gastroduodenal artery
Duodenal bulb (cap)
First part of duodenum
Second part of duodenum
Duodenum

Stomach
Fundus
Cardia
Greater curve
Body
Incisura
Lesser curve
Antrum

Right gastro-epiploic artery
Pyloric sphincter   Right gastric artery

• **Fig. 21.2** Surgical Anatomy of Stomach and Duodenum Showing Common Sites of Peptic Ulceration. Acid secretion by the gastric mucosa is controlled by two mechanisms: (1) the vagus nerve stimulates acid secretion by the parietal cells (cholinergic stimulation) and (2) gastrin (produced by the APUD (amine precursor uptake and decarboxylation) cells in the antrum) promotes secretion of acid and pepsin by the parietal and peptic cells of the fundus and body. The second is mediated via H_2-receptors. *(1)* Marks the common site for duodenal ulcers, which may be anterior or posterior; *(2)* the common site of lesser curve gastric ulcers; and *(3)* the site of pyloric channel ulcers.

Sites of Peptic Ulceration (Fig. 21.2)

Stomach and Duodenum

The most common sites for chronic peptic ulcers are in the **first part of the duodenum** (the duodenal bulb) or the **gastric antrum**, particularly along the lesser curve. A chronic **stomal ulcer** may also appear at the margin of a surgically created communication between stomach and intestine (gastroenterostomy).

In the rare **Zollinger–Ellison syndrome**, a gastrin-secreting tumour of pancreatic origin overstimulates acid–pepsin production and causes severe and widespread peptic ulceration. The ulcers commonly involve stomach and duodenum and extend into the second part of the duodenum or even further distally.

Oesophagus

Peptic inflammation and superficial ulceration may involve the lower oesophagus. It is almost always secondary to acid–pepsin reflux, and is often associated with hiatus hernia. *H. pylori* infection (see later) is probably not an important factor here. Reflux causes intermittent destruction of the lower oesophageal mucosa by acid or bile (or both), causing **linear ulceration** and prompting vigorous attempts at healing. One outcome is replacement of the normal squamous epithelium with metaplastic columnar mucosa. This is known as **Barrett oesophagus** and is one of the few known predisposing factors for adenocarcinoma of the lower oesophagus, a condition that has increased by 70% over the last 25 years (see Ch. 22, p. 336). Chronic peptic ulcers, similar to gastroduodenal ulcers, may also develop at the lower end of the oesophagus.

Aetiological Factors in Peptic Disease

Helicobacter pylori Infection

The importance of *H. pylori* infection as the main initiating factor in peptic ulceration has finally been universally accepted following the pioneering work of Dr Barry J. Marshall and Dr J. Robin Warren in Perth, Australia in the early 1980s. In a dramatic demonstration of Koch's postulates, Marshall produced a duodenal ulcer in himself a few days after ingesting cultured *H. pylori*. The ulcer proved to be *H. pylori*-positive on biopsy and was cured by anti-*Helicobacter* antibiotic therapy. The pair won the Nobel Prize in Physiology or Medicine for 2005 for their discovery of the bacterium and its role in gastritis and peptic ulcer disease. Before their work, it had been believed that microorganisms could not live in the highly acid environment of the normal stomach. However, gastric biopsies had frequently shown intramucosal bacteria, which they were eventually able to culture in vitro. These spiral-shaped organisms appear able to penetrate protective surface mucus and then accumulate in the region of intercellular junctions. There, they may excite inflammation, stimulating excess acid–pepsin production or compromising normal protective mechanisms.

The jigsaw began to fit together when it was found that peptic ulcers could regularly be successfully treated with a combination of bismuth and antibiotics. Later work showed that *H. pylori* infection in duodenal ulcer patients was associated with a sixfold increase in gastric acid production which remitted when the infection was eliminated. There is now evidence that *H. pylori* is sometimes carcinogenic, initiating certain types of gastric lymphoma and some cases of gastric cancer. The broad picture is now evident: *H. pylori* causes a chronic infection with complications that include gastric and duodenal ulcer, gastric mucosa-associated lymphoma and gastric cancer. Only a small percentage of patients with duodenal or gastric ulcers are *H. pylori* negative. Tests for *H. pylori* infection include stool antigen tests, serum anti-*H. pylori* immunoglobulin G and hydrogen breath tests. However, the most reliable method of diagnosis is endoscopic biopsies with immediate testing for urease produced by the organism (see later, Fig. 21.7) and histological examination of biopsy specimens.

Further details of this fascinating story remain to be worked out; for example, why not all patients with *H. pylori* infection develop upper gastrointestinal lesions, and why not all patients with certain gastric cancers have been exposed to *H. pylori*. There is even speculation that elimination of *H. pylori* may predispose some patients to gastric cancer.

Acid–Pepsin Production

Parietal cells secrete acid in direct or indirect response to acetylcholine, gastrin and histamine. It is likely that the common mediator is histamine via H_2-receptors. The final common pathway for hydrogen ion secretion is via activation of a specific enzyme, H^+/K^+ adenosine triphosphatase, which exchanges hydrogen ions generated in the parietal cell for potassium ions in the gastric lumen, using a mechanism known as the ***proton pump***. In **duodenal ulceration**, the fundamental abnormality appears to be excessive production of acid–pepsin by the stomach, both basal (i.e., overnight) and stimulated. This may be a defensive response to *H. pylori* infection.

In patients with **gastric ulcers**, measured acid secretion is either normal or low, and the essential problem seems to be diminished resistance to acid–pepsin attack, probably related to the quantity or quality of mucus produced. Nevertheless, reduction of acid production by medical or surgical means is effective in healing gastric ulcers.

Mucosal Resistance

There are several mechanisms which protect the upper gastrointestinal mucosa against autodigestion. Somatostatin and cyclooxygenase (COX)1 induced prostaglandins are inhibitors of parietal cell secretion and the latter have other cytoprotective properties. Two forms of mucus, soluble and insoluble, are secreted continuously by gastric and duodenal mucosa; they contain bicarbonate and together maintain the cell surface pH at neutrality.

NSAIDs prescribed for arthritic disorders are commonly identified as the causative factor for acute presentations of peptic ulceration. NSAIDs probably have their greatest effect systemically rather than locally, via their blocking effects on prostaglandin production. Indeed, in elderly patients presenting with upper gastrointestinal bleeding or perforation, ulceration may occur after only a few NSAID tablets have been taken or at any time during their use. This risk is not diminished by enteric-coated preparations, nor by administration by routes other than orally, for example, as suppositories. The risk of NSAID-induced ulceration increases steeply in later life. All NSAIDs have been incriminated and their power to provoke peptic ulceration is in direct proportion to their effectiveness at relieving arthritic symptoms. A history of 'indigestion' in patients taking NSAIDs must be taken seriously.

Other Mucosal Irritants

Aspirin and other NSAIDs are known to induce acute mucosal inflammation directly (**acute gastritis**). In a susceptible individual, inflammation may persist, resulting in chronic ulceration. Prolonged heavy alcohol intake is also a recognised risk factor. The junction between parietal and antral cells on the lesser curvature of the stomach has been noted to be particularly vulnerable to gastric ulceration, although the reason is not understood. Cigarette smoking is twice as common in patients with chronic peptic ulcer disease as in the general population. Its pathogenic role is attributed to increased vagal activity, and its effect on producing relative gastric mucosal ischaemia. Ceasing smoking greatly assists in the healing of peptic ulcers.

Investigation and Clinical Features of Peptic Disorders

Investigation of Suspected Peptic Ulcer Disease

The diagnosis and management of peptic disorders relies mainly on flexible endoscopy, which revolutionised the process after its introduction in the late 1960s. Barium meal contrast radiography has largely been superseded by endoscopy.

Endoscopy

Oesophago-gastro-duodenoscopy, also known as OGD or gastroscopy, involves visual examination of the mucosa using a steerable, flexible endoscope. Gastroscopy enables direct and comprehensive examination of the whole of the upper gastrointestinal tract prone to peptic ulcer disease.

In peptic ulcer disease, gastroscopy has definite advantages over contrast radiography, which by its nature can only demonstrate substantial structural abnormalities and then only as two-dimensional images. Benign gastric or oesophageal ulceration can be reliably distinguished from malignancy if endoscopic biopsies are taken from several places around the ulcer edge. In patients with peptic disorders, biopsies of distal gastric mucosa are now taken routinely to investigate *H. pylori* infection.

In acute upper gastrointestinal haemorrhage, gastroscopy is almost mandatory, as described in Chapter 19. Gastroscopy can identify the site of the bleeding and is particularly useful if gastrooesophageal varices are suspected to be the source of bleeding but are found not to be. Gastroscopy also allows recognition of features, which can help stratify patients into low or high risk of rebleeding and it provides an important means of treating bleeding sites by injection of vasoconstrictors or sclerosants.

Contrast Radiology

Contrast radiography of the upper gastrointestinal tract is used largely to determine swallowing function, to define anatomy, particularly with large hiatus hernias, and to give an idea of the effectiveness of gastric emptying. It involves the patient swallowing barium suspension (**barium meal**). During the investigation, the patient is tilted and rolled in various directions to demonstrate the whole region of interest. Effervescent tablets are given to produce gaseous distension of the stomach and duodenum and spread the contrast in a thin, even layer over the mucosal surface. This standard **double contrast technique** improves the imaging of mucosal detail.

Presenting Features of Peptic Ulcer Disease

The various ways in which peptic inflammation affects the oesophagus, stomach and duodenum are summarised in Table 21.1.

TABLE 21.1	Clinical Consequences of Peptic Ulcer Disease in Different Anatomical Sites	
Pathological Process	**Clinical Lesion**	**Symptoms**
Oesophagus		
Transient acid–pepsin reflux	Mild reversible acute inflammation, that is, transient oesophagitis	Burning retrosternal pain (i.e., 'heartburn')
Recurrent acid–pepsin reflux or failure of oesophagus to expel acid by peristalsis (often found in hiatus hernia)	Episodes of acute inflammation, that is, reflux oesophagitis—probably reversible with no scarring	Recurrent epigastric and retrosternal pain. Chronic iron deficiency anaemia may occur
Persistent severe reflux	Chronic low-grade blood loss. Continuous severe inflammation with superficial ulceration. May lead to chronic ulceration and/or stricture	Severe retrosternal pain, dysphagia and sometimes recurrent small haematemeses
Stomach		
Acute gastric irritation, for example, by NSAIDs or alcohol	Acute (reversible) mucosal inflammation, that is, acute gastritis or erosive/haemorrhagic gastritis	Epigastric pain, vomiting, acute upper gastrointestinal bleeding
Acute reduction in mucosal resistance provoked by visceral ischaemia or the systemic inflammatory response syndrome (usually in intensive therapy unit patients or after burns)	Widespread superficial gastric ulceration (gastric erosions)	May bleed uncontrollably or perforate
Chronic *Helicobacter pylori* infection, probably with longstanding diminished resistance to acid–pepsin attack, with or without extrinsic irritation	Chronic or recurrent gastric ulceration	Epigastric pain—characteristically exacerbated by food (especially if acid or spicy), anorexia and weight loss. Symptoms of chronic anaemia
Duodenum		
Episodic acid–pepsin attack	Acute (reversible) mucosal inflammation, that is, duodenitis	Episodic epigastric pain
Chronic *H. pylori* infection, probably with persistent acid–pepsin attack	Duodenal ulceration (may involve pyloric canal)	Epigastric pain—typically relieved by food and occurring several hours after food, especially at night
Preexisting duodenal scarring causing pyloric stenosis with superadded acute inflammation and mucosal swelling	Complete pyloric obstruction	Symptoms of chronic anaemia. Severe vomiting, dehydration, shock, gross electrolyte disturbance (hypochloraemic alkalosis)
Both Stomach and Duodenum		
Periodic loss of protective equilibrium	Recurrent ulceration	Intermittent symptomatic episodes
Erosion of a major vessel in ulcer floor	Severe haemorrhage	Massive haematemesis or melaena
Unchecked ulceration	Perforation and peritonitis	Acute severe abdominal pain and shock

NSAIDs, Nonsteroidal anti-inflammatory drugs.

Epigastric pain (usually described as 'boring', 'gnawing' or 'burning') is the principal presenting symptom and is common to peptic disorders whatever the site. Pain is often accompanied by other forms of discomfort, often described by the patient as 'indigestion' or 'dyspepsia'. A more specific description may suggest particular diagnostic entities. Retrosternal pain ('heartburn') and bitter regurgitation ('waterbrash') suggests reflux oesophagitis. Nausea or vomiting, anorexia (loss of appetite) and abdominal fullness or bloating are common in gastric ulcer and pyloric stenosis, but may also occur in a variety of other upper gastrointestinal disorders, for example, gallstone disease and irritable bowel syndrome.

The relationship of symptoms to food intake may help to distinguish gastric from duodenal ulceration; gastric ulcer pain is typically exacerbated by food and duodenal ulcer pain relieved by it.

Peptic ulcers may be virtually asymptomatic, particularly those caused by NSAIDs. Diagnosis may then only occur on acute presentation with bleeding or perforation or on investigation of iron deficiency anaemia.

Nonacute Presentations of Peptic Ulcer Disease

Peptic Disorders of the Oesophagus

All peptic disorders of the oesophagus are associated with reflux of gastric contents. These disorders range from mild reversible inflammation, through moderate acute inflammation with superficial ulceration (**reflux oesophagitis**), to severe persistent inflammation, which may lead to **fibrotic scarring and stenosis** (see Fig. 21.3) and sometimes **chronic peptic ulceration**. In many patients, reflux is associated with hiatus hernia (see Ch. 22).

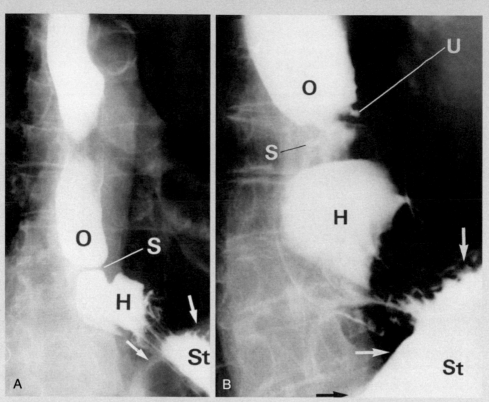

• **Fig. 21.3** Peptic Strictures of the Oesophagus. **(A)** A barium swallow in a 60-year-old woman who complained of burning retrosternal pain when lying flat (present for several years) and the recent onset of pain and difficulty when swallowing solid foods. The x-rays show the lower end of the oesophagus (O) and stomach (St), part of which lies above the level of the diaphragm (position arrowed), forming a sliding hiatus hernia (H). There is a tight stenosis in the last 2 cm of the oesophagus caused by a peptic stricture (S). **(B)** At greater magnification, barium can be seen filling the crater of a chronic peptic ulcer (U) immediately above the stricture.

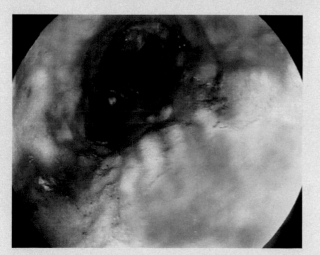

• **Fig. 21.4** Reflux Oesophagitis. Gastroscopic view of the lower end of the oesophagus in a woman of 62 years with a long history of reflux. Note the patchy ulceration (U) and the irregular fibrotic cardia caused by recurrent ulceration and attempts at healing. Further scarring may cause stricture formation.

On gastroscopy, reflux oesophagitis is characterised by mucosal reddening and, in more severe cases, by typical linear superficial ulceration (see Fig. 21.4). Peptic strictures occur in the distal oesophagus and are usually located just above the oesophagogastric junction, which itself often lies above the diaphragm because of inflammatory shortening of the oesophagus. The normal oesophagogastric junction is about 40 cm from the incisor teeth when seen on endoscopy. Specialised intestinal metaplasia, dysplasia and carcinoma must be excluded by biopsies because the visual appearances may not be characteristic. Occasionally, a deep chronic ulcer occurs in the lower oesophagus; this looks and behaves like an often linear gastric or duodenal ulcer. When squamous oesophageal epithelium is repeatedly damaged by reflux, it may be replaced by metaplastic columnar epithelium. This is known as **Barrett oesophagus** and there is strong evidence that it predisposes to malignant change. If found, it should be biopsied to exclude dysplasia. When dysplasia is severe, there is about a 1% annual risk of malignant change and endoscopic resection or surgery is necessary. Standard protocols are usually used for surveillance of Barrett oesophagus with repeated endoscopy every 2 to 3 years.

Peptic Disorders of the Stomach

Peptic disorders of the stomach range from mild inflammation (**gastritis**) to **chronic gastric ulcers** and most often occur in the antral region and along the lesser curve beyond the incisura.

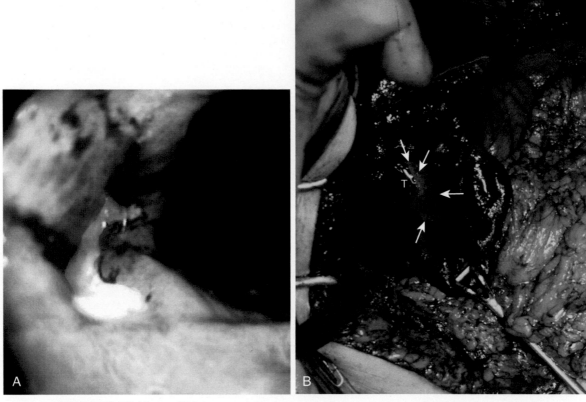

• **Fig. 21.5** Peptic Ulcers. (A) Lesser curve benign gastric ulcer as seen through a gastroscope. At the original examination, the ulcer could be viewed from several directions and biopsies taken of the edge to exclude malignancy. (B) Photograph taken at emergency laparotomy for bleeding duodenal ulcer. The pylorus has been opened longitudinally and a deep chronic posterior ulcer crater is identified *(arrowed)*. Thrombus *(T)* overlying an eroded artery is visible. A bleeding artery in the ulcer crater was underrun with sutures to arrest the haemorrhage.

Chronic gastric ulcers must be distinguished from malignant ulcers. The site may aid recognition of a benign ulcer, but carcinoma may occur in any part of the stomach, with the region of the gastrooesophageal junction now the most common. Malignancy can only be excluded by histological examination of multiple representative biopsies taken from around the ulcer circumference (not the base). In most cases, carcinoma probably arises de novo but occasionally a benign ulcer may undergo malignant transformation.

Gastritis

Gastritis appears as widespread reddening of the mucosa. If biliary reflux from the duodenum into the stomach is evident, the condition is sometimes referred to as *biliary gastritis* on the assumption that it is caused by the irritant effect of biliary and pancreatic secretions. Acute gastritis, often caused by alcohol (chronic alcoholism or single alcoholic binges) or aspirin/NSAID ingestion, can cause symptoms of sufficient severity to warrant gastroscopy. The mucosa often exhibits patchy shallow ulceration (**erosive gastritis**) and is friable and easily traumatised, causing bleeding.

Stress Ulcers

Acute 'stress' ulcers are single or multiple small discrete superficial lesions that may develop rapidly in seriously ill patients, often in intensive care units. The condition may be a complication of extensive burns, systemic sepsis (possibly via visceral hypoperfusion),

multiple trauma, major head injuries, uraemia or terminal illness. Stress ulcers typically present with haemorrhage (**haemorrhagic gastritis**), which is sometimes catastrophic, and occasionally with perforation. There is minimal mucosal inflammation around the ulcers and the aetiology may be primarily mucosal ischaemia rather than peptic. The risk of this life-threatening complication can be minimised in vulnerable patients by prophylactic treatment with proton-pump inhibitors.

Chronic Gastric Ulceration

Chronic gastric ulcers vary greatly in size but the majority are small (less than 2 cm in diameter). **Giant ulcers** (up to 10 cm) are occasionally seen in the elderly; if posteriorly situated, they may erode through the stomach wall, obliterating the lesser sac and adhering to the surface of the pancreas. In these cases, the ulcer base or floor is composed of pancreatic tissue and erosion may cause catastrophic haemorrhage.

Benign gastric ulcers are typically regular in outline with a base consisting of white fibrinous slough. The ulcer gives the impression of having been punched out of the gastric wall, and there is no heaping-up of the mucosal margin, as seen in malignant ulcers. The surrounding mucosa is surprisingly normal, although there may be radiating folds resulting from chronic fibrotic contractures. The typical endoscopic appearance of a gastric ulcer is shown in Fig. 21.5A.

Peptic disorders of the stomach typically cause severe, often disabling, epigastric pain, which tends to be exacerbated by food, especially if acidic or spicy. The pain may be so severe that patients lose weight and develop a fear of food. Symptoms tend to persist for weeks or months, fluctuating in intensity and then disappearing completely, only to recur weeks or months later. Symptoms are a poor guide to disease activity or response to treatment. Indeed, major ulcers may be silent. Both can be monitored only by repeated gastroscopy until healing. A rare complication of peptic disease is perforation of a gastric ulcer into the transverse colon. The resulting gastrocolic fistula causes true faecal vomiting.

Peptic Disorders of the Duodenum

Duodenitis

Duodenitis, a nonulcerative form of duodenal inflammation, has a similar endoscopic appearance to gastritis. It is commonly discovered in patients suspected of having duodenal ulceration, and probably represents a mild form of peptic disease.

Chronic Duodenal Ulceration

Chronic duodenal ulcers almost exclusively occur in the pyloric channel and the first part of the duodenum. The latter area is known endoscopically as the 'duodenal bulb' and radiologically as the 'duodenal cap'. On endoscopy, duodenal ulcers have a range of appearances similar to chronic gastric ulcers. There is usually a single ulcer but two or more ulcers at one time are common ('kissing ulcers' occur on opposing walls of the duodenum). Malignancy is very rare in the duodenal bulb, so biopsy of the ulcer for this purpose is seldom necessary; biopsy of the gastric antrum for confirmation of *H. pylori* infections is, however, indicated. The endoscopic characteristics of a duodenal ulcer are shown in Fig. 21.6.

CASE HISTORY

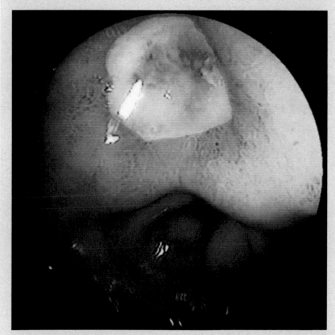

• **Fig. 21.6 Duodenal Ulceration.** Endoscopic view of lesser curve gastric ulcer. This ulcer has probably only been present for about 4 months, as it does not show surrounding scarring and distortion of the gastric wall that would be characteristic of longstanding ulcers.

• BOX 21.1 Principles of Management of Peptic Disorders

Control of Predisposing or Aggravating Causes
- Modify diet, reduce alcohol intake, cease smoking, avoid irritant and ulcer-provoking drugs (aspirin and other NSAIDs), avoid stress, reduce oesophageal reflux by losing weight and attention to posture

Elimination of Proven *Helicobacter pylori* Infection
- Combined therapy with antacid and antibiotic combinations

Diminishing of Irritant Effects of Acid–Pepsin
- Simple antacid drugs, alginate preparations, liquorice derivatives, bismuth preparations

Administration of Mucosal Protective Agents
- Sucralfate

Reduction of Acid Secretion
- H_2-receptor-blocking drugs (cimetidine, ranitidine), proton-pump inhibitors (PPIs, e.g., omeprazole), surgical vagotomy (rarely employed nowadays)

Surgical Removal of Intractable Ulcers and Gastrin-Secreting Tissue
- Partial gastrectomy

Correction of Secondary Anatomical Problems
- Dilatation of oesophageal strictures, operations for pyloric stenosis and hiatus hernia

NSAIDs, Nonsteroidal anti-inflammatory drugs.

Duodenal ulcer symptoms follow the same general pattern as gastric ulcer but with important exceptions. The pain tends to appear several hours after a meal ('hunger pain') and is relieved by eating. A typical history includes episodic early morning waking (often around 2 a.m.) with epigastric pain; this pain is relieved by drinking milk and eating bland foods. Consequently, undiagnosed patients tend to gain weight from the increased intake of food and milk. This is in contrast to the weight loss often associated with gastric ulcer. Symptoms in duodenal ulcer are more useful as a guide to disease activity and response to treatment than in gastric ulcer.

Management of Chronic Peptic Ulcer Disease

Both the nature and the management of peptic ulcer disease have undergone extraordinary changes over the past four decades. Back then, medical management was relatively ineffective and was largely confined to simple antacid drugs, bland diets and bed rest. The only definitive treatment was major surgery and it was widely used, often after a long period of chronic symptoms. Surgery was deferred as long as possible in the hope of spontaneous remission, and patients often had to 'earn' their operations by years of suffering! Partial gastrectomy offered the best cure rate and was thus the most common operation despite its mortality of 2% to 10% and its serious long-term complication rate. Later, various versions of surgical vagotomy were shown to be almost equally effective, but with fewer complications.

The principles of modern management of peptic disorders are summarised in Box 21.1.

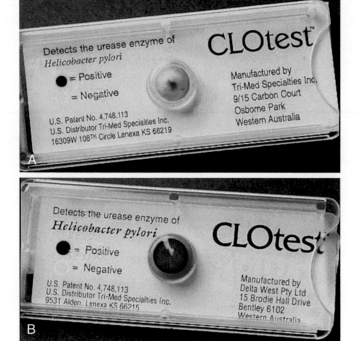

• **Fig. 21.7** Proprietary Urease Testing Kit for *Helicobacter pylori*. Biopsies of gastric or duodenal mucosa are placed in the well and the result read after a set period. A positive result is indicated by the colour change from **(A)** to **(B)**.

Control of Predisposing or Aggravating Causes

The patient's history may reveal adverse factors, which can be easily eliminated. These are summarised at the start of Box 21.1. Radical dietary modification is unnecessary; patients should merely be advised to avoid food which they find aggravates the symptoms. Spicy or acidic foods are often blamed.

Aspirin and other NSAIDs should be avoided, although this is often difficult in patients with arthritic disorders. The ulcerogenic effect of these drugs is directly proportional to their effectiveness and relates largely to their systemic anti-COX1 activity, an agent protective of gastroduodenal mucosa. There is therefore little to be gained from changing drugs within the group or by using them in enteric-coated or suppository form. If NSAIDs cannot be avoided in patients with a predisposition to peptic ulceration, concurrent use of cytoprotective drugs may be indicated.

Patients with oesophageal reflux, especially if associated with hiatus hernia, can minimise the damage by simple mechanical measures, such as losing weight, elevating the head end of the bed and being aware of posture in daily activities.

Elimination of Proven *Helicobacter pylori* Infection

Once *H. pylori* has been confirmed, treatment involves a course of acid inhibition combined with antibiotic treatment. Eradication usually produces long-term ulcer remission, and *H. pylori* reinfection is rare. A triple regimen including a proton-pump inhibitor (e.g., omeprazole) and two antibiotics (clarithromycin plus either amoxicillin or metronidazole) given for 1 week eliminates *Helicobacter* in over 90% of cases, although increasingly strains of *H. pylori* are demonstrating antibiotic resistance and local antibiotic protocols should be followed. Longer courses give potentially higher elimination rates but produce more side effects and lower compliance. Confirmation of eradication can be achieved by reendoscopy and rapid urease testing (Fig. 21.7), or by breath testing.

Diminishing of Irritant Effects of Acid–Pepsin

An array of proprietary antacid preparations is available over the counter and on prescription. When used assiduously, they promote ulcer healing almost as effectively as any other drug, although more slowly. They all use a few main active ingredients. **Sodium bicarbonate** offers rapid but temporary relief of symptoms, while **magnesium trisilicate** or **aluminium hydroxide** promotes ulcer healing. Some of these agents, however, interfere with proton-pump inhibitors. **Colloidal bismuth compounds** have been in use for many years. They have an antacid action and have been found to be active against *H. pylori*.

Alginate preparations form a foamy layer on the surface of gastric contents, coating the upper stomach and lower oesophagus and protecting it from oesophageal reflux.

Administration of Mucosal Protective Agents

Sucralfate is a complex of aluminium hydroxide and sulphated sucrose that is minimally absorbed from the gastrointestinal tract. It is believed to act by binding to denuded areas of mucosa and protecting them from acid–pepsin attack. It has been shown to be as effective as H_2-blockers in providing symptom relief and healing when given in the dose of 2 g twice daily. It does not interfere with other drugs and is safe in pregnancy. It is also effective for preventing stress ulcers in seriously ill patients.

Reduction of Acid Secretion

Acid secretion by the gastric mucosa is normally controlled by two mechanisms:

- Direct cholinergic stimulation of parietal cells mediated via the **vagus nerve.** This is under reflex control originating in the cerebral cortex triggered by the sight and taste of food.
- Gastrin is secreted by APUD (amine precursor uptake and decarboxylation) cells in the gastric antrum and promotes acid secretion via histamine released from mast cells, in the vicinity of the parietal cells. The histamine receptors on the parietal cells are distinct from those elsewhere in the body and are designated as **type 2 (H_2) receptors**; these receptors are not blocked by standard 'antihistamine' drugs, such as chlorphenamine. Gastrin secretion is partly controlled by the vagus and partly by local (vagally independent) reflexes initiated by gastric distension and the presence of food or alcohol in the stomach.

From this, two practical methods have been found to reduce acid secretion: drugs which selectively block H_2-receptors or the proton-pump mechanism (described earlier), and surgical division of the vagus nerve.

H_2-Receptor Blockade and Proton-Pump Antagonists

H_2-receptor blocking drugs were developed in the 1970s and were the first 'medical' revolution in the management of peptic disorders. **Cimetidine** was the first but was joined by **ranitidine**, which has a few minor advantages but is no more effective for healing ulcers. H_2-receptor antagonists are highly effective in reducing gastric acid secretion. Symptomatic response is rapid, usually within a day or two, and healing follows within a few weeks in 70% to 90% of cases. Recurrence rates, however, are high even with maintenance therapy, with 50% to 75% of patients developing further symptoms within 2 years. Long term use of these drugs is now recognised as causing potentially adverse effects on the colonic microbiome.

A newer group of drugs, the substituted **benzimidazoles**, are extremely potent and reduce acid production to near zero by direct inhibition of the proton pump. **Omeprazole** and other variants are now often the first-line treatment for most peptic ulcer disorders. In all cases where *H. pylori* infection is present, the use of these drugs must be combined with eradication antibiotic therapy.

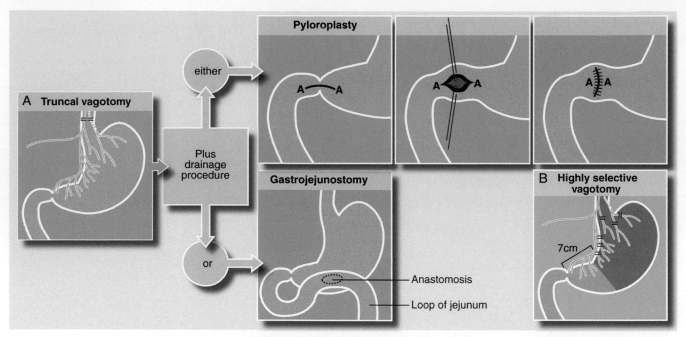

• **Fig. 21.8** The Vagotomies and Gastric Drainage Procedures (rarely performed nowadays but of historical interest). (A) Truncal vagotomy is followed by a drainage procedure, either pyloroplasty (Heinecke–Mikulicz is illustrated) or gastrojejunostomy. In gastrojejunostomy, an anastomosis is created to the most dependent part of the stomach; a short efferent loop of jejunum is brought up either in front of the transverse colon and sutured to the anterior wall of the stomach (antecolic), or behind the transverse colon via an incision in the mesocolon and sutured to the posterior wall of the stomach (retrocolic). (B) Highly selective vagotomy does not require a drainage procedure. Only the parietal cell mass is denervated, preserving the innervation of the pylorus and antrum plus the rest of the abdominal viscera.

Vagotomy

Vagotomy was first performed in the 1920s and popularised by Dragstedt from 1943. It gradually superseded classic partial gastrectomy as the surgical treatment of choice for chronic duodenal ulcer. The vagotomy operations illustrated in Fig. 21.8 are now only of historical interest. The simplest involved dividing the anterior and posterior vagal trunks close to the abdominal oesophagus, just below the diaphragm (**truncal vagotomy**). The operation is effective in promoting ulcer healing but paralyses gastric motility and slows pyloric emptying. A surgical **drainage procedure**, usually **pyloroplasty** ('V & P'), or less commonly **gastrojejunostomy**, was therefore a necessary part of the operation.

Attempts to reduce the gastric emptying complications of truncal vagotomy led to operations designed to preserve the innervation of the distal antrum and pylorus, whilst denervating the proximal acid-secreting portion of the stomach. **Highly selective vagotomy** preserved the nerves of Latarjet and avoided the need for a gastric drainage procedure. Early postoperative side effects were fewer but ulcer recurrence rates were higher than for truncal vagotomy.

Surgical Removal of Intractable Ulcers and Gastrin-Secreting Tissue

Partial gastrectomy was occasionally used for patients where medical management had failed to heal a benign **gastric ulcer** or to treat repeated recurrences. The operation had the dual role of removing the ulcer and the gastrin-secreting mucosa. The classic gastrectomy for chronic gastric ulcer was known as the *Billroth I type* (Billroth, 1881) and involved removing the distal stomach. The gastric remnant was then anastomosed to the first part of the duodenum (Fig. 21.9).

The standard partial gastrectomy for **duodenal ulcers** was a **Polya-type gastrectomy** (Polya, 1911), also involving resection of the distal stomach but anastomosing the cut end of the stomach to the side of a loop of proximal jejunum (gastrojejunostomy). This is also known as a *Billroth II* operation. The cut end of the duodenum (duodenal stump) was closed and the ulcer left in situ to heal (see Fig. 21.9). Numerous variations on gastrectomy have been described over the years, but the essential difference is whether the gastric remnant is anastomosed to the duodenum (Billroth I-type) or to a jejunal loop (Polya-type).

In general, partial gastrectomy was highly effective in relieving symptoms and preventing recurrence of peptic disease, but long-term side effects were a serious problem affecting 30% to 40% of patients.

Complications and Side Effects of Partial Gastrectomy

The main complications of partial gastrectomy occur in the long term and may not become manifest for years (Box 21.2). Recurrent ulceration after partial gastrectomy was rare and occurred in the gastric remnant or at the stomal margin. The usual reason was that insufficient stomach had been removed, but occasionally malignant change was responsible (3% risk over 15 years). Abnormally high acid production was another cause, sometimes caused by Zollinger–Ellison syndrome or hyperparathyroidism.

Correction of Secondary Anatomical Problems

The main anatomical problems secondary to peptic disease are oesophageal stricture and pyloric stenosis.

Oesophageal strictures can usually be managed by periodic dilatation and medical or surgical treatment of the underlying cause.

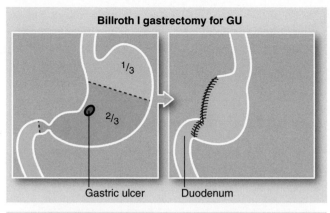

Billroth I gastrectomy for GU

Gastric ulcer   Duodenum

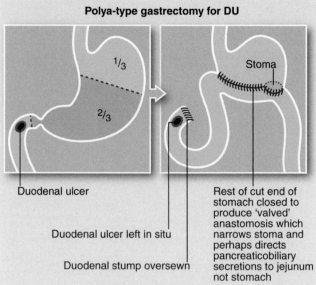

Polya-type gastrectomy for DU

Stoma

Duodenal ulcer

Duodenal ulcer left in situ

Duodenal stump oversewn

Rest of cut end of stomach closed to produce 'valved' anastomosis which narrows stoma and perhaps directs pancreaticobiliary secretions to jejunum not stomach

• **Fig. 21.9** Types of Partial Gastrectomy Formerly Performed for Peptic Ulcer Disease. *GU,* gastric ulcer; *DU,* duodenal ulcer

---

• BOX 21.2   Side Effects of Partial Gastrectomy

- Inability to eat normal-sized meals because of reduced gastric capacity
- 'Dumping' caused by rapid emptying of stomach contents—common but most patients adapt with time
- Episodic bilious vomiting because of reflux of bile into stomach via the anastomosis
- Tendency to bolus obstruction of the gastric outlet stoma
- Weight loss caused by a combination of aforementioned factors and malabsorption—especially common in women
- Vitamin B_{12} deficiency caused by loss of gastric intrinsic factor; may present as macrocytic anaemia or subacute combined degeneration of the spinal cord—potentially catastrophic, occurring many years after operation and preventable by regular vitamin B_{12} (hydroxycobalamin) injections
- Iron deficiency anaemia caused by reduced iron absorption—common but easily prevented by taking iron tablets, for example, once weekly
- Malignant change in gastric remnant possibly caused by bacterial production of carcinogens—rare

---

With the patient intravenously sedated, a guidewire is inserted across the stricture endoscopically, and then metal, plastic or balloon dilators are inserted over it. Occasionally, reflux continues to cause damage and stricturing; it may then become necessary to perform antireflux surgery.

Emergency Presentations of Peptic Ulcer Disease

The emergency presentations of peptic ulcer disease are acute haemorrhage, perforation and, much less commonly, pyloric stenosis. Peptic ulcer disease was responsible for much major emergency abdominal surgery until the early 1970s. Since then there has been a remarkable reduction in emergency presentations of peptic ulcer, and emergency surgery is now uncommon. This change was well under way in the West before the introduction of effective modern drug therapy and can probably be attributed to the progressive improvement in living standards after the Second World War.

Haemorrhage From a Peptic Ulcer

Acute bleeding from a peptic ulcer presents with haematemesis or melaena or both. Management is discussed in detail in Chapter 19.

Perforation of a Peptic Ulcer

Perforation of a gastric or duodenal ulcer into the peritoneal cavity causes peritonitis. Perforations of peptic ulcers occur most commonly in elderly patients taking NSAIDs and in patients consuming excess alcohol.

Duodenal ulcer perforations are two or three times more common than gastric ulcer perforations. The perforation typically occurs on the anterior surface of the duodenal bulb just beyond the pylorus. About half the patients with a peptic ulcer perforation have had recent ulcer symptoms but the other half are asymptomatic.

Gastric ulcer perforations virtually always occur in the elderly. About a third of these are caused by perforation of a gastric carcinoma. Thus standard surgical treatments for gastric perforation include excision or extensive biopsy of the ulcer.

Clinical Presentation of Perforated Peptic Ulcer

Perforation of a gastric or duodenal ulcer usually presents as a sudden onset of epigastric pain, rapidly spreading to the whole abdomen. The pain is continuous and is aggravated by moving about. Paradoxically, there may be vomiting of brownish or even blood-stained fluid. On examination, the patient is in obvious pain but is not shocked or toxic.

There is generalised involuntary abdominal guarding, which in younger patients is so tense as to be described as '**board-like rigidity**', although this may be absent in the elderly. There is also generalised abdominal tenderness but this may be difficult to detect because of guarding. After several hours, abdominal wall rigidity tends to relax although tenderness remains. Peptic ulcer perforation initially causes a chemical, as opposed to bacterial, peritonitis, unlike more distal bowel perforations. This explains the lack of general toxicity in the early stages. If untreated for more than 24 hours, secondary infection may take place and systemic signs appear.

If posterior wall gastric ulcers perforate, they leak gastric contents into the lesser sac, which tends to confine the peritonitis. These patients thus present with less marked symptoms.

Diagnosis of Perforated Peptic Ulcer

Diagnosis of an upper gastrointestinal perforation can usually be made from the symptoms and signs alone. A plain erect radiograph of the chest often reveals gas under the diaphragm, confirming the perforation of a hollow viscus but not its origin. This radiographic evidence of perforation, however, is not always present. If perforation is suspected but the signs are equivocal, an abdominal radiograph or computed tomography (CT) scan may be taken after the patient has swallowed 25 mL of water-soluble contrast; this may confirm the leakage. Diagnostic gastroscopy is contraindicated because the stomach must be inflated during this examination and air and gastric contents would erupt into the peritoneal cavity. CT scanning is commonly used and reveals free gas within the abdomen together with free fluid, although again the origin may not be clear. Laparoscopy is increasingly used to diagnose perforated ulcers.

Surgical Management of Peptic Perforation

Emergency surgery is indicated in nearly all cases of upper gastrointestinal perforation. The patient is first resuscitated and a nasogastric tube inserted. The operation is most commonly performed at laparotomy, but laparoscopic management of perforated duodenal ulcers is now well established with equally good results. The principles are similar in either case. At surgery, the abdomen is inspected and the diagnosis confirmed. 'Peritoneal toilet' is performed to remove fluid and food contaminating the peritoneal cavity. A perforated duodenal ulcer is usually obvious as a punched-out hole near the pylorus. An anterior gastric perforation is also obvious, but a posterior gastric ulcer is not visible unless the lesser sac is opened, usually along the greater curve.

In duodenal perforation, simple closure of the perforation by suturing a vascularised flap of omentum over the defect is the treatment of choice. This should be followed by *Helicobacter* eradication therapy as 90% of duodenal ulcers are associated with *H. pylori* infection.

In perforated gastric ulcer, the classic operation was Billroth I gastrectomy, including the whole ulcer in the resection. However, local excision of the ulcer and simple closure are safely used, provided the ulcer is believed to be benign. In any case, the ulcer edge must be biopsied in several places to be certain.

Conservative Management of Perforated Duodenal Ulcer

If an elderly, unfit patient presents late with a perforated duodenal ulcer, many surgeons treat this conservatively. This involves nasogastric aspiration, intravenous fluids, gastric acid suppression and antibiotics. Many of these patients who might otherwise have succumbed with major surgery recover satisfactorily.

Pyloric Stenosis (Fig. 21.10)

The pyloric canal and the immediate prepyloric area are common sites of chronic ulceration. There may be typical symptoms of chronic duodenal ulcer or the presentation may be with pyloric stenosis and a minimal history of ulcer pain. Chronic ulceration near the pylorus causes fibrosis, which may progress to stricture formation. In the early stages, this leads to partial gastric outlet obstruction. An acute exacerbation of the ulcer leads to mucosal swelling and pyloric sphincter spasm, which then precipitates complete luminal obstruction.

Clinical Features of Pyloric Stenosis

These patients rarely give any history of peptic ulcer pain but tend to present with a short history (a few weeks at most) of episodic and sometimes projectile vomiting. This is unrelated to eating, and the vomitus typically contains foul-smelling semidigested food eaten a day or more previously. It does not contain green bile. Often patients do not seek medical advice until they have become severely dehydrated with gross electrolyte disturbance.

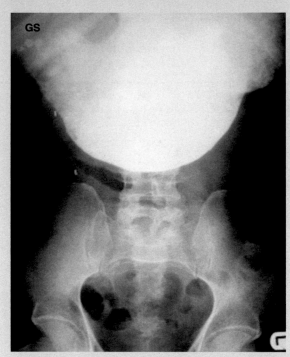

GS

• **Fig. 21.10 Gastric Outlet Obstruction.** Barium meal examination in a woman of 78 years who presented with a 2-week history of vomiting. She was grossly dehydrated with a hypochloraemic alkalosis. She was resuscitated and a nasogastric tube passed. This film shows huge gastric dilatation and no flow of barium beyond the pylorus. She also has incidental gallstones *(GS)*. The obstruction proved to be caused by chronic duodenal ulceration, but a diagnosis of carcinoma of the gastric antrum must be considered in such a patient.

On clinical examination, undernourishment, dehydration, constipation, weakness and weight loss may dominate the picture. Because the stomach is full of residual fluid and food, shaking the patient's abdomen from side to side produces an audible **succussion splash**. Gastric peristalsis may be visible in longstanding cases, and a dilated stomach full of residual food may be palpable. On plain abdominal x-ray, it may be possible to see the grossly dilated stomach filled with mottled food material.

Several gastric washouts, using a large-bore oral tube, may be necessary to clear the gastric residue before endoscopy or barium meal is attempted.

The differential diagnosis of gastric outflow obstruction also includes carcinoma of the head of the pancreas (with or without obstructive jaundice) and, rarely, chronic pancreatitis.

Biochemical Abnormalities in Pyloric Stenosis

The biochemical disturbances in these patients are complex and depend on the volume and composition of fluid lost by vomiting and on the body's compensatory mechanisms. Hydrogen and chloride are the principal ions lost in the vomitus. In response, the kidney conserves hydrogen ions by exchanging them for sodium ions (and some potassium ions), which are necessarily lost in the urine. The kidney also conserves chloride ions by exchanging them for bicarbonate ions. The net result may be a profound depletion of total body sodium (which is not accurately reflected in the plasma sodium level), profound hypochloraemia and profound metabolic alkalosis (**hypochloraemic alkalosis**). The plasma urea level is often high as a result of dehydration. Finally, the proportion of ionised calcium in the serum may fall as a result of the alkalosis, inducing tetany.

Management of Pyloric Stenosis

The first management priority in gastric outlet obstruction is resuscitation. Fluid and electrolyte deficiencies are corrected by infusion of physiological saline with added potassium chloride. The volume required often amounts to 10 litres or more. Rehydration will usually return the blood urea level to normal, but may unmask anaemia serious enough to require blood transfusion.

Often the obstruction has a significant inflammatory element, and acid suppression and *Helicobacter* eradication will produce a significant clinical response. If these fail or malignancy is suspected, endoscopy should be repeated and careful balloon dilation of the stenosis may achieve the desired result. If the obstruction persists, operative treatment may then become necessary in the form of either a gastrojejunostomy to bypass the obstruction, or more rarely a partial gastrectomy.

22

Disorders of the Oesophagus

CHAPTER OUTLINE

Introduction

Benign oesophageal diseases form a small but significant part of upper gastrointestinal (GI) surgeons' workload. Most are managed by medical gastroenterologists except those likely to require surgery; in which case close collaboration is needed between medical and surgical specialists. Oesophageal cancer surgery is largely performed in specialised units.

Difficulty in swallowing, **dysphagia**, is the most common presenting symptom. **Reflux oesophagitis** and other peptic disorders of the lower oesophagus (often associated with hiatus hernia) and **oesophageal carcinomas** are the most common conditions encountered. **Achalasia** and **pharyngeal pouch** are occasionally seen; **oesophageal web** (as in Plummer–Vinson syndrome), **leiomyomas** and **GI stromal tumours** (GIST) are extremely rare.

Oesophageal varices, secondary to cirrhosis, usually present as massive haematemesis and are usually managed with nonsurgical therapy.

Carcinoma of the Oesophagus

Pathology and Clinical Features

The oesophagus is lined by stratified squamous epithelium. Historically, the majority of oesophageal malignancies were **squamous carcinomas**. The rest were **adenocarcinomas** in the lower third, probably derived from metaplastic intestinal mucosa, that is, Barrett oesophagus. However, over the last few decades, there has been a slow but steady reversal in these proportions; currently, adenocarcinoma makes up 60% to 70% of new cases. Both forms tend to behave aggressively.

Tumours at the gastrooesophageal junction originate from three areas: the distal oesophagus (type 1), the gastric cardia (type 2) or the subcardial gastric wall (type 3). Oesophageal cancers may fungate into the lumen but more often infiltrate diffusely along and around the oesophageal wall. Once through the wall, the tumour invades adjoining mediastinal organs.

Difficulty in swallowing (dysphagia) is the classic symptom, but it tends to develop insidiously. Patients initially have trouble with solids but tend to compensate (liquidising their food, for example) before seeking medical advice. Later, they have trouble swallowing liquids. By the time dysphagia manifests, the cancer is often incurable and lymphatic spread has already occurred to mediastinal nodes. Sometimes, involvement of other mediastinal organs, for example, recurrent laryngeal nerve invasion or an oesophagotracheal fistula, produces the first symptoms. Low oesophageal lesions tend to metastasise to upper abdominal nodes and the liver.

Epidemiology and Aetiology

The incidence of oesophageal cancer in Western countries is relatively low compared with cancer of the colon or stomach. It accounts for about 5% of all deaths from cancer, with men at twofold greater risk than women. The disease is usually advanced by the time of presentation, hence the mortality rate is appalling, with 70% dying within a year and only 8% surviving 5 years (Fig. 22.1). Recently, outcomes have improved because of centralisation to specialist centres, neoadjuvant treatments and better patient selection through improved imaging tests.

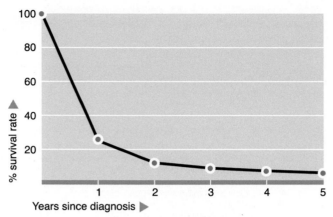

• **Fig. 22.1** Survival After Diagnosis of Oesophageal Carcinoma.

Dyspepsia Alone
- Patients over 55 years with recent onset, unexplained and persistent dyspepsia

Dyspepsia Plus Any of the Following 'Alarm Symptoms' at Any Age. Note: Patients With Symptoms Marked ‡ Should Be Referred Even Without Dyspepsia
- Progressive unintentional weight loss‡
- Persistent vomiting‡
- Iron deficiency anaemia‡
- Epigastric mass‡
- Dysphagia
- Chronic gastrointestinal bleeding
- Suspicious barium meal result

Dyspepsia—Unexplained Worsening, Plus
- Anaemia
- Known Barrett oesophagus, dysplasia, atrophic gastritis or intestinal metaplasia
- Surgery for peptic ulcer over 20 years before

Unexplained Upper Abdominal Pain and Weight Loss
- May need urgent ultrasound

Obstructive Jaundice
- May need urgent ultrasound

Oesophageal carcinoma is uncommon before the age of 50 years. At least 50% occur in the lower third and only about 15% in the upper third. Heavy alcohol intake is associated with at least 20 times greater risk and smokers have five times the risk of non-smokers; however, these risk factors classically predispose only to squamous cell carcinoma. Frequent hot drinks over 65°C are also believed to be a factor.

Since 1980, adenocarcinomas have increased by 70% relative to squamous carcinomas in many Western countries. This may be associated with the widespread use of acid-suppressing medication and possibly with dietary changes. There is no familial predisposition but people with structural and functional disorders, such as peptic oesophagitis and stricture, achalasia, oesophageal web or pharyngeal pouch, are at considerably greater risk. Areas of exceptionally high incidence have been reported in China, elsewhere in the Far East, and around the Caspian Sea. There is some evidence that a fungus, *Aspergillus,* which grows on food grain may be responsible. These epidemiological patterns suggest that chronic tissue irritation is an important aetiological factor. One common finding in dietary studies is an association with low fruit and vegetable intake.

Investigation of Suspected Oesophageal Carcinoma

Dysphagia or pain on swallowing (**odynophagia**) in a middle-aged or elderly patient demands urgent investigation to exclude carcinoma (Box 22.1). General physical examination is usually unrewarding except in advanced disease. In these cases, there may be signs of **wasting**, **hepatomegaly** because of metastases, a **Virchow node** in the left supraclavicular fossa or sometimes **hoarseness** from recurrent laryngeal nerve involvement. Oesophago-gastro-duodenoscopy allows direct inspection of the oesophagus using a flexible endoscope and biopsies are taken of any suspicious areas (Fig. 22.2).

Staging the Cancer

Once oesophageal carcinoma is diagnosed, it is important to establish the extent of local invasion and whether metastasis has occurred to thoracic or abdominal lymph nodes, liver or peritoneum; this will determine whether potentially curative treatment is appropriate. Computed tomography (CT) scanning of chest and abdomen is the principal investigation but it often understages the disease. **Staging laparoscopy** for lower third tumours can show peritoneal or visceral metastases not seen on CT scan;

some units use staging **thoracoscopy** to assess the pleural cavity for similar reasons. **Endoscopic ultrasound (EUS)** clearly demonstrates the different layers of the oesophageal wall and thus helps to delineate the tumour more accurately in length and, importantly, depth of invasion (T stage). It also has high sensitivity and specificity for involvement of local lymph nodes and can enable biopsy of suspicious nodes in otherwise inaccessible locations (**EUS-guided biopsy**), enhancing the staging process and in some cases preventing unnecessary surgery. The greater the number of involved nodes, the lower the chances of surgical cure. Increasingly, patients also undergo fluorodeoxyglucose positron emission tomography, known as PET scans, which localise any cancerous tissue more accurately than CT scanning alone.

Management of Carcinoma of the Oesophagus

The ideal treatment would be to completely resect the cancer. In practice, this can rarely be achieved because of overt or occult spread. Even if cure is impossible, oesophageal obstruction must be relieved to allow the patient to eat and to prevent the appalling consequences of complete obstruction, namely inability to swallow even saliva.

The choice of treatment depends on the patient's fitness and the stage, but surgical resection of the tumour is only used when the aim is curative. Comorbidity, such as chronic lung disease or cirrhosis (often from the adverse effects of cigarettes and alcohol) may influence the decision. Cardiac fitness is assessed clinically and by electrocardiography (ECG), echocardiography, and cardiopulmonary exercise testing. In addition, spirometry and blood gases should be performed to assess fitness for thoracotomy. If the forced expiratory volume in 1 second (FEV_1) is less than

CASE HISTORIES

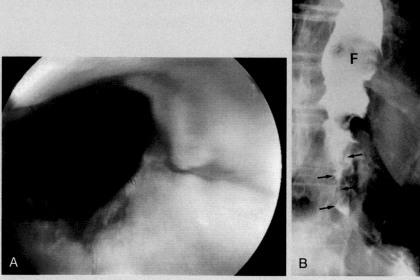

• **Fig. 22.2 Barrett Oesophagus and Oesophageal Carcinoma. (A)** Endoscopic view of Barrett oesophagus demonstrating linear ulceration and deeper red mucosa with chronic ulceration at the oesophagogastric junction. Diagnosis is confirmed on biopsy. This condition is potentially premalignant. **(B)** Barium swallow in an elderly man who presented with almost complete dysphagia. The film shows the lower end of the oesophagus, which has an irregular narrowing of the lumen *(arrowed)*. This appearance did not alter in several views of the same area and is characteristic of malignancy. Nevertheless, endoscopy is usually performed to obtain histological confirmation by biopsies. The oesophagus aforementioned is moderately dilated and contains a bolus of food *(F)*, which cannot pass onwards.

2 L, single lung ventilation used during thoracotomy is unlikely to be tolerated. Adjuvant therapy in addition to surgery has a role in some patients, although clinical trials are continuing to determine precise indications. More often, chemotherapy is given alone or in combination with radiotherapy (chemoradiotherapy) before surgery (**neoadjuvant therapy**), in an attempt to shrink or downsize the tumour.

Radiotherapy in combination with chemotherapy can been given as the sole form of treatment for squamous carcinoma. However, radiotherapy-induced inflammation tends to result in oedema, which may make swallowing difficult initially. Nowadays, radiotherapy alone tends to be reserved for palliation.

For incurable patients with dysphagia, palliative procedures to restore swallowing, such as argon plasma tissue coagulation, laser treatment or stent insertion, can be effective and are preferable to major surgery, particularly if life expectancy is short.

Surgery

Once a decision has been made to operate, the choice of operation depends on the level of the lesion. In general, the aim is to remove the tumour with an appropriate safety margin, to perform a two-field lymphadenectomy (removing mediastinal and abdominal lymph nodes) and to achieve a leak-free anastomosis.

Lesions above the carina (tracheal bifurcation) are usually dealt with by a three-stage **oesophagectomy,** known as the *McKeown operation*, with all stages performed at the same operation. The first stage is to mobilise the tumour and oesophagus via a right thoracotomy with the patient in the left lateral position. The second stage involves rolling the patient into a supine position and performing a laparotomy to allow the stomach to be mobilised

and fashioned into a conduit. A third incision is then made in the neck through which oesophagus and tumour are delivered. The tumour is resected and the gastric conduit anastomosed to the cervical oesophagus. A cervical anastomosis is safer than an intrathoracic one, as the consequences of anastomotic leakage are less devastating.

If the tumour arises lower in the oesophagus, a two-stage **Ivor Lewis operation** is usually performed. The abdomen is opened first, and the stomach mobilised and fashioned into a conduit. The patient is then turned into a left lateral position and the right chest opened, the oesophagus mobilised and the tumour and lymph nodes excised. Finally, the gastric conduit is drawn up into the chest and anastomosed to the proximal oesophageal remnant. If the stomach cannot be used to create a conduit, a conduit can be formed with the right or the left side of colon. Very rarely, it may be possible to bring up a single end of jejunum (Rouxen-Y) to make the connection (Fig. 22.3). Controversy exists about whether extending lymphadenectomy into the neck, socalled three-field lymphadenectomy, is beneficial. The procedure increases operative risks and only appears to benefit a subgroup with proximal tumours.

An operation that gained popularity is the **transhiatal oesophagectomy**. A thoracotomy is avoided by mobilising the oesophagus and the cancer by blunt dissection from below via the diaphragmatic hiatus and from above via a neck incision, performing the anastomosis in the neck after resection. However, interest is waning because the safety margins of excision may be insufficient for potential cure and adequate lymphadenectomy is impossible to achieve in the chest. There is also a risk of damaging veins during dissection (particularly the azygos) and causing catastrophic haemorrhage.

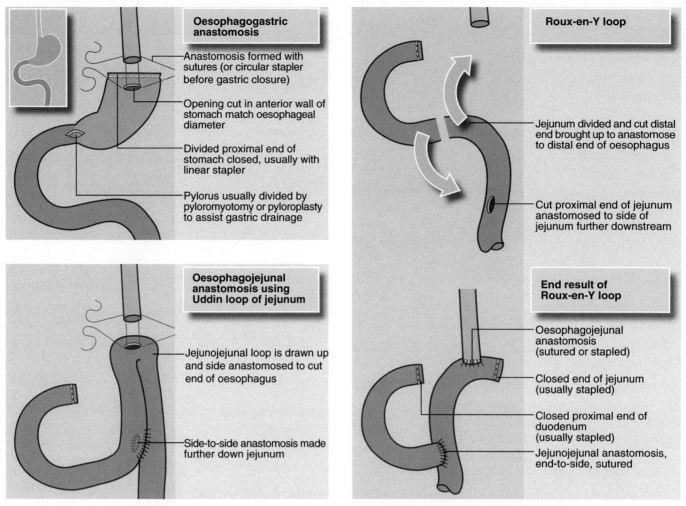

• **Fig. 22.3** Methods of Reconstruction After Distal Oesophagectomy and Partial or Total Gastrectomy.

There is increasing interest in laparoscopic approaches to these cancers, and many units now regularly perform laparoscopic oesophagectomies. Techniques involve combined laparoscopic and thoracoscopic approaches. Perioperative morbidity and mortality and cancer recurrence rates appear to be at least comparable with open surgery, and there are the additional benefits of minimal access surgery.

Oesophagectomy is always a major undertaking and carries the potentially fatal risk of anastomotic breakdown. This may lead to mediastinitis, lung abscess or oesophagopleural fistula. Patients need to be made aware of the risks in relation to the benefits, as well as the likely prolonged convalescent period and the long-term morbidity. Postoperative problems include dysphagia, small capacity for food (early satiety), and reflux.

Inoperable Lesions

If operation is inappropriate, oesophageal patency can often be restored by palliative ablation of the tumour with laser therapy or argon plasma coagulation via a gastroscope. These treatments can be repeated as the tumour regrows. Alternatively, the oesophagus can be intubated with an expanding metal stent (see Fig. 22.4) through the lesion. This is usually done under intravenous sedation, using the endoscopic technique of **pulsion intubation**. First the oesophageal lesion is dilated, then the stent inserted using x-ray guidance. Oesophageal stents can also be inserted entirely under x-ray guidance without the need for endoscopy. Stents relieve symptoms, but

food has to be liquidised and the tube kept 'clean' by taking fizzy drinks after eating. Patients are more susceptible to acid reflux, for which antacid medication may need to be prescribed. Chemotherapy, external beam radiotherapy and intraluminal brachytherapy (local radiotherapy) are increasingly used for palliation.

Hiatus Hernia and Reflux Oesophagitis

Pathophysiology

The oesophagus is essentially a tube of smooth muscle conveying food to the stomach by peristalsis. At the lower end, there is a tonically active sphincter mechanism. Its contraction coordinates with oesophageal peristalsis, relaxing to allow food to enter the stomach. The purpose of the sphincter mechanism is to prevent reflux of stomach contents into the oesophagus. After passing through the diaphragm, the oesophagus continues for about 2 cm within the abdomen before joining the stomach. The sphincter mechanism is not completely understood, but it probably involves several components as follows: a functional (but not anatomical) sphincter of the oesophageal wall immediately above the diaphragm and the smooth muscle at the gastric cardia. This mechanism is reinforced by diaphragmatic crural contraction, by the acute angle at which the oesophagus enters the stomach and by the **'flutter valve'** effect of intraabdominal pressure on the abdominal oesophagus causing luminal collapse.

Hiatus hernia occurs when the proximal part of the stomach passes through the diaphragmatic hiatus up into the chest (Fig. 22.5). Around 90% of hiatus hernias are of the **sliding type**, in which the gastrooesophageal junction is drawn up into the chest and a segment of stomach becomes constricted at the diaphragmatic hiatus. The hernia tends to slide up into the chest with each peristaltic contraction. These hernias may become huge and, rarely, may contain the whole stomach including pylorus and first part of the duodenum, sometimes with part of the colon as well. In the 10% of nonsliding cases, the gastrooesophageal junction remains below the diaphragm and a bulge of stomach herniates through the hiatus beside the oesophagus. These are described as paraoesophageal or rolling hiatus hernias. In reality, most rolling hiatus hernias also have a sliding component.

In sliding hiatus hernia, the lower oesophageal sphincter mechanism often becomes defective, causing reflux of acid–peptic stomach contents. This is not a problem with rolling hiatus hernias, which more usually present with pain or dysphagia. Extremely large rolling hiatus hernias can also present with breathlessness owing to compression of the adjoining lungs.

Hiatus hernia in adults is commonly associated with smoking and obesity. The pressure of intraabdominal fat may be contributory. Hiatus hernia can also be a congenital abnormality presenting in early infancy.

Clinical Features of Reflux Oesophagitis

Hiatus hernia is common, especially in women, and becomes more common with advancing years. Only a small proportion of patients with hiatus hernia experience symptoms of **acid–peptic reflux**, that is, 'heartburn'; moreover, reflux can occur without a hiatus hernia. Reflux causes acute inflammation (**oesophagitis**), experienced as burning retrosternal pain (**heartburn**), bitter-tasting regurgitation or other forms of 'indigestion'. Symptoms are typically worse at night when the patient lies flat or on bending forward during the day.

If reflux is severe and persistent, mucosal destruction is recurrent and inflammation becomes chronic. Progressive scarring leads to fibrosis of the wall and this may lead to luminal narrowing (stricture) and dysphagia. Longstanding oesophageal reflux predisposes to **Barrett ocsophagus**, with normal squamous oesophageal epithelium being replaced by metaplastic columnar mucosa. Barrett oesophagus is the only known predisposing factor for adenocarcinoma of the lower oesophagus. Histological examination of biopsies may reveal **specialised intestinal metaplasia**. The presence of dysplastic epithelium on biopsy, in the background of Barrett should be a cause for concern as it is a marker of malignant change. This supports the metaplasia/dysplasia/carcinoma model for evolution of lower oesophageal cancer.

CASE HISTORY

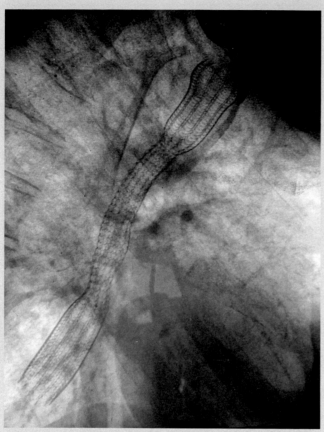

• **Fig. 22.4** Intubation of Oesophageal Cancer: Cloth-Covered Metal Stent in Situ. This 70-year-old man presented with inoperable carcinoma of the middle third of the oesophagus. The malignant stricture was dilated via a flexible gastroscope and a Dacron-covered metal stent inserted to keep the stricture open as a palliative measure. This lateral chest x-ray shows the stent in situ.

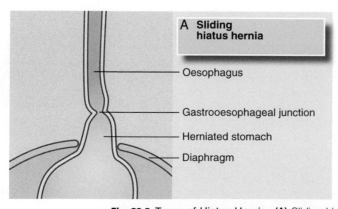

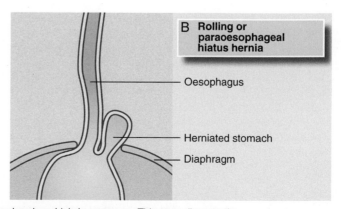

• **Fig. 22.5** Types of Hiatus Hernia. **(A)** Sliding hiatus hernia, which is common. This type disrupts the physiological antireflux mechanism. **(B)** Rolling or paraoesophageal hiatus hernia, which is rare. The antireflux mechanism is usually left intact

Occasionally, oesophageal reflux symptoms are severe and acute, causing chest pain, which can easily be mistaken for angina or even myocardial infarction. There is often an element of **oesophageal spasm** which, like angina, is relieved by glyceryl trinitrate and similar drugs, which may confuse the diagnosis.

In general, hiatus hernias are assessed at endoscopy, with biopsy if necessary. The latter is important to exclude carcinoma, especially in patients with dysphagia. In specialised units, **oesophageal manometry studies** can assess the oesophageal muscular function and **oesophageal pH studies** assess the extent and severity of reflux. These studies help determine which patients are likely to benefit from surgery. Rarely barium swallow examination (Figs 22.6 and 22.7) may be necessary to delineate complicated anatomy.

CASE HISTORIES

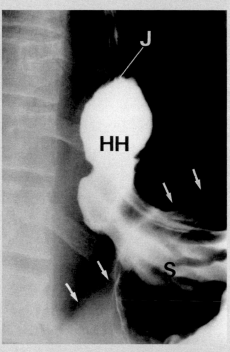

• **Fig. 22.6** Sliding Hiatus Hernia. Sliding hiatus hernia in a 63-year-old woman. The hiatus hernia is marked *(HH)*, the stomach *(S)* and the oesophagogastric junction *(J)*; the position of the diaphragm is *arrowed*.

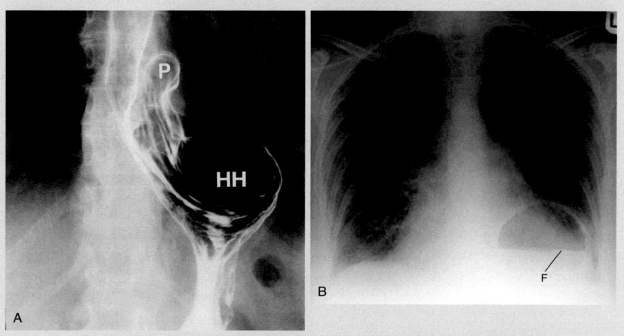

• **Fig. 22.7** Sliding Hiatus Hernia. **(A)** Large incarcerated (irreducible) sliding hiatus hernia *(HH)* in an elderly woman with few symptoms. Note there is also a small paraoesophageal 'rolling' hiatus hernia *(P)*. **(B)** Plain chest x-ray of the same patient showing a fluid level *(F)* strongly suggestive of a hiatus hernia.

Management of Hiatus Hernia and Reflux Oesophagitis

Most patients can be managed conservatively, with surgery reserved for intractable cases. Treatment is aimed at reducing acid–pepsin activity and preventing reflux.

Reducing Reflux

Weight reduction, where appropriate, is the most effective long-term antireflux measure. Changes in diet often of themselves improve symptoms of reflux. For example, **alcohol** causes the sphincter to relax and many medical students can personally vouch for the combined effect of alcohol and spicy food. Other foods known to precipitate reflux are caffeine, high fat foods and chocolate. Reflux can be substantially reduced by taking smaller, more frequent and drier meals, by using blocks to elevate the head of the bed at night on bricks and by sleeping on two or more pillows in an upright position. **Smoking** induces sphincter relaxation, and quitting often reduces reflux dramatically. Patients should also be advised to wear loose-fitting clothing, and avoid bending or straining soon after meals. **Alginate drugs**, available in liquid or chewable tablet form, produce a foamy surface layer on the stomach contents and are said to coat the lower oesophagus, protecting it from reflux effects. These drugs are most effective if taken soon after food.

Prokinetic Agents

Drugs that stimulate motility can have a useful effect in reflux. **Metoclopramide** and **domperidone** are dopamine antagonists that stimulate oesophageal clearance and gastric emptying and increase small bowel transit, as well as enhancing contraction of the oesophageal sphincter.

Reducing Acid–Pepsin Production

This is probably the mainstay of treatment for reflux disease. Simple antacid drugs and H_2-receptor antagonists are sometimes effective, but in most cases **omeprazole** or another proton-pump inhibitor (PPI) is the drug of choice.

Management of Strictures

Inflammatory fibrous strictures used to be regularly dilated with gum-elastic **bougies** of progressively increasing size, under general anaesthesia, via a rigid oesophagoscope. Nowadays, dilatation is usually performed under intravenous sedation using flexible gastroscopy under x-ray control, with a balloon to dilate the stricture. If the stricture recurs (which it usually does) and causes dysphagia despite conservative treatment for reflux, an antireflux operation may be indicated. This usually allows healing of mucosal damage and may prevent further stricture formation.

Surgery for Hiatus Hernia and Reflux Oesophagitis

Surgery has historically been reserved for intractable symptoms, recurrent stricture and chronic oesophagitis, which fails to respond to PPI therapy. This especially includes patients with Barrett oesophagus (having excluded those with a high risk of malignancy by biopsy). Surgery may also be indicated for the young or middle-aged patient in whom PPIs produce a response but who do not wish to take long-term medication. The traditional operations for formal repair of hiatus hernia, performed via chest or abdomen (e.g., Belsey Mark IV), have largely been superseded by laparoscopic **Nissen fundoplication**. This operation involves dissection of the gastrooesophageal junction at the hiatus, tightening the crura (which may have become lax, allowing the hiatus hernia to develop) and wrapping the gastric fundus around the intraabdominal portion of the oesophagus to recreate a flutter valve.

In experienced hands, this is the operation of choice and allows the patient a rapid return to normal activity. Clinical trials have shown that the laparoscopic approach gives results comparable to open fundoplication. Typical side effects of any Nissen operation include temporary dysphagia, gas-bloat syndrome (because of retained air and decreased ability to belch) and consequently increased flatus. These problems usually settle in time, but must be clearly explained to the patient before obtaining consent for operation. The most significant (but fortunately rare) postoperative complication is that of a **slipped wrap**. In this case, the fundal wrap slips down onto the stomach, or up through the hiatus into the chest (usually after a bout of excessive vomiting). In either case, the patient usually presents with acute onset chest and/or upper abdominal pain and dysphagia. This complication should be managed as a surgical emergency with diagnostic confirmation followed by early reoperation.

Achalasia

Pathophysiology and Clinical Presentation

Achalasia is an uncommon disorder of oesophageal motility. In pathological terms, there is a poorly understood neurological defect involving Auerbach myenteric plexus, with loss of inhibitory neurons. Peristalsis is disrupted throughout the entire oesophagus, causing uncoordinated contractions and inadequate relaxation of the lower oesophageal sphincter.

The condition presents in two main age groups, young adults and the elderly. In the latter, the cause may be a central rather than a local neurological deficit. Achalasia, as with any structural oesophageal abnormality, predisposes to cancer with a 5% lifetime risk of developing squamous oesophageal carcinoma, usually 15 to 20 years after diagnosis of achalasia.

Clinically, the cardiac sphincter becomes constricted and the proximal oesophagus dilates with accumulated fluid and solids. Difficulty in swallowing is the usual presenting symptom, together with halitosis, weight loss, reflux of food into the back of the throat. Solids tend to sink to the lower end of the dilated oesophagus, whereas fluids spill over into the trachea causing **spluttering dysphagia** (see Ch. 18, p. 276) and coughing, particularly at night. Recurrent aspiration pneumonias can be the first presentation in some elderly patients. Vomiting and retrosternal pain may occur in more severe cases.

Investigation of Suspected Achalasia

Chest x-ray may show the mediastinal shadow is widened by a dilated oesophagus; sometimes a fluid level in the oesophagus is visible behind the heart (see Fig. 22.7B). At endoscopy, the typical appearance is of a capacious distal oesophagus, usually with food and fluid residue, and a tight lower oesophageal sphincter that may or may not admit the tip of the gastroscope. It is important to see the oesophagogastric junction to exclude an occult neoplasm masquerading as achalasia (**pseudoachalasia**). Barium swallow examination reveals gross dilatation of the oesophagus with a tapering constriction (often described as a 'bird's beak') at the lower end. The constriction barely allows contrast to enter the stomach (see Fig. 22.8). Under fluoroscopic screening, uncoordinated purposeless peristaltic waves can often be seen; these are described as **tertiary contractions**, distinct from normal coordinated primary and secondary contractions. Oesophageal manometry is the cardinal test for achalasia, demonstrating excessive lower oesophageal sphincter pressure that fails to relax on swallowing, and absent peristalsis in patients with a more chronic history.

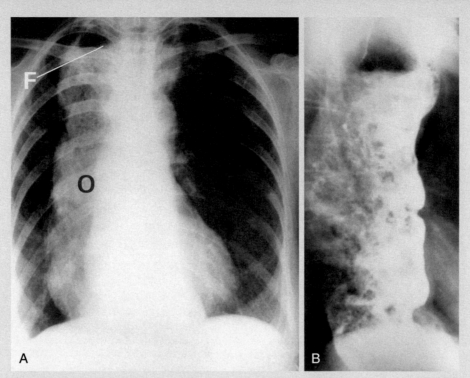

• **Fig. 22.8** Late-Stage Achalasia in a 60-Year-Old Man. **(A)** The chest x-ray shows gross mediastinal widening caused by a massively dilated oesophagus *(O)* filled with food debris. Note the mottled appearance of the oesophagus and the fluid level *(F)* at its upper end. Note also the absence of a gastric air bubble below the diaphragm. This is characteristic of achalasia. **(B)** Barium swallow in the same patient. This confirms the findings on the chest x-ray.

Management of Achalasia

The condition is by its nature incurable, and treatment aims to relieve the distal obstruction. The standard operation is a laparoscopic abdominal procedure involving a longitudinal incision of the lower oesophageal and upper gastric muscle wall, until the mucosa bulges through (**Heller cardiomyotomy**); this is best combined with a partial fundoplication to overcome the almost inevitable reflux that will result. Balloon dilatation is sometimes used as an alternative but often needs to be repeated. Botulinum toxin (Botox) is now often used to relax the lower oesophageal sphincter and is an excellent temporising measure, but needs to be repeated after 3 to 6 months, as the effect wears off. Patients with achalasia should be followed up and periodically endoscoped to exclude developing squamous carcinoma (see Fig. 22.9). The latest technique is an endoscopic myotomy (Per-Oral Endoscopic Myotomy or POEM).

Pharyngeal Pouch

Pharyngeal pouch is a rare cause of dysphagia. It arises at the junction of the pharynx and oesophagus, and probably results from lack of coordination between the inferior constrictor muscle and cricopharyngeus during swallowing. At this point, there is an area of relative weakness known as *Killian dehiscence*. The result is a progressive mucosal outpouching between the two muscles. The condition is best diagnosed by barium swallow (see Fig. 22.10). Pharyngeal pouch can be easily perforated during endoscopy, and

therefore in patients undergoing endoscopy to investigate 'high' dysphagia, the procedure should be performed by an experienced endoscopist. Treatment of pharyngeal pouch is by surgical excision from the side of the neck, or via a completely endoluminal approach using a stapler to join the pouch to the oesophagus.

Oesophageal Web

Circumferential mucosal folds (or webs) in the oesophagus may produce annular narrowing and cause dysphagia. They also predispose to carcinoma in the long term. In the upper oesophagus, webs are associated with severe iron deficiency anaemia, particularly in women. The triad of dysphagia, anaemia and atrophic glossitis is known as **Plummer–Vinson** or **Paterson–Brown–Kelly syndrome**.

Gastrooesophageal Varices

Pathophysiology

Gastrooesophageal varices result from **portal venous hypertension**. The most common cause is cirrhosis of the liver, usually linked with alcohol abuse. Less common causes include portal vein thrombosis, hepatic vein thrombosis (**Budd–Chiari syndrome**) and schistosomiasis.

With resistance to flow, the pressure rises in the portal venous system, which leads to abnormal communications developing

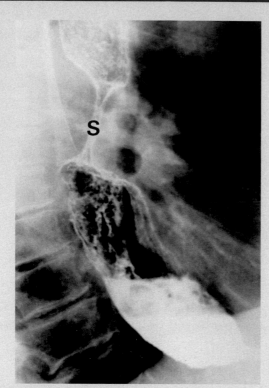

• **Fig. 22.9** Oesophageal Carcinoma Secondary to Achalasia. Malignant stricture *(S)* in the middle third of the oesophagus in a 60-year-old woman with achalasia of long standing. She had a Heller myotomy at the age of 26 years. Note that this surgery does not reduce the inherent predisposition to carcinoma.

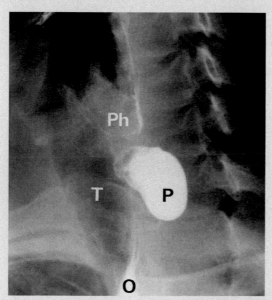

• **Fig. 22.10** Pharyngeal Pouch. Lateral view during barium swallow examination in a 41-year-old man complaining of mild dysphagia; the x-ray shows a contrast-filled pouch *(P)* extending from the pharynx *(Ph)*. Note the gas-filled trachea *(T)* lying anteriorly. *O*, oesophagus.

between the peripheral portal system and the systemic venous circulation. This is known as **portal-systemic shunting**. Multiple large veins appear in the peritoneal cavity and retroperitoneal area, making any form of abdominal surgery hazardous. Large submucosal veins also appear at the lower end of the oesophagus and gastric fundus, and are known as **gastrooesophageal varices** (see Fig. 22.11). These varices can cause massive GI haemorrhage, possibly related to rises in intravariceal pressure. Up to 40% of cirrhotic patients suffer variceal haemorrhage at some stage.

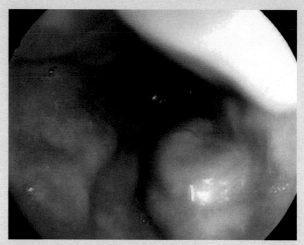

• **Fig. 22.11** Endoscopic View of Oesophageal Varices. This man of 63 years was known to have alcoholic cirrhosis and had suffered one acute gastrointestinal haemorrhage, treated successfully by injection of bleeding varices. The bulging blue masses can be seen protruding into the oesophageal lumen.

Elective Management

Gastrooesophageal varices are not usually treated unless they have bled. Occasionally, elective treatment is carried out in cases where haemorrhage is considered highly likely, with the improving efficacy of banding and sclerotherapy. After recovery from an acute bleed, varices should be treated at planned intervals by banding or injection sclerotherapy, until they are eliminated.

Management of Bleeding Gastrooesophageal Varices

Diagnosis and Resuscitation

When a patient with known cirrhosis or varices presents with massive upper GI haemorrhage, the first priority is resuscitation. The source of haemorrhage is next sought by endoscopy. Only about half of these patients will be bleeding from oesophageal varices. The rest have bleeding gastric varices, gastric erosions, a peptic ulcer or Mallory–Weiss tears of the lower oesophagus. In this last condition, arterial bleeding is the cause and it does not respond to measures designed to treat bleeding varices, but is usually self-limiting. Whatever treatment is undertaken, it must be remembered that cirrhotic patients often have defective clotting, further exacerbated by massive haemorrhage. It is prudent to perform clotting studies and give specific coagulation factors.

Treatment

If bleeding is from varices, an attempt may be made at endoscopy to band or inject them with a sclerosant (e.g., ethanolamine or sodium tetradecyl sulphate). The mainstay of initial treatment is an **infusion of vasopressin** or an analogue, such as terlipressin. Octreotide has also been used successfully. More than 75% of patients initially respond to this therapy. Meanwhile, resuscitation continues with blood volume replacement, fresh-frozen plasma and platelets. Excess water and sodium should be avoided as this rapidly migrates into the peritoneal cavity as ascites. Hepatic encephalopathy should be anticipated as a result of the protein load of blood in the bowel and oral neomycin or lactulose should be administered. Delirium tremens may also require treatment if the patient is an alcoholic.

In patients not responding to octreotide, an attempt is made to apply tamponade. After endotracheal intubation to protect the airway, a special tube is passed through the mouth into the stomach and a balloon inflated. Traction is exerted on the upper end for up to 4 hours to arrest the haemorrhage. Several varieties of tube are in use: the **Sengstaken–Blakemore tube** has separate intragastric and oesophageal balloons. Most cases cease bleeding with inflation of the gastric balloon alone in combination with traction. The **Linton balloon** is an alternative comprising a single large intragastric balloon (300–600 mL) which allows simultaneous endoscopy and banding or injection sclerotherapy of varices.

If variceal haemorrhage continues despite effective conservative therapy, **transjugular intrahepatic portal-systemic stenting** is sometimes used. This involves cannulating the internal jugular vein and placing an angiography catheter within the intrahepatic vena cava. Using combined fluoroscopy and ultrasound, the catheter is guided into the portal system within the liver. Then an

TABLE 22.1	Child Criteria for Assessing Operative Risk in Portal Hypertension		
	SCORE POINTS		
Risk Factor	**1**	**2**	**3**
Encephalopathy	None	Minimal	Marked
Ascites	None	Slight	Moderate
Bilirubin (μmol/L)	<35	36–50	<50
Albumin (g/L)	>35	28–35	>28
Prothrombin ratio	<1.4	1.4–2.0	>2.0

Each criterion is scored and the total added:
Child grade A (good risk) scores 5–6
Grade B (moderate risk) scores 7–9
Grade C (bad risk) scores 10–15

expanding metal stent is placed to connect the intrahepatic portal system to the vena cava.

As a last resort, emergency surgical treatment is performed, but all operations carry high mortality in such seriously ill patients. The simplest operation is **transgastric oesophageal stapling**. A circular stapler is passed into the oesophagus via a gastrotomy, a ligature tied around the oesophagus between the staple cartridge and the anvil, and the gun fired. This places two rows of staples through the full thickness of the oesophageal wall, disconnecting the longitudinal veins. Operative risk in these patients has been calculated using **Child criteria**, shown in Table 22.1.

23

Tumours of the Stomach and Small Intestine

CHAPTER OUTLINE

Introduction

Most gastric tumours are malignant: nearly all are adenocarcinomas; the rest are lymphomas or rarely, carcinoid tumours or sarcoma. True adenomatous **gastric polyps** are rare; most gastric polypoid lesions are small benign hyperplastic nodules.

Tumours of small bowel are rare. Of the malignant tumours, lymphomas and gastrointestinal stromal tumours (GIST) are much more common than adenocarcinomas. **Peutz–Jeghers syndrome** is a rare inherited disorder characterised by multiple benign polyps in the small bowel and perioral pigmentation plus increased risk of breast, colorectal and other cancers. Patients are fairly commonly encountered at student examinations (see Ch. 27, p. 378).

Carcinoma of Stomach

Pathology of Gastric Carcinoma

Gastric carcinomas are almost exclusively adenocarcinomas. Two distinct histopathological groups are recognised, each with its own epidemiological associations. The **intestinal type** has histological features similar to intestinal epithelium. Cells grow in clumps and there is marked inflammatory infiltrate. The second variety is the **diffuse type**. Here, the cells are singular, often arranged in single file and surrounded by a marked stromal reaction. Tumour cells have large intracellular **mucin** droplets, which displace the nucleus to the cell periphery, giving the characteristic **signet ring appearance** (Fig. 23.1). Intestinal-type carcinomas have a better prognosis than mucin-producing signet ring carcinomas.

Gastric carcinomas develop in three morphological forms described later; the **intestinal type** largely produces fungating tumours and malignant ulcers, and the **diffuse type** causes infiltrating carcinomas:
- **Fungating tumours**—these polypoid lesions may grow to a huge size.
- **Malignant ulcers**—these probably result from necrosis in broad-based solid tumours. Malignant ulcers are often larger than peptic ulcers (except for giant benign ulcers of the elderly) with a heaped-up indurated (hardened) margin.
- **Infiltrating carcinomas**—this form spreads widely beneath the mucosa, and diffusely and extensively invades the muscle wall. This causes thickening and rigidity and the entire stomach contracts to a very small capacity. This is known as **linitis plastica** and its appearance likened to a 'leather bottle'. Linitis plastica affects a slightly younger age group than intestinal-type cancer and has a very poor prognosis. Diagnosis may be delayed because endoscopic changes are often subtle and standard biopsies of mucosa may not show malignancy.

'Early gastric cancer' is defined as cancer limited to the mucosa and submucosa. This is found most often as a result of endoscopic screening or whilst investigating possible peptic ulcer. Results of surgery in this group are excellent, with a surgical cure rate of about 90%.

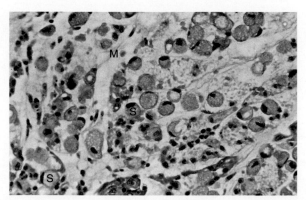

• **Fig. 23.1** Signet-Ring Carcinoma of the Stomach—Histopathology. High-power view of typical infiltrating type of gastric carcinoma showing numerous signet ring cells *(S)*. This appearance is caused by the presence of intracellular mucin *(M)*.

Epidemiology of Gastric Carcinoma

Gastric cancer is the fifth most common cancer in the world, causing 14% of cancers, and is the fifth most frequent cause of cancer deaths at 11% (2012 figures: see http://www.cancerresearchuk.org/sites/default/files/cs_report_world.pdf). The disease is rare before the age of 50 years and increases in frequency thereafter. Males have two to three times the risk of females, and the disease is more common in lower socioeconomic groups. Korea has overtaken Japan in having the highest annual incidence—a crude rate of 62 per 100,000 per year in men and 25 in women (2015). In the United Kingdom, equivalent rates are 13.6 for men and 7.2 for women (2015). The offspring of Japanese immigrants to America carry no greater risk than other Americans, evidence that environmental rather than racial factors are central in the aetiology. In much of the Western world, the incidence and death rates of gastric cancer have steadily decreased over recent years, and this is almost entirely because of a decline in the intestinal type. In Japan, the age standardised incidence for men has fallen from 80 per 100,000 per annum in 1975 to 46 in 2012.

The epidemiology gives enticing clues as to the causes of the disease. There are marked regional variations in incidence, largely explained by disparities in the rate of intestinal-type carcinomas. This, and the fact that this type is more prevalent in lower socio-economic groups, suggests that environmental factors are important in its genesis. There is probably no universal aetiological factor but rather a combination of cofactors that bring about malignant change. Japan, with its very high incidence of this disease, continues to play a leading role in research into early detection and management.

Aetiology of Gastric Carcinoma and Premalignant Conditions

Atrophic Gastritis

Multifocal atrophic gastritis (type B) is a condition that precedes intestinal-type gastric cancer. It probably represents one step of a sequence running from superficial gastritis, via atrophic gastritis to intestinal and colonic metaplasia, dysplasia and eventually to cancer. Multifocal atrophic gastritis is the result of **chronic inflammation**. Risk factors for type B gastritis include *Helicobacter pylori* infection and certain items of diet. The **diffuse corporeal type of gastritis (type A)** of pernicious anaemia is a much weaker aetiological factor for cancer. Patients with this have a three- to sixfold increase in risk, but the absolute risk remains low.

Helicobacter pylori Infection

H. pylori is known to initiate peptic ulceration, and chronic *H. pylori* infection has become a prime suspect for initiating intestinal-type gastric cancer. The organism can colonise gastric mucosa over long periods and cause chronic gastritis, which may progress to type B multifocal atrophic gastritis. In one biopsy study of gastric cancers, *H. pylori* was found in 90% of intestinal-type cancers, whilst only 30% of the diffuse type were infected. The carcinogenic mechanism of *H. pylori* may involve alterations to the gastric acid–pepsin environment, with increased cell turnover and possibly enhanced mucosal susceptibility to ingested carcinogens. *H. pylori* eradication does not reverse gastric atrophy but does improve the enzymic and hormonal secretory capacity of the stomach. *H. pylori* also appears likely to be involved in **gastric lymphoma** of the **mucosa-associated lymphoid tissue (MALT)** type (see p. 346).

Dietary Factors

Dietary factors shown to increase the incidence of gastric cancer include excess intake of salt and nitroso compounds and a low intake of ascorbic acid. In this respect, diets high in dried and salted fish and salt-cured and smoke-cured meats appear to be a particular risk. Lettuce grown in temperate climates appears to offer some protective effect.

Clinical Features of Gastric Carcinoma

Symptoms are often minimal until late in the course of the disease so that 70% of patients present with advanced local and/or metastatic disease. Lesions at the inlet or outlet of the stomach cause **obstructive symptoms** earlier than those elsewhere where the diameter allows for substantial growth before encroachment. Vomiting occurs if the gastric outlet becomes obstructed, typically by tumours of the antrum, and dysphagia occurs with tumours just below the gastrooesophageal junction.

In **advanced disease**, up to half the patients are asymptomatic and the rest have pain, nausea, vomiting, anorexia or a feeling of fullness after small meals (**early satiety**). Sometimes, these symptoms are there months before the patient presents. **Anaemia** from chronic occult blood loss is common and one-third have positive stool tests for occult blood. One-third have **cachexia** (severe weight loss and wasting). This usually indicates metastatic disease and may be the only manifestation of cancer at the time. Of the 70% who present with advanced local disease (stage T_3), more than half have extensive abdominal nodal spread and half have distant metastases. The presenting features of gastric carcinoma are summarised in Box 23.1.

Spread of Gastric Cancer

Invasive gastric cancer progresses to involve submucosal lymphatics, and the depth of penetration through the gastric wall correlates closely with the likelihood of nodal metastases. The tumour node metastasis (TNM) system is now the standard staging structure agreed internationally, with additional Japanese nomenclature designating particular groups of lymph nodes draining the stomach as **stations**, numbered 1–16. Lymphatic metastatic spread initially involves nodes in the perigastric and periduodenal area; these are known as *perigastric stations 1–6*. Involvement of these is considered N1 in the TNM system; their clearance along with gastrectomy is known as a *D1 resection*. Positive nodes along the main arteries of the coeliac axis, splenic hilum and porta hepatis constitute the N2 stations (6–12).

- Often asymptomatic until a late stage
- Nonspecific epigastric pain and dyspepsia
- Iron deficiency anaemia
- Nausea and vomiting
- Anorexia and early satiety
- Feeling of abdominal fullness or discomfort
- Marked weight loss (cachexia)—late stage
- Epigastric mass (late stage)
- Left supraclavicular mass (metastasis in Virchow node)
- Obstructive jaundice (metastases in the porta hepatis)
- Pelvic mass (metastases to ovaries)

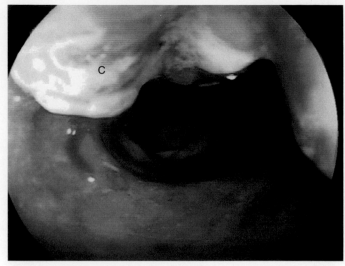

• **Fig. 23.2** Endoscopic View of Carcinoma of the Stomach. Gastroscopic view of large fungating intestinal-type carcinoma of stomach in the prepyloric region (C). Diagnosis was confirmed by endoscopic biopsy.

Nodes in the retroduodenal and paraaortic area constitute N3 or even M1 stations. Clearance of N1 and N2 lymph node stations is achieved by the radical D2 gastrectomy (pioneered in Japan). Histological examination of the resected lymph nodes enhances the accuracy of TNM staging and improves the ability to predict long-term survival after surgery.

Direct Spread and Metastasis

- **Direct spread** into the transverse colon is not unusual in advanced cases and sometimes results in **gastrocolic fistula** formation, with true faecal vomiting.
- **Transperitoneal (or transcoelomic) spread** may involve the surface of the ovaries (**Krukenberg tumour**) or form masses in the pouch of Douglas; a mass is often palpable on rectal examination. Transcoelomic spread can result in peritoneal disease and rarely an umbilical nodule (Sister Mary Joseph nodule).
- **Remote lymph node spread**—the left supraclavicular (**Virchow**) lymph node classically becomes invaded via the thoracic duct, giving a palpable mass (**Troisier sign**) sometimes found at initial presentation.
- **Haematogenous spread** to involve liver, lungs, brain and bone is common.

Investigation of Suspected Gastric Carcinoma

Initial Diagnosis

Early detection radically increases the chances of curing the condition. A high index of suspicion and early endoscopy for nonspecific symptoms improve these chances. In one American series where early endoscopy was the rule, only 15% of gastric cancers were unsuitable for operation at initial diagnosis, and half the operations were performed with the aim of cure.

In areas with a high incidence of gastric cancer, **endoscopic screening** (Fig. 23.2) is an effective and popular method of detecting early disease. It is widely used in Japan, with the result that over 40% of cancers operated upon after screening have been in a presymptomatic stage and can truly be defined histologically as 'early gastric cancer'. About 90% of these patients undergo potentially curative operations.

Barium meal used to be the standard investigation, but it was difficult to differentiate between benign gastric ulcer and carcinoma. The radiological appearances of a typical gastric malignancy is shown in Fig. 23.3 for historical reasons. **Endoscopy**, which allows visual inspection and biopsy, is now the standard investigation. The site of a lesion may be important as benign ulcers are usually found on the lesser curve or in the prepyloric area, whereas carcinomas arise in any part of the stomach. The initial endoscopy in a patient found to have carcinoma gives an accurate diagnosis in

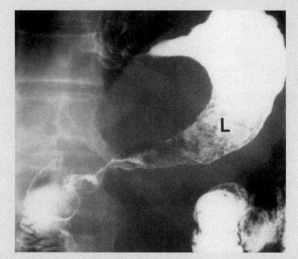

• **Fig. 23.3** Barium Meal Showing Linitis Plastica. Linitis plastica-type infiltrating carcinoma of the stomach (L). Note the shrunken appearance of the whole stomach caused by widespread submucosal invasion of the tumour. Endoscopic biopsy may not give the correct diagnosis because the mucosa is often intact. This 60-year-old woman presented with anorexia. She had a total gastrectomy but died 5 months later of widespread metastases.

90% of those with **exophytic** lesions (where the tumour grows out into the lumen) but only 50% for **infiltrating** lesions (Fig. 23.3). Multiple biopsies improve these rates, as do repeat endoscopy and rebiopsy of suspicious lesions.

Staging

Once cancer is diagnosed, knowing the stage helps determine the most appropriate treatment and whether surgery is likely to benefit the patient. Computed tomography (**CT**) **scanning of chest and abdomen** is often the first investigation, and many patients are found to already have local tumour invasion, lymph node involvement and hepatic metastases already by this stage. Staging

laparoscopy is essential as CT scanning can miss small nodules on the stomach serosa, peritoneum, omentum and liver surface. **Endoscopic ultrasonography** (EUS) via a flexible endoscope is highly accurate for determining the depth of penetration of small gastric cancers, and hence the 'T' (tumour) stage. Local spread (e.g., into pancreas), nodal involvement, left hepatic lobe metastases and ascites are also demonstrable by this method. Finally, fluorodeoxyglucose positron emission tomography (PET), known as **PET scanning**, is increasingly used to search for metastatic disease not identified by any other modality.

Management of Gastric Carcinoma

Like oesophageal cancer, gastric cancer is increasingly managed in specialist centres. This consolidates surgical, radiological and oncological expertise and ensures that other professionals, such as anaesthetists, theatre staff, intensive care and high-dependency unit staff, dieticians and physiotherapists become experienced in managing these cases and can all contribute to a multidisciplinary team.

Radical Surgery

As described, metastasis from gastric cancer is often early, widespread and occult. For this reason, **radical surgery** offers the only prospect of cure even when the tumour appears small. Radical gastrectomies are very major operations and careful staging is needed to ensure that there is a realistic chance of cure, together with thorough assessment of general fitness.

Japanese surgeons have developed radical D1 and D2 gastrectomies for patients where cure is the intention. Both involve total or subtotal gastrectomy; D1 involves N1 nodal stations, whilst D2 removes N1 and N2 nodal stations. In Japan, if the cancer proves to be confined to mucosa and submucosa, 5-year survival approaches 90%; with local node involvement, survival is about 50%. With more distant spread, survival falls dramatically to 5%. Western results are gradually approaching Japanese survival figures. Just as in oesophageal cancer, survival is improving because of better patient selection, improved perioperative care, centralisation of care in specialist centres and the advent of neoadjuvant treatment.

Chemotherapy and Radiotherapy

Gastric cancers respond to both chemotherapy and radiotherapy. The epirubicin–cisplatin–5-fluorouracil regimen is effective against gastric cancer and the MAGIC (Medical Research Council Adjuvant Gastric Infusional Chemotherapy) trial published in 2006 improved 5-year survival from 23% for surgery alone to 36% for preoperative chemotherapy and surgery. Combined pre- and postoperative treatment is now the standard of care for resectable gastric cancer.

Radiotherapy has not been regularly used in gastric cancer but may have a place in palliation, particularly for local recurrence.

Palliative Procedures

For patients with advanced cancer, it is wrong to perform palliative surgery where modern methods of palliation are available. Palliative surgical resections or bypasses are then rarely necessary. If tumour bleeding, necrosis or encroachment on the gastric lumen results in distressing symptoms, such as nausea, anorexia, vomiting or symptoms of anaemia, palliative chemotherapy or radiotherapy may be required. Gastric outlet obstruction may be relieved by placing a self-expanding intraluminal stent across the obstructing pyloric cancer, but a laparoscopic bypass (gastrojejunostomy) procedure may occasionally be required.

Gastric Polyps

Most gastric polyps are benign **hyperplastic nodules** of gastric mucosa. They may be single or multiple and can occur anywhere in the stomach. They almost never become malignant.

Genuine **adenomatous polyps** are rare. These are true neoplasms, with histological and morphological forms similar to adenomatous polyps of the large intestine (see Ch. 27). Adenomas are usually single, large and asymptomatic. Most are found incidentally on endoscopic examination. Up to 40% show histological features of malignancy. Treatment is by endoscopic excision (**endoscopic mucosal resection**).

Gastrointestinal Stromal Tumours

GISTs are rare mesenchymal tumours that can arise anywhere in the GI tract. They were once thought to be leiomyomas because of the histological similarity but immunocytochemical markers can now distinguish mesenchymal tissue types and differentiate them from muscle and nerve tumours. GISTs have now been identified as originating from the **interstitial cells of Cajal**, the so-called pacemakers of gut motility. GISTs are most frequently found in the stomach and can range from <1 cm to >20 cm. The risk of malignancy is determined partly by tumour location but mostly by size and histological mitotic index (Table 23.1). Most gastric GISTs are small (<5 cm) and have a low mitotic index.

GISTs are often diagnosed incidentally at endoscopy or in patients having abdominal CT scans for other reasons. They can be sessile (domed) or pedunculated intramural lesions covered by normal mucosa (Fig. 23.4B). Small lesions may be asymptomatic; large lesions produce symptoms or signs of any abdominal mass. Gastric tumours are prone to haemorrhage via a central 'umbilicated' ulcer (Fig. 23.4A); these are typically found after an acute episode of haematemesis or melaena. Following diagnosis and before surgery, the patient may need to be staged by CT to confirm the size and exclude metastases (usually hepatic, rarely nodal). Suitable biopsies allow immunocytochemical analysis, but it can be difficult to obtain sufficiently deep samples. Deeper biopsies are facilitated EUS. Local resection, usually in the form of a wedge resection, is appropriate if the lesion has low malignant potential. Unlike, gastric adenocarcinomas, malignant GISTs do not require a more extensive lymphadenectomy.

GIST tumours are highly resistant to traditional chemotherapy; however, the c-kit tyrosine kinase inhibitor, imatinib (Gleevec), is highly effective for advanced and metastatic disease and has improved 2-year survival rates to 75% to 80%.

TABLE 23.1	Risk of Aggressive Behaviour of Gastrointestinal Stromal Tumours (GIST)	
Risk of Aggressive Behaviour (Malignant Potential)	Greatest Dimension (cm)	Mitoses Per 50 Microscope High-Power Fields
Very low	<2	<5
Low	2–5	<5
Intermediate	<5	6–10
	5–10	<5
High	>5	>5
	>10	Any number
	Any size	>10

CASE HISTORIES

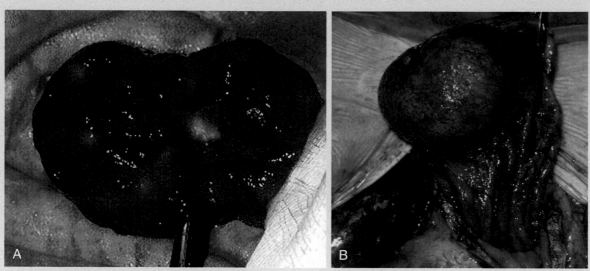

• **Fig. 23.4** Gastrointestinal Stromal Tumour (GIST). **(A)** This 64-year-old woman presented with recurrent iron deficiency anaemia. A large ulcerated polyp had been seen at endoscopy. Here, the stomach has been opened at laparotomy and the polyp is held up in the surgeon's hand. Deep peptic ulcers can be seen on its surface. Histologically, it proved to be a GIST. **(B)** Another GIST, which had become impacted in the pylorus causing gastric outlet obstruction. It was delivered through the gastrotomy, excised and the defect closed with sutures.

CASE HISTORY

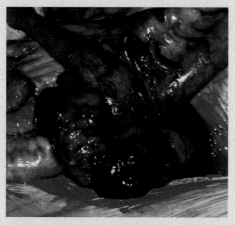

• **Fig. 23.5** Malignant Gastrointestinal Stromal Tumour (leiomyosarcoma) of the Jejunum. This operative specimen shows a large fleshy lesion on the outer surface of the upper jejunum. The patient was a 33-year-old woman who presented with iron deficiency anaemia refractory to oral iron. An abnormality was finally seen on a barium small bowel study after many fruitless investigations. This tumour was histologically well differentiated and amenable to resection; after 5 years, there was no recurrence.

Small Bowel Gastrointestinal Stromal Tumours

GISTs of small bowel are histologically similar to gastric tumours but may present by obstructing the lumen or growing out from the serosal surface of the bowel (Fig. 23.5). Primary resection and anastomosis is the usual treatment and survival is influenced by the size and mitotic index.

Gastric and Small Bowel Lymphomas

Pathology and Clinical Features of Lymphomas

Primary lymphomas sometimes arise in the stomach or small bowel. They constitute about 10% of gastric malignancies. As with peptic ulcer and intestinal-type gastric adenocarcinoma, *H. pylori* infection is an important initiating factor. In non-Hodgkin lymphoma, small bowel lymphoid tissue may become involved.

In the stomach, most lymphomas are non-Hodgkin lymphomas of B-cell origin. They may become extensive, diffusely infiltrating the stomach wall or, less often, projecting into the lumen as bulky ulcerating masses. The symptoms and endoscopic appearances closely resemble gastric adenocarcinoma but recognising lymphoma is important because the treatment is very different and the prognosis much better. Unlike gastric carcinoma, lymphomas tend to occur in children and young adults. Some cases of low-grade lymphoma involving the MALT or 'MALTomas' have been reported to resolve following *Helicobacter* eradication, but this is only successful if the disease is detected early.

In the small intestine, lymphomas also produce bulky lesions, which may obstruct, ulcerate, bleed or even perforate. Occasionally, a lymphoma provides the focus for an intussusception (see Figs 23.6 and 23.7 and also Fig. 50.12, p. 645). Small bowel lymphoma may be a complication of coeliac disease but the risk is only about six times higher than for the general population.

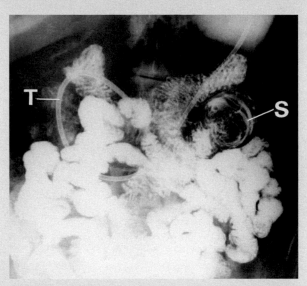

• **Fig. 23.6** **Intussuscepting Tumour of Small Bowel.** This 35-year-old woman suffered several self-limiting episodes of small bowel obstruction. During one of those episodes, this small bowel barium enema was performed by placing the tip of a nasojejunal tube *(T)* just distal to the duodenojejunal flexure and instilling barium. A small bowel intussusception is demonstrated by the 'coiled spring' sign *(S)*, caused by the presence of barium between the telescoping layers of bowel. At surgery, a gastrointestinal stromal tumour was found to be responsible.

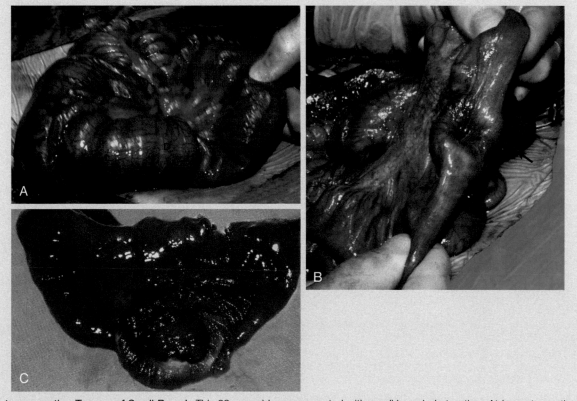

• **Fig. 23.7** **Intussuscepting Tumour of Small Bowel.** This 22-year-old man presented with small bowel obstruction. At laparotomy, the obstruction was found to be caused by an ileoileal intussusception. This set of operative photographs **(A)** shows how the proximal ileum *(P)* had intussuscepted into the distal ileum *(D)*. When this was reduced **(B)**, an abnormality of the bowel wall could be seen to have formed the apex of the intussuscipiens *(arrowed)*. In **(C)**, a polypoid tumour can be seen on the luminal surface, which proved histologically to be a lymphoma.

Management of Lymphomas

Gastric lymphomas are usually treated with primary chemotherapy using the cyclophosphamide, doxorubicin, vincristine, and prednisone regimen, sometimes with the addition of rituximab, and subtotal gastrectomy is rarely needed unless the tumour bleeds persistently or perforates. Primary **small bowel** lymphomas are often localised lesions, amenable to surgical excision. Postoperative radiotherapy or chemotherapy or both may be necessary. Treatment gives a 5-year survival rate of around 50%.

Carcinoid Tumours

Pathology of Carcinoid Tumours

Carcinoid tumours probably arise from APUD cells of the GI endocrine system. Thus they can arise anywhere in the GI tract or in tissues embryologically derived from it, including the pancreas and biliary system. More than 50% of carcinoid tumours are found in the appendix, and most of the rest occur in the small intestine.

Clinical Presentation of Carcinoid Tumours

Appendiceal carcinoid tumours are usually discovered incidentally in appendicectomy specimens and virtually always remain small and benign. In contrast, carcinoid tumours elsewhere spread locally in the bowel and mesentery, later becoming disseminated to the liver and other sites. The bowel lesions themselves usually present with symptoms of partial or complete obstruction.

Carcinoid tumours secrete a variety of catecholamines, including **serotonin**. When there is a large volume of tumour, usually in the form of liver metastases, enough catecholamines are secreted to cause the **carcinoid syndrome**. This is characterised by an array of clinical phenomena including transient 'hot flushes', hypotension, asthma and diarrhoea. A metabolite of serotonin, **5-hydroxy-indoleacetic acid**, can be measured in the urine as a diagnostic marker.

Management of Carcinoid Tumours

Treatment usually involves excising the primary lesion along with local lymph nodes. An appendiceal carcinoid present at the tip only and less than 2 cm in diameter can be treated by simple appendicectomy. In patients with metastatic disease, the condition progresses very slowly. It responds well to surgery, and in the typical young patient a more radical approach can be recommended than for other intraabdominal malignancies. Metastatic carcinoid is not curable by radiotherapy or chemotherapy.

The full carcinoid syndrome is usually associated with large volume hepatic metastases. It is uncommon and symptoms can be controlled with the help of drugs, such as **octreotide**, a somatostatin analogue. Radiotherapy is useful if pain is caused by massive liver enlargement as it may induce some shrinkage.

Other Tumours of the Small Intestine

Small bowel tumours include **solitary benign angiomas**. These are usually found incidentally at operation or autopsy but sometimes present with intussusception or chronic haemorrhage.

Adenocarcinomas do occur in the small intestine, especially in the duodenum, but are rare compared with stomach and large bowel. Small bowel adenocarcinomas present with bowel obstruction, biliary obstruction when in the periampullary region, bleeding or symptoms of metastases. Barium follow-through examination or an abdominal CT scan for chronic symptoms may demonstrate the lesion, but more commonly it is found and resected at a laparotomy for acute obstruction, only being recognised on histological examination. Unfortunately, metastasis to regional lymph nodes or the liver has already occurred in many patients by the time of presentation.

Peutz–Jeghers syndrome is described in Chapter 27 (p. 378).

24

Tumours of the Pancreas and Hepatobiliary System; the Spleen

Introduction

More than 90% of pancreatic cancers are adenocarcinomas derived from exocrine ductal cells. These have the worst survival of all gastrointestinal (GI) malignancies, with only about 12% surviving 1 year and 2% surviving 5 years. Much less commonly, neoplasia arises from **exocrine acinar (secretory) cells** (2%) or from **endocrine islet cells** (8%). Most endocrine tumours present with excess hormone secretion, for example, insulin, glucagon or gastrin. Around 90% of insulinomas are benign but most others are malignant, although survival is often prolonged.

Ductal adenocarcinoma typically presents late, with intractable abdominal pain, weight loss and obstructive jaundice caused by common bile duct compression, also a frequent presentation of the uncommon **periampullary carcinomas**. These include biliary cholangiocarcinomas and adenocarcinomas of the ampulla of Vater and duodenum.

Primary sclerosing cholangitis (PSC) is a rare, nonmalignant liver disease involving inflammatory fibrosis of bile ducts. It presents similarly to pancreatic cancer and is therefore included in this chapter. The uncommon **carcinoma of gall bladder** often presents with cholecystitis symptoms, with jaundice developing later.

Primary liver tumours are infrequent in developed countries but common in some developing countries, where hepatitis B and C are the main predisposing factors. **Secondary liver tumours** are common everywhere from haematogenous spread of many types of cancer. Surgical disorders of the spleen are covered at the end of this chapter.

Carcinoma of the Pancreas

Pathology

This is usually an adenocarcinoma arising from cells lining the ducts. About 60% to 70% arise in the head (the largest part) and 30% to 40% in the body or tail. Cancers often form a well-differentiated ductular pattern but despite this, it is a highly malignant tumour. It metastasises early to lymph nodes, to peritoneum, and to liver via the portal vein (Fig. 24.1). At presentation, less than 20% are resectable and the overall prognosis is dire.

Pancreatic cancer presents at a mean age of 65 years and is rare under 50 years. The incidence is similar in males and females, and in the Western world, ranks equal third with oesophageal cancer among GI cancers, after large bowel and stomach. In absolute numbers, it is uncommon, being responsible for about 7000 deaths each year in the United Kingdom, although numbers in developed countries continue to rise. Risk factors include cigarette smoking (2–3 times the risk and presenting 15 years earlier), chronic pancreatitis (18 times risk, increasing to over 50 times in hereditary pancreatitis), obesity/type II diabetes (twice the risk), and positive family history.

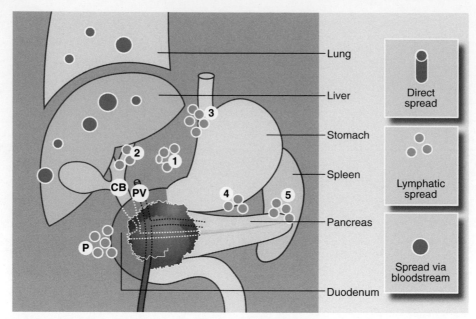

• **Fig. 24.1** Spread of Carcinoma of the Pancreas. Direct spread may involve the common bile duct (CB) where it traverses the pancreas, the duodenum and the portal vein (PV). Lymphatic spread may reach the paraduodenal peritoneum (P) and the nodes of the coeliac axis (1), the porta hepatis (2), the lesser and greater curves of the stomach (3, 4) and the hilum of the spleen (5). Spread may also occur via the bloodstream to the liver, lungs, etc.

• BOX 24.1 Presenting Features Of Pancreatic Carcinoma

Common Presenting Features
- Substantial weight loss (about 80% of cases)
- Abdominal pain (about 60%)
- Obstructive jaundice, often without pain (about 50%)

Less Common Presenting Features
- Acute pancreatitis (rare)
- Diabetes mellitus (preceding or following diagnosis)
- Gastric outlet obstruction (because of external compression)
- Thrombophlebitis migrans (recurrent superficial venous thromboses)
- Pancreatic steatorrhoea (because of pancreatic duct obstruction)

Clinical Features of Ductal Pancreatic Carcinoma

There are no useful screening tests and so pancreatic cancer nearly always presents with symptoms and signs. The main features are substantial weight loss (80%), abdominal pain (60%) and obstructive jaundice (50%). Ascites and an abdominal mass are uncommon (Box 24.1).

Pain and Other Abdominal Symptoms and Signs

The **pain** of advanced pancreatic carcinoma is severe and continuous and typically described as 'deep' and 'gnawing'; it may drive patients to suicide. It is often nocturnal and poorly relieved by analgesics but sometimes alleviated by leaning forwards from sitting ('the pancreatic position'). Severe pain usually represents locally advanced disease, with extrapancreatic invasion into retroperitoneal nerves around the coeliac axis. There are often ill-defined **dyspeptic symptoms**, such as

anorexia, nausea or sporadic vomiting and usually profound **weight loss**.

Obstructive Jaundice

Jaundice, often without pain early on, develops over several weeks, and is associated with pale stools and dark urine. These clinical features are dramatic and never ignored. The jaundice is caused by common bile duct compression in its course through the pancreatic head. As a result, the proximal bile duct dilates and the gall bladder may become palpable (**Courvoisier law**, see Ch. 18, p. 285). Bile duct obstruction may also be caused by metastases in porta hepatis lymph nodes. Liver metastases alone rarely cause jaundice.

Note that pancreatic cancer and other obstructing biliary tumours typically produce a painless and progressive jaundice. In contrast, that of gallstone disease is less intense and fluctuates in intensity, and there is usually typical biliary pain.

Approach to Investigation of Suspected Pancreatic Carcinoma (Box 24.2)

A patient with obstructive jaundice should be investigated as described in Chapter 18, p. 286. If pancreatic cancer is likely, optimum management is via a streamlined diagnostic pathway carried out in a specialised, high-volume pancreatic centre.

When investigations are complete, the multidisciplinary team considers whether curative treatment is feasible and how to plan and implement it, or if not appropriate, what palliative treatment is needed.

Computed Tomography and Ultrasound Imaging

Ultrasound seeks masses in pancreas and liver, dilated bile ducts and stones in the gall bladder (abdominal ultrasound is

If patient jaundiced—suspect diagnosis from age, typical history, signs, liver function tests.
If patient not jaundiced—suspect diagnosis on abnormal ultrasound or computed tomography (CT, differential diagnosis is often pancreatitis).

- **Primary imaging**—usually CT scan
- **Confirm histology**—CT-guided biopsy, endoscopic ultrasound-guided needle aspiration cytology
- **Assess primary tumour in detail**—site, size, local invasion especially of blood vessels using ultrasound, high-definition CT
- **Assess metastatic spread**—liver, nodes, peritoneum using CT, laparoscopy, ± laparoscopic ultrasound

unreliable for common bile duct stones). Additional detail about a mass comes from high-resolution computed tomography (CT) scans, ideally before endoscopic retrograde cholangiopancreatography (ERCP) to ensure an artefact-free field. CT can show tumour extent and the presence and volume of liver metastases. It can demonstrate **vascular invasion** of superior mesenteric and portal veins, and superior mesenteric artery and coeliac axis, any of which lessen the feasibility of surgical resection. The extent of primary and/or metastatic disease on imaging may indicate the tumour is **inoperable** (i.e., not resectable with intent to cure). Palliation can then be used and the patient saved a fruitless attempt at resection.

Endoscopic Ultrasound and Needle Aspiration Cytology

Where ultrasound and/or CT indicate a pancreatic head carcinoma may be resectable, **endoscopic ultrasound** (EUS) can give added detail. In this, an ultrasound probe is positioned in the second part of the duodenum via a gastroscope. This allows precise examination of the pancreatic head and associated vessels, as well as duodenum and ampullary region.

Ultrasound-guided **needle aspiration** sampling of suspicious lesions can be performed via the gastric lumen for cytology, either before surgery or to guide oncological management. EUS is the gold standard for assessing tumour size, site and vascular involvement and thus potential operability. However, its accuracy is severely impaired if a stent has already been placed to relieve jaundice.

Magnetic Resonance Cholangiopancreatography

In biliary obstruction, magnetic resonance cholangiopancreatography (MRCP) produces images similar to ERCP in diagnostic usefulness, but is particularly useful for confirming choledocholithiasis (bile duct stones) or for obstructive lesions of the bile duct itself, such as cholangiocarcinoma or PSC.

Endoscopic Retrograde Cholangiopancreatography and Therapeutic Intervention

ERCP is now largely used for therapeutic intervention. For obstructive jaundice caused by stone, ERCP is the main mechanism for removing duct stones. For inoperable carcinoma of the pancreatic head, placing a tubular stent across the obstruction allows palliation of jaundice by draining the biliary tree. Plastic stents eventually become encrusted and occluded so wider bore expanding metallic stents are now more often used.

Lesions in the Body and Tail of the Pancreas

When pancreatic cancer is suspected in a nonjaundiced patient, abdominal CT can confirm the diagnosis more reliably than ultrasound, although small tumours may be missed (see Fig. 24.2A and B). CT scanning also indicates retroperitoneal and portal vein invasion; it shows metastases in liver and lymph nodes and CT-guided needle biopsy can obtain histopathology specimens, all of which can determine resectability. CT scanning can understage the disease, chiefly because it does not detect small-volume hepatic and peritoneal deposits.

CASE HISTORIES

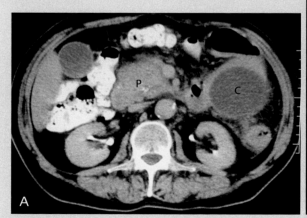
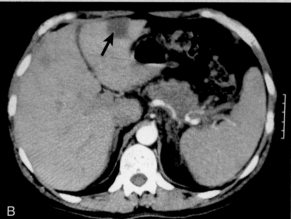

• **Fig. 24.2 Carcinoma of the Head of the Pancreas.** **(A)** Computed tomography (CT) scan showing enlargement of the head of the pancreas *(P)* most suspicious of carcinoma. The dark circular lesion within the tail of the pancreas is a secondary cyst or pseudocyst *(C)*. **(B)** CT scan further cephalad (towards the head) of the same patient showing one obvious low-attenuation lesion in the liver consistent with a metastasis *(arrowed)*. The diagnosis of carcinoma of the pancreas was confirmed on percutaneous biopsy of the pancreatic lesion. Thus this 54-year-old man had inoperable disease. Unfortunately, this is all too common a presentation.

EUS via the stomach can examine the pancreatic body and tail and allow aspiration cytology. Cancers here do not cause the early warning sign of jaundice and hence tend to present so late that resectability is highly unlikely.

Staging laparoscopy may be included as a final evaluation before resection, allowing inspection and biopsy of peritoneum for small metastases; diagnostic laparoscopic ultrasound has largely been superseded by high-definition CT and EUS. Accurate staging means resection can be offered to those most likely to benefit, whilst avoiding unnecessary surgery in the rest.

Cystic Neoplasms of the Pancreas

Cystic neoplasms are sometimes discovered incidentally on CT or ultrasonography, with the investigation prompted by nonspecific upper abdominal symptoms. Cystic neoplasms can be difficult to differentiate from pancreatic pseudocysts but CT and endoscopic ultrasound (EUS) can define morphology and allow aspiration for cytology and biochemical analysis (e.g., carcinoembryonic antigen, CA19.9 and amylase). After excluding pseudocyst, the differential diagnosis includes **serous** and **mucinous cystadenomas** and **cystadenocarcinomas**. If EUS-guided aspiration confirms a **serous** cystadenoma, then no further intervention is required as these exhibit benign behaviour despite becoming quite large in some cases. Mucinous cystadenomas and intraductal papillary mucinous neoplasms (IPMNs) carry significant malignant potential and, where feasible, resection is recommended. IPMNs arising within the pancreatic ductal side branches have indeterminate malignant risk and in the absence of adverse radiological, biochemical or cytological features, surveillance with regular imaging is undertaken.

Management of Pancreatic Carcinoma

Surgical Resection and Adjuvant Therapy

It is an unfortunate truth that most patients with pancreatic cancer present at an incurable stage. Only about 15% to 20% have apparently localised disease with a potential for surgical cure. **Whipple operation** (pancreaticoduodenectomy, see Fig. 24.6, p. 355) is the standard type of operation where resection of the pancreatic head is indicated. It is a major undertaking with high operative morbidity and mortality; even in specialist centres, mortality is 1% to 2% with a 15% to 20% morbidity (pancreatic leaks, delayed gastric emptying, wound infections) and a 5-year survival of only 15% to 20%.

Postoperative combination chemotherapy with gemcitabine and capecitabine confers a modest survival advantage. Clinical trials investigating the role of chemoradiation, neoadjuvant therapy and immunotherapy are ongoing and newer combinations (e.g., Folfirinox) and other agents (e.g., NAB Paclitaxel) are showing promise in clinical practice.

Palliation of Pancreatic Cancer

When there is obvious widespread disease, the patient should be allowed to die with minimal surgical interference but with careful attention to symptom control. Good analgesia is fundamental; severe pain can often be relieved by permanent **coeliac ganglion blockade**, performed percutaneously. **Obstructive jaundice** can usually be relieved by inserting a biliary stent at ERCP. If unsuccessful, a percutaneous transhepatic cholangiogram can help pass a guidewire to the duodenum to facilitate ERCP or else place a stent from earlier; techniques are illustrated in Fig. 24.3. Surgical bypass (usually a **'triple bypass'**, see Fig. 24.3) may provide longer-lasting relief from jaundice and duodenal obstruction than stenting. Duodenal obstruction alone can be bypassed by endoscopic stent placement or laparoscopic gastroenterostomy.

Endocrine Tumours of the Pancreas

Neuroendocrine cells of the islets of Langerhans give rise to several uncommon tumours. These often produce excess hormone secretions responsible for the presenting features. Islet cells make up 2% of the pancreatic mass and comprise cells of four types: **alpha cells** secrete glucagon, **beta cells** secrete insulin, **delta cells** secrete somatostatin and **F** or **PP cells** secrete pancreatic polypeptide.

Insulinomas

The most common endocrine tumours are **insulinomas** derived from beta cells, but they occur in only 1.7 per million people per year. The main symptoms are cerebral disturbances caused by hypoglycaemic attacks, often when fasting or exercising and relieved by oral or intravenous glucose (Fig. 24.4). About 90% of insulinomas are single and 90% are benign and amenable to curative resection. They occur with equal frequency in the head, body and tail of the pancreas. Malignancy is only diagnosed if metastases appear.

The diagnosis is usually made late, often after hypoglycaemic attacks have caused accusations of alcoholism or referrals for psychiatric or neurological advice for abnormal behaviour or epilepsy. When inappropriate hyperinsulinaemia has been confirmed, CT scanning, magnetic resonance imaging (MRI) and EUS usually identify the lesion. If unsuccessful, venous sampling may help and intraoperative ultrasound and palpation can usually locate otherwise invisible lesions. Insulinomas are usually small and can be treated by enucleation, although larger or deep lesions may need pancreatic resection.

Glucagonomas

Alpha cells may give rise to **glucagonomas**; these are very rare and present with diabetes mellitus and a characteristic skin rash known as **migratory necrolytic erythema**.

Gastrinomas

Gastrin-secreting tumours (**gastrinomas**) occur once per million people per year. They arise in pancreatic islets or in ectopic cells in the duodenal wall. About 25% occur in patients with multiple endocrine neoplasia type 1 (MEN 1), described later. Gastrinomas cause severe and intractable peptic ulceration and diarrhoea known as **Zollinger–Ellison syndrome**.

The diagnosis is made by demonstrating persistently high serum gastrin. The tumour is localised and staged by CT, MRI, EUS and octreotide scan. Many lesions are too small to show on standard imaging and can only be located by intraoperative ultrasonography at laparotomy. About 60% are malignant but they grow slowly and metastasise late, so excision is often curative. If the primary tumour is inoperable, palliation with high-dose **proton-pump inhibitors** often prevents peptic ulcer symptoms and complications.

Multiple Endocrine Neoplasia Syndromes

Pancreatic neuroendocrine tumours sometimes occur in inherited autosomal dominant multiple endocrine neoplasia syndromes (MEN). Two main types are recognised, MEN 1 and MEN 2.

- MEN 1—islet cell tumours, pituitary adenomas and parathyroid hyperplasia
- MEN 2a—medullary thyroid carcinoma (often in childhood), phaeochromocytoma and parathyroid adenoma or hyperplasia
- MEN 2b—medullary thyroid carcinoma, phaeochromocytoma, mucosal neuromas and GI ganglioneuromas and Marfanoid features

CASE HISTORY

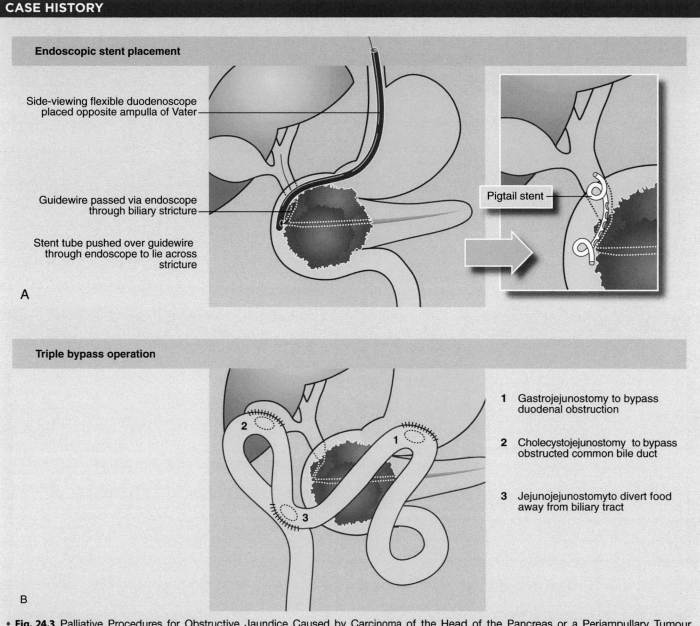

Endoscopic stent placement

Side-viewing flexible duodenoscope placed opposite ampulla of Vater

Guidewire passed via endoscope through biliary stricture

Stent tube pushed over guidewire through endoscope to lie across stricture

A

Pigtail stent

Triple bypass operation

1 Gastrojejunostomy to bypass duodenal obstruction

2 Cholecystojejunostomy to bypass obstructed common bile duct

3 Jejunojejunostomyto divert food away from biliary tract

B

• **Fig. 24.3** Palliative Procedures for Obstructive Jaundice Caused by Carcinoma of the Head of the Pancreas or a Periampullary Tumour. **(A)** Endoscopic stent placement. The sphincter of Oddi may require a preliminary endoscopic sphincterotomy before intubation. A self-retaining plastic stent, placed endoscopically or percutaneously, lies in situ across the biliary stricture. Note the 'pig-tail' ends of this type of stent which curl up when the wire is removed, retaining the stent in the correct position. **(B)** Triple bypass operation, less commonly performed nowadays because of the efficacy of endoscopic stenting and the short-life expectancy of patients with pancreatic cancer.

Biliary and Periampullary Tumours

Adenocarcinomas originating from biliary duct epithelium are known as **cholangiocarcinomas**. They develop anywhere in the intra- or extrahepatic duct system but are more common near the confluence of right and left hepatic ducts (Klatskin tumour). The less common **intrahepatic cholangiocarcinomas** present like primary hepatocellular carcinomas but most of the biliary system remains patent so jaundice is rare. In contrast, **extrahepatic cholangiocarcinomas** usually obstruct bile drainage and present with painless progressive jaundice. Cholangiocarcinomas are more frequent in **PSC**. Distinguishing cholangiocarcinoma from the hallmark multiple strictures of sclerosing cholangitis can be taxing.

Cholangiocarcinomas have a dense fibrous stroma and grow along ducts rather than producing focal proliferative lesions. The resulting smooth elongated stricture can be demonstrated by ERCP, MRCP or transhepatic cholangiography (see Fig. 24.5). Histological proof of malignancy may be elusive owing to the fibrous nature of the tumour. Unlike pancreatic cancer, cholangiocarcinomas are often slow-growing and metastasise late. Despite this, lymph node involvement at presentation is common, and extension along bile ducts and involvement of portal vein and hepatic arterial branches results in a low operability rate and an even lower long-term survival. Radical procedures combining partial hepatectomy with excision of the involved biliary tree and 'en bloc' portal vein resection and reconstruction may offer better clearance and improved survival for selected patients.

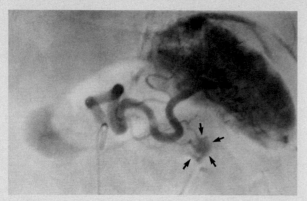

• **Fig. 24.4** Insulinoma as Seen on a Selective Arteriogram (Subtraction Film). This 31-year-old woman suffered from bouts of faintness, which proved to be caused by intermittent hypoglycaemia. Selective splenic arteriography demonstrated an abnormal mass of blood vessels about 1.5 cm in diameter *(arrowed)* in the tail of the pancreas representing an insulinoma. The tail of the pancreas was excised and the patient's symptoms disappeared.

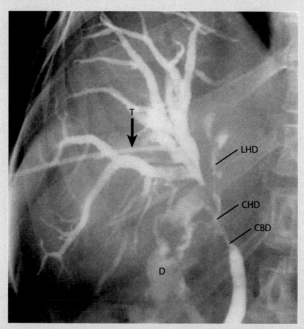

• **Fig. 24.5** Cholangiocarcinoma. Percutaneous transhepatic cholangiogram in a 66-year-old man with painless progressive jaundice from an inoperable cholangiocarcinoma; this x-ray shows a long stricture of the common bile duct *(CBD)*, common hepatic duct *(CHD)* and left hepatic duct *(LHD)*. Some contrast has flowed through into the duodenum. The cystic duct is obliterated, preventing filling of the gall bladder. A percutaneous drainage tube *(T)* has been inserted into the right hepatic duct system before an attempt to place a stent across the stricture by the same route. Some contrast has flowed through into the duodenum (D). Nowadays, most stents are placed endoscopically (see Fig. 24.3).

An unusual lesion is adenocarcinoma of the ampulla of Vater. Here it forms a polypoid lesion projecting into the duodenum and obstructing biliary drainage causing jaundice. Tumours are friable and bleed persistently, giving positive faecal occult bloods. An association with intestinal polyposis syndromes has been described. Diagnosis is made at endoscopy by inspection and biopsy. Very rarely, adenocarcinoma arises in the duodenal mucosa and causes obstructive jaundice if close to the ampulla. Again, the lesion is readily diagnosed at ERCP/ EUS and biopsy.

Management of Extrahepatic Cholangiocarcinoma and Periampullary Carcinoma

Extrahepatic and periampullary cancers can often be successfully treated by Whipple pancreaticoduodenectomy, Fig. 24.6.

Carcinoma of the Gall Bladder

Carcinoma of the gall bladder is predominantly a disease of old age and is nearly always associated with stones. Chronic inflammation is the likely carcinogenic factor. Early diagnosis is usually made incidentally at cholecystectomy and in this special case, wide excision of the gall bladder bed plus hilar lymphadenectomy may offer a chance of cure. In most, the diagnosis is late with advanced disease and jaundice. Direct invasion of liver plus lymphatic spread make resection impracticable and survival is usually short.

Primary Sclerosing Cholangitis

This is a rare condition, probably of autoimmune origin, causing progressive fibrosis and multiple biliary strictures. Luminal narrowing causes gradual and progressive obstructive jaundice and, later, secondary cirrhosis. It may arise sporadically but often occurs in longstanding ulcerative colitis. Bile duct stenosis is usually diffuse, with a characteristic MRCP/ERCP appearance (see Fig. 24.7), but just occasionally, it is localised to the extrahepatic biliary system. Here the radiological appearance is indistinguishable from cholangiocarcinoma, causing a diagnostic predicament. 'Spy-glass' endoscopy of the biliary tree via ERCP can be useful in such cases, allowing direct visualisation of strictures and biopsy for histology. Management is by endoscopic dilatation of clinically significant strictures and prescribing choleretic drugs to improve bile flow. In advanced cases, liver transplantation is an option; interestingly, up to a third demonstrate cholangiocarcinoma in the excised liver.

Liver Tumours and Abscesses

Primary malignant liver tumours are uncommon in developed countries; most are **hepatocellular carcinomas** derived from hepatocytes. Even less commonly, other elements give rise to tumours, such as **angiosarcoma**. Benign liver lesions are increasingly found incidentally during ultrasound for gallstones. The most frequent are benign cysts and haemangiomas, which need no treatment.

Less commonly, benign solid areas of **focal nodular hyperplasia** (FNH) are discovered. These are more prevalent in women.

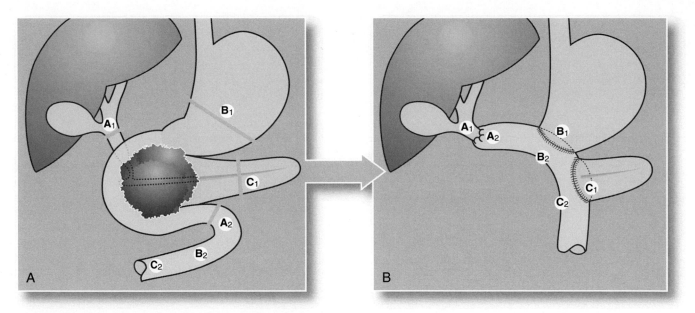

• **Fig. 24.6** Whipple Operation (Pancreaticoduodenectomy). **(A)** Structures are divided at the lines A_1, A_2, B_1, C_1. **(B)** The distal half of the stomach, the entire duodenal loop, the head and body of the pancreas and the lower end of the common bile duct are all removed, then reconstruction is performed with anastomoses between A_1 and A_2, B_1 and B_2 and C_1 and C_2.

CASE HISTORY

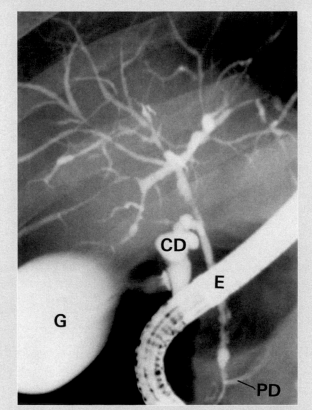

• **Fig. 24.7** Primary Sclerosing Cholangitis. Endoscopic retrograde cholangiopancreatography in a 52-year-old man with longstanding ulcerative colitis who developed painless jaundice. There is widespread irregular narrowing of both the intrahepatic and extrahepatic bile ducts typical of sclerosing cholangitis. Note the endoscope *(E)*, the normal gall bladder *(G)* and the cystic duct *(CD)* filling with contrast. The proximal part of the pancreatic duct *(PD)* also contains contrast.

Other benign solid lesions include **hepatic adenomas, which may be associated with oral contraceptive pill use**. FNH is more common than adenoma (ratio of 9:1) but adenoma may lead to hepatoma, so most liver surgeons recommend resection, whilst hyperplasia can safely be left. Both look similar on standard imaging, but FNH may have a characteristic central scar. A combination of multimodal imaging and biopsy can confirm the diagnosis in most cases.

Liver Abscesses

These usually present symptomatically with pyrexia, malaise and upper abdominal pain or tenderness. The most important cause worldwide is **amoebiasis**; about 10% of the world population is chronically infected with *Entamoeba histolytica*. Simple pyogenic abscesses can arise from biliary infection (e.g., ascending cholangitis), through the portal venous system (e.g., appendix or diverticular abscess) or generalised bacteraemia (e.g., endocarditis). Most liver abscesses are managed effectively with combined radiological drainage and long-course antimicrobial therapy. The key exception is **hydatid cysts** arising from *Echinococcus* infection, a zoonosis transmitted through contact with dogs or sheep. Draining hydatid cysts carries a serious risk of peritoneal dissemination and anaphylaxis, so complete surgical excision is undertaken with cover from an antihelminthic agent, such as mebendazole.

Hepatocellular Carcinoma

Hepatocellular carcinomas (also known as **hepatomas**) are malignant, slowly-growing tumours that often arise multicentrically and synchronously throughout the liver. Hepatocellular carcinoma is the sixth most prevalent cancer worldwide and the third cause of cancer-related death. More than 700,000 cases were diagnosed in 2008, so it represents a substantial global burden. Unusually for malignancy, an aetiological factor can be identified in nearly all cases; factors include infection with hepatitis B and especially hepatitis C, alcoholic cirrhosis, haemochromatosis and chronic active hepatitis. Around 80% to 90% have some form of preexisting cirrhosis. In developed countries, **alcoholic cirrhosis** and nonalcoholic fatty liver disease (associated with the metabolic syndrome) are the usual aetiological factors; indeed, hepatoma occurs in about 25% of patients with cirrhosis of more than 5 years' standing. The risk in patients with **haemochromatosis** and **chronic active hepatitis** is even higher.

Hepatocellular carcinoma is very common in parts of Africa and the Far East. Here, the usual cause is hepatitis B-induced cirrhosis, but environmental carcinogens have also been implicated including **aflatoxin** from *Aspergillus* growing on stored grains and peanuts. Various **parasitic infestations**, for example, schistosomiasis, *Echinococcus* (tapeworm) and *Clonorchis sinensis* (liver fluke), also predispose to it. In developed countries, the peak incidence is between the ages of 40 and 60 years, but in developing countries, most cases occur between 20 and 40 years.

Clinical Features and Management of Hepatocellular Carcinoma

The presenting features are anorexia, weight loss, abdominal pain and distension, often with jaundice and ascites, plus nonabdominal stigmata of cirrhosis. A liver mass may be palpable. Multiple modality imaging, combining ultrasound, CT or MRI scanning (along with markedly elevated α-fetoprotein) can establish the diagnosis and delineate the size and position of the liver mass or masses. Radiologically guided needle biopsy is used for indeterminate lesions but has a false negative rate of 30% to 40% and so a negative result should not rule out malignancy.

By the time of initial diagnosis, carcinoma is usually widespread in the liver, rendering curative resection impossible. However, in developed countries, asymptomatic tumours are often discovered incidentally, allowing potentially curative therapeutic intervention. Occasionally, smaller lesions are resectable but only in patients with less severe or well compensated cirrhosis. At one time, liver transplantation appeared to offer the necessary radical resection, but results with large tumours proved unsatisfactory as recurrence was the rule. Transplantation is more promising when there are fewer than three tumours, each smaller than 3 cm, or a single tumour smaller than 5 cm *(the Milan criteria)*. In these, outcomes are comparable to those for liver transplantation for cirrhosis alone, with 5-year survival around 70%.

Patients with known cirrhosis should ideally be in a 6-monthly ultrasound surveillance programme to identify developing hepatocellular carcinoma early. If tumours are discovered, the patient may be considered for transplantation or for palliation to curb tumour growth. Palliation may involve local cytotoxic drugs given by 'chemoembolisation' via a hepatic intraarterial cannula. Where resection or transplantation are not practicable (e.g., because of advanced age, comorbidities or patient choice), radiofrequency ablation can manage neoplasms in cirrhotic livers, and in some centres, is the first-line treatment for small lesions. Chemoembolisation and radiofrequency ablation can give many years of disease control.

Secondary Liver Tumours

Secondary liver tumours are extremely common and arise from a wide variety of primary sources, especially stomach, pancreas, large bowel, breast and bronchus. Liver metastases are initially asymptomatic but the patient begins to feel ill with anorexia and weight loss, as the parenchyma is progressively destroyed.

Jaundice is unusual and appears only at a terminal stage when the biochemical picture tends to be a mixed hepatitic and obstructive pattern.

Many colorectal cancer patients can be cured by primary surgery, but those that eventually die almost all have metastatic liver disease. Whilst there is no benefit in resecting metastatic disease in most other sites, colorectal liver metastases (along with lung metastases) are a special case, with a real chance of cure. Some 10% to 20% may be suitable for curative resection; recent optimistic outcome reports mean increasing numbers are considered for liver resection, now that better surgical techniques are available and surgeons more willing to undertake extensive or multiple resections.

The liver has a large reserve capacity and a remarkable regenerative capability. This means that up to 75% of liver tissue can be surgically resected, provided there is no other liver disease. Resection is sometimes combined with chemotherapy and/or radiofrequency ablation to 'downsize' the tumour in advance. This surgery is a major undertaking, best practised in specialised units with operative mortality of around 1% to 2% and 5-year survival of 40% to 60%. If further metastases appear in the hypertrophied regenerating liver, further resection or radiofrequency ablation can sometimes be done. In this context, a similar approach is adopted with lung metastases and patients may have both lung and liver resection in addition to primary surgery.

In other primary cancers, such as oesophagogastric and bronchus, liver metastases usually indicate surgically incurable disease, reflecting the systemic nature of the malignancy. Occasionally, however, metastases from renal cell carcinoma, breast or neuroendocrine tumours have been successfully resected. If liver metastases are painful, palliation by systemic chemotherapy may retard growth and suppress symptoms. Multiple inoperable metastases can often be controlled by a range of physical methods including local cryotherapy, radiofrequency ablation, laser destruction and percutaneous alcohol injection. Such treatments are unlikely to extend survival and controlled clinical trials of benefit are notably lacking.

The Spleen

The spleen plays a major role in defence against infections, particularly involving encapsulated organisms. It also filters and removes senescent or defective blood cells. Primary splenic diseases are uncommon but a range of haematological disorders may involve the organ and usually manifest as splenomegaly (see Ch. 18, p. 289). Historically, splenectomy was common in myeloproliferative disorders and often used for diagnosis, but is now rarely indicated except to treat hypersplenism, that is, excessive consumption of cellular blood components, or for symptom control in pain associated with massive splenomegaly. The surgeon is most frequently involved in repair, partial resection or removal of a normal spleen after trauma or iatrogenic injury (Ch. 15, p. 220).

Elective Splenectomy

Patients undergoing elective (and emergency) splenectomy require immunisation against common encapsulated pathogens (*Pneumococcus, Haemophilus influenzae* type B and *Meningococcus*, ideally given at least 2 weeks before operation) and are advised to take lifelong antibiotic prophylaxis.

Laparoscopic splenectomy has become the standard technique for most elective cases and is outlined in Chapter 10, p. 146. The most common elective indication for splenectomy is **immune thrombocytopenic purpura**, in which antiplatelet antibodies lead to platelet destruction and an increased risk of spontaneous haemorrhage. Splenectomy is curative in about 85% of cases.

When erythrocyte loss is severe or resistant to medical management, splenectomy is sometimes required for haemolytic anaemias, including hereditary spherocytosis, thalassaemia and autoimmune haemolytic anaemia. It is common to perform simultaneous cholecystectomy for secondary pigment gallstones. In addition, in sickle cell anaemia, splenic infarction or abscess formation may require splenectomy.

Rarely, primary lesions of the spleen may require partial or total splenectomy; these include haemangiomas, primary angiosarcoma and cysts.

25
Pancreatitis

CHAPTER OUTLINE

Introduction

Pancreatitis is a common inflammatory disorder of the pancreas characterised by abdominal pain. Most cases present in an acute form known as **acute pancreatitis** and attacks range between mild to severe. Severe attacks can be life threatening, with a mortality of around 20%.

A small proportion of patients suffer a persistent form known as **chronic pancreatitis**; this is much more common in men and is often associated with high alcohol intake.

Acute Pancreatitis

Aetiology and Epidemiology of Acute Pancreatitis

Gallstones and alcohol together account for about 80% of acute pancreatitis worldwide. These and the other main causes of acute pancreatitis are listed in Table 25.1 (also Boxes 25.1 and 25.2). **Opie** in 1901 first pointed out the relationship between gallstones and pancreatitis based on autopsy evidence. Small gallstones may cause transient obstruction as they pass through the ampulla via the bile ducts, or larger stones may impact at the lower end of the common bile duct, resulting in **pancreatic duct obstruction**. The resultant back pressure in the pancreatic ductal system leads to intrapancreatic enzyme activation through impeding of acinar exocytosis. In normal exocytosis, vesicles are carried to the cell membrane and their contents secreted into the extracellular environment.

The proportion of acute pancreatitis caused by alcoholism varies from country to country; in the United Kingdom about two-thirds of patients have a gallstone aetiology, whereas in parts of the United States of America and continental Europe about two-thirds have an alcohol aetiology. Longstanding high intake for at least 2 years is usually required to cause alcoholic pancreatitis but can result from a single session of heavy drinking—students finishing exams beware! Chronic alcohol exposure causes microtubular dysfunction in acinar cells leading to accumulation of intracellular enzymes. Alcohol also decreases the stability of zymogen and lysosomal membranes and enhances acinar cell sensitivity to cholecystokinin (CCK) further increasing pathological enzyme activation. Genetic susceptibility plays an important role in alcohol-induced pancreatitis and several high-risk genetic mutations have been identified.

In developed countries, the annual incidence of acute pancreatitis requiring hospital admission is about 1:2000 population and mortality is between 2% and 6%. About 20% fall into the category of **severe pancreatitis**. Women are affected more than men, but men are more likely to suffer recurrent attacks. The peak incidence is between 50 and 60 years. The reported incidence appears to have risen by a factor of 10 over the last 50 years, with only part of this attributable to improved diagnosis. Other factors are unknown.

Pathophysiology of Acute Pancreatitis

Acute pancreatitis is characterised by the sudden onset of diffuse inflammation of the pancreas. A range of diverse factors initiate disturbances of cellular metabolism, chiefly concerned with membrane stability, which lead to inappropriate activation of zymogens (preenzymes) within the pancreas. Activation of **trypsin** is probably the key initiating event and this overwhelms intrinsic antitrypsin activity, leading to **interstitial oedematous pancreatitis**. Fortunately, the extent and severity of inflammation remain mild and self-limiting in most patients and systemic effects are mild. In the least severe cases, there is minimal peritoneal exudation and no pancreatic changes detectable on contrast-enhanced computed tomography (CT) scanning. In more severe disease, the pancreas becomes swollen and oedematous but remains viable. If laparotomy is inadvertently performed at this stage, clear, noninfected peritoneal fluid is found, with whitish patches on great omentum and mesentery representing areas of **fat saponification** ('fat necrosis'). If it is extensive, calcium becomes sequestered in these areas and this is incriminated in the drop in blood calcium, characteristic of severe acute pancreatitis.

TABLE 25.1	Aetiology of Acute Pancreatitis	
Condition		**Frequency**
OBSTRUCTION		
Gallstones		30%–70% of cases
Congenital abnormalities: pancreas divisum with accessory duct obstruction; choledochocoele; duodenal diverticula		5% of cases
Ampullary or pancreatic tumours		3% of cases
Abnormally high pressure in the sphincter of Oddi (over 40 mmHg)		1%–2% of cases
Ascariasis (second most common cause in endemic areas, e.g., Kashmir)		Depends on locality
DRUGS AND TOXINS		
Alcohol excess		30%–70% of cases
Drugs: ('**SAND**'—**S**teroids and sulphonamides, **A**zathioprine (and 6-mercaptopurine), **N**SAIDs, **D**iuretics, such as furosemide and thiazides, and didanosine); also antibacterials, such as metronidazole and tetracycline, H_2 blockers and many other classes of drug		1%–2%
Scorpion venom		Very rare
Snake bites		Very rare
IATROGENIC AND TRAUMATIC CAUSES		
Following endoscopic retrograde cholangiopancreatography (ERCP) or endoscopic sphincterotomy		2%–6% of patients having the procedure
Following cardiopulmonary bypass		0.5%–5% of patients having bypass
Blunt pancreatic trauma, usually caused by motor vehicle accidents		Very rare
Repeated marathon running		Very rare
METABOLIC CAUSES		
Hypertriglyceridaemia (>11 mmol/L)		2% of cases
Hypercalcaemia		Rare
Hypothermia		Rare
Pregnancy		Rare
INFECTION		
AIDS: secondary infection with cytomegalovirus and others		About 10% in patients with AIDS
Other viruses: mumps, chickenpox, Coxsackie viruses, hepatitis A, B and C		Very rare
IDIOPATHIC PANCREATITIS		
No definable cause after thorough diagnostic evaluation including ERCP; research studies show about two-thirds of 'idiopathic' cases have gallstone microlithiasis		10%–12% of cases

AIDS, Acquired immunodeficiency syndrome; *NSAIDs*, nonsteroidal anti-inflammatory drugs.

As severity increases, trypsin and other enzymes cause increasingly extensive local damage, as well as activation of complement and cytokine systems leading on to systemic inflammatory response syndrome (SIRS) and organ failure. Manifestations include shock, acute respiratory distress syndrome (ARDS), kidney failure and disseminated intravascular coagulation (DIC; see Ch. 2). At this stage, **acute peripancreatic fluid collections** become detectable on CT. The most severe pancreatitis is associated with **pancreatic necrosis**. Ischaemia within the gland plus reperfusion injury are likely mechanisms in transforming acute oedematous pancreatitis into this necrotising disease.

Complications are common and mortality in this group (even without infection) is as high as 10%.

A substantial proportion of these patients develop **infection** of the necrotic pancreas, usually with gram-negative organisms translocated from bowel. This occurs within 2 weeks of the onset and greatly increases mortality (up to 25%).

In patients dying of acute necrotising pancreatitis, the peritoneal cavity becomes filled with dark, blood-stained inflammatory exudate containing fine lipid droplets. This is known as **acute haemorrhagic pancreatitis**. The peritoneal surface is grossly inflamed and semidigested, and the pancreas is a necrotic mass.

• BOX 25.1 Mnemonic for the Causes of Acute Pancreatitis: 'I Get Smashed'

- I Idiopathic
- G Gallstones
- E Ethanol
- T Trauma
- S Steroids
- M Mumps
- A Autoimmune
- S Scorpion/snakes
- H Hyperlipidaemia/hypercalcaemia
- E Endoscopic retrograde cholangiopancreatography
- D Drugs

• BOX 25.2 History and Investigations Helpful in Determining the Cause of Acute Pancreatitis

History
- Previous gallstones
- Alcohol intake
- Family history
- Drug intake
- Exposure to known viral causes or prodromal symptoms

Initial Investigations (Acute Phase)
- Pancreatic enzymes in plasma
- Liver function tests
- Ultrasound of gall bladder

Follow-up Investigations (Recovery Phase)
- Fasting plasma lipids
- Fasting plasma calcium
- Viral antibody titres
- Repeat biliary ultrasound
- Magnetic resonance cholangiopancreatography (MRCP)
- Computed tomography (multislice with pancreas protocol)

Clinical Features of Acute Pancreatitis (Box 25.3)

Acute pancreatitis presents as a patient with an acute abdomen who has severe abdominal pain coming on suddenly and continuously from the outset. Initially, it is poorly localised in the central and upper abdomen and is often described by the patient as 'going through to the back'. Vomiting may be an early feature. In the early stages, the patient is restless and constantly changes posture in a search for a comfortable position. Pain is most often relieved by leaning forward in the '**pancreatic position**'. With the onset of chemical peritonitis, movement becomes increasingly painful and the patient lies very still. Clinical signs depend on the severity of the inflammatory process and the stage it has reached.

Investigation of Suspected Pancreatitis

Acute pancreatitis must be excluded in any adult presenting with acute abdominal pain, and in any child with peritonitis not readily attributable to appendicitis. Several organisations have produced comprehensive guidelines on the management of acute pancreatitis, for example: https://www.uptodate.com/contents/management-of-acute-pancreatitis.

• BOX 25.3 Clinical Features of Acute Pancreatitis

Mild Attack
- Acute abdominal pain
- Minimal or rapidly resolving abdominal signs, for example, abdominal distension, some abdominal tenderness and guarding, absent bowel sounds
- Minimal systemic illness
- Moderate tachycardia

Severe Attack
- Severe acute abdominal pain
- Severe toxaemia and shock
- Generalised peritonitis (diffuse abdominal tenderness, guarding, rigidity, absent bowel sounds)
- Acute respiratory distress syndrome (may develop during the first few days)

Plasma Amylase

Amylase is one of the enzymes released into the circulation in pancreatitis; measurement is a simple laboratory investigation and is generally a reliable diagnostic test. A level above 1000 IU/mL is usually regarded as diagnostic of acute pancreatitis but levels are often lower in alcoholic pancreatitis, particularly during recurrent attacks. Any inflammatory upper abdominal condition near the pancreas (e.g., cholecystitis, perforated peptic ulcer or strangulated bowel) can cause a moderate rise in amylase, although this rarely reaches 1000 IU/mL. Levels rise rapidly at the outset of an attack, and readings of 10,000 IU/mL or more may be recorded on admission to hospital. However, levels fall rapidly after 3 to 5 days, so a diagnosis of pancreatitis should not rely on an arbitrary threshold; rather the amylase level should be interpreted in relation to how much time has elapsed since the onset.

Serial amylase levels correlate poorly with disease severity; C-reactive protein (CRP) levels are more useful. Note that false negative amylase results may occur in lipaemic serum, although modern assays are less susceptible to this problem.

On rare occasions, plasma amylase may be normal in acute pancreatitis. This occurs where most of the gland has been destroyed by severe pancreatitis. It may also occur if a patient presents several days into an attack. If pancreatitis is strongly suspected but the amylase is normal, the diagnosis may be confirmed by radiological imaging (see next section).

Plasma lipase estimation has been recommended for diagnosing acute pancreatitis as it is more sensitive than amylase and has a longer half-life, so is easier to detect later in the disease. It is not as widely used but can be useful in difficult or late-presenting cases. In addition, elevated alanine aminotransferase levels are highly specific for gallstone pancreatitis.

Once the patient is in the recovery phase, fasting bloods should be taken for calcium levels and for plasma lipids, particularly triglycerides. Viral antibody titres may be useful in cases of idiopathic pancreatitis.

Imaging

Plain x-rays of chest (erect) to look for free gas under the diaphragm, and abdomen (supine) are often performed during the initial investigation. The latter may show a featureless 'groundglass' appearance. Bowel gas tends to be absent except perhaps for a '**sentinel loop**' of dilated adynamic small bowel in the centre. Note that these signs are not specific for pancreatitis and are often absent. Rarely, radiopaque gallstones are visible.

An **ultrasound scan** of the biliary tree is essential but good images are not always obtained early; a delay of 48 to 72 hours may improve image quality. The goal is to look for small calculi in the gall bladder or bile ducts typically responsible for gallstone pancreatitis. If no definite cause for the pancreatitis is found, a repeat ultrasound should be performed following recovery.

CT scanning has a limited role in the diagnosis of acute pancreatitis. Initially, it is indicated only when clinical and biochemical findings are equivocal, particularly if amylase is normal and intraabdominal pathology, such as perforation or infarction need to be excluded. CT scans performed too early cannot predict the final severity and are unlikely to influence management during the first week. In **severe pancreatitis**, contrast-enhanced CT is valuable for demonstrating necrosis, but this cannot be identified until at least 4 days after the onset of symptoms.

Endoscopic Retrograde Cholangiopancreatography, Endoscopic Ultrasound and Magnetic Resonance Cholangiopancreatography

In patients with severe acute gallstone pancreatitis, urgent endoscopic retrograde cholangiopancreatography (ERCP) and sphincterotomy should be carried out within 72 hours of the onset of pain. This is especially important in patients with cholangitis, jaundice or a dilated common bile duct. If a cause for the pancreatitis has not become evident from the history or initial investigation, magnetic resonance cholangiopancreatography (MRCP) and endoscopic ultrasound (EUS) have important diagnostic roles once the patient has recovered from the acute attack. In this group, less common causes can often be revealed, including small pancreatic or periampullary tumours, pancreatic duct stricture, microlithiasis or congenital pancreas divisum.

Clinical Classification

To provide **early warning** of severity, each patient with acute pancreatitis is sorted into one of two categories, **mild** or **severe**. This provides an indicator of prognosis within the first 48 hours, and is central to formulating a management strategy. Categorisation is based on thoroughly tested scoring systems originally developed by **Ranson** in the United States (Box 25.4) and modified by **Imrie** (Glasgow criteria—Table 25.2). If three or more of the factors listed are present, the patient is diagnosed as having severe pancreatitis and should be admitted to a critical care unit for close monitoring. The more adverse factors present, the worse the prognosis. Even if a patient is initially placed in the mild group, continued observation is essential as deterioration to severe pancreatitis can occur at any time. The clinical features of acute pancreatitis are summarised in Box 25.3. The Atlanta classification can be used to group patients by severity, but is often most useful in retrospect.

Mild Acute Pancreatitis

Mild attacks are common. The patient looks generally well with minimal systemic features. Nevertheless, there is often considerable pain. The abdomen is usually distended and diffusely tender but with little guarding. Bowel sounds may be absent as a result of inflammatory ileus. The patient may be mildly jaundiced from periampullary oedema. The differential diagnosis includes biliary colic, acute cholecystitis, an acute exacerbation of a peptic ulcer or even a perforation of a peptic ulcer. Lower lobe pneumonia or an inferior myocardial infarction may sometimes present like this. Sometimes the pancreatitis diagnosis is made after elevated plasma amylase is unexpectedly found.

• BOX 25.4 Criteria for Early Identification of Severe Pancreatitis (After Ranson)

Severe pancreatitis, with a high risk of major complications or death, is defined by the presence of three or more of the following features:

On Admission
- Age over 55 years (nongallstone pancreatitis) or 70 years (gallstone pancreatitis)
- Leucocyte count greater than $16,000 \times 10^9$/L
- Blood glucose greater than 10 mmol/L in a patient who is not diabetic
- Lactate dehydrogenase (LDH) greater than 350 IU/L
- Serum glutamic oxaloacetic transaminase (SGOT) >100 u/L

During the Next 48 Hours
- Haematocrit increase of more than 10%
- Plasma urea increase of more than 10 mmol/L despite adequate intravenous therapy
- Hypocalcaemia (corrected serum Ca <2.0 mmol/L)
- Low arterial pressure of oxygen
- (<8 kPa or 60 mmHg)
- Metabolic acidosis (base deficit more than 4 mEq/L)
- Estimated fluid sequestration more than 6 L

TABLE 25.2 A Mnemonic ('PANCREAS') for Remembering the Modified Glasgow Scoring System of Severity Prediction in Acute Pancreatitis (After E M Moore, With Permission[a])

Mnemonic Letter	Criterion	Positive When
P	PaO_2	<8 kPA or 60 mmHg
A	Age	>55 years
N	Neutrophil count	$>15 \times 10^9$/L
C	Calcium (blood)	<2 mmol/L
R	Raised plasma urea	>16 mmol/L
E	Enzyme (plasma lactate dehydrogenase, LDH)	>600 IU/L
A	Albumin (plasma)	<32 g/L
S	Sugar (plasma glucose)	>10 mmol/L

[a]Moore, E. A useful mnemonic for severity stratification in acute pancreatitis. *Ann R Coll Surg Engl.* 2000;82:16–17.

PaO_2, Partial pressure of oxygen in arterial blood.

Severe Acute Pancreatitis

In a severe attack, the patient looks apathetic, grey and shocked and there are typical abdominal signs of generalised peritonitis, that is, extreme tenderness, guarding and rigidity. In this case, the differential diagnosis includes other major abdominal catastrophes, especially faecal peritonitis from perforated large bowel and concealed haemorrhage from a leaking aortic aneurysm or ruptured ectopic pregnancy. Massive bowel infarction caused by arterial occlusion may present like this but abdominal signs are less marked. An important early and dangerous complication of severe acute pancreatitis is **ARDS**.

Management of Acute Pancreatitis

Mild Attacks

The management of acute pancreatitis has been the subject of several international consensus conferences, the most important of which took place in Atlanta in 1992. This codified many definitions and circumstances within acute pancreatitis. Numerous sets of guidelines are available but all are based on similar evidence (see example earlier).

Mild attacks require no further emergency investigation once diagnosed on plasma amylase, and are managed by fluid resuscitation and analgesia: recovery is usually rapid. These patients need no dietary restriction. Later management is aimed at treating predisposing factors. Gallstones should be sought by ultrasonography; if present, cholecystectomy is the definitive treatment and is ideally performed on the same admission or at worst 2 to 4 weeks after recovery. Ductal stones should be removed at operation or endoscopically before discharge from hospital. Alcohol abuse must be discouraged.

Severe Attacks

A severe attack is defined by referring to a specified list of criteria and should be evaluated on admission and over the next 48 hours (see Table 25.2 and Box 25.4). Patients with severe pancreatitis may die early in the attack because of profound systemic toxaemia (SIRS), shock and multiple organ dysfunction syndrome (MODS); see Chapter 3, p. 48. ARDS develops rapidly with little warning but a deteriorating arterial partial pressure of oxygen may herald its onset. This is an indication for urgent ventilatory support before the condition becomes established.

Even when pancreatitis is severe, supportive measures are still the mainstay of treatment. These include **oxygen** supplementation and goal directed intravenous **fluid resuscitation**. A nasogastric tube is only passed to aspirate the stomach if gastroparesis causes troublesome vomiting. Enteral fine-bore nasogastric or nasojejunal feeding has been reported to significantly decrease morbidity. If enteral feeding is not tolerated because of ileus, then total parenteral nutrition may become necessary.

Gross fluid and electrolyte disturbances, as well as hypocalcaemia are also likely to occur. Fluid balance in the shocked patient is complicated by massive losses of protein-rich fluid into the peritoneal cavity and interstitially ('third space losses'). This sequestration of fluid needs to be countered by large amounts of intravenous fluids, carefully monitored by measuring cardiac output by transoesophageal Doppler and/or central venous pressure and hourly urine output. Any patient with severe pancreatitis, or anyone with acute pancreatitis who develops signs of serious deterioration, should be admitted to a critical care unit for close monitoring and vigorous treatment of cardiovascular, pulmonary, renal and septic complications. Box 25.5 lists recommended investigations to guide management.

There is probably little benefit in measuring plasma amylase again once the diagnosis is made. CRP is more useful, as it is a good indicator of systemic inflammation and hence developing necrosis and other complications. If the CRP is elevated >150 mg/L after 48 hours, complications are more likely. Biochemical estimations, particularly liver transaminases and bilirubin, are charted regularly, looking chiefly for evidence of biliary obstruction; renal function tests are performed for evidence of acute kidney failure.

> **• BOX 25.5 Recommended Frequent Investigations in Severe Acute Pancreatitis**
>
> - Haemoglobin estimation and white cell count
> - Arterial blood gas estimations
> - Blood sugar
> - Plasma electrolytes, creatinine and urea
> - 'Liver function tests' (i.e., bilirubin, alkaline phosphatase, lactate dehydrogenase [LDH], transaminases, plasma proteins)
> - Plasma calcium and phosphate
> - C-reactive protein

Prophylactic parenteral antibiotics are no longer recommended as there is no evidence that they reduce infective complications or mortality.

Endoscopy and Surgery in Severe Acute Pancreatitis

All patients suspected of having or proven to have a gallstone aetiology should undergo urgent therapeutic ERCP, which should take place within 72 hours of the onset of pain. This applies whether severe pancreatitis is predicted or confirmed. All of these patients require **sphincterotomy** of the sphincter of Oddi, whether or not stones are found in the common bile duct. If stones are seen or if cholangitis or jaundice is present, biliary stenting may be required.

There is no role for surgery during the acute attack but in patients with stones, laparoscopic cholecystectomy with operative cholangiography should be performed before discharge because deferring it increases the risk of another attack. In the small group of critically ill patients with infected necrotic tissue and infected peripancreatic fluid collections, minimally invasive necrosectomy can be safe and effective. Open laparotomy may rarely be required in the face of catastrophic secondary complications, such as mesenteric infarction or colonic perforation, but is associated with an extremely high mortality.

Complications of Acute Pancreatitis

Mortality

About 15% of patients admitted to hospital with acute pancreatitis have severe disease, which carries a high risk of potential complications. However, about a further 10% initially diagnosed with mild pancreatitis deteriorate markedly during admission and become severe. In severe pancreatitis, mortality is 10% to 30%, that is, 2% to 5% of all cases, and obese patients have a higher mortality. About half of those that die, do so within the first week, usually of ARDS and pulmonary failure. Other early life-threatening complications are associated with **MODS**. Manifestations include cardiovascular collapse aggravated by fluid shifts, kidney failure made worse by hypotension, and DIC. If death occurs after the first week, infective complications of pancreatic necrosis added to existing organ failure are the usual cause.

Pancreatic Necrosis and Infection

In severe pancreatitis, **pancreatic and peripancreatic necrosis** may manifest during the first 2 weeks of the attack (Fig. 25.1). Necrosis is identified using intravenous contrast-enhanced CT scanning in which the necrotic pancreas does not opacify, having lost its blood supply. Infection of devitalised pancreatic and peripancreatic tissues occurs in about one-third of patients with severe pancreatitis, and is often lethal. Infection may be suspected on CT by gas bubbles in pancreatic fluid collections but can only

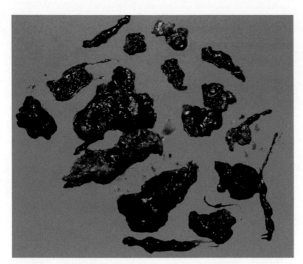

• **Fig. 25.1** Pancreatic Necrosis. Necrotic pancreas removed 16 days after a severe attack of pancreatitis complicated by peripancreatic infection. The patient made a slow recovery but became diabetic in the convalescent period.

CASE HISTORY

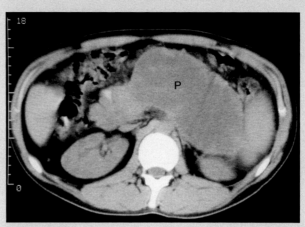

• **Fig. 25.2** Pancreatic Pseudocyst. This 57-year-old man was admitted to hospital with an acute abdomen 3 weeks before this scan. He was found to have acute pancreatitis caused by gallstones. The symptoms and signs of pancreatitis smouldered on and the C-reactive protein and plasma amylase failed to return to normal. This computed tomography scan of his upper abdomen shows the cause of the persistent symptoms, a pseudocyst arising from the tail of the pancreas *(P)*.

be confirmed by percutaneous aspiration (with microscopy and culture of the aspirate), usually performed under CT guidance. It is important the patient is treated with both broad-spectrum antibiotics and antifungals, as infection is usually polymicrobial and at least 40% contain fungi. In proven infected cases, operative debridement with minimally invasive **necrosectomy** may be appropriate after several weeks delay to allow the necrotic area to demarcate into a clear 'walled off' cavity.

Fluid Collections Around the Pancreas

During the initial attack, **acute peripancreatic fluid collections** may develop. Most resolve spontaneously, but for those that do not, CT-guided percutaneous drainage is valuable. Fluid collections persisting for longer than 6 weeks are termed **pancreatic pseudocysts** (see later). Late in the course of the disease, a **pancreatic abscess** or 'walled-off' pancreatic necrosis may appear. This is a well-localised collection of pus within the gland, and contrasts with **infected necrotising pancreatitis**, which appears earlier and is not localised.

Pancreatic Pseudocyst

A pancreatic pseudocyst is a collection of pancreatic enzymes, inflammatory fluid and necrotic debris, usually encapsulated within the lesser sac. Pseudocysts appear in 1% to 8% of cases of acute pancreatitis and are less likely to resolve spontaneously than early acute fluid collections. A pseudocyst is not a true cyst (i.e., there is no epithelial lining) although the surrounding tissues become thickened by the inflammatory response. Pseudocysts may occur after even a moderate attack of pancreatitis and sometimes reach the size of a football. An upper abdominal mass may be palpable. If a pseudocyst is suspected, CT scanning is the investigation of choice (Fig. 25.2).

Management varies according to size. Larger cysts, especially those larger than 10 cm, are unlikely to resolve. Those around 6 cm can be safely observed for up to 6 months, provided they have a typical appearance on CT scanning and are asymptomatic. If the cyst has failed to resolve by then, intervention should be considered. Operation, either by laparoscopy or an open approach, involves 'marsupialising' the pseudocyst into the posterior wall of the stomach. This can be performed after about 6 weeks, when

the wall of the pseudocyst has 'matured' enough to hold sutures. EUS-guided gastrocystomy using large bore stents is increasingly used in specialist centres, although their efficacy is not yet proven.

Pancreatic Abscess

Pancreatic abscesses occur in 1% to 4% of cases of acute pancreatitis. Certain patients remain systemically well despite pancreatic necrosis, with an illness that may grumble on for several weeks. There is a recurrent high swinging fever indicating the presence of an abscess. By that time, the necrotic pancreas is likely to have formed a discrete grey mass lying free within the pancreatic bed and bathed in pus. Pus may extend widely in retroperitoneal tissues. Surgery is then required to remove the necrotic tissue and drain the abscesses.

Complications of Severe Acute Pancreatitis

Severe acute pancreatitis can cause wide-ranging complications in almost every body system:
• Multiorgan failure may lead to kidney failure, respiratory failure, cardiac failure, and haematological and coagulation disorders.
• Direct pressure effects, inflammation and hypotension may cause portal vein thrombosis.
• Local pressure plus hypotension may cause bowel ischaemia—the transverse colon is commonly affected because of the position of the middle colic artery.
• Pseudoaneurysms may form in vessels, such as the splenic artery because of inflammatory damage to the arterial wall and fluid collections around them and can result in life-threatening haemorrhage.
• Internal pancreatic fistulae may form, particularly if necrosis causes disruption of the pancreatic duct or the wall of a pseudocyst. The result may be pancreatic ascites, mediastinal pseudocysts, enzymatic mediastinitis or pancreatic pleural effusions.

Late Complications of Acute Pancreatitis

Diabetes mellitus, and intestinal malabsorption caused by loss of pancreatic secretions sometimes occur after severe attacks that have caused substantial pancreatic necrosis and loss of pancreatic tissue.

Recurrent and Chronic Pancreatitis

Recurrent Acute Pancreatitis

Some patients suffer recurrent attacks, usually resulting from alcohol abuse or gallstone disease. The first and second attacks may be severe, but attacks after that almost never have lethal complications. The patient is entirely well between attacks. Attacks vary in severity in different patients but are rarely extreme.

Chronic Pancreatitis

Some patients suffer persistent and severe upper abdominal pain, similar in character to a prolonged attack of acute pancreatitis. These patients do not develop the other features of acute pancreatitis and may not have elevated amylase levels. The pain is so severe and so persistent as to drive some patients to suicide. Carcinoma of the pancreas and chronic pancreatic inflammation should both be considered in this pattern of pain. Inflammatory swelling of the pancreatic head occasionally causes obstructive jaundice but carcinoma in this position is a far more common cause of jaundice.

Despite the pain, there are usually no abnormal abdominal signs. Plasma amylase may be moderately elevated on occasions; the diagnosis of chronic pancreatitis may, however, be missed if raised amylase is not detected (because tests are not done at an appropriate time or the patient never has elevated levels). There is a danger these patients may be dismissed as suffering from psychosomatic pain.

In chronic pancreatitis, ultrasound or CT scans may show glandular swelling (sometimes difficult to differentiate from pancreatic carcinoma), pancreatic atrophy, parenchymal calcification (see Fig. 25.3) and a dilated pancreatic duct. If ERCP is performed, the pancreatic duct system may look normal or else may be distorted and irregular in calibre, confirming chronic inflammation and fibrosis (Fig. 25.4). Sometimes pancreatic duct stones are shown.

CASE HISTORY

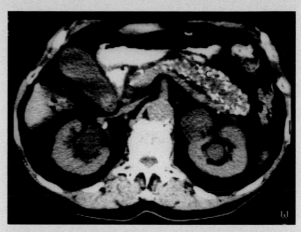

• Fig. 25.3 Pancreatic Calcification in Chronic Pancreatitis. This obese 55-year-old man had a long history of severe abdominal pain and alcohol abuse. Pancreatic calcification was not visible on a plain abdominal x-ray but extensive calcification is clearly seen on this computed tomography scan.

Chronic pancreatitis may cause years of misery, perhaps eventually 'burning out' as the gland atrophies completely. It is important to make the diagnosis early, so pain can be relieved. In the long term, malabsorption or diabetes is more likely to develop than after acute pancreatitis.

Treatment of chronic pancreatitis is far from satisfactory. Surgery is only useful if structural abnormalities can be found. Procedures include removal of pancreatic duct stones, partial pancreatectomy of body and tail for duct stenosis, sphincteroplasty of the pancreatic duct opening, or occasionally total pancreatectomy. Chemical coeliac ganglion blockade provides useful (and often permanent) pain relief, but does nothing to prevent inflammation. If there are multiple duct strictures, the pancreatic duct can be surgically split along its whole length and the side of a loop of jejunum sutured to it to allow unrestricted drainage. Interventional endoscopy can be used for dilatation and stenting of isolated pancreatic duct strictures.

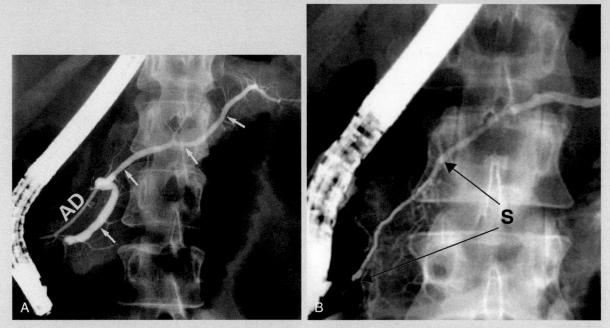

• **Fig. 25.4 Retrograde Pancreatography.** These films were both obtained by injecting contrast into the pancreatic duct using a flexible duodenoscope (it should be noted that these images could now be obtained using magnetic resonance cholangiopancreatography as a noninvasive alternative). **(A)** This pancreatogram is normal. The main duct *(arrowed)* narrows regularly towards the tail of the pancreas and there are no strictures or dilatations along its length. The accessory pancreatic duct *(AD)* also fills in this patient. **(B)** This pancreatogram is from a man of 26 years with a history of severe upper abdominal pain. There is a long stricture *(S)* of the main duct, between the *red arrows*, of unknown origin. Typical changes of chronic pancreatitis, that is, irregularity of the wall with dilatations and poor filling of small ducts, are seen in the duct distal to the stricture.

26

Appendicitis

Introduction

Acute appendicitis is the most common cause of intraabdominal infection in developed countries and appendicectomy, the most common emergency operation. In the United Kingdom, 1.9 females per 1000 have the operation each year compared with 1.5 males, and about one in seven people eventually undergo the operation. Surprisingly, the incidence of appendicitis fell by about 30% between the 1960s and the 1980s, for reasons unknown.

Appendicitis can occur at any age but is most common below 40 years, especially between 10 and 20 years. It is rare below the age of 10 years and very rare below 2 years, but more likely to present with a perforation with a greater than 65% incidence in 0- to 4-year-olds. Appendicitis is believed to be less common in rural parts of developing countries, but the incidence approaches that of the West in the cities. Different susceptibility in similar people may be related to reduced dietary fibre in city dwellers.

Acute appendicitis should be considered in any patients presenting to hospital with acute abdominal pain. Even previous appendicectomy does not absolutely rule out the diagnosis. Despite lay impressions, a positive diagnosis is often difficult to make; this is partly because of the lack of specific tests to confirm or exclude appendicitis. At open operation, a noninflamed appendix is sometimes found but a small number of 'negative' operations may be unavoidable. Laparoscopy improves diagnostic accuracy, particularly in young women, and is used therapeutically to remove an inflamed appendix; it also has lower complication rates.

Anatomy of the Appendix

The appendix is a blind-ending tube arising from the caecum at the meeting point of the three taenia coli, just distal to the ileocaecal junction. The appendix base thus most commonly lies in the right iliac fossa, close to **McBurney point**. This is two-thirds of the way along a line from umbilicus to anterior superior iliac spine (see later, Fig. 26.6, p. 373). In most cases, the appendix is mobile within the peritoneal cavity, suspended by its mesentery (**mesoappendix**), with the appendicular artery in its free edge. This is effectively an end-artery, with anastomotic connections only proximally.

The appendix is described as lying in several 'classic' sites, but apart from the true retrocaecal appendix, the organ probably floats in a broad arc about its base (Fig. 26.1); only inflammation will fix it in a particular place. Its position then determines the clinical presentation. In about 30% of appendicectomies, it lies over the pelvic brim the ('**pelvic appendix**'). In some cases, the appendix lies retroperitoneally behind the caecum and often plastered to it by fibrous bands. Thus an inflamed retrocaecal appendix may irritate the right ureter and psoas muscle, and may even lie high enough to simulate gall bladder pain.

Histologically, the appendix has the same basic structure as the colon. It is covered by serosa (visceral layer of peritoneum) becoming continuous with the mesoappendix serosa. A retroperitoneal appendix has no serosal covering. A prominent feature of the appendix is its collections of lymphoid tissue in the lamina propria. This often has germinal centres and is prominent in childhood, but diminishes with increasing age.

The mucosa contains a large number of cells of the gastrointestinal endocrine amine precursor uptake and decarboxylation (APUD) system. These secrete mainly serotonin and were formerly known as **argentaffin cells**. Carcinoid tumours commonly occur in the appendix and arise from these cells.

Pathophysiology of Appendicitis

Appendicitis is probably initiated by luminal obstruction caused by impacted faeces or a faecolith. This explanation fits the epidemiological observation that appendicitis is more common with a low dietary fibre intake.

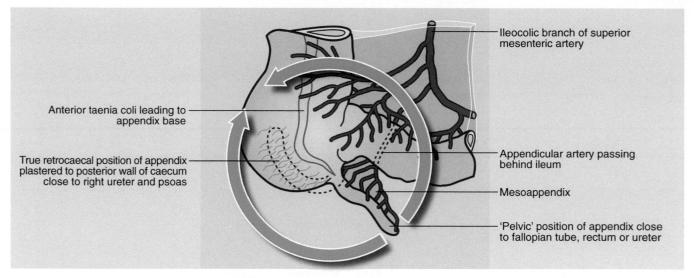

• **Fig. 26.1** Surgical Anatomy of the Appendix. The appendix can be positioned anywhere on the circumference shown by the *arrowed arc*.

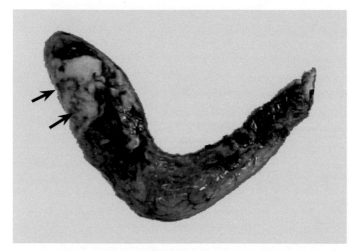

• **Fig. 26.2** Acute Appendicitis. Macroscopic photograph showing acutely inflamed appendix. The distended tip shows a purulent exudate on the serosal surface *(arrowed)*.

In the early stages of appendicitis, the mucosa becomes inflamed first. Inflammation eventually extends through the submucosa to involve the muscular and serosal (peritoneal) layers. A fibrinopurulent exudate on the serosal surface extends to any adjacent peritoneal surface, for example, bowel or abdominal wall, causing localised peritonitis.

By this stage, the necrotic glandular mucosa sloughs into the lumen, which becomes distended with pus. Finally, the end-arteries supplying the appendix thrombose and the infarcted appendix becomes necrotic or **gangrenous** at the distal end and the appendix begins to disintegrate. Perforation soon follows and faecally contaminated contents spread into the peritoneum. If the spilled contents are enveloped by omentum or adherent small bowel, a localised **abscess** results; otherwise spreading peritonitis develops. Acute appendicitis is illustrated histologically in Fig. 26.2.

Clinical Features of Appendicitis

The pathophysiological evolution of appendicitis and corresponding symptoms and signs are illustrated in Fig. 26.3.

Classic Appendicitis

Acute appendicitis classically begins with poorly localised, colicky central abdominal **visceral pain**; this results from smooth muscle spasm as a reaction to appendiceal obstruction. Anorexia and vomiting often occur at this stage.

As inflammation advances over the ensuing 12 to 24 hours, it progresses through the appendiceal wall to involve the parietal peritoneum (innervated somatically). Then pain typically becomes **localised** to the right iliac fossa. Signs of local peritonitis can be elicited, that is, tenderness, guarding and rebound tenderness. This classic picture is seen in less than half of all cases, largely because localising symptoms and signs vary with the anatomical relations of the inflamed appendix and the vigour of the body's defences.

Other Presentations of Acute Appendicitis

If the inflamed or perforated appendix lies in the pelvis near the rectum, it may cause local irritation and diarrhoea. Consider a pelvic collection secondary to appendicitis in children with abdominal pain, associated with diarrhoea, persisting longer than 5 days. If it lies near the bladder or ureter, inflammation may cause urinary frequency, dysuria and (microscopic) pyuria, that is, leucocytes in the urine. These findings may be mistakenly interpreted as urinary tract infection. An inflamed retrocaecal appendix produces none of the usual localising symptoms or signs, but may irritate the psoas muscle, causing involuntary right hip flexion and pain on extension. A high retrocaecal appendix may cause pain and tenderness below the right costal margin. An inflamed appendix near the Fallopian tube causes pelvic pain suggestive of an acute gynaecological disorder, such as salpingitis or torsion of an ovarian cyst.

The early phase of poorly localised pain typically lasts for a few hours until peritoneal inflammation produces localising signs. If untreated, the inflamed appendix may become gangrenous after 12 to 24 hours and perforate, causing peritonitis unless sealed off by omentum. The whole abdomen becomes rigid and tender and there is marked systemic toxicity. Perforation is common in young children. Sometimes, the pathological sequence is extremely rapid and the patient presents with sudden peritonitis.

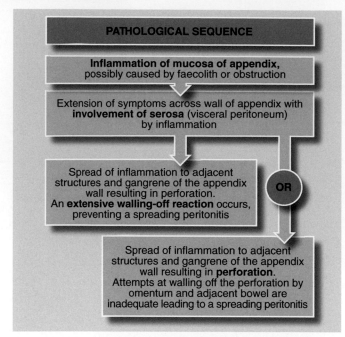
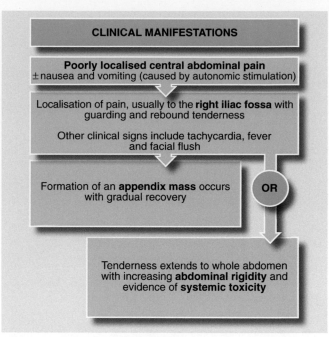

• **Fig. 26.3** Pathophysiology and Clinical Manifestations of Acute Appendicitis.

In older patients, a gangrenous or perforated appendix is more likely to be contained by greater omentum or loops of small bowel. This results in a palpable **appendix mass**. This may contain free pus and is then known as an **appendiceal abscess**. As with any significant abscess, there is a tachycardia and swinging pyrexia. An appendix mass usually resolves spontaneously over 2 to 6 weeks. In the elderly, an appendix abscess is often walled off by loops of small bowel. There may be no palpable mass and the symptoms and signs may not suggest appendicitis. These include nonspecific abdominal pain and features of small bowel obstruction caused by localised paralytic ileus. Occasionally, appendicitis may present in a most unusual way. Examples include discharge of an appendix abscess into the Fallopian tube presenting as a purulent vaginal discharge, or appendicitis within an inguinal hernia presenting as a groin abscess.

Making the Diagnosis of Appendicitis

Acute appendicitis is a clinical diagnosis, relying almost entirely on history and examination. Investigations are only useful in excluding differential diagnoses. Ideally, the diagnosis should be made and the appendix removed before it becomes gangrenous and perforates. This markedly reduces the risk of infective complications. However, unnecessary appendicectomies must be kept to a minimum.

Diagnosis of acute appendicitis poses little difficulty if the patient exhibits the classic symptoms and signs summarised in Box 26.1. However, the patient may present at a very early stage, or the signs may have some other pathological cause. At least two out of three children admitted to hospital with suspected appendicitis do not have the condition.

If evidence for acute appendicitis is insufficient and no other diagnosis can be made, the patient should be kept under observation, admitted to hospital if necessary and reexamined periodically. Eventually, the symptoms settle or the diagnosis becomes clear. Diagnostic laparoscopy may be needed in equivocal cases.

• **BOX 26.1** **Cardinal Features of Acute Appendicitis**

- Abdominal pain for less than 72 hours
- Vomiting one to three times
- Facial flush
- Tenderness concentrated on the right iliac fossa
- Anterior tenderness on rectal examination
- Fever between 37.3°C and 38.5°C
- No evidence of urinary tract infection on urine microscopy

Special Points in the History and Examination

Acute appendicitis typically runs a short course, between a few hours and about 3 days. If symptoms have been present for longer, appendicitis is unlikely unless an 'appendix mass' has developed. A recent or current sore throat or viral-type illness, particularly in children, favours a diagnosis of **mesenteric adenitis** (inflammation of mesenteric lymph nodes analogous to viral tonsillitis). Urinary symptoms suggest **urinary tract infection** but may also occur with pelvic appendicitis.

The patient with appendicitis is typically quiet, apathetic and flushed with limited abdominal wall movement; the lively child doing jigsaw puzzles almost never has appendicitis! Oral foetor may be present but is not a reliable sign. Cervical lymphadenopathy may suggest a viral origin for the abdominal pain. Mild tachycardia and pyrexia are typical of appendicitis, but a temperature much over 38°C makes the diagnosis of acute viral illness or urinary tract infection more likely. A perforated appendix may be the exception to this rule.

Signs of peritoneal inflammation in the right iliac fossa are often absent in the early stages. The patient should be asked to cough, blow the abdominal wall out and draw it in; these all cause pain if parietal peritoneum is inflamed. In children, it may be difficult to interpret apparent tenderness, especially if the child cries and refuses to cooperate. This can usually be overcome by distracting the child's attention, whilst palpating the abdomen through the bedclothes, or even with the child's own hand under the examiner's hand. Several signs (e.g., Rovsing sign—pressure in the left iliac fossa causing pain in the right iliac fossa) are said to point to a diagnosis of appendicitis but all are unreliable. One useful test is to ask the child to stand, then to hop on the right leg. If this can be achieved, there is unlikely to be significant peritoneal inflammation.

Rebound tenderness was traditionally demonstrated by palpating deeply, then suddenly releasing the hand. However, this can cause excessive and unexpected pain. A kinder and more precise method is to perform gentle percussion in the right iliac fossa. This displaces and irritates inflamed peritoneum in a controlled way; if this is painful, then rebound is present. Anterior peritoneal tenderness on rectal examination (i.e., pelvic peritonitis) supports the diagnosis of appendicitis, provided other signs are consistent, but note the appendix itself cannot be palpated. In pelvic appendicitis, rectal tenderness may be the only abdominal sign. Lack of this sign does not, however, exclude appendicitis.

Differential Diagnosis

This theoretically includes all the causes of an acute abdomen. However, the conditions of practical importance are summarised in Box 26.2. These other conditions rarely need operation. Certain uncommon conditions, such as *Yersinia* ileitis and inflamed Meckel diverticulum (Fig. 26.4) are included in the list but they can only be distinguished from appendicitis at laparoscopy or operation.

The Equivocal Diagnosis

If acute appendicitis can be confidently diagnosed clinically, no further investigations are needed except for potential comorbidity, anaemia or dehydration. It is worth emphasising there are no specific diagnostic tests; where the diagnosis is in doubt, the patient **must** be reexamined every few hours to detect clinical changes to ensure deterioration is detected early. Missing an evident clinical diagnosis and sending the patient home causes unnecessary problems and is likely to prompt a claim for medical negligence.

Certain investigations may be useful where the diagnosis is in doubt. The white blood cell count is usually unhelpful, as a modest rise occurs in many conditions. If there is a great rise (say to over 16×10^3), appendicitis is usually already clinically obvious, but a low white blood cell count helps exclude nonsuppurative gynaecological pathology. Urinalysis must be performed if urinary tract infection is possible. A **pregnancy test** should be performed in females of childbearing age.

Various **scoring systems** have been devised to improve the accuracy of clinical diagnosis. The best known is the Alvarado score (Table 26.1) but results are too variable for it to be of much clinical benefit. The Alvarado scoring system is an objective, structured means of assessing patients with right iliac fossa pain but has proved unreliable in diagnosing acute appendicitis. However, its value lies with patients with an initial score of 4 or less who are very unlikely to have appendicitis and do not need hospital admission unless symptoms worsen. In patients with appendicitis, 40% have rising scores, confirming this as a progressive disorder in which symptoms and signs evolve with time.

Abdominal x-rays are not needed unless there is confusing evidence of abdominal pathology after a period of observation. A single right iliac fossa fluid level or even widespread small bowel

• BOX 26.2 Main Differential Diagnoses of Acute Appendicitis

Urinary Tract Infection (Cystitis or Pyelonephritis)
- Unlikely if nitrites are absent from dipstick testing of the urine and can be excluded if there are not significant numbers of white blood cells or bacteria on urine microscopy

Mesenteric Adenitis
- Common in children and often associated with an upper respiratory infection or sore throat
- Inflammation and enlargement of the abdominal lymph nodes, probably viral in origin
- Fever is typically higher than in appendicitis (i.e., greater than 38.5°C) and settles rapidly
- A firm diagnosis can only be made at laparotomy or laparoscopy, but gradual resolution favours this diagnosis

Large Bowel Disorders
- Constipation may cause colicky abdominal pain and iliac fossa tenderness. There is no fever and the rectum is loaded with faeces
- Diverticulitis affecting the caecum or the sigmoid colon (when lying in the right iliac fossa) is usually diagnosed only at operation

Gynaecological Disorders
- The pain of ovulation about 14 days after the last menstrual period (mittelschmerz) may cause right iliac fossa pain. There is often a history of similar pain in the past. There are no signs of infection and the pain settles quickly
- Salpingitis (most commonly chlamydial) causes lower abdominal pain, often with a vaginal discharge. Digital vaginal examination typically reveals adnexal tenderness, and moving the cervix from side to side induces pain ('cervical excitation')
- Torsion of, or haemorrhage into a right ovarian cyst may produce symptoms like appendicitis, but there is no fever. A tender mobile mass may be palpable in the right suprapubic region or on vaginal examination. This diagnosis can be confirmed with ultrasound
- Ectopic pregnancy. May present with anaemia and/or hypotension. A pregnancy test is mandatory

Small Bowel Pathology
- An inflamed or perforated Meckel diverticulum (see Fig. 26.4) may present exactly like appendicitis
- Terminal ileitis because of Crohn disease (or, more rarely, *Yersinia pseudotuberculosis*)
- Necrotic small bowel from strangulation usually presents with intestinal obstruction

Acute Pancreatitis
- Pain is predominantly central
- If there is tenderness in the right iliac fossa, it will also be present in the epigastrium
- If in doubt, the serum amylase should be measured

Gastroenteritis
- Vague abdominal pain and tenderness, which may be associated with vomiting and diarrhoea
- Usually improves steadily during a period of observation

dilatation suggests local adynamic bowel disorder caused by appendicitis causing functional obstruction, but this is an uncommon finding. Even less commonly, a perforated appendix may allow sufficient free gas to escape to show on plain x-rays. In adults with an equivocal diagnosis of appendicitis, the plasma amylase should be measured to exclude acute pancreatitis. Abdominal ultrasound can

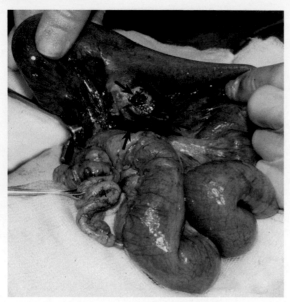

• **Fig. 26.4** Perforated Meckel Diverticulum. This man of 28 years presented with a typical history and clinical findings of acute appendicitis. However, at operation he was found to have a normal appendix but a perforated Meckel diverticulum *(arrowed)*. The diverticulum was resected and the appendix also removed to prevent future confusion and the patient made a good recovery. On histological examination, the Meckel's diverticulum was found to contain gastric mucosa.

TABLE 26.1	Paediatric Appendicitis Scoring (PAS) System in Suspected Acute Appendicitis Based on the Alvarado Score	
Clinical Variable		**Point Value**
Migration of pain to RIF		1
RIF tenderness		2
Nausea/vomiting		1
Anorexia		1
Pain with cough/percussion/hopping		2
Fever >38°C		1
Leucocytosis (WBC >10,000 cells/mL)		1
Neutrophils left shift increase in immature forms		1
MAXIMUM TOTAL SCORE		10
<4 = low risk; >6 = high risk of acute appendicitis		

be helpful to detect an abscess or mass, or nonappendiceal pathology, but cannot be relied upon to show uncomplicated appendicitis. Computed tomography scanning is claimed to be accurate, but submits the patient to a high radiation dose and greatly increases the cost of investigation. In patients over 50 years, this disadvantage must be balanced against the fact that incidental pathology, such as tumours may be diagnosed before operation. Laparoscopy is increasingly used in women of menstruating age in whom gynaecological pathologies are common. However, this is an invasive investigation requiring a general anaesthetic and is best used when an operation is clearly indicated but the diagnosis is still ambiguous.

Problems in the Diagnosis of Appendicitis

The Very Young

Appendicitis is rarely seen below 2 years of age, but when it does occur, the 'typical' abdominal symptoms and signs are obscure or absent. An infant or toddler may display signs of infection without revealing an abdominal origin. Abdominal x-rays may demonstrate dilated loops of bowel and fluid levels. Generalised peritonitis supervenes all too rapidly in this age group because abdominal defences are rudimentary, in particular the greater omentum 'wrapping' effect. Laparotomy is usually indicated in an ill infant with abdominal signs. Children under 5 years often present with peritonitis and should ideally be referred to a specialised Paediatric Surgical Unit.

The Elderly

Appendicitis usually develops more slowly in the elderly. The appendix wall becomes fibrotic with age and the area is more readily walled off by omentum and adherent small bowel. Indeed, many cases probably resolve spontaneously. In those who reach hospital, the history is often as long as 1 week. Features of obstruction may be present, including vomiting, colicky abdominal pain and obstructed bowel sounds. A mass may be palpable if the patient is relaxed and not too tender but often it can be palpated only under general anaesthesia. Abdominal x-rays may reveal fluid levels in the right iliac fossa.

Pregnancy

Appendicitis occurs at least as often during pregnancy as at other times but the diagnosis can be difficult. The appendix is displaced upwards by the enlarging uterus and abdominal pain and tenderness are in a higher position. The management of the pregnant patient must be shared with an obstetrician. Laparoscopy may be indicated, but becomes technically difficult beyond 26 weeks. Mortality from appendicitis for both mother and foetus rises as the pregnancy progresses and can be as high as 9% for the mother and 20% for the foetus in the third trimester.

The 'Grumbling' Appendix

Recurrent bouts of right iliac fossa pain are often labelled 'grumbling appendix'. Appendicular pathology is probably not the cause in most. Persistent chronic appendiceal inflammation probably does not occur, but recurrent bouts of appendicular colic or low-grade acute appendicitis undoubtedly do. These children may have several abortive admissions for abdominal pain and it may eventually be justifiable to remove the appendix to allay parental anxiety. A noninflamed appendix containing a faecolith or threadworms (assumed to have caused the pain) is often found. The pain will be cured in no more than half.

The management of suspected appendicitis is summarised in Fig. 26.5.

Appendicectomy

The annual death rate from appendicitis has fallen dramatically since 1960. There were 3193 deaths in 1934 in the United Kingdom, whereas by 1982 this had fallen to 110 and to 9 by 1997. This results from better general nutrition, earlier presentation, better preoperative preparation and better anaesthesia. Deaths that now occur are usually caused by dehydration and electrolyte changes unrecognised or ineffectively treated before surgery, often as a result of a late or missed diagnosis. Infective complications of appendicitis have fallen dramatically since the 1970s because of the widespread use of prophylactic antibiotics.

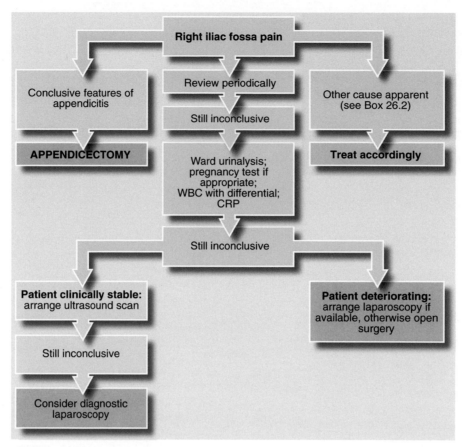

• **Fig. 26.5** Summary—Management of Suspected Appendicitis. *CRP,* C-reactive protein; *WBC,* white blood cell.

Antibiotic Prophylaxis

In appendicitis, most intraabdominal infective complications and wound infections occur in perforated or gangrenous appendicitis (Box 26.3). Most uncomplicated infecting organisms are anaerobes and infections can largely be prevented by prophylactic metronidazole. Rectal suppositories are as effective as intravenous metronidazole and are cheaper, but are best given 2 hours before operation. Aerobic organisms are involved in fewer cases and some surgeons advocate additional prophylaxis with an antibiotic, such as a cephalosporin. In adults with moderate appendicitis, trials of antibiotic treatment alone compare favourably with appendicectomy but about a quarter present later with recurrent appendicitis.

Technique of Appendicectomy

The principal steps are illustrated in Fig. 26.6 and should be understood by any doctor assisting with the operation. Increasingly, laparotomy is being replaced by laparoscopic diagnosis and surgery, but the principles are similar. Surgeons performing appendicectomy need to be aware of possible appendiceal neoplasms, present in 0.5% to 0.9% of appendectomies. Most are innocent carcinoid-type tumours but others are mucinous adenocarcinomas.

Open Appendicectomy

A low skin-crease incision (**Lanz**) rather than a higher and more oblique one centred on McBurney point is now favoured, as it gives a better cosmetic result. The superficial (Scarpa) fascia (well marked in children) is incised and the three musculoaponeurotic abdominal wall layers split along the line of their fibres. This produces the '**gridiron**' **incision**, described as such because the fibres of external oblique and internal oblique run at right angles to each other. Peritoneum is then lifted and opened and may reveal pus or mucopurulent watery fluid; a swab is taken for microscopy and culture. The appendix is located with a finger and delivered into the wound; further exploration may be needed if it does not lie nearby. A retrocaecal appendix requires mobilisation of the caecum by dividing the peritoneum along its lateral side.

Once the appendix has been delivered, its blood supply in the mesoappendix is divided between clips and ligated. The appendix base is crushed with a haemostat, which is then reapplied more distally. An absorbable ligature is tied around the crushed area. After this preparation, the appendix is then excised. A 'purse-string' suture may be placed in the caecum near the appendix base to invert the appendix, although this is not used in laparoscopic surgery and patients have not suffered from its omission. If the appendix is perforated or gangrenous, or if pus was found, thorough peritoneal toilet is performed. A sump sucker is guided down into the pelvis with a finger to aspirate fluid, and the area is gently swabbed with gauze to remove adherent infected material. Any pus or a faecolith left behind predisposes to a pelvic abscess.

The peritoneum, internal oblique and external oblique are each closed with two or three absorbable sutures. Drainage is not usually recommended unless there is a thick-walled abscess cavity, which will not collapse. If the appendix is perforated or gangrenous, delayed primary closure of the skin is advisable as this reduces the high risk of wound infection. The superficial layers are left open initially and closed after 48 hours if the wound is clean.

After operation, oral fluids, followed by solids, are gradually increased unless vomiting or other complications occur, and most patients can be discharged on the second or third postoperative day.

Laparoscopic Appendicectomy

Laparoscopy is a valuable technique that allows the appendix to be found wherever it lies. It also permits visual examination of the rest of the abdominal cavity and pelvis, improving diagnostic accuracy over open operation and minimising negative appendicectomies. It is strongly indicated in patients who are clearly unwell and in need of an operation but in whom the diagnosis is not clear. It is also useful in women of menstruating age and in any patient with pelvic symptoms. If the appendix is abnormal or if there is free fluid in the peritoneal cavity for which no other cause can be found, appendicectomy is performed. Laparoscopic appendicectomy is valuable in the obese, obviating the need for a large incision and a high risk of wound infection. Some surgeons use laparoscopy as a diagnostic tool and then convert to an open operation but laparoscopic appendicectomy may be performed if appropriate skills and instruments are available.

The principles and techniques are similar to open surgery, but laparoscopy is more technically demanding. The mesoappendix may be clipped or divided by diathermy and the appendix base is ligated using preformed 'endo-loop' sutures. The appendix base is rarely buried and must never be diathermied. Superior visualisation and good access allow a thorough washout to be performed. Laparoscopic removal of the appendix has a lower wound infection rate and may allow an earlier return to normal activities.

The 'Lily-White' Appendix

If the appendix is found not to be inflamed at open operation (colloquially termed *lily-white*), it should always be removed because an appendicectomy scar would lead future doctors to assume the appendix has been removed. The abdomen is explored as allowed by the incision to search for a cause for the symptoms:
- **Mesenteric lymph nodes** in children may be grossly enlarged by mesenteric adenitis—probably viral in origin.
- **The terminal ileum** may be thickened and reddened by Crohn disease or, more rarely, by *Yersinia* ileitis. The latter is a self-limiting condition caused by the organism *Yersinia pseudotuberculosis* and requires no specific treatment. The appendix is removed but the bowel left untouched. If possible, an enlarged mesenteric node is removed for histological examination.
- **A Meckel diverticulum** may be found within 60 cm of the ileocaecal valve—if inflamed, this is removed but a wide-mouthed noninflamed diverticulum is usually left alone.
- **Both ovaries can usually be palpated**—ovaries may be twisted, inflamed or enlarged or an inflamed Fallopian tube may be seen.
- **Cholecystitis, sigmoid diverticulitis** (with the sigmoid displaced to the right), **inflammation of a caecal diverticulum, hydronephrosis**, a perforated peptic ulcer with fluid tracking via the right paracolic gutter or a **leaking aneurysm** are rarely found.

The Appendix Mass

A vigorous response to appendicitis may result in a right iliac fossa mass, often with fever. Usually the patient has few systemic symptoms or signs of ill health. A conservative regimen followed by interval appendicectomy 6 weeks later (**Ochsner–Sherren regimen**) was advocated in preantibiotic days, but is now less favoured. Early operation under antibiotic cover is now performed more frequently.

PAS Score

<5	Appendicitis unlikely
5	Appendicitis possible
≥6	Appendicitis probable

RIF, Right Iliac Fossa; *WBC*, white blood cell.

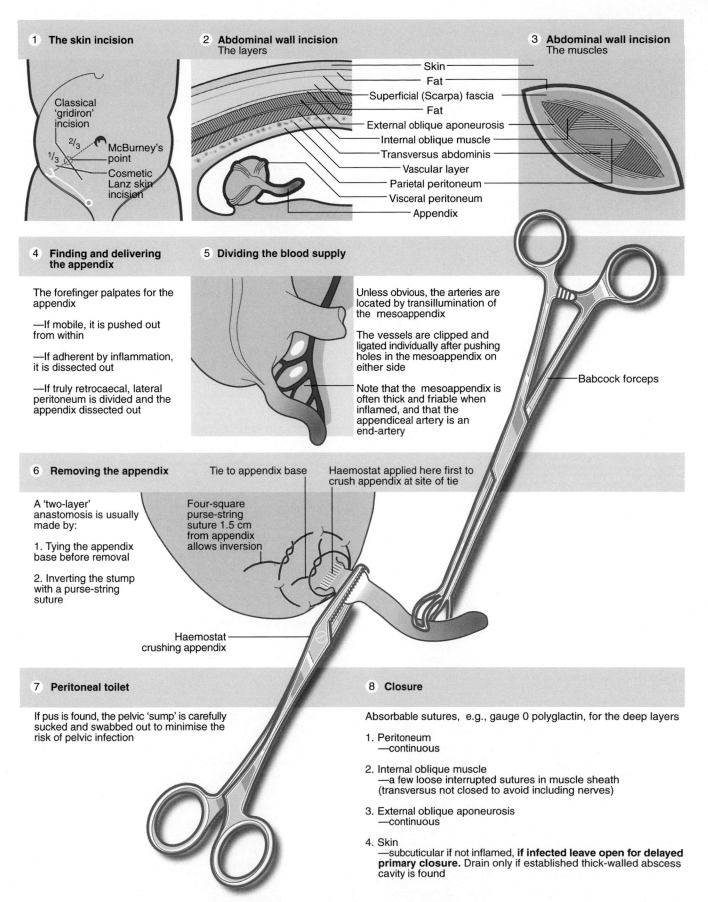

1 The skin incision

Classical 'gridiron' incision

2/3

1/3

McBurney's point

Cosmetic Lanz skin incision

2 Abdominal wall incision
The layers

Skin
Fat
Superficial (Scarpa) fascia
Fat
External oblique aponeurosis
Internal oblique muscle
Transversus abdominis
Vascular layer
Parietal peritoneum
Visceral peritoneum
Appendix

3 Abdominal wall incision
The muscles

4 Finding and delivering the appendix

The forefinger palpates for the appendix

—If mobile, it is pushed out from within

—If adherent by inflammation, it is dissected out

—If truly retrocaecal, lateral peritoneum is divided and the appendix dissected out

5 Dividing the blood supply

Unless obvious, the arteries are located by transillumination of the mesoappendix

The vessels are clipped and ligated individually after pushing holes in the mesoappendix on either side

Note that the mesoappendix is often thick and friable when inflamed, and that the appendiceal artery is an end-artery

Babcock forceps

6 Removing the appendix

A 'two-layer' anastomosis is usually made by:

1. Tying the appendix base before removal

2. Inverting the stump with a purse-string suture

Tie to appendix base

Four-square purse-string suture 1.5 cm from appendix allows inversion

Haemostat applied here first to crush appendix at site of tie

Haemostat crushing appendix

7 Peritoneal toilet

If pus is found, the pelvic 'sump' is carefully sucked and swabbed out to minimise the risk of pelvic infection

8 Closure

Absorbable sutures, e.g., gauge 0 polyglactin, for the deep layers

1. Peritoneum
   —continuous

2. Internal oblique muscle
   —a few loose interrupted sutures in muscle sheath (transversus not closed to avoid including nerves)

3. External oblique aponeurosis
   —continuous

4. Skin
   —subcuticular if not inflamed, **if infected leave open for delayed primary closure.** Drain only if established thick-walled abscess cavity is found

• **Fig. 26.6** Appendicectomy—Operative Technique.

Introduction

Carcinoma of the colon and rectum is the third most common malignancy in both men and women in Western countries. In the United Kingdom, the lifetime risk of colorectal cancer is 5%, although the condition is less common in the developing world. It is rare below the age of 50 years but the diagnosis must be considered in symptomatic patients as this remains an important group. Colorectal cancer is not only extremely common, it is also potentially preventable by screening the colon for premalignant or early malignant lesions, particularly **adenomatous polyps**, in people over 50 years. Surgery for large bowel cancer is generally rewarding, with high rates of cure achieved by timely resection.

Most cancers arise as a result of a complex interaction between genetic and environmental factors. The Western diet in particular with its high red meat content has been incriminated in much of the geographic variation in incidence. About 5% of colorectal cancer is strongly genetically linked. It is important to recognise patients in this small group of **inherited colorectal cancer syndromes**, as there are effective guidelines available for screening and treatment of patients with these high-risk syndromes.

Most colorectal cancers originate in the glandular mucosa and are therefore histologically **adenocarcinomas**. Other forms of malignancy in the large bowel, such as **carcinoid tumour** or **lymphoma** are rare. Squamous carcinomas occur at the anus or in anal canal skin, as do malignant melanomas, but these have an entirely different aetiology and different methods of management; they are discussed in Chapter 30.

Surgery is the mainstay of treatment for colorectal cancer. The common procedures and the complications of large bowel surgery are outlined in this chapter and the different types of intestinal stomas and their indications are described.

Colorectal Polyps

The term **polyp** is simply a morphological description and describes any localised lesion protruding from the bowel mucosa into the lumen; it does not imply any specific pathology. This conforms to the use of the term elsewhere, for example, allergic nasal polyps. A simple pathological classification of large bowel polyps is shown in Box 27.1, emphasising the range of polyp types that can occur there.

Adenomatous Polyps and Adenomas

Polyps are common in the large bowel (Fig. 27.1). The most significant are **adenomas** (i.e., benign neoplasms) and all have potential for **malignant change**. In general, it takes 5 to 10 years to progress to invasive cancer. Early removal prevents the progression from adenoma to adenocarcinoma. The process by which the epithelial cells acquire increasingly severe genetic mutations is termed the **adenoma–carcinoma sequence**. Thus if adenomas are found at endoscopy, all of them should be meticulously removed (see Fig. 27.1C) and subjected to histological examination.

Most adenomas are typically **pedunculated** or **sessile** (stalkless), allowing easy recognition and removal by diathermy snare. The much less common **flat adenomas** are found particularly in the Far East. These can be small and meticulous colonoscopy increases detection rates. Recognition may require special dye-spray techniques. Flat adenomas can be removed by endoscopic mucosal resection, injecting saline into the submucosa to 'lift' the flat lesion before excising the abnormal mucosa with diathermy, sometimes in several pieces.

Adenomatous lesions examined histologically display a range of epithelial abnormalities from low- to high-grade dysplasia, to early invasive cancer. In invasive cancer, the cellular abnormality has breached the muscularis mucosa, from where extension progressively occurs into the submucosa. As a rule, the larger the lesion, the more likely it is to be malignant: only 1% of polyps smaller than 1 cm are malignant, whereas about half of those larger than 2.5 cm are malignant.

Even in apparently benign lesions, there may be discrete areas of frank malignancy, so thorough histological examination is needed. When pedunculated lesions are removed by colonoscopic snaring, it is crucial to establish whether there is stalk invasion: if the stalk is clear of cancer, further treatment is not usually required. The Haggitt classification for stalked and the Kikuchi classification for flat cancers give indications of their malignant potential.

Classification of Colonic Adenomas

Three patterns of lesion are recognised histologically: tubular adenomas, villous adenomas and tubulovillous adenomas.

Tubular adenomas are small pedunculated or sessile lesions, in which the adenoma cells retain a tubular form similar to normal colonic mucosa. Tubular adenomas have the least potential for malignant transformation.

Villous adenomas are usually sessile (no stalk) and frond-like (papilliferous) lesions which tend to secrete mucus. The epithelial component of villous adenoma is more dysplastic than tubular adenoma and there is a correspondingly greater potential for malignancy; as with tubulovillous adenomas, this potential is proportional to size.

Tubulovillous adenomas are intermediate between tubular and villous and make up most colonic polyps (see Fig. 27.1D). Most are low-grade, pedunculated, and the stalk is covered with normal colonic epithelium. The stalk probably develops by peristalsis dragging the tumour mass distally and can range from about 0.5 to 10 cm long. The Paris classification helps determine their potential for malignancy.

Distribution of Colorectal Adenomas

Although adenomatous polyps can occur in any part of the large bowel, three-quarters of them arise in rectum and sigmoid colon. This exactly parallels the distribution of carcinomas and provides verification that most cancers develop from polyps.

Adenomas often arise singly (particularly villous adenoma) but more than 20% of patients with colonic polyps have **multiple polyps,** most often tubulovillous. Patients with proven carcinoma often have coexisting benign adenomas (**synchronous**), likely to become malignant later if not removed (Fig. 27.2). This explains why the whole colon should ideally be examined before colectomy, preferably by colonoscopy, and why long-term follow up after treatment of large bowel cancer should include regular colonoscopy.

Symptoms and Signs of Colorectal Polyps

Many polyps cause no symptoms, and are found incidentally on colonoscopy, barium enema or computed tomography (CT) colonography. Symptomatic polyps typically present with **rectal bleeding** and sometimes **iron deficiency anaemia** from occult blood loss. **Mucus production**, especially from villous adenomas, may be so copious as to be the main presenting complaint. Very occasionally, symptomatic **hypokalaemia** may develop because so much potassium-containing mucus is lost. Distal lesions occasionally produce **tenesmus** (a painful urge to defaecate) or may **prolapse** through the anus. Rarely, large polyps can cause obstructive symptoms or intussusception.

Diagnosis and Management of Colorectal Polyps

For symptomatic patients, visualisation of the entire colon is needed. Most colorectal investigation is somewhat invasive and uncomfortable and the benefits have to be explained to patients, whilst respecting their dignity and privacy as far as possible. In the outpatient clinic, **rigid sigmoidoscopy** (which actually visualises the rectum not the sigmoid) is often performed initially, as nearly half of all polyps lie within 15 cm, the realistic reach of the instrument. **Flexible sigmoidoscopy**, usually performed with bowel preparation or after a phosphate enema, reaches past the sigmoid and descending colon to the splenic flexure, covering 75% of the area at risk, but to view the remainder of the bowel requires **colonoscopy**. Well performed colonoscopy is the 'gold standard' investigation: it allows visualisation of the entire large bowel mucosa, and polyps may be removed at the same time. For this reason, it is the first-line investigation in virtually all centres. However, there are disadvantages: it requires a full day's bowel preparation and the procedure often requires sedation because of the discomfort. Furthermore, colonoscopy carries a 1:1000 risk of major haemorrhage or perforation. Sessile, small or flat adenomas in any location can be difficult to recognise, even at colonoscopy, and these potentially malignant lesions can be missed, especially if bowel preparation has been poor.

An alternative investigation growing in popularity and accuracy is **CT colonography**. Some studies have shown it to be virtually as sensitive for detecting polyps, but if positive, colonoscopy should follow. It is less invasive and does not require sedation but bowel preparation is needed. Other alternative investigations include double contrast barium enema or rarely, unprepared CT scan, although this is unreliable for detecting polyps, it may be useful in excluding cancers in the frail and elderly.

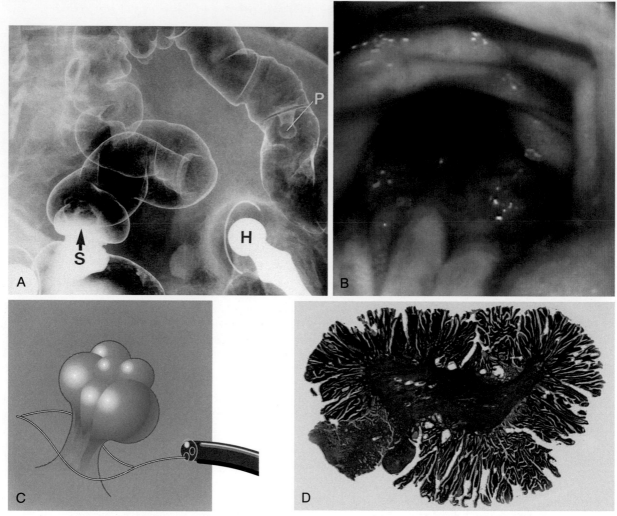

• **Fig. 27.1** Colorectal Polyps. **(A)** This 65-year-old man was found to have positive faecal occult blood on colorectal cancer screening. This computed tomography colography image shows a solitary polyp (S) in the sigmoid colon, later removed by colonoscopic snaring. It proved to be a benign adenoma. (P) indicates another smaller polyp in the descending colon, also removed. (H) indicates a hip prosthesis **(B)** A 2-cm polyp on a long stalk in the sigmoid colon. **(C)** The snare loop is tightened around the stalk of the polyp before applying diathermy current to remove it and coagulate the blood vessels in the stalk. **(D)** Adenomatous polyp having mainly villous glandular architecture. The example shown in **(A)** has a well-defined stalk *(S)*, although this is more typical of tubular or tubulovillous polyps, villous adenomas often having a broad base.

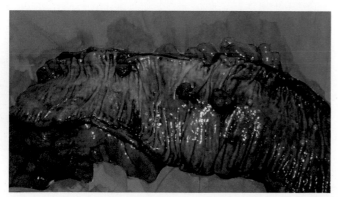

• **Fig. 27.2** Multiple Colonic Adenomatous Polyps. This length of opened descending colon is from a 64-year-old man who presented with an invasive carcinoma of the rectum *(not shown here)*. Several adenomatous polyps of various sizes can be seen in this part of the bowel; the larger polyps have greater malignant potential.

Once an adenomatous polyp is found or a colorectal cancer has been treated, that patient is at risk of forming further polyps elsewhere in the large bowel and needs follow-up colonoscopies. Intervals between colonoscopies are set according to guidelines determined by the number, size and pathology of polyps at each investigation and vary between 1 and 5 years.

Ideally, everyone at risk (by age or predisposing factors) would undergo colonoscopic surveillance (screening) to detect asymptomatic polyps (as well as invasive cancers) so polyps can be removed before undergoing malignant change. The UK National Health Service national bowel cancer screening programme uses faecal occult blood (FOB) testing every 2 years for people between 60 and 74years of age and more recently, bowel scope screening at 55 years. FOB testing aids detection of about 50% of asymptomatic cancers and is predicted to reduce mortality from colorectal cancer by at least 15%. FOB is to be superseded by the faecal immunochemical test, which is more sensitive. Greater reductions will be achieved if patient compliance can be improved, and by the more recent single flexible sigmoidoscopy offered to people aged 55 years.

Adenocarcinoma of Colon and Rectum

Epidemiology of Colorectal Carcinoma

Table 27.1 shows that colorectal cancer is the third most common cause of death from cancer in the developed world; one in 20 people in the United Kingdom suffers from it at some point in their lives and almost a third arise in the rectum. The disease is rare before the age of 50 years (except in inherited colorectal cancer syndromes, see later) but common after the age of 60 years. There is little difference in incidence between the sexes.

Apart from increasing age, **diet** seems to be an important factor. Since colorectal cancer is more common in developed countries, the Western low-fibre, high-fat diet may increase risk. High intake of red meat and alcohol may increase risk, whilst fish, fibre, and antioxidants in fruit and vegetables may reduce it. Other protective agents may include **aspirin** and resistant dietary starch.

Ulcerative colitis and Crohn disease, chronic inflammatory conditions of the large bowel (see Ch. 28), carry independent risk of bowel neoplasia. After 10 years of active disease, the cancer risk rises by 1% each year.

TABLE 27.1 Death Rates From Colorectal Cancer Compared With Other Malignancies (United Kingdom, 2004). Cancers Are Listed in Order of Frequency			
Males (United Kingdom)	Number of Deaths in 2010	Rate per Million Population	% of All Male Cancer Deaths in 2010
1. Lung	19,410	479	23.5
2. Prostate	10,721	238	13
3. Colon and rectum	8574	209	10.4
4. Oesophagus	5105	130	6.2
5. Pancreas	3872	98	4.7
6. Bladder	3294	75	4
7. Stomach	3102	75	3.8
8. Leukaemia	2526	62	3.1
9. Kidney	2451	62	3
10. Non-Hodgkin lymphoma	2394	59	2.9
Other sites	21,032		25.5
All male cancers	**82,841**		
Females (United Kingdom)	Number of Deaths in 2010	Rate per Million Population	% of All Female Cancer Deaths in 2010
1. Lung	15,449	313	20.7
2. Breast	11,556	244	15.5
3. Colon and rectum	7134	127	9.5
4. Ovary	4295	91	5.7
5. Pancreas	4029	77	5.4
6. Oesophagus	2505	45	3.3
7. Non-Hodgkin Lymphoma	2042	38	2.7
8. Leukaemia	1978	36	2.6
9. Uterus	1937	39	2.6
10. Stomach	1858	33	2.5
Other sites	22,011		29.4
All female cancers	**74,794**		

Cancer mortality is decreasing in the United Kingdom, thanks to earlier diagnosis and improved treatments. For all cancers combined, mortality has fallen by approximately 26% and 20% in males and females, respectively, since 1990. The largest falls in mortality have occurred for stomach cancer (by 36% and 32% in males and females respectively), cervical cancer (by 28%) and breast cancer (by 19%). Mortality from lung cancer has fallen by 19% in males but increased by 6% in females, attributable to changes in patterns of smoking.

Finally, some **inherited genetic conditions** give rise to colorectal cancer. This explains the higher risk in first-degree relatives of patients with early-onset cancers, and why it is important to ask about family history of bowel or other potentially inherited cancers in patients presenting with bowel symptoms.

Inherited Conditions Causing Bowel Cancer

A small proportion of bowel cancers result from inherited conditions but they account for a disproportionate number of those presenting when young. Identifying these 'at risk' families allows counselling, surveillance and cancer prevention, best done through referral to specialist Familial Colorectal Cancer clinics. These inherited conditions may be divided into the **polyposis syndromes**, in which sufferers develop large numbers of polyps early in life, likely to undergo malignant change, and **hereditary non polyposis colorectal cancer (HNPCC)**, in which sufferers have 'normal' or low numbers of adenomatous polyps, which tend to progress to cancer. The latter is the most common inherited condition predisposing to bowel cancer.

Polyposis Syndromes

The most important is **familial adenomatous polyposis**, because it is reasonably common (1:30,000 people) and because large bowel cancer is inevitable if untreated. An autosomal dominant defect in the *adenomatous polyposis coli* gene causes 100 or more adenomatous polyps to develop in the large bowel by the mid-teens. Affected patients usually have one parent with the condition, but new mutations can occur spontaneously. Each affected individual is certain to develop colorectal cancer by the age of 40 years, unless preventive measures are taken. Ideally, prophylactic surgery should be performed in early adulthood to remove the area at risk. One option is subtotal colectomy and ileorectal anastomosis, which removes nearly all the large bowel but retains the rectum. This requires very careful very long-term surveillance for malignancy. The alternative is to remove the rectum as well (**panproctocolectomy**) and perform an ileostomy or an **ileal pouch** restorative procedure.

Another polyposis syndrome is **Peutz–Jeghers** syndrome, which causes hamartomatous polyps throughout the gastrointestinal tract. Patients often have freckles around the mouth and on hands, feet and genitalia. Half of these patients are likely to die by the age of 50 years because of polyp-related emergencies, such as bowel intussusception or cancer. Patients are prone to develop cancers of small and large bowel, stomach, pancreas, testis and breast.

Hereditary Nonpolyposis Colorectal Cancer. HNPCC syndrome (also known as *Lynch syndrome*) results from defects in mismatch repair genes, which mend damaged deoxyribonucleic acid. The condition carries a 70% lifetime risk of colorectal cancer, but also a substantially increased risk of one or more of other 'indicator' cancers, such as endometrium, ovary, urothelium, small bowel and brain. Families can be difficult to identify because of the diversity of cancers and incomplete genetic penetrance (i.e., not everyone carrying the defect will develop cancer). When HNPCC is suggested by histological characteristics, young age of tumour onset, cooccurrence of tumours or family history, tumour tissue can be screened by immunohistochemistry and assessment of microsatellite instability. If abnormal, formal genetic tests are then undertaken. Those carrying a mutation are best offered colonoscopy every 2 years from the age of 25 years.

Pathophysiology of Colorectal Carcinoma

Colorectal carcinomas exhibit a wide range of differentiation, which broadly correlates with their clinical behaviour and prognosis (see Fig. 27.4). Most carcinomas are initially **exophytic** (i.e., protruding into the lumen) and later ulcerate on the surface and progressively invade the muscular bowel wall. Eventually, the tumour involves serosa and surrounding structures. Stromal fibrosis may cause luminal narrowing, responsible for the common acute presentation of **large bowel obstruction**.

Large bowel carcinomas metastasise via lymphatics and the bloodstream, and by the time of diagnosis, as many as 25% of patients already have distant metastases (Fig. 27.3). Lymphatic spread is sequential, first to mesenteric nodes and then onward to paraaortic nodes. Occasionally, lymph node involvement is directly responsible for the clinical presentation. For example, paraaortic nodes may present as a palpable mass or cause **duodenal obstruction**. Other enlarged nodes may compress bile ducts in the porta hepatis causing **jaundice**.

Haematogenous spread usually occurs later than lymphatic spread and is predominantly to the liver and less commonly to other sites, such as lung or bone. Systemic manifestations may also occur.

Presentation of Large Bowel Carcinoma

Late presentations with metastases have been discussed. For local disease, the mode of growth and clinical presentation of large bowel cancer depend to some extent on the site.

Blood Loss and Anaemia

Carcinomas of caecum and ascending colon rarely obstruct unless the ileocaecal valve is involved. This is because the right colon has a larger diameter than the left and the faecal stream is more fluid. However, occult **bleeding** from the tumour surface commonly causes iron deficiency **anaemia**, and these patients typically present with anaemia and a palpable mass in the right iliac fossa.

Change of Bowel Habit and Large Bowel Obstruction

Colorectal cancers usually secrete mucus and bleed into the lumen, which tends to change the bowel habit towards a looser stool. Thus a recent history of loose stool is more likely to predict cancer than increasing constipation, especially since constipation is so common in the elderly population. Faeces in the left colon are more solid and the intraluminal pressure is higher, thus distal cancers here are more likely to obstruct. Colonic cancers tend to progressively encircle the bowel wall, encroaching on the lumen and producing an **annular stenosis**, taking perhaps a year to involve each quarter of the circumference.

Large bowel obstruction may be partial or complete. **Partial obstruction** may present as a change in bowel habit, often noticed as constipation with intermittent 'overflow' diarrhoea. **Complete obstruction** precipitates emergency hospital admission (see Ch. 19).

Rectal Bleeding

Carcinomas distal to the splenic flexure often cause visible blood to be passed per rectum. The character of the blood and the nature of its mixing with stool depend on how far proximally the lesion is from the anus.

Tenesmus

Carcinomas or polyps in the lower two-thirds of the rectum may be perceived as masses of faeces. This stimulates a persistent defaecation response, causing an unpleasant sensation of incomplete evacuation known as *tenesmus*.

CASE HISTORY

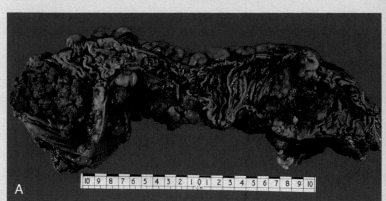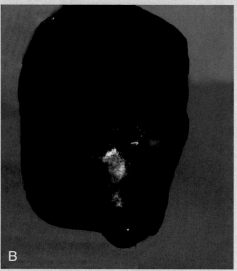

• **Fig. 27.3** Cancers of the Colon and Rectum. **(A)** Synchronous cancers of the transverse colon. This elderly man presented with a change in bowel habit, with constipation and overflow diarrhoea. Preoperative colonoscopy revealed two cancers that were biopsied and later resected at operation and the ends anastomosed. **(B)** This 49-year-old man presented with a 9-month history of rectal bleeding, found to be caused by a sigmoid colon carcinoma, which was resected. Two years later, he was found on ultrasound screening to have a single metastasis in the right lobe of the liver. No other metastases were found, so he underwent a resection of the right lobe of the liver; the resected specimen is seen here. Unfortunately, he returned 3 years later with a malignant paraduodenal mass and widespread peritoneal metastases, from which he died.

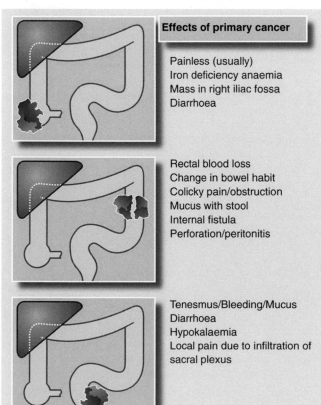

Effects of primary cancer

Painless (usually)
Iron deficiency anaemia
Mass in right iliac fossa
Diarrhoea

Rectal blood loss
Change in bowel habit
Colicky pain/obstruction
Mucus with stool
Internal fistula
Perforation/peritonitis

Tenesmus/Bleeding/Mucus
Diarrhoea
Hypokalaemia
Local pain due to infiltration of sacral plexus

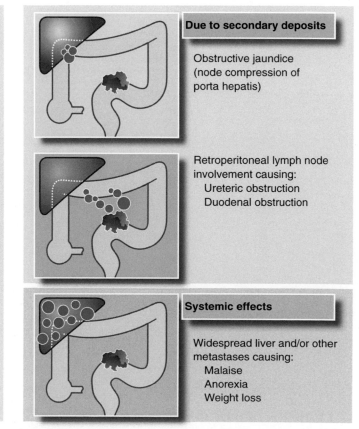

Due to secondary deposits

Obstructive jaundice
(node compression of porta hepatis)

Retroperitoneal lymph node involvement causing:
    Ureteric obstruction
    Duodenal obstruction

Systemic effects

Widespread liver and/or other metastases causing:
    Malaise
    Anorexia
    Weight loss

• **Fig. 27.4** Symptoms and Signs of Colorectal Cancer.

Perforation

A cancer penetrating the bowel wall may stimulate a vigorous local inflammatory process resulting in a **pericolic abscess**, which contains the perforation, at least for a while. This most often occurs in the rectosigmoid area and usually presents with left iliac fossa pain and tenderness and a swinging fever. The differential diagnosis is acute diverticulitis or a diverticular abscess.

A carcinoma anywhere in the colon (but rarely in the rectum) may perforate and present as an acute abdomen with **peritonitis**. Occasionally a carcinoma may erode into a nearby organ creating a malignant **fistula**. Fistulation can occur into stomach, bladder, uterus or vagina, or direct to the skin. Perforated cancers tend to carry a poor long-term prognosis even after successful treatment.

Clinical Signs in Suspected Colorectal Carcinoma

These are illustrated in Fig. 27.4. General examination may show features suggesting disseminated malignancy, for example, obvious cachexia or supraclavicular node enlargement. Abdominal examination is usually unremarkable but may reveal a mass in the colon, hepatomegaly caused by metastases, or ascitic fluid. Unfortunately, all these signs represent late and often incurable disease.

Rectal examination is mandatory in all suspected cases, as a high proportion of carcinomas occur in the lowest 12 cm and can be reached with an examining finger. In addition, intraperitoneal tumour spread into the pouch of Douglas may be palpable anteriorly through the rectal wall. The degree of **fixation** of a rectal tumour to surrounding structures can also be evaluated digitally to give some indication of the need for neoadjuvant radiotherapy and operative difficulty. Finally, the glove should be inspected for stool colour and consistency, as well as blood and mucus.

Investigation of Suspected Colorectal Carcinoma

Proctoscopy and rigid or flexible sigmoidoscopy are usually performed at the initial consultation for anyone complaining of bowel symptoms. About 50% of colorectal cancers lie within reach of a rigid sigmoidoscope and 75% within reach of a flexible sigmoidoscope. Lesions can be biopsied through either instrument.

A history of rectal bleeding should be fully investigated in patients over about 45 years and in any patient if the symptoms or signs suggest malignancy. This applies even if a local cause, such as haemorrhoids is found, since these are so common that they will often be found coincidentally. **Flexible sigmoidoscopy** is the minimum initial investigation for rectal bleeding because the causative lesion is probably in the left side of the colon. If a tumour is found, the rest of the bowel must still be examined for synchronous tumours or further polyps.

Where a change in bowel habit (particularly looser stools) or unexplained anaemia is present, any bowel lesion could be left or right sided, and thus the entire colon must be examined by colonoscopy or radiological imaging (Fig. 27.5).

Blood Tests

Bowel neoplasms often cause anaemia but liver function tests remain normal, until almost all parenchyma is replaced by tumour. Hypokalaemia rarely results from lesions producing excess mucin. Tumour markers are neither sensitive nor specific for a primary diagnosis of colorectal cancer but **carcinoembryonic antigen** (CEA) is used to monitor cancer recurrence.

Imaging for Staging

When colorectal malignancy is diagnosed, colonic surgery is likely to be necessary to relieve symptoms irrespective of distant spread. **Staging** is performed to guide oncological planning and

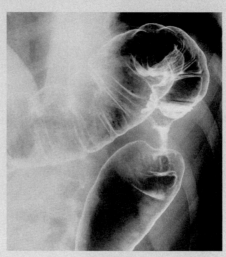

• **Fig. 27.5** Colonic Carcinoma: Barium Enema Examination. Typical 'apple-core' lesion just distal to the splenic flexure of a man of 39 years who complained of rectal bleeding. With this degree of stenosis, it was surprising that he had had no change in bowel habit. Acute obstruction would probably soon have occurred if the tumour had not been recognised and resected. The patient is unusually young for colorectal carcinoma in the Western world.

counselling. Liver and lung metastases are sought (and may be amenable to curative resectional surgery) along with other evidence of spread within the abdomen or to bone. CT thorax, abdomen and pelvis is the most useful investigation. Magnetic resonance imaging (MRI) is performed if liver metastases are suspected (or ultrasound if unavailable). CT positron emission tomography scanning is occasionally used. MRI scanning adds essential information about the precise extent of local spread of rectal cancer.

In a patient presenting as an emergency with complete large bowel obstruction, plain abdominal x-rays often show large bowel dilated by gas, down to the level of obstruction and empty of gas beyond it. The level is often at the sigmoid colon or rectosigmoid junction. CT scanning is essential to confirm the likely diagnosis of carcinoma. An 'instant' Gastrografin enema (i.e., without bowel preparation) can confirm the diagnosis and at the same time exclude **pseudoobstruction**.

Management of Colorectal Carcinoma

Surgical excision is the main treatment. For tumours localised to the bowel wall, resection offers an excellent chance of complete cure; for tumours at a more advanced stage, chemotherapy and radiotherapy may increase the chance of cure. For rectal cancers, chemoradiotherapy (long course), or short-course radiotherapy alone, may be given preoperatively (known as **neoadjuvant therapy**) to shrink the tumour to improve the chances of successful surgical removal. Management plans are ideally formulated by multidisciplinary team discussion, where surgeons, oncologists, radiologists, geneticists, palliative care physicians and colorectal specialist nurses discuss all aspects of the case.

For advanced disease, even with very extensive tumours, palliative resection may be worthwhile to relieve obstruction or to prevent continuing blood loss. In frail patients with metastatic disease, in whom any surgery is too risky, a **stent** can often be placed endoscopically on the left side of the colon to hold the

TABLE 27.2 Staging and Survival Rates From Treated Colorectal Carcinoma

UICC Stage	Tumour/Node/Metastasis (TNM) Stage	Modified Dukes stage	Approximate 5-Year Survival
Stage 0	Dysplasia only		
Stage I	Tumour invades submucosa (T1) Tumour invades muscularis propria (T2) No lymph node metastases	A	85%–95%
Stage II	Tumour invades beyond muscularis propria (T3) Tumour invades into other organs (T4) No lymph node metastases	B	60%–80%
Stage III	1–3 regional lymph nodes involved—any T (N1) 4 or more regional lymph nodes involved—any T (N2) No distant metastases	C C1: apical node not involved (node furthest from tumour) C2: apical node involved	30%–60%
Stage IV	Distant metastasis (M1) Any T stage, any N stage	D	<10%

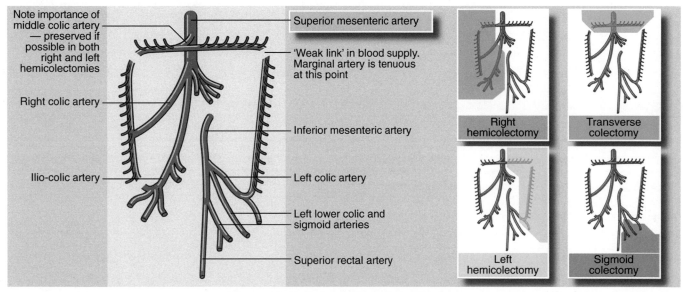

• **Fig. 27.6** Standard Operations for Colonic Cancer.

bowel open and relieve obstruction. There is an increasing role for liver resection and also to a lesser degree pulmonary resection for metastases where there is a curative (not palliative) intent.

Staging of Colorectal Carcinoma

Staging of colorectal carcinoma influences the desirability of further treatment by chemotherapy or radiotherapy. It also gives an estimate of the statistical probability of surviving 5 years and the likelihood of cure. Final staging of colorectal cancer depends on information from several sources: the findings at laparotomy, histological examination of the resected specimen and the radiological and other imaging for distant organ spread. The two most widely used staging systems are the tumour/node/metastasis (**TNM**) and **Dukes classification**, outlined in Table 27.2.

Approximately a quarter of all patients with colorectal cancer have metastases at presentation; most of these die within 5 years. Of those that undergo radical surgery with the aim of cure, 50% are alive and well 5 years later. Very few patients surviving 5 years die later of recurrent disease.

Operations for Colorectal Cancer

The principles of colorectal tumour resection are as follows:
- Before elective operations, the bowel may be prepared by giving a low residue diet and enemas. Oral purgatives are no longer given for right-sided tumours, but most surgeons prepare patients with low left tumours. However, beware of the risk of dehydration. Oral antibiotics are increasingly being given, having been shown to reduce surgical site infection and anastomotic leak rate.
- Perioperative prophylactic antibiotics (e.g., gentamicin, penicillin and metronidazole) are given.
- Operative access is achieved laparoscopically, or by laparotomy, usually via a midline incision.
- The affected segment of bowel is removed with a margin of normal bowel, usually 5 cm clear each side of the tumour. There must be a good blood supply to the cut ends of bowel to ensure healing so, in practice, lines of resection are determined by the distribution of mesenteric blood vessels (Fig. 27.6). For example, ascending colon lesions are treated by

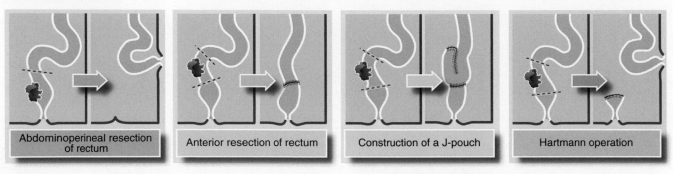

| Abdominoperineal resection of rectum | Anterior resection of rectum | Construction of a J-pouch | Hartmann operation |

• **Fig. 27.7** Standard Operations for Rectal Cancer. Hartmann procedure is described in Fig. 27.11.

removing the whole right colon (right hemicolectomy), as the ileocolic artery must be ligated to remove a section of the right colon.

• A broad section of colonic mesentery is removed with the bowel. This contains the primary field of lymph node drainage. If there are other obvious lymph node metastases, these are usually included in the resection specimen.

• **Rectal cancers** are a special case and an outline of standard operations is given in Fig. 27.7. The preferred operation is a sphincter-saving **anterior resection of rectum**; provided the lower edge of the tumour is 1 to 2 cm above the anal sphincters, the sphincter can usually be preserved. This operation involves excising the tumour with an appropriate length of bowel, plus an intact envelope of fat around it (the **mesorectum** containing local lymph nodes). The proximal end of bowel is then anastomosed to the distal stump. Occasionally, a pelvic reservoir is created using a **J-pouch** technique (see Fig. 27.7), when performing a coloanal anastomosis. This has been shown to reduce the frequency and urgency of defaecation without increasing surgical complications. A temporary defunctioning ileostomy or colostomy is generally used for operations below the peritoneal reflection to aid healing of a low anastomosis. If the sphincter is involved, the entire rectum and anus have to be removed via an **abdominoperineal excision**, with the proximal end of bowel brought out as a colostomy.

• In most colonic cases, the two cut ends of bowel can be anastomosed without the need for a temporary or permanent colostomy, though this is not so for rectal cases (the indications for stomas and their types and management are described later). The method used to rejoin the bowel depends on the site of the anastomosis, the preference of the surgeon and whether there is much disparity in diameter between the ends to be joined. Methods of large bowel anastomosis are shown in Figs 27.8 and 27.9.

• Postoperatively, an 'enhanced recovery' program may be used to encourage early eating and mobilisation (see Ch. 2, p. 17). These have been shown to lower complication rates and shorten hospital stays.

The Role of Adjuvant Radiotherapy and Chemotherapy

Neoadjuvant radiotherapy is usually offered to patients with locally advanced rectal cancer, together with postoperative chemotherapy if there is lymph node involvement or vascular invasion, to increase the chance of prolonged survival. Neoadjuvant radiotherapy is particularly relevant for rectal tumours tethered in the pelvis, where shrinking a large tumour can make it operable. Radiotherapy after surgery is less effective and reflects incorrect preoperative staging. It risks radiation damage to small bowel now lying in the pelvis.

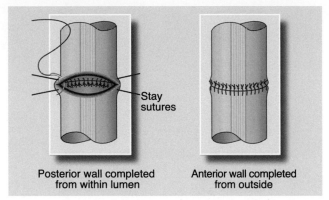

Posterior wall completed from within lumen — Stay sutures — Anterior wall completed from outside

• **Fig. 27.8** Single-Layer Method of Bowel Anastomosis. A single-layer anastomosis using interrupted absorbable sutures is the safest and most commonly used method of anastomosis for nearly all types of bowel. If the bowel cannot be rotated, the posterior layer sutures are placed from inside the bowel and knotted within the lumen. Sutures usually incorporate the muscle wall and submucosa but not the mucosa.

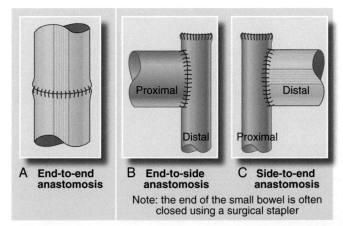

| A End-to-end anastomosis | B End-to-side anastomosis | C Side-to-end anastomosis |

Note: the end of the small bowel is often closed using a surgical stapler

• **Fig. 27.9** Safe and Reliable Methods of Matching the Diameter of the Bowel Ends to Effect a Safe Anastomosis. (A) An end-to-end anastomosis is used when bowel ends are of similar diameter. (B) An end-to-side anastomosis is used where the proximal end is greater in diameter than the distal end, for example, in small bowel obstruction. (C) A side-to-end anastomosis is used where the distal end is greater in diameter than the proximal end, for example, in right hemicolectomy.

For chemotherapy in large bowel cancer, **5-fluorouracil (5-FU)** is the chief adjuvant agent; it is often given in combination with a range of newer agents.

Management of Advanced Disease and Recurrence

In advanced disease, primary tumour is sometimes resected to relieve its local effects even with distant metastases. Most of these patients die within 1 or 2 years and only about one in 10 survives 3 years. The exception is metastasis confined to the liver (see later), where partial liver resection is enabling prolonged survival in up to 40% of patients.

The **liver** is the most common site of distant metastasis. Liver metastases may be discovered at imaging for staging before operation, at operation or later as a result of surveillance with CT or blood tumour marker (CEA) estimation. Occasionally, there may be one or two metastases (or even multiple metastases) confined to a resectable anatomical lobe, sometimes after downstaging chemotherapy and reassessment. Given the relatively good outcome, liver resections for metastases are increasingly performed. MRI scanning should be used to look for occult metastases before attempting liver resection.

Patients with liver metastases seldom become jaundiced until the parenchyma is almost completely destroyed or major bile ducts are compressed at the porta hepatis. Specific treatment for this late event is rarely effective, although oral dexamethasone may temporarily reduce metastatic tissue oedema and relieve symptoms. Liver transplantation is fruitless. Colorectal tumours sometimes metastasise to **bone**, particularly the lumbar spine, and painful lesions may be palliated by radiotherapy.

Metastatic colorectal carcinomas are most often treated with 5-FU, with oxaliplatin as a second-line agent. This can substantially prolong survival and improve quality of life.

'Recurrences' within the colon usually represent new cancers arising metachronously from preexisting or new adenomas. Careful examination of the entire colon before the first operation is likely to reduce such disease. Local recurrence in rectal cancer is now seen less than 10%, but this was more common before neoadjuvant radiotherapy and before the importance of total mesorectal excision in anterior resection was realised (Fig. 27.10). In abdominoperineal excision, some surgeons use a prone patient position in theatre, which can give a clearer view of the anatomy and allows wider, more oncological margin clearance to be obtained. Recurrences often cause intractable perineal pain; occasionally a fungating mass grows in the anal region or buttocks. These very distressing complications may be palliated to a degree with radiotherapy.

Complications of Large Bowel Surgery

Complications of large bowel surgery include mortality, morbidity, anastomotic leakage and pelvic nerve damage and are summarised in Box 27.2. Infection arising from faecal contamination is the main early complication of large bowel surgery. Contamination may result from perforation before operation, inadvertent faecal spillage during the operation or postoperative anastomotic leakage or breakdown.

Three main types of surgical site infection occur: wound infection and/or dehiscence, intraperitoneal abscesses and generalised peritonitis. Intraabdominal infection carries a high risk of sepsis and multiorgan dysfunction, particularly after emergency operations. Most of these infective complications are radically reduced by appropriate use of prophylactic antibiotics.

Stomas

Indications and General Principles

It is often necessary to divert the faecal stream to the anterior abdominal wall via a stoma. The effluent is collected in a removable plastic bag attached by adhesive to the abdominal skin. Stomas are named according to the part of the bowel opening on to the abdominal wall, that is, **ileostomy** or **colostomy**. The term **urostomy** is used for the ileal conduit that connects ureters to the skin surface in patients whose bladder has been removed.

Stomas may be permanent or temporary. Wherever possible, the need for a stoma should be anticipated before operation and

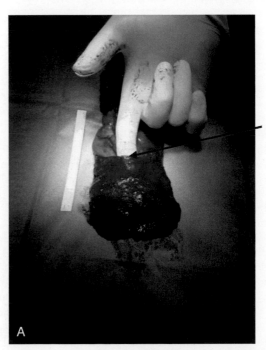

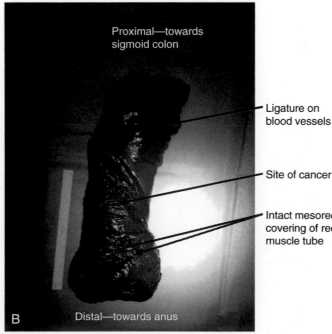

• **Fig. 27.10** Total Mesorectal Excision for Low Rectal Carcinoma. Low carcinoma of rectum in a 70-year-old woman, who presented with rectal bleeding and a change of bowel habit. A low anterior resection was performed with a covering loop ileostomy. The bowel was rejoined using the circular stapler. Two complete 'doughnuts' of tissue indicated successful firing of the stapler (see also Fig. 27.4).

discussed with the patient. This is done to obtain informed consent and to prepare the patient for what is often perceived as worse than it is. Specialised **stoma therapists** assist in planning and aftercare. Before the operation, they counsel the patient, who is encouraged to try out a dummy appliance and talk to other stoma patients. The stoma therapist also identifies and marks the most suitable and comfortable site for the stoma appliance. This takes into account the patient's occupation and leisure activities, clothing and ability for self-care. Colostomies are usually fashioned in the left iliac fossa and ileostomies in the right iliac fossa.

Permanent Stomas

These are necessary when there is no distal bowel segment remaining after resection or when for some reason the bowel is not to be rejoined. A **colostomy** is required after **abdominoperineal excision** of a low rectal or anal canal tumour. An **ileostomy** (see Fig. 27.12) is used after excision of the whole colon and rectum (panproctocolectomy) unless a pouch reconstruction is performed. Sometimes in patients with severe and permanent incontinence, a colostomy may make a better life possible.

Emergency Procedures

A temporary stoma may be created (even by an inexperienced surgeon) as an emergency measure to relieve complete distal large bowel obstruction, causing proximal bowel dilatation. If the ileocaecal valve remains competent in complete obstruction, the caecum can rupture and cause death by peritonitis. Thus if a patient with large bowel obstruction has a dilated caecum but no small bowel dilatation on plain abdominal x-ray, the ileocaecal valve is likely to be competent. If the patient develops right iliac fossa pain, perforation is imminent. Perforation can be prevented by a timely diverting stoma; the obstructing lesion may be removed at the same operation or later.

• BOX 27.2   Complications of Large Bowel Surgery

Early Complications

Local
- Inadvertent damage to other organs, for example, ureter, bladder, duodenum or spleen—usually recognised at operation
- Haemorrhage, for example, slipped ligature
- Wound infection—cellulitis, abscess or wound edge necrosis
- Intraabdominal abscess—at site of surgery, pelvic or subphrenic

Regional
- Anastomotic leak or breakdown—local or general peritonitis
- Stoma problems—sloughing or retraction
- Compartment syndrome in legs caused by prolonged elevation during perineal surgery (rare)

Systemic
- New onset atrial fibrillation or flutter—often indicates anastomotic breakdown
- Systemic sepsis leading to multiorgan dysfunction syndrome

Later Complications
- Diarrhoea—because of short bowel
- Division of pelvic parasympathetic nerves—causes sexual/bladder dysfunction
- Small bowel obstruction—because of pelvic peritoneal adhesions or tangling of small bowel with colostomy or ileostomy, or later as a complication of radiotherapy causing small bowel damage

---

Defunctioning Stomas

A 'defunctioning' stoma (ileostomy or colostomy) may be used to protect a more distal anastomosis at particular risk of leakage or breakdown, by preventing intraluminal pressure rises and by diverting the faecal stream. Common examples are most low rectal anastomoses (flatus and faeces may leak through the anastomosis), an anastomosis performed after resection of an obstructing lesion (distension may compromise the blood supply), or emergency resection involving unprepared bowel (solid faeces may remain impacted in the lumen). Reversing the temporary stoma to restore bowel continuity is often a relatively simple procedure, usually performed after 3 to 4 months. Most surgeons like to perform a limited contrast enema to demonstrate anastomotic integrity before closing the stoma.

Bowel Rest

A temporary colostomy may be used to 'rest' a more distal segment of bowel or a perineum involved in an inflammatory process, by diverting the faecal stream. Examples include pericolic abscess, complex anorectal fistulae and major surgical perineal wounds.

Types of Stoma

The way in which a stoma is fashioned depends on its purpose. The main types of stoma are described later and illustrated in Fig. 27.11. Colonic stomas are designed with the bowel mucosa lying almost flush with the skin. Small bowel stomas are fashioned with a 'spout' of bowel protruding about 3 cm, to ensure that the irritant small bowel contents enter the ileostomy appliance directly rather than flowing on to the skin (Fig. 27.12).

Loop Stoma

This type of stoma is designed so that both proximal and distal segments of bowel drain onto the skin surface (see Fig. 27.11A). This deflects proximal effluent to the skin surface and provides a 'blow-off' valve for the distal loop. Loop stomas are used mainly for temporary defunctioning to protect a distal anastomosis. It is straightforward to reanastomose the ends at reversal; the loop is then dropped back into the abdomen. The most common form of loop stoma is the **loop ileostomy**; occasionally a **loop transverse colostomy** is used.

Split or 'Spectacle' Stoma

This is the ultimate form of defunctioning stoma but has been largely superseded by the loop stoma. After resection, both proximal and distal bowel ends are brought separately to the skin surface. The proximal end stoma passes stool into a stoma appliance; the distal stoma (or **mucous fistula**) defunctions the bowel beyond it and produces just a little mucus.

End Stoma

This type of stoma is usually permanent. An end **colostomy** is most commonly used to 'resite the anus' on to the abdominal wall after removal of the rectum and anal sphincter (i.e., abdominoperineal excision—see Fig. 27.11B). An **ileostomy** may be used after subtotal or panproctocolectomy, particularly in fulminant colitis (see Fig. 27.11C). Later, some form of reconstruction may be considered, involving an ileal pouch or reservoir in the pelvis composed of loops of ileum sutured side-to-side connected to the anus. The anal sphincter mechanism is preserved so that the patient is usually continent and can control evacuation.

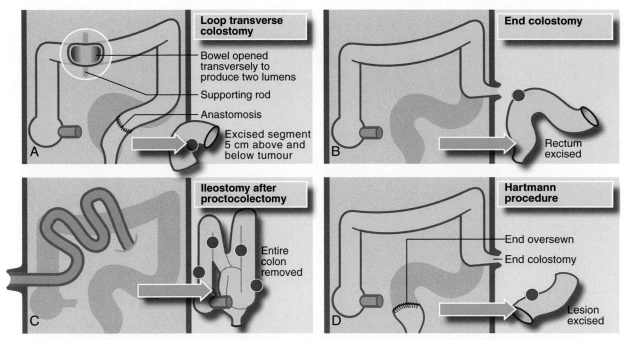

• **Fig. 27.11 Principal Types of Ileostomy and Colostomy. (A)** Loop transverse colostomy is usually temporary, and is used to defunction the distal bowel. **(B)** End colostomy is usually permanent. **(C)** Ileostomy after proctocolectomy is permanent. Note the protruding 'spout' produced by everting the ileum. **(D)** End colostomy in Hartmann procedure sometimes becomes permanent.

CASE HISTORY

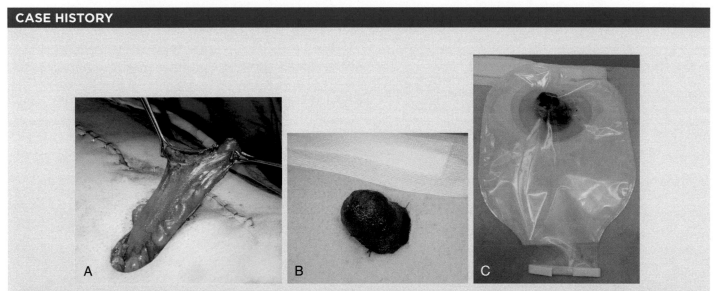

• **Fig. 27.12 End Ileostomy.** This man of 45 years had suffered remittent ulcerative colitis for 12 years, which could only be managed with high doses of steroids. He underwent subtotal colectomy and formation of this end ileostomy. Later, he will be considered for a pouch reconstruction. **(A)** Formation of ileostomy. The end of the ileum is brought to the surface via an opening made in the right iliac fossa at a point predetermined by the stoma therapist. **(B)** The end of the ileum has been turned back on itself like a cuff to form a spout or Brook ileostomy. **(C)** The stoma bag placed in the operating theatre

Hartmann Procedure: End Colostomy and Rectal Stump

Hartmann procedure is a relatively safe technique, particularly for less experienced surgeons, and carries less overall risk than primary anastomosis. It is used after emergency resection of rectosigmoid lesions, where primary anastomosis is inadvisable because of obstruction, inflammation or faecal contamination or surgical inexperience. It may be the choice of treatment for frail or debilitated patients. At Hartmann operation, the lesion is resected, the proximal bowel is made into an end colostomy (the same as that used after an abdominoperineal excision) and the cut end of the distal remnant is closed with sutures or staples (see Fig. 27.11D). Secretions from the residual rectum still pass through the anus. Several months later, when local inflammation has resolved, a decision may be made to reconnect the bowel, depending on fitness and the preference of the patient. However, the colostomy is so well tolerated that some patients prefer to keep

TABLE 27.3	Complications of Ileostomy and Colostomy	
Complication	**Treatment**
Early Complications	
Mucosal sloughing or necrosis of the terminal bowel caused by ischaemia	Reoperation and refashioning of the stoma
Obstruction of stoma caused by oedema or faecal impaction	Exploration with a gloved finger and sometimes glycerol suppositories or softening enemas
Persistent leakage between skin and appliance causing skin erosion and patient distress, often caused by inappropriate location of stoma (e.g., over skin crease)	May respond to stoma nursing care or require a resiting operation
Late Complications	
Parastomal hernia caused by abdominal wall weakness	Resiting of stoma ± mesh reinforcement of abdominal wall
Prolapse of bowel	Refashioning of stoma
Parastomal fistula	Refashioning of stoma, or local repair, possibly laparoscopic
Retraction of 'spout' ileostomy	Reoperation and refashioning of a new ileostomy
Stenosis of stomal orifice	Refashioning of stoma
Perforation after colonic irrigation	Emergency operation
Psychological and psychosexual dysfunction	May require counselling or measures to reverse stoma

it permanently rather than undergo another major operation. A staple technique makes reversal substantially easier than a hand sewn technique.

Irrigation Technique for Managing a Colostomy

An ileostomy tends to work continuously during the day, whereas a colostomy is intermittent. Some patients with a colostomy prefer to dispense with a stoma bag by using a technique of colonic irrigation. Once every few days, the patient passes a litre or more of water into the colostomy via a special spout, then the water is allowed to drain out, with the aim of emptying the entire colon. After this, the stoma is covered with a dry dressing, as a stoma bag is not needed until the next irrigation.

Complications of Colostomy and Ileostomy

These are summarised in Table 27.3.

28

Chronic Inflammatory Disorders of the Bowel

Introduction

Substantial inflammation in any part of the small or large bowel usually presents with diarrhoea (i.e., frequent passage of loose stools). When inflammation affects the large bowel, the diarrhoea often contains blood. **Chronic diarrhoea** is defined as lasting for longer than 6 weeks, different from the acute diarrhoea of gastroenteritis, which is usually of viral origin or related to food poisoning and is usually self-limiting, though often fatal in infants in the developing world.

A chronic change of bowel habit to looser and more frequent stools, whether containing blood or not, raises the possibility of three categories of diagnosis: **infective** (bacillary or amoebic), **inflammatory bowel diseases** (ulcerative colitis, Crohn disease or rarer forms of noninfective colitis) and **neoplasms** (covered in the previous chapter).

The term *inflammatory bowel disease* usually means the two chronic bowel disorders, **ulcerative colitis** or **Crohn disease**. They share many pathophysiological and clinical features. However, Crohn disease can involve any part of the gastrointestinal (GI) tract, whilst ulcerative colitis is confined to the large bowel. When the large bowel alone is inflamed, it is important to differentiate between these conditions because

management and the spectrum of complications differ substantially (Table 28.1).

These diseases are chronic and relapsing by nature. They have variable responses to treatments, with a potential for complications after major surgery. The most effective management and best outcomes result from cooperation between medical and surgical gastroenterologists. Patients can mostly be managed on an outpatient basis but acute exacerbations or complications may require admission. Surgery is usually indicated when medical management has failed or when complications, such as fulminant colitis, obstruction, toxic dilatation of the colon or perforation occur. In addition, ulcerative colitis and Crohn disease are long-term risk factors for **colorectal cancer**.

In developing countries, **infections** that cause chronic large bowel inflammation are more common and may also be contracted by travellers. **Amoebiasis**, in particular, may mimic ulcerative colitis, and **tuberculosis** may mimic Crohn disease even in the UK.

Pseudomembranous and other forms of **antibiotic-related colitis** are increasingly common in hospitalised patients after antibiotic treatment; they are discussed in Chapter 12. Whilst typical cases can be readily diagnosed and treated, severe forms may require emergency colectomy and may cause fatality in elderly patients. Symptoms may occur as long as 6 months after antibiotic use.

Infective causes must be excluded before inflammatory bowel disease is diagnosed because life-threatening complications can result from treating infective conditions with immunosuppressive drugs used for inflammatory bowel disease.

Epidemiology and Aetiology of Inflammatory Bowel Disease

Ulcerative colitis and Crohn colitis are considered to be separate entities but in 10% to 15% of cases, no clear distinction can be made—this is termed **indeterminate colitis** on resection specimens. It is possible that the diseases share aetiological factors or even represent different facets of the same disease.

Ulcerative colitis and Crohn disease are relatively common in developed countries but the diseases seem rare in most of Africa, Asia and South America. In the West, the incidence of Crohn disease appears to have increased over the past few decades (to 100 per 100,000 population per year), whilst ulcerative colitis (200 per 100,000) has remained static or may have even declined.

TABLE 28.1   Comparative Features of Ulcerative Colitis and Crohn Disease

	Ulcerative Colitis	Crohn Disease
Pathology		
Inflammation	Recurrent acute inflammation with intervening quiescent phases	Chronic relapsing inflammation
General distribution	Continuous involvement of affected part of colon	Skip lesions in any part of gastrointestinal tract
Rectal involvement	Always	About 25%
Ileal involvement	Backwash ileitis only	Involved in 80% of cases; exclusive to ileum in 50% of cases
Depth of wall involved	Mucosa only	Transmural, including serosa
Mucosal changes	Widespread irregular superficial ulceration with or without pseudopolyps	Fissured ulceration causing 'cobblestone' appearance
Granuloma formation	Absent	Characteristic but not always present
Mesenteric adenopathy	Reactive hyperplasia only	Lymph nodes often enlarged; granulomas may be present
Fibrosis of wall	Minimal	Marked
Main Clinical Features		
Diarrhoea	Severe during acute attacks, often causing incontinence	Less prominent
Rectal bleeding	Very common	Less common
Abdominal pain	Mild cramping 'predefaecation' pain with diarrhoeal attacks	Dominant feature—persistent or grumbling pain with severe acute attacks
Abdominal mass	No	Relatively common
General debility	Less marked	Characteristic
Complications		
Strictures	Rare	Common and often multiple
Fistulae	Rare	Common
Anal and perianal lesions	Uncommon	Common
Massive haemorrhage	Occurs in fulminant disease	Rare
Pathology		
Intestinal obstruction	Rare	Incomplete obstruction is common
Perforation	Complication of toxic megacolon	Free perforation rare but perforation causing local abscess formation or internal fistula common
Toxic megacolon	May occur in fulminant attacks	Rare
Malignant change	High risk with severe/longstanding disease	Low risk
Management		
Local 5-aminosalicylic acid (ASA)/ steroids	Left-sided active disease	Less effective
Systemic steroids	Severe exacerbations	Severe exacerbations
Oral 5-ASA	To treat mild attacks Long-term maintenance	Less effective
Immunosuppressives	In severe cases, unresponsive to steroids As steroid-sparing agent	'Steroid sparing' in intractable cases
Surgery	Less common —in longstanding disease with evidence of dysplasia or malignancy —in fulminant colitis —in uncontrolled chronic disease	Commonly required

Most inflammatory bowel disease develops in the late teen years or 20s. Gender, social class and urban living seems to be irrelevant. In the United States of America, white people are three times more susceptible to ulcerative colitis than black people and five times more susceptible to Crohn disease.

The aetiology of these diseases remains obscure. There is a familial incidence: 6% to 8% of patients with ulcerative colitis and about 20% of those with Crohn disease have first-degree relatives with the same condition. It is likely that both conditions are genetically heterogeneous and polygenic. For Crohn disease, implicated genes include *NOD2/CARD15*. For ulcerative colitis, genes *IBD1, IBD2* and *IBD3* have been identified. It is postulated that the presence of more than one of these genetic mutations may result in Crohn disease.

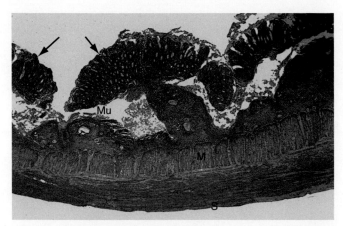

• **Fig. 28.1** Ulcerative Colitis—Histopathology. Erosion and undermining of the mucosa *(Mu)* by the inflammatory process has produced typical pseudopolyps *(arrowed)*. Inflammation spares the muscle wall *(M)* and serosa *(S)*. Mucosal glands show reactive and regenerative changes.

Another similarity between the two diseases is the association with a range of non-GI autoimmune disorders involving eyes, joints, skin and liver. The most common for both ulcerative colitis and Crohn disease is **ankylosing spondylitis**, which is usually associated with the lymphocyte surface antigen human leucocyte antigen (HLA)-B27. In contrast, pericholangitis occurs often in ulcerative colitis but is rare in Crohn disease, and occasionally progresses to **sclerosing cholangitis**.

Infection is believed to play a part in initiating some cases of both ulcerative colitis and Crohn disease, as many cases follow an acute attack of gastroenteritis. Importantly, tobacco smoking is more common in patients with Crohn disease, and smoking increases disease recurrence. Ulcerative colitis, by contrast, is more prevalent in nonsmokers.

Ulcerative Colitis

Ulcerative colitis is an inflammatory disorder of the mucosa and submucosa of the **large bowel** only. It is characterised by recurrent acute exacerbations and intervening periods of quiescence or chronic low-grade activity. The symptom severity corresponds to the level of disease activity. Extracolonic features affect a small proportion of patients and include anaemia, inflammation of joints (**arthropathy**) and inflammation of eyes, skin and biliary tract. The disease always involves the rectum, but often extends proximally in continuity to involve a variable length of colon. In nearly 20% of cases (but only those with pancolitis, i.e., colitis involving the whole large bowel), the distal end of the ileum becomes secondarily affected; this is described as **backwash ileitis**.

Pathophysiology of Ulcerative Colitis

Initially, the colonic mucosa becomes acutely inflamed. Neutrophils accumulate in the lamina propria and within the tubular colonic glands to form small, highly characteristic **crypt abscesses**. Sloughing of the overlying mucosa produces small superficial ulcers. If the inflammatory process persists, the ulcers coalesce into extensive areas of irregular ulceration. Residual islands of intact but oedematous mucosa project into the bowel lumen; these inflammatory lesions are called **pseudopolyps** (Fig. 28.1). The inflammation is usually confined to the mucosa and submucosa, only extending into the muscular wall and peritoneal surface in **fulminating colitis**.

Acute inflammatory episodes range from several days' to several months' duration. After subsiding, they can recur months or even years later. During quiescent periods, the acute inflammation resolves and the mucosa regenerates. The lamina propria, however, remains swollen by a chronic inflammatory infiltrate of lymphocytes and plasma cells. The colonic glands show a marked reduction in the number of mucin-secreting goblet cells, histologically termed **goblet cell depletion**.

After the disease has been present for some time, **dysplastic changes** can appear in the epithelium. Dysplasia (Latin for 'bad form') involves recognisable changes indicating early transformation to neoplasia. After prolonged or repeated episodes of inflammation, dysplasia may progress to **adenocarcinoma**. The risk of malignancy is greatest for those with early onset and extensive disease, and is approximately 5% after 10 years of colitis. Endoscopic surveillance is necessary, with intervals determined by the duration and extent of disease. Cancer diagnosis may be delayed if symptoms are mistaken for a relapse of colitis and are not investigated. Cancers in these patients are often particularly aggressive and occur on average 20 years earlier than in the general population.

In longstanding colitis, the mucosa and submucosa undergo fibrosis, resulting in smoothing out of haustrations and a shortened colon, which has a characteristic radiological appearance, the so-called **lead pipe colon** (Fig. 28.2).

Clinical Features of Ulcerative Colitis

Acute inflammatory attacks are marked by loose blood-stained stools streaked with mucus. This mucus results from inflammation of rectosigmoid colonic mucosa. As the extent of inflammation increases, the diarrhoea may become severe. The patient may pass 20 or more loose stools a day, each time preceded by cramping abdominal pain. In many patients, the urge to defaecate is so precipitate that incontinence occurs unless a lavatory is immediately available.

Any attack of ulcerative colitis may progress to the severe form of **fulminant colitis**; the patient may become prostrated by dehydration, severe electrolyte disturbance and blood loss. Occasionally, the colon dilates massively and patchy necrosis eventually occurs. The patient is systemically ill with high fever, marked tachycardia and dehydration. This process, known as **toxic megacolon**, culminates in perforation and fatal peritonitis, unless emergency colectomy is performed.

Ulcerative colitis should probably be regarded as a systemic disorder. It is sometimes accompanied by extra-GI manifestations, summarised in Box 28.1. During active phases, inflammatory markers (erythrocyte sedimentation rate [ESR] and C-reactive protein [CRP]) are elevated and moderate anaemia and hypoalbuminaemia is common. Associated arthropathy, eye and skin disorders usually flare up in parallel with the colitis (although they may rarely precede the intestinal symptoms). However, the liver-related conditions—sclerosing cholangitis, chronic active hepatitis and bile duct carcinoma—are often independent of colitic activity and are therefore difficult to treat.

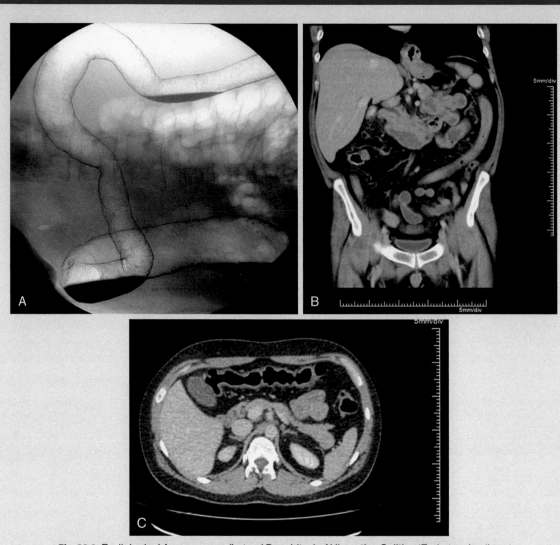

• **Fig. 28.2** Radiological Appearances (Lateral Decubitus) of Ulcerative Colitis. 'End-stage' or 'burnt-out' ulcerative colitis in a 49-year-old office worker. He had suffered episodic, but not incapacitating, diarrhoea for 34 years, but presented on this occasion because of urgency and incontinence. Sigmoidoscopy showed only moderate rectal ulceration. **(A)** This barium enema shows a typical smooth, shortened 'lead pipe' colon, with complete loss of haustration. Note that the film is orientated in the lateral decubitus position. He failed to respond to medical treatment and underwent proctocolectomy and ileostomy. **(B)** Coronal section of computed tomography (CT) scan in a different patient with burnt-out ulcerative colitis showing the loss of haustral pattern and thickened colonic wall. **(C)** Transaxial CT demonstrating thickened transverse colon.

Clinical Examination and Investigation of Suspected Ulcerative Colitis

The typical patient referred for investigation of suspected ulcerative colitis is a young adult with a history of several weeks of frequent loose stools, later streaked with blood and mucus. The attack often starts with an attack of gastroenteritis or traveller's diarrhoea, which fails to settle. There is sometimes a history of non-GI symptoms, such as arthropathy or uveitis.

General examination often reveals anaemia but abdominal examination is usually unremarkable. Rectal examination, followed by proctoscopy and flexible sigmoidoscopy, is mandatory to palpate, inspect and, if necessary, biopsy the rectal mucosa. The affected mucosa ranges in appearance from mildly hyperaemic and easily traumatised to extensive patchy ulceration.

At least three separate fresh stool samples should be analysed to exclude bacterial or parasitic causes or cytomegalovirus, as these conditions may closely simulate ulcerative colitis but require entirely different treatment.

Proctitis

Some patients with ulcerative colitis have inflammation confined to the lower rectum. The mucosa often has a granular appearance and the condition is described as **proctitis** or **granular proctitis**.

• BOX 28.1   Systemic Manifestations of Ulcerative Colitis

Weight Loss
- Frequent during exacerbations

Anaemia
- Typically chronic and nonspecific (normochromic, normocytic)

Arthropathy
- Sacroiliitis/ankylosing spondylitis or rheumatoid-like arthritis, especially of large joints (approximately 20% of cases)

Uveitis and Iritis
- Painful red eye or eyes (approximately 10%)

Skin Lesions
- Erythema nodosum, that is, tender red nodules on the shins (uncommon), pyoderma gangrenosum, that is, purulent skin ulcers (rare)

Sclerosing Cholangitis
- Progressive fibrosis of intrahepatic biliary system leading to cirrhosis, progressive liver failure, jaundice and eventually death (rare)

Its cause is unknown and its course is self-limiting. It tends to recur at times of stress, often at protracted intervals. Proctitis usually responds to short courses of local 5-aminosalicylic acid (5-ASA) suppositories (see later), but can occasionally progress into a distal or even a total colitis.

Contrast Radiology

If the clinical picture and histological findings are consistent with inflammatory bowel disease, the extent and degree of colonic involvement can be assessed by barium enema examination. Radiological appearances are illustrated in Figs 28.2 and 28.3. CT scanning is usually performed in acute disease.

Endoscopy

In an acute situation, an unprepared flexible sigmoidoscopy is usually performed. In nonacute situations, colonoscopy enables direct inspection of the entire colonic mucosa and the taking of multiple biopsies (Fig. 28.4). Furthermore, in patients with longstanding total colitis, colonoscopy with narrow band imaging and multiple biopsies is used for annual surveillance for dysplastic change.

Fulminant Ulcerative Colitis

Fulminant attacks sometimes occur, with extremely frequent watery, blood-stained stools and severe systemic illness. An attack may progress to toxic dilatation and eventual colonic perforation. Urgent colectomy may be judged necessary to treat fulminant colitis resistant to medical therapy, or to treat toxic megacolon, once infective causes have been excluded.

Whatever the cause, patients with acute colitis require urgent hospital admission and resuscitation including fluid, electrolyte and blood replacement. Sigmoidoscopy and biopsy are performed to establish the diagnosis. Stool is sent for microscopy and culture. Plain abdominal radiography is performed to monitor for dilatation, which might indicate toxic megacolon (defined as a colonic diameter greater than 6 cm in the presence of pyrexia or tachycardia). In the absence of megacolon, plain radiography may demonstrate other features of acute ulcerative colitis as shown in Fig. 28.5.

CASE HISTORY

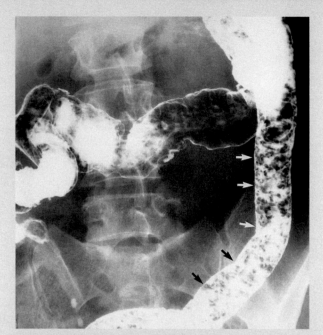

• **Fig. 28.3** Radiological Appearances of Ulcerative Colitis. Severe and longstanding ulcerative colitis in a man of 50 years. The whole colon is affected (pancolitis) with loss of the normal haustral pattern. There is extensive pseudopolyp formation, particularly in the descending and sigmoid colon, manifest by multiple small filling defects *(arrowed)*. Prolonged severe ulceration stimulates mitotic activity and is probably responsible for dysplastic changes and eventual malignant change in longstanding severe ulcerative colitis.

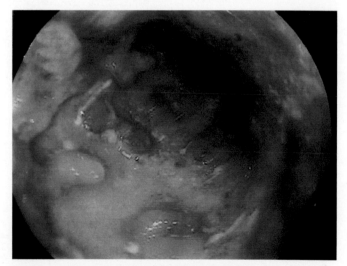

• **Fig. 28.4** Colonoscopic View of Ulcerative Colitis. This colon is quiescent with no evidence of current ulceration but inflammatory polyps are seen as memorials to past severe inflammation and ulceration.

Management of Ulcerative Colitis

The choice of treatment depends on the severity of individual attacks, the amount of colon involved, the extent of chronic symptoms and the risk of long-term complications. The treatment options are summarised in Box 28.2.

CASE HISTORY

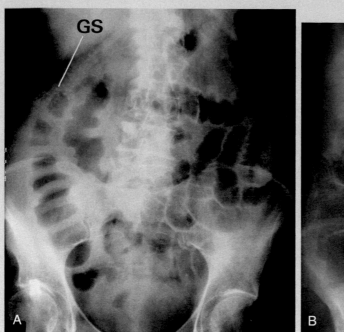
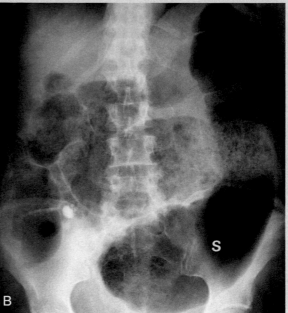

• **Fig. 28.5** Acute Ulcerative Colitis and Toxic Megacolon. **(A)** This 44-year-old woman presented with fulminant ulcerative colitis. She was prostrated by frequent diarrhoea and consequent electrolyte abnormalities. This plain supine radiograph shows acute right-sided colitis. The caecum, ascending colon and proximal transverse colon are affected. In this area, there is absence of the normal 'convex outward' pattern and there are thick folds crossing the bowel lumen. This appearance is caused by oedema of the bowel wall; note the incidental finding of gallstones *(GS)*. **(B)** This patient presented in a similar way but became toxic, while in hospital undergoing intensive medical treatment. There was an increasing tachycardia, fever and abdominal tenderness. Serial plain abdominal radiographs showed an increasing diameter of the left colon. This film shows the sigmoid colon *(S)* dilated to 10 cm and in imminent danger of perforation. This is known as *toxic dilatation of the colon*; it occurs most commonly in ulcerative colitis and usually affects the transverse colon.

• **BOX 28.2** **Main Treatment Measures for Ulcerative Colitis**

Local Corticosteroid or 5-ASA Preparations (Suppositories, Foam or Liquid Enema)
• Used in cases of left-sided active disease

Systemic Corticosteroids
• Suppress moderate or severe exacerbations (oral or intravenous administration according to severity of disease)

Oral (or Sometimes Rectal) Aminosalicylate Preparations (e.g., Sulfasalazine, Mesalazine [Asacol or Pentasa] or Olsalazine)
• Long-term maintenance therapy to minimise relapse

Surgical Removal of the Colon
• Emergency operation: incipient or actual perforation, serious haemorrhage, failure of fulminant colitis to improve on medical treatment
• Elective operation: failure of medical treatment, risk of malignancy

---

Aminosalicylate Preparations

Mild attacks of proctitis or proctosigmoiditis are treated locally with 5-ASA suppositories or enemas, which are more effective in acute proctitis than steroids. Mild attacks of pancolitis are treated initially with oral 5-ASA preparations, which are also used as maintenance therapy in ulcerative colitis to prevent relapse. Although aspirin and other nonsteroidal anti-inflammatories are chemically related to 5-ASA compounds, these drugs should be avoided as they may worsen inflammatory bowel disease. The 5-ASA compounds are discussed later in this chapter, as they are also used in the management of Crohn disease.

Corticosteroids

Steroid suppositories or enemas (foam or liquid) can be used for local treatment of rectal inflammation. Short courses of high-dose oral corticosteroids are used for more severe exacerbations (e.g., prednisolone 40 mg daily for 2 weeks then reducing the daily dose by 5 mg weekly). Intravenous administration is advisable in seriously ill patients. There is no evidence that 'bowel rest' (i.e., nil by mouth) and total parenteral nutrition are of any value in ulcerative colitis. Immunosuppressive drugs, including **ciclosporin** and **azathioprine**, are often tried in patients who fail to respond to corticosteroids. Azathioprine is also used as a 'steroid-sparing' agent in patients whose disease settles on steroids but flares again as steroids are reduced.

Other Supportive Measures

In the acute case, antidiarrhoeal agents, such as codeine phosphate or loperamide should be avoided as they can precipitate toxic dilatation.

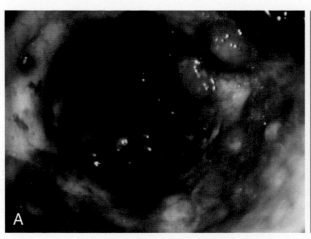
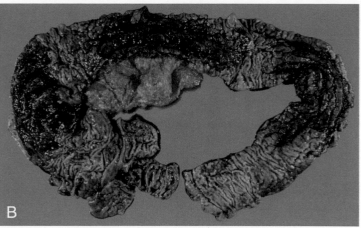

• **Fig. 28.6** Appearances of Crohn Colitis. **(A)** This is a typical colonoscopic view of florid Crohn colitis. Note the nodular appearance producing a 'cobblestone' surface with linear ulcers between the nodules. **(B)** This subtotal colectomy specimen was removed from a man of 54 years with a long history of weight loss, diarrhoea and abdominal pain (see barium enema, Fig. 28.11). There are three 'skip lesions' typical of Crohn disease, in the ascending colon, the transverse colon and the hepatic flexure showing thickening of the wall, cobblestone mucosal surface and narrowing of the lumen.

Patients with moderately severe chronic disease frequently become anaemic and lose weight, in part because of persistent stool loss of protein. These problems may be helped by medical treatment, a diet high in calories and protein, and oral iron supplements.

Surgery for Ulcerative Colitis

Surgery is required in only about 20% of patients with ulcerative colitis. Colectomy may be needed in the following:

- Urgent treatment of fulminant cases, which fail to respond to intensive medical treatment. 'Failure to respond' has no precise definition but there should normally be symptomatic improvement after a week of intensive management.
- Acute cases, which progress to toxic megacolon, perforation or major haemorrhage.
- Patients with chronic disabling symptoms of intractable diarrhoea with urgency, recurring anaemia and failure to maintain adequate weight and nutrition.
- Children with failure to thrive and retardation of growth (both are exacerbated by corticosteroid therapy).
- Patients with longstanding colitis who develop dysplasia or malignancy.

As a principle, surgery for ulcerative colitis requires removal of the entire large bowel and is curative. There are three main surgical options:

- **Subtotal colectomy with ileostomy** is the safest operation in the emergency situation when the patient is sick and on high-dose corticosteroids. Most of the diseased colon is removed, but the patient is left with an inflamed rectal stump. Months later, when the patient is well, this may be revised to one of the other surgical options. Alternatively, the rectum may be retained and treated with local therapy plus endoscopic surveillance, although the cancer risk remains.
- **Proctocolectomy with permanent ileostomy** (includes removal of rectum) is generally recommended for elderly patients in whom sphincter-preserving procedures are inadvisable.
- **Restorative proctocolectomy (ileoanal pouch, Parks pouch)** is a sphincter-preserving operation, which avoids a permanent

ileostomy (see Fig. 27.8). The entire colon and rectal mucosa is excised and a **pouch** reservoir is fashioned from a loop of terminal ileum. The pouch is brought into the pelvis and anastomosed to the upper anal canal. A temporary ileostomy is usually retained for a few months to allow healing. Many patients have excellent continence and can evacuate their bowels in the normal way.

Crohn Disease

Crohn disease is a chronic relapsing inflammatory disorder of **any part** of the GI tract (though nearly always small or large bowel), which predominantly affects younger people. About 60% of patients are under 25 years at the time of initial diagnosis, and on average, symptoms will have been present intermittently for 5 years. A useful website is <http://www.crohns.org.uk/>.

The disease often affects one or more discrete segments of bowel with intervening parts completely spared, unlike the continuous nature of ulcerative colitis. These discontinuous affected areas are known as **skip lesions** (Fig. 28.6).

The small bowel alone is affected in 50% of patients, the large bowel alone in 20% and both together in 30%. The terminal ileum is affected most commonly; in up to half of all cases, the disease is confined to the terminal ileum. In the original description of this disease, it was named *terminal ileitis*. Later, when it became clear that other segments of bowel could be affected, the name was changed to **regional enteritis**, a term still used in the United States of America. Crohn disease also commonly affects the perianal region, whether or not large bowel is involved. Occasionally, the disease involves the stomach, duodenum, oesophagus or mouth.

In contrast to ulcerative colitis, the inflammation involves the entire thickness of the bowel wall (**transmural inflammation**). Because of this, affected bowel may partially obstruct, fistulate or perforate, whereas this rarely occurs in ulcerative colitis. See Table 28.1 for comparisons between Crohn disease and ulcerative colitis.

With each exacerbation, previously affected or new areas may become involved. The disease tends to run a protracted and unpredictable course.

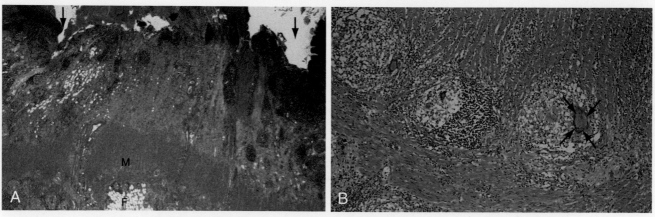

• **Fig. 28.7** Crohn Disease Affecting the Colon—Histopathology. **(A)** Inflammation has produced fissure ulcers *(arrowed)* which extend into the muscle wall *(M)*. Lymphoid aggregates are also present and the inflammatory process extends into serosal fat *(F)*. **(B)** High-power view showing well-formed granulomas with typical giant cells *(arrowed)*.

Pathophysiology and Clinical Consequences of Crohn Disease

The essential pathological feature is chronic inflammation of bowel, with inflammation extending diffusely through the entire bowel wall. The wall becomes markedly thickened by inflammatory oedema, especially in the submucosa. The epithelium remains largely intact but is criss-crossed by deep **fissured ulcers**. These large serpiginous ulcers and the intervening areas of dome-shaped mucosa and submucosa give a typical 'cobblestone' surface appearance (see Fig. 28.6).

Granulomas containing multinucleate giant cells (Fig. 28.7) are usually scattered throughout the inflamed bowel wall, as well as in local lymph nodes. (Although these noncaseating granulomas are typical of Crohn disease, they are not always found, and ruptured crypt abscesses in ulcerative colitis may also cause them.) Longstanding inflammation leads to progressive **fibrosis** of the thickened bowel wall, which encroaches on the lumen, producing **elongated strictures**.

Effects of Mucosal Inflammation

Mucosal inflammation causes diarrhoea which, if the colon is involved, may be streaked with mucus and blood. Luminal narrowing in the small bowel results in partial obstruction that causes grumbling, colicky abdominal pain, sometimes with acute episodes. Pain is a prominent feature in Crohn disease in contrast to ulcerative colitis, since inflamed large bowel does not obstruct in this way.

If small bowel is inflamed, diarrhoea occurs and digestive and absorptive functions may be compromised. Extensive disease results in general malabsorption causing protein-calorie malnutrition, iron and folate deficiency and anaemia. In children, Crohn disease may cause marked growth retardation. Ileal inflammation disrupts **bile salt reabsorption**. Excess bile salts in the faeces cause colonic irritation (and more diarrhoea), while diminished recirculation of bile salts may result in gallstone formation. Involvement of the terminal ileum may reduce vitamin B_{12} absorption but serious deficiency usually occurs only after surgical resection.

Effects of Transmural Inflammation

Crohn disease causes added problems if serosal inflammation extends to adjacent structures. If inflamed bowel impinges on **parietal peritoneum**, pain becomes localised and more severe and signs of local peritonitis develop. Indeed, Crohn disease of the terminal ileum may mimic acute appendicitis. At appendicectomy, the terminal ileum is visibly inflamed and the bowel wall abnormally thick to palpation. In this case, the terminal ileum should not be excised as a firm diagnosis of Crohn disease requires histological and microbacterial exclusion of *Yersinia* ileitis, as well as tuberculosis. Both may simulate Crohn, but are completely reversible with medical treatment.

Serosal inflammation may cause a diseased segment of bowel to adhere to adjacent abdominal structures. Several complications may occur if these become matted together by the inflammatory process:
- **Adhesions.** These tough, fibrotic postinflammatory adhesions are rarely symptomatic but constitute a formidable obstacle if operation is needed later.
- **Perforation.** Free perforation is rare but a contained perforation may occur, which causes localised pericolic or pelvic abscess formation.
- **Fistulae.** These may develop between diseased bowel and other hollow viscera causing unusual clinical phenomena. For example, a gastrocolic fistula may result in true faecal vomiting; an ileorectal fistula may aggravate diarrhoea. Enterovesical fistulae cause severe urinary tract infections and pneumaturia (passage of urine containing air bubbles), and fistulae between bowel and uterus or vagina lead to vaginal passage of faeces. Enterocutaneous fistulae between bowel and skin occasionally develop as a complication of bowel resection for Crohn disease, or spontaneously.

Perianal Inflammation

Perianal inflammation occurs in 15% of patients with Crohn disease. Symptoms include recurrent perianal abscesses, characteristic blueish, boggy 'piles' (Fig. 28.8) and anterolateral anal fissures. The last two are quite distinct from ordinary haemorrhoids and posterior anal fissures. Multiple fistulae commonly develop between rectum and perianal skin and can extend into the labia or scrotum. Fistulae are sometimes so numerous as to cause a 'pepper-pot' or 'watering-can' perineum (see Fig. 28.9). Paradoxically, this is more often associated with small bowel disease than colorectal disease.

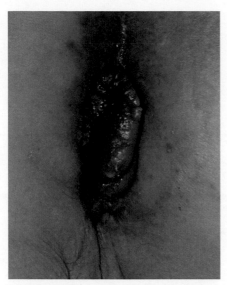

• **Fig. 28.8** Crohn 'Piles'. This appearance is typical of Crohn 'piles'. They are pale and oedematous in contrast to ordinary haemorrhoids.

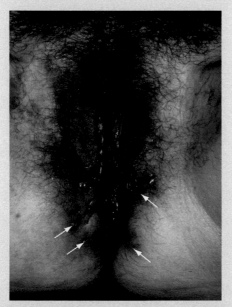

• **Fig. 28.9** Multiple Anal Fistulae in Crohn Disease. This 30-year-old woman had several 'skip lesions' of Crohn disease in her small bowel and was troubled by recurrent perianal sepsis. This photograph shows a typical 'pepper-pot perineum', with several fistulous openings *(arrowed)* seen around the circumference of the anus. Anal skin tags are also visible.

Systemic Features

Like ulcerative colitis, Crohn disease is a systemic disorder and has a similar range of non-GI manifestations (see Box 28.1). In contrast with ulcerative colitis, it is usual for patients to feel generally ill during an acute attack. Specific systemic features affecting skin, joints or the eye are relatively uncommon and not necessarily related to bowel disease activity.

Symptoms and Signs in Crohn Disease

Symptoms of Crohn disease can be similar to those of ulcerative colitis, particularly when large bowel is involved (see Table 28.1). Diarrhoea is usually less distressing and less likely to contain blood. Other characteristic symptoms include cramp-like abdominal pain, weight loss and general malaise. As an aide memoire, think of **pain, weight loss** and **diarrhoea** as symptomatic of Crohn.

Physical examination may reveal generalised wasting and anaemia and sometimes other features like arthropathy. On abdominal examination, there may be areas of tenderness, an inflammatory mass in the right iliac fossa, where omentum wraps around inflamed terminal ileum or the scars of previous surgery. The perianal skin should be examined for fissures, fistulae, Crohn 'piles' or stenotic scarring from previous disease. Diseased rectal mucosa, with its typical firm surface nodularity, may be felt on digital examination. Sigmoidoscopic examination is usually normal but there may be mucosal oedema if the rectum is involved. In more severe cases, the typical 'cobblestone' appearance with fissured ulceration may be seen. Biopsies may be positive even when the mucosa is apparently normal.

Approach to Investigation of Suspected Crohn Disease

Investigation of suspected Crohn disease is similar to that for ulcerative colitis in respect of the large bowel, but follows a different pattern when there is suspected small bowel disease.

Colonoscopy enables a histological diagnosis to be obtained in colonic disease, and also allows biopsies of terminal ileum to be taken, which are often diagnostic. Barium 'follow-through' is the traditional method of examining small bowel but better images are sometimes obtained by controlled instillation of barium into the duodenum, via a nasogastric tube. Typical radiological appearances of Crohn disease include narrowing of the lumen caused by mural oedema and fibrosis, nodularity and cobblestoning of the mucosal surface, deep fissured ulceration extending into the muscular wall, spiky 'rose thorn' ulcers and possibly evidence of fistula formation. Radiological changes in small and large bowel are shown in Figs 28.10 and 28.11. Note that large bowel abnormalities on barium enema may be difficult or impossible to distinguish from ulcerative colitis.

As in ulcerative colitis, full blood count, inflammatory markers (ESR and CRP) and liver function tests also give an indication of the disease activity; stool microscopy and culture is always undertaken to exclude an infective cause for diarrhoea.

Appearances of Crohn colitis are shown in Fig. 28.11.

Management of Crohn Disease

The aim of medical therapy in active Crohn disease is to bring about and maintain remission. The treatments available may be broadly divided into three classes of medication.

Anti-inflammatory Agents

• **5-ASA compounds**, as used in ulcerative colitis. These act locally, making it a challenge to deliver oral medication to inflamed small bowel without gastric inactivation. **Sulfasalazine** (a combination of 5-ASA and a carrier, sulfapyridine) is useful in ulcerative colitis and large bowel Crohn disease

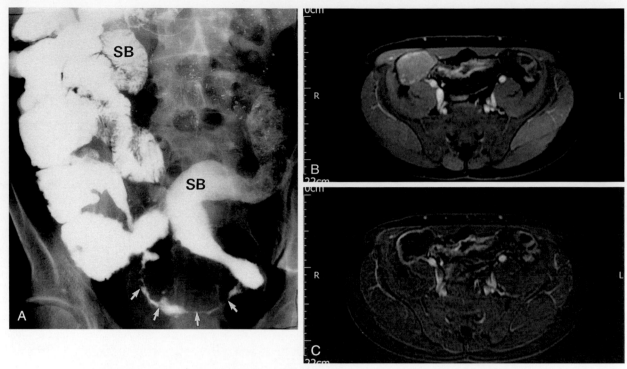

• **Fig. 28.10** Radiological Appearances in Crohn Disease. This man of 51 years had recurrent attacks of colicky abdominal pain, with diarrhoea and loss of weight. **(A)** This barium follow-through examination shows one of the characteristic radiological appearances of Crohn disease. The terminal ileum is extremely narrowed by inflammation of the whole wall thickness *(arrowed)*; this is known as the 'string sign of Kantor' and causes the symptoms and signs of partial obstruction. This film also shows dilatation of small bowel *(SB)* proximal to the stricture. **(B)** Transaxial magnetic resonance imaging (MRI) slice showing contrast enhancement of terminal ileum with characteristic thickening of bowel wall at this site. **(C)** Transaxial MRI demonstrating contrast enhancement at terminal ileum characteristic of Crohn disease.

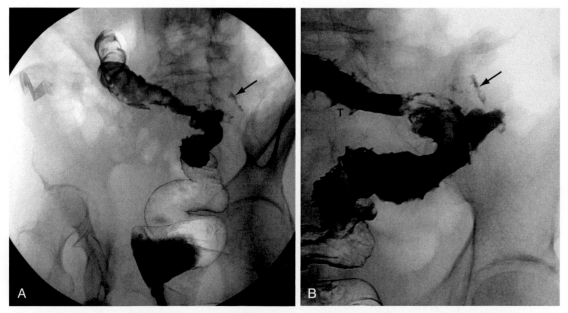

• **Fig. 28.11** Radiological Appearances in Crohn disease. **(A)** Double contrast barium enema in a 28-year-old woman who complained of 8 months' history of recurrent abdominal pains and diarrhoea. She had not lost weight. This film shows a 'ragged' segment in the sigmoid colon with narrowing and 'rose thorn' ulcers *(T)*, better seen in the close-up view in **(B)**. In both views, contrast is visible outside the colon *(arrowed)*. In fact, this is in small bowel because of a fistula between colon and small bowel.

because the active ingredient is released by colonic bacteria. However, some patients suffer side effects related to the sulfapyridine. Mesalazine is useful for more proximal Crohn disease as the active compound is released earlier. Rectal Crohn disease can be treated with 5-ASA suppositories or enemas, as in ulcerative colitis. 5-ASA compounds can be used as maintenance therapy in Crohn disease but large doses are required.

- **Corticosteroids** can act as systemic agents (e.g., prednisolone) or locally. Budesonide is a new oral steroid, which is mostly released in the terminal ileum then rapidly inactivated by the liver after absorption, minimising systemic effects. Corticosteroids act rapidly to control flare-ups, but are rarely used for long-term maintenance.

Immunomodulators

- **Azathioprine and 6-mercaptopurine** are immunosuppressants, sometimes used in more severe Crohn disease. They can spare the need for damaging steroids, or they can help maintain remission in patients who relapse on 5-ASA compounds. About 10% of those treated are at risk of bone marrow suppression, but those at risk can be predicted by pretreatment testing.
- **Methotrexate** acts both as an anti-inflammatory agent and an immunomodulator but has potentially serious side effects upon liver and bone marrow.
- **Infliximab** is a chimeric monoclonal antibody to tumour necrosis factor α, an inflammatory mediator. It is given by intravenous infusion for acute disease and is usually effective within 2 weeks. The drug can be given at 8-weekly intervals to maintain remission. Risks include developing antibodies to the drug. It should not be used where there is active infection or an abscess.

Other Supportive Treatments

- Antidiarrhoeal drugs (e.g., loperamide) and antispasmodics are used in chronic symptoms.
- Dietary modification: liquid/low-fibre diets for those with obstructive symptoms, and supplementary calories, iron and vitamins.

The Role of Surgery in Crohn Disease

Surgery should not be considered curative in Crohn disease, unlike ulcerative colitis. This is because operating on one section of bowel does not affect later recurrences elsewhere. Up to 70% of patients with Crohn disease will eventually need surgery, of whom half will need further surgery within 5 years.

The main indications for surgery can be summarised as follows:
- acute complications, for example, abscess, perforation;
- persistent local ileal disease;
- intolerable long-term obstructive and other symptoms, for example, abdominal pain, perianal disease, general ill-health;
- enterocutaneous fistulae and symptomatic internal fistulae.

The choice of operation depends on the site and extent of disease. The former belief that all disease must be resected has been abandoned. Given the diffuse nature of the disease and likelihood of further operations, as much bowel as possible should be preserved. Surgery for multiple small bowel strictures now involves **stricturoplasty** of each lesion, a technique of enlarging the lumen of diseased bowel without losing potential absorptive length. If

disease is limited, resection of the diseased segment with a small margin of normal tissue may be performed, followed by wide side-to-side anastomosis. **Abscesses** are usually treated by simple drainage, with resection of the affected bowel at the same time or later.

Fistulae between abdominal viscera are treated by removing the diseased bowel. In contrast, enterocutaneous fistulae, usually a complication of recent surgery, are a more formidable problem since they are often associated with complicating factors like intraabdominal infection, gross fluid and electrolyte abnormalities and a hypercatabolic state. Patients with enterocutaneous fistulae require intensive preparatory medical care and strategic surgical intervention before definitive treatment is possible.

For severe **large bowel disease**, the entire colon is generally removed (panproctocolectomy with ileostomy). This is because there are usually several colonic 'skip lesions' and recurrence is likely. Pouch procedures are not recommended because of the risk of recurrent disease in the small bowel reservoir.

Recurrent disease often necessitates further surgery. Careful medical treatment to reduce disease recurrence and hence increase intervals between reoperations is imperative: stopping smoking, 5-ASA preparations, and even azathioprine may be used, particularly if the patient has been left with a short bowel.

Other Chronic Inflammations of the Colon

Amoebic Colitis

Entamoeba histolytica is a protozoan parasite responsible for amoebic colitis. It is an endemic bowel commensal in many developing countries. Most of those infected have no symptoms but they are all carriers; less than 5% suffer amoebic colitis. In these, the organism invades the large bowel mucosa, causing chronic relapsing symptoms similar to ulcerative colitis. Encysted parasites are shed by carriers in faeces and infection is readily transmitted to new individuals via the faecal–oral route, contaminated hands or uncooked food.

The incidence of amoebiasis is likely to increase in the West as tourism expands into endemic areas. If sufferers are mistakenly treated with systemic steroids for inflammatory bowel disease, the result may be fatal. Occasionally, rampant invasion progresses to local perforation and a pericolic abscess or toxic megacolon.

In any case of amoebic colitis, amoebae passing to the liver in the portal veins sometimes produce **hepatic abscesses**, most frequently in the right lobe. These are usually solitary and are filled with reddish-brown necrotic material, said to resemble anchovy sauce.

Clinical Features of Amoebic Colitis

The disease usually affects the proximal colon, causing colicky abdominal pain, erratic bowel habit with episodes of blood-stained loose stools and right iliac fossa tenderness. If the distal colon is involved, the patient suffers chronic watery diarrhoea with blood and mucus. When the entire colon is involved, there is generalised abdominal tenderness, as well as systemic features, for example, pyrexia and progressive weight loss. Large granulomatous colonic lesions known as **amoebomas** may be palpable and must be differentiated from carcinoma or diverticular disease.

If the patient develops an amoebic liver abscess, systemic features become more marked, with general ill-health and a swinging pyrexia with sweating attacks. There is pain in the liver area and an enlarged tender liver on palpation. The abscess may rupture spontaneously into the peritoneal cavity (causing peritonitis) or through the diaphragm into the chest. Secondary lung abscesses may then rupture into the bronchi and the patient coughs up 'anchovy sauce' sputum.

Diagnosis of Amoebiasis

In developed countries, amoebic colitis should always be considered in the differential diagnosis of ulcerative colitis or Crohn colitis. Amoebic colitis is best diagnosed by microscopic examination of fresh stool specimens; this may reveal trophozoites containing ingested red cells.

Liver abscesses cause serological tests for amoebiasis to become positive. The lesions are readily demonstrated by hepatic ultrasound and the diagnosis is confirmed by needle aspiration.

Treatment of Amoebiasis

Metronidazole is the drug treatment of choice for amoebic dysentery and is given orally, 800 mg three times daily for 5 days, followed by diloxanide 500 mg three times daily for 10 days to eradicate cysts. Liver abscesses are treated with metronidazole 400 mg three times daily for 5 to 10 days followed again by diloxanide. Emergency surgery is occasionally necessary in fulminating amoebic colitis or less urgently for large liver abscesses.

Microscopic Colitis

This recently described condition is so called because the histology is abnormal but the macroscopic appearance may be normal. It causes chronic watery diarrhoea and is thought to be the cause in up to 5% of patients complaining of this symptom. Its aetiology is still unknown, but a link with nonsteroidal anti-inflammatory drugs has been noted. Specific histological findings (collagenous and lymphocytic types) are seen in biopsy specimens, although the colon may look macroscopically normal at colonoscopy. Treatment is not very effective: budesonide and bismuth may be tried for patients unable to control symptoms with antidiarrhoeal agents.

29

Disorders of Large Bowel Motility, Structure and Perfusion

CHAPTER OUTLINE

Introduction

Irritable bowel syndrome (IBS), chronic constipation and **diverticular disease** all arise from disordered peristaltic function and are at least partly attributable to the highly refined Western diet. These disorders could be regarded as endemic in developed societies.

IBS causes distressing abdominal discomfort in younger patients, whilst chronic constipation affects people of all age groups.

Diverticular disease is probably caused by long-term dietary factors. These disorders make substantial demands on the professional time of family practitioners, physicians and surgeons, yet they are largely preventable. A hundred years ago, they were largely unknown in the West (apart from an obsession with constipation), as they still are in rural communities in many developing countries.

In addition to treating symptoms, the main surgical significance is that these conditions must be distinguished from inflammatory bowel diseases in the young, and large bowel cancer in the older population. They have several symptoms in common:
- intermittent attacks of abdominal pain, which can be severe;
- erratic bowel habit;
- abdominal bloating and passage of excessive flatus.

Sigmoid volvulus is an acute condition resulting from chronic dilatation of the sigmoid colon plus an acute twisting of the sigmoid loop on a narrow mesentery, resulting in obstruction and massive dilatation (see later, Fig. 29.1).

Angiodysplasia of the large bowel and **ischaemic colitis** are vascular conditions of the ageing gut, and both usually present with rectal bleeding and pain. Again, colorectal cancer has to be excluded as the cause of bleeding.

Modern Diet and Disease

Epidemiological Observations

Little scientific attention was paid to diet-related disease until the 1970s, although Gaylord Hauser had written about fibre in the diet in the 1930s. In the 1970s, the ideas of Surgeon Captain T. L. Cleeve, a Royal Navy physician, and later the remarkable epidemiological observations of Denis Burkitt, a long-time missionary surgeon in Africa, emerged. Now the subjects of diet, and latterly, the colonic microbiome are respectable in surgical circles and have contributed to the understanding, prevention and management of many common diseases. Diseases, such as IBS, diverticular disease and appendicitis, common in Western society, appear to be far less common in much of the developing world and this difference is almost certainly diet related. Thus it follows that a dietary history is important in evaluating patients with these disorders, and dietary changes are often a fundamental part of management.

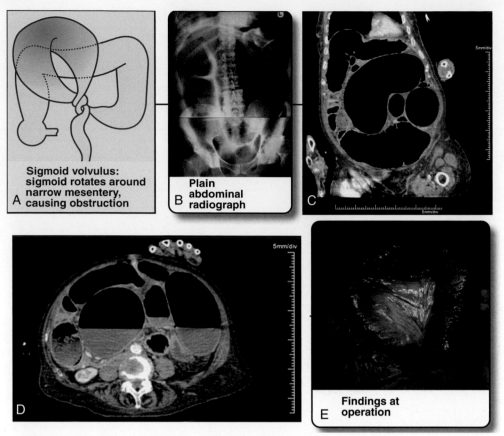

• **Fig. 29.1** Normal Colon, Megacolon and Sigmoid Volvulus. **(A)** Schematic diagram showing a grossly distended fluid-filled sigmoid colon twisted about its narrow neck, producing a 'closed-loop' obstruction; the loop is beginning to undergo necrosis. **(B)** and **(C)** This 35-year-old man with Down syndrome presented with a massively swollen abdomen and total constipation. **(B)** Plain abdominal radiograph showing the abdomen filled with the dilated sigmoid loop, confirming the clinical diagnosis of sigmoid volvulus. Note the abdomen was so distended that two films were required to cover the area. The volvulus could not be relieved by gentle passage of a flatus tube. **(C)** Coronal computed tomography (CT) showing 'coffee bean' shape of volved large bowel. **(D)** Transaxial CT showing sigmoid volvulus in a frail patient who cannot place their hands by their side during scanning. At operation **(E)**, the hugely distended sigmoid emerged from the laparotomy wound. The loop had twisted three times around its narrow base and the colon was of doubtful viability. This sigmoid colon was resected without untwisting the volvulus.

Over millions of years as 'hunter-gatherers', humans subsisted on a staple diet of an extensive variety of vegetables and fruits, grains, legumes and nuts, supplemented by occasional meat or fish. The modern human gastrointestinal (GI) and metabolic systems are thus perfectly adapted to that diet. During the brief period (in evolutionary terms) of the last 100 years, the average Western diet has changed dramatically, caused by a move to farming and by affluence, fashion, convenience, food processing and advertising. Since the 1980s, there have been similar dietary changes in the more prosperous parts of developing countries, particularly in the cities. The modern diet contains many more calories than the hunter-gatherer diet. These are largely in the form of refined carbohydrates, sugars and fats, especially saturated animal fats and 'trans' fats in artificially hydrogenated vegetable oils (though these are gradually being phased out). Perhaps equally important, the modern diet contains far less absorbable and nonabsorbable fibre residue.

Mechanisms of Disease Caused by Modern Diet

Whilst the increase in calories and nutrients has brought benefits, it has also brought problems. The modern diet adversely affects both bowel function and metabolism, particularly of lipids. Box 29.1 outlines the important ways in which modern diet can induce disease and dysfunction. With regard to bowel diseases, the most important diet-related factors are likely to be faecal volume and consistency, together with GI transit time. The average Western adult passes between 80 and 120 g of firm stool each day with a transit time of about 3 days, although transit time can be as long as 2 weeks in the elderly. In contrast, rural dwellers in the developing world, with a diet similar to the hunter-gatherer, pass between 300 and 800 g of much softer stool each day, with an average transit time of less than a day and a half.

Dietary Fibre Content

An essential part of managing many bowel conditions (other than IBS) and preventing others is a substantial increase in dietary fibre intake, along with good oral fluid intake to allow fibre to be effective. Fibre appears essential to maintaining a healthy microbiome. Box 29.2 lists foods with a high fibre content that can be eaten regularly with little effort or extra expense. Increasing the fibre content almost inevitably leads to reduced consumption of refined

Slowed Gastrointestinal Transit Time

- Increases duration of contact between stool and bowel mucosa; this increases duration of contact of carcinogens, predisposing to colorectal cancer

Increased Intraabdominal Pressure Caused by Straining at Stool

- Obstructs venous return making haemorrhoids and varicose veins more likely
- Predisposes to hiatus hernia, inguinal hernia and rectal prolapse

Reduced Bulk and More Solid Consistency of Faeces

- Make peristalsis less effective and constipation more likely
- Increase intraluminal pressure, perhaps predisposing to diverticular disease
- Hard stool increases friction, causing anal fissure and perhaps haemorrhoids
- Small stool bulk increases concentration of carcinogens
- May contribute to pathogenesis of appendicitis by obstructing appendiceal orifice

Decreased Loss of Bile Salts in the Faeces

- Increased bile salt pool predisposes to gallstone formation
- Increased bile salts in lumen may result in formation of carcinogens

Changes in Bacterial Flora of the Bowel

- May result in formation of carcinogens
- May be implicated in appendicitis

Increased Refined Carbohydrate Intake

- Predisposes to diabetes
- Contributes to excess calorie intake causing obesity

Increased Dietary Fat Intake, Particularly Saturated Animal Fats

- Predisposes to atherosclerosis
- Predisposes to gallstone formation
- Contributes to excess calorie intake and obesity

Increased Absorption of Dietary Fat Because of Reduced Binding by Fibre

- Increases fat absorption and blood lipid levels

Obesity

- Weakens abdominal wall muscles predisposing to hiatus hernia, abdominal wall hernias and vaginal prolapse
- Predisposes to thromboembolism
- Contributes to musculoskeletal and joint disorders

- Wholegrain and bran-enriched breakfast cereals, for example, muesli, All-Bran, Weetabix (not cornflakes, puffed rice, etc.)
- Wholemeal bread (not white or 'brown')
- Other wholewheat products, for example, wholewheat pasta, wholemeal pastry, digestive biscuits
- Other wholegrain, for example, brown rice, cracked wheat
- Pulses of any kind, for example, haricot beans (including canned baked beans), kidney beans, chick peas, other dried beans and lentils
- Potatoes (skins should be left on)
- Unpeeled fruit and vegetables (actually low in fibre compared with grains and pulses)

carbohydrates and saturated animal fats, and lower total energy intake. Patients should introduce dietary fibre gradually because a sudden increase is likely to cause abdominal discomfort and distension and more flatus. Bulking agents (**ispaghula husk** preparations) can be taken in the early stages for a rapid result, whilst avoiding unpleasant side-effects.

Irritable Bowel Syndrome

IBS has only been accepted as a pathological entity in recent years, although Osler coined the term *mucous colitis* in 1892 to describe mucorrhoea (excess mucus in the stool) and abdominal colic, often found in patients with psychological problems. Another common name is '**spastic colon**'. The condition is widespread, particularly in young and middle-aged women.

Clinical Features of Irritable Bowel Syndrome

IBS is a functional GI disorder characterised by abdominal pain and altered bowel habit without identifiable organic pathology. IBS can only be diagnosed clinically (after excluding organic causes) as there are no specific diagnostic tests. A group of experts formalised a diagnostic set of symptoms known as the **Rome II Criteria**. To fulfil a diagnosis of IBS, a patient must have the following symptoms continuously or recurrently for at least 3 months in a year: abdominal pain relieved by defaecation, and a change in stool frequency and consistency. Symptoms supporting the diagnosis include altered stool form, mucorrhoea and abdominal bloating.

The patient typically complains of episodic 'cramping' abdominal pain at any time of day and lasting from 15 minutes to several hours. The pain is unrelated to meals or other obvious provoking factors. It occurs anywhere in the abdomen but tends to arise peripherally, that is, in either iliac fossa or epigastrium, and usually recurs in the same general area in any one patient.

Symptoms occur daily for weeks at a time and then resolve for weeks or months, only to return later. The patient may recognise that symptoms are worse at times of stress and are absent during weekends and holidays. The pain may provoke an urge to open the bowels, and evacuation may bring relief. An erratic bowel habit is characteristic of IBS: passage of loose stools alternates with constipation, with small hard stools described as looking like rabbit pellets; but patients are divided into those for whom either diarrhoea or constipation is the predominant problem. Sufferers often complain of abdominal distension and excess flatus.

Pathophysiology and Aetiology of Irritable Bowel Syndrome

The pathophysiology is poorly understood. Colonic motility studies show abnormal rises in intraluminal pressure and disordered peristalsis with segmenting, nonpropulsive contractions. The small volume of faeces (because of little residual fibre) becomes excessively dehydrated and fragmented. However, some patients with IBS appear to be hypersensitive to gut distension and their symptoms may be made worse by a high-fibre diet. These in particular, may benefit from a low-fibre diet plus methylcellulose fibre substitutes that do not ferment, for example, Celevac. Thus the patient avoids constipation without the fermentation and excess gas produced by a high-fibre diet. There is growing support for the view that at least some IBS is caused by specific food intolerance, particularly wheat protein, and it is worth excluding this in a trial of treatment.

Management of Irritable Bowel Syndrome

The diagnosis is made on the basis of a typical history and often after a trial of treatment, but the diagnosis can only be considered after excluding organic pathologies. In the younger patient in the Western world, where carcinoma is unlikely, abdominal and rectal examination (probably including flexible sigmoidoscopy) is all that is required. In IBS, these are normal except perhaps for mild tenderness in the area of pain. In parts of the developing world where colonic cancer can occur in younger patients, more complete colonic examination may be required. Other factors helping to exclude inflammatory bowel disease are an absence of weight loss, general ill-health, troublesome diarrhoea and rectal bleeding. A normal erythrocyte sedimentation rate and C-reactive protein suggests no systemic inflammation, and normal **faecal calprotectin** estimation can exclude inflammatory bowel disease in favour of IBS.

Persistent upper GI pain should be investigated, with gallstones or peptic ulcer disease in mind. In a patient over 50 years with new symptoms, IBS is less likely, and cancer and diverticular disease must be excluded before IBS can be confirmed.

Treatment involves reassurance, adjusting the diet to test for wheat intolerance, treating the predominant symptom of constipation or diarrhoea, and antispasmodic drugs, such as mebeverine and peppermint oil. Mebeverine plus codeine phosphate (as an analgesic) given immediately an attack comes on produces rapid relief and confirms the diagnosis. There is probably little benefit in giving continuous treatment. For selected patients, relaxation therapy or antidepressants, such as amitriptyline may be beneficial.

Constipation

Clinical Features of Constipation

Many patients suffer from chronic constipation, whether or not they consider it a problem. Constipation is difficult to define but the essence is a subjective inability to evacuate the bowels with sufficient frequency, ease, completeness or satisfaction. Perception of normality varies greatly; some patients insist that daily evacuation is essential, whilst others tolerate a bowel movement only once a week.

Constipation is often considered in two groups. The first is **slow transit** with a general failure of colonic propulsion. The second, much smaller group includes patients with an **evacuation disorder**. These patients often complain of incomplete evacuation and a sensation of obstructed defaecation: some disorders responsible (like rectal intussusception) can only be demonstrated on a dynamic x-ray study known as an **evacuation proctogram**. These patients also require specialised anorectal physiological assessment.

From a medical viewpoint, evacuation less than twice a week is abnormal. In the uncomplaining elderly, defaecation may occur infrequently, causing vague discomfort and anorexia, and predisposing to urinary retention, incontinence and urinary tract infection. Severe constipation alone may lead to **faecal impaction** and **complete bowel obstruction** necessitating hospital admission. Faecal fluid may intermittently escape past the impacted faecal mass and cause soiling, overflow incontinence or apparent ('**spurious**') diarrhoea.

Abdominal pain may be the presenting symptom of constipation. The pain may be sufficiently severe to precipitate emergency admission with suspected appendicitis (usually children) or suspected intestinal obstruction (usually the elderly). As many as 25% of patients in these age groups admitted with abdominal pain is eventually diagnosed as suffering from constipation. There is no fever, tachycardia or vomiting, and signs of peritoneal inflammation are absent. There may be mild abdominal tenderness. The faecally loaded left side of the colon often forms a palpable column, which indents on palpation with a putty-like consistency. Rectal examination usually reveals a palpable faecal mass, although in the elderly the faeces may be impacted higher up, so an empty rectum does not exclude constipation.

Pathophysiology of Chronic Constipation

For surgeons, chronic constipation is mainly a problem of children and the elderly. Patients present as emergencies and in the clinic. In most, the cause is a combination of low-fibre diet, poor fluid intake, obesity, inactivity and persistent failure to respond promptly to the urge to defaecate. Long-term use of **purgative drugs,** such as senna may have an adverse effect on peristalsis. Some drugs, particularly **codeine** and **opiates,** slow large bowel motility, whilst yet other drugs, such as **aluminium hydroxide mixtures** and **iron preparations** solidify the stool. Constipation is a characteristic feature of **hypothyroidism** and is also seen in hypo- and **hypercalcaemia.**

Management of Constipation

Diagnosis of constipation in children is usually made on the history and examination; successful treatment confirms the diagnosis. If chronic severe constipation persists in infants despite treatment, a diagnosis of **ultra-short segment Hirschsprung disease** (see Ch. 50) should be considered. In the elderly, a dietary, fluid intake and drug history should be obtained, and blood tests performed to exclude metabolic causes of constipation. It is vital to differentiate constipation from early large bowel obstruction in these patients. Carcinoma or the complications of diverticular disease should be excluded by sigmoidoscopy and barium enema, colonoscopy or computed tomography (CT) pneumocolon.

In severe constipation, treatment involves a series of measures used progressively:

- Discontinue constipating medication.
- Rectal measures: lubricant glycerine suppositories, small phosphate enemas, stool-softening arachis oil enemas, manual disimpaction (may require general anaesthesia).
- Oral agents (Box 29.3): senna, bisacodyl or osmotic laxatives containing macrogol (polyethylene glycol 3350). A more radical method is to use oral sodium picosulfate (as used in surgical bowel preparation), along with adequate oral or intravenous

---

• BOX 29.3 **Oral Laxative Agents**

- Stimulant/irritant laxatives, for example, dantron, bisacodyl, senna derivatives
- Faecal softeners and lubricants, for example, Dioctyl, liquid paraffin
- Osmotic laxatives, for example, lactulose, mixtures of magnesium hydroxide or magnesium sulphate
- Proprietary preparations, for example, Milpar (liquid paraffin and magnesium hydroxide emulsion)
- Strong laxatives for single-dose use for bowel preparation or very stubborn constipation, for example, sodium picosulfate (stimulant), mannitol solution (osmotic)

Note: bulking agents do not have a laxative effect in the short term

fluids to avoid dehydration. Note that if powerful oral laxatives are given to an obstructed patient, life-threatening perforation of the bowel can occur.

- Oral 'maintenance' medications: sodium docusate as a stool softener, lactulose, Fybogel.

In milder long-term constipation, dietary measures should be used. Many patients take a high-fibre diet but do not drink enough, failing to recognise that both are necessary to produce the benefits of fibre. Many women fail to gain from a high-fibre diet; clearly, increasing their fibre even more would not improve matters. If the condition is not severe, then eating more figs, apricots and prunes may solve the problem. Otherwise, a low dose of a stimulant laxative taken intermittently may be needed.

Sigmoid Volvulus (See Fig. 29.1)

Pathophysiology of Sigmoid Volvulus

Patients with longstanding chronic constipation tend to develop a capacious, elongated and relatively atonic colon, especially in the sigmoid region. This is sometimes described as **acquired** or **idiopathic megacolon**. The condition is more common in cultures with a very high fibre intake.

Occasionally, a huge sigmoid loop, heavy with faeces and distended with gas, becomes twisted on its mesenteric pedicle (often abnormally narrow) to produce a closed-loop obstruction (see Fig. 29.1A–C). If this volvulus is not corrected, venous infarction ensues, followed by perforation and potentially catastrophic faecal peritonitis. This full picture is uncommon, but there is often a history of transient episodes of abdominal pain diagnosed as constipation. Note that volvulus elsewhere, of the caecum, small bowel or stomach is unrelated to constipation.

Clinical Features of Sigmoid Volvulus

In Western countries, sigmoid volvulus is rare except in the elderly, those with severe learning difficulties, and long-stay patients in mental institutions; these groups all readily become faecally loaded. In contrast, it is very common in parts of the world where diet is extremely high in fibre (e.g., parts of Chile, rural Zambia).

The patient with sigmoid volvulus is mildly unwell with abdominal distension and a variable degree of abdominal pain. There is absolute constipation (of both faeces and flatus) that has persisted for at least 24 hours. On digital examination, the rectum is empty but capacious. The abdomen is visibly distended and tympanitic to percussion but rarely tender. This is true even if the colon has reached the stage of venous infarction. Once perforation occurs, the full clinical picture of faecal peritonitis will be evident.

Management of Sigmoid Volvulus

Plain abdominal x-ray usually shows a single grossly dilated sigmoid loop, often reaching the xiphisternum (see Fig. 29.1). An erect film may reveal a characteristic 'inverted U' or 'coffee-bean sign' of bowel gas in the upper abdomen, with fluid levels at the same height in the two bowel limbs in the lower abdomen; a lateral decubitus x-ray may reveal two parallel fluid levels running the length of the abdomen. Ideally, the diagnosis should be confirmed with CT in the acute setting.

If sigmoid volvulus is diagnosed, a flexible sigmoidoscope is gently passed as far as possible into the rectum and a flatus tube inserted through it. The end of the **flatus tube** is then gently manipulated through the twisted bowel into the obstructed loop.

If this is successful, there is a gush of liquid faeces and flatus, relieving the obstruction. The flatus tube can be left in situ for 24 hours to maintain decompression, discourage retwisting and allow recovery of the vascular supply of the bowel wall. Despite this, volvulus is likely to recur.

If plain x-ray and sigmoidoscopy do not confirm volvulus but large bowel obstruction is still suspected, CT scanning with reconstructed images is performed, or else an 'instant' **Gastrografin enema examination** without bowel preparation. These tests differentiate volvulus from other obstructions, such as cancer and diverticular disease, and from pseudoobstruction. In volvulus, pressure from the enema may cause the bowel to untwist, releasing a torrent of faeces and flatus.

If a volvulus cannot be released, operation is performed urgently. In most cases, the bowel is still viable but sigmoid colectomy is usually required to prevent recurrence. A safe alternative procedure is to excise the sigmoid and bring the divided ends of bowel out to form a **double-barrelled colostom**y, rather than risk a primary anastomosis in this dilated and unprepared colon. For recurrent volvulus, **sigmoid colectomy** or suturing the bowel to the abdominal wall to prevent twisting may be performed electively. There may be a role of percutaneous endoscopic colostomy in the elderly and frail but this carries significant morbidity.

Diverticular Disease

Diverticular disease is largely caused by too low an intake of dietary fibre. It causes substantial morbidity in the older population, particularly in the West, and is a very common reason for hospital admission and operation. In developed countries, localised outpouchings or diverticula are present in the bowel wall in at least one-third of people over the age of 60 years, and greater than 50% of people over the age of 80 years. There is strong evidence that this can be caused or aggravated by a chronic lack of dietary fibre but there may also be a genetic element. Females are affected more often than males. (Note: the singular noun is *diverticulum* and the plural *diverticula*, not *diverticulae*; the adjectival form is *diverticular*.)

Pathophysiology of Diverticular Disease

In diverticular disease, the colonic circular muscle is thickened because of an excess of elastic tissue between muscle fibres rather than muscle hypertrophy. The likely mechanism for diverticular formation is functional **hypersegmentation**. In this, adjoining segments of colon contract at the same time, sending peristaltic waves towards each other. This causes very high luminal pressure in short segments, which forces mucosa to herniate through weak points in the wall. These potential defects occur where mucosal blood vessels penetrate the wall from outside, between longitudinal muscle bands (**taeniae coli**). The sigmoid colon is the section most commonly affected by diverticular disease and the condition extends for a variable distance proximally. Right-sided diverticular disease is more common in Japanese, Chinese and Polynesian races and is common in Hawaii. In the West, isolated caecal diverticula sometimes occur and may become inflamed or perforate; these are probably congenital rather than acquired.

The presence of uncomplicated diverticula is unimportant; this asymptomatic condition is known as '**diverticulosis**'. An individual diverticulum may, however, become inflamed as a result of obstruction of its narrow outlet. This causes a **diverticular abscess**. The abscess lies outside the bowel wall and leads to complications described later.

Complications of Diverticular Disease

Diverticular disease may lead to a range of complications, including:

- spreading pericolic inflammation
- pericolic abscess
- intraperitoneal perforation
- fistula formation into other abdominal or pelvic viscera
- bowel-to-bowel adhesions
- fibrous strictures of bowel
- acute haemorrhage (which tends to occur without inflammation)

Clinical Presentations of Diverticular Disease and Their Management

The consequences of diverticular inflammation are collectively described as **diverticulitis** and are summarised in Fig. 29.2. Most people with diverticula are asymptomatic, and diverticula are a common incidental finding when the colon is investigated by barium enema or colonoscopy. Typical appearances are shown in Figs 29.3 and 29.4.

Chronic Grumbling Diverticular Pain (See Fig. 29.2B)

This is probably the most common manifestation of diverticular disease and is usually managed in family practices. Peridiverticular inflammation is chronic, low-grade and recurrent. Local irritation provokes bowel wall spasm, causing pain and erratic bowel habit. There is chronic constipation with small pellet-like faeces and episodic diarrhoea. There are few abnormalities on clinical examination, except perhaps mild left iliac fossa tenderness and faecal loading. Endoscopy or radiological imaging is often performed to confirm the diagnosis and exclude malignancy.

In most patients, symptoms can be relieved by taking a high-fibre diet and bulking agents, although some patients find symptoms are better on a low-fibre intake.

Acute Diverticulitis (i.e., Spreading Pericolic Inflammation; See Fig. 29.2C)

This represents local extension of the inflammation described earlier. It involves pericolic tissues and parietal peritoneum. Typically, the patient complains of continuous left iliac fossa pain and is systemically ill with a pyrexia and tachycardia, often requiring hospital admission. Abdominal findings range from mild left iliac fossa tenderness to obvious local peritonitis.

Antibiotic treatment is directed against the usual faecal organisms. In severe cases, a combination of intravenous antibiotics, such as ciprofloxacin and metronidazole is used, and the bowel 'rested' by stopping oral intake and giving intravenous fluids. Less severe cases can be managed at home with supportive treatment. Antibiotics have been shown to bring no benefit in mild cases.

Hinchey Classification of Abscesses and Perforation

Four stages are described: stage 1 is a small pericolic or mesenteric abscess <4 cm; stage 2 is a large, often pelvic, abscess; stage 3 is a small perforation causing gaseous and purulent peritonitis; and stage 4 is free rupture with faecal peritonitis. Mortality rate for stages 1 and 2 is <5%, for stage 3, 13% and for stage 4, 43%.

In patients admitted with complicated diverticular disease, initial imaging is with CT scan. Stage 1 patients nearly all settle with antibiotics; stage 2 patients can often be drained percutaneously; stage 3 patients usually need operation but this may be limited to a laparoscopic washout, and stage 4 patients need urgent laparotomy. Endoscopy to exclude malignancy should not be performed until inflammation has settled, after several weeks.

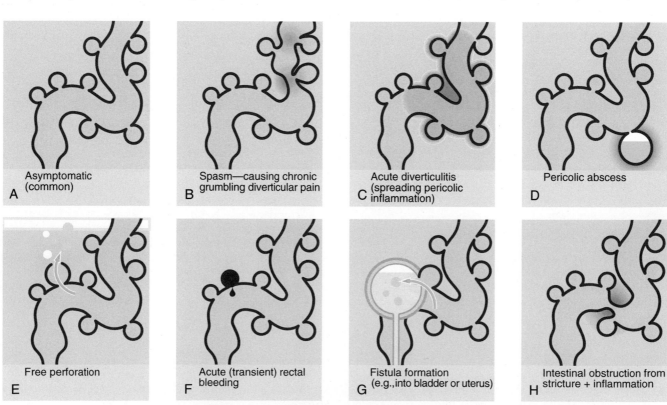

A Asymptomatic (common)

B Spasm—causing chronic grumbling diverticular pain

C Acute diverticulitis (spreading pericolic inflammation)

D Pericolic abscess

E Free perforation

F Acute (transient) rectal bleeding

G Fistula formation (e.g., into bladder or uterus)

H Intestinal obstruction from stricture + inflammation

• **Fig. 29.2** Clinical Presentations of Diverticular Disease.

Pericolic Abscess (See Fig. 29.2D)

Pericolic abscess represents a further extension of the pathological process just described. The clinical presentation is similar at first but fails to resolve with antibiotics. The patient suffers persistent pain and tenderness, a swinging pyrexia and incomplete struction aused by spasm of bowel wall muscle. Sometimes, a pericolic abscess presents as 'pyrexia of unknown origin' or even sepsis (septicaemia). A pericolic abscess may drain spontaneously into bowel, producing an attack of purulent diarrhoea; the condition then resolves. Diagnosis of a pericolic abscess is made on CT scan. A contrast enema may show leakage of contrast into the abscess cavity (Fig. 29.5).

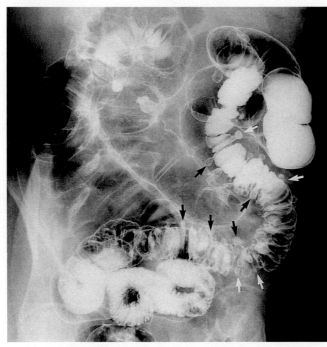

• **Fig. 29.3** Diverticular Disease. Barium enema showing the typical appearance of multiple diverticula *(arrowed)* in the sigmoid and descending colon in a 77-year-old woman. A few diverticula are also present in the transverse colon.

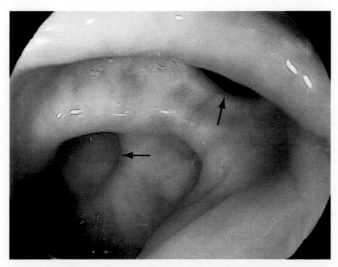

• **Fig. 29.4** Colonoscopic View of Diverticula *(arrowed)*.

Antibiotic therapy is the first line of treatment for abscesses <4 cm. Ideally, this allows the abscess to be contained, and then resolve or drain spontaneously into bowel. Abscesses >4 cm can be drained percutaneously under radiological guidance. If this treatment fails, operation is required. This is often a major procedure usually involving exploration and drainage of the abscess and diverting the faecal stream via a colostomy. The affected segment of bowel must be removed to prevent recurrence. Note that perforated carcinoma can present in a similar way and histological diagnosis is mandatory. The surgical options are to leave a rectal stump for later reanastomosis (Hartmann operation, see Fig. 27.7, p. 382), a safe operation for nonspecialists, or to primarily reanastomose the bowel ends. Reanastomosis is not attempted in faecal peritonitis or in a frail patient, as the chances of success are remote.

Diverticular Perforation (See Fig. 29.2E)

A small, asymptomatic diverticular abscess may rupture spontaneously, that is, perforate, resulting in escape of gas and minimal bowel contents into the peritoneal cavity. The patient presents with an acute abdomen, with the severity of clinical signs depending on the size of perforation and degree of peritoneal contamination. Perforations vary from pinhole size to a hole of 1 cm or more causing generalised faecal peritonitis and potentially fatal sepsis. With small perforations, symptoms and signs may be similar to acute diverticulitis; diagnosis of perforation is confirmed by finding free subdiaphragmatic gas on CT or erect chest x-ray.

Conservative treatment using percutaneous drain placement and bowel rest is appropriate for minimal perforations but Hinchey stage 4 perforations require immediate parenteral antibiotics, followed by laparotomy for peritoneal toilet, diversion of the faecal stream and resection of diseased bowel. Recent data suggests laparoscopic washout may be as effective as segmental resection in selected cases.

Fistula Formation Into Other Abdominal or Pelvic Structures (See Fig. 29.2G)

Fistula formation can occur when an inflamed diverticulum lies close to another hollow viscus. Inflammatory adhesions develop and the diverticulum then ruptures into the other viscus. A fistula between large bowel and small bowel (see Fig. 29.6) causes diarrhoea. A vesicocolic fistula causes **pneumaturia** and severe urinary tract infection. A fistula into the vagina after a previous hysterectomy causes a purulent vaginal discharge. Diverticular disease is the most common cause of these types of fistula but they may also be caused by Crohn disease and sometimes colorectal cancers. Fistulae rarely show up on barium enema examination. CT scanning may reveal a loss of normal tissue planes between bowel and viscus, and/or gas in the bladder. Diagnosis can also be made on the history, at operation or, in the case of bladder fistula, at cystoscopy. Surgery involves excision and histological examination of the affected segment of bowel and repair of the viscus.

Intestinal Obstruction (See Fig. 29.2H)

Diverticular disease occasionally presents with large bowel obstruction caused by acute inflammatory thickening, muscle hypertrophy and spasm. **Incomplete obstruction** is more common and presents as severe constipation. Chronic diverticular inflammation sometimes causes local fibrous strictures, particularly in the sigmoid, which cause intermittent bouts of constipation when the stool is dry. These strictures should be distinguished from malignancy or Crohn disease but this may not be possible radiologically

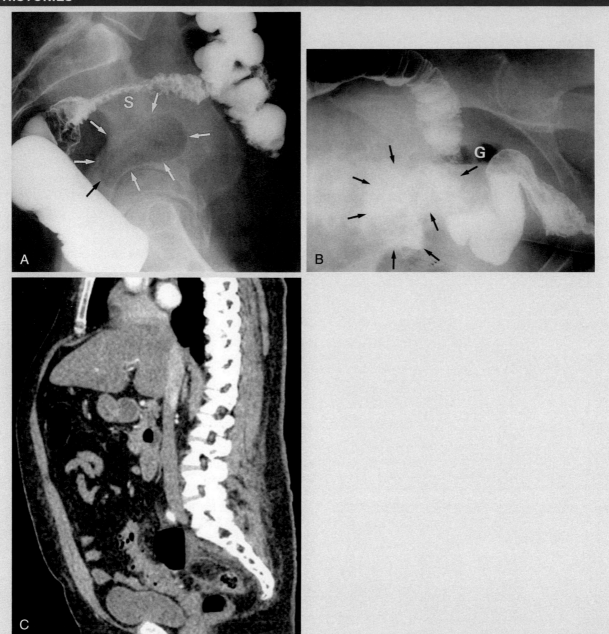

• **Fig. 29.5 Pericolic Abscess Caused by Perforated Diverticular Disease.** Barium enema films from a 49-year-old woman who presented with abdominal pain and tenderness, a mass in the left iliac fossa and a swinging pyrexia. She was treated with antibiotics but the pyrexia failed to settle. **(A)** Right lateral view of the rectosigmoid region showing marked narrowing of the distal sigmoid *(S)* caused by spasm and inflammatory oedema. The radiolucent area anteroinferiorly *(outline arrowed)* represents a bubble of gas in a large pelvic abscess. **(B)** Lateral decubitus film (left side upwards) of the same patient taken later during the same examination. This shows barium which has leaked into the abscess cavity *(outline arrowed)*. Note also a fluid level with a gas bubble *(G)* above it, within the abscess. At laparotomy, a large pericolic and pelvic abscess was found to be walled off. This was drained surgically, the sigmoid colon excised and the end of the descending colon brought out as a terminal colostomy in the left iliac fossa. The rectal stump was oversewn; 3 months later, the bowel was reconnected. **(C)** Sagittal computed tomography of the abdomen and pelvis showing thickened sigmoid colon with pericolic abscess and pericolic abscess with air fluid level.

or endoscopically, with the diagnosis being made at histology following resection, (see Fig. 29.5; Fig. 29.7).

When acute diverticular inflammation involves the pericolic tissues, small bowel may become involved. Thus (secondary) small bowel adynamic disorder may be the presenting feature, with obstruction-like symptoms.

Acute Rectal Haemorrhage (See Fig. 29.2F)

Diverticular disease may present with acute rectal bleeding, which, unlike the other complications of diverticula, is not usually the result of inflammation. Blood loss is variable but the bleeding almost always stops spontaneously. The patient typically complains of having passed a mass of fairly fresh blood instead of the expected stool and is admitted to hospital urgently. The main differential diagnosis is **ischaemic colitis** but other causes of rectal bleeding, such as carcinoma and haemorrhoids, must be considered.

Management is rarely surgical but an angiogram (or CT) and embolisation is sometimes performed by a specialist radiologist if the bleeding is severe. After necessary resuscitation, the patient is kept under observation for several days, after which it is safe to perform further investigations.

For further reading please see: http://www.nejm.org/doi/full/10.1056/NEJMcp073228.

Colonic Angiodysplasias

Colonic angiodysplasias have been recognised as a common cause of acute or chronic rectal bleeding and iron deficiency anaemia since the mid-1970s. The lesions are tiny tortuous dilated veins in the colonic wall, usually in the ascending colon, and produce bleeding out of proportion to their size (Fig. 29.8). They may also occur in the stomach and small bowel. The origin of colonic angiodysplasias is unknown but since they occur later in life, they are probably acquired and degenerative (Fig. 29.9).

If bleeding is acute and is occurring rapidly, CT angiography or selective mesenteric arteriography may demonstrate the source of bleeding and it may be possible to occlude the vessel angiographically. In chronic or recurrent haemorrhage, large bowel lesions can be visualised by colonoscopy. This underlines the importance of

CASE HISTORY

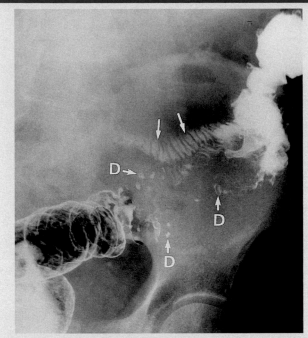

• **Fig. 29.6 Diverticular Fistula Into the Distal Ileum.** Barium enema of a 61-year-old man with a recently erratic bowel habit, who presented with pain and tenderness in the left iliac fossa. The x-ray shows the sigmoid colon, although part of it is poorly filled with barium, which is only seen in the diverticula (D). There is a loop of small bowel which contains contrast (arrowed), indicating the presence of a coloileal fistula caused by peridiverticulitis.

CASE HISTORY

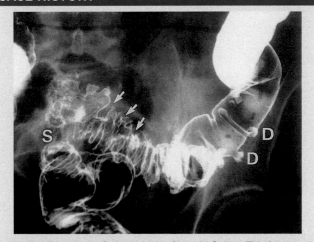

• **Fig. 29.7 Diverticular Stricture in the Sigmoid Colon.** This 64-year-old man suffered several attacks of diverticulitis, which settled with antibiotics. This frontal view of a barium enema shows diverticula (D) in the upper sigmoid colon and circular muscle hypertrophy in the distal sigmoid colon (arrowed) typical of diverticular disease. There is a stricture (S) near the rectosigmoid junction. This stricture does not show the typical 'shouldering' of a carcinoma, although carcinoma could not be excluded on barium enema. Colonoscopy confirmed that it was benign. This patient later had a severe attack of diverticulitis, which required surgery and a Hartmann operation was performed.

CASE HISTORY

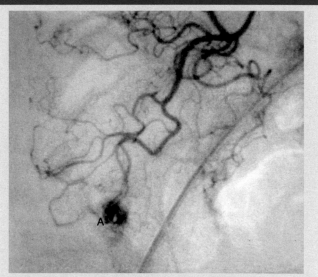

• **Fig. 29.8 Caecal Angiodysplasia.** This 66-year-old man had been admitted to hospital on 12 occasions for rectal bleeding or anaemia and received a total of 77 units of blood by transfusion. This selective arteriogram was performed on the most recent admission and shows an abnormal mass of blood vessels (A) in the caecum typical of angiodysplasia. This part of the bowel was resected and the patient had not rebled 3 years later.

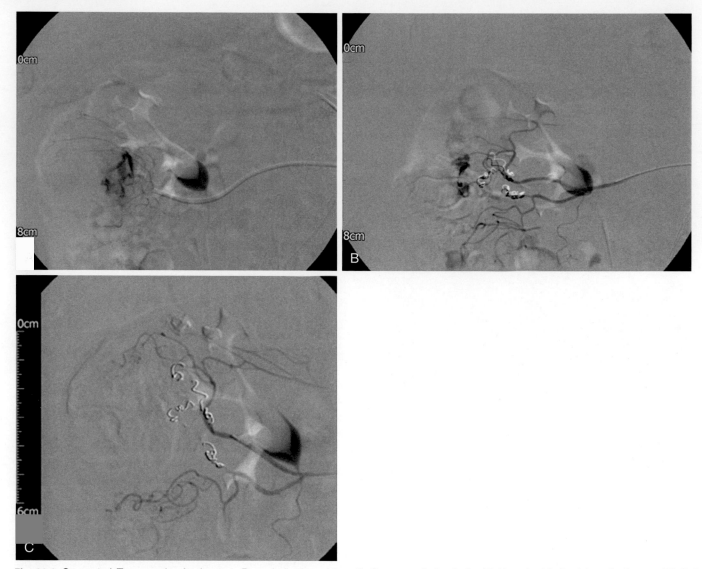

• **Fig. 29.9** Computed Tomography Angiogram. Preembolisation of hepatic flexure angiodysplasia. (A) Vascular blush at hepatic flexure. (B) Coils deployed into lesion with incomplete embolisation. (C) Postembolisation of hepatic flexure angiodysplasia.

thorough colonoscopy in patients with unexplained GI blood loss. Lesions can often be treated by electrical coagulation via a colonoscope. If unsuccessful, the affected segment is excised. Similar lesions occur more rarely in small bowel and bleed in the same way.

Ischaemic Colitis

Ischaemic colitis is a condition of the elderly, which usually presents with rectal bleeding. The history is characteristic; there is a bout of cramp-like abdominal pain lasting a few hours, followed by an attack of rectal bleeding. Usually the bleeding is dark red,

often without faeces, and occurs one to three times over about 12 hours. The episode then ceases spontaneously. The differential diagnosis includes acute bleeding from diverticular disease. The cause is transient ischaemia of a segment of large bowel, followed by sloughing of the mucosa. The splenic flexure is the most vulnerable. Further attacks occasionally occur but most patients have no further trouble. Investigation by CT in the acute stage may reveal colonic oedema in the affected segment (Fig. 29.10). A rare late complication is fibrotic stricturing of the area affected by ischaemia. Endoscopic examination has a role if the patient does not have an acute abdomen.

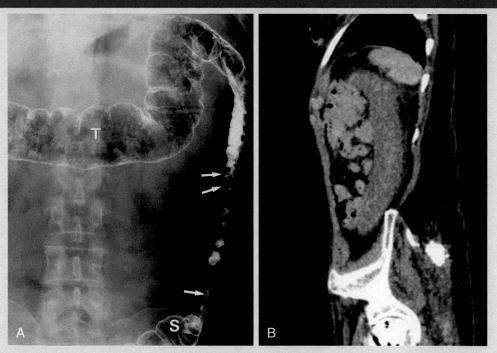

• **Fig. 29.10** Ischaemic Colitis. This 72-year-old man presented with a bout of severe abdominal pain 48 hours before this barium enema was performed. Soon after the pain, there was a single episode of fresh rectal bleeding. This film shows typical (though extensive) changes of acute ischaemic colitis, which characteristically involved the proximal descending colon. The transverse colon *(T)* and sigmoid colon *(S)* are normal. Note the extremely narrowed lumen of the ischaemic segment and the characteristic thumb-printing *(arrowed)* caused by mucosal oedema. (B) Sagittal computed tomography of thickened segment of left colon indicating ischaemic colitis.

30

Anal and Perianal Disorders

CHAPTER OUTLINE

must be distinguished from rectal carcinoma and the rare anal carcinoma. Most anal and perianal conditions can be treated on an outpatient basis, although abscesses, and haemorrhoids that have become strangulated or thrombosed may present as surgical emergencies.

Anatomy of the Anal Canal

At the anal verge outside the anal canal, there is normal skin composed of **stratified squamous epithelium** with skin appendages—sweat glands, hair follicles and sebaceous glands. The anal canal proper is about 4 to 5 cm in a male and 3 cm long in a female, extending from the lower to the upper border of the internal sphincter (Fig. 30.2). There are three zones, each with different lining epithelium:

- The lowest or **distal zone** lies between the squamous–mucocutaneous junction and the level of the anal valves at the **dentate (pectinate) line.** This is lined by **nonkeratinising** squamous epithelium without skin appendages or glands; the epithelium contains some melanocytes. This area is exquisitely sensitive, for example, to injection.
- The **anal transitional zone.** This lies between the zone of squamous epithelium below and the columnar mucosal zone above, and extends a distance varying between 0.3 and 2 cm. It consists of transitional epithelium resembling urothelium, four to nine cell layers thick. Anal glands are present in the submucosa but there is minimal mucin production. A unique type of anal carcinoma develops from it with a viral aetiology.
- The upper part of the anal canal is lined by rectal mucosa. On proctoscopic inspection, it is a dark reddish-blue where it overlies the submucosal venous plexus, becoming the typical pink of colorectal mucosa more proximally. This area of mucosa is relatively insensitive.

The mucosa of the upper part of the anal canal is thrown into 6 to 10 longitudinal folds, the **columns of Morgagni,** each containing a terminal branch of the superior rectal artery and vein. The folds are most prominent in the left lateral, right posterior and

Introduction

Anal and perianal disorders make up about 20% of general surgical outpatient referrals. These conditions can be distressing or embarrassing and patients often tolerate symptoms for a long time before seeking medical advice. The common anal symptoms are summarised in Box 30.1 and interpretation is discussed in Chapter 18.

The range of anal and perianal disorders is illustrated in Fig. 30.1. Haemorrhoids and other common benign conditions

---

• BOX 30.1 Common Anal Symptoms

- Anal bleeding
- Anal itching and discomfort
- Pain on defaecation
- Perianal itching and irritation
- 'Something coming down'
- Perianal discharge

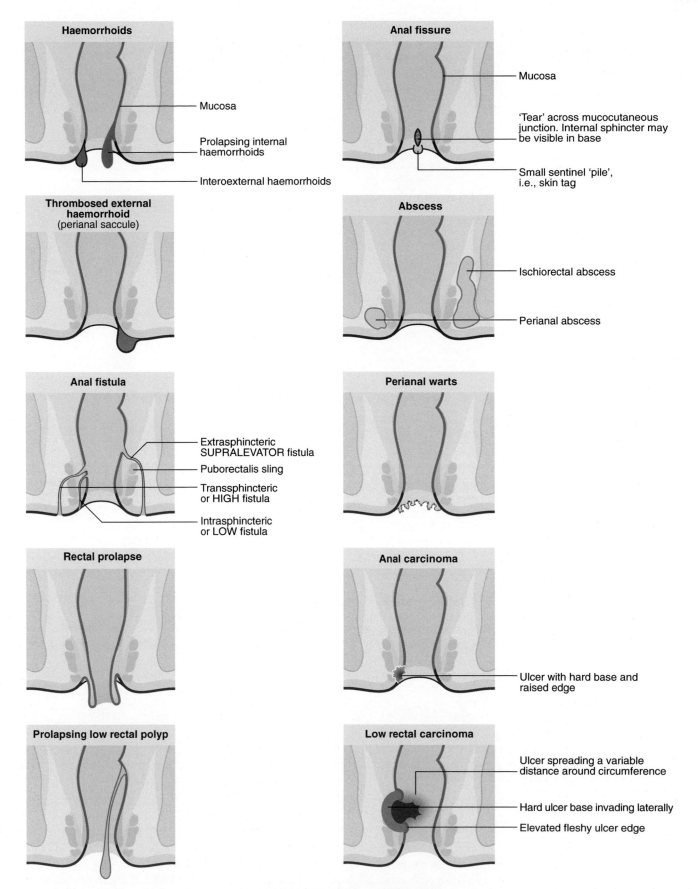

• **Fig. 30.1** Anal and Perianal Disorders.

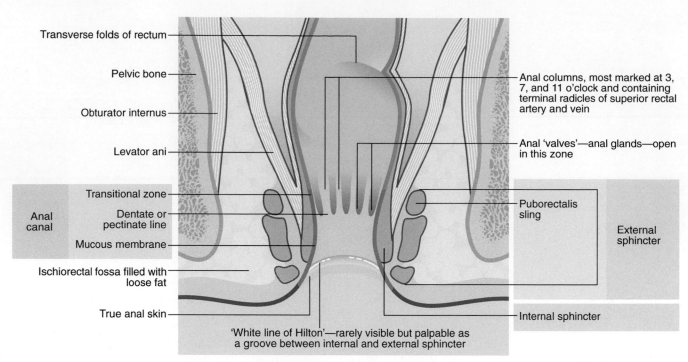

• **Fig. 30.2** Anatomy of the Anal Canal.

right anterior sectors where the vessels form prominent **anal cushions**. These are important in fine control of continence. They may become pathologically enlarged to form **haemorrhoids**, which are complex collections of arterioles, arteries, venules, venous saccules and connective tissue. The anal columns are not readily visible on proctoscopy but the transition between glandular rectal mucosa and anal skin is clearly visible. The lymphatics of the upper anal canal drain to the pelvic and abdominal lymph node chain, whereas the lower part of the anal canal drains to inguinal lymph nodes.

The anal sphincter mechanism has three constituents: the **internal sphincter**, the **external sphincter** and the **puborectalis muscle**. The internal sphincter represents a downward but thickened continuation of the rectal wall musculature. The encircling external sphincter and the puborectalis sling (part of levator ani) arise from the pelvic floor. Continence is maintained principally by the anal sphincters squeezing the three anal cushions together to occlude the lumen. Continence is assisted by the rectum forming a compliant reservoir to accumulate faeces.

Haemorrhoids

Haemorrhoids (piles) are extremely common, affecting nearly half of the population at some time. Men tend to suffer more often and for longer periods, whereas women are particularly susceptible in late pregnancy and the puerperium.

Pathogenesis of Haemorrhoids

Constipation and pregnancy are the most common triggers for development of haemorrhoids. Lack of fibre in the modern Western diet is a likely factor. Straining during constipation raises intraabdominal pressure, which obstructs venous return, causing the venous plexuses to engorge. The bulging mucosa is then dragged distally by the hard stool. Furthermore, persistent

straining causes the pelvic floor to sag downwards, extruding the anal mucosa and causing a small degree of prolapse. Haemorrhoids are usually located in the 3, 7 and 11 o'clock positions when viewed with the patient in the supine lithotomy position. These correspond to the anatomical positions of the anal cushions. The venous component causes a problem only if it becomes thrombosed to form a **thrombosed external venous saccule** (sometimes inaccurately labelled a perianal haematoma).

In pregnancy-related haemorrhoids, venous engorgement and mucosal prolapse are probably the main mechanisms. Progesterone mediates venous dilatation, and the foetus obstructs pelvic venous return.

Classification of Haemorrhoids

Haemorrhoids (piles) are classified into first, second and third degrees according to the extent of prolapse through the anal canal. **First degree (or grade I) piles** never prolapse; **second degree (grade II) piles** prolapse during defaecation and then return spontaneously; **third degree (grade III) piles** remain outside the anal margin unless replaced digitally (Fig. 30.3). Most haemorrhoids can be described as *internal* because they are covered by glandular mucosa. Large neglected haemorrhoids may extend beneath the stratified squamous epithelium so their lower part becomes covered by skin. These are correctly described as **interoexternal haemorrhoids**, or more commonly 'external piles'.

Symptoms and Signs of Haemorrhoids

Haemorrhoids often produce symptoms intermittently. Attacks last from a few days to a few weeks, often with complete freedom from trouble between times. Episodes of constipation are often a precipitating factor.

Any haemorrhoid may **bleed** from stool trauma during defaecation. Bleeding from the arterial component of the anal cushion

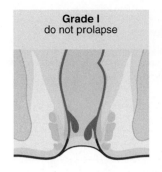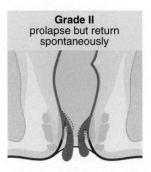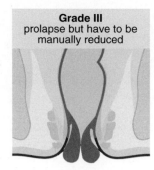

• **Fig. 30.3** Classification of Haemorrhoids

results in the characteristic bright red rectal bleeding. Large haemorrhoids may **prolapse** and then **thrombose**, causing acute severe pain if venous return is obstructed by sphincter tone. Longstanding haemorrhoids eventually atrophy, probably by thrombosis and fibrosis, leaving small **skin tags** at the anal margin.

The common chronic or intermittent symptoms of haemorrhoids are:

- Perianal irritation and itching (pruritus ani) caused by mucus leakage. Scratching exacerbates the problem.
- Rectal bleeding (fresh blood, on the paper or separate from stool).
- Mucus leakage caused by imperfect closure of the anal cushions.
- Mild incontinence of flatus also caused by imperfect closure of the anal cushions.
- Haemorrhoidal prolapse.

Most patients reaching the surgeon have tried various anaesthetic or soothing creams and suppositories, either self-administered or prescribed by the family practitioner. The usual reasons for referral are persistent symptoms or the need to exclude malignancy as a cause of bleeding.

On examination, external piles or skin tags may be visible in the anal area. Digital examination is essential to exclude carcinoma and provides a useful measure of anal tone. Haemorrhoids are not palpable unless they are large since the contained blood empties with finger pressure. **Proctoscopy** is needed to demonstrate internal piles, which are seen bulging into the lumen as the proctoscope is withdrawn. **Sigmoidoscopy**, rigid or ideally flexible, is important in patients over 40 years, if there is a history of bleeding or any symptoms suspicious of malignancy; occasionally a rectal polyp will be diagnosed in this way. Since haemorrhoids are so common, they can mask an unrelated diagnosis of cancer.

Acute Presentations of Haemorrhoids

Thrombosed or strangulated haemorrhoids present with acute severe pain and many patients are admitted to hospital as emergencies. These complications are common in the late stages of pregnancy and soon after delivery. The diagnosis of **thrombosed haemorrhoids** is usually obvious on inspection as an oedematous, congested purplish mass at the anal margin. Tight spasm of the anal sphincter makes digital rectal examination extremely painful. **Strangulated haemorrhoids** are even more painful, and the strangulated mass may become necrotic or even ulcerated. Symptomatic relief is provided by several days of bed rest and application of ice packs and topical anaesthetic gel; this conservative treatment may be the best that can safely be offered in late pregnancy. Some surgeons favour urgent haemorrhoidectomy for thrombosed or

strangulated piles, accepting the slightly higher risk of complications in exchange for a more rapid recovery and a shorter hospital stay. Prophylactic antibiotics should be given to cover the operation because of the risk of infection in necrotic tissue.

Conservative Management and Prevention of Haemorrhoids

The most important means of preventing and treating haemorrhoids is avoiding constipation and ensuring a bulky stool. This is best achieved by taking a diet high in fibre with adequate fluid intake. The patient should be advised to always heed the call to evacuate. This appears to be associated with a reflex release of lubricating mucus, which may be absent later. Sufferers should be strongly encouraged to avoid straining and to spend minimal time defaecating. A prolonged ritual often leads to further straining at the end of defaecation, when a mild prolapse can be experienced as incomplete evacuation of faeces. In many patients, these simple measures are enough to relieve symptoms. Note that repetitive straining occasionally leads to the formation of a '**solitary ulcer**' on the anterior wall of the proximal anal canal, which may be clinically indistinguishable from a malignant ulcer. With third degree haemorrhoids, symptoms can often be relieved by the patient replacing the prolapsing haemorrhoids digitally after defaecation.

Creams, suppositories and other topical preparations available with or without prescription are very widely used. Some contain local anaesthetic agents or steroids. They are useful for temporary symptomatic relief but do nothing to treat the underlying condition. Overuse may cause allergic reactions, maceration of the perianal skin and secondary infections.

Surgical Treatments for Haemorrhoids

Injection of Sclerosants or Banding

First-degree haemorrhoids, which do not regress with dietary change and avoiding straining, and most second-degree haemorrhoids, can be treated on an outpatient basis by sclerosant injections or banding.

In **sclerotherapy**, with the aid of a proctoscope, 1 to 3 ml of a mildly irritant solution of 5% phenol in oil is injected submucosally around the pedicles of the three major haemorrhoids in the insensitive upper anal canal. This provokes a fibrotic reaction, effectively obliterating the haemorrhoidal vessels and causing atrophy of the haemorrhoids (Fig. 30.4). Injections are painless if the needle is placed correctly; direct injection into the haemorrhoid would be extremely painful. Sclerotherapy is usually repeated on two to three occasions at intervals of 4 to 6 weeks.

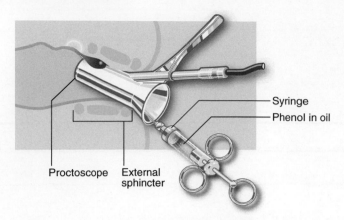

- **Fig. 30.4** Sclerotherapy or Injection of Haemorrhoids. A mildly irritant solution of 5% phenol in oil is injected submucosally around the pedicle of the haemorrhoid.

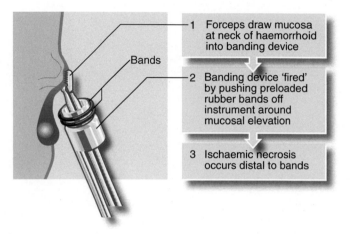

- **Fig. 30.5** Rubber Banding Technique for Haemorrhoids. Note that the haemorrhoid itself is not banded but the band is applied to the blood vessels at its base.

Note: sclerotherapy is **not** suitable for patients with nut allergies because of the nut origin of the carrier oil, and should ideally be avoided in males because of the risk of prostatitis and impotence.

An alternative and much more commonly used treatment is **banding**. A cone of mucosa just above the haemorrhoidal neck is drawn into a banding instrument, often by suction, and tight elastic bands released around the base of the cone, constricting the haemorrhoidal vessels (Fig. 30.5). Importantly, the bands are not placed around the stalks of prolapsing haemorrhoids; this would be unbearably painful because of the somatic innervation of anal skin. The result of banding is that the haemorrhoid gradually shrinks. The bands separate with time and are passed. Of note, both sclerotherapy and banding techniques can and may need to be repeated.

Haemorrhoidectomy

Haemorrhoidal excision is indicated for third-degree haemorrhoids and for lesser degrees when other treatments have failed. The most common operation is that described by **Milligan and Morgan**, in which the haemorrhoidal masses are excised with overlying mucosa and some skin (Fig. 30.6). This leaves skin and mucosal defects, which heal by secondary intention and wound contraction. A skin bridge **must** be preserved between each wound

to prevent the serious late complication of anal stenosis. **Stapled haemorrhoidectomy** enjoyed some popularity for large haemorrhoids, particularly when mucosal prolapse is a feature. It aims to restore the anatomy of the anal cushions by excising a ring of low rectal mucosa, including the engorged necks of the piles. The metal staple line remains permanently in situ, palpable digitally and sometimes causing pain. This operation requires great skill and occasionally results in serious complications; this fact plus the residual staple line are contributing to a decline in interest in the operation, although it may have a role in the treatment of prolapsed circumferential haemorrhoids.

Before haemorrhoidectomy, stool softeners, such as bulking agents and gentle laxatives should be given to avoid constipation afterwards. The painful early postoperative period can be greatly eased by caudal analgesia given at operation.

Haemorrhoidal Artery Ligation Operation

This is a promising new procedure without an incision. It involves locating the artery supplying each haemorrhoid using ultrasound, then encircling it with a stitch, via the insensitive lower rectal mucosa, to cut off its blood supply and may be accompanied by a mucopexy. Over the following few days the haemorrhoids shrink, bleeding and local symptoms abate, although skin tags remain.

Thrombosed External Haemorrhoids

A thrombosed external haemorrhoid or **thrombosed external venous saccule** is an acutely painful anal condition (Fig. 30.7). The onset is sudden and, if untreated, there is persistent pain lasting 1 to 2 weeks, worse on defaecation. On examination, a blue-black hemispherical bulge is seen in the skin near the anal margin. This is sometimes called a *perianal haematoma*, but this is inaccurate. The condition can occur in patients with haemorrhoids but is usually seen in isolation.

Most thrombosed external haemorrhoids subside over a few days and patients need only oral analgesia. If pain is severe or prolonged, the thrombosis may be incised and drained under local anaesthesia; some surgeons favour this as first-line therapy.

Anal Fissure

An anal fissure is a longitudinal tear in the mucosa and skin of the anal canal, sometimes caused by passing a large, constipated stool. The tear is nearly always in the posterior midline of the anal margin. The fissure causes acute pain during defaecation and sphincter spasm, both of which persist for an hour or longer. There is often a small amount of fresh bleeding at defaecation. The result is fear of defaecation and this aggravates the constipation. This history alone is diagnostic of an anal fissure. On inspection, the fissure is concealed by the anal spasm but a small skin tag (sentinel pile) may be seen at the superficial end of the fissure (Fig. 30.8). Rectal examination is extremely painful and rarely possible unless the fissure has become chronic.

Patients sometimes tolerate the pain of an acute fissure by using local anaesthetic creams and then present much later with a chronic anal fissure, prevented from healing by internal sphincter spasm and repeated tearing open of the fissure during passage of stools.

Management of Anal Fissure

Anal fissure can be managed conservatively or operatively. Modern conservative treatment involves the use of topical glyceryl trinitrate

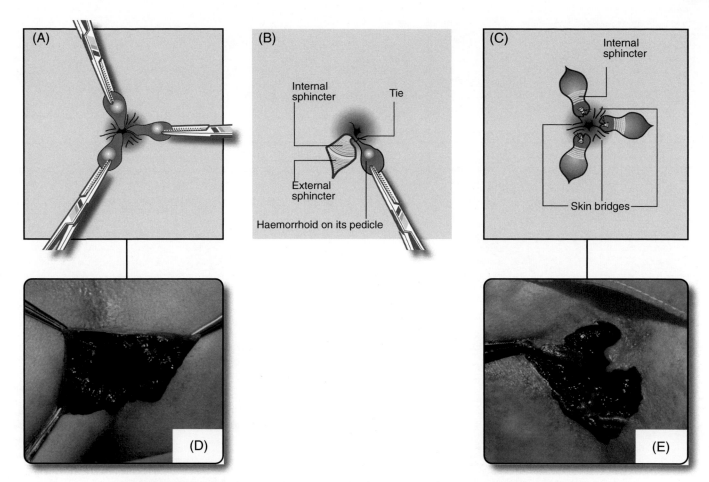

• **Fig. 30.6** Milligan–Morgan Open Haemorrhoidectomy. **(A)** and **(D)** Identification of the main haemor-rhoids; the external part of each is clamped with a haemostat and retracted outwards. **(B)** Scissors are used to incise the skin around the external haemorrhoid, excess skin being excised at the same time. The haemorrhoid is then raised on its pedicle by dissecting it from the external and internal sphincters. The skin is not closed. **(C)** and **(E)** The process is repeated for the other primary haemorrhoids, ensuring that **skin bridges** are preserved at the anal margin between the areas resected or anal stenosis will occur as healing proceeds ('if it looks like a dahlia, it's a failure'). The completed haemorrhoidectomy has a 'clover-leaf' appearance ('if it looks like a clover, it's all over'). After haemostasis is ensured, wounds are dressed with a nonadherent dressing (e.g., Mepitel) and a surgical pad applied, held in place by elasticated net underpants.

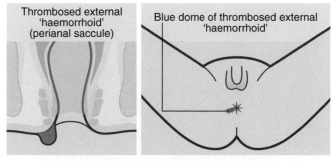

• **Fig. 30.7** Thrombosed External Haemorrhoid.

(GTN) ointment 0.2% to 0.4%, applied twice a day for 2 months. This relaxes the sphincter spasm and increases blood supply to the fissure, allowing healing. Patients need to be warned that it may cause headaches. This treatment can cure most anal fissures. For the rest, diltiazem 2% ointment, a calcium-channel blocker, may be successful and a good alternative if side effects are experienced with GTN. Injection of botulinum toxin into the sphincter complex is another way to cause a temporary 'chemical sphincterotomy'.

Surgery in the form of **lateral submucous (internal) sphinc-terotomy** brings more immediate relief, but there is a 10% to 15% incidence of incontinence of flatus following this proce-dure. Surgeons tend to be reluctant to offer sphincterotomy to women because their sphincters are shorter and less robust, and because occult sphincter injury from childbirth may already have occurred. However, if conservative treatments fail and the patient is suitably informed of the risks, an internal anal sphincterotomy may be offered. This operation involves dividing just under 1 cm of the lower rim of the internal sphincter via a small lateral inci-sion. For chronic refractory fissures, anal advancement flap opera-tions are sometimes performed; this avoids the sphincter muscle damage caused by sphincterotomy. **Lord anal stretch**, which involved manual dilatation of the sphincter, led to unacceptable rates of incontinence caused by sphincter damage and has long been abandoned.

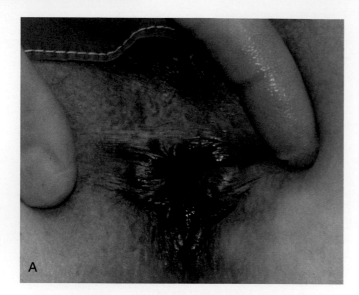

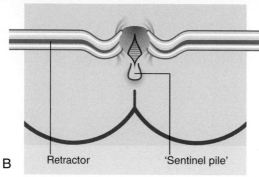

B   Retractor   'Sentinel pile'

• **Fig. 30.8** Anal Fissure. **(A)** Chronic anal fissure with a 'sentinel pile'. Simple fissures are typically posteriorly located, as in this patient. **(B)** Explanatory diagram.

Anorectal Abscesses

Pathophysiology and Clinical Features

Abscesses in the anorectal area are common surgical emergencies. They present with constant and often severe perineal pain and local tenderness.

Anorectal abscesses begin as acute purulent infections of **anal glands**. These lie in the **intersphincteric space** between the internal and external sphincters and drain into tiny pits, the anal crypts, near the dentate line. The ducts are very narrow and duct obstruction may be what initiates the infection. Rarely, an abscess remains confined between the sphincters and an **intersphincteric abscess** results. The only symptom may be chronic anal pain, and there is often little to find on clinical examination. The only clue may be localised tenderness on rectal palpation.

From the intersphincteric plane, infection tends to spread in one or more of three directions (Fig. 30.9):

- **Downwards** between the sphincters towards the anal verge, forming a **perianal abscess.** This is the most common presentation and accounts for 80% of anorectal abscesses. The patient presents acutely with a painful, tender, red swelling close to the anal verge.
- **Outwards** through the external sphincter into the loose fibrofatty tissue of the ischiorectal fossa, forming an **ischiorectal abscess.** There is little barrier to spread of infection once it has entered this space and a neglected or inadequately treated abscess may become

enormous. Ischiorectal abscesses make up about 15% of anorectal abscesses. The patient presents with perineal pain and systemic signs of infection. There is tenderness over the ischiorectal fossa lateral to the anus but there may be no visible redness or swelling; rectal palpation reveals a tender mass lateral to the rectum.

- **Upwards** between the sphincters to form a **supralevator abscess**, involving the pararectal tissues above the pelvic floor. These make up less than 5% of anorectal abscesses and present with systemic signs of infection, rectal pain and difficulty in micturition. On rectal examination, a tender mass is often palpable near the tip of the finger.

Treatment of Anorectal Abscesses

If perianal infection is seen very early, oral antibiotic treatment may abort it. Antibiotics used in this way by general practitioners, coupled with early referral, has reduced the number and severity of cases reaching the surgeon. However, once an abscess is diagnosed, **surgical drainage** is needed; antibiotics are only indicated in addition when there is spreading infection. Drainage is performed after careful examination (examination under anaesthetic [EUA]) to determine the extent of the abscess under regional or general anaesthesia. **Perianal** and **ischiorectal abscesses** are drained via the perianal skin, ensuring all loculations are broken down. An **intersphincteric abscess** is drained via an internal sphincterotomy. A swab of the pus is sent for microbiological diagnosis to differentiate infection by skin pathogens (e.g., *Staphylococcus*), which occur spontaneously, from infections of bowel origin (e.g., *Escherichia coli*), which suggest an underlying fistula. Large ischiorectal abscesses require packing or placement of a drain to keep the neck of the cavity open, whilst granulation tissue gradually fills the space from its depths. Further examinations under anaesthesia after a few days are usually planned to ensure complete drainage and to inspect for fistulae. Supralevator abscesses are more complicated and require complex staged surgical procedures.

Incising a perianal abscess results in complete resolution in about 50% of cases; the other half develop an **anal fistula** (see later). The fistula is usually undetectable at the time of drainage but is recognised by a persistent discharge near the skin incision for several weeks afterwards (see Fig. 18.6).

Differential diagnosis of abscesses in the perianal area includes:

- **Crohn disease**—may cause multiple abscesses and complex fistulae (see Ch. 28) and must be excluded.
- **Hidradenitis suppurativa**—originates in perianal apocrine glands in the skin; it is easily distinguished from deeper perianal abscesses by careful inspection and palpation. There may be multiple infected glands in the natal cleft, groins and sometimes axillae.
- **Pilonidal abscess**—occurs in the skin of the natal cleft (see Fig. 30.9) but may mimic a true perianal abscess if near the anal margin; careful examination shows no communication with the anal canal and often the presence of embedded hairs. Treatment is by incision and drainage but further procedures may be required to treat the associated pilonidal sinus (see p. 418).
- **Tuberculous abscess and fistula**—very rare.

Anal Fistula

Anal fistulae usually develop as a complication of perianal, ischiorectal or supralevator abscesses. A fistula is an abnormal connection between two epithelial surfaces and consists of a chronically

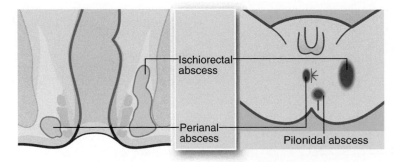

• **Fig. 30.9** Abscesses in the Anorectal Region.

infected tract, which may eventually become epithelialised. It extends from an **internal opening** at the level of the dentate line, and passes through the site of previous abscess to an external opening on the perianal skin, near the old drainage scar. The communication between abscess cavity and bowel is established by spontaneous discharge of the enlarging abscess into the bowel, before surgical drainage or after incomplete surgical drainage. To minimise the risk of fistula, any abscess in the anal region should be drained early and thoroughly.

The patient with a fistula typically complains of intermittent discharge of mucus or pus in the perianal region, often faecally stained. On examination, a small papilla of granulation tissue is seen on the skin within 2 to 3 cm of the anal margin (see Fig. 18.6). Pus may be expressed from it by compressing the underlying tract digitally between papilla and anus. This clinical picture is diagnostic of an anal fistula, but this apparently trivial skin lesion is often dismissed as a pustule or an incompletely healed perianal abscess.

Most anal fistulae are simple and relatively superficial, with the internal opening located in a crypt at the level of the dentate line (well below puborectalis), most often in the posterior midline. These are known as **low anal fistulae** (Fig. 30.10). For successful treatment, it is essential to locate the internal opening so the entire tract can be dealt with.

Goodsall rule helps to predict the course of a low fistula:

- If the external opening is **in front** of an imaginary transverse line across the anus, the fistula is likely to have a short **direct** tract to the anal canal.
- If the external opening is **behind** the transverse line, the tract is likely to have a **curved** course towards an internal opening in the posterior midline.

Assessment and treatment of fistulae requires general or regional anaesthesia. EUA is performed first. A malleable probe is gently manipulated through the fistula to try to demonstrate the internal orifice. If this is not found, hydrogen peroxide diluted with saline can be gently injected into the external opening. Provided the fistula is superficial and involves less than half of the sphincter bulk, treatment is by laying open the entire tract by cutting down on to the probe with diathermy, transecting the anal margin and opening the whole length of the fistula. This should be less than 0.5 cm in total. This is known as **fistulotomy** and involves dividing some of the internal and external sphincter. The wound heals gradually by secondary intention. There should be no loss of faecal continence, but flatus may be less well controlled. Attempts have been made to deal with some fistulae by using tissue glues or fibrin packs but results so far are unimpressive although they cause little harm.

If the fistula involves more than half the length of the anal sphincter complex, surgical treatment is difficult and highly

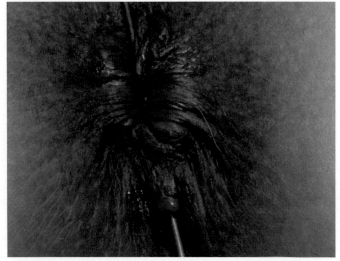

• **Fig. 30.10** Anal Fistula. A probe has been passed from the skin surface through a low anal fistula to emerge in the anal canal at the level of the dentate line. Treatment consisted simply of cutting down onto the probe, laying open the fistula along its length. The wound was left to heal by secondary intention.

specialised because of the need to retain the functional integrity of the sphincters to preserve continence. Where complex or recurrent fistulae are suspected, the anatomy can be defined well by **magnetic resonance imaging** so that careful staged surgery and/ or appropriate conservative measures can be planned.

In many of the more severe cases, primary surgical cure is not attempted and infection is controlled long term by placing a soft **Seton** or thread through the tract and out through the anus, where it is tied loosely to form a ring. This maintains free drainage of pus and reduces the risk of abscess formation, whilst the Seton goes largely unnoticed by the patient. After a long period of quiescence, the Seton may be removed and minimally invasive techniques may be used to deal with the tract. In the worst cases, where there is extensive destructive involvement of the anal sphincters in the infective process, the only surgical cure is perineal excision of the whole anal canal and lower rectum, and a permanent end colostomy. In exceptional cases, patients may choose this option to improve their quality of life, for example in Crohn disease.

Anal fistulae sometimes occur as a manifestation of **Crohn disease**. Such fistulae tend to be multiple and in the most extreme cases form a 'pepper-pot' perineum (see Fig. 28.9, p. 395). There is a significant role for medical therapy with biologics and Seton drainage, which can then be removed.

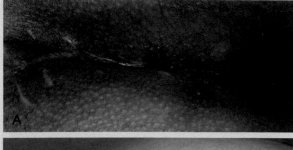
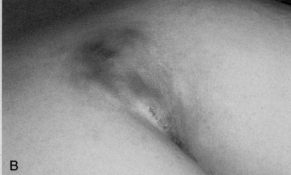

• **Fig. 30.11** Pilonidal Sinus and Abscess. **(A)** Recurrent pilonidal sinuses. The scar from a previous operation for this condition is visible. There are several tufts of hair emerging from sinuses in the midline and a typical sinus opening *(S)* to one side. **(B)** Pilonidal abscess in a different patient of 24 years. This is a common presentation and usually requires formal surgical drainage and curettage of the sinuses.

Pilonidal Sinus and Abscess

These conditions arise from the skin of the natal cleft rather than the anus. As the name implies, pilonidal sinuses, cysts and abscesses contain **'a nest of hairs'**. They are common in young adults, particularly hirsute men, and are found at the upper end of the natal cleft. Here, between the buttocks, there is often a congenital dimple or pit. Fragments of hair falling from the back or head accumulate in this nidus. The hairs slowly work their way into the dermis, with the cuticular scales on the hairs acting like barbs of an arrow. The process is encouraged by the massaging effect of sitting for long periods; pilonidal sinus is thus common in truck and tractor drivers. Sinuses also occur between the hairdresser's fingers from implantation of their clients' hair (see later).

Pilonidal sinuses tend to run a long indolent course with chronic or intermittent purulent discharge to the skin surface, via one or more sinuses. Periodic acute exacerbations may progress to abscesses (Fig. 30.11).

Pilonidal Abscess

The mass of hairs and other skin debris in a pilonidal sinus excites a foreign-body inflammatory reaction, often resulting in a mildly or intermittently discharging sinus. If the cavity becomes secondarily infected, an abscess develops and causes acute pain and swelling. Pilonidal abscesses are often multilocular. They sometimes drain spontaneously but rarely heal completely. Many require surgical drainage because of pain.

Treatment of Pilonidal Sinus

Definitive treatment aims to eliminate the nidus of hairs and associated cystic cavities, chronic abscesses and sinuses. At operation,

obvious plugs of hair are first removed and then the sinus network is explored with probes. In the past, surgical excision left large tissue defects extending to the sacral fascia, which took months to heal. Currently, the favoured surgical treatment is the **Bascom** 'cleft lift' procedure, which may have the secondary advantage of flattening the cleft to minimise recurrence (Fig. 30.12).

Despite surgery, pilonidal lesions commonly recur, although the Bascom procedure is promising in this respect. More recently, there has been interest in minimally invasive endoscopic pilonidal sinus treatment, which appears to have healing rates as high as 85%. Recurrence may also be reduced by careful attention to hygiene. Daily baths and regular shaving of the area are recommended.

Rectal Prolapse

Rectal prolapse is a herniation of the rectum through the pelvic floor, so the mucosa and muscle wall effectively intussuscept through the anal canal (Fig. 30.13). It is mainly seen in the elderly although some presentations with different aetiologies occur in the young.

In childhood, prolapse usually occurs around the age of 2 years. It tends to occur during toilet training and causes parental anxiety. Parents should be reassured that the prolapse will return spontaneously after defaecation or if not, gentle manipulation using water-soluble lubricant jelly may be required. These children should be given a high-fibre diet and taught not to strain during defaecation. More sophisticated treatment is rarely required.

In the elderly, rectal prolapse initially occurs only with defaecation and retracts spontaneously. Sometimes, the patient has to reduce the prolapse manually, often with little complaint. At a later stage, prolapse may occur when the patient merely stands up. This can lead to incontinence because of dilatation of the internal anal sphincter. The patient becomes reluctant to leave home and often becomes socially isolated and is then likely to require surgical treatment.

Management of Rectal Prolapse

Rectal prolapse can be treated by abdominal or perineal procedures, or a combination of both. The **abdominal** operations, which may be performed laparoscopically, include two main types:

• **Suture fixation rectopexy**, where the rectum is mobilised through a laparoscopic approach and the mesorectum sutured to the sacral promontory and presacral fascia.
• **Resection rectopexy**, where the rectum is mobilised and sutured in the same way, but a sigmoid colectomy is also performed to try to prevent the constipation that often accompanies suture fixation alone. This is now rarely required.

The most popular **perineal** procedure is **Delorme operation**, which is appropriate for most elderly patients because of its low morbidity and mortality, although there is a high recurrence rate. It involves excising redundant **rectal mucosa**, plicating the rectal wall and replacing the prolapsed rectum. More radical abdominal procedures or any procedure involving an anastomosis (e.g., Altemeier perineal sigmoidectomy) is usually contraindicated because of greater risk.

Faecal Incontinence (Table 30.1)

The process of maintaining continence is complex, involving higher behavioural control, sensory and motor pathways and the anal sphincter mechanisms. In addition, the rectal reservoir must function effectively. The continence mechanism has evolved to

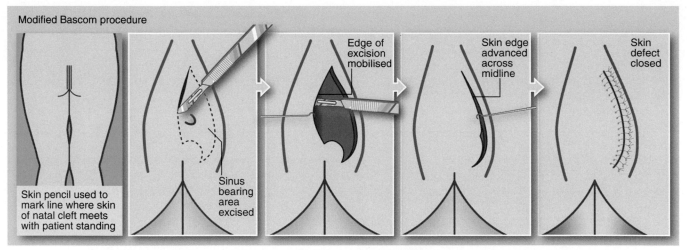

Modified Bascom procedure

Skin pencil used to mark line where skin of natal cleft meets with patient standing

Sinus bearing area excised

Edge of excision mobilised

Skin edge advanced across midline

Skin defect closed

• **Fig. 30.12** Modified Bascom Procedure.

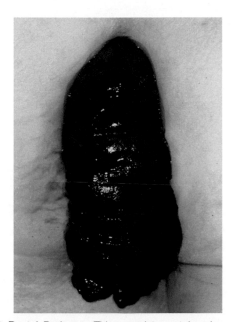

• **Fig. 30.13** Rectal Prolapse. This complete rectal prolapse was in an 80-year-old woman. It emerged spontaneously whenever she stood, causing considerable discomfort and inconvenience, to say the least!

TABLE 30.1	Causes of Faecal Incontinence	
Underlying Problem	**Disorders**	
Anorectal incontinence—pudendal neuropathy (previously known as '*idiopathic faecal incontinence*'), anal sphincter and pelvic floor damage	Obstetric damage, operative damage, radiation damage, rectal prolapse, high anal fistula	
Colorectal disease	Inflammatory bowel disease; polyps and tumours in rectum and anal canal	
Faecal quality	Diarrhoea from any cause including infective; faecal impaction with overflow diarrhoea and incontinence	
Rectal reservoir and sensation	Inflammatory bowel disease	
Brain and higher cerebral functioning	Neurological disorders—dementias, psychological disturbances, impaired consciousness	
Sensorimotor pathways	Spinal injury; neurological disorders	
Mobility and access to toilet	Enforced bed rest or impaired mobility	

cope principally with semisolid faeces and may fail if the stool is fluid. Incontinence presents in varying degrees: first for flatus, then for fluid and finally for solids as control is progressively lost. Declining mobility may also be a factor: mild incontinence that would otherwise be manageable may become a problem, where debility and immobility impair the patient's ability to move to the toilet when required.

Incontinence is socially debilitating. It is surprisingly common but often concealed. It particularly affects some younger parous women and many elderly people. Social embarrassment forces patients to alter their lifestyles, so that they never stray far from a lavatory, using constipating agents like loperamide or simply staying at home all day. Assessment of the severity of incontinence should include enquiring about these coping strategies, as patients or carers may be too embarrassed to volunteer them. Standard rating scales can be used to assess incontinence and compare treatments, for example, the Cleveland Clinic faecal incontinence scale.

Young faecally incontinent patients are mostly female and usually suffer from **anorectal incontinence**. In the elderly, the aetiology is usually multifactorial.

Anorectal Incontinence

The main functional abnormality in anorectal incontinence is weakness of the external anal sphincter and pelvic floor muscles. This is sometimes caused by direct injury from trauma or surgery, but most cases were labelled idiopathic. It is now recognised that the most important cause of sphincter dysfunction in women is obstetric injury. Repeated childbirth, episiotomies or difficult forceps deliveries increase the risk. The mechanism is probably via traumatic **pudendal neuropathy**, leading to atrophy of sphincteric and pelvic floor muscles. Even chronic straining at stool may cause pudendal neuropathy. In old age, degenerative

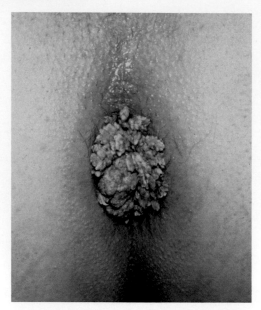

• **Fig. 30.14** Anal Warts (Condylomata Acuminata).

changes in the spinal cord appear to be the principal cause of muscle atrophy.

If sphincters have been physically damaged, surgical sphincter repair may be undertaken but results are not always predictable or long lasting. Continuous sacral nerve stimulation, where an implanted 'pacemaker' promotes increased sphincter tone, has been shown to be effective. As a last resort, a colostomy may allow the patient a better quality of life.

Anal Warts (Condylomata Accuminata)

Warts in the perianal region (Fig. 30.14) have a viral aetiology (human papillomavirus [HPV] types 6 and 11) and are generally transmitted by sexual activity. Just as cervical cancer is linked to specific strains of HPV infection, anal warts indicate an increased risk of anal canal carcinoma by virtue of their common aetiology. Immune suppression, for example in patients with organ transplants or with HIV infection, can lead to rapidly developing anal warts and progression to malignant change.

In small numbers, anal warts can be treated by topical applications of **podophyllin**. When large numbers are present, surgical excision under general anaesthetic is the only practical option. This involves meticulous excision of each individual wart by electrocautery. The normal skin between the warts is carefully preserved to avoid delayed healing or the disastrous complication of anal stenosis. Carefully mapped biopsies can also be undertaken to monitor for dysplastic change. In the future, prevention will come from HPV vaccines in both sexes, shown to prevent papillomavirus-induced cervical cancer, genital warts, and some oral cancers.

Squamous Cell Carcinoma of the Anus

Epidemiology

The annual incidence of anal cancer in women and the general population is about 1:100,000; however, in men who have sex with men and who are HIV negative, the incidence markedly increases to 35:100,000 and it doubles if the men are HIV

positive. The sharp increase of mainly nonkeratinising cancers arising in the transitional zone in these groups is largely caused by heightened rates of infection with HPV and the effects of immunosuppression fostering its progress. An effective vaccine has now been developed for HPV and, if administered in the early teens, should prevent infection and its consequences.

Clinical Features

The symptoms of anal carcinoma are similar to those of haemorrhoids and other familiar benign anal conditions, namely fresh rectal bleeding, anal pain, discomfort and discharge. Later, incontinence can result from involvement of the anal sphincter. The patient may ignore the symptoms for a period and the doctor may initially overlook the diagnosis. On digital rectal examination, a localised firm or hard ulcer or a growth with an irregular surface and edge may be palpable and there may be surrounding woody induration. The lesion is usually visible on proctoscopy and the diagnosis confirmed by biopsy. Palpation of the groins may reveal hard, matted involved inguinal nodes. Anal canal carcinoma also metastasises to intraabdominal superior rectal nodes, reflecting the mixed drainage of the anal canal.

Chemoradiotherapy has now largely superseded abdominoperineal excision because of demonstrably better cure rates for nonsurgical therapy, although abdominoperineal resection of the rectum may be required to salvage residual or recurrent disease.

Other Rare Anal Neoplasms

The anal canal is the third most common site for **malignant melanomas** after skin and the eye. These cause nonspecific anal symptoms of discomfort and bleeding and diagnosis may thus be delayed. These melanomas are usually nonpigmented and biopsy evidence is needed to make a firm diagnosis. Treatment outcomes are poor. **Adenocarcinoma** of the rectum may extend distally into the anal region, and rarely **basal cell carcinomas** may occur here.

Proctalgia Fugax

Proctalgia fugax is a neuropathic type of pain, which often manifests as brief episodes of severe lancinating pain in the perineum with sphincter spasms. It occurs at unpredictable times but often at night. It usually occurs independently of conditions such as anal fissure, complicated piles and anal or rectal neoplasms; the patient may be convinced that cancer is the cause and may suspect that the doctor thinks it is 'all in the mind'. The cause is unknown but is believed not to be psychological. Whilst it is difficult to cure, reassurance and recommending ice packs or warm baths may help. If this fails, therapy with amitriptyline or gabapentin may control symptoms.

Pruritus Ani

Anal itching can be distressing. It is generally caused by mucus leakage and may occur without significant haemorrhoids; even a minute quantity of leaking mucus or faecal material causes profound irritation. Patients generally try to self-medicate with various creams but these tend to increase skin maceration and worsen the problem. Pruritus can be helped greatly if all topical creams are stopped and the perineum is washed and dabbed dry after defaecation using plain water. Even soap can aggravate the symptoms. Good defaecatory habits are encouraged along with fluids and bulking agents.

31

Thoracic Surgery

Introduction

Thoracic surgery traditionally covers the diagnosis and management of all noncardiac disease within the chest. However, the practice varies between countries. For example, in the United Kingdom, unlike North America, most oesophageal disease is now managed by gastroenterologists and upper gastrointestinal (GI) surgeons rather than thoracic surgeons. This chapter will review the management of benign and malignant conditions of the chest and mediastinal disorders that are commonly managed by UK thoracic surgeons. The principles of oesophageal surgery are covered separately in Chapter 22 and chest trauma in Chapter 15.

Investigative Techniques

Imaging

Chest x-ray, computed tomography (CT), magnetic resonance imaging (MRI), ultrasound (US) and synchronised CT-positron emission tomography (CT-PET) are the most commonly used modalities. Chest x-ray is useful as a baseline and also for early

postprocedure follow-up. Contrast enhanced CT of the chest and upper abdomen provides the best anatomical information and is used for both preoperative planning and follow up. Low radiation-dose protocols are being used successfully in some lung cancer screening projects and there is some evidence suggesting that screening certain groups may lead to longer survival and this may become common practice. CT-PET can be used to identify potential spread to local lymph nodes, as well as distant metastases outside the chest. MRI is most useful to study soft tissues, and in malignancy, in particular, to determine the extent of chest wall and diaphragm invasion, spinal invasion and for distant spread to the liver or brain. US is useful to guide drainage of collections, siting of chest-drains and for guiding biopsy of superficial or pleural-based lesions. In some cases, before placing a nonemergency chest drain, US or CT scanning is performed to minimise the risk of complications.

Lung Function Tests

Lung function tests give a detailed portrait of the physiological effects of individual chest diseases, and can track changes over time or as a result of treatment. When surgery is contemplated, lung function tests help assess the patient's capacity. Tests include:
- Measurement of **air flow** into and out of the alveoli, that is, forced expiratory volume in 1 second, forced vital capacity, peak air flow, total lung capacity, alveolar ventilation.
- Measurement of **gas diffusion** across the alveolar–capillary interface, usually involving measuring rates of carbon monoxide diffusion.
- Assessing the amount of dead space by calculating the **residual volume** and **total lung capacity.**
- Assessing exercise capacity, for example, by the 6-minute walk test or by formal cardiopulmonary exercise testing.
- Baseline arterial or capillary blood gases.

Bronchoscopy

Flexible bronchoscopy can be performed with topical local anaesthesia and minimal or no sedation. It is possible to examine down to segmental bronchi, obtain small biopsies and clear secretions.

For cancer staging, transbronchial US (endobronchial US, EBUS) allows biopsy of lymph nodes close to the airway to the level of the lobar bronchi. This can be combined with transoesophageal US (EUS) to allow more lymph node stations and the left adrenal gland to be biopsied.

Rigid bronchoscopy is performed under general anaesthesia and allows passage of larger instruments, including a flexible bronchoscope, for removal of foreign bodies, obtaining large biopsies, opening of the airway and control of bleeding.

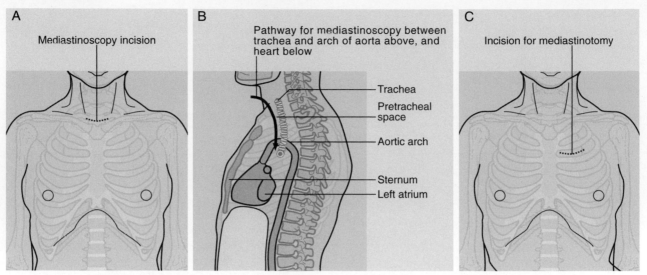

• **Fig. 31.1** Mediastinoscopy and Mediastinotomy. (A) and (B) Mediastinoscopy for investigation of the posterior mediastinum. (C) Mediastinotomy.

Pleural Aspiration and Percutaneous Biopsy

Aspiration of pleural effusions for cytological examination can be performed using a standard wide-bore needle and syringe. Blind pleural biopsy is now discouraged because of its relatively low yield and high complication rate. Many thoracic masses are amenable to percutaneous biopsy under US or CT guidance, although thoracoscopy or direct surgical cut-down to the lesion (or a procedure that combines both) has the best yield.

Video-Mediastinoscopy

A mediastinoscope is used to biopsy paratracheal and subcarinal lymph nodes. The instrument is a rigid tube incorporating fibreoptic light guides; it is inserted via a skin incision above the suprasternal notch and passed caudally along the plane of the pretracheal fascia (Fig. 31.1A and B). The route passes close to the azygos vein, superior vena cava, innominate artery, arch of the aorta, pulmonary artery and the recurrent laryngeal nerves posterolaterally on each side. These structures and the oesophagus are at risk of damage and, although rare, this must be explained to the patient. Mediastinoscopy gives access to the mediastinum except for the subaortic fossa (below the aortic arch and often containing lymph nodes). Access to this area is obtained by anterior mediastinotomy or video-assisted thoracic surgery.

The number of mediastinoscopies has fallen because of the yield from CT-PET scanning and Endoscopic US (EBUS and EUS).

Thoracoscopy

This is more commonly known as **video-assisted thoracoscopic surgery** or **VATS**. It is usually performed under general anaesthesia but basic procedures may use local anaesthesia with sedation. In addition, some units perform VATS under deep sedation with spontaneous ventilation, even for major resections. Instruments for viewing and operating are inserted through small incisions in the chest wall.

Thoracoscopy is the preferred technique for pleural biopsy, pneumothorax treatment and evacuation of early empyema and is

also used to sample mediastinal lymph nodes and perform cervical (thoracodorsal) sympathectomy. In the United Kingdom, VATS is also becoming increasingly common for a range of more complex procedures, for example, lobectomy. In some units, the rate of VATS lobectomy is more than 60% overall and >90% for stage 1 lung cancer.

VATS procedures may be performed via a multiportal or uniportal approach. In both, there is a nonrib-spreading 'utility' incision of about 2 to 8 cm. In the uniportal approach, all instruments and the camera are passed through the single utility port and this incision can also be used for the drain at the end of the procedure. In the multiportal approach, one to three further port incisions are made for a video-telescope and surgical instruments. In this approach, drains can be placed in suitable ports. Any resected specimen is placed in an extraction bag so it can be removed intact via the utility incision. The position of the ports depends on the procedure being performed and surgeon preference. The most performed VATS is via lateral chest wall incisions but a subxiphoid incision is used by some surgeons for selected procedures, for example, thymectomy, lung volume reduction surgery or lobectomy.

Anterior Mediastinotomy

Anterior mediastinotomy (see Fig. 31.1C), a form of minithoracotomy, may be used to obtain biopsies from anterior mediastinal lesions, for example, thymic tumours. The approach can be left or right of the sternum, either intercostally or with costal cartilage resection. Left anterior mediastinotomy affords good access for biopsy of subaortic fossa masses. VATS is increasingly replacing anterior mediastinotomy as the preferred method of accessing these sites.

Thoracotomy

Thoracotomy, described later, gives full access to the paratracheal, subcarinal and hilar lymph node groups, the great vessels, oesophagus, lung and pericardium and is used when less invasive procedures are inappropriate or have failed.

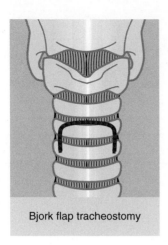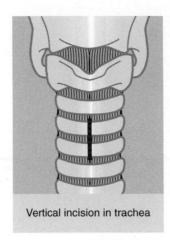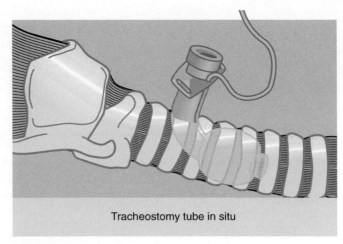

Bjork flap tracheostomy	Vertical incision in trachea	Tracheostomy tube in situ

• **Fig. 31.2** Tracheostomy Placement.

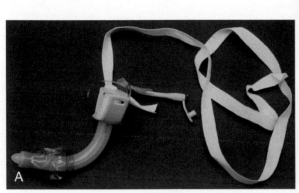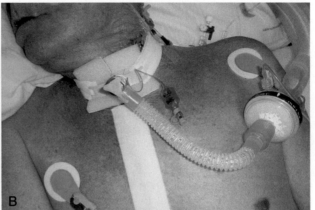

• **Fig. 31.3** Tracheostomy. (A) Disposable tracheostomy tube. Note the distal balloon, which is inflated via the small tube to provide a snug fit inside the trachea. (B) Patient being ventilated via an elective tracheostomy after cardiac surgery.

Therapeutic Procedures

Tracheostomy

Principles of Tracheostomy

A tracheostomy (Figs 31.2 and 31.3) is an artificial opening into the trachea to provide a secure airway when the pharyngeal airway or larynx needs to be bypassed. With time, an epithelialised fistula develops between the skin and trachea, which allows tracheostomy tubes to be changed and the airways cleaned with ease. In many units 'percutaneous tracheostomy' is performed using a 'Seldinger-type' technique. However, the technique of 'open' tracheostomy should be familiar to most surgeons.

Indications for tracheostomy include:
- Permanent functional obstruction of the upper airway, for example, carcinoma of larynx.
- Temporary or potential upper airway obstruction, for example, facial fractures, major head and neck operations or injuries.
- Long-term ventilatory support, when prolonged endotracheal intubation would otherwise be likely to cause permanent significant tracheal damage. Tracheostomy also provides continuous access to the lower airways for bronchial aspiration and toilet.

Tracheostomy should be a planned procedure performed in the operating room under general anaesthesia. It is *not* an emergency procedure for patients with upper airway obstruction. For these, endotracheal intubation or cricothyroidotomy (Fig. 31.4) should be used.

Complications of Tracheostomy

- **Haemorrhage** caused by erosion of the innominate (brachiocephalic) artery or vein
- **Tracheooesophageal fistula**
- **Displacement of the tracheostomy tube** may occur before the desired 'fistula' becomes established, making it difficult to reintubate the trachea
- **Tracheal stenosis**, usually the result of prolonged use of a high-pressure cuff causing pressure necrosis and then scarring and narrowing of the trachea (now rare because of the introduction of low-pressure cuffs)

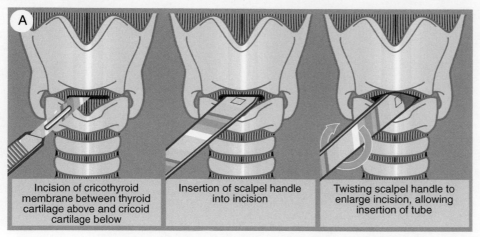

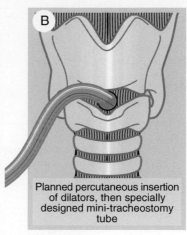

• **Fig. 31.4** Cricothyroidotomy. (A) In a dire emergency, this life-saving procedure can be rapidly used to gain time. (B) Modern mini-cricothyroidotomy can be performed percutaneously by making a small incision through the cricothyroid membrane and progressively dilating it with graduated dilators before insertion of a specially constructed small-diameter tube, for example, Minitrach or Quicktrach. These are used in accident victims and often in intensive care units.

Thoracotomy

Most thoracotomies are now devised to spare at least some muscles from being divided.

Posterolateral Thoracotomy

Posterolateral thoracotomy is the traditional approach for lung and oesophageal resections. as well as for surgery of the descending aorta (left side). In general, a curved incision passes below the inferior angle of the scapula, latissimus dorsi is divided and the chest is entered through the fourth to sixth intercostal space. If necessary, the incision can be extended into the abdomen (thoracoabdominal incision), for example, for oesophagogastrectomy or thoracoabdominal aortic aneurysm. With smaller incisions, latissimus dorsi and serratus anterior may be spared.

Lateral Thoracotomy

Lateral thoracotomy involves an incision extending between anterior and posterior axillary lines. In some cases, it is possible to spare both latissimus dorsi and serratus anterior from being divided.

Anterolateral Thoracotomy

This approach is becoming increasingly common for open lung resections. It provides good access to the hilum. Latissimus dorsi is spared but the serratus anterior muscle is often divided. The skin incision extends anteriorly from the anterior axillary line towards the lateral border of the sternum. The division of the intercostal muscles and parietal pleura can be extended posteriorly towards the spine to allow greater retraction without rib division.

Anterior Thoracotomy

This can be used for diagnostic biopsy or pericardial window. It can also be used for lung transplantation and emergency resuscitative thoracotomy (for cardiac massage).

Median Sternotomy

Median sternotomy gives wide access to the heart and the entire anterior mediastinum, including the great vessels. It is the standard incision for cardiac surgery, as well as for open excision of thymic lesions and large retrosternal parathyroid tumours and, occasionally, resection of a goitre with substantial retrosternal extension.

Specific Thoracic Disorders

Problems Affecting the Pleural Space

Introduction

The pleural cavity is a potential space between the chest wall and lung, lined by a continuous sheet of mesothelium. The lining of the chest wall is the **parietal pleura** and that covering the lung is the **visceral pleura**. The pleural space normally contains a minute amount of serous fluid causing it to adhere by surface tension. This, and the negative pressure arising from the tendency of the chest wall to expand, keeps the lungs expanded. Disease or injury may result in accumulation of air (**pneumothorax**) or liquid (**effusion**) in the pleural cavity. Pleural effusions are classified as transudates or exudates. Fluid collections can be subdivided into pus (empyema), blood (haemothorax), chyle (chylothorax) and, rarely, lymph (lymphothorax).

The pleural space is not essential to life, and a principle of managing pleural problems is often to eliminate this space. This is achieved by draining the space, ensuring the lung abuts the chest wall, and stimulating the lung to adhere to it. This is known as **pleurodesis**. Pleural adhesions may occur spontaneously or following episodes of infection/inflammation or postsurgery.

Pneumothorax

Pneumothorax is classified as primary or secondary. Primary refers to 'spontaneous' pneumothorax, occurring without obvious lung disease. It is most common in people between the ages of 15 and 30 years, and is characteristically (but not exclusively) seen in tall, thin males. Secondary pneumothorax occurs in patients with other lung disease, most often chronic obstructive pulmonary disease (COPD). It is most common after 50 years of age in patients with a smoking history but can occur in a range of conditions, including *Pneumocystis* pneumonia and collagen disorders.

Primary or 'spontaneous' pneumothorax most often results from rupture of a 'bleb' on the pleural surface of the lung. A bleb is a subpleural small air-filled cavity that communicates with lung parenchyma. Rupture allows air to escape into the pleural space and the lung collapses. **Traumatic pneumothorax** usually results

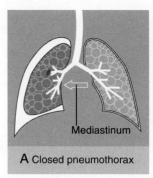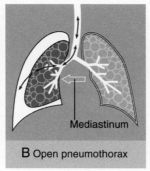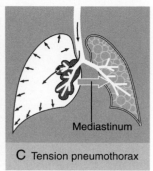

• **Fig. 31.5** Classification of Pneumothorax. (A) In closed pneumothorax, the pleural defect closes spontaneously, leaving a fixed amount of air in the pleural space. (B) In open pneumothorax, there is free passage of air via an open defect in the visceral pleura. (C) In tension pneumothorax, the pleural defect acts as a flap valve allowing progressive entry of air into the pleural space, collapsing the lung and pushing the mediastinum to the opposite side.

from blunt chest injury, often from rib fractures penetrating visceral pleura. Penetrating chest injury, such as stab wounds, may also be responsible. Different types of pneumothorax are illustrated in Fig. 31.5. An open pneumothorax is one in which the chest wall is breached and air can come in and out of the chest through it. A tension pneumothorax can complicate a closed or open pneumothorax. It occurs when the pressure outside the lung in the chest increases to that above the venous pressure. This impedes venous return, leading to a fall in cardiac output and respiratory distress. The mediastinum also shifts away from the side of the pneumothorax. Untreated, it can be rapidly fatal.

Sometimes, after trauma, if the site of air leakage acts as a one-way valve, a **tension pneumothorax** is created and this is an emergency.

Treatment of a pneumothorax is required under the following circumstances:

- where there is a tension pneumothorax;
- when the lung volume is compromised by more than about 25% as calculated on a postero-anterior (PA) chest x-ray;
- if the pneumothorax is increasing;
- when a small pneumothorax is having a disproportionate effect on lung function because of preexisting lung disease.

Treatment of Pneumothorax

Aspiration. An uncomplicated pneumothorax in an otherwise fit patient can be treated by aspiration. A 50-ml syringe is connected to a three-way tap or one-way valve and a needle. The needle is inserted intercostally into the pneumothorax and air aspirated or allowed to blow out. Progress is later monitored by chest x-ray. The process can be repeated, but formal tube drainage may be needed if the pneumothorax recurs.

In **tension pneumothorax**, rapid emergency relief can be obtained by passing a large needle into the pleural space. A relatively safe point is just lateral to the midclavicular line in the second intercostal space although newer trauma guidelines advise just anterior to the midaxillary line, 5th intercostal space. A formal chest drain should be inserted soon afterwards.

Intercostal Tube Drainage. The technique of intercostal chest drainage is described in Fig. 31.6; see also Fig. 31.7. If a pneumothorax needs a drain, a single small apical drain is used, for example, 16 F gauge. Smaller drains are used by nonsurgeons but these have a high failure rate because of kinking and blockage.

Any intercostal tube drain must be connected to an apparatus to prevent lung collapse from air being drawn into the chest, by negative intrapleural pressure. The traditional arrangement is to connect the chest drain to a rigid tube, secured below the water level in a bottle, to form an **underwater seal**. This allows air and fluid to leave the chest cavity but not return. The bottle is kept below patient level so gravity assists. As the patient breathes, excess pleural air and liquid are gradually expelled into the bottle. If there is a lung air leak via a breach in the visceral pleura, this is manifest by continued bubbling in the bottle and failure of the lung to expand. Continuous suction may then be applied to the underwater seal outlet for a few days; this usually helps the lung to expand and adhere to the chest wall, thereby remaining inflated and blocking the air leak. Newer, digital, drainage systems have a valve rather than an underwater seal. They are self-contained units, which can apply suction directly from the drain box and so allow greater mobility for the patient. They can also provide a measurement of air flow (in ml/min) as well as liquid drainage volumes.

Patients with underwater seal intercostal drains must be transported with care to ensure the drainage bottle does not tip over, and always remains below patient level, to prevent fluid reflux into the chest. This is not required with newer drainage systems. It is no longer recommended that chest tubes be clamped when patients are moved, as this is potentially dangerous (an exception to this is after pneumonectomy).

Intercostal drains are removed when the lung is fully expanded. For pneumothorax, cessation of bubbling in the bottle for 24 hours is an indication for removal; for liquid drainage, the duration varies with the underlying problem.

Treatment of Persistent or Recurrent Pneumothorax

More extensive surgical intervention may be required for persistent or recurrent pneumothorax. The general rule is that surgery is offered for an unresolving pneumothorax, two pneumothoraces on the same side or one on each side. Patients in high-risk occupations, such as pilots, must be offered surgery after a single pneumothorax. Approaches include stapling of bullae to prevent air leakage and pleural abrasion or pleurectomy. In patients with fragile lungs, as in secondary pneumothorax, lung resection is sometimes avoided by insufflating sterile surgical talc to encourage a chemical pleurodesis (Fig. 31.8). Most of this surgery is now performed by VATS.

Excess Pleural Fluid

Excess pleural fluid may be a watery transudate (e.g., in heart failure) or an exudate of variable viscosity (e.g., because of pleural infection).

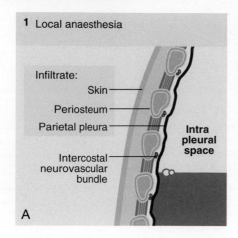

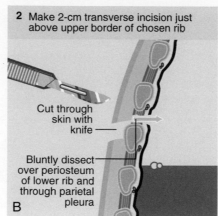

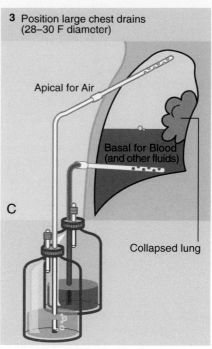

- **Fig. 31.6** Technique of Intercostal Tube Drainage of Chest (Tube Thoracostomy).
- Inject local anaesthetics to block sensitive structures and intercostal nerve and give time for this to take effect.
- Make 2-cm incision near upper border of rib and parallel to it.
- Bluntly dissect intercostal muscles down to parietal pleura with artery forceps. Stay near upper border of rib to avoid intercostal vessels.
- Palpate lung with gloved index finger to free adhesions and ensure free entry for the drain
- Remove trocar from large-bore chest drain tube (at least 28 F gauge); 16 F can be used for pneumothorax alone. Grasp distal end with artery forceps and guide drain into chest in an apical or a basal direction according to purpose. Never insert a chest drain with the trocar in position as this is highly dangerous.
- Attach drain to an underwater seal and suture drain to chest wall. Snug the skin around the drain with a purse string suture. Apply airtight dressing around the tube and tape tube to chest wall. Sit patient up to 45 degrees.
- Take a chest x-ray to confirm position of tube.

Indications for draining a pleural effusion include:
- **Diagnostic**
  - o empyema
  - o suspected malignancy
  - o traumatic haemothorax
- **Therapeutic**
  - o removing the compressive effects of a large pleural fluid collection on the lung
  - o draining pus from an empyema
  - o arresting haemorrhage from damaged intercostal vessels causing haemothorax

Uncomplicated pleural effusions are usually drained via a large-bore tube (28 F gauge or larger) inserted towards the base of the pleural cavity in the most practical dependent position. If fluid collections are loculated, more than one drain may be required.

Malignant Effusions
Malignant effusions (e.g., from breast cancer) usually recur after simple drainage and need to be treated in other ways including:
- Stimulating **adhesion formation** between visceral and parietal pleura (**pleurodesis**). This can be achieved by aspirating the fluid, insufflating an irritant, such as sterile talc and maintaining tube drainage until permanent adhesions develop.

- **Parietal pleurectomy.** Traditionally performed by thoracotomy but now usually by VATS, this involves stripping the parietal pleura to cause diffuse adhesion of the lung surface to the chest wall (see Fig. 31.8B).
- **Pleuroperitoneal shunting** using a tubular device connecting the two cavities. This is implanted beneath the skin and incorporates a one-way valve. Excess pleural fluid is manually 'pumped' from the pleura into the peritoneum by the patient several times a day, where it is resorbed. Unfortunately, the pumping can be uncomfortable and devices can become blocked so this is rarely performed.
- **Tunnelled intrapleural catheter.** A small catheter is tunnelled a few centimetres from the skin to the pleural space and can be opened to intermittently drain the pleural space. The catheter can be inserted under local anaesthesia. Tunnelling reduces the infection risk. The persistent drainage encourages pleural apposition and eventually pleurodesis.

Empyema
When pleural fluid becomes infected, pus accumulates in the pleural cavity and becomes known as an **empyema**. Early on, this can be treated by dependent intercostal tube drainage with irrigation if necessary. Some empyemas respond to treatment with fibrinolytics. In chronic cases, a thick fibrous wall or **cortex** gradually

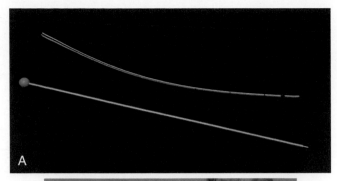

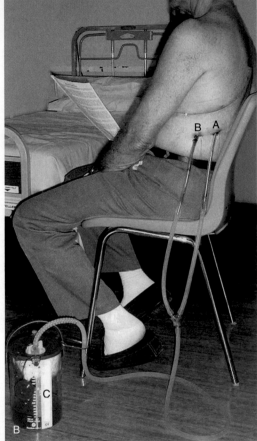

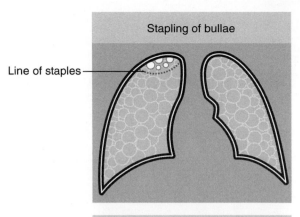

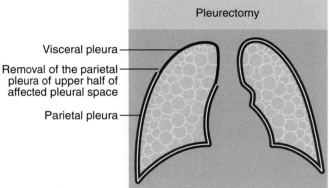

• **Fig. 31.8** Surgical Approaches for Treatment of Persistent Pneumothorax.

• **Fig. 31.7** Chest Drain. **(A)** 30 F gauge tube (10 mm) with stylet removed (and thrown away!). Note the radiopaque line and the side holes near the tip. **(B)** Postthoracotomy and lobar resection of lung for cancer. This patient has two chest drains in situ, *(A)* an **A**pical drain for **A**ir and *(B)* a **B**asal drain for **B**lood. Both are connected to an underwater seal, *(C)*, to prevent inflow of air that would cause a pneumothorax.

forms around the pus-filled space. Treatment options then include prolonged closed tube drainage, open tube drainage (sometimes involving removing a small segment of rib), and surgical 'decortication' (Figs 31.9 and 31.10), which releases entrapped lung and tethered chest wall and diaphragm, allowing the lung to reexpand.

Haemothorax

Following chest trauma, blood can accumulate in the pleural space. This usually needs draining via a large bore drain. A similar strategy is used after open chest surgery. Traditionally, two wide-bore drains are placed, although many surgeons now place only a single posteroapical drain (sometimes with extra basal holes). If there is particular concern about bleeding, then two drains may be placed.

Clotted blood does not drain well and usually needs evacuation by VATS or thoracotomy. Removing blood allows the lung to expand against the chest wall, and this helps to arrest continuing haemorrhage from intercostal vessels. Persistent or increasing drainage of blood indicates continuing intrathoracic bleeding and requires intervention. Continued bleeding is usually from the systemic circulation (e.g., internal mammary, intercostal or great vessels) rather than from lung parenchyma.

Lung Abscess

Lung abscesses have become much less common with effective antibiotic treatment of pulmonary infections. Onset of symptoms may be insidious, with clinical features including a swinging pyrexia, foul-smelling sputum and a cavitating shadow on chest x-ray. Primary lung abscess may follow bacterial lung infection, most commonly with *Staphylococcus aureus, Streptococcus, Pseudomonas* or *Klebsiella*.

Secondary lung abscess may follow aspiration of GI contents or occur in lung segments distal to bronchial obstruction, by a centrally placed neoplasm or inhaled foreign body.

Lung abscesses are usually treated with antibiotics alone but occasionally a cavity requires drainage. Drains are usually placed percutaneously under US or CT guidance. Surgery by deroofing ('marsupialisation') or resection of the abscess may be required. Good chest drainage is vital after the procedure.

Cancer of the Lung

Cancers in the lung are either primary or metastatic deposits from elsewhere. Smoking is the commonest cause of primary lung

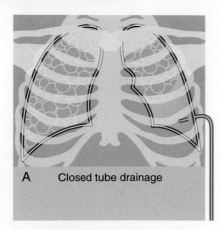

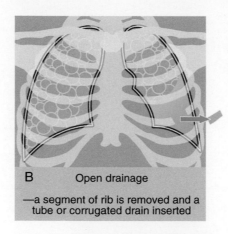

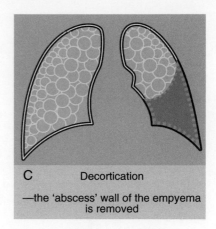

| A | Closed tube drainage | B | Open drainage | C | Decortication |

B —a segment of rib is removed and a tube or corrugated drain inserted

C —the 'abscess' wall of the empyema is removed

• **Fig. 31.9** Treatment of Empyema Thoracis.

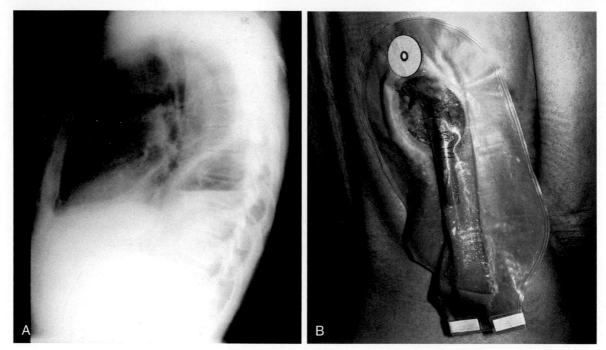

• **Fig. 31.10** Empyema Thoracis. This 51-year-old man underwent a thoracoabdominal oesophagogastrectomy for proximal gastric cancer. He suffered a small intrathoracic anastomotic leak and developed an intrapleural empyema, shown by the fluid level in (A). (B) Drainage of empyema. A section of rib overlying the cavity was resected, and a large red rubber tube was inserted to give dependent drainage into a bag. The drain was gradually shortened as the cavity closed. This patient was alive and well 15 years later.

cancer. Owing to smoking controls, rates of lung cancer are starting to plateau in developed countries but continue to increase elsewhere, usually in line with the number of cigarettes smoked. Many primary tumours will have metastasised by the time of presentation to locoregional lymph nodes, as well as to distant sites, such as the liver, adrenal glands, bone and brain.

Primary lung cancers are classified into **small cell tumours** (10%–15%) and **non-small cell lung cancers** (NSCLC). Early stage small cell lung cancer can be resected in suitable patients but they will still require chemotherapy because of the very high risk of metastases. Most small cell cancers are treated nonsurgically, as they have metastasised by the time of diagnosis. Small cell lung cancers are generally more responsive to chemoradiotherapy than NSCLC.

Non-small cell cancers are further subdivided: the two commonest types are squamous cell cancer and adenocarcinoma, but there are other less common histological subtypes. Many lung cancers grow rapidly, so assessment must not be delayed, if curative treatment with surgery or chemo-/radiotherapy is envisaged. Neuroendocrine tumours of the lung also occur, covering a spectrum from **typical carcinoid** (often slow growing with minimal chance of metastases), to atypical carcinoid and large cell neuroendocrine tumours, the latter of which are closer in behaviour to small cell lung cancer. They are still usually removed by surgery.

Once a lung cancer is suspected it should be promptly diagnosed and staged and sometimes the same test provides diagnostic and staging information.

Diagnosis

This rests on obtaining tissue for cytological or histological examination. This is generally obtained by bronchoscopic biopsy or brushings, EBUS/EUS aspiration or CT-guided biopsy.

For a primary lung cancer, staging is normally done after contrast enhanced CT of chest and upper abdomen, CT-PET and head scan but these can be omitted in selected cases.

Staging of Lung Cancer and Its Implications

Tumour/node/metastasis (TNM) staging of lung cancer is fundamental to planning appropriate treatment. This is periodically reviewed and the most recent classification (the eighth version) became applicable in 2018. It is highly detailed and technical and not easily simplified to illustrate here. In staging, contrast-enhanced CT scanning of chest and upper abdomen is usually the first step. The likelihood of enlarged lymph nodes being malignant increases with size. The order of further tests varies with local practice but generally includes a CT-PET scan, brain imaging with CT or MRI and evaluation of enlarged or PET-positive sites by biopsy/EBUS/EUS. If histological confirmation has not been achieved by biopsy of a suspicious node, the primary site may need biopsy.

If the lung cancer is confirmed to be 'early', that is, stage I or II and selected patients with IIIa disease, fit patients are offered surgery. Stage 1a NSCLC can have a 5-year survival of >90%, but very few patients present this early.

If preoperative staging of mediastinal lymph nodes is negative but N_2 disease is discovered at surgery (i.e., occult N_2 disease), around 50% can undergo a histologically complete resection; this subgroup would expect a 5-year survival of about 30%.

Some patients with more advanced disease are also offered surgery, including patients with limited mediastinal node involvement, and very occasionally patients with a removable isolated distant metastasis.

Palliative Treatment

Patients whose disease is too extensive for surgery can be offered radiotherapy with curative intent, usually accompanied by chemotherapy, provided the tumour and lymph nodes can be encompassed within a radiotherapy field with acceptable toxicity. For advanced disease, radiotherapy can provide effective palliation, with increased life expectancy, as well as treatment for troublesome complications, such as lobar collapse, haemoptysis, superior vena caval obstruction or symptomatic metastases in brain or bone. Modern radiotherapy techniques, such as stereotactic radiotherapy, are becoming available and can be used with radical intent in patients unfit for surgical resection.

Chemotherapy adds around 5% on average to postsurgery 5-year survivals and can be offered to appropriate patients, particularly those found to have node-positive disease on postresection histological analysis, or patients with tumours larger than 4 cm (even without positive nodes).

New molecular therapies have been introduced and can have benefits. For example, patients with certain epidermal growth factor receptor mutations respond very well to modulator drugs of those pathways. Immunotherapy also shows promise and will doubtless become more important as methods improve.

Surgical Treatment of Lung Cancer

The role of surgery varies according to cell-type, known responsiveness to other therapies, respiratory function, age and fitness of the patient for major surgery. Surgery is usually reserved for potentially curable ('operable') patients. Surgery involves wide resection of the primary with sampling of locoregional (mediastinal) lymph nodes to establish accurate pathological TNM staging; this influences whether to offer adjuvant chemotherapy or radiotherapy.

Surgical resection involves removing one or more affected lung lobes (**lobectomy**) or the whole lung (**pneumonectomy**), sometimes with resection of involved chest wall. In patients with impaired lung function, sublobar resection (**segmentectomy** or nonanatomical 'wedge' resection) may be justified with the aim of preserving lung function. In patients with synchronous primary lung cancers, sequential segmentectomies/wedge resections may be offered (with a recovery period between operations).

The traditional surgical approach is posterolateral thoracotomy, although VATS is becoming increasingly common. The right lung has upper, middle and lower lobes, the left has upper and lower lobes. The empty thoracic space left by resection is soon taken up by hyperinflation of the remaining lung tissue, mediastinal shift, and elevation of the hemidiaphragm.

After pneumonectomy, there is a space, which may become partially or sometimes fully occupied by mediastinal shift, fibrosis and reduced dimensions of that side of the chest.

Nonmalignant Indications for Lung Resection

- **Trauma**—major sharp injury to a lobe or lung, or blunt trauma, where a bronchus has been ruptured.
- **Infection**—consequences of infection, including bleeding caused by bronchiectasis or secondary fungal infection of a persistent, antibiotic 'sterilised' abscess cavity.
- **Benign tumours**—if curative excision via bronchotomy is impracticable.
- **Lung transplantation**—transplantation of a single lung is sometimes performed for nonmalignant disease when there is minimal respiratory reserve and one lung is substantially more affected than the other. Bilateral lung transplantation is performed in patients with lung diseases involving infection, for example, cystic fibrosis or bronchiectasis. Heart–lung transplantation is offered when both lungs and heart are irreparably damaged, for example, Eisenmenger syndrome (see Ch. 14).

Lung Volume Reduction Surgery

In severe emphysema, the considerable destruction of lung tissue actually causes hyperinflation of the lung. This pushes the diaphragm down, stretching it. Increasing intrathoracic volume to lower pressure needed for inspiration becomes difficult. Also in COPD, the lung has less compliance and does not deflate easily, so the work of breathing goes up and the patient experiences progressive breathlessness. In lung volume reduction surgery, the most affected parts of the lung are resected. This allows the diaphragm to take up a more physiological position, work of breathing is reduced and the patient is less breathless. In selected patients, this gives better survival and a range of other health improvements, such as increased exercise capacity, weight gain and improved quality of life measures.

Malignant Mesothelioma

This is a malignant proliferation of mesothelial cells and can arise in pleura (or less commonly in peritoneum). There is usually extensive local spread, restriction of the lung and pleural effusion. Spread is usually late and can be to local lymph nodes and eventually more distantly. There are three main histological forms

Anterior mediastinum (between sternum and pericardium)	Middle mediastinum (pericardium and its contents and lymph nodes)	Posterior mediastinum (posterior to pericardium)
• Retrosternal thyroid • Parathyroid hypertrophy or tumour • Thymoma • Lymph node enlargement • Aneurysm of ascending aorta • Hernia through foramen of Morgagni • Germ cell tumour (seminoma/teratoma)	• Lymph node enlargement • Mediastinal cysts	• Neurogenic tumours • Aneurysm of descending aorta • Hiatus hernia • Congenital hernia through foramen of Bochdalek

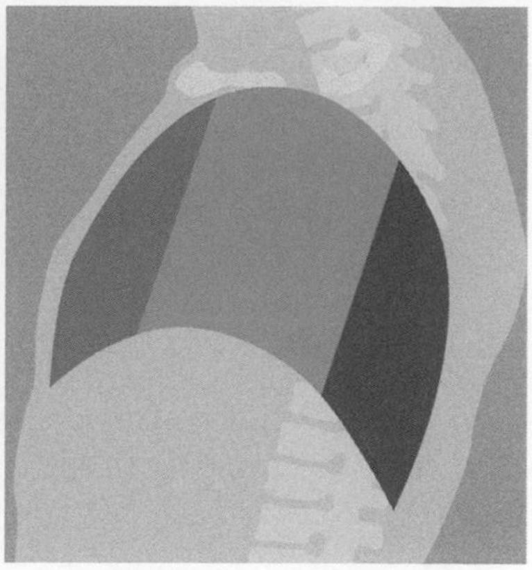

• **Fig. 31.11** Disorders of the Mediastinum.

somewhat correlated with disease behaviour: **epithelioid**, which is the least aggressive, **biphasic** or mixed (histologically a mixture of epithelioid and sarcomatoid types), and **sarcomatoid**, which is the most aggressive.

Malignant mesothelioma is strongly associated with **asbestos** exposure, either direct, as in a building industry worker, or indirect, such as from a family member. There is generally a long interval between exposure and development of the disease (20–40+ years). The carcinogenic agent is the blue asbestos fibre that provokes chronic inflammation that may eventually become malignant. Asbestos exposure is also associated with increased rates of lung cancer. Mesothelioma is likely to peak around 2020 in developed countries, because of the elimination of asbestos from buildings, but is still rising in other parts of the world. Unfortunately, asbestos is still widely used in less developed countries.

In some countries, such as in the United Kingdom, mesothelioma is considered an occupational disease and financial support is available from the government or other bodies.

Presentation of Malignant Mesothelioma

This usually presents with chest pain caused by irritation of intercostal nerves, or shortness of breath caused by loss of lung volume from the tumour, the pleural effusion or both.

Investigation

A chest x-ray is usually followed by a CT scan. A tissue diagnosis can then be obtained by percutaneous radiologically guided biopsy or thoracoscopy.

Treatment

Mesothelioma is rarely curable. Occasionally, a localised malignant mesothelioma can undergo complete resection with hope of cure, but the more usual aim of surgery is maximum debulking ('cytoreduction') in advance of adjuvant therapy, or pure palliation.

Extrapleural pneumonectomy (EPP) involves removing pleura, lung, usually pericardium, and diaphragm, which then requires reconstruction. The Mesothelioma and Radical Surgery (MARS) trial showed that EPP is potentially more detrimental than chemotherapy and so EPP is rarely performed. Extended pleural decortication (EPD) involves removal of the pleura and lung cortex to allow lung reexpansion but without resection of the lung itself. Depending on the extent of the disease, the diaphragm and/or pericardium may also be resected and replaced with patches. Currently, the MARS2 trial is evaluating EPD and

chemotherapy versus chemotherapy alone. In specialist centres, approximately 5% to 10% 5-year post-EPD survival can be expected.

Palliative procedures include thoracoscopic pleurectomy (rarely performed), simple talc pleurodesis, pleuroperitoneal shunts and insertion of tunnelled intrapleural catheters.

Cisplatin (or carboplatin is the current, standard first-line chemotherapy regime for mesothelioma. Newer immunotherapy agents are being trialled as adjuncts to conventional chemotherapy. The place of radiotherapy is also controversial. 'Port-site' radiotherapy has been used to reduce the growth of mesothelioma through previous incisions, and high-dose hemithoracic radiotherapy to the operated side has previously been used after pneumonectomy with the aim of reducing recurrence.

Benign Asbestos Diseases of the Chest

Asbestos exposure may be associated with pleural effusions, pleural plaques, 'infolded lung' and lung fibrosis. These are not of themselves premalignant, but are markers of exposure. They may cause major problems, culminating in respiratory failure.

Disorders of the Mediastinum

Disorders of the mediastinum of surgical importance are summarised in Fig. 31.11.

Anterior Mediastinum

Retrosternal Thyroid

Rarely, the thyroid gland is wholly ectopically located in the anterior mediastinum, where it can become enlarged by any of the processes discussed in Chapter 49. Sometimes, an inferior extension of a normally located thyroid gland may spread retrosternally into the anterior mediastinum. The adverse effects of retrosternal thyroid enlargement are usually related to progressive displacement of the trachea. Sudden enlargement of retrosternal thyroid tissue caused by haemorrhage into it can threaten the airway. Most retrosternal thyroids can be removed through a standard thyroidectomy collar incision and only rarely is a median sternotomy or thoracotomy required.

Thymus

The thymus causes few pathological problems except for uncommon benign or malignant tumours. For benign thymomas or low-grade cancers, surgery alone may be sufficient and 5-year survival can be as good as 70% or better following complete resection.

Thymic cancers are also often sensitive to chemotherapy and radiotherapy and large, aggressive or invasive thymic cancers may benefit from neoadjuvant or adjuvant treatment.

Myasthenia gravis is an unusual clinical condition associated with certain thymic tumours or thymic hyperplasia. After thymectomy, some patients with myasthenia gravis improve, but this is unpredictable.

Parathyroid

Benign and malignant parathyroid tumours usually occur in the neck, but sometimes occur anywhere between the retrothyroid area and the aortic arch. If retrosternal lesions are suspected, exploration of the anterior mediastinum accompanied by thymectomy usually enables the abnormal parathyroid tissue to be removed. Modern methods of localisation and intraoperative parathormone levels to check removal are usually used.

Lymph Node Enlargement

Lymphoma can occur here and good quality biopsies are needed for diagnosis. The usual treatment is chemotherapy with or without radiotherapy.

Germ Cell Tumours

The anterior mediastinum is a relatively common site for these uncommon tumours. These tumours can be approached surgically by sternotomy, a collar incision or VATS.

Middle Mediastinum

This contains the pericardium and hila of both lungs. Disorders requiring surgical intervention include:

- Lymph node enlargement—lung cancer or lymphoma are the most common causes. Tumour type may be defined by biopsy, and the extent by CT scanning. Nonmalignant granulomatous diseases can also manifest here (e.g., sarcoid).
- Aneurysms—those of the ascending aorta or the arch of the aorta are usually degenerative but may also appear as a late complication of aortic trauma or dissection. Syphilitic aneurysm is now rare.
- Developmental cysts—these include pericardial, bronchogenic, enterogenous and cysts of uncertain origin. Mediastinal cysts occasionally become infected and even more rarely undergo malignant change.
- Germ cell tumours—primary or secondary teratoma or seminoma occasionally occur. These are diagnosed by histology or raised serum markers and can usually be treated successfully with chemotherapy.

Posterior Mediastinum

The posterior mediastinum lies behind the pericardium. Surgery may be required for the following conditions:

- Aneurysms of the descending aorta.
- Tumours of neurological origin—these may be bilobed and extend into the spinal canal. These are usually benign.
- Diaphragmatic hernia—hiatus hernia is common but is not always associated with gastric reflux. Most sliding hernias can now be treated with acid-reducing drugs, weight loss and other simple advice (see Ch. 22). The more unusual paraoesophageal or rolling hiatus hernia may lead to gastric infarction and many believe its presence is an indication for surgery. Congenital herniation into the posterior mediastinum (hernia of Bochdalek) is very rare. Thoracic or abdominal approaches for hiatus hernia are performed. The commonest operation for hiatus hernia with reflux is a laparoscopic fundoplication.

32

Hernias and Other Groin Problems

Introduction

This chapter describes the clinical presentation and diagnosis of lumps and swellings in the groin along with specific conditions causing these problems. Other hernias of the anterior abdominal wall (ventral hernias) are considered at the end of the chapter.

Groin lumps and swellings account for about 10% of general surgical outpatient referrals. In both sexes, the most common lumps in the groin are **hernias**, mainly inguinal but also femoral. Both are caused by abdominal contents protruding through an abdominal wall defect. The normal testicular descent is from the abdomen to the scrotum via the inguinal canal, and this area remains vulnerable throughout life; consequently, inguinal hernias are much more common in males. If large, an **inguinal hernia**

may present as a scrotal rather than a groin lump, but it is obvious that it arises in the groin. In the female, the uterine round ligament pursues a similar course, which explains inguinal hernias in females. The femoral canal, below the inguinal ligament, is another potential weakness and may give rise to a **femoral hernia**, particularly in women.

Enlarged lymph nodes caused by infection or malignancy also cause groin lumps or swellings. Less common are vascular abnormalities, such as a **saphena varix** or a **femoral artery aneurysm**. Very rarely nowadays, a **psoas abscess** may track down beneath the inguinal ligament to present in the groin. This used to be a common complication of spinal tuberculosis, but is now more often a result of infection tracking down from a perforation in the left colon, caused by diverticulitis or Crohn colitis.

The anatomy of the groin provides a good starting point for understanding surgical problems in this area and is explained in Fig. 32.1.

Lumps in the Groin

Clinical Examination

Groin and scrotum must be examined to discover the anatomical origin of the swelling. Lumps in the groin are examined as lumps elsewhere but there are some special points to note:
- examine the patient both standing and lying;
- examine for the presence of a cough impulse and test the reducibility of the lump;
- demonstrate the relationship of the **origin** of the lump to the inguinal ligament and the pubic tubercle.

Position for Examination

The patient must first be examined whilst standing. This increases intraabdominal pressure and makes any hernia more visible. Ask the patient to cough, while palpating the lump: intraabdominal pressure transmitted through the abdominal wall causes an expansile **cough impulse** in a hernia. Small inguinal hernias may reduce on lying down, and a scrotal varicocoele (see Ch. 33) will empty.

Consistency and Reducibility

Hernias are usually soft and 'squishy' but the most reliable diagnostic sign is if the lump reduces when the patient lies flat or can

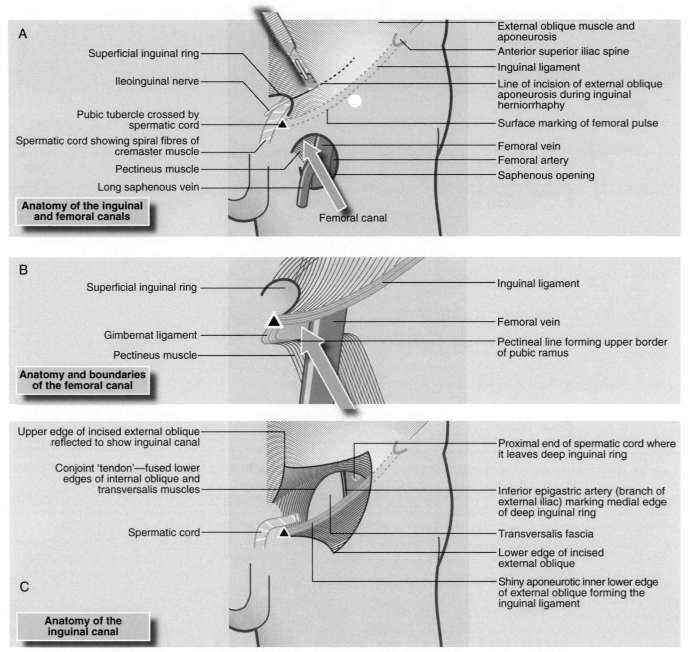

A

Superficial inguinal ring
Ileoinguinal nerve
Pubic tubercle crossed by spermatic cord
Spermatic cord showing spiral fibres of cremaster muscle
Pectineus muscle
Long saphenous vein

External oblique muscle and aponeurosis
Anterior superior iliac spine
Inguinal ligament
Line of incision of external oblique aponeurosis during inguinal herniorrhaphy
Surface marking of femoral pulse
Femoral vein
Femoral artery
Saphenous opening

Anatomy of the inguinal and femoral canals

Femoral canal

B

Superficial inguinal ring
Gimbernat ligament
Pectineus muscle

Inguinal ligament
Femoral vein
Pectineal line forming upper border of pubic ramus

Anatomy and boundaries of the femoral canal

C

Upper edge of incised external oblique reflected to show inguinal canal
Conjoint 'tendon'—fused lower edges of internal oblique and transversalis muscles
Spermatic cord

Proximal end of spermatic cord where it leaves deep inguinal ring
Inferior epigastric artery (branch of external iliac) marking medial edge of deep inguinal ring
Transversalis fascia
Lower edge of incised external oblique
Shiny aponeurotic inner lower edge of external oblique forming the inguinal ligament

Anatomy of the inguinal canal

• **Fig. 32.1** Structure of the Inguinal and Femoral Canals. (A) **The entire groin area**. The surface marking of the femoral pulse is shown, midway between the pubic symphysis and the anterior superior iliac spine; the deep ring lies 2.5 cm above it. (B) **Structure of the femoral canal**—the abdominal opening seen from below. (C) **Structure of the inguinal canal**. The inguinal canal displayed by incising the anterior wall (external oblique aponeurosis) as in the first stage of open repair; the spermatic cord has been removed for clarity.

be reduced by gentle manipulation by patient or clinician. Most inguinal hernias are at least partly reducible, although longstanding hernias gradually become irreducible because of adhesions within the sac. These are said to be **incarcerated**, that is, chronically irreducible. In contrast, femoral hernias are nearly always **irreducible** and have no cough impulse as the femoral canal is so narrow (Table 32.1), a common trap for the unwary.

A **strangulated** inguinal hernia can be readily diagnosed by finding an irreducible hernia in the correct anatomical position;

the lump is tender and often red. Conversely, strangulated femoral hernias are usually very small and unimpressive, often no more than the size of a grape, yet have serious consequences. Strangulated hernias, particularly femoral hernias, sometimes present with abdominal pain or signs of obstruction but without localised pain in the groin. This emphasises the importance of examining the hernial orifices in every patient with an acute abdomen, and being aware of the femoral hernia trap described earlier.

TABLE 32.1	Summary of Groin Lumps and Swellings and Their Clinical Features	
Disorder	**Anatomical/Developmental Basis**	**Clinical Features**
a. **Inguinal hernia** Direct	Simple bulging of abdominal contents resulting from inadequate support by weak or ruptured posterior wall of inguinal canal (transversalis fascia)	Discomfort; lump usually disappears on lying down; risk of incarceration if large but low risk of strangulation
Indirect	Passage of abdominal contents, often including bowel, through inguinal canal towards scrotum or labium majus	Potential for incarceration and strangulation; much more common in men
b. **Femoral hernia**	Abdominal contents, often including bowel, migrate into femoral canal	Rarely has a cough impulse; rarely reducible; high rate of strangulation; more common in women
c. **Inguinal lymphadenopathy**	Inguinal nodes drain lower limb, abdominal wall below umbilicus, anal canal, scrotal skin, penis (but not testes, which drain to paraaortic and parailiac nodes)	Enlarged nodes indicate infection, lymphoma or metastases from primary lesion in drainage area
d. **Saphena varix**	Dilatation of long saphenous vein superficial to deep fascia before it enters the femoral vein	Can be mistaken for femoral hernia but empties on pressure and disappears on lying down, unlike femoral hernia; varicose veins present in the leg
e. **Femoral artery aneurysm**	Dilatation of common femoral artery just below inguinal ligament	Found in patients over 65 years, mostly male; classic clinical sign is expansile pulsation; could be mistaken for femoral hernia
f. **Psoas abscess**	Classically, a tuberculous abscess of lumbar vertebra tracking down inside sheath of psoas muscle; occasionally a pyogenic abscess originating within the abdomen presents via the same route	Tuberculosis presents as swelling or 'cold abscess' below inguinal ligament; rare nowadays but may be confused with lymph nodes; pyogenic abscess typically 'hot'; rarely may be caused by abscess from renal stones

Enlarged inguinal lymph nodes vary in consistency, number and size depending on the pathological cause; they are of course not reducible. A **saphena varix** is very soft and disappears completely on palpation or if the patient lies down, refilling when pressure is released or if the patient stands. The leg on that side nearly always has obvious varicose veins. A saphena varix also exhibits a cough impulse. **Femoral artery aneurysms**, however, are firm but pulsatile. These vascular conditions must be diagnosed correctly as injudicious operation could be catastrophic!

Relationship to the Inguinal Ligament

The site of the lump in relation to the inguinal ligament needs to be identified. The ligament is not visible but stretches between two palpable bony prominences, the **anterior superior iliac spine** laterally and the **pubic tubercle** medially (see Fig. 32.1A). The pubic tubercle is higher than might be imagined from the skin contour, lying 2 to 3 cm above the groin crease. The iliac spine is easy to locate but the pubic tubercle can be difficult, especially in obese patients. It is best found by palpating along the upper border of the pubic symphysis, outwards from the midline (care is needed in the male as the spermatic cord can be tender, where it crosses the pubic tubercle).

As shown in Fig. 32.2, inguinal hernias always originate **above** the inguinal ligament, whereas femoral hernias, saphena varices and femoral artery aneurysms always arise **below** it. Enlarged inguinal **lymph nodes** are usually situated below the inguinal ligament.

Direct and Indirect Inguinal Hernias (Fig. 32.3)

Distinguishing between direct and indirect inguinal hernias may be clinically difficult, but it is a useful exercise in eliciting clinical signs and frequently comes up in student examinations! By definition, an **indirect inguinal hernia** is one in which the hernial sac lies within the spermatic cord, leaving the abdomen via the deep (internal) inguinal ring to pass along the inguinal canal, exiting through the superficial (external) ring. Thus if the hernia can be completely reduced, finger pressure over the deep ring will prevent it reappearing on coughing (the deep ring is midway between the pubic symphysis and the pubic tubercle, 2.5 cm above the femoral pulse; see Fig. 32.1A). In contrast, a **direct inguinal hernia** leaves the abdomen through a weakness or split in the **transversalis fascia**, the posterior wall of the inguinal canal, emerging directly through the superficial ring, and cannot be controlled by digital pressure over the deep ring. In practice, this test is difficult and often unreliable. The patient's age is perhaps the most useful indicator of the likely type of inguinal hernia, with indirect hernias most frequent under the age of 50 years and direct hernias more common after that age.

Inguinal and Femoral Hernias

Differentiating an inguinal from a femoral hernia may sometimes be problematic but is important, as it will determine the surgical approach and the operation performed. The key is the position of the hernia in relation to the inguinal ligament. An inguinal hernia, emerging from the superficial ring, has its origin above the inguinal ligament, often descending over or medial to the pubic tubercle. A femoral hernia originates below the inguinal ligament and lies lateral to the pubic tubercle. Rarely, it becomes large, and tends to be deflected upwards and may seem to arise above the inguinal ligament. This explains the importance of careful examination to determine the origin of the neck of any groin hernia.

Inguinal Hernia

Inguinal hernia is one of the most common conditions seen in general surgical clinics. In a typical district general hospital,

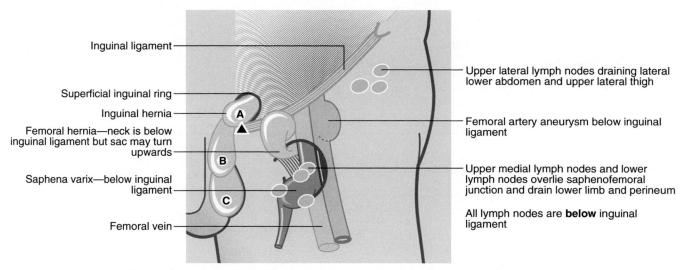

• **Fig. 32.2** Significance of the Relationship of Groin Lumps to the Inguinal Ligament. *(A–C)* are stages in the enlargement of an indirect inguinal hernia. Note that the neck is above the inguinal ligament. A direct inguinal hernia enlarges forwards in position *(A)*, but occasionally extends into the scrotum.

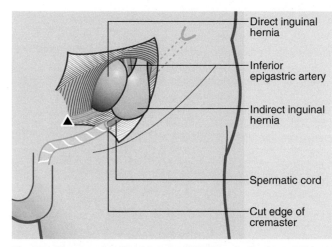

• **Fig. 32.3** Direct and Indirect Inguinal Hernias. A direct inguinal hernia bulges medially to the inferior epigastric artery and is not usually attached to the spermatic cord. An indirect inguinal hernia leaves the deep inguinal ring lateral to the artery and lies within the cremaster muscle covering the cord.

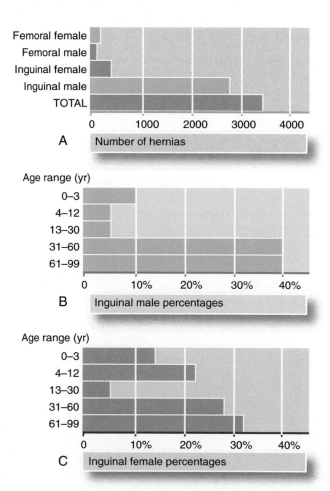

• **Fig. 32.4** Relative Annual Incidence of Inguinal and Femoral Hernias in East Anglia (United Kingdom). (A) Number of hernias by type and (B) incidence of inguinal hernias in males by age. (C) Incidence of inguinal hernias in females by age.

inguinal hernias account for about 7% of surgical outpatient consultations and about 12% of operating theatre time.

As shown in Fig. 32.4, inguinal hernias in males are by far the most common type of groin hernia. Inguinal hernias occur eight times more often in males because of the abdominal wall deficiency caused by testicular descent. Femoral hernias are rare in males, comprising only 2.5% of groin hernias. Even in females, inguinal hernias are the most frequent (twice as common as femorals). Femoral hernias are twice as common in females as in males.

Inguinal hernias occur at any age. In childhood, they always have a developmental origin and are common in premature infants. In males, hernias appear most often before the age of 5 years or after middle age. A smaller peak occurs in the late teens and early 20s. Hernias in these young men probably result from a congenital predisposition, exacerbated by work or sport. Most inguinal hernias should be repaired early to reduce the long-term

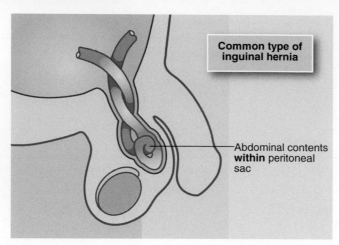

Common type of
inguinal hernia

Abdominal contents
within peritoneal
sac

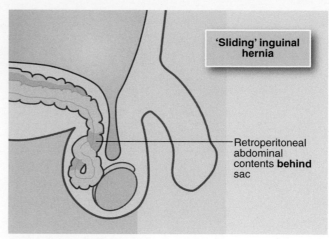

'Sliding' inguinal
hernia

Retroperitoneal
abdominal
contents **behind**
sac

• **Fig. 32.5** Common and Sliding Inguinal Hernias.

risk of strangulation and the need for emergency operation. The exception is small, easily reducible painless direct hernias in elderly men or those with substantial comorbidity, where watchful waiting is a reasonable strategy.

Anatomical Considerations

The surgical anatomy of the inguinal canal is shown in Fig. 32.1C. The external oblique aponeurosis (or fascia) forms the anterior wall of the inguinal canal. In the diagram, it has been split obliquely from the external ring along the line of its fibres, for about 5 cm laterally, and the cut edges reflected upwards and downwards to expose the inguinal canal. This is how it would appear after the first stage of an inguinal hernia repair operation.

The internal oblique and transversus abdominis muscles are deficient above the medial half of the inguinal ligament, with the D-shaped defect normally filled with the **transversalis fascia**. Normal transversalis is particularly strong here and forms the posterior wall of the inguinal canal, providing the only restraint to herniation of the abdominal contents. Arching over this, the inferior borders of the two muscles fuse to form the conjoint musculature and 'tendon', which extends from the lateral half of the inguinal ligament to the pubic crest.

The spermatic cord passes through the deep ring, a defect in the transversalis fascia at the most lateral part of the muscular defect. The **inferior epigastric artery** passes upwards from the external iliac immediately medial to it. Thus the **deep (internal) ring** is bounded by the inguinal ligament below, conjoint musculature above and laterally, and the inferior epigastric artery medially. At operation, its relationship to the inferior epigastric artery defines whether an inguinal hernia is direct or indirect.

Mechanisms of Inguinal Hernia Formation

Inguinal herniation may be direct or indirect. In either case, the herniated abdominal contents are contained within a sac of peritoneum. In an **indirect hernia**, the peritoneal sac may represent a patent or reopened processus vaginalis and may extend as far as the tunica vaginalis and surround the testis.

Direct hernias tend to bulge forwards and rarely enter the scrotum. They are usually found in older patients with deficient muscles and weak transversalis fascia. The neck of a direct sac is broad, in contrast to the narrow neck of an indirect sac,

confined as it is by the borders of the deep ring. Consequently, indirect inguinal hernias are more liable to strangulate. A direct hernia may occur suddenly after physical strain. In this case, the transversalis fascia has split, causing the appearance of a 'rupture'.

An indirect and a direct hernia can occur together on the same side—a **pantaloon hernia**. A hernia may consist merely of peritoneum and associated extraperitoneal fat, but if larger, the sac usually contains omentum or small bowel, or less commonly large bowel or appendix. Occasionally, the contents of the sac are diseased, for example, large bowel carcinoma, an inflamed appendix (acute appendicitis) or peritoneal tumour metastases. Sometimes, a retroperitoneal viscus 'slides' down the posterior abdominal wall and herniates directly (occasionally indirectly) into the inguinal canal, dragging its overlying peritoneum with it. Thus the visceral contents of a **sliding hernia** lie behind and outside the peritoneal sac (Fig. 32.5). This most commonly occurs in the left groin involving the descending and sigmoid colon or in larger direct hernias, may involve the bladder.

Spigelian Hernia

Rarely, herniation occurs through a fascial defect in the linea semilunaris at the lateral border of rectus abdominis. The hernial sac comes to lie interstitially, that is, between the layers of internal and external oblique or transversus abdominis. This is a **Spigelian hernia**. It has some clinical characteristics of an inguinal hernia, but the bulge lies higher than an inguinal hernia and may be difficult to palpate, because it is covered by one or more layers of the abdominal wall (Fig. 32.6).

Natural History of Inguinal Hernia

Inguinal hernias usually develop slowly. Lifetime risk of developing an inguinal hernia is high (>1 in 4 men; >1 in 30 women) and men account for ~90% of all inguinal hernia repairs. Inguinal hernias have a bimodal distribution, with peaks aged 1 year (indirect) and in those aged 70 to 80 years (direct). Women with affected first degree relatives are at much higher risk of developing an inguinal hernia. Hernia repairs remain one of the most common general surgical operations in the world with an estimated 20 million repairs per year.

Several factors have been highlighted as being important for the development of inguinal hernias (Table 32.2).

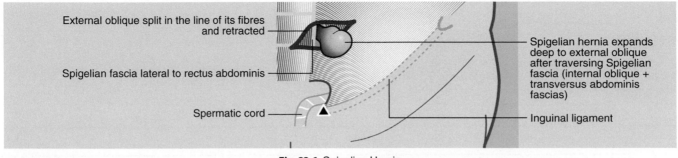

• **Fig. 32.6** Spigelian Hernia.

TABLE 32.2	Important Factors for the Development of Inguinal Hernias
Risk Factor	**Influence**
Inheritance	Increased risk in first degree relatives, connective tissue disorders
Age	Increasing risk of direct hernia with age
Gender	Incidence in men approximately 10 times more than in women
Obesity	BMI inversely related to inguinal hernia risk
Collagen metabolism	Reduced type I:III ratio and increased systemic MMP-2
Open prostatectomy	Increased risk of inguinal hernia

BMI, Body mass index; *MMP-2*, matrix metallopeptidase 2.

The association of any condition which persistently raises intraabdominal pressure, for example, constipation, straining at micturition or chronic coughing, with inguinal hernia development is weak. The evidence surrounding the influence of heavy lifting on inguinal hernia development is contradictory. In infants, a period of severe coughing or crying may precipitate an acute indirect hernia, which may become irreducible.

A chronically irreducible hernia that is not strangulated is described as **incarcerated**. However, the term is often used inaccurately when a clinician is uncertain if an acutely irreducible hernia is strangulated. In patients presenting as emergencies, it is safer to assume such a hernia is strangulated until proved otherwise.

Hernial Strangulation

Inguinal hernias that are difficult to reduce or which intermittently cause pain are at particular risk of strangulation. Strangulation occurs if the hernial contents become constricted by the neck of the sac or by twisting. Obstruction of venous return then leads to swelling and later to arterial obstruction. If strangulation is not relieved by manual or operative reduction, **infarction** follows. A strangulated inguinal hernia first becomes irreducible and then tender and later red. Symptoms and signs of bowel obstruction develop over the next few hours, followed by peritonitis, if the bowel perforates (Fig. 32.7). Strangulation is a surgical emergency.

Management of Inguinal Hernias

Inguinal hernias in adults should ideally be repaired by **mesh patching** or by **herniorrhaphy**, although there is evidence that small, reducible direct hernias in older men can safely be left alone.

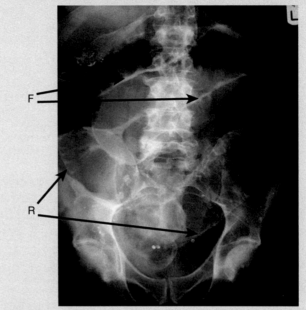

• **Fig. 32.7** Strangulated Inguinal Hernia. This 40-year-old man presented with symptoms and signs of distal small bowel obstruction evidently caused by a strangulated inguinal hernia. At first, the abdomen, though distended and tympanitic, was not tender. However, during resuscitation, the abdomen became tender. This x-ray shows a clear outline of the outside of parts of the small bowel (R), representing Rigler sign. A false Rigler sign is seen in other parts (F); this is where two loops of thickened small bowel lie in contact. Rigler sign indicates free peritoneal gas due to a perforation.

Hernia operations are often performed under general anaesthesia, although epidural or spinal or local anaesthesia is becoming the norm, particularly in patients with poor cardiovascular or respiratory function. Many surgeons favour an open repair, under local anaesthesia, for such cases; certainly if age or infirmity makes anaesthesia hazardous, this is a safe option.

Some hernias become intermittently irreducible, often with local pain and tenderness or even symptoms of bowel obstruction (vomiting, colicky abdominal pain, distension and absolute constipation). Such warning episodes are an indication for early operation. More severe and prolonged symptoms of this nature precipitate emergency admission to hospital, in which case strangulation must be assumed and operation performed urgently, preferably within 4 hours to maximise the chance of saving ischaemic bowel. In any patient with an obstructed or strangulated hernia,

CASE HISTORY

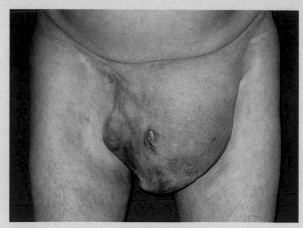

• **Fig. 32.8** Inguinoscrotal Hernia. This man of 76 years lived alone and only presented to a doctor when he had increasing difficulty controlling the direction of his micturition. His penis had disappeared altogether as the hernia had enlarged. The right testis is visible in the scrotum, but the left side of the scrotum is filled with a large hernia. At operation, the abdominal wall defect was surprisingly small and was easily repaired by a standard method.

the first step is to ensure that the patient is fully resuscitated; more patients die of fluid and electrolyte problems than of delaying an operation by a few hours.

Very large 'wheelbarrow' hernias are invariably of long standing and are found mainly in elderly men (see Fig. 32.8). They only present when size becomes a handicap, if bowel strangulates within the hernia or if the anatomical distortion interferes with micturition. Bowel adhesions may make operation difficult and postoperative wound infections are common. If the hernia is not strangulated, a bag truss to support the hernia may be an appropriate treatment.

Inguinal Herniorrhaphy and Herniotomy

Until recently, the standard open techniques of herniorrhaphy were mostly based on Bassini's 19th century extraperitoneal approach, which removed the peritoneal sac or reduced it into the abdomen and then used nonabsorbable sutures or mesh to repair the abdominal wall.

In 1989 **Lichtenstein** described his mesh implant technique, which rapidly became the standard operation. This uses a 'tension-free' technique, using a patch of nonabsorbable, open-weave, mesh to repair and reinforce the defect rather than pulling together muscle and fascial layers together under tension. Fig. 32.9 shows the principles of the Lichtenstein type of inguinal hernia repair.

The mesh technique has several distinct advantages:
• This technique is easily learned and trainee surgeons can reliably produce good results.
• Postoperative pain is substantially less, allowing increased mobility and early return to normal activities, such as work and driving.
• Recurrence rates appear to be exceptionally low.
• It is relatively cheap and cost effective.

Having a foreign body implanted might be expected to increase the risk of infection but in practice, it is exceptionally rare. The mesh used does not have to be expensive—studies are

being published of successful hernia repairs in developing countries using sterilised mosquito netting!

In infants, the patent processus vaginalis is merely ligated and excised (**herniotomy**); formal repair of the abdominal wall defect is usually unnecessary. If the defect is enormous, a single stitch should be used on the medial side to narrow the deep ring.

Complications of Hernia Repair

Early complications of hernia repair include scrotal haematoma and wound infection. Most surgeons use prophylactic antibiotics for mesh repairs but there is little evidence of benefit. Late complications include recurrence (see later), chronic **groin pain** caused by inadvertent trapping of the ilioinguinal or another nerve in the repair, and **testicular atrophy** caused by inadvertent damage to the testicular artery, usually with diathermy, or overtightening of the deep ring.

Recurrence

Inguinal hernias recur in 2% to 25% of cases over a lifetime. The rate is greatly increased when inadequate attention has been given to good operative technique.

The causes of inguinal hernia recurrence include:
• Inappropriate technique—suture darn (Bassini) type repairs have a high recurrence rate.
• Operator inexperience—some techniques, especially laparoscopic repairs, have a long learning curve.
• Technical failure—failure to recognise and remove an indirect sac at operation; insufficient coverage of the defect; suture or mesh failure.
• Missed diagnosis of a concomitant femoral hernia.
• Inherently poor musculature or connective tissue, chronic cough, urinary obstruction, constipation or resumption of heavy work too soon after repair.
• Underlying physiological problems that impair healing, such as poorly controlled diabetes or smoking—smokers have twice the recurrence rates of nonsmokers. It is important to screen for problems of this type and address them before hernia surgery.

Laparoscopic Inguinal Hernia Repair (See also Ch. 10)

Laparoscopic repair of inguinal hernias by a transperitoneal or retroperitoneal route is now the standard operation for hernia repair in many centres. It is strongly recommended as the technique of choice in women, as it allows coverage of the whole myopectineal orifice, thus allowing repair of inguinal and femoral hernias simultaneously. It offers less postoperative pain and a slightly quicker return to normal activities, but has a slightly higher risk of major complications and recurrences compared to open techniques for primary hernia repair. The method is particularly recommended for repair of recurrent hernias, having the advantage of allowing the mesh to be placed in virgin territory, and also for bilateral repair, when both sides can be repaired through the same three small incisions. There is a long learning curve for laparoscopic repair and the recurrence rate may be slightly higher than the Lichtenstein technique.

Mesh

Open and laparoscopic repairs of inguinal hernias both use mesh. Modern meshes were developed in the late 1950s and support the defective abdominal wall and eventually become incorporated by fibrosis. Mesh repairs are proven to reduce recurrence

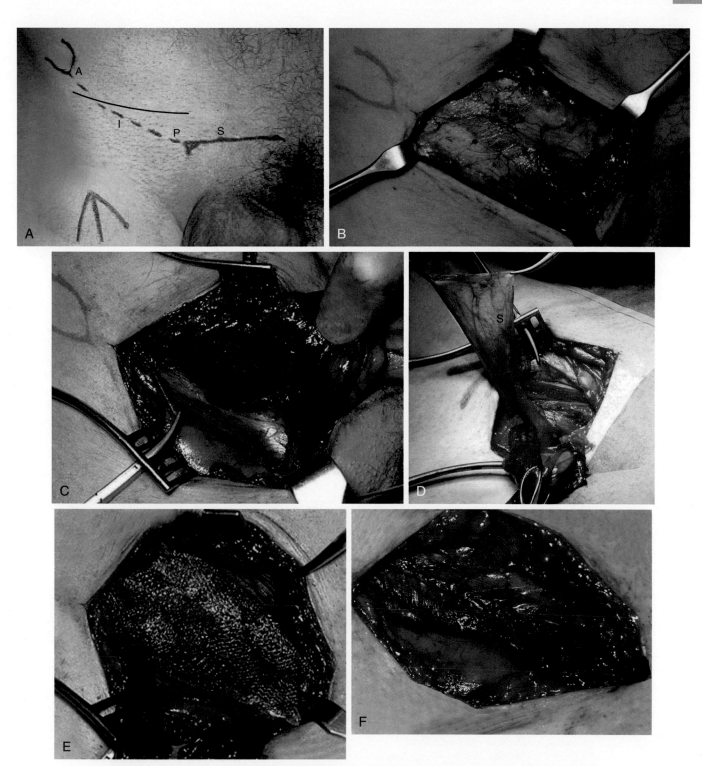

• **Fig. 32.9** **Technique of Mesh Hernia Repair.** (A) Skin markings demonstrating the upper border of the pubic arch *(S)*, the anterior superior iliac spine *(A)*, the pubic tubercle *(P)* and the inguinal ligament *(I)*. Note the side of the planned operation has been marked with an *arrow* on the thigh to ensure the correct side is operated upon. The line of incision is shown as a *solid line*. (B) The dissection down to the external oblique aponeurosis. The external (superficial) ring is *arrowed*. (C) External oblique aponeurosis opened, demonstrating the shiny inguinal ligament, which is its inturned lower edge. (D) The indirect hernia sac *(S)* dissected out from the spermatic cord and held upwards before ligation and excision. The inferior epigastric artery and vein lie at the medial border of the deep inguinal ring. (E) Polypropylene mesh is cut to shape before insertion and sutured in place along the inguinal ligament and, in this case, tacked to the surface of the internal oblique with 'starry sky' sutures. (F) External oblique closed to recreate the inguinal canal before skin closure.

rates compared to nonmesh, although the optimal mesh design remains unknown. Many mesh varieties are available but they can broadly be classified into synthetic polymers and biological tissue. Synthetic meshes are the most common type and are designed for clean cases. Polymer types may be absorbable or nonabsorbable and vary in their porosity or size of hole between individual polymer fibres. Macroporous meshes may promote better healing and cause less chronic pain. Polypropylene and polyester are the most common synthetic meshes used and these dominate the market because of low cost and good performance. Absorbable mesh materials undergo hydrolysis and degrade over different periods and are selected to fit individual clinical situations. Common types include polylactic acid and polyglycolic acid.

Biological meshes are derived from tissue and may be allografts (human derived) or xenografts (animal derived—bovine, porcine or ovine). They may be made from dermis, pericardium or intestinal submucosa. The intention is to provide a collagen scaffold for scar tissue to grow into. Indications for their use are unclear, but have been proposed for contaminated or infected cases, as they may be more resistant to infection than synthetic meshes. However, they are much more expensive than synthetic meshes.

Mesh implants are safe and effective for most patients, but a few patients have complications, particularly with synthetic nonabsorbable mesh. Complications may not manifest for several years or even decades until after the operation. The most common reported problem is chronic pain, which may be caused by several factors, but it is worth noting that nonmesh repairs (e.g., Shouldice technique) do not have a lower rate of chronic groin pain. Other complications include erosion, fistulation, dysejaculation, chronic infection and mesh fragmentation. These complications have made mesh use controversial in the eyes of some, but with such generally good outcomes, current professional guidelines universally recommend mesh for use in hernia repair.

Postoperative Care and Return to Normal Activities

Most inguinal hernias are now repaired on a day case basis, although some patients with comorbidities may need to stay in hospital overnight.

During the first postoperative week, patients should avoid activities likely to strain the repair, such as heavy lifting or driving a car. Over the next 2 or 3 weeks, they should gradually return to normal activity, including usual sexual activity. Time to return to work depends on the physical nature of the job and whether activities cause pain, but usually varies from 2 to 4 weeks.

Trusses

A truss made of padded webbing may control certain types of hernia, when surgery is inappropriate or unacceptable to the patient. They can safely be used only if the hernia is easily reducible and can be kept reduced and free of symptoms. For very large irreducible hernias, a 'bag truss' can support the hernia. Most trusses are ill fitting and ineffective and are better avoided if possible. There is some evidence that trusses increase fibrosis and inflammation and may make repair more difficult—early repair is the best option if practicable.

Femoral Hernia

A femoral hernia is formed by a protrusion of peritoneum into the potential space of the femoral canal. The sac may contain abdominal viscera (usually small bowel) or omentum. Around 40% of femoral hernias present with strangulation. The incidence is

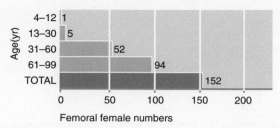

• **Fig. 32.10** Annual Incidence of Femoral Hernias in Females by Age in East Anglia (United Kingdom).

higher in women and increases with age (see Figs 32.4 and 32.10). Increased intraabdominal pressure, and other factors related to pregnancy, may be important in females, since the incidence of femoral hernia is higher in parous than nulliparous women.

Clinical Features of Femoral Hernia

The anatomy of the femoral canal is shown in Fig. 32.1B, page 433. A femoral hernia is usually small, appearing as a lump immediately below the inguinal ligament and just lateral to its medial attachment to the pubic tubercle. Since the femoral canal is narrow, a cough impulse can rarely be detected, and the hernia is usually irreducible. Thus small femoral hernias may be difficult to distinguish from other lumps arising in the femoral canal, such as a lipoma or enlarged Cloquet lymph node. However, a hernia is deeply fixed, whereas the others tend to be more mobile.

Strangulated Femoral Hernia

In contrast to strangulated inguinal hernia, there are often no obvious localising symptoms and signs in strangulated femoral hernia, and the classic presenting features are those of distal small bowel obstruction. The diagnosis of strangulated femoral hernia is easily missed, unless the femoral region is carefully and expertly examined for a lump. A femoral hernia can easily be missed in an obese patient and computed tomography scanning of the abdomen may be required to clarify the diagnosis.

In nearly 30% of strangulated femoral hernias, only a portion of the bowel circumference is trapped in the hernial sac. Although the bowel lumen remains patent and the patient continues to pass flatus, peristalsis is sufficiently disrupted for other signs of obstruction to occur, notably vomiting. This is known as **Richter hernia** (see Fig. 32.11). Resuscitation and urgent operation are required, as for completely strangulated hernias.

Management of Femoral Hernia

The abdominal orifice of the femoral canal is small and indistensible, so abdominal contents finding their way into the canal strangulate much more readily than in inguinal hernias. Thus all femoral hernias, even if asymptomatic, should be repaired without delay.

Elective repair is performed by first isolating, emptying and excising the peritoneal sac (Fig. 32.12). The femoral canal is then closed with nonabsorbable sutures or with a plug placed between pectineus fascia and inguinal ligament. The canal can be exposed by several different methods. The most common are: (1) the **femoral** or low approach; (2) the **Lotheissen** or high approach, via the posterior wall of the inguinal canal and (3) the **McEvedy** or pararectus extraperitoneal approach. The last is virtually a laparotomy and is rarely used. Occasionally a femoral hernia containing bowel cannot be safely reduced via a local approach, or bowel of doubtful

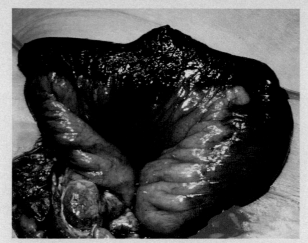

• **Fig. 32.11** Richter Hernia. This 71-year-old woman presented with symptoms and signs of incomplete small bowel obstruction; these included vomiting, abdominal distension and colicky abdominal pain, but she continued to pass flatus. She had a 2-cm femoral hernia, which was not tender. At operation, only a part of the wall of the ileum was trapped in the hernia. The photograph shows bruising around the area trapped in the hernia. Luckily, the bowel was viable and did not need resection. The hernia was repaired before closure.

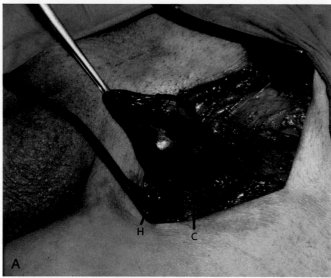

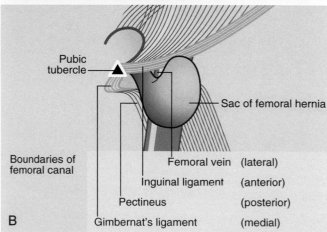

• **Fig. 32.12** Femoral Hernia. (A) An average-sized femoral hernia (H) at operation. The patient's genitalia are to the left of the photograph. The line of the inguinal ligament is marked with an *interrupted line* and the opening of the femoral canal is seen at (C). (B) The four margins of the femoral canal.

viability escapes back into the abdominal cavity. In either case, a laparotomy incision is required to safely complete the operation.

Enlarged Inguinal Lymph Nodes

The lymph nodes of the inguinal region are clustered into the three anatomical groups shown in Fig. 32.13. These drain the lower abdominal wall and lower back, perineum (including vulva and vagina), anal canal, penis and scrotal skin and the whole lower limb. The testes are derived from the retroperitoneal area and hence drain to the upper paraaortic nodes within the abdomen rather than inguinal nodes.

Inguinal lymph nodes may become secondarily enlarged as a result of local disease in their field of drainage. Examples include infections of the foot, skin diseases, sexually transmitted infection or tumours. Inguinal node enlargement may also be part of a generalised lymphadenopathy in lymphoma or a systemic infection, such as glandular fever or acquired immunodeficiency syndrome (AIDS). Inguinal nodes may also become involved in tuberculosis (TB). Multiple small firm ('shotty') nodes are commonly found and are accepted as normal if less than 1 cm in diameter. These nodes probably result from minor infections of the lower limb.

Clinical Features of Enlarged Inguinal Lymph Nodes

Enlarged inguinal lymph nodes present with pain or a lump in the groin but are often discovered incidentally. Enlarged lymph nodes are recognised by their anatomical position and by excluding hernias or vascular abnormalities. Enlarged nodes are usually mobile but become fixed to the surrounding tissues, when infiltrated by tumour. If doubt exists as to whether nodes are enlarged, ultrasound scanning usually gives a definitive answer and can guide

percutaneous needle biopsy. In general, nodes smaller than 1 cm are unlikely to be malignant.

The history may need to be reviewed for clues as to the origin of any nodes. A history of systemic manifestations of lymphoma, TB or AIDS should be sought. These include malaise, periodic fevers and weight loss. There may be a history of a 'mole' or 'wart' having been removed, even many years before. If this was a malignant melanoma or squamous carcinoma, it could now have metastasised. Other symptoms of tumours that metastasise to inguinal lymph nodes should be sought; for example, anal pain or bleeding might indicate an anal carcinoma, and an unretractable foreskin may hide a penile carcinoma.

Examination should include palpating lymph nodes in the neck and axillae, and palpating the liver and spleen. The skin of the whole drainage field should be examined closely, paying particular attention to the back, perineum and feet, including between the toes and beneath the toenails, and beneath the foreskin. The examination may reveal infection, squamous cell carcinoma or malignant melanoma. Rectal examination is mandatory to exclude anal carcinoma. A blood test for human immunodeficiency virus antigen may be indicated.

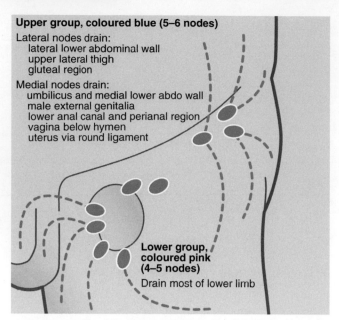

Upper group, coloured blue (5–6 nodes)

Lateral nodes drain:
    lateral lower abdominal wall
    upper lateral thigh
    gluteal region

Medial nodes drain:
    umbilicus and medial lower abdo wall
    male external genitalia
    lower anal canal and perianal region
    vagina below hymen
    uterus via round ligament

Lower group,
coloured pink
(4–5 nodes)

Drain most of lower limb

• **Fig. 32.13** Superficial Inguinal Lymph Nodes of the Groin. The lower group lie around the termination of the long saphenous vein. Both upper and lower groups drain to the external iliac nodes.

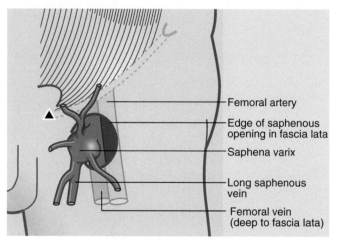

Femoral artery

Edge of saphenous opening in fascia lata

Saphena varix

Long saphenous vein

Femoral vein (deep to fascia lata)

• **Fig. 32.14** Saphena Varix.

If enlarged lymph nodes cannot be explained by simple local factors or a systemic illness, nodes should be sampled for histology. If metastatic malignancy is suspected, fine-needle aspiration or needle core biopsy is appropriate, but if lymphoma is likely, a node should be surgically removed or be subject to an open biopsy to obtain substantial tissue for histological typing.

Saphena Varix

A saphena varix is a dilatation of the long saphenous vein in the groin, just proximal to its junction with the femoral vein (Fig. 32.14). The varix is caused by valvular incompetence at this point; there are usually substantial varicose veins elsewhere in the long saphenous system.

The varix can reach the size of a golf ball or even larger. On examination, the swelling is soft and diffuse. The diagnostic feature is that it empties with minimal pressure and refills on release

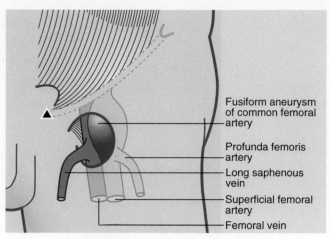

Fusiform aneurysm of common femoral artery

Profunda femoris artery

Long saphenous vein

Superficial femoral artery

Femoral vein

• **Fig. 32.15** Femoral Artery Aneurysm.

('the sign of emptying'). A cough impulse is invariably present and a fluid thrill can be felt if varicosities further down the thigh are tapped lightly. Treatment is high saphenous ligation, as for saphenofemoral reflux associated with varicose veins (see Ch. 43).

Femoral Artery Aneurysm

Femoral aneurysms are uncommon as a cause of lumps in the groin. They may occur as part of a generalised aneurysmal disease, involving the abdominal aorta, iliac and lower limb arterial system, but can also occur in isolation. Diagnosis is made on clinical examination; the lump lies below the midpoint of the inguinal ligament (Fig. 32.15) and has a characteristic expansile pulsation. Distinguishing an aneurysm from a femoral hernia is clearly vitally important. The management of aneurysms is discussed in Chapter 42.

Chronic Groin Pain

Chronic groin pain without any clues in the history and without swelling is difficult to diagnose and treat. Groin pain may be caused by **inflamed inguinal lymph nodes** secondary to infection in their field of drainage. **Strained muscle attachments** to the bony pelvis sometimes cause groin pain; this particularly affects the hip adductor attachments near the pubic tubercle and usually follows extreme physical activity. Groin pain may also be **referred** from a diseased hip joint. 'Groin strain' (a.k.a. athletic pubalgia or sportsman's groin) is a difficult entity to understand and often affects professional sports people. It starts acutely but often becomes chronic; the diagnosis is one of exclusion. A newly appeared inguinal hernia may cause groin pain, often on sitting, yet be too small to detect clinically. Unfortunately, there is no dependable test for an early hernia other than laparoscopy, although ultrasound in experienced hands is fairly reliable. There is increasing interest in the use of magnetic resonance imaging for investigating chronic groin pain but the science is still young.

Ventral Hernias

Ventral hernias include epigastric, umbilical and paraumbilical hernias. Ventral incisional hernias occurring through previous surgical or traumatic wounds are considered in Chapter 12.

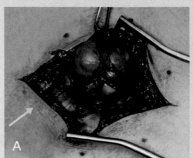 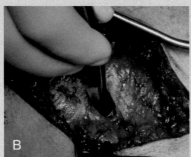 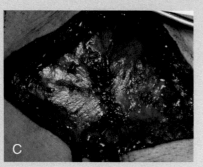

• **Fig. 32.16** Epigastric Hernia. This man of 28 years had an unusually large epigastric hernia that caused pain on exercise. It was situated in the midline, midway between the xiphisternum and the umbilicus. (A) 'Mushroom-like' epigastric hernia mass protruding through the linea alba (fibres indicated by *arrow*). (B) Relatively small defect in linea alba after mobilising and reducing the hernia. (C) After edge-to-edge repair of defect using continuous nonabsorbable nylon suture.

Epigastric Hernias

These are midline herniations through defects in the linea alba, anywhere between xiphoid process and umbilicus. They are four times more common in males and are often tiny, with a defect less than 0.5 cm. Most are symptomless and the presence of a lump and sometimes episodic sharp pain on exertion are the usual presenting complaints. Treatment is by surgical repair—closing the hernial defect and usually reinforcing the closure with mesh (Fig. 32.16).

Umbilical and Paraumbilical Hernias

Umbilical hernias in children are discussed in Chapter 51. **Paraumbilical hernias** are acquired rather than congenital. They occur in all age groups but are five times more common in females. The abdominal wall defect is in the linea alba, generally above or below the umbilical cicatrix. The swelling lies adjacent to the umbilicus, with the umbilicus itself pushed to the side to produce the characteristic 'smile' of a paraumbilical hernia.

True umbilical hernias are the third most common abdominal hernia in adults and appear directly through the umbilical cicatrix. They also occur more commonly in females, and obesity and poor muscle tone are predisposing factors. Hernias range from asymptomatic small protrusions, through larger and occasionally painful lumps, to very large, irreducible and intermittently painful swellings. Both paraumbilical and umbilical hernias become progressively larger and surgical repair is the treatment of choice. This is by suture closure of the hernial defect and reinforcement with mesh.

33

Disorders of the Male Genitalia

CHAPTER OUTLINE

Disorders of the Scrotal Contents

Introduction

Abnormalities of the scrotal contents include disorders of the testis and its coverings, the spermatic cord and inguinoscrotal hernias (see Ch. 32). Distinguishing between them usually requires only clinical examination. Diagnoses that must not be missed are testicular tumours and testicular torsion. Other problems include inflammation, infection, hydrocoeles and cysts, maldescent and testicular trauma, as well as varicocoele. Male sterilisation and disorders of the penis are also covered in this chapter.

Clinical Examination of Scrotal Lumps and Swellings

A lump or swelling in the scrotum may be:
- A solid or cystic mass arising from a component of scrotal contents or spermatic cord. These include testis, epididymis, epididymal appendage, vas deferens and dilation of pampiniform plexus.
- A collection of fluid in the tunica or processus vaginalis (**hydrocoele**).
- An indirect inguinal hernia extending along the embryological path of testicular descent into the scrotum.

The important disorders of the scrotum and contents are summarised in Table 33.1, with their anatomical and clinical significance.

The Origin of a Scrotal Lump

The first objective is to determine whether the swelling arises in the groin, the spermatic cord or the scrotum, and is achieved by palpating the cord at the scrotal neck. In a hernia, the cord is broader than normal and the hernia can be shown to communicate with the abdominal cavity by a cough impulse or by reducing the hernia. Spermatic cord swellings (varicocoele or cyst) are usually easily recognised (examine with the patient standing). In purely scrotal lumps, the spermatic cord is normal in diameter.

Testicular and Epididymal Lumps

With a scrotal abnormality, an attempt should be made to palpate testis and epididymis separately, and to determine their relationship to the lump. If the testis is enlarged or has a lump within it, this is a tumour until proven otherwise. Patients with testicular swellings caused by lymphoma may have systematic symptoms and 10% have bilateral tumours. Any testicular pathology may cause a little fluid to accumulate in the tunica vaginalis, producing a small **secondary hydrocoele**, but this rarely interferes with testicular palpation.

Lumps in the epididymis (cysts, chronic epididymitis or, rarely, tuberculous granulomata) are discrete from, but attached to, an otherwise normal testis. Tiny focal lumps in the epididymis are rarely clinically important. Infective lesions (i.e., abscesses) cause diffuse and usually painful thickening of the epididymis, whereas epididymal cysts are almost always located at the upper pole. Epididymal cysts are filled with clear fluid and therefore transilluminate. **Transillumination** (see Fig. 33.1) is demonstrated by shining a strong beam of light through the scrotum in a partly darkened room. If the lesion is fluid-filled, it will glow (except in the case of blood). About 10% of cysts in the epididymis, and most in the cord, are filled with an opalescent fluid containing spermatozoa (**spermatocoeles**), which can also transilluminate. Scrotal ultrasound can confirm the diagnosis.

TABLE 33.1   Summary of Disorders of the Scrotum and Its Contents and Their Clinical Features

Disorder	Anatomical/Developmental Basis	Clinical Features
1. Testicular Disorders		
a. **Maldescended testis** (see also Ch. 51)	Failure of complete descent from retroperitoneal site into scrotum; testis may be arrested at any point of descent or in an ectopic site	Mainly a problem of infancy and childhood and requiring orchidopexy; differential diagnosis of lump in groin with an empty ipsilateral hemiscrotum; slightly increased predisposition to malignancy; fertility may be impaired; increased risk of torsion
b. **Torsion of testis**	Rotation of testis in scrotum; twisting of the spermatic cord results in venous obstruction, which may culminate in infarction; extravaginal in neonates and intravaginal in adults; recurrent incomplete (intermittent) torsion may occur	Complete torsion causes severe acute scrotal pain (and sometimes abdominal pain); partial torsion may cause episodic pain
c. **Inflammation of epididymis and/or testis**	Epididymitis, caused by common urinary tract pathogens or sexually transmitted organisms; often associated with pain or swelling of the testis Acute orchitis is often viral (mumps) Chronic orchitis may be caused by tuberculosis or syphilitic gumma	Acute epididymitis is painful; must be distinguished from testicular torsion; usually associated with UTI Testicular pain and swelling Usually presents as painless testicular enlargement
d. **Malignant testicular tumours**	Majority are derived from germ cells of testis; metastasise via lymphatics to parailiac and paraaortic nodes or via bloodstream, commonly to lung	Majority present as painless swelling of testis; 20% present with pain
2. Disorders of Other Scrotal Contents		
a. **Hydrocoele**	Collection of fluid in space around testis and within the tunica vaginalis; in children may still be in communication with peritoneal cavity (communicating hydrocoele)	Presents as a painless scrotal swelling, which transilluminates; testis may be difficult to palpate within it until fluid is drained
b. **Haematocoele**	Collection of blood around testis; usually early result of trauma or surgery	Presents like a hydrocoele after trauma but does not transilluminate
c. **Varicocoele**	Dilatation of pampiniform venous plexus of spermatic cord; left side most commonly affected	Presents as a scrotal swelling separate from testis and epididymis; can feel like a 'bag of worms'; less prominent on lying down, thus patient must be examined standing
d. **Epididymal cyst and spermatocoele**	Cysts derived from epididymal tissue	Epididymal cyst presents as a scrotal swelling, which transilluminates; separate from the testis, often multilocular. Spermatocoele is unilocular, sometimes bilateral, in cord or epididymis and may be transilluminable
e. **Torsion of hydatid of Morgagni**	Torsion of epididymal appendage	Occurs in children; may present late as a small hydrocoele; in the acute phase, presents as scrotal pain and may simulate testicular torsion; sometimes seen as a 'blue spot'
f. **Indirect inguinal hernia**	Herniation of abdominal contents along the embryological path of testicular descent	Presents as a scrotal swelling, often with a cough impulse, that can be reduced back into the abdomen

UTI, Urinary tract infection.

Scrotal Pain

Acute Pain (Box 33.1)

In acute scrotal pain, **testicular torsion** *must* be excluded, since the torted testis can be saved if an operation is performed promptly; an exploratory operation is mandatory if torsion cannot be confidently excluded. Torsion occurs mainly in adolescents but occasionally in young adults. Recurrent, incomplete (intermittent) torsion may cause transient episodes of severe testicular pain. In these cases, the anatomical relationship of the testis to the tunica vaginalis is often abnormal so the testes lie horizontally rather than vertically when standing. These **'bell-clapper'** testes are susceptible to torsion. The main differential diagnosis at all ages is acute epididymitis. Torsion of an epididymal appendage (hydatid of Morgagni) produces symptoms similar to testicular torsion in children but less severe; surgical

exploration is usually still required to exclude it. A traumatic haematocoele also causes acute pain but the trauma or surgery that preceded it points to the likely diagnosis.

Chronic Pain

Chronic scrotal pain is often caused by **inflammation**. It can be related to previous surgery (i.e., vasectomy, hydrocoele repair). Patients present weeks or months after the vasectomy operation, complaining of localised tenderness at the operation site or a general ache in one side of the scrotum. If there is a small tender lump caused by a stitch granuloma, this is usually cured by excision. Sperm leakage (**sperm granuloma**) following vasectomy may also cause chronic pain. Pain is a feature of chronic bacterial epididymitis, which usually follows an acute episode.

CASE HISTORY

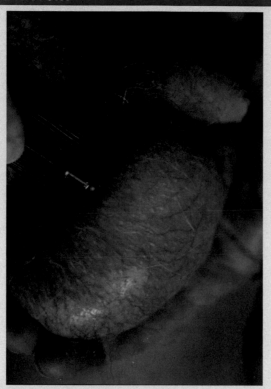

Fig. 33.1 Transillumination of a Cyst in the Scrotum. This 30-year-old man complained of a swelling in the right scrotum. On clinical examination, there is a 3 cm soft rounded swelling at the upper pole of the epididymis. A confident diagnosis of epididymal cyst can thus be made.

BOX 33.1 Common Causes of Acute Pain in the Scrotum

Torsion of the Testis

- Sudden onset of unilateral scrotal pain with or without poorly localised abdominal pain
- In early cases, the testis is high in the scrotum and exquisitely tender, and the cord is thickened; later these signs are often obscured by oedema
- The opposite testis may lie horizontally (bell-clapper testis)

Torsion of the Epididymal Appendage (Hydatid of Morgagni)

- Nearly always in children
- Sudden onset of unilateral scrotal pain; the testis hangs normally. There is tenderness only at its upper pole and minimal overlying oedema
- May see a blue spot sign

Acute Epididymitis

- Moderate or severe scrotal pain and tenderness with marked redness and oedema
- Often preceded by symptoms of urinary tract infection; urine usually contains white cells, nitrites and organisms

Haematocoele Following Trauma or Scrotal Surgery (e.g., Vasectomy)

- History may be diagnostic, although torsion is sometimes precipitated by trauma

Inflammation of the Epididymis and Testis

Epididymitis

Bacterial epididymitis is the most common inflammatory disorder of scrotal contents. It is usually secondary to urethral infection that ascends via the vas deferens. The source is usually a urinary tract infection with coliforms, such as *Escherichia coli* (in the 50–65 years age group), or a sexually transmitted infection with *Chlamydia* or *Neisseria gonorrhoeae* (common in the 15–30 years age group). Epididymitis is often incorrectly called *orchitis* or *epididymoorchitis*. The testis is rarely infected, although the inflammation may cause testicular tenderness.

In epididymitis, pain usually begins acutely. It may present as a surgical emergency and be clinically indistinguishable from testicular torsion. On examination, the affected side of the scrotum and its contents are swollen, oedematous and tender, and the scrotal skin can be red and warm. It may be difficult to palpate the testis and epididymis separately once infection is established. In boys and young men, epididymitis must never be diagnosed in the absence of urinary symptoms, a proven urinary infection or urethritis. Such an 'acute scrotum' must be explored to exclude torsion (see p. 451).

Treatment of acute epididymitis is initial bed rest and pain relief and 2 to 4 weeks of an appropriate broad-spectrum antibiotic. The infecting organism is often not identified but attempts should be made to do so using urine or blood cultures. Current guidance recommends a 14-day course of oral doxycycline and a single intramuscular injection of ceftriaxone for patients at risk of *Chlamydia* and *N. gonorrhoeae*. Oral levofloxacin, ciprofloxacin or ofloxacin are recommended for epididymitis caused by gram-negative organisms (i.e., *E. coli*). Persistent or chronic epididymitis may cause the patient to suffer chronic scrotal tenderness. Chronic epididymitis may also result from inadequate antibiotic treatment of an acute episode.

Tuberculous Epididymitis

Tuberculosis may involve the epididymis via bloodstream spread from a pulmonary or other focus. A tuberculous urinary tract infection can spread to the epididymis, with swelling as the presenting complaint. Typically, the whole length of the epididymis is thickened, nontender and 'cold', with a beaded cord (i.e., involvement of the vas in the spermatic cord). In contrast to bacterial epididymitis, a tuberculous epididymis can be readily distinguished from the testis on palpation. If untreated, the testis may also become involved.

Diagnosis requires analysis of serial early morning urine specimens for mycobacteria or, more reliably, histological examination of percutaneous needle biopsies. Patients will have sterile pyuria (white cells in the urine in the absence of bacterial infection) and a raised erythrocyte sedimentation rate on blood testing. Where available, polymerase chain reaction urine testing can provide a rapid diagnosis of tuberculosis. If tuberculosis is confirmed, a search must be made for pulmonary and urinary tract disease (see Ch. 38).

Orchitis

Primary bacterial orchitis is rare and may result from pyogenic infection in the genital tract or elsewhere. **Tertiary gummatous syphilis** may involve the testis, producing diffuse nontender enlargement. This is now rare and there is usually a history of primary and secondary lesions.

Viral orchitis is most often caused by **mumps**. In postpubertal males, bilateral mumps orchitis produces infertility in

50%; elevated follicle-stimulating hormone (FSH) blood levels following orchitis may indicate subfertility. Mumps orchitis manifests 4 to 6 days after the onset of parotitis, with unilateral or bilateral enlarged, tender testes and an inflammatory hydrocoele. Treatment is directed at symptomatic relief. Other viruses affecting the testis include Coxsackie, human immunodeficiency virus (HIV) and Epstein–Barr. Lymphatic filariasis can be a cause of orchitis in endemic parts of Africa and Asia, and is associated with hydrocoele, scrotal oedema and genital elephantiasis.

Hydrocoele

Primary Hydrocoele

A hydrocoele is an excessive collection of fluid within the tunica vaginalis, that is, in the serous space surrounding the testis. Like the peritoneal cavity, the tunica normally contains a little serous fluid, which is produced and reabsorbed at an equivalent rate (Fig. 33.2).

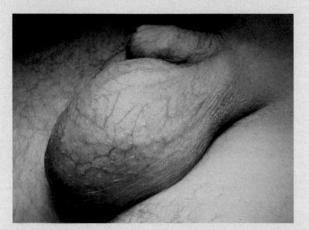

CASE HISTORY

• **Fig. 33.2 Testicular Hydrocoele.** This man of 67 years had a painless swelling of the left side of the scrotum for several years that was slowly enlarging. On examination, the swelling was confined to the scrotum and did not involve widening of the cord at the scrotal neck, which might indicate a hernia. The testis was not palpable separately from the swelling, and the swelling transilluminated, confirming the diagnosis.

In infants and children, a hydrocoele is usually an expression of a patent processus vaginalis (PPV). In some, the scrotal swelling disappears overnight, and is known as a **communicating hydrocoele**. Provided there is no hernia, hydrocoeles in boys below the age of 1 year usually resolve spontaneously. For older children, ligation of the PPV is required; surgical repair is recommended if the hydrocoele fails to resolve by age 2 years.

Primary hydrocoeles may develop in adulthood, particularly in the elderly, by slow accumulation of serous fluid, presumably by impaired reabsorption. These can reach a huge size, containing several hundred millilitres of fluid and may feel heavy or uncomfortable when large. The swelling is soft and nontender and the testis cannot usually be palpated. The presence of fluid is confirmed by transillumination.

Note that a secondary hydrocoele may develop in response to a testicular tumour or inflammation. In most, the hydrocoele is small and the testis can easily be palpated to reveal the primary abnormality.

Management

For symptomatic patients, a hydrocoele operation can be performed by everting the sac and oversewing the edges (Jaboulay procedure) or plicating the sac (Lord method). If the sac is thick, it is best excised. Alternatives include observation alone or periodic aspiration if the patient is unsuitable for surgery. If a testicular tumour is a possibility, a hydrocoele must not be aspirated as malignant cells can be disseminated via the scrotal skin to its lymphatic field.

Hydrocoele of the Cord

Rarely, a hydrocoele develops in a remnant of the processus vaginalis somewhere along the course of the spermatic cord. This hydrocoele also transilluminates, and is known as an **encysted hydrocoele of the cord** (Fig. 33.3).

Fournier Gangrene

Fournier Gangrene is a form of **necrotising fasciitis** of genitalia and perineum and usually causes systemic sepsis. It does not involve the testes. The underlying causes include genitourinary trauma (skin injury, paraphimosis, urethral disruption from urethral instrumentation or catheter), surgery (circumcision), perirectal abscess and urethral stricture. Predisposing factors include diabetes mellitus, corticosteroid use, and chronic alcohol excess. The principal infecting organism is an anaerobe but there is often synergistic aerobic infection. This is a urological emergency. Treatment includes resuscitation, broad spectrum intravenous antibiotics and surgical excision of all necrotic tissue, and this is likely to require repeat procedures. After complete resection, vacuum dressings are applied to assist with wound healing. The extent of the debridement usually requires later reconstruction by a plastic surgery team.

Epididymal Cyst and Spermatocoele

Multiple cysts can develop in the upper pole of the epididymis and present as a painless scrotal swelling (see Fig. 33.3). Epididymal cysts affect a slightly younger age group than hydrocoeles. The testis can be palpated separately from the cysts, which transilluminate.

Less common is a **spermatocoele**, a single cyst containing spermatozoa. Spermatocoeles usually occur in the head of the epididymis. They are clinically similar to epididymal cysts but may or may not transilluminate. Occasionally, they occur in the spermatic cord and surgical excision may cause obstruction to passage of sperm. If a patient wishes to remain fertile and the cysts are bilateral, excision may be contraindicated.

Varicocoele

A varicocoele (see Fig. 33.3 and Fig. 33.4) represents dilatation and tortuosity of the pampiniform venous plexus of the spermatic cord. The condition is much more common on the left (90%), and results from the different venous drainage of the two sides: on the left, the testicular vein drains into the higher-pressure renal vein, whereas the right testicular vein drains directly into the inferior vena cava.

Varicocoele is common, affecting about 15% of young adult males. It is usually asymptomatic but is often discovered during examination for infertility. Varicocoele increases scrotal temperature, which may inhibit sperm numbers and function and cause possible loss of testicular volume. When lying flat, the distended veins often collapse and become impalpable. Varicocoele is best

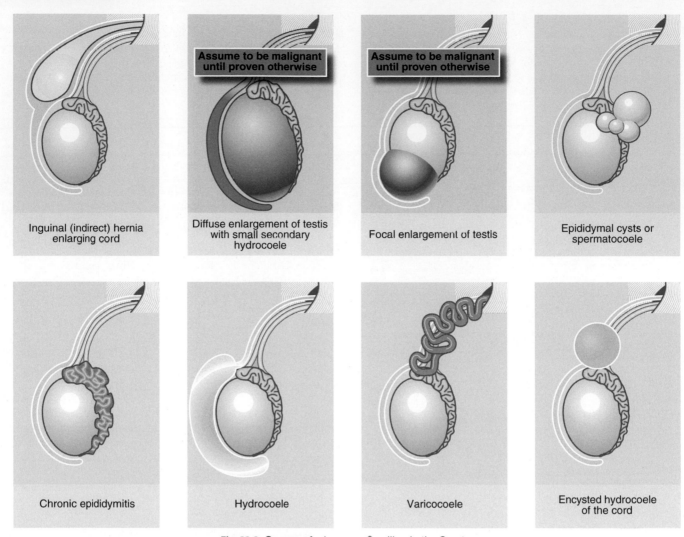

Inguinal (indirect) hernia enlarging cord

Assume to be malignant until proven otherwise

Diffuse enlargement of testis with small secondary hydrocoele

Assume to be malignant until proven otherwise

Focal enlargement of testis

Epididymal cysts or spermatocoele

Chronic epididymitis

Hydrocoele

Varicocoele

Encysted hydrocoele of the cord

• **Fig. 33.3** Causes of a Lump or Swelling in the Scrotum.

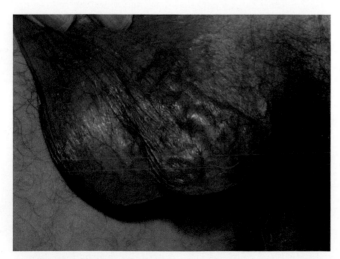

• **Fig. 33.4** Varicocoele. Note the 'bag of worms' appearance.

diagnosed with the patient examined standing. A small varicocoele (grade 1) is only felt with a Valsalva manoeuvre; moderate sized varicocoele (grade 2) can be felt as thickened veins in the spermatic cord, and a large varicocoele (grade 3) feels like 'a bag of worms'.

Rarely, a left-sided varicocoele may be caused by an invading renal cell carcinoma obstructing the left renal vein. A new onset right-sided varicocoele can be caused by renal cell carcinoma obstructing the vena cava or compression from other retroperitoneal masses; such varicocoeles do not collapse when the patient lies flat. These all warrant urgent investigation with upper tract ultrasound.

In adults, surgical treatment of varicocoele is indicated for relief of pain or treatment of low sperm count (oligospermia). In the child or adolescent, treatment may be advised if there is evidence of delayed testicular growth, and to preserve spermatogenesis. The treatment of choice is percutaneous embolisation. The optimal surgical technique is open microsurgical varicocoelectomy. Alternatively, laparoscopic ligation of internal spermatic veins in the retroperitoneum can be performed.

Testicular Tumours

Testicular tumours are relatively uncommon, making up about 1.5% of male cancers and 5% of all urological cancers; however, they are the most common cancer in men in their third and fourth decades. Curative treatment is now available for most of them, even when metastatic. Testicular lymphatic drainage and the route of lymphatic metastases is towards intraabdominal nodes, which

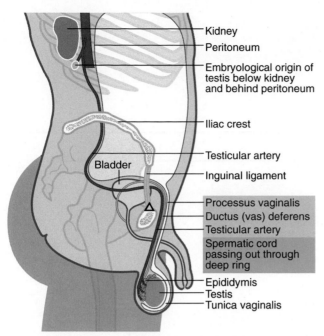

• **Fig. 33.5** Embryological Descent of the Testis. The testicular artery marks the line of descent of testis towards the scrotum. In the embryo, the arterial supply is direct from the aorta and this persists even when the testis has reached the scrotum.

is determined by the embryology of testicular descent (Fig. 33.5). Note that this is different from scrotal skin, which drains towards inguinal nodes.

The incidence of new testicular malignancies is rising to 15 per 100,000 males per annum (peaking in the 25- to 29-year-old group). Around half have already metastasised by the time of presentation. Risk factors include a history of ipsilateral undescended testis, subfertility, a positive family history (first-degree relative affected) or a personal history of tumour affecting the other testis. The relative risk of cancer is at least eight times higher in undescended testes, with an absolute risk of around 2% to 3%, and these tumours are usually seminomas.

More than 90% of primary testicular tumours are derived from **germ cells**, categorised into seminoma (48%) and nonseminomatous (42%) germ cell tumours. The remainder are classified as **sex cord/gonadal stromal** and **miscellaneous stromal tumours**. The World Health Organization histopathological classification is shown in Box 33.2. Germ cell testicular tumours are generally fast-growing tumours that metastasise to intraabdominal lymph nodes and later to the lungs via the bloodstream.

Nongerm cell tumours include **Leydig cell tumours**, which are derived from the gonadal stroma and tend to be well circumscribed; only 10% are malignant. Whilst patients may identify a testicular lump, they may also present with features of excess androgens/oestrogens secretion. This can precipitate precocious puberty in a child and feminisation in an adult male (gynaecomastia).

Testes may become involved in more widespread malignancies, such as lymphoma and chronic lymphocytic leukaemia. Metastases to testes from solid organ malignancies are rare though occasionally their first presentation can be with testicular enlargement or lumps. Surgeons may be asked to perform a testicular biopsy to help confirm a diagnosis.

• **BOX 33.2** World Health Organization Histopathological Classification of Testicular Tumours (Adapted)

1. Germ Cell Tumours (90%)
Noninvasive germ cell neoplasia (germ cell neoplasia in situ)
Seminoma
Teratoma
Embryonal carcinoma
Yolk sac tumour
Trophoblastic tumours (choriocarcinoma)
Mixed nonseminomatous germ cell tumours
Mixed germ cell tumours

2. Sex Cord/Gonadal Stromal Tumours
Leydig cell tumours
Sertoli cell tumours
Mixed

3. Miscellaneous Tumours
Ovarian epithelial tumours

4. Haematolymphoid Tumours
Lymphoma

5. Tumours of the Collecting Ducts and Rete Testis

Pathology of Common Testicular Germ Cell Tumours
Seminomas
More than half of malignant testicular tumours are seminomas, derived from spermatocytes (see Fig. 33.6). They occur predominantly between the ages of 20 and 45 years, with a peak incidence at 35 years. A distinct but rare form of seminoma, **spermatocytic seminoma**, occurs between the ages of 50 and 70 years and almost never metastasises.

CASE HISTORY

Testis: upper and lower poles are indicated by the thin arrows

The tumour is the hypoechoic area indicated by the thick arrow

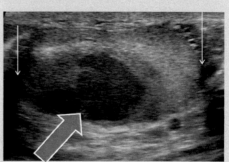

• **Fig. 33.6** Seminoma. This ultrasound scan was performed on a 23-year-old man with a short history of an enlarged testis. There was no clinical sign of a hydrocoele. The scan shows a solid mass involving the whole testis, with no evidence of fluid. The scan is fairly homogeneous, suggesting seminoma. Teratomas tend to be more variegated but making a definitive diagnosis requires surgical exploration.

Nonseminomatous Germ Cell Tumours
Teratomas are slightly less common than seminomas and their peak incidence is a decade earlier. Since they are derived from multipotent cells, teratomas may contain tissue from all germ cell layers: for example, squamous epithelium (ectoderm), cartilage

and smooth muscle (mesoderm), and respiratory epithelium (endoderm). Other common histologies in nonseminomatous tumours are embryonal carcinoma (which is deemed aggressive), choriocarcinoma and yolk sac elements.

Clinical Features of Testicular Tumours

A malignant testicular tumour usually presents as a painless, progressively enlarging testicular lump. If the testicular capsule becomes involved, a **secondary hydrocoele** may appear but this is usually small and does not hinder palpation.

Seminomas and nonseminomatous germ cell tumours both spread via lymphatics to paraaortic nodes at about the level of L1/2. Spread is then proximally along the lymphatic chain, then via the thoracic duct to supraclavicular nodes and the systemic circulation. Lung secondaries are common. Poorly differentiated testicular tumours tend to metastasise early and may present as enlarged abdominal or cervical lymph nodes, or with symptoms of lung metastases.

A solid testicular lump **must** be assumed to be malignant until proven otherwise. The history will highlight the duration of the problem, any risk factors and symptoms of metastatic disease. On examination, the testis is either diffusely enlarged or contains a discrete lump, which is firm and nontender. Systemic examination may reveal evidence of metastases (e.g., a palpable abdominal mass). Examination should include palpation for malignant cervical nodes.

Investigation and Treatment of Testicular Tumours

The outlook for treated testicular tumours, even with metastases, is usually excellent with 5-year survivals exceeding 95%. Investigation and treatment usually take place in parallel. The aims are to confirm the diagnosis, detect any metastases and stage the disease, then to treat according to the stage.

The first investigation for a well man with a testicular lump/mass is scrotal **ultrasonography** (see Fig. 33.6). If this confirms a solid testicular mass, surgical removal of the affected testis (radical orchidectomy) is required. Preliminary staging investigations are usually performed next, including chest x-ray/computed tomography (CT) (to detect hilar node or lung involvement), and CT abdomen and pelvis (to assess retroperitoneal nodes and other possible metastatic sites). Blood levels of **tumour markers** also contribute to both diagnosis and staging, and can be monitored postorchidectomy to assess response to treatment. A standard method of staging testicular tumours is shown in Figs 33.7 and 33.8, and Box 33.3.

Tumour Markers

Overall, tumour markers are raised in around only 50% of patients with testicular tumours (i.e., negative markers do not exclude a diagnosis of testicular cancer), but they do influence treatment choice. **Human chorionic gonadotrophin** (beta-hCG) is secreted by syncytiotrophoblastic cells and levels may rise in any type of testicular germ cell tumour. **Alpha-fetoprotein** (AFP) is produced by yolk sac cells. About 70% of patients with metastatic teratoma have elevated AFP levels, but this marker is not expressed in pure seminoma. **Lactate dehydrogenase** is a useful tool in assessing tumour burden, and is also important in dictating optimal treatment.

Semen Cryopreservation Preoperatively

In addition to orchidectomy, patients commonly need adjuvant treatments postoperatively, including chemotherapy, which can adversely affect fertility. Patients need to be counselled carefully and, if requested, semen can be collected and stored before surgery

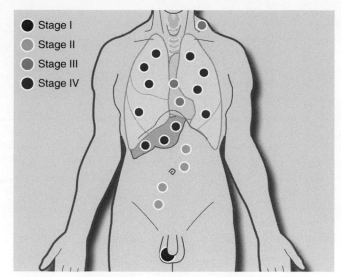

Stage I
Stage II
Stage III
Stage IV

• **Fig. 33.7** Typical Course of Lymph Node Involvement in Testicular Cancer.

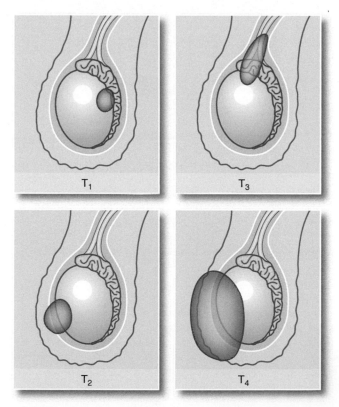

T_1 T_3

T_2 T_4

• **Fig. 33.8** Pathological Staging of Testicular Cancer. T_1 Tumour limited to testis and epididymis and no vascular/lymphatic invasion. T_2 Tumour limited to testis with vascular/lymphatic invasion or invading tunica vaginalis. T_3 Tumour invades spermatic cord. T_4 Tumour invades scrotum.

• **BOX 33.3** **Typical Progression of Metastatic Involvement in Testicular Cancer**

I   Tumour confined to testis
II Retroperitoneal lymph node involvement
III Metastasis above the diaphragm confined to lymph nodes
IV Extralymphatic metastases (usually lungs and liver)

to allow artificial insemination or in-vitro fertilisation later. Patients must undergo testing for HIV, and hepatitis B and C, before semen sample transfer to a long-term frozen storage facility.

Surgery

Radical orchidectomy is the only appropriate treatment for the primary tumour and is usually performed as part of the diagnostic process. The surgical approach is via an inguinal incision to avoid involving scrotal skin. The spermatic cord is temporarily clamped to prevent lymphatic and venous spread of tumour cells and the testis is brought out. If there is diagnostic doubt, a testicular biopsy can be taken and examined immediately by frozen section before proceeding. Otherwise, orchidectomy is performed, dividing the cord at the internal inguinal ring. The other testis is usually unaffected and can be preserved, however biopsy is offered to men at higher risk of a contralateral noninvasive germ cell neoplasm (small testis <12 mL, history of undescended testis or subfertility). Further treatment is planned according to tumour type and stage. A testicular prosthesis can be inserted at the time of orchidectomy or at a later date.

Management of Seminoma

For stage I seminoma, that is, disease confined to the testis, one option is surveillance with intensive follow-up for patients at low risk. However, as up to 20% of men have microscopic metastases that cause relapse after orchidectomy alone, adjuvant chemotherapy with one to two cycles of carboplatin is offered, particularly with higher risk disease (e.g., primary tumours >4 cm, or with rete testis invasion).

For stage IIA disease (i.e., abdominal lymphadenopathy up to 2 cm diameter with satisfactory tumour markers), radical radiotherapy to the ipsilateral paraaortic and iliac nodes gives a cure rate of about 95%. Chemotherapy is an alternative to radiotherapy using BEP (bleomycin, etoposide and cisplatin) or EP (etoposide and cisplatin).

Management of Teratomas and Other Nonseminomatous Germ Cell Tumours

Up to 30% of these patients with stage I disease would relapse within a year of orchidectomy without further treatment. Radiotherapy has no curative role in these types of tumour. There are three options for further treatment for stage I disease, each with similar outcomes.

- Intensive surveillance if low risk (no vascular invasion)
- Immediate adjuvant chemotherapy for high-risk patients (e.g., vascular invasion or a high percentage of embryonal components) with BEP
- Retroperitoneal lymph node dissection for high-risk patients that wish to avoid chemotherapy (but instead risks ejaculatory failure from autonomic nerve damage)

Metastatic disease is treated with chemotherapy; BEP or EP in patients with lower risk disease and BEP or VIP (etoposide, ifosfamide and cisplatin) for patients with intermediate or high-risk disease. Residual disease postchemotherapy should be resected if surgically feasible. The treatment of testicular tumours is summarised in Box 33.4.

Absent Scrotal Testis (Cryptorchidism)

Failure of testicular descent (also known as *undescended testis* or *cryptorchidism*), occurs in 3% to 4% of male infants at birth, falling to about 1% by 12 months. It can be classified as:

- **Retractile**—intermittent active cremasteric reflex, which draws the testis out of scrotum. The testis can be gently 'milked' back

---

- **BOX 33.4 General Principles of Treatment of Testicular Tumours**

1. Removal of the affected testis—usually performed as part of the diagnostic process.
2. Stage I disease (i.e., no metastases)—intensive surveillance or adjuvant chemotherapy (carboplatin for seminoma, BEP for nonseminoma).
3. For seminomas, radiotherapy can be considered for adjuvant treatment of stage I and II, disease.
4. Metastatic disease. For good prognosis patients—three cycles of BEP, or four cycles of EP chemotherapy. For intermediate or poor risk patients—four cycles of BEP chemotherapy.
5. Surgical resection of all residual masses postchemotherapy, where feasible.
6. Retroperitoneal lymph node dissection for residual retroperitoneal disease after treatment for metastatic disease.

BEP, Bleomycin, etoposide and cisplatin; *EP,* etoposide and cisplatin.

---

into the scrotum. Predisposes to 'testicular ascent' (a testis previously in the scrotum retracting into the groin—seen in boys aged 7 to 9 years).

- **Incomplete descent**—testis lies along the normal line of descent; intraabdominal, inguinal or prescrotal (see Fig. 33.5).
- **Ectopic**—abnormal line of testicular descent outside the external ring; testis may be palpable in the perineum, femoral region or base of penis.
- **Absent**— anorchia is rare but can be caused by antenatal intraabdominal torsion.
- **Atrophic**— secondary to trauma or iatrogenic (hernia operation or scrotal surgery).

Management of Maldescent of the Testis

In developed countries, maldescent is usually identified at screening during early childhood and surgically corrected by orchidopexy at a young age (see Ch. 51); to best preserve spermatogenesis, the testis should be surgically placed in the scrotum between 6 months and 1 year. There is some evidence that orchidopexy before the age of 10 years decreases the risk of testicular cancer.

Torsion of the Testis or Epididymal Appendage

Testicular Torsion (Figs 33.9 and 33.10)

In infants, the newly descended testis and its investing tunica vaginalis are mobile within the scrotum. These testes may undergo **extravaginal torsion**, which presents as a hard, swollen testis; those of acute onset should have urgent surgery. Later in childhood, the testis becomes suspended in a near vertical position, anchored by the spermatic cord and by attachments to the posterior scrotal wall. This attachment prevents rotation. Minor anatomical variations can produce a narrow-based pedicle with a horizontal ('bell-clapper') testicular lie that allows the testis to twist about its axis within the tunica (**intravaginal torsion**). When this occurs, pampiniform plexus veins become compressed causing venous congestion. After a few hours, venous infarction occurs unless the torsion is corrected. Thus torsion is an emergency demanding prompt diagnosis and urgent surgical treatment to save the testis.

Torsion presents with a sudden onset of severe testicular pain, often with poorly localised central abdominal pain (because the testis retains its embryological nerve supply) and sometimes vomiting. In the early stages, the affected testis is tender, slightly swollen and drawn up into the neck of the scrotum, where the cord may be palpably thickened. With these features, the diagnosis is seldom in doubt. At a later stage, the scrotal skin becomes red and oedematous, making accurate palpation difficult. At this point, torsion may be difficult to distinguish from acute epididymitis and the scrotum **must** be explored surgically.

Torsion of the Epididymal Appendage (Hydatid of Morgagni)

The hydatid of Morgagni is a small embryological remnant at the upper pole of the testis (see Fig. 33.10). This may undergo torsion and produce symptoms similar to testicular torsion, out of proportion to the small size of the infarcted tissue. Infarction of the hydatid is of no consequence except that it must be distinguished from testicular torsion.

CASE HISTORY

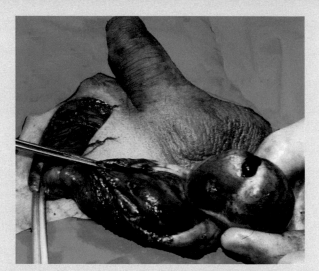

• **Fig. 33.9** Torsion of the Testis. This 15-year-old boy experienced sudden severe lower abdominal pain extending to the scrotum during a football match. A provisional diagnosis of torsion was made and the scrotum explored within 2 hours of the onset of pain. At operation, the testis was twisted 2½ times around on its cord and was near infarction. On untwisting, however, it soon regained normal colour. Both testes were fixed to prevent future torsion.

Management of Suspected Testicular Torsion

Differentiating between acute epididymitis and torsion can be difficult. If a firm diagnosis cannot be reached, surgical exploration is mandatory. Investigations are of little value; Doppler ultrasound examination may be used to show testicular blood flow but results can be misleading.

Urgent operation is usually imperative as delay leads to a risk of testicular necrosis after about 6 hours. A scrotal incision is made and the testis is examined and untwisted. If the testis is black and fails to recover its colour, it is necrotic and should be removed. If some colour is restored, the testis is best left, although it may later atrophy. After untwisting, the testis is sutured to the midline septum and/or inner layer of the scrotal wall with three nonabsorbable sutures placed at different points. In children, it can be placed in a surgically created dartos pouch, under the scrotal skin. Both testes should be secured, as predisposition to torsion is usually bilateral.

Trauma to the Testis

The testes may be injured during contact sports or as a consequence of trauma from a road traffic collision. The dense fibrous capsule investing the testis (tunica albuginea) may remain intact or it may split, but the testis is extremely painful in either case. If the tunica remains intact, a **testicular haematoma** results; if it splits, there is testicular rupture and protrusion of seminiferous tubules. Bleeding into the tunica vaginalis cavity forms a **haematocoele**. Scrotal ultrasound will confirm the diagnosis.

Recommendations are that testicular rupture should be repaired by closing the testicular tunica albuginea capsule after excising nonviable tissue. Large symptomatic haematocoeles should be explored and evacuated where possible to achieve quicker resolution of symptoms, although this is often difficult, as blood infiltrates the adjoining tissues.

Male Sterilisation

Male sterilisation by vasectomy is a simple, effective method of birth control, and can be performed under local anaesthesia. The essential prerequisite is that the couple involved should have

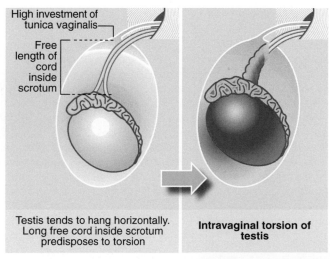

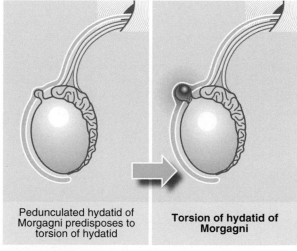

High investment of tunica vaginalis

Free length of cord inside scrotum

Testis tends to hang horizontally. Long free cord inside scrotum predisposes to torsion

Intravaginal torsion of testis

Pedunculated hydatid of Morgagni predisposes to torsion of hydatid

Torsion of hydatid of Morgagni

• **Fig. 33.10** Torsion of the Testis and Hydatid of Morgagni.

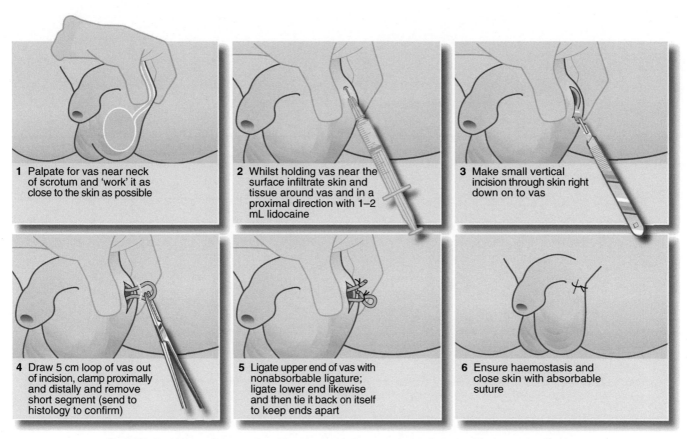

1 Palpate for vas near neck of scrotum and 'work' it as close to the skin as possible

2 Whilst holding vas near the surface infiltrate skin and tissue around vas and in a proximal direction with 1–2 mL lidocaine

3 Make small vertical incision through skin right down on to vas

4 Draw 5 cm loop of vas out of incision, clamp proximally and distally and remove short segment (send to histology to confirm)

5 Ligate upper end of vas with nonabsorbable ligature; ligate lower end likewise and then tie it back on itself to keep ends apart

6 Ensure haemostasis and close skin with absorbable suture

• **Fig. 33.11** Technique of Vasectomy. Note that in this figure, each side is dealt with separately with separate skin incisions. An alternative is to make a midline incision to access both vasa.

completed their family, since reversal is technically difficult and unreliable (vasectomy should be considered irreversible). A technique of vasectomy is illustrated in Fig. 33.11.

Most procedures involve removing a section of the vas (ductus) deferens and ligating and/or cauterising the cut ends. For medicolegal reasons, the nature of the excised portion can be confirmed histologically. Spermatozoa remain in the proximal duct system for several months after vasectomy, and so couples should use alternative forms of contraception until at least two successive sperm counts are negative. These need to be performed 1 month apart, at 16 and 20 weeks postoperatively, and after 20 to 25 ejaculations. Early failure rate is one in 200. Despite correct operative technique and negative sperm counts, there is also a late failure rate of about one case in every 2000 (caused by recanalisation of the vasa).

Early complications of vasectomy include postoperative scrotal haematoma and wound infection. Later, failure of sterilisation may become apparent, or a **sperm granuloma** may present as a tender scrotal swelling near the cut end of the vas for which further excision may be required. Chronic pain can occur in the testis (in up to 10%) and the patient must be warned of this possibility at the time of consent.

Disorders of the Penis

Problems with the foreskin (prepuce) are common and form most penile surgical disorders. Other disorders are uncommon in adults but the most serious is **carcinoma of the penis**. In children, penile disorders are either developmental or minor inflammatory conditions, discussed in Chapter 51. Disorders of the foreskin include **balanoposthitis** (inflammation of the glans and foreskin), **phimosis** (stricture of the preputial meatus resulting in an inability to retract the foreskin), **paraphimosis** (acute constriction of the glans by a tight retracted foreskin) and **balanitis xerotica obliterans** (BXO, idiopathic sclerosis of the foreskin). **Peyronie disease** (idiopathic fibrosis of the corpora cavernosa) is now a frequent presentation in urological clinics (see later). Exclusion of cancer is usually the first step.

Foreskin Problems in Adults

Phimosis

A physiological phimosis is present at birth and during childhood until adhesions between the inner foreskin and glans penis release and the foreskin becomes retractile. Less than 1% will persist into adulthood, and most do not need treatment, unless there are complications, such as recurrent balanitis, urinary infections or BXO, see later.

Adult males present to clinic with a foreskin that will not fully retract, causing pain on erection and intercourse. Such phimosis is usually caused by fibrosis of the foreskin and may be caused by chronic or recurrent low-grade *Candida* infection or BXO (see later). The condition may be accompanied by stenosis of the urethral meatus, also caused by recurrent inflammation and fibrosis. Topical steroids can be tried, but definitive treatment usually involves circumcision; a preputioplasty (or foreskin widening operation) is sometimes successful.

Balanoposthitis (Balanitis)

The term balanoposthitis refers to overt inflammation of the glans penis and foreskin (Greek: *balanos* gland, *posthe* foreskin); it is the

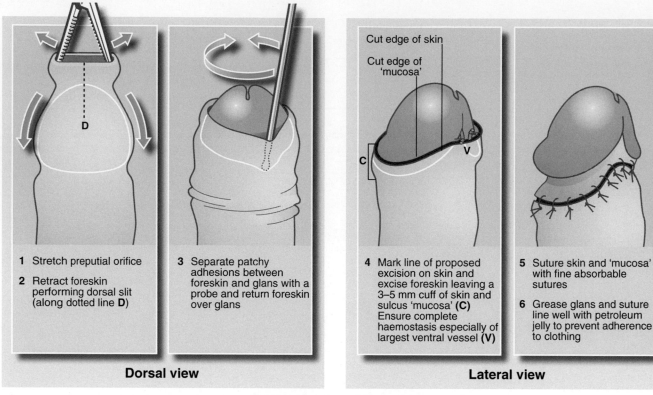

1 Stretch preputial orifice

2 Retract foreskin performing dorsal slit (along dotted line **D**)

3 Separate patchy adhesions between foreskin and glans with a probe and return foreskin over glans

Dorsal view

Cut edge of skin

Cut edge of 'mucosa'

4 Mark line of proposed excision on skin and excise foreskin leaving a 3–5 mm cuff of skin and sulcus 'mucosa' **(C)** Ensure complete haemostasis especially of largest ventral vessel **(V)**

5 Suture skin and 'mucosa' with fine absorbable sutures

6 Grease glans and suture line well with petroleum jelly to prevent adherence to clothing

Lateral view

• **Fig. 33.12** Technique of Circumcision.

correct term but the short form 'balanitis' has passed into common usage. The condition occurs most commonly in children. Inflammation alone is most often caused by *Candida* or faecal bacteria, but this problem rarely reaches the surgeon.

BXO (also known as *lichen sclerosus et atrophicus*) is a fibrotic condition of the foreskin of unknown aetiology. It produces a thickened, stenosed, often depigmented foreskin, which is often adherent to the glans. Circumcision is usually curative. As many as 25% of children with phimosis have this condition. The process can involve the urethral meatus and may cause stenosis, sometimes requiring meatotomy or meatoplasty at the time of circumcision. More rarely, it results in a urethral stricture likely to require urethroplasty.

Paraphimosis

If a phimotic foreskin is forcibly retracted, the tight meatal band may lodge in the coronal sulcus making reduction impossible; this is known as *paraphimosis*. Progressive oedema of the glans penis and foreskin then exacerbates the difficulty of reduction. It may occur at any age, but is particularly common in elderly men, in whom the foreskin is not correctly pulled forwards after retraction for catheterisation or washing the glans. Paraphimosis also occurs in children and adolescents experimenting with foreskin retraction or cleaning beneath it. In most cases, the foreskin can be reduced by firm manual compression of the glans and foreskin. Local anaesthetic jelly is applied first for lubrication and pain relief. A local anaesthetic penile subcutaneous ring block is sometimes needed—of note, remember **never** to use adrenaline in the penis, as this can cause necrosis. Sometimes, incising the tight ring may be necessary under local or general anaesthesia to effect reduction (a dorsal slit). If reduced manually, a circumcision or preputioplasty (in which the phimotic band is incised longitudinally and the skin sutured transversely), is usually offered at a later

date, when the oedema and inflammation have resolved, to avoid recurrence of the problem.

Circumcision

Circumcision has been a widespread practice in many communities for religious or cultural reasons. However, in many healthcare settings, it is no longer offered routinely to infants and children, to avoid unnecessary complications in boys, who will generally gain a fully retractile foreskin in adulthood.

Circumcision is reserved for unresolved phimosis, recurrent balanitis and BXO. Reported benefits of circumcision include reduction in the risk of penile cancer and transmission of HIV, and it can be beneficial in some boys with recurrent urinary tract infections associated with anatomical risk factors such as significant vesicoureteric reflux or posterior urethral valves. A surgical technique is shown in Fig. 33.12. Remember to use only **bipolar** diathermy on the penis. During the operation, the urethral meatus should be checked for stenosis. If present, a meatotomy may be required. An occasional early postoperative complication is haemorrhage, which usually requires surgical re-exploration. Postoperative bleeding can best be prevented by meticulous haemostasis at operation.

Peyronie Disease

This disease of unknown aetiology occurs most commonly in men aged 40 to 60 years. Some cases are thought to result from penile trauma during sexual activity and others are associated with Dupuytren contracture of the palmar fascia. Slowly progressive asymmetrical fibrotic plaques develop in the fascia surrounding the corpora cavernosa. The corpus spongiosum, including the glans, is spared. The plaques may become calcified. The condition causes the penis to bend towards the affected side on erection, making intercourse difficult and painful. There may be spontaneous partial resolution

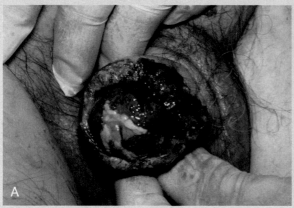
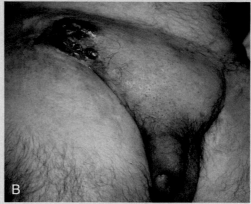

• **Fig. 33.13** Carcinoma of the Penis. (A) An obvious carcinoma of the penis, revealed when the foreskin is retracted. (B) Unfortunately, this patient already had extensive spread to the inguinal lymph nodes.

with time, therefore surgery is usually deferred for 12 months after initial presentation. Medical treatments are sometimes used in the early stages of Peyronie disease, such as vitamin E or Potassium parraminobenzoate (POTABA), but are of limited benefit.

Severe persistent cases require surgery. **Nesbit operation** involves creating pleats in the corpus on the contralateral side; this results in unavoidable penile shortening. The Lue procedure involves excision of the plaques, which are replaced by a patch of tissue, such as processed human or bovine pericardium or small intestinal submucosa; tunica vaginalis and saphenous vein grafts were used previously. The Lue operation is reserved for more significant curvature and preserves penile length but has a higher risk of impotence. Either procedure may restore symmetrical erection. Penile prosthetic implants may be required if there is associated erectile dysfunction not responsive to medication.

Carcinoma of the Penis

Carcinoma of the penis is rare in developed countries and almost unknown in circumcised males. Poor hygiene and accumulation of smegma are suspected aetiological factors, but there is growing evidence of a viral aetiology linked to that of carcinoma of the uterine cervix in females (human papilloma virus).

Histologically, the tumours are predominantly squamous cell carcinomas, usually well differentiated, which arise from the inner surface of the foreskin or the glans penis near the coronal sulcus. The tumour invades locally and tends to penetrate the corpora cavernosa and distal urethra (Fig. 33.13A). Metastatic spread is to inguinal lymph nodes (see Fig. 33.13B). **Erythroplasia of Queyrat** is the term given to severe dysplasia and carcinoma-in-situ of the glans or inner surface of the foreskin that may represent a precursor of invasive carcinoma.

Most cases of carcinoma of the penis are found in older men, with a peak in the sixth decade of life. The disease is usually well advanced before an irregular lump, bleeding or discharge is noticed. In uncircumcised males, the lesion may be hidden by the foreskin. Fig. 33.14 illustrates staging of the disease.

Local surgical excision or 'glansectomy' is often performed, with reconstructive surgery if feasible. Circumcision is used to treat prepucial lesions. In advanced cases, partial or complete penile amputation (with formation of a perineal urostomy to pass urine or suprapubic catheter) and dissection of involved inguinal lymph nodes, may be required. Radiotherapy is a nonsurgical alternative for all stages. Palliation in stage IV disease can be with radiotherapy or chemotherapy with salvage surgery.

Priapism

Priapism is an abnormally prolonged penile erection lasting 4 hours or more. It can occur without sexual stimulation, and does not resolve after ejaculation. The abnormality affects only the **corpora cavernosa** and is caused by a disturbance of mechanisms that control penile detumescence. The corpus spongiosum surrounding the urethra and forming the glans penis is not affected, and the glans remains flaccid.

There are three types of priapism. **High-flow (arterial or non-ischaemic) priapism** occurs when an artery ruptures into the lacunar spaces of the corpora cavernosa. This is often associated with trauma and is relatively uncommon and painless. Compared with venous priapism, there is less tumescence and it is less painful. **Low-flow (venous or ischaemic) priapism** is caused by prolonged corporeal venous stasis caused by occlusion of the venous outlet mechanism ('veno-occlusive' priapism). This is a urological emergency as it eventually results in penile ischaemia. It is painful and, unless treated, results in long-term fibrosis and impotence (loss of the ability to achieve an erection). In veno-occlusive priapism, tissue changes that will lead to fibrosis are already evident within 24 hours, whereas there is no such change in arterial priapism. The most common cause is a side-effect of injected intracavernosal drugs used to treat erectile dysfunction.

Treatment of veno-occlusive priapism must be prompt to avoid long-term erectile problems. Ice packs and external compression are a useful temporising measure but usually will not give long-term relief. Aspiration of blood from the cavernosa using a butterfly needle is the next step. Intracavernous injection of an alpha-adrenergic agonist (phenylephrine) or oral terbutaline, a beta-2-adrenergic receptor agonist, usually produces detumescence. If these measures are unsuccessful, operative management by means of a surgical shunt may be necessary but results are sometimes disappointing.

Recurrent or stuttering priapism is uncommon and associated with sickle cell disease. It presents with intermittent,

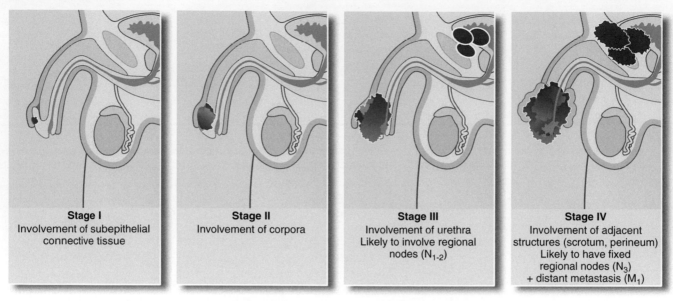

Stage I	Stage II	Stage III	Stage IV
Involvement of subepithelial connective tissue	Involvement of corpora	Involvement of urethra Likely to involve regional nodes (N_{1-2})	Involvement of adjacent structures (scrotum, perineum) Likely to have fixed regional nodes (N_3) + distant metastasis (M_1)

• **Fig. 33.14** Stages in the Spread of Carcinoma of the Penis.

ischaemic short-lived episodes of priapism, which become painful if prolonged. Management involves optimising the underlying sickle cell condition and prevention of future episodes.

Erectile Dysfunction

Erectile dysfunction (or impotence) is the persistent or recurrent inability to gain or maintain an erection sufficient for satisfactory sexual intercourse. It becomes more common with increasing age and is usually multifactorial in aetiology. Erectile dysfunction is not only distressing, but can be the first symptom of a significant underlying, but as yet unrecognised, medical condition, such as coronary heart disease, new onset diabetes, dyslipidaemia or hypogonadism (testosterone deficiency). A clear history will identify any known risk factors for erectile dysfunction, such as pre-existing diabetes mellitus, smoking, cardiovascular disease, hypertension, pelvic and penile surgery, trauma, low testosterone and previous radiotherapy. Basic assessment includes a blood pressure check, examination of the external genitalia and rectal examination. Blood testing for early morning testosterone levels, fasting glucose and lipid profile levels are important; further tests

are considered on an individual risk basis and include prostate specific antigen to assess for prostate cancer risk, and sex hormone binding globulin, luteinising hormone, FSH and prolactin levels to look for contributing hormonal abnormalities. After any reversible factors have been treated, the first-line drug therapy is with phosphodiesterase type-5 inhibitors, such as sildenafil (Viagra) and tadalafil (Cialis), usually taken on demand. If these fail at their maximal doses or are not tolerated, alternatives include intraurethral therapy with alprostadil pellet (MUSE) or intracavernosal injection therapy with alprostadil (Caverjet). If pharmacotherapy fails or is contraindicated, vacuum erection devices can be applied to encourage blood flow into the penis, and the erection is then maintained with a constriction band at the base of the penis. Surgical options are considered after other treatments are ineffective or unsuitable. They include insertion of a malleable or inflatable penile prosthesis, which consists of expandable cylinders inserted into the corpora cavernosa, and an activation pump placed in the scrotum to use on demand. Whilst success and satisfaction rates are high, complications can be significant with infection, mechanical failure and erosion requiring implant removal.

34

Symptoms, Signs and Investigation of Urinary Tract Disorders

Introduction

Urinary tract disorders are common and comprise a significant part of the workload of General Practitioners, general physicians, paediatricians and surgeons. Prostate disorders account for at least half of the work in urological surgery. The main conditions are benign prostatic enlargement (BPE) caused by prostatic hyperplasia, affecting about 10% of ageing males in Western countries, and prostatic carcinoma, which is now the second most common cancer in men worldwide and the commonest cancer diagnosed in men in developed countries. The remaining surgical disorders of kidney and urinary tract can be divided into five broad groups: tumours, stone disease (**urolithiasis**), infections, congenital abnormalities and finally, local and systemic disorders secondarily involving the urinary tract.

This chapter deals with the symptoms, signs, approach to investigation and diagnosis of urinary tract disease. The various disease entities are then discussed in the five following chapters.

Symptoms of Urinary Tract Disease

Urinary symptoms may be caused by intrinsic disease of the urinary tract or by disease of other structures.

Symptoms Caused by Intrinsic Disease of the Urinary Tract

Outflow of urine from the kidney may become impeded by urinary tract obstruction, and this may secondarily interfere with renal function. Chronic obstruction to bladder outflow or bilateral upper tract obstruction may lead to renal failure, often without any localising symptoms.

BPE (also referred to as *benign prostatic hyperplasia* or *BPH* once the histology is known) is the most common prostatic disorder, and usually presents with symptoms of bladder outflow obstruction (i.e., hesitancy or straining to initiate voiding, poor flow, incomplete emptying or urinary retention) and sometimes with haematuria. Prostatic obstruction predisposes to bladder infections and stones secondary to incomplete bladder emptying, and the patient may present with the consequent symptoms.

Prostate cancer may present with bladder outflow obstruction similar to BPE or it may be discovered at an asymptomatic stage at a medical check-up, by digital rectal examination (DRE) or by a blood test (prostate specific antigen, PSA). Some cases are first diagnosed because of symptoms of metastases, such as bone pain.

Chronic prostatitis may be bacterial or abacterial and usually presents with a chronic perineal ache. In the acute form, bacterial prostatitis can present as a systemic illness (or even gram-negative sepsis) with urinary symptoms and an exquisitely tender prostate. Occasionally, a prostatic abscess develops.

The important urinary tract tumours, stone diseases and infections are outlined in Table 34.1. Any of these may present with haematuria. Disorders which cause urinary stasis also predispose to urinary tract infection.

TABLE 34.1 | **Pathophysiology and Clinical Features of Urinary Tract Tumours, Stones and Infections**

Disease	Pathophysiology	Clinical Features
TUMOURS		
Renal cell carcinoma —fairly common	Occurs in adults. Derived from renal tubular cells	Presents either incidentally (e.g., on CT scan) or with symptoms of haematuria, a mass, or constitutional signs, such as pyrexia or polycythaemia or is asymptomatic
Nephroblastoma (Wilms tumour; see Ch. 51)—rare	Developmental origin; usually diagnosed before age 5 years	Presents as an abnormal mass with or without pain and haematuria
Urothelial carcinoma (UC) —common	May arise in transitional epithelium anywhere in urinary tract from pelvicalyceal system to urethra, but most common in bladder	Usually presents with haematuria. Predisposes to urinary tract infections. May cause ureteric obstruction
Squamous cell carcinoma (SCC)—very rare	Arises in metaplastic squamous epithelium. Secondary to chronic stone or schistosomal irritation, especially in bladder. Also arises de novo in squamous epithelium of distal urethra	Bladder SCC is often asymptomatic until it reaches an advanced stage; tends to be muscle-invasive at presentation with urinary symptoms, infection, haematuria, and pain
Adenocarcinoma of bladder—very rare	Arises from columnar epithelium of urachal remnant	Features include haematuria and urinary symptoms; around a third have lymph node metastases at presentation
Stone Disease		
In general	Stones in situ may cause irritation of urinary tract epithelium	Present as pain or haematuria or recurrent infection
Stones may develop in pelvicalyceal system or bladder. Pelvicalyceal stones can pass into the ureter—very common	Chronic—renal stones may cause chronic pelviureteric or ureteric obstruction either directly or by causing fibrotic strictures Acute—renal stones may cause ureteric obstruction as they pass down the tract	Present with chronic pain (caused by back pressure) or recurrent infection Present as acute colicky pain often with renal tenderness (renal or ureteric colic). Infection may supervene, destroying the kidney if untreated
Infections		
'Common' infections caused by bowel organisms	Infection develops either via bloodstream (haematogenous) or lower urinary tract stasis predisposes to infection	Typically, present with dysuria and frequency with or without haematuria. Any urinary tract abnormality or stasis predisposes to infection Ascending infection may cause pyelonephritis, that is, infection of kidney and renal pelvis
Tuberculosis—uncommon	Kidney involvement via bloodstream from pulmonary or other primary disease. May spread via urine to ureters and bladder	May present as haematuria, persistent sterile pyuria, or as an incidental finding in pulmonary tuberculosis
Urinary schistosomiasis (also known as bilharzia)—very common in some developing countries; probably the world's most common cause of haematuria	Induces chronic inflammation and fibrosis in bladder wall leading to gross bladder distortion, stones and sometimes squamous cell carcinoma	Presents with haematuria and various symptoms of infection and bladder fibrosis
Urethritis	Commonly caused by sexually transmitted infections, for example, gonococcus or *Chlamydia*	Presents with urethral discharge and dysuria

CT, Computed tomography.

Congenital abnormalities may involve the kidneys, ureters, bladder, urethra and genitalia, either alone or in combination. Most of the serious abnormalities are recognised antenatally by ultrasound, at birth or in early childhood. The exceptions are **polycystic disease** and **medullary sponge kidney**, which usually present in adulthood. Less serious congenital abnormalities, such as duplex systems, may predispose to urinary tract infections because of abnormal flow dynamics. These abnormalities may be discovered at any age during investigation of recurrent urinary infections. Congenital disorders, which present mainly in adulthood, are discussed in Chapter 39 and those presenting mainly in childhood in Chapter 51.

Urinary Symptoms Caused by Non-urinary Disease

The urinary tract sometimes becomes secondarily involved in local inflammatory conditions, such as Crohn disease or diverticular disease. Fistulae may form, resulting in passage of flatus and/or faeces in the urine (pneumaturia and faecuria). Pelvic tumours in women can present with urinary retention. Retroperitoneal fibrosis, diverticulitis, tumours of the prostate, cervix or colon, and sometimes aortic or iliac aneurysms may secondarily involve the ureters and cause upper urinary tract obstruction.

The Common Symptoms of Urinary Tract Disease

These fall into eight categories:
- abdominal pain
- passage of blood in the urine (**haematuria**)
- pain associated with micturition (**dysuria**)
- disorders of micturition, such as frequency or hesitancy
- retention of urine (acute or chronic)
- urinary incontinence
- passage of bowel gas in the urine (**pneumaturia**)
- passage of blood in the semen (**haemospermia**)

Abdominal Pain

Urinary tract disorders may cause abdominal pain with or without urinary symptoms.

Pain Arising From the Kidneys and Upper Tract

Both renal inflammation and stretching of the renal capsule cause pain in the renal angle, the posterior gap between the lowest rib and iliac crest. This area may also become tender to palpation or percussion. Renal stones, tumours or polycystic disease may cause dull and persistent loin pain even without obstruction.

In acute infections, such as pyelonephritis (affecting renal pelvis and kidney) or bladder infection, the pain is severe and is usually associated with systemic features and urinary tract symptoms.

Acute upper ureteric obstruction and distension of the pelvicalyceal system produce excruciating loin pain. The pain is colicky (resulting from powerful ureteric peristalsis) and often radiates to the hypochondrium (right or left upper quadrant of the abdomen) or groin (Fig. 34.1). This pain is known as *renal* or *ureteric colic*. When obstruction is low in the ureter, the pain may radiate to the genitalia.

Pain Arising From the Bladder and Lower Tract

Pain originating in the bladder (e.g., in cystitis) is experienced in the suprapubic area. Pain may be referred to the penis or vulva if the bladder trigone is involved. In adults, urinary symptoms, such as dysuria and frequency, are usually present as well, but children may have no localising symptoms or complain only of pain, making the diagnosis less obvious. Dysuria is usually the predominant symptom of urethral disorders, but pain arising in the male urethra (e.g., in sexually transmitted infections) is usually referred to the tip of the penis. Finally, the pain of prostatic inflammation (prostatitis) is usually felt deep in the perineum. The prostate is tender on rectal examination.

Pain Simulating Urinary Tract Disease

Pain from other abdominal pathology may sometimes mimic pain arising from the urinary tract. Acute appendicitis may present with suprapubic pain, and biliary tract pain may be referred to the right thoracolumbar region, while posterior duodenal ulcers and pancreatic disease may cause pain in the central lumbar region. An expanding or leaking abdominal aortic aneurysm may sometimes mimic urinary tract disease, particularly if a ureter is compressed, causing flank pain, which can be mistaken for renal colic. Diseases of the thoracolumbar spine, such as metastatic cancer, tuberculosis, spondylosis and disc lesions may also simulate upper urinary tract disorders. Suspected renal colic with a local rash is usually caused by shingles (herpes zoster); the rash may not appear for several days after the onset of pain; perineal zoster may cause retention of urine. In women, pain arising from the ovaries or

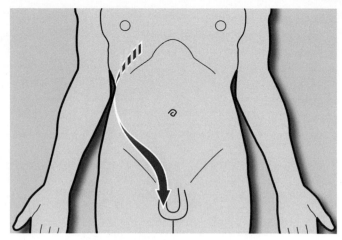

• **Fig. 34.1** Renal Pain and Its Referral.

genital tract (e.g., pelvic inflammatory disease) may be confused with bladder pain.

Haematuria

Patients may notice blood or even clots in the urine (**frank or visible haematuria**) and this needs to be distinguished from vaginal bleeding. More often, blood is discovered on 'dipstick' testing or microscopy of a midstream urine specimen (**microscopic or nonvisible haematuria**). Haematuria is often episodic rather than persistent, whatever the cause. 'Dipstick' testing for haematuria is extremely sensitive and hence yields many false positive results.

Causes of Haematuria (Fig. 34.2 for Renal Causes)

Tumours are a common cause of visible and non-visible haematuria and must be suspected even if another possible cause is found. Haematuria from tumours is typically painless, although upper urinary tract bleeding can cause 'clot colic'. However, carcinoma-in-situ of the bladder, a dysplastic condition with a high probability of progression to invasive carcinoma, usually presents with irritative voiding, dysuria, and haematuria, often with a finding of sterile pyuria (pus cell without proven bacteria) on urine testing. Irritation from infection or stones may also cause bleeding, but is usually accompanied by pain or dysuria. If the urethra is obstructed by prostatic enlargement, straining at micturition may cause bleeding from dilated veins at the bladder neck.

Trauma to a normal kidney may cause frank haematuria if substantial force has been applied, but non-visible haematuria is common after minor trauma in contact sports and rarely indicates significant injury. Enlarged kidneys are more susceptible to trauma, whatever the primary pathology. In hydronephrosis or polycystic kidneys, minor blunt trauma may cause gross haematuria.

Sometimes, urine becomes red with haemoglobin rather than blood. In young people this may be induced by vigorous exercise, such as jogging (**exercise haemoglobinuria** and **haematuria**). These patients are believed to have defective red cell membranes, which makes them more vulnerable to trauma. Exercise haemoglobinuria is self-limiting and requires no treatment.

Haematuria also occurs in renal parenchymal inflammation, such as glomerulonephritis or arteritis. Haematuria may be caused by microemboli impacting in the kidneys, as in atrial fibrillation or infective endocarditis. Any urinary tract disorder with a potential for haematuria is more likely to be revealed when a patient is on anticoagulant therapy or develops a bleeding diathesis.

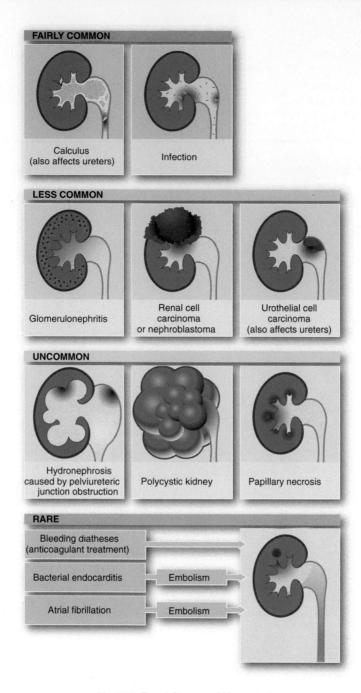

FAIRLY COMMON

Calculus (also affects ureters)

Infection

LESS COMMON

Glomerulonephritis

Renal cell carcinoma or nephroblastoma

Urothelial cell carcinoma (also affects ureters)

UNCOMMON

Hydronephrosis caused by pelviureteric junction obstruction

Polycystic kidney

Papillary necrosis

RARE

Bleeding diatheses (anticoagulant treatment)

Bacterial endocarditis → Embolism

Atrial fibrillation → Embolism

• **Fig. 34.2** Renal Causes of Haematuria.

Diagnostic Features of Haematuria

The stage of micturition at which blood appears is sometimes diagnostically useful. Blood from the kidneys, ureters or bladder wall will completely mix with the urine, and be present throughout the urinary stream. Urethral bleeding may leak out independently of micturition, or be seen only at the beginning or end of the urinary stream. Blood arising from the bladder neck or posterior urethra may sometimes present as terminal haematuria. Gross bleeding may result in the passage of clots.

Haematuria on dipstick testing can be confirmed by urine microscopy for red blood cells, and checked for infection by culture and sensitivity. Microscopic haematuria may represent a noteworthy lesion anywhere in the urinary tract and must be taken seriously; however, a significant cause is found in only 5% to 25% of patients.

Dysuria

Dysuria describes pain or discomfort on micturition, often accompanied by difficulty in voiding. The pain is often described as 'burning' or 'like passing shards of glass'. Any irritation of the urethra may cause dysuria. The most common cause is urinary tract infection, but recent urethral instrumentation or catheterisation can also cause dysuria.

Disorders of Micturition

The normal bladder has a capacity of 350 to 500 mL. When capacity is reached, there is a conscious perception of bladder fullness (mediated via the periaqueductal grey matter in the pons),

TABLE 34.2   Symptoms of Disorders of Micturition

Symptom	Description	Causes
Urinary frequency	Frequent passage of small quantities of urine but with normal daily urine volume (unlike in polyuria)	**Bladder irritation** — infection (common), carcinoma-in-situ of bladder **Incomplete bladder emptying** — bladder outlet obstruction, neurological (e.g., multiple sclerosis) **Overactive bladder (detrusor overactivity)** **Small or indistensible bladder** — surgery, fibrosis (e.g., tuberculosis, schistosomiasis, radiotherapy) **Inflammatory cystitis**—for example, bladder pain syndrome/interstitial cystitis, which is also associated with chronic pain.
Nocturia	The need to pass urine at night, usually accompanied by frequency or polyuria	**Prostatic enlargement** **Cardiac failure** — peripheral oedema returning to systemic circulation when supine (nocturnal polyuria) **Old age** — enhanced renal blood flow when recumbent **Drugs** — for example, some calcium channel blockers
Urgency	Sudden desire to void, may result in incontinence	**Cystitis** — bladder neck irritation **Overactive bladder** **Prostatic enlargement** — abnormal entry of urine into proximal urethra, high detrusor pressure caused by bladder outlet obstruction
Hesitancy	Difficulty in initiating micturition	**Prostatic enlargement** — insufficient urine entry into proximal urethra to cause sphincter relaxation **Psychosomatic** — often situational (e.g., in a urinal) in young males
Poor urinary stream	Slow or interrupted urine stream	**Urethral compression** — prostatic enlargement, bladder neck hypertrophy **Urethral stricture** — because of inflammation and scarring **Underactive bladder** —increased risk with age
Postmicturition dribbling	Continuous flow of urine drops at the end of micturition and may amount to incontinence	**Weak bulbospongiosus muscle** — incomplete emptying of urethra; pooling of urine in bulbar urethra **Abnormal sphincter function**
Urinary incontinence	Involuntary loss of urine	**Overactive bladder** —causes urgency incontinence **Urethral sphincter weakness or defect** —causes stress incontinence **Anatomical defect** —iatrogenic fistula between bladder and vagina causing continuous urine leak

and at a socially acceptable time, the voiding reflex is triggered via the pontine micturition centre in the brain stem. Micturition is normally initiated by sphincter relaxation coupled with detrusor contraction, and the bladder empties. There are seven common symptoms of disorders of micturition:

- urinary frequency
- nocturia
- urgency
- hesitancy
- poor urinary stream
- postmicturition dribbling
- urinary incontinence

Features and common causes of these symptoms are summarised in Table 34.2.

Lower Urinary Tract Symptoms

These are divided into voiding (or obstructive) symptoms: hesitancy, poor stream, incomplete bladder emptying and terminal dribbling; and storage (or irritative) symptoms: frequency, nocturia, urgency and urge incontinence. Combinations of these symptoms can occur in prostatic obstruction; similar symptoms also occur in bladder neck obstruction, urethral stricture, bladder calculi and lower urinary tract infection. The severity of symptoms in men is assessed using the International Prostate Symptom Score (see Box 35.1, p. 473).

Retention of Urine

Urinary retention is the inability to void when the bladder is full. It occurs when the sphincter is unable to relax or when there is a prostatic or urethral obstruction, and the causes may coexist. Less commonly, it can occur when the bladder smooth muscle (detrusor) is unable to generate a contraction. This is termed **bladder underactivity** and contributing causes include increasing age, neurological disorders (such as multiple sclerosis, spinal cord injury (SCI), Parkinson disease, stroke), diabetes, a consequence of prolonged bladder outlet obstruction or pelvic surgery, and as a side effect of medication (i.e., anticholinergic drugs used to relax the detrusor muscle in bladder overactivity).

Acute Retention

Acute urinary retention is often very painful and occasionally occurs in normal individuals, usually males, particularly postoperatively, when fluid overload, drugs, pain, the supine posture, anxiety or embarrassment are responsible. Similar factors may precipitate an episode in men with asymptomatic prostatic enlargement. Occasionally, acute retention is caused by an obstructing blood clot (**clot retention**) or stone.

In females, acute urinary retention may also occur in pregnancy, if the enlarging uterus becomes wedged in the pelvis at about 14 weeks' gestation. Large ovarian cysts or uterine fibroids may cause similar obstruction. Other possible causes include neurological disorders, such as sacral nerve injury, multiple sclerosis, and following stress incontinence surgery (which increases the resistance of the bladder outlet and urethra). **Fowler syndrome** is an uncommon condition, which presents in young women as acute urinary retention caused by an underactive bladder, but is caused by a hypercontractile, non-relaxing external urethral sphincter. It is associated with urethral or pelvic pain, which limits the ability to tolerate urethral catheterisation. Alternative options to drain the bladder include insertion of a suprapubic catheter, or formation of a Mitrofanoff channel, which uses the appendix to provide a route to pass a catheter from the umbilicus or abdominal wall directly into the bladder, bypassing the urethra. Sacral nerve neuromodulation techniques can also be used to relax the sphincter to allow spontaneous voiding.

Chronic Retention

Chronic retention is often painless and occurs with structural or functional abnormalities of bladder muscle or the sphincter mechanism. Less commonly, it is caused by persistent urethral obstruction. In chronic retention, voiding of urine is often incomplete. The problem progresses until the residual volume approaches maximum bladder capacity. Voiding then usually occurs by 'overflow' and the bladder usually becomes abnormally distended. When obstruction is prolonged and severe, the bladder muscle hypertrophies, bladder diverticula may develop, and back pressure on the kidneys can cause uraemia and renal failure (high-pressure chronic retention). At any stage, complete cessation of flow, that is, **acute-on-chronic retention**, may be precipitated by overfilling (often alcohol induced), urinary tract infection or constipation. The most common cause of chronic retention is bladder outlet obstruction caused by a hypertrophied bladder neck or prostatic enlargement. It may also be caused by lower spinal neurological problems, for example, central protrusion of lumbar intervertebral discs damaging the S2, 3, 4 detrusor muscle innervation.

Urinary Incontinence

Involuntary passage of urine is a distressing and socially debilitating symptom. During filling, the detrusor muscle relaxes so the intravesical pressure does not rise until bladder capacity is

> • **BOX 34.1** Causes of Incontinence of Urine
>
> **Loss of Cortical Control (Suprapontine) Causing Neurogenic Bladder Overactivity**
> - Stoke
> - Dementia
> - Multiple sclerosis
>
> **Suprasacral Spine Disorders (Between Pons and L5) Causing Neurogenic Bladder Overactivity**
> - Spinal cord injury
> - Disc prolapse
> - Myelomeningocele
>
> **Sacral and Peripheral Nerve Abnormalities Causing Stress Incontinence**
> - Low spinal cord injury
> - Cauda equina
> - Diabetes
> - Pelvic surgery
>
> **Sphincter Abnormalities Causing Stress Incontinence**
> - Pregnancy and childbirth
> - Prostatectomy
> - Tumour invasion
> - Urethral trauma
>
> **Bladder Abnormalities**
> - Contracted (high pressure, stiff) bladder
>
> **Anatomical Abnormalities**
> - Vesicovaginal fistula
> - Rare congenital abnormalities (i.e., ectopic ureter)

approached. Once the bladder is filled, voiding occurs by coordinated detrusor contraction and sphincter relaxation. Both are mediated via a spinal reflex at the level of S2, 3, 4. Superimposed on this system is an inhibitory mechanism under cortical (conscious) control, to delay voiding, if it is socially inappropriate. Conscious control, including nocturnal control, develops during early childhood. Night-time incontinence is known as **nocturnal enuresis**.

The pathophysiology of incontinence can be divided into categories based on disorders of structure and function, which are described later and summed up in Box 34.1. Some disease processes may produce incontinence by more than one mechanism. Urinary incontinence can be caused by a known underlying neurological problem (i.e., 'neurogenic'), or 'idiopathic' for non-neurogenic patients, or where the cause is unknown.

Loss of Cortical Control (Suprapontine Injury)

Loss of inhibitory control over reflex voiding may occur in disease of the cortex, such as the dementias, stroke and multiple sclerosis. This results generally in a low pressure, 'safe' bladder, however, patients can experience bladder overactivity and inappropriate voiding caused by loss of coordination of bladder and sphincter function.

Suprasacral Cord Conditions

These include disorders, such as SCI, spina bifida and disc prolapse, which can result in an 'unsafe', high-pressure bladder with risk to the upper tracts. Patients can experience neuropathic bladder overactivity, a stiff (poorly compliant) bladder, autonomic dysreflexia (in SCI at T6 level or above), or detrusor sphincter dyssynergia, whereby the bladder and external urethral sphincter both contract at the same time, resulting in dysfunctional or obstructed voiding. Careful assessment of both bladder function and upper urinary tracts is required in neuropathic patients, and treatment of any high bladder pressures (with medication, surgery or catheterisation) is essential to manage symptoms and preserve renal function.

Disorders of Sacral Reflex Control of Detrusor and Sphincter Function by Sacral Cord or Peripheral Nerve Damage

If the sacral reflex arc is damaged on either afferent or efferent sides, reflex contraction of the detrusor and relaxation of the sphincter are lost. This may occur in low SCI, cauda equina, diabetic neuropathy, pelvic organ surgery or invasive pelvic tumours. This results in a low pressure, 'safe' bladder with poor innervations of the external urethral sphincter, resulting in bladder distention, risk of urinary retention and urinary incontinence. The large residual urine volume predisposes to infection and should be emptied regularly if possible, by techniques such as clean intermittent self-catheterisation.

Idiopathic Bladder Overactivity and Urge Incontinence

With increasing age, overactive bladder symptoms (urinary frequency, urgency and leak of urine before reaching the toilet) become more common in both sexes. This results from uninhibited contractions of the detrusor muscle during the filling/storage phase of micturition when the bladder is not at full capacity, resulting in irritative symptoms and urgency incontinence.

Untreated **bladder infection** produces excessive sensory irritation resulting in similar overactive bladder symptoms, usually with other systemic symptoms, such as fever and dysuria.

Persistent bladder outflow obstruction caused by prostatic enlargement can initially produce both voiding symptoms and storage symptoms, but over time, can result in progressive stretching of the bladder and damage to the voiding reflex. The result can be a hugely distended, flaccid, **underactive bladder**, with or without dribbling overflow incontinence. New onset **nocturnal enuresis** is a 'red flag' symptom in adult men, as it may signify high-pressure chronic retention and risk of renal impairment. The treatment is bladder disobstruction (initially, with a catheter and later, with bladder outlet surgery).

Structural Abnormalities of the Bladder or Sphincter

The most common condition in this category is **stress incontinence**, in which there is usually a combination of a weak sphincter coupled with a degree of bladder neck and urethral hypermobility in women. Any sudden increase in pressure on the bladder (such as coughing, sneezing or laughing) causes small quantities of urine to leak out. Stress incontinence is usually more common in parous women and can result from pelvic floor damage during pregnancy and childbirth. There is often a degree of uterine prolapse and cystocoele. Various operations can alleviate this.

Transurethral resection of prostate for urinary symptoms or radical prostatectomy for prostate cancer can result in damage to the sphincter in men, as may locally invasive tumours or pelvic fractures involving the proximal urethra. Tuberculosis, radiotherapy and bladder pain syndrome (interstitial cystitis) in its severest form may cause severe bladder contraction and frequency to the point of incontinence.

Incontinence is a feature of several rare congenital abnormalities, such as epispadias or an ectopic ureter opening below the

---

> #### ● BOX 34.2 Causes of Vesicocolic Fistula and Pneumaturia
>
> - Diverticular disease and pericolic abscess bursting into bladder (most common cause)
> - Carcinoma of bladder invading colon
> - Colonic carcinoma invading bladder
> - Crohn disease inflammation fistulating into bladder

sphincter mechanism. These should be excluded in a child who fails to develop continence. An iatrogenic cause of complete incontinence in women (the patient reports never having a dry pad) is a fistula between the bladder and vagina (**vesicovaginal fistula**), which can be caused by prolonged labour without medical or midwife assistance, injury during assisted vaginal delivery or hysterectomy, or following radiotherapy for cervical cancer. A **urethral diverticulum** is a cyst, which communicates with the urethra. In women, it can manifest as urinary incontinence, dyspareunia (painful sexual intercourse) and is a cause of recurrent urinary tract infections.

Pneumaturia

Pneumaturia is the passage of gas mixed with urine. It is caused by abnormal communication between bowel and urinary tract resulting in fistula formation. The most common causes are diverticular disease and Crohn disease, although it can also occur in carcinoma of the colon or bladder (Box 34.2). Gross urinary tract infection is inevitable. The patient typically complains of symptoms of urinary infection (dysuria and frequency) and may also describe bubbles or even faeces in the urine.

Haematospermia

Haematospermia describes the presence of blood in semen. It is most commonly caused by infection, but can be caused by a stone in an ejaculatory duct. In the older male patient, it is a rare presenting symptom of prostatic carcinoma.

Approach to the Diagnosis of Urinary Symptoms

Special Points in the History

A detailed history of the urinary tract symptoms should be taken, together with a general history to elucidate any systemic causes or contributing factors, for example, diabetes or multiple sclerosis. A full history of medication, past and present, should be recorded.

In patients with haematuria, the occupational history may be important. Exposure to aniline dyes and other industrial chemicals that were once widely used in the rubber and cable industries greatly increase the risk of urothelial carcinoma (previously termed *transitional cell carcinoma*) of the urinary tract. Tobacco smoking is estimated to cause 50% of bladder cancers.

Haematuria can also be caused by infestation with *Schistosoma*, which is endemic in parts of the Middle East and Africa, and is transmitted by water snails. A history of residence or travel in affected regions should therefore be sought. Similarly, a history of exposure to tuberculosis, which is common in developing countries, should be sought from patient populations at increased risk who present with haematuria.

Physical Examination

General Examination

A full general examination should pay special attention to a sallow complexion and signs of weight loss, which could indicate uraemia, particularly if accompanied by a uriniferous smell and scratch marks indicating itching. Blood pressure must be measured in every case, as hypertension may be a feature of pyelonephritis, renal artery stenosis, polycystic kidneys or glomerulonephritis.

Abdominal Examination

Abdominal inspection may reveal asymmetry caused by a large renal mass; this may be a nephroblastoma in a child or polycystic kidneys in an adult. In chronic retention, a large, sometimes asymmetrical bladder may be visible. The loins should be carefully inspected from the back; a subtle fullness may indicate a renal mass or a perinephric abscess.

A bimanual technique is used when examining the abdomen for kidney enlargement. One hand palpates the subcostal region anteriorly, while the other hand is placed posteriorly in the renal angle to push the kidney forward on to the palpating hand. The kidneys are impalpable, unless they are enlarged or displaced, except in a very thin patient. A renal mass may move with respiration and, because it is retroperitoneal, with bowel anteriorly, should also have an area of resonance on percussion overlying it. The main causes of an enlarged kidney are hydronephrosis, polycystic disease, renal cell carcinoma and nephroblastoma (Wilms tumour) in children. Loin tenderness is uncommon in non-acute renal disorders except in chronic perinephric abscess. Tenderness is usually found in acute conditions, such as pyelonephritis or acute obstruction. Renal tenderness can be distinguished from vertebral tenderness by gently tapping the spinous processes. This will cause pain if the tenderness is vertebral.

The lower abdomen is palpated for an enlarged or distended bladder, which is felt as a soft mass arising from the pelvis, sometimes asymmetrically. It is dull to percussion and pressure on it may induce an urge to void; bladder distension is easily confirmed on ultrasound examination. A suprapubic mass in the male usually indicates urinary retention, but occasionally, it is a colonic carcinoma or a large bladder tumour or stone (all firm to palpation). In the female, ovarian masses, pregnancy or uterine fibroids are more common causes of a suprapubic mass than urinary retention. Finally, auscultation along the 12th rib posteriorly may reveal the bruit of renal artery stenosis.

Rectal Examination

Rectal examination should be performed in both sexes guided by the clinical history. In females, a vaginal examination may also be indicated. In the male, the prostate is palpated per rectum for size, shape and consistency (Fig. 34.3). The normal prostate is about 3 cm in diameter and weighs 20 to 25 g; it can become massively enlarged and weigh over several hundred grams, so that its upper edge may be out of reach of the examining finger. Most transurethral prostatectomy operations for urinary symptoms leave a capsular remnant, so that the prostate appears palpable after prostatectomy, and may be of a firmer consistency.

The severity of prostatic obstructive symptoms depends not on the prostatic diameter but on the extent of encroachment upon the urethra. In some cases, an enlarged median lobe lying posteriorly above the bladder outlet may act as a flap valve, intermittently obstructing urine outflow.

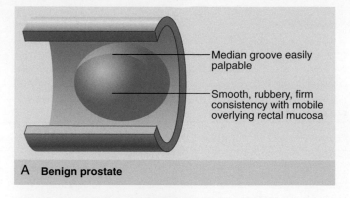

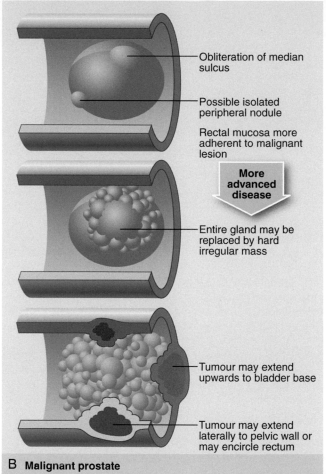

- **Fig. 34.3** Palpation Characteristics of the Prostate. **(A)** Benign. **(B)** Malignant.

On palpation, the normal prostate has a smooth surface and a firm consistency and is divided into two lateral lobes by a midline groove (median sulcus). In prostatic hyperplasia, enlargement is usually symmetrical, and the midline groove is maintained. Consistency remains normal. In contrast, a prostate infiltrated with carcinoma is irregular and asymmetrical. There are often hard nodules, and the median groove may be lost. In advanced cases, the tumour may be felt invading laterally into the pelvis or posteriorly around the rectum (Fig. 34.4). Digital examination can help distinguish benign from malignant prostatic enlargement in gross cases, but if carcinoma is suspected, **transrectal ultrasound scanning (TRUS)** using a rectal probe is performed, together

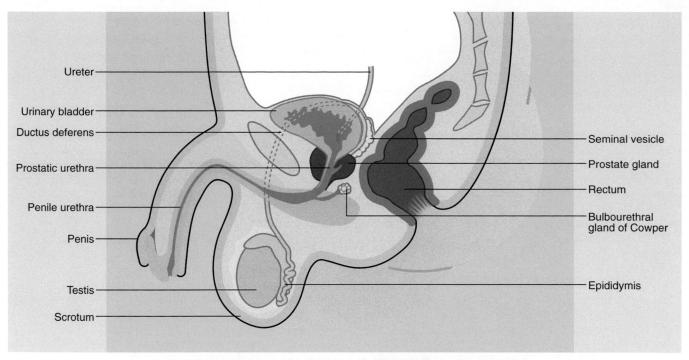

• **Fig. 34.4** Relationship of the Prostate to the Rectum and Peritoneal Cavity.

with multiple needle biopsies, under ultrasound guidance. Note, however, that there is a 2% risk of systemic sepsis and the procedure needs to be covered with a short course of antibiotics, for example, ciprofloxacin. Increasingly, magnetic resonance imaging (MRI) prostate is being used as a non-invasive and accurate method of diagnosis and as tool to guide accurate prostate biopsy. The symptom of prostatic tenderness is uncommon and may indicate prostatitis.

Investigation of Suspected Urinary Tract Disease

In common conditions, like BPE or urinary tract infection, the diagnosis is usually evident from the history and examination. 'Red flag' symptoms, such as haematuria, however, suggest several diagnostic possibilities and other diagnoses must be excluded.

A simple approach to investigation of urinary tract disease is to consider the following questions:

- Are any blood tests likely to be helpful in diagnosis?
- What urine tests are indicated?
- Where is the lesion?

Are Any Blood Tests Likely to Be Helpful in Diagnosis?

Blood tests that can be useful are summarised in Box 34.3.

When prostate cancer is suspected, **PSA** levels should be estimated and fractionated into **free PSA**, **total PSA** and their **ratio**. The free PSA is more likely to be raised in carcinoma and is a reliable indicator if the level is markedly elevated; the higher the level, the greater the volume of cancer. In biopsy-proven prostatic cancer, persistently raised PSA levels above 20 ng/ml are likely to indicate metastatic disease. However, the level may be normal in the presence of a small-volume cancer.

> • **BOX 34.3** **Blood Tests Useful in Diagnosing Urinary Tract Disease**
>
> **Full Blood Count**
> - Hypochromic microcytic anaemia—chronic iron deficiency anaemia caused by haematuria (rare)
> - Normochromic normocytic anaemia—chronic renal failure (lack of erythropoietin), chronic inflammatory disorders, for example, tuberculosis
> - Polycythaemia—renal adenocarcinoma
> - Leucocytosis—infection
>
> **Erythrocyte Sedimentation Rate (ESR) and C-Reactive Protein (CRP)**
> - Raised in chronic and acute infections, renal adenocarcinoma and retroperitoneal fibrosis
>
> **Urea, Electrolytes and Creatinine**
> - Impaired renal function in bilateral obstructive uropathy or chronic renal failure associated with hypertension, diabetes, etc.
>
> **Prostate-Specific Antigen (PSA)**
> - Raised in carcinoma of prostate but a normal level does not exclude it. Moderate elevations occur in benign disease. PSA is also temporarily raised with acute retention of urine, urinary tract infection and following urethral instrumentation or prostatic biopsy. In these scenarios, avoid PSA testing in the acute setting; instead, check PSA 4–6 weeks later.
>
> **Alkaline Phosphatase (Bone Isoenzyme)**
> - Raised in multiple bony metastases from any type of tumour
>
> **Calcium, Phosphate, Uric Acid and Parathyroid Hormone Levels**
> - Useful investigations in stone disease

Total PSA rises with age and, in benign hyperplasia, tends to rise in proportion to prostate mass. Acute retention, urinary tract infection, any urethral instrumentation or biopsy of the prostate causes elevation of the PSA for up to 6 weeks; standard DRE does not affect PSA level.

What Urine Tests Are Indicated?

Any urinary symptoms should prompt collection of a clean **mid-stream urine specimen** for microscopy and bacteriology. Microscopy will show the presence or absence of significant numbers of red blood cells (**microscopic haematuria**), white cells (**pyuria**) and bacteria (**bacteriuria**). However, the cells can lyse if the specimen is kept overnight at room temperature.

Bacteriuria of more than 10^5 colony-forming units per ml is considered to indicate significant infection. The urine is cultured to identify the organisms, and organisms are tested for antibiotic sensitivity. Culture-negative urine (**sterile pyuria**) is characteristic of urinary tract tuberculosis, urinary stone, bladder tumour, prostatitis or (most commonly), a partially treated urinary tract infection. In selected patients, with sterile pyuria, where the diagnosis of tuberculosis is being considered, three early morning urine specimens should be examined for acid-fast bacilli and cultured. **Bacteriuria without significant pyuria** usually indicates contamination of the urine specimen. **Casts** found on microscopy suggest a nephritic (renal inflammatory) process. The presence of epithelial cells indicates perineal contamination of the specimen, a common problem in females and infants.

Urine cytology is a useful screening test for urothelial tumours in people who have risk factors for urothelial carcinoma (smokers, positive family history, exposure to industrial carcinogens). The test has a high positivity in carcinoma-in-situ and high grade (poorly differentiated) tumours. Cytology needs to be performed on freshly voided urine. Some centres with an efficient local service use cytology for long-term follow-up of patients with treated bladder cancer.

Where Is the Lesion?

Investigations for localising urinary tract pathology are summarised in Table 34.3.

Suspected Upper Tract Lesions

Ultrasound
Renal ultrasound is a valuable noninvasive technique for investigating suspected renal masses. It is particularly useful in differentiating solid from cystic lesions and for demonstrating renal pelvis dilatation (hydronephrosis). Ultrasonography can also define the size, shape and position of stones in the kidney, but can rarely demonstrate a stone in the ureter. If bladder pathology is suspected, the bladder can easily be examined at the same time.

Computed Tomography Scanning
Computed tomography (CT) scanning is now the gold standard for imaging the urinary tract, although it provides limited assessment of function. It will also allow assessment of other organs. Modern spiral and multislice CT machines give rapid image capture and better definition; non-contrast CT is indicated for investigation of stone disease, particularly ureteric colic. CT with intravenous contrast helps distinguish renal malignancy from hamartomas and other benign diseases by measuring attenuation using Hounsfield units (or uptake of contrast and change of enhancement of the renal lesion). Delayed images can also be taken (CT urogram) to assess for ureteric obstruction caused by tumour or extrinsic compression from other disease processes. CT can also diagnose **angiomyolipoma** of the kidney. In renal cell carcinoma, CT can demonstrate direct spread along the renal vein and into the inferior vena cava so that surgery can be better planned. Enlarged lymph nodes may be diagnosed and biopsied

percutaneously and the liver examined for metastases. In bladder or prostatic cancer, CT can aid staging by demonstrating whether the disease is **organ-confined**.

Intravenous Urography
In most centres, CT has superseded intravenous urography (IVU) for renal tract investigation. IVU involves intravenous injection of a contrast medium, which is rapidly filtered by the glomeruli and excreted. This radiopaque solution opacifies the urinary system, demonstrating renal parenchyma, renal pelvis and the ureteric anatomy. The cortical concentration of contrast (**nephrogram**) gives an indication of the size, shape, thickness and bilateral symmetry of the renal cortex.

Cysts and tumours of the kidneys are usually revealed by the distortion of normal anatomy, but may be indistinguishable by this investigation. Tumours opacify with contrast to a variable extent and sometimes show a characteristic 'vascular blush'.

A dilated collecting system (renal pelvis, calyces and ureter) is usually easily seen on IVU and the level of an obstruction can often be demonstrated. When obstruction is almost complete, films may have to be taken at long intervals as back pressure delays cortical excretion.

Urothelial carcinoma may show as filling defects in the collecting system or bladder. If an abnormality is seen in the kidney or renal pelvis, **renal CT with contrast** is recommended to reveal more detail (see Ch. 5). If renal excretion is poor, as in chronic renal failure, contrast studies will yield poorer images (i.e., IVU and CT urogram). In addition, the contrast material may lead to further impairment of renal function. Intravenous contrast is liable to precipitate acute renal failure in diabetic nephropathy. In such cases, retrograde pyelography may be a suitable alternative.

Special Contrast Investigations
Retrograde pyelography, in which contrast is injected directly up the ureters, via a cystoscope, is especially useful for defining ureteric tumours, ureteric stricture, pelviureteric junction obstruction and radiolucent ureteric stones (where CT has not already made the diagnosis). It is also used to define anatomy before ureteric stent insertion.

Radionuclide Scanning
Dynamic radionuclide scanning with mercaptoacetyl-triglycerine (MAG3) renogram can be used to assess differential renal function and is particularly useful in monitoring function and renal drainage, after relief of obstruction. If the patient is then screened, whilst emptying the bladder of radioactive tracer, it can also provide a non-invasive assessment of vesicoureteric reflux by capturing an indirect micturating cystourethrogram image. Dimercapto-succinic acid (DMSA) renogram is used to accurately assess the split function of the kidneys and can also demonstrate renal scars.

Suspected Lower Tract Lesions
Radiography and Ultrasound
Ultrasound examination is the standard investigation. Modern high-resolution equipment can demonstrate tumours, cysts, stones and other abnormalities of bladder and prostate shape and volume, but can seldom define lesions smaller than 5 mm. The bladder is best seen if it is distended with urine; patients should be advised to drink copious fluids before the investigation.

It can also be used to estimate the bladder residual urine volume in outlet obstruction. **Transrectal ultrasound** can help assess the size of the prostate, enable directed biopsy of abnormal areas, or help achieve representative biopsies of all areas of the prostate.

TABLE 34.3 **Summary of Investigations for Localising Urinary Tract Pathology**

Investigation	Indications	Findings
Plain erect abdominal x-ray ('KUB' film)	Follow-up of radiopaque stones	Renal calcification; stones in kidney, ureter and bladder
Ultrasound scanning	Renal masses	Abnormal renal size, shape and position Differentiates solid from cystic renal lesions
	Suspected upper tract obstruction	Shows dilatation of renal pelvis or ureters
	Symptoms of bladder outlet obstruction	Estimates bladder volume after micturition; bladder wall thickness; complications of upper tract obstruction
	Transrectal ultrasound (TRUS) for assessing prostatic symptoms or enlargement	Useful for assessing the size of the gland and guiding biopsy needles for prostate cancer diagnosis
	Chronic renal disease and chronic urinary obstruction	Thickness of renal cortex
	General investigation of urinary symptoms	Morphology of upper tracts and bladder
	Investigation of urethral strictures	Definition of penile urethral strictures
CT scanning (plus intravenous contrast)	Renal mass suspicious of tumour	Abnormal mass and blood supply typical of renal tumour
	Palpable loin mass; differentiation of a pelvic mass from a prostatic or bladder tumour	Size, nature of lesions and extent of invasion
	Loin pain (CT without contrast may be used specifically to detect renal and ureteric stones)	Definition of cause particularly in calculus disease
Intravenous urography (with or without tomography)	Haematuria	If tumour present, may show non-functioning part of cortex and/or distorted anatomy
	Suspected urinary tract stone	Back pressure effects of obstruction on upper tract; position of stone
Special contrast examinations of upper tract, for example, retrograde or percutaneous (antegrade) ureterography	Obstruction of upper urinary tract not shown by other means	Site and perhaps nature of obstruction
Micturating cystography	Recurrent urinary tract infections or 'failure to thrive' in children	Severity of vesicoureteric reflux
Radionuclide renal scans	Definition of renal blood flow, function or morphology Diagnosis or follow-up of upper tract obstruction	Renal morphology, excretory function (total and differential), presence and sites of obstruction
	Vesicoureteric reflex	Indirect evidence of vesicoureteric reflux
Radionuclide bone scans	Bone pain in (suspected or diagnosed) prostatic carcinoma	Bony metastases
Cystourethroscopy (with or without biopsy or bladder resection)	Haematuria	Urothelial tumours of urethra or bladder
	Investigation of bladder neck obstruction and treatment, for example, transurethral resection of bladder neck or prostate	Visual inspection of bladder neck and prostate
	Treatment of bladder stones	Litholapaxy (stone fragmentation)
Ureteroscopy	Ureteric problems—stones and tumours	Direct visualisation of ureter and guidance for instrumentation to destroy or retrieve stones
Urine flow rate	Measurement and charting of urinary flow in bladder outlet obstruction Poor flow indicates obstruction or poorly functioning detrusor	Assessment before and after prostatectomy or bladder neck incision
Cystometrography (urodynamics with or without contrast)	Investigation of incontinence, assessment of bladder outlet obstruction and results of treatment	Nature of incontinence To confirm bladder outflow obstruction in equivocal outlet obstruction To demonstrate overactive bladder (detrusor overactivity) in irritative voiding
Renal arteriography	Occasional use in renal tumours	Demonstrating abnormal tumour blood supply (rarely used nowadays) Therapeutic embolisation for bleeding or pain in inoperable tumours or before surgery

CT, Computed tomography; *KUB,* kidney, ureter, bladder.

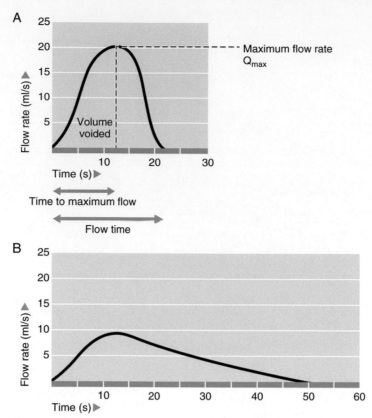

• **Fig. 34.5** Male Urinary Flow Rate. **(A)** Normal pattern flow rate. **(B)** Obstructed flow rate from a man with benign prostatic enlargement.

Cystourethroscopy

Cystourethroscopy (cystoscopy), using rigid or flexible instruments, is an important diagnostic and therapeutic tool for disease of the urethra, prostate and bladder. Flexible cystoscopy can usually be performed under local anaesthesia on an outpatient basis.

A similar but longer rigid instrument, the **ureteroscope**, is used for fragmenting and retrieving stones from the ureter; a flexible ureteroscope allows passage to the kidney and treatment of calyceal stones by laser lithotripsy (see Fig. 37.6, p. 495); a flexible uretero-scope allows passage to the kidney and treatment of calyceal stones by laser lithotripsy (Fig. 37.5B, p. 494). Both can be used to biopsy ureteric tumours and provide laser ablation therapy for small ureteric cancers in patient otherwise unfit to undergo a nephroureterectomy.

When a bladder tumour or urethral pathology is suspected, **cystoscopy** is the investigation of choice. Flexible cystoscopy under local anaesthetic allows direct visual examination, but if biopsy and immediate treatment are known to be required, rigid cystoscopy is usually performed under general or regional anaesthesia; anaesthesia also permits deep bimanual palpation (EUA, examination under anaesthesia).

Other Investigations

If clinical examination suggests local spread of a bladder or prostatic tumour, **CT** or **MRI scanning** can assess the extent of invasion. In carcinoma of prostate, **radionuclide (bone) scanning** is the most accurate non-invasive method for diagnosing and locating bony metastases.

In perineal injuries and pelvic fractures, **urethrography** is best for assessing suspected urethral rupture and may be combined with **suprapubic contrast cystography**. It is also used for urethral stricture examination. For suspected urethral obstruction, **contrast urethrography** or urethral ultrasound can localise the site of obstruction or stricture. If a colovesical fistula is suspected, **barium enema** may demonstrate the colonic lesion responsible (but rarely the fistula itself).

Urine flow rate provides a rapid assessment of the amount of outflow obstruction and can also assess response to treatment. It is easily measured and can be plotted on a graph as voiding progresses (Fig. 34.5). The patient passes urine into a funnel leading to the machine, although volumes voided below 150 mL can be misleading. When incontinence and bladder overactivity are being investigated, **urodynamic studies** can assess the relationship between bladder pressure and volume. They are particularly useful in the case of high-pressure bladders with outlet obstruction and in diagnosing urgency and stress incontinence.

35

Disorders of the Prostate

Introduction

Benign hyperplasia and carcinoma are the most common prostatic disorders and have an increasing importance in an ageing population. Inflammation and infection of the prostate (**prostatitis**) is a less common condition that occurs in a younger age group and is rather poorly defined clinically.

Anatomy

The normal prostate gland is about 3 cm long and 3 cm in diameter and weighs 20 to 25 g. The gland is situated immediately below the bladder neck so that the first 3 cm of the urethra lies within the gland (Fig. 35.1), so the proximal urethral walls (the **prostatic urethra**) are composed of glandular tissue. This contributes to the continence mechanism in men and is referred to as the internal sphincter mechanism. The urethra then passes through the pelvic floor muscle sheet, where it becomes the membranous urethra, and at this level is surrounded by the external urethral sphincter muscle. Prostatic hyperplasia or carcinoma may cause local urethral obstruction and carcinoma may invade and disrupt the sphincter mechanism.

The posterior aspect of the gland is palpable rectally (see Fig. 35.1) and a **median groove** can usually be identified. This groove (or sulcus) is described as dividing the gland into two lateral lobes and tends to be obliterated in advanced prostatic cancer but is usually exaggerated in benign prostatic enlargement.

When the prostatic urethra is examined cystoscopically (see Fig. 35.3, p. 475), an important landmark is an elongated mound on the ventral (or posterior) wall of the prostatic urethra known as the **verumontanum** (urethral crest), which can be variable in size and prominence. At its midpoint is a small depression, sometimes visible, into which the two **ejaculatory ducts** open. The posterior part of the gland above the ejaculatory ducts is known as the **median lobe**. If this becomes hypertrophied it may extend into the floor of the bladder (the surgical 'middle lobe'); this may act as a flap valve and obstruct the bladder outlet.

As seen in Fig. 35.1, the bulk of the normal prostate consists of up to 50 peripheral **glandular lobules**. These converge into about 20 separate ducts opening into the prostatic urethra, lateral to the verumontanum. As well as this glandular tissue proper, there is a zone of small paraurethral glands adjacent to the urethra, the **transition zone**. From middle age onwards, the transition zone tends to enlarge to cause **benign prostatic hyperplasia** (**BPH**). At the same time, the **peripheral** glandular tissue is compressed to form a fibrous outer 'surgical capsule'. In contrast, prostate cancer arises most often in the peripheral glandular tissue, tending to spread outwards into bordering structures more often than obstructing the centrally located urethra. Even after transurethral prostatectomy, cancer can arise in the residual peripheral zone.

The normal prostate gland is surrounded by a filmy **true capsule** of little surgical significance; external to this, is a rich venous plexus which, in turn, is invested by a dense fascial sheath. During radical or endoscopic prostatectomy, it is important not to disturb this venous plexus, as it is a common source of bleeding during and after the operation. There are direct venous connections between the plexus and the vertebral extradural plexus, which provide a direct route for blood-borne dissemination of prostate cancer. Posteriorly, the prostatic fascial sheath is fused with the dense **fascia of Denonvilliers**. This provides a barrier against direct spread of cancer from the prostate to the rectum and vice versa.

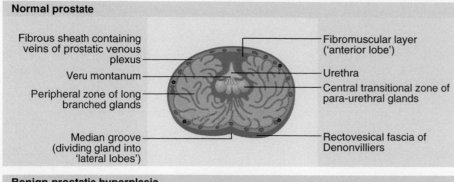

Normal prostate

Fibrous sheath containing veins of prostatic venous plexus

Veru montanum

Peripheral zone of long branched glands

Median groove (dividing gland into 'lateral lobes')

Fibromuscular layer ('anterior lobe')

Urethra

Central transitional zone of para-urethral glands

Rectovesical fascia of Denonvilliers

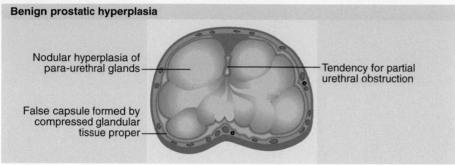

Benign prostatic hyperplasia

Nodular hyperplasia of para-urethral glands

False capsule formed by compressed glandular tissue proper

Tendency for partial urethral obstruction

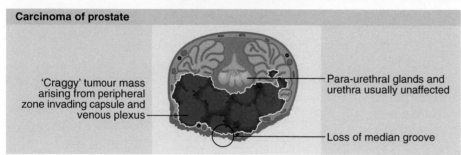

Carcinoma of prostate

'Craggy' tumour mass arising from peripheral zone invading capsule and venous plexus

Para-urethral glands and urethra usually unaffected

Loss of median groove

• **Fig. 35.1** Horizontal Sections Through Normal, Hyperplastic and Malignant Prostate Glands.

Benign Prostatic Hyperplasia

Clinically-evident growth of the prostate, which may be associated with voiding (obstructive) urinary symptoms is termed **benign prostatic enlargement (BPE)**. BPH is the histological diagnosis and the cause of the enlargement, and the terms are often used interchangeably. This condition affects half of all men over 50 years, and the proportion increases with advancing age so that BPH is almost universal at 70 years. Approximately half of those with BPH are asymptomatic or have only mild symptoms. In about 50% of men over 60 years, however, hyperplasia produces enough symptoms for treatment to be considered.

Pathophysiology of Benign Prostatic Hyperplasia

In pathological terms, the paraurethral transition zone glands undergo **nodular hyperplasia**. This causes progressive symmetrical enlargement of the gland up to several times its normal size.

The prostate volume cannot be reliably estimated by digital examination and is best assessed by ultrasound. However, there is little relationship between prostatic volume and symptoms; the presence of a large prostate without symptoms is not an indication for treatment. Urine flow rate is determined by the calibre and length of the prostatic urethra and by detrusor contractility, not by prostatic bulk. Prostatic urethroscopy provides further anatomical detail, but no functional information.

> • **BOX 35.1** Symptoms of Bladder Outlet Obstruction
>
> Symptoms formally assessed using the International Prostate Symptom Score (I-PSS). Each symptom is graded from 0 to 5 for the previous month. The total indicates the severity of symptoms: 0–7 = mild; 8–19 = moderate; 20–35 = severe.
> - Incomplete bladder emptying after urination
> - Frequency—need for urination again after less than 2 hours
> - Intermittent flow—stopping and starting during urination
> - Urgency—difficult to postpone urination
> - Weak stream—often made worse by a full bladder or by straining
> - Straining to begin urination
> - Nocturia—number of times needing to urinate per night
> It also includes a separate question on how this problem affects the patient's quality of life, graded from 0 (delighted) to 6 (terrible).
> Other symptoms (not scored)
> - Hesitancy, worse with a full bladder or at night
> - Postmicturition dribbling
> - Double micturition ('pis-à-deux')

Clinical Features of Benign Prostatic Hyperplasia

Symptoms and signs of bladder outflow obstruction (summarised in Box 35.1) are usually gradual in onset. Benign causes are prostatic hyperplasia and the apparently independent disorder of **bladder neck hypertrophy and fibrosis**. **Acute retention** of urine may occur suddenly at any time and is commonly

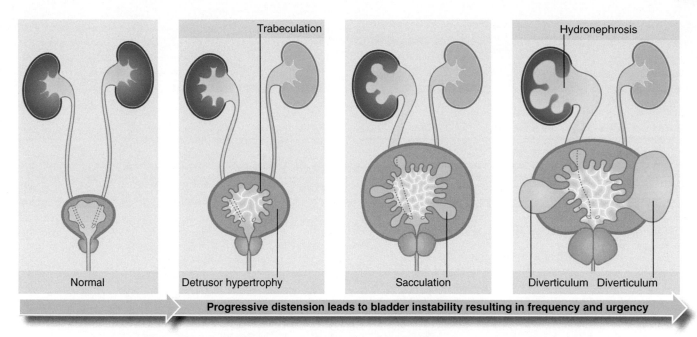

• **Fig. 35.2** Back-Pressure Effects on the Bladder and Kidneys Caused by Prolonged and Increasing Bladder Neck Obstruction. Note that upper tract dilatation tends to be bilateral; the left kidney (*in blue*) in this figure is included in its normal state to allow comparison with the right kidney, pelvicalyceal system and ureter, as they progressively dilate under the effects of increasing bladder pressure and retention of urine.

precipitated by bladder overfilling after excessive fluid intake. It is also a risk after general surgical or orthopaedic operations on older men, and also of any pelvic or perineal operations after adolescence. In some patients, the severity of prostatic symptoms fluctuates from month to month (and even perhaps with the season), making it difficult to decide whether an operation is necessary.

Complications of Bladder Outlet Obstruction

Prostatic obstruction can progressively interfere with the patient's ability to empty his bladder, but only 20% to 30% of patients have progressive symptoms, and 50% remain unchanged over 5 years. In progressive cases, the volume of **residual urine** gradually increases over weeks and months (i.e., chronic retention) and in a minority, this leads to a rise in intravesical pressure. In the latter, the threshold for the voiding reflex is reached more quickly and calls to void become more frequent. The stagnant residual urine is prone to infection, which exacerbates the symptoms. In chronic retention, the bladder becomes vastly distended and atonic, which can lead to **overflow incontinence**. In other cases, the detrusor muscle undergoes hypertrophy in an attempt to overcome the outflow obstruction (Fig. 35.2). The normally smooth bladder lining then becomes trabeculated. Eventually, muscle fibre bundles are replaced by noncontractile fibrous tissue; this may explain why some patients fail to improve after obstruction is relieved. With a further rise in pressure, the depressions between the muscle bands deepen (sacculation) and eventually form **bladder diverticula**. Urinary stasis in the diverticula predisposes to stone formation.

A small proportion of patients with bladder outlet obstruction experience few local symptoms. In these, rising intravesical pressure can be transmitted back into the ureters and kidneys causing hydronephrosis and **progressive renal parenchymal damage**. Patients often present with systemic illness or symptoms, such as anorexia, apparently of non-renal origin. The renal failure may be accompanied by anaemia, dehydration, acidosis and infection.

Bladder outflow obstruction in these patients is easily overlooked unless the bladder is examined for distension and plasma creatinine and urea measured. The symptom of nocturnal enuresis (i.e., incontinence at night) is a warning sign for high-pressure chronic retention. Emergency intervention is catheterisation, with later definitive treatment being bladder outlet surgery.

Management of Benign Prostatic Enlargement

The principles of management of bladder outlet obstruction believed to be caused by BPE are outlined in Box 35.2.

Diagnosis

A detailed history is first taken to assess the nature of the symptoms and how much they interfere with the patient's life. The International Prostate Symptom Score sheet helps in assessing the overall impact of symptoms in a standardised way (see Box 35.1). This, and the patient's general condition, are the principal factors determining whether treatment is needed. The abdomen is examined for an enlarged bladder and the prostate palpated rectally. These clinical examinations, however, reveal only gross abnormalities.

The next step is to investigate the effects of outlet obstruction on the bladder by measuring **urinary flow rate** and estimating the **volume of residual urine** using ultrasound. This is reliable, quick, noninvasive, safe and cheap. When urinary symptoms are severe but residual volume is insignificant, the alternative diagnosis of an **overactive bladder** should be considered. Twin-channel **urodynamic studies** are more complex and involve measuring the filling and emptying pressures of the bladder, but may be valuable if diagnostic doubts remain.

Renal function is assessed by estimating plasma urea, creatinine and electrolytes. If these are abnormal, further metabolic investigations may be necessary and renal tract ultrasound is mandatory.

A **midstream specimen of urine** should be examined by microscopy and culture as urinary infection alone may be

Management of Chronic Bladder Outflow Obstruction

- Assess the symptoms and the likely need for treatment from the history, particularly how much the symptoms bother the patient.
- Estimate the severity of bladder outlet obstruction by ultrasound and by measuring urine flow rate (± urodynamics).
- Investigate any disturbance of upper tract function and structure with renal function tests and ultrasound.
- Exclude urinary tract infection by urine microscopy and culture.
- Exclude prostatic carcinoma clinically, biochemically (prostate specific antigen) and by transrectal diagnostic ultrasound; if necessary, perform guided-needle biopsy of abnormal areas.
- Treat renal failure and other systemic problems.
- Consider whether catheter drainage of the bladder is required.
- Cystoscope the patient to rule out other pathology and to define the anatomical problem.
- Discuss with the patient what can be offered and at what risk, that is, drug treatment is first-line followed by bladder outlet surgery if symptoms fail to improve (transurethral resection of prostate or holmium laser enucleation of the prostate), or, as a last resort, long-term catheterisation.
- Implement appropriate nonsurgical treatments.

If operation becomes necessary, diagnose the cause and extent of obstruction by cystoscopy, then either:
- Resect or laser benign prostatic hyperplasia, divide bladder neck hypertrophy transurethrally (bladder neck incision), or obtain biopsy material by transurethral resection of prostate if carcinoma seems likely and prior confirmation has been negative.
  or
- Consider any other alternative operative measures, such as Urolift implants to expand the prostatic urethral cavity for small to moderate sized prostates, open simple (Millen) prostatectomy for large prostates, or excision of diverticula (once bladder outlet obstruction has been treated).

responsible for the symptoms or may have precipitated an episode of urinary retention. In addition, if surgery is intended, it is important that infection is eradicated to minimise risk of perioperative infection and secondary haemorrhage.

If the prostate feels nodular on palpation, cancer should be suspected, particularly if the serum **prostate-specific antigen** (PSA) is elevated. Transrectal ultrasound scanning (TRUS) and needle biopsy should be performed even if prostatectomy is planned, because a preoperative diagnosis of cancer is likely to alter the plan of management. Magnetic resonance imaging (MRI) is an additional investigation used to diagnose, stage and target biopsies for prostate cancer (although this tends to be reserved for guiding repeat biopsies, where previous results have been benign but clinical suspicion persists). Marked elevation of serum PSA is diagnostic of prostatic cancer but a mildly elevated PSA may be caused by benign disease or infection. A normal result does not, however, exclude cancer.

Relief of Retention and Obstructive Effects on the Kidney

Immediate catheterisation should be offered to patients presenting with large volume urinary retention (750 mL or more) associated with abnormal renal function or upper tract dilatation on renal tract ultrasound. Bladder drainage allows any reversible component of renal failure to self-correct. This commonly corrects in days, but in some chronic cases, it may take up to 3 weeks to improve biochemical renal function tests. After that, spontaneous improvement is unlikely. Initially, fluid and electrolyte balance is monitored and normalised, if necessary by intravenous fluids. In patients with chronic outflow obstruction and obstructive renal

failure, catheterisation may produce a **massive diuresis** and this should be anticipated and treated appropriately. Where there has been any evidence of renal compromise caused by bladder outlet obstruction, the catheter must not be removed until definitive treatment has been performed (i.e., bladder outlet surgery) or the patient accepts a long-term catheter.

Cystoscopy

The anatomical nature of the bladder outlet obstruction can be further assessed by direct cystoscopic examination. It also provides an opportunity to examine for other problems, such as trabeculation, diverticula, tumours and stones. In patients with complications from bladder outlet obstruction or severe symptoms not responding to medical treatment, transurethral resection or holmium laser enucleation of the prostatic obstruction is performed, under the same anaesthetic (see transurethral resection of prostate [TURP], later). In elderly or unfit patients, placement of a **urethral stent** may be considered, however, they are rarely used, as these devices are prone to displacement, haemorrhage, local irritation and blockage. Only very occasionally are patients too unfit for some form of intervention. It is now rarely necessary to leave a patient with a long-term catheter, but in this event, a suprapubic catheter is preferable to a urethral catheter, because of the ease of changing it, greater patient comfort, and avoidance of urethral trauma, which can result in traumatic hypospadias long term.

Drug Treatments

Alpha-adrenergic A_1 receptors are present in the bladder neck and prostate. Selective alpha-1a subtype adrenergic blocking drugs (**tamsulosin** and **alfuzosin**) enable the prostatic urethra to open more readily by blocking prostatic smooth muscle contraction, so relieving symptoms.

Finasteride and **dutasteride** block the enzyme 5-alpha reductase from converting testosterone to dihydrotestosterone (a more potent androgen) and thus reduce the size of hyperplastic prostate glands. A 6-month trial of treatment is required; if successful, symptoms may improve to the extent that surgery can be delayed or avoided. Some herbal remedies, such as **saw palmetto**, contain naturally occurring 5-alpha reductase inhibitors. Combination therapy with alpha-adrenergic blockers and 5-alpha reductase inhibitors may be beneficial in patients with larger glands.

Minimally Invasive Options

Prostate artery embolisation is not commonly offered but does provide an alternative option for those who have failed medical therapy and wish to avoid surgery. Under fluoroscopy guidance and using local anaesthetic, interventional radiologists access the femoral artery to selectively block the prostate artery using microparticles. This results in prostatic necrosis and a reduction in prostate size. Risks include urinary retention, pain, and dysuria. Whilst urinary symptoms are improved and sexual function is generally preserved, results are inferior to TURP.

Transurethral Resection of Prostate and Other Transurethral Treatments

Transurethral prostatectomy remains the gold standard therapy for bladder outlet obstruction caused by an enlarged prostate. With the widespread introduction of bipolar TURP (Gyrus), it can achieve significantly reduced blood loss as compared to monopolar devices, allowing this operation to be performed as a day case procedure. Holmium laser enucleation of prostate (HoLEP) yields at least equivalent results to TURP, and is particularly useful for larger glands, thus avoiding the need for open retropubic prostatectomy. Laser ablation techniques (using KTP-green light and holmium lasers) can be appropriate in special circumstances, such as a patient on warfarin. For patients with smaller prostates, without an obstructing median lobe, the Urolift device can be inserted under local anaesthetic or sedation as a day case. This uses cystoscopy to deploy small implants into the prostate to retract the lateral lobes away from the urethral lumen. Whilst less effective than TURP, it is an option for those wishing to defer larger surgery and avoid the small risk of sexual dysfunction.

The aim of transurethral prostatectomy is to remove the bulk of the prostate but leave the compressed normal peripheral tissue. This protects the subcapsular venous plexus that might otherwise bleed catastrophically. In TURP, a series of 'chips' or strips of tissue are excised with a resectoscope using a cutting diathermy wire loop; the chips drift into the bladder. The enlarged gland is progressively sliced away as shown in Fig. 35.3, taking great care to preserve the sphincter mechanism immediately distal to the verumontanum. Bleeding points are carefully cauterised. The prostatic chips are always examined histologically and may reveal unsuspected (incidental) carcinoma. Normal saline is used to irrigate bipolar procedures; a transparent isotonic irrigation solution is used during monopolar TURP, which washes away blood and debris to allow continuous visibility. Since some irrigation fluid is inevitably absorbed, sterile **glycine solution** is most often used for monopolar TURP instead of water, as it does not cause haemolysis. If large volumes of glycine are absorbed, this causes dilutional hyponatraemia and hyperammonaemia, along with drastic plasma electrolyte changes, producing the **TUR syndrome**.

When obstruction is caused by bladder neck hypertrophy, the prostate is not usually resected but the bladder neck muscle is divided by making a longitudinal incision (bladder neck incision, BNI) using a diathermy point (Collin knife) or holmium laser via the resectoscope. This operation is also effective where the obstruction is caused by a small prostate (<30 g).

Retropubic Prostatectomy

Open simple (Millen) prostatectomy, now rarely performed, is used mainly when the gland is so large that transurethral resection is not practicable, or occasionally when there are accompanying bladder diverticula or huge stones that also require treatment.

Complications of Transurethral Resection of Prostate, HoLEP and Open Prostatectomy

Prostatectomy usually disrupts the bladder neck mechanism that normally prevents semen entering the bladder during ejaculation. Patients risk failure to ejaculate through the penis after prostatectomy (**retrograde ejaculation**), although the sensation of orgasm is unaffected. This affects up to 75% of patients. Maintaining fertility is not usually important in this older age group, but should the need arise, urine can be filtered to recover sperm for artificial insemination. **Erectile impotence** follows TURP in 5% to 10%, a rate similar to other major operations in the pelvis or perineal area. Some degree of erectile function deterioration is also seen in up to 10% of HoLEP patients. However, as quality of life generally improves once urinary symptoms are treated, sexual satisfaction rates can become better in some men postoperatively. **Urethral strictures** develop in 5% of cases, reflecting the use of relatively large instruments and potentially harmful urethral catheters.

Minor **haematuria** can be expected during the first few weeks after prostatectomy. Secondary haemorrhage (caused by infection) can be more profuse and may cause **clot retention**, that is, retention of urine caused by obstructing blood clot. Recovery of complete urinary continence is sometimes delayed following prostatectomy, but permanent damage to the sphincter mechanism is rare (<1%).

Long-Term Catheterisation or Stenting

Operation greatly improves the quality of life in most patients. Even in patients over 80 years, perioperative morbidity and mortality are acceptably low. Nevertheless, a small proportion of severely debilitated, immobile or frail patients are better managed by long-term suprapubic (or urethral) catheterisation, changed regularly by the local practitioner team. In situ urethral stenting is an alternative, although it has a high rate of failure and other complications.

Acute Urinary Retention and Its Management

Acute urinary retention may occur in patients with longstanding symptoms of bladder outlet obstruction; indeed, in the majority of men with chronic retention, acute retention is the first presentation. It is often precipitated by overfilling of the bladder, faecal loading or urinary tract infection. Acute retention is a common cause of emergency surgical admission and a frequent early complication after any major operation, especially in males; it may therefore occur at any age even without bladder neck hypertrophy or prostatic enlargement. Management of postoperative acute retention is described in Chapter 7.

Diagnosis of Acute Retention

In a patient with no urine output, acute retention must be distinguished from anuria. However, the diagnosis is not usually difficult—the patient in retention is acutely distressed with abdominal or perineal pain and a readily palpable bladder. A history of previous similar episodes, urological surgery or accidental injury should be sought in case special treatment is required.

Catheterisation

Acute retention is usually treated by urethral or suprapubic catheterisation using an aseptic technique (Fig. 35.4). Urethral catheterisation may prove challenging in patients with a history of difficult catheterisation, prostatectomy or urethral stricture, or the finding of a nonretractile foreskin. If the problem appears complex, an experienced opinion should be sought early before risking urethral damage by unwise attempts at urethral catheterisation. Urologists can perform local anaesthetic flexible cystoscopy and insertion of an open-ended catheter over a guidewire if the urethra is patent. Inserting a suprapubic catheter is the alternative. Puncture technique (preferably ultrasound guided) can be performed provided the bladder is palpably distended. If the patient has undertaken previous abdominal or pelvic surgery, open cystotomy and insertion of suprapubic catheter is safer and reduces the risk of bowel injury (which is 1%–2% with every technique). Suprapubic catheter insertion should be avoided if there is a history of bladder cancer or if the patient is on anticoagulants. A surgeon with urological training may elect to carry out cystourethroscopy and appropriate surgical treatment as a single scheduled procedure, if catheterisation is not urgent.

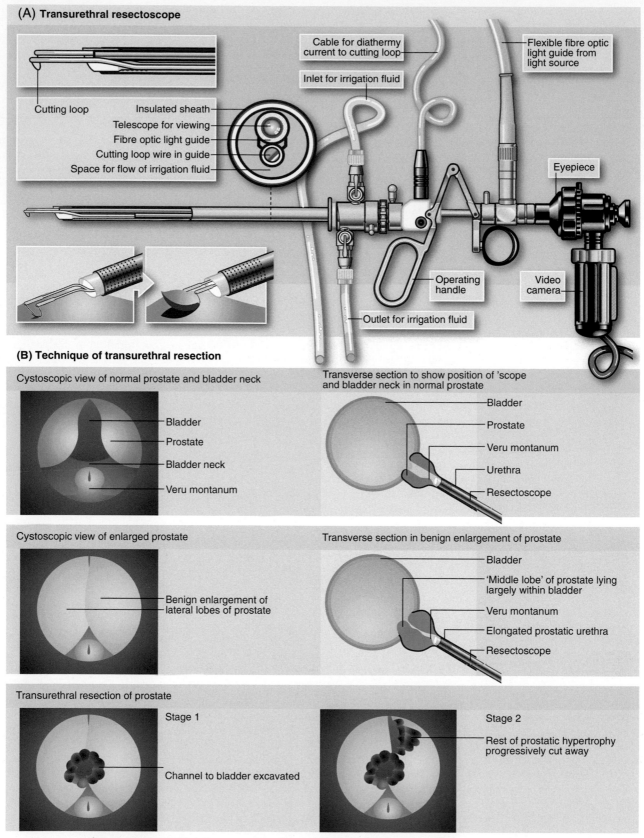

(A) Transurethral resectoscope

Cable for diathermy current to cutting loop

Inlet for irrigation fluid

Flexible fibre optic light guide from light source

Cutting loop
Insulated sheath
Telescope for viewing
Fibre optic light guide
Cutting loop wire in guide
Space for flow of irrigation fluid

Eyepiece

Operating handle

Video camera

Outlet for irrigation fluid

(B) Technique of transurethral resection

Cystoscopic view of normal prostate and bladder neck

Bladder
Prostate
Bladder neck
Veru montanum

Transverse section to show position of 'scope and bladder neck in normal prostate

Bladder
Prostate
Veru montanum
Urethra
Resectoscope

Cystoscopic view of enlarged prostate

Benign enlargement of lateral lobes of prostate

Transverse section in benign enlargement of prostate

Bladder
'Middle lobe' of prostate lying largely within bladder
Veru montanum
Elongated prostatic urethra
Resectoscope

Transurethral resection of prostate

Stage 1

Channel to bladder excavated

Stage 2

Rest of prostatic hypertrophy progressively cut away

• **Fig. 35.3** Transurethral Prostatectomy. **(A)** Transurethral resectoscope. 'Divots' or chips are cut by squeezing the handle towards the eyepiece, while turning the diathermy current on. This 'cheese-wires' the cutting loop through tissue. **(B)** Technique of transurethral resection.

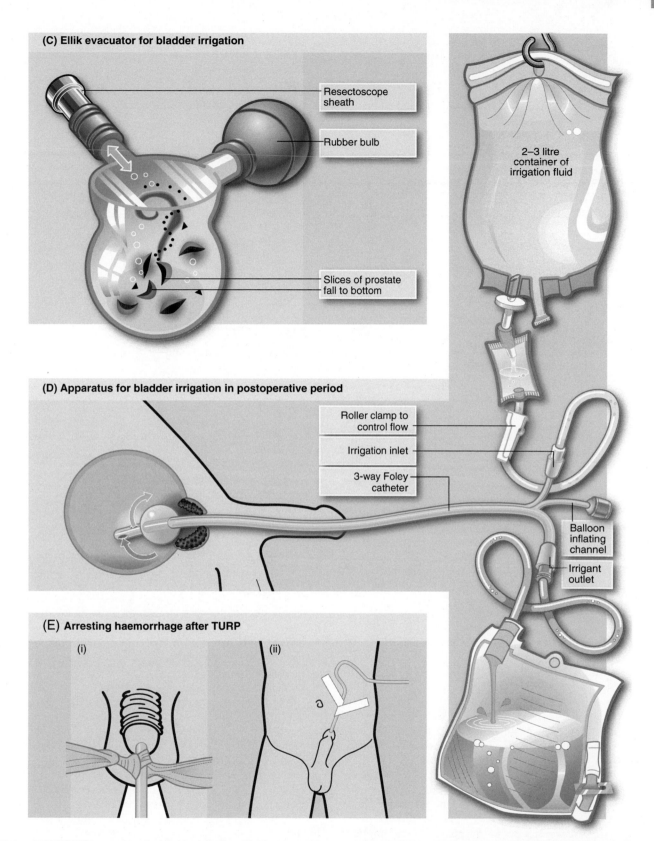

(C) Ellik evacuator for bladder irrigation

Resectoscope sheath

Rubber bulb

Slices of prostate fall to bottom

2–3 litre container of irrigation fluid

(D) Apparatus for bladder irrigation in postoperative period

Roller clamp to control flow

Irrigation inlet

3-way Foley catheter

Balloon inflating channel

Irrigant outlet

(E) Arresting haemorrhage after TURP

(i)

(ii)

Fig. 35.3, cont'd (C) Ellik evacuator for bladder irrigation. The instrument is completely filled with irrigation fluid and then attached to the resectoscope sheath, which is left in the bladder after withdrawal of the main instrument. Squeezing the bulb flushes fluid alternately in and out of the bladder, bringing the cut prostatic slices with it, which then settle to the bottom of the container. **(D)** Apparatus for bladder irrigation in the postoperative period. The rate of fluid flow is adjusted to be fast enough to prevent clotting within the bladder. In practice the effluent should be pink rather than red. **(E)** Arresting haemorrhage after TURP. Excessive bleeding after transurethral resection can often be controlled by exerting traction on the catheter for 20 minutes (but not more). Tension is maintained by (1) tying a swab around the catheter, or (2) attaching the catheter to the anterior abdominal wall with adhesive tape. *TURP,* Transurethral resection of prostate.

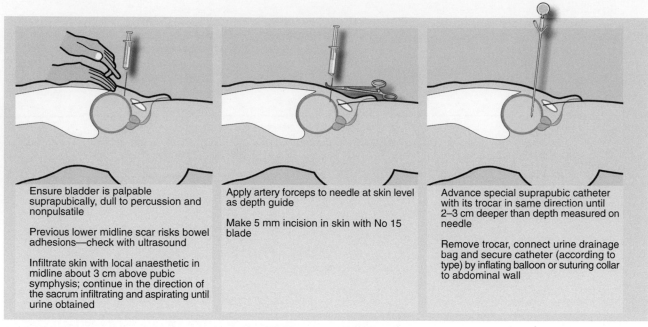

Ensure bladder is palpable suprapubically, dull to percussion and nonpulsatile

Previous lower midline scar risks bowel adhesions—check with ultrasound

Infiltrate skin with local anaesthetic in midline about 3 cm above pubic symphysis; continue in the direction of the sacrum infiltrating and aspirating until urine obtained

Apply artery forceps to needle at skin level as depth guide

Make 5 mm incision in skin with No 15 blade

Advance special suprapubic catheter with its trocar in same direction until 2–3 cm deeper than depth measured on needle

Remove trocar, connect urine drainage bag and secure catheter (according to type) by inflating balloon or suturing collar to abdominal wall

• **Fig. 35.4** Suprapubic Catheterisation.

Evaluating the Underlying Cause and Any Precipitating Factors

A catheter is usually left in situ for 1 or 2 days after relieving the acute retention. The patient should be fully assessed, and after establishing the likely cause (commonly BPE) and ensuring that renal function has not been impaired, a decision is whether to attempt a **trial without catheter (TWOC)** in hospital or in the community, that is, test whether the patient can void urine satisfactorily when the catheter is removed, or clamped off, in the case of a suprapubic, or whether to proceed directly with surgical or other treatment. Any urinary tract infection, constipation or other reversible contributing cause must be treated before any trial without catheter or operation.

'Trial Without Catheter'

If appropriate, the catheter should be removed either around midnight or very early in the morning so that a catheter can be replaced before the patient's bedtime if the trial is unsuccessful. Success is if the patient can pass reasonable volumes of urine with each void, that is, more than about 100 mL. Even if passing good volumes, the patient must be examined at intervals to ensure that the bladder is not distending with retained urine, indicating chronic retention with overflow. Prescribing an alpha-adrenergic blocker, such as tamsulosin for 48 hours before TWOC can increase success rates. Unsuccessful TWOC is an indication for cystourethroscopy and probable surgical treatment, or investigation with urodynamics if there is concern that the retention is caused by bladder underactivity (for which TURP may not necessarily guarantee resumption of spontaneous voiding). Approximately 50% will pass urine successfully, although up to 50% will have a further episode of retention within 1 year. Men with low urinary flow rates, large residual volumes and palpably large prostates are more likely to develop further retention.

In addition to failed TWOC, other common indications for cystourethroscopy and prostatectomy or BNI are:

- a huge volume of retained urine released by catheterisation—indicating chronic retention (if urodynamics confirm the presence of bladder outlet obstruction);
- raised plasma urea and creatinine, which improve after catheterisation—indicating chronic obstructive uropathy;
- previous episodes of acute retention;
- bladder outflow obstruction caused by carcinoma of prostate;
- presence of bladder calculi;
- acute retention in combination with a history of lower urinary tract symptoms, sufficient in themselves to warrant surgery (in patients who are already on and hence failed with medication).

Indwelling Catheters and Their Management

Indications for permanent urethral or suprapubic catheterisation include:

- patients unfit for prostatectomy;
- incontinent patients who are severely debilitated, frail or immobile;
- incontinence caused by external sphincter damage caused by previous prostatectomy or invading carcinoma;
- 'sacral neurogenic bladder', for example, in multiple sclerosis (with poor manual dexterity);
- patients unable to perform intermittent self-catheterisation.

Recurrent catheter blockage and **infection** are the major problems of long-term catheterisation. Catheters readily become blocked by epithelial debris or by gradual accretion of calculus. Modern silicone or silicone-coated 'long-term' catheters are better but must still be changed regularly every 10 to 12 weeks. In most cases, they can be changed at home by the community nurse, using full sterile precautions, because if infection becomes established in the presence of a catheter, it is difficult to eradicate. However, low-grade infection is almost always present with indwelling catheters and usually does not cause symptoms or discomfort. Antibiotics should be prescribed only if local symptoms become troublesome or if systemic signs of infection develop.

Catheters in Paraplegic Patients

In paraplegic patients, ureteric reflux predisposes to recurrent upper urinary tract infections. Established infections can lead to progressive renal failure. For these patients, special care must be taken to avoid introducing infection, and urine microscopy and culture should be performed regularly and any infections treated promptly. **Intermittent catheterisation**, rather than an indwelling catheter, may be a better form of management, provided it is performed correctly; in many cases, patients successfully perform this themselves. Patients can still suffer problems because of bladder overactivity and poor compliance, which can manifest as catheter bypassing or recurrent blockages. Anticholinergic medications or injection of botulinum toxin A into the bladder wall is needed to manage this in some patients.

Carcinoma of the Prostate

Pathophysiology

Carcinoma of the prostate is common after the age of 65 years and is becoming increasingly common in the two decades before that. The rising incidence is partly explained by many more early cases discovered because of increasing public awareness, and screening using PSA testing, particularly in the United States of America. The rise may also be related to high meat and fat consumption: East Asians living on a predominantly vegetarian diet have the lowest incidence of prostate cancer.

Cancer most commonly arises in the **peripheral** prostatic glands rather than in the paraurethral tissue (transition zone) and thus is often slow to intrude on the urethra and cause obstruction. Prostate cancers are nearly all **adenocarcinomas,** with a variable degree of differentiation, reflected in their behaviour and aggressiveness of local and metastatic spread.

Most adenocarcinomas are well differentiated and contained within the capsule, slowly invading adjacent prostatic tissue and sometimes involving the bladder neck or sphincter mechanism. In many cases, the prostate is already enlarged by benign hyperplasia. Prostate cancer metastasises to pelvic lymph nodes and via the bloodstream to bone (for which it has a particular affinity) and other organs. Tumour cells enter the subcapsular venous plexus then the spinal venous system, which may explain the frequency of bone metastases in the pelvis and spinal column. The 5-year survival rate for patients with distant metastases (stage IV) is about 30% as compared to nearly 100% in men with localised cancer (stages I–II).

The prostate produces a glycoprotein enzyme called **PSA**. The role of PSA is to liquefy the ejaculate to assist with fertility. Increased levels of PSA are released into the bloodstream as a result of tissue architecture destruction from prostate cancer, and more advanced tumours with greater tumour mass produce greater amounts and hence higher blood levels of PSA. Other prostatic conditions (e.g., hyperplasia, prostatitis) may cause elevation of PSA, but levels over 10 to 15 ng/mL are more likely to be caused by cancer, provided urinary infection can be eliminated as a cause.

The main prognostic indicators for prostate cancer are its PSA level at presentation, tumour grade and stage. Routine prostate cancer screening with PSA however, is not recommended owing to the proven risks of overtreating patients with localised asymptomatic disease who become exposed to unnecessary risks of therapy (see Ch. 6).

Many patients have asymptomatic, localised or dormant disease diagnosed incidentally at TURP, for presumed benign disease.

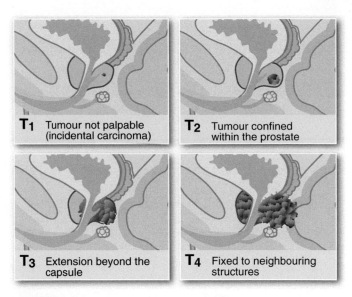

T₁ Tumour not palpable (incidental carcinoma)	**T₂** Tumour confined within the prostate
T₃ Extension beyond the capsule	**T₄** Fixed to neighbouring structures

• **Fig. 35.5** Tumour, Node, Metastasis (TNM) Staging System for Prostatic Cancer.

At autopsy, one-third or more of men over 50 years and 90% of men over 90 years dying of other causes have microscopic cancer in the prostate and it can be assumed that this is true for the population at large. The natural history of these occult cancers is unknown and many clearly do not progress to become clinically relevant. Even after characteristic local symptoms appear, the disease often pursues a prolonged course. Many patients over 70 years die *with* their prostate cancer rather than *from* it. On the other hand, 50% of patients under 70 years with moderately or poorly differentiated cancers will eventually die from the disease and a greater proportion will develop significant morbidity. A **'watchful waiting'** approach can be adopted for some men with prostate cancer, with observation using PSA blood tests; treatment is usually only offered if symptoms occur. This tends to be reserved for older men with significant comorbidities. **Active surveillance**, in comparison, is the close monitoring of slow-growing prostate cancer with serial PSA blood tests, digital rectal examination, and repeat prostate biopsies. The aim of active surveillance is to defer definitive cancer treatment until progression is evident to avoid the side effects of treatment until necessary.

Symptoms and signs of prostatic cancer depend on the degree of local and systemic spread. Clinical staging is most commonly based on the Tumour, Node, Metastasis (TNM) system (Fig. 35.5). Incidence of pelvic lymph node involvement varies from 2% in T_1 tumours to 85% in T_4 tumours. The palpation characteristics of the malignant prostate are illustrated in Fig. 35.1

Symptoms and Signs of Prostatic Cancer

Patients with stage T_1 or T_2 tumours may be asymptomatic. They may be discovered incidentally or on a routine health check, or present with lower urinary tract symptoms difficult to differentiate from those caused by BPH. Those with T_3 and T_4 tumours may also develop other local symptoms from advancement of the primary tumour, for example, encirclement of the rectum or occlusion of ureters and presenting with renal failure. Patients with nodal disease (N⁺) may have symptoms from local compression (swollen legs) and impaired lymphatic drainage (penile and genital oedema). Unfortunately, advanced disease (such as some T_3 and most T_4 lesions) have often metastasised by the time of

- Asymptomatic—screening by rectal examination and prostate specific antigen (PSA)
- Asymptomatic—incidental finding of nodular prostate on digital rectal examination
- Symptoms of bladder outflow obstruction—tumour suspected by finding nodular prostate on rectal examination or a suspiciously raised serum PSA or found on histology after transurethral resection of prostate
- Symptoms of spread to surrounding pelvic tissues, for example, change in bowel habit, urinary retention, loss of continence, recent impotence, ureteric obstruction, acute kidney injury (AKI)
- Symptoms of bony metastases, for example, bone pain, malaise, anaemia, pathological fractures

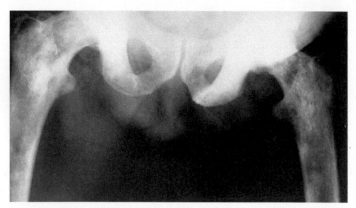

• **Fig. 35.6** Osteosclerotic Bony Metastases From Prostatic Carcinoma.

presentation (M^+) and can present with bone pain, pathological fractures (e.g., of the femur) or spinal cord compression. Thus older men presenting with **backache** should always have a rectal examination and PSA examination. In more advanced cases, non-specific symptoms of malaise, fatigue, weight loss and anaemia may also develop and escape recognition for many months.

Rectal examination can sometimes reveal the primary diagnosis. On palpation of a T_1 tumour, the prostate appears normal or smoothly enlarged by benign hyperplasia; stage T_2, typically presents with a nodular, asymmetrical surface, and stage T_3, with a large, hard, irregular gland with evidence of extension beyond the capsule or into the seminal vesicles. A tumour fixed to bone or adjacent pelvic organs is stage T_4. Local spread may involve the rectum (causing changes in bowel habit) or the bladder neck and ureters (causing incontinence, impotence or rarely obstructive renal failure). At this late stage, the tumour is obvious on rectal palpation as a hard, craggy mass. In very advanced cases, where cancer has invaded laterally to involve the pelvic walls or encircle the rectum, the pelvis may appear 'frozen' solid with tumour. Some patients develop major deep venous thrombosis, affecting the lower limb. Modes of presentation of carcinoma of the prostate are summarised in Box 35.3.

Approach to Investigation of Suspected Prostatic Carcinoma

Unless the prostate feels malignant or there are obvious bony metastases, it may be impossible to distinguish clinically between benign disease and prostatic carcinoma. Serum **PSA** should be measured, and this usually directs further investigation, although results must be interpreted with caution, as modestly rising levels with advancing age are accepted as normal (an age-related range is provided by local biochemistry laboratories). A normal PSA result cannot exclude carcinoma confined to the gland; PSA is normal in 25% of these cases. Substantially elevated PSA usually indicates aggressive local disease or more often, metastatic disease, although false positive results can occur in BPH or inflammation (caused by prostatitis or urinary tract infections).

Transrectal ultrasonography is used to image the prostate irrespective of the findings on palpation and to guide **transrectal needle biopsy** if necessary, where typically 10 to 12 cores of prostate are sampled (see Fig. 35.7, p. 479). Alternatively, transrectal ultrasound can be used to guide **transperineal (saturation) prostate biopsy**—this is commonly performed under general anaesthetic but has the advantage of sampling the prostate greater than 20 times, increasing the accuracy of diagnosis. Risks of prostate biopsy include urosepsis, urinary retention, haematuria, haemospermia and rectal bleeding. The prostate cancer tissue retrieved is given a Gleason score rated according to how well differentiated the tissue appears on microscopy. The two commonest histological patterns are expressed as a total value out of 10 (and associated with a grade group score). Gleason score 6 is well differentiated, 7 is moderately differentiated; whilst 8–10 is poorly differentiated. The grade influences treatment options and prognosis.

Multiparametric MRI prostate plays a role in staging of disease. It is helpful in identifying prostate lesions when clinical suspicion of a prostate cancer persists even though biopsies have been negative. MRI has been particularly helpful in improving the accuracy of prostatic biopsies by allowing the real-time fusion of MRI and transrectal ultrasound images during the biopsy procedure, enhancing the detection of prostate cancer.

Computed tomography is used to detect (and stage) lymph node disease and metastasis for high risk patients (see Fig. 35.7A).

If a patient has skeletal pain, x-rays and radionuclide bone scans are indicated. On x-ray, prostatic bony metastases are typically **sclerotic** or osteoblastic (i.e., dense, appearing white on x-rays) rather than **lytic** (as in most other bony secondaries), giving the characteristic patchy 'cotton-wool' appearance shown in Fig. 35.6. Some lesions, however, are radiolucent. An isotope bone scan can reveal metastases even when a plain x-ray is normal.

Management of Prostatic Carcinoma

Early-Stage Disease (Stages T_1 or T_2; no Lymph Node Involvement N_0; no Metastasis M_0)

One treatment option for patients with low-grade, impalpable, organ-confined prostate cancer, with a life expectancy of >10 years, is **active surveillance**, until there is evidence of increased disease activity (rising PSA or detectable nodule on palpation). This can give outcomes equivalent to radical treatment and spares many of the side-effects of radical treatment. There is, however, evidence of improved survival with early radical treatment in patients with moderate to high-grade organ-confined disease, compared to active surveillance, and a lower risk of metastasis of disease at 10 years.

Radical prostatectomy or radical radiotherapy is potentially curative for organ-confined disease, that is, disease confined to the prostate or 'true' stage T_1 and T_2. If external beam radiation therapy is chosen, it is delivered so as to provide a high local tumour dose without adversely affecting the rectum. An alternative is the use of radioactive seed implants (**brachytherapy**),

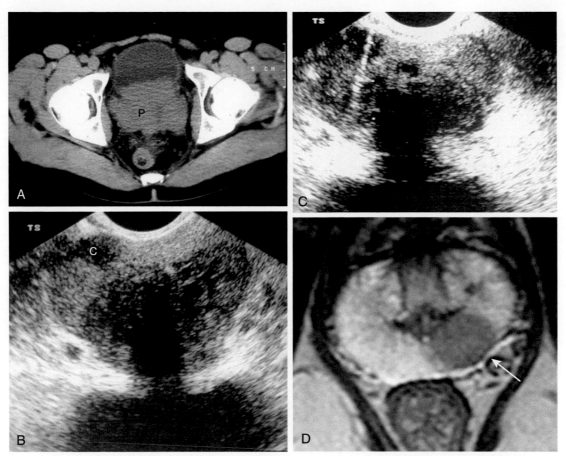

• **Fig. 35.7** Carcinoma of the Prostate. (A) Computed tomography scan showing a large carcinoma of the prostate *(P)* invading extensively into the bladder anteriorly and posteriorly towards the rectum. This was a late and aggressive form of the disease and the patient lived less than 1 year. (B) and (C) Ultrasound-guided biopsy. (B) Transrectal ultrasound scan of prostate showing a small cancer *(C)* within the peripheral zone and an acoustic shadow beyond it. The larger central zone is enlarged by benign hypertrophy. (C) After transrectal biopsy. The white line represents bubbles of air left after successful needle biopsy of the tumour. (D) T2 weighed magnetic resonance image showing focal low signal consistent with a prostate carcinoma (shown by *arrow*) in the left peripheral zone of the prostate.

whereby the seeds are placed accurately within the prostate under ultrasound control. These deliver the necessary high but localised dosage. Brachytherapy, however, may worsen urinary symptoms in some men and is therefore not recommended for patients who already have urinary symptoms or have a significantly enlarged prostate gland.

Radical prostatectomy entails risks, such as incontinence and impotence, although complication rates are lower using advanced surgical techniques, including robotic-assisted radical prostatectomy (RARP); RARP or non-robotic laparoscopic prostatectomy have become the operation of choice in many centres. Patient selection for radical treatment is important in terms of the cancer characteristics (staging, PSA level and tumour volume), as well as patient characteristics (comorbidity, age, sexual function and patient preference). Patients must be fully counselled in the range of treatment options (including no treatment) and their complications.

Other minimally invasive options available for localised prostate cancer, offered in selected research centres, include cryosurgery and high-intensity focused ultrasound (HIFU). Cryosurgery is a technique, which freezes the prostate using probes to induce cell death. HIFU uses focused ultrasound waves to kills cancer cells by thermal and mechanical effects on the tissue. These can provide focal therapy, which treats only the part of the prostate affected by cancer rather that the whole gland.

Locally Advanced Nonmetastatic Disease (Stages T_3, N_0, M_0)

Locally advanced primary stage T_3 disease is usually treated by radiotherapy with additional hormone (androgen deprivation) therapy. Radical prostatectomy (with pelvic lymph node dissection) may be offered to younger men, as part of multimodal treatment (with adjuvant radiotherapy).

Metastatic Disease (Stage T_4, N^+ and/or M^+)

Many patients still present with metastatic disease. In these, the aim of treatment is to control symptoms and to retard the progression of disease. For patients presenting with bladder outlet symptoms, standard transurethral resection or 'channel TURP' usually restores urinary flow.

Most prostatic cancers are androgen-dependent, at least initially, and hormonal manipulation is the mainstay of treatment of advanced disease. Local radiotherapy is frequently effective for treating painful metastases. Pathological fractures in the sclerotic metastases of prostatic cancer are much less common than in the lytic metastases of other cancers. This is fortunate, since the dense bone is more difficult to cut and drill than normal bone, should internal fixation be needed.

Hormonal Therapy

Most cancers depend on the presence of male sex hormones (e.g., testosterone) for their growth and are rendered quiescent, at least for a time, by pharmacological or surgical castration. This is referred to as androgen deprivation therapy. Three main treatment options are available:

- **Luteinising hormone-releasing hormone (LHRH) agonists, such as goserelin.** These drugs need to be injected at 4 to 12 weekly intervals and result in medical castration (i.e., undetectable levels of testosterone in serum). Therapy initially causes **stimulation** of luteinising hormone (LH) release from the pituitary, which in turn causes increased testicular testosterone secretion for up to 2 weeks. This is followed by **inhibition** of LH release by competitively blocking the receptors, resulting in an 'anorchic' state. Hot flushes and sexual dysfunction are the major side-effects. Many patients experience a 'flare' of symptoms in the first 2 weeks, aggravating bone pain or spinal cord compression. For this reason, the first 2 to 3 weeks are covered by antiandrogen therapy (e.g., cyproterone acetate or bicalutamide).

 LHRH antagonists, such as degarelix, are suitable for advanced prostate cancer. These drugs work by blocking gonadotrophin-releasing hormone receptors (GnRH) directly at the pituitary and thus do not cause the initial testosterone-induced flare, as seen with LHRH agonists. The main advantages therefore are that it is fast acting and avoids the need for antiandrogen therapy in the first few weeks.

- **Removal of both testes by subcapsular orchidectomy.** This is a quick and simple scrotal operation and removes about 95% of testosterone synthesised (the rest is from the adrenals), producing an immediate fall in plasma testosterone. The testicular capsules are left in situ and these fill with blood clot and preserve the scrotal contour. There are few side-effects other than hot flushes and sexual dysfunction, and no serious long-term sequelae. With the advent of medical castration (in the form of LHRH agonists or antagonists), surgical castration is now performed increasingly rarely.

- **Antiandrogen drugs, such as bicalutamide.** These block the binding of dihydrotestosterone to its receptor at cellular level and, in contrast to LHRH agonists, block both testicular and adrenal testosterone. Bicalutamide is often used in combination with LHRH agonists to prevent the initial 'testosterone flare', or as part of a strategy to maximally inhibit serum testosterone levels known as *maximum androgen blockade*. Side effects include gynaecomastia, breast tenderness and risk of liver dysfunction.

Almost inevitably, prostatic cancer eventually escapes its androgen dependency and becomes **refractory** to hormonal treatment (**castrate-resistant prostate cancer**). The mechanism is complex and is not completely understood, but occurs at a mean of 2 years after commencing treatment in M$^+$ and 5 years in N$^+$ M^0 disease. When this occurs, secondary or salvage treatment with diethylstilbestrol may be of value. This is a synthetic androgen suppresses LHRH secretion from the hypothalamus,

• **BOX 35.4** Management of Prostatic Carcinoma—Summary

Histological Diagnosis
- By ultrasound-guided transrectal or transperineal prostate biopsy or after transurethral resection of prostate for symptoms of bladder outlet obstruction

Staging
- If radical treatment is contemplated—rectal examination, prostate-specific antigen, transrectal ultrasound, computed tomography or magnetic resonance imaging scanning for local spread and lymph node involvement

Treatment by Stage
- Stages T$_1$ and T$_2$—a choice of active surveillance or radical local treatment, that is, prostatectomy or radiotherapy
- Stage T$_3$—radiotherapy, often with neoadjuvant or adjuvant hormonal therapy or radical prostatectomy with pelvic lymph node excision as part of multimodal approach with adjuvant radiotherapy
- Stage T$_4$
  — antiandrogen therapies (e.g., bilateral orchidectomy), plus radiotherapy for painful bony metastases or spinal cord compression
  or
  — drug treatment with luteinising hormone-releasing hormone analogues or antagonists
  or
  — *if castrate-resistant*
  — drug treatment with oestrogens resulting in testosterone suppression, for example, diethylstilbestrol
  or
  — Systemic chemotherapy, for example, docetaxel

but has a high rate of serious thromboembolic side-effects. Bone metastases can sometimes be palliated by intravenous radioactive strontium. Systemic chemotherapy is offered to men with low volume disease, who have failed radical local treatment and hormone therapy, and for symptoms control in palliative patients. The principles and techniques of palliative care are described in Chapter 13. The management of prostatic carcinoma is summarised in Box 35.4.

Prostatitis

Bacterial prostatitis is an uncommon inflammatory disorder of the prostate usually caused by gram-negative organisms (most often *Escherichia coli*). Less common causes include gram-positive bacteria (enterococci) and occasionally sexually transmitted infections (*Neisseria gonorrhoeae*). It occurs in acute and chronic forms. Urinary tract infection or instrumentation may be a predisposing factor.

Acute Prostatitis

Acute prostatitis is caused by bacterial infection, and is characterised by perineal pain and fever. Prostatic swelling may also cause bladder outflow obstruction and urinary frequency. The prostate is exquisitely tender on rectal examination.

Initial treatment is with intravenous antibiotics, such as gentamicin, until the patient is apyrexial and then an oral quinolone antibiotic for 6 weeks.

Chronic Prostatitis

Chronic prostatitis is most commonly inflammatory in nature and presents with chronic, low-grade perineal and suprapubic pain, and urinary frequency, urgency, dysuria and poor flow. Symptoms and signs can be vague and the diagnosis is sometimes made on insufficient grounds. Around 5% of cases are caused by chronic bacterial infection, most commonly by coliforms, whereas in 95%, no infective cause can be found (a condition named *chronic pelvic pain syndrome*). Other theories of causation, such as autoimmunity and intraprostatic urinary reflux have been proposed.

Treatment is with appropriate antibiotics according to culture and sensitivity of prostatic fluid obtained after prostatic massage. Anti-inflammatory drugs may be used in addition to or instead of antibiotics, particularly in the non-infective cases. Other common strategies include pelvic floor relaxation physiotherapy, alpha-adrenergic blockers (tamsulosin has a role in newly diagnosis patients and those with lower urinary tract symptoms), 5-alpha reductase inhibitors (finasteride can help urinary symptoms and improve intraductal reflux) and amitriptyline for chronic pain. Therapeutic prostatic massage is rarely offered now. Patient with refractory pain symptoms are referred to a chronic pain team.

36

Tumours of the Kidney and Urinary Tract

Introduction

Two types of cancer arise from the renal parenchyma: renal cell carcinomas and nephroblastomas. **Renal cell carcinomas** (also known as *renal adenocarcinomas* and previously as *hypernephromas*) are confined to adults. **Nephroblastomas** (Wilms tumours) are developmental in origin and present in infancy or early childhood (see Ch. 51). Occasional benign renal tumours occur, for example, oncocytoma, adenoma and angiomyolipoma (Box 36.1).

Tumours of the transitional cell epithelium lining the urinary tract (urothelium) are very common. They may arise anywhere in the tract, including the renal pelvicalyceal system, the ureters, the bladder and occasionally the urethra. Pelvicalyceal tumours are uncommon. These **urothelial carcinomas (UCs)**, previously known as **transitional cell carcinomas**, occur exclusively in adults and most commonly in the bladder. **Squamous cell carcinomas** (SCCs) sometimes occur in the urinary tract and probably arise from metaplastic squamous epithelium, caused by chronic irritation from stones or schistosomiasis. SCCs also arise occasionally in squamous epithelium at the urethral meatus. Very rarely, an **adenocarcinoma** develops in the bladder from glandular epithelial remnants of the embryological **urachus,** or a **sarcoma** may develop from connective tissue elements.

Renal Cell Carcinoma

Pathology of Renal Cell Carcinoma

Renal cell carcinoma accounts for about 3% of adult malignancies and is twice as common in males as females. It rarely develops before puberty, but may occur at any age thereafter, with the peak incidence between 60 and 70 years. Renal cell carcinoma mainly occurs sporadically, but there are rare familial forms, such as von Hippel–Lindau disease. The only proven environmental risk factor is tobacco use.

The main types of renal cell carcinoma are clear cell, papillary and chromophobe. C**lear cell carcinoma** is the most common form and originates in renal tubules. They are well circumscribed; the cut surface is yellow (caused by lipid accumulation), often associated with haemorrhage or necrosis.

Renal cell carcinomas vary in grade of malignancy. Small isolated tumours are often found incidentally at autopsy. Tumours of less than 2 cm rarely display invasion or metastasis. Bilateral tumours are present in about 5%. Large tumours invade surrounding tissues and may metastasise to paraaortic lymph nodes. Advanced renal cell carcinoma characteristically extends into the lumen of the renal vein and into the inferior vena cava ('tumour thrombus'—Fig. 36.1). Distant spread is typically to lung, liver and bone. Lung metastases are often typical discrete **'cannonball secondaries'** (see Fig. 36.4). Isolated metastases occasionally develop in the brain, bone and elsewhere.

Staging of Renal Cell Carcinoma

Stage I tumours are ≤7 cm and confined by the renal capsule; stage II tumours are ≥7 cm and still limited to the kidney; stage

---

> **BOX 36.1** **Histological Classification of Adult Renal Tumours**

A. Malignant
   1. Conventional clear cell carcinoma (70%–80%)
   2. Papillary or tubulopapillary renal carcinoma (10%–15%)
   3. Chromophobe renal carcinoma (5%)
   4. Collecting duct carcinoma (rare)
   5. Medullary carcinoma (rare)
B. Benign
   1. Oncocytoma
   2. Papillary or tubular adenoma
   3. Angiomyolipoma

III tumours have renal vein or perinephric tissues involvement but remain confined by Gerota perinephric fascia, and may have regional nodal spread; stage IV tumours invade beyond Gerota fascia, have nodal spread and may have metastatic spread (see Fig. 36.1).

Clinical Features of Renal Cell Carcinoma

The classic presentation is with the triad of **haematuria**, a **mass** and **flank pain**; although all three features only occur in about 15% of cases, one is present in 40% of patients (see Figs. 36.2 and 36.3). Commonly, diagnosis is made **incidentally** by discovering a tumour on ultrasonography or computed tomography (CT) scanning. Renal cell carcinomas often become large before diagnosis owing to their retroperitoneal position; tumours larger ≥7 cm have a 17% chance of having already metastasised. Common and uncommon presenting features of renal cell carcinoma are summarised in Box 36.2.

Approach to Investigation of Suspected Renal Cell Carcinoma

Ultrasound investigation reliably distinguishes simple benign cysts from solid masses most likely to be tumours, and can demonstrate tumour thrombus in the inferior vena cava. CT scanning (with images before and after administration of intravenous contrast) is used to diagnose and stage the disease by assessing invasion of perinephric tissues and by demonstrating regional lymph node or liver metastases (see Fig. 36.3). In addition, imaging can confirm a normal contralateral kidney before planning nephrectomy of the affected kidney. Triple phase CT is also used to clarify the nature of abnormal renal cysts; the Bosniak classification defines complex cysts as containing thick septations, calcium deposition and soft tissue enhancement. Bosniak type III and IV cysts are treated as malignant.

Arteriography can be used in the case of solitary unilateral or bilateral tumours to assess the prospects for segmental resection, although contrast-enhanced CT angiography has generally replaced it as the investigation of choice. Renal tumours have a characteristic circulatory pattern distinct from normal kidney (see Fig. 36.4A). Arteriography is more commonly used, if therapeutic embolisation is being considered, to reduce the vascularity of a tumour before surgery.

A full blood count is performed to look for anaemia or polycythaemia; serum creatinine to assess baseline renal function, and a CT chest or x-ray taken to look for pulmonary metastases (Fig. 36.4B and C). No other preoperative investigations are usually required unless there is concern over postoperative renal function, when renal scintigraphy (i.e., dimercaptosuccinic acid [DMSA] renogram) can be used to assess the individual function of each kidney, to predict potential problems postoperatively.

Management of Renal Cell Carcinoma

In most patients, the kidney involved by tumour is excised (**nephrectomy**). **Partial nephrectomy** is suitable for smaller tumours (stage T_1); this facilitates preservation of as much renal function as possible. Surgical techniques are open, laparoscopic or robotic-assisted laparoscopic nephrectomy. Laparoscopy has the benefit of reduced blood loss and pain, shorter hospital stay and earlier return to normal activity. Traditionally, open renal surgery was via a loin incision (supra-12th rib incision), however, as an open approach is now usually reserved for large tumours, many surgeons prefer an anterior transperitoneal approach, which allows clinical staging, permits control of the inferior vena cava and provides access to the renal artery and vein during extensive resections. Alternatively, a posterolateral thoracoabdominal approach allows early access to the inferior vena cava and renal arteries. In radical nephrectomy, the kidney and perinephric fat should be taken *en bloc*, with excision of any enlarged lymph nodes. For small renal masses, in older patients or those with significant comorbidities, less invasive options, such as active surveillance, cryotherapy (tissue freezing therapy) and radiofrequency ablation can be considered.

Renal cell carcinoma is unusual in that surgical removal of isolated pulmonary or cerebral metastases occasionally results in cure. These isolated metastases may present years

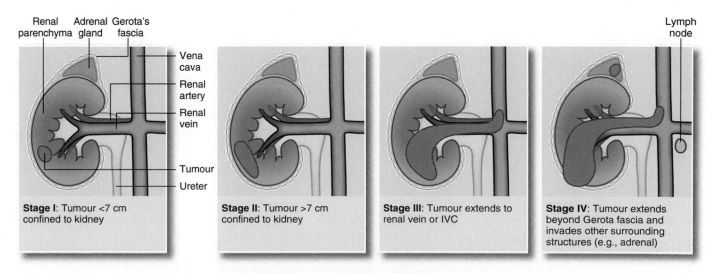

• **Fig. 36.1** Renal Cancer Staging. *IVC,* Inferior vena cava.

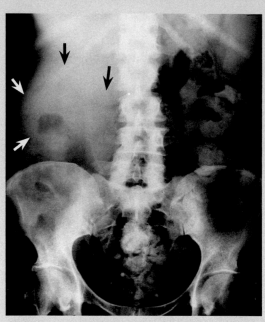

• **Fig. 36.2** Renal Cell Carcinoma: Plain Radiography. This 50-year-old man presented with painless haematuria. The plain abdominal film shows a large soft-tissue mass in the right loin, which obscures the psoas shadow *(arrowed)*. Later investigation showed this to be a renal cell carcinoma.

• BOX 36.2 **Presenting Features of Renal Cell Carcinoma**

Common Presentations
- Visible (frank) haematuria
- Non-visible (microscopic) haematuria often discovered incidentally
- Loin pain
- Renal mass
- Incidental finding on imaging

Uncommon Presentations
- Iron deficiency anaemia[a]
- Polycythaemia caused by erythropoietin production[a]
- Hypertension caused by renin production[a]
- Hypercalcaemia caused by parathormone-like protein production[a]
- Pyrexia of unknown origin
- Elevated erythrocyte sedimentation rate
- Symptoms of metastatic disease (bone pain, weight loss, night sweats)
- Secondary lesions (e.g., 'cannonball' lesions on chest x-ray, pathological fractures)
- Acute varicocoele

[a]*These are paraneoplastic syndromes caused by ectopic hormone release by the tumour.*

after the primary surgery. Therapeutic options for metastatic clear cell renal carcinoma include immunotherapy (bevacizumab and interferon-α) and tyrosine kinase inhibitors (sunitinib); radiotherapy has a role in treating bone or brain metastases.

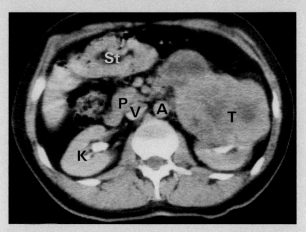

• **Fig. 36.3** Renal Cell Carcinoma: Computed Tomography (CT) Scan. A 62-year-old man presented with left loin pain and a palpable loin mass. This CT scan shows a huge left renal tumour *(T)*; note the variable density of the tumour caused by areas of necrosis and haemorrhage. Note also the normal right kidney *(K)*, aorta *(A)*, pancreas *(P)*, inferior vena cava *(V)* and distal stomach *(St)*.

Urothelial Carcinoma (Transitional Cell Carcinoma)

Epidemiology and Aetiology of Urothelial Carcinoma

Tumours of urothelium are common. Histologically, they are nearly all UCs; other than rarities, the rest are SCCs (7%) or adenocarcinomas (1%). Most arise primarily in the bladder (90%–95%), but they also occur in the pelvicalyceal system and ureters, and rarely in the urethra. Urothelial tumours are uncommon below the age of 50 years and the incidence increases with age. Men are affected three times more often than women. Bladder cancer is the ninth most commonly diagnosed cancer worldwide.

Cigarette smoking is associated with a fourfold increase in the incidence of urothelial tumours; this is probably mediated by urinary excretion of inhaled carcinogens. The proportion of bladder cancer caused by smoking is 50%. Urothelial cancers have been strongly associated with exposure to industrial carcinogens, once widely used in the rubber, cable, dye and printing industries. The likely carcinogens, benzidine, nigrosine and beta naphthylamine, are now banned in most countries, but tumours can develop as long as 25 years after exposure and so a detailed occupational history should be taken in suspected cases. Prolonged exposure to carcinogens causes a 20 to 60 times increased risk of developing urothelial cancer. These carcinogens are excreted in the urine and the more prolonged presence of urine in the bladder compared with the rest of the tract probably explains why urothelial tumours most often arise in the bladder. Occupational exposure accounts for around 10% of bladder cancers.

Pathology of Urothelial Carcinoma

Well-differentiated UCs histologically resemble normal transitional epithelium. Less well-differentiated tumours become increasingly unlike their tissue of origin, so that the most

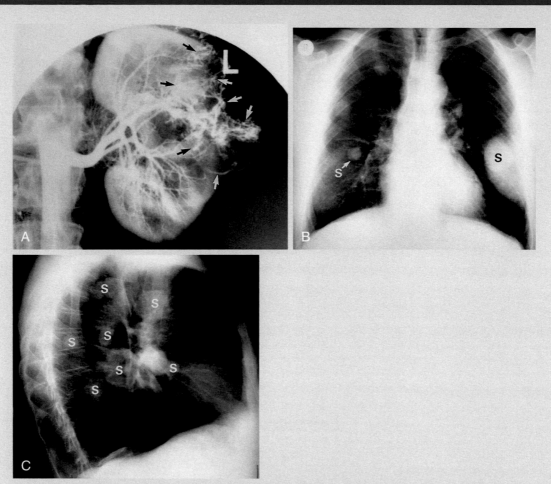

• **Fig. 36.4** Renal Cell Carcinoma: Arteriography and Radiography. This 68-year-old woman presented with haematuria and imaging confirmed a left renal tumour. Before computed tomography scanning was developed, renal arteriography was often used in the diagnosis of renal cell carcinoma and to display its arterial supply as an aid to surgery, but is now mainly used for planning of renal embolisation. **(A)** This left renal arteriogram outlines the normal renal vessels but also shows a large crescentic mass of abnormal vessels (outline *arrowed in white*) typical of renal cell carcinoma. Only the residual part of the tumour vasculature is demonstrated, the rest having been destroyed by necrosis within the tumour. Unfortunately, this patient had already developed pulmonary metastases, as shown in the chest x-rays **(B)** and **(C)**. **(B)** Posterior to anterior (PA) and **(C)** lateral view chest x-rays showing multiple 'cannonball' secondary lesions *(S)* of various sizes. These are typical of renal cell carcinoma.

anaplastic tumours can only be classified as urothelial because they are known to have arisen in the urinary tract. The degree of differentiation tends to be reflected in the tumour morphology as visualised at cystoscopy. Well-differentiated tumours form papillary frond-like lesions, whereas more aggressive tumours form plaque-like lesions, which invade underlying muscle and surrounding tissues.

Most aetiological factors act on the whole urothelium, predisposing it to malignant transformation. Consequently, urothelial tumours can be **multifocal** and there may already be multiple tumours at presentation. When the primary tumour is in the pelvicalyceal system or ureter, there is a high risk of tumours developing later in the urothelium distal to the primary. Around 20% to 50% of patients, with upper tract urothelial tumours, will ultimately develop bladder urothelial tumours. In contrast, only 2% to 6% of patients with bladder UC will develop upper tract UC.

A high-risk form of nonmuscle-invasive UC of the bladder is **carcinoma-in-situ (CIS)**. This presents with urinary frequency and dysuria; urine analysis may demonstrate sterile pyuria and haematuria. Symptoms can be misdiagnosed as prostatitis in men. The lesions desquamate easily and have a high pick-up rate on urine cytology. Untreated, they infiltrate rapidly.

Clinical Features of Urothelial Carcinoma

UC usually presents with painless haematuria (Fig. 36.5). Upper tract lesions can cause obstruction caused by tumour growth, or very occasionally may cause **ureteric colic** (clot colic) and long stringy clots are seen in the urine. If bleeding is gross, clots may cause ureteric obstruction. Rapid bleeding from a bladder tumour may cause **clot retention**, that is, acute retention of urine caused by clot obstruction. Bladder tumours arising near a ureteric orifice can obstruct one ureter, causing **hydronephrosis**. Rarely,

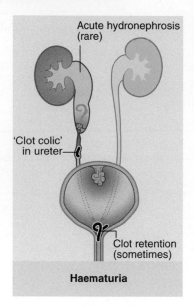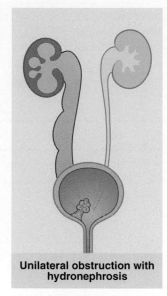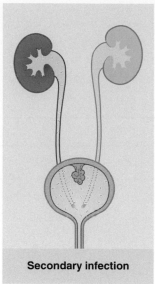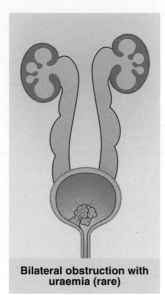

Haematuria **Secondary infection** **Unilateral obstruction with hydronephrosis** **Bilateral obstruction with uraemia (rare)**

• **Fig. 36.5** Presenting Features of Urothelial Tumours.

CASE HISTORY

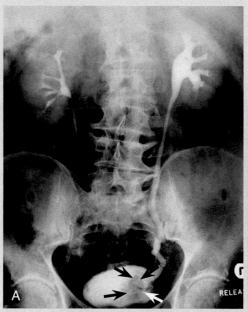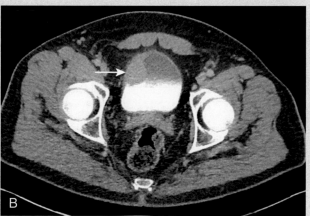

• **Fig. 36.6** Urothelial Tumours at Different Sites. **(A)** This 67-year-old man complained of loin pain and haematuria. On the left side of this intravenous urogram, there is hydronephrosis and ureteric obstruction caused by a bladder tumour visible at the vesicoureteric orifice *(arrowed)*. **(B)** This 62-year-old man presented with visible haematuria, urinary frequency and urgency. A delayed phase contrast computed tomography shows contrast *(white)* half filling the bladder, and a tumour on the right bladder wall *(arrow)*.

bilateral obstruction causes renal impairment. Bladder tumours also predispose to infection; unexplained recurrent urinary tract infections need investigating to exclude UC as a cause. Tumour invasion near the bladder neck may cause obstructive lower urinary tract symptoms, or incontinence, but this is usually preceded by haematuria or infection. Lower urinary tract storage symptoms (urinary frequency and urgency) may also be the presenting feature of bladder cancer, usually associated with visible or nonvisible haematuria.

Investigation of Suspected Urothelial Carcinoma

Confirmed haematuria in the absence of infection must be investigated. Ultrasound examination may reveal hydronephrosis if there is ureteric involvement by UC. Contrast CT scanning will outline the upper tract, as well as the renal parenchyma. Intravenous urogram can also outline the upper tract, but is becoming obsolete (see Fig. 36.6). Imaging is followed by cystoscopy, the only reliable method of examining the lining of the bladder and

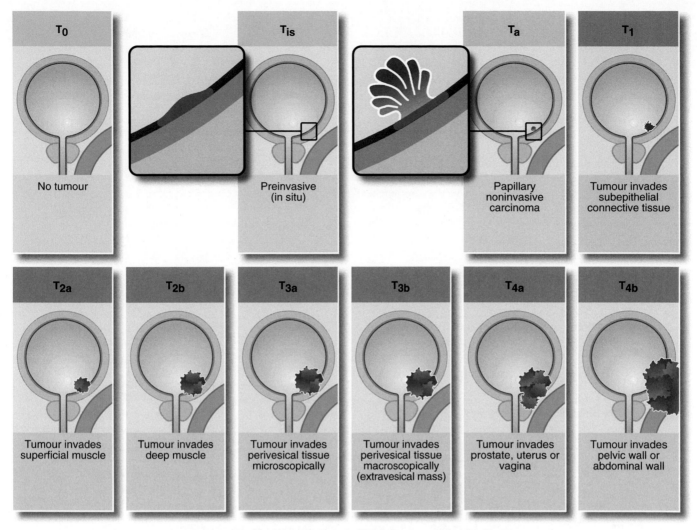

• **Fig. 36.7** Tumour Node Metastasis (TNM) Staging of Bladder Cancer.

urethra. If there is an upper tract tumour, cystoscopy may reveal blood emerging from a ureteric orifice. Urine cytology is useful, but most accurate for identifying high-grade cancer cells and carcinoma in situ.

Staging of Urothelial Tumours of the Bladder

Staging is achieved by cystoscopic examination and examination under anaesthesia, combined with histological examination of resected specimens, and imaging with CT or magnetic resonance imaging. For small and superficial lesions, histology shows the extent of bladder wall invasion, degree of tumour differentiation and whether the tumour has been completely removed. For larger or deeper lesions, palpation of the bladder under general anaesthesia bimanually between a finger in the rectum (or vagina) and a hand on the anterior abdominal wall should be performed before and after resection of the tumour. This gives an idea of the extent of bladder wall penetration and spread into the pelvis (which would create a fixed mass). CT scanning is a more reliable indication of spread into the bladder wall or beyond. Note, however, that CT scanning can be misleading, if performed soon after resection of a bladder tumour.

The Tumour Node Metastasis (TNM) clinical system widely used in **staging** bladder tumours is illustrated in Fig. 36.7 (the 'T' is the clinical stage of the tumour). Tumours are also **graded** according to the degree of histological differentiation: G1, which is well differentiated (also known as papillary urothelial neoplasm of low malignant potential or PUNLMP); G2, which is moderately differentiated (divided into low and high grade); G3, which is poorly differentiated (or high grade). In addition, some pathologists grade bladder tumours according to P and G pathological criteria. **The 'P' system** (small p for the biopsy specimen and capital P for the whole specimen) classifies the extent of invasion on gross anatomical and histological grounds. Thus as an example, a pathologist may report a biopsy as pT_2G3.

Management of Urothelial Carcinoma

Bladder Tumours

UCs of the bladder display a variety of morphological types ranging from small, discrete, often multiple, frond-like lesions through to extensive papilliferous or flat solid tumours. The first type is usually at a very early invasive stage and such lesions were formerly known as *papillomas* before their malignant potential was fully realised. If papillary tumours coexist with CIS, however, the long-term prognosis is ominous. These patients are usually offered immunotherapy, with a course of intravesical Bacillus Calmette-Guerin (BCG) to stimulate local immunity. However, if CIS persists, then total (radical) cystectomy is the treatment of choice.

The initial management of bladder tumours is usually aimed at complete removal of tumour tissue by cystoscopic **transurethral resection of bladder tumour (TURBT)**, even with large lesions. Further management then depends on the stage of tumour spread determined by examination under anaesthesia, CT scanning and histological staging.

As shown in Fig. 36.8, bladder tumours, classified as T_a or T_1, can usually be completely resected. Single-dose **intravesical chemotherapy** with mitomycin C has been shown to reduce the recurrence rate after the initial TURBT in T_a or T_1 disease. T_1 lesions are notoriously recurrent and if they recur repeatedly, weekly courses of intravesical chemotherapy (mitomycin C) or BCG is the treatment of choice. For T_2/T_3 lesions, the preferred treatment in a fit patient is **radical cystectomy**. The tumour can sometimes be downstaged before surgery by neoadjuvant systemic chemotherapy. Radiotherapy is a good alternative for the unfit or older patient, in those unwilling to undergo cystectomy, or for relapse after initial cystectomy or initial systemic chemotherapy.

When radical cystectomy is necessary, some method of **urinary diversion** is required. The classic operation involves isolation of a segment of ileum; both ureters are then anastomosed onto the ileal segment, creating an **ileal conduit**, whilst the other end is opened onto the abdominal wall as a urostomy. An earlier operation, in which both ureters were diverted into the sigmoid colon (ureterosigmoidostomy), has generally been abandoned because of electrolyte disruption and a high risk of carcinoma at the ureterocolic anastomoses. An alternative to ileal conduit is the formation of a **continent pouch** (neobladder). If the urethra and bladder neck are clear of cancer, this can be constructed from a refashioned segment of ileum and anastomosed to the urethra (**orthotopic neobladder**). A **heterotopic neobladder** is formed from colon and ileum and uses a continent catheterisable channel (i.e., Mitrofanoff channel using the appendix), to empty the pouch with intermittent self-catheterisation.

T_4 tumours are usually incurable; even total cystectomy rarely eliminates the entire lesion. Radiotherapy offers palliation and is valuable for controlling pain and haematuria.

Urothelial Tumours of the Upper Tract

UCs of the pelvicalyceal system and ureter are uncommon. Treatment usually requires excision of the whole upper tract on the affected side including kidney, ureter and a cuff of bladder wall surrounding the distal ureter (nephroureterectomy). However, some small, isolated low-risk renal pelvic tumours can be dealt with endoscopically, by laser ablation, via a fibreoptic flexible ureteroscope, and very occasionally, via a nephroscope passed percutaneously into the pelvicalyceal system.

Unusual Urinary Tract Tumours

The uncommon SCC of the urinary tract is diagnosed and treated along similar lines to UC, although generally bladder SCC has a worse prognosis, with many presenting with muscle-invasive disease. It can develop as a complication of chronic inflammation caused by indwelling catheters, stones or caused by schistosomiasis in Egypt and the Middle East, where the parasite infection is endemic. Distal urethral SCC lesions are managed in the same way as penile carcinoma (see Ch. 33). Adenocarcinoma is rare but can occur anywhere in the bladder, most often in a urachal remnant at the vault. Tumours of this type can often be removed by segmental resection of the bladder (partial cystectomy).

Follow-Up and Control of Recurrent Disease

Patients who have had potentially curative treatment for urothelial tumours (i.e., bladder stages T_1 to T_3 and all upper tract lesions) must be followed up longer term. The goal is to detect recurrence of the original tumour and to diagnose new primary lesions at an early stage, bearing in mind that environmental factors that induced the initial lesion predispose the remaining urothelium to malignant change. It is not always easy to distinguish between

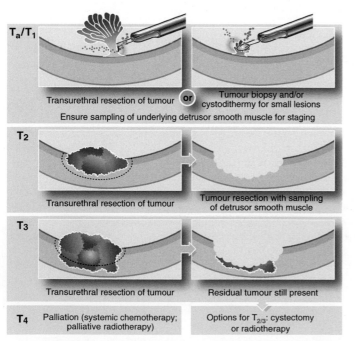

• **Fig. 36.8** Cystoscopic Management of Bladder Tumours—Summary. Note that repeat resection is indicated for: high-grade, noninvasive tumours ($G3pT_a/1$) to ensure original tumour was not understaged; if no muscle present in initial specimen; and if first resection was incomplete. Bladder chemotherapy (mitomycin C single dose) is commonly given in theatre after the primary resection.

• BOX 36.3 **Surveillance of Nonmuscle Invasive Bladder Cancer With Cystoscopy**

Bladder Cancer Risk Category	Follow-Up Regimen
Low risk (i.e., small, low-grade pTa G1/G2 solitary tumour)	Cystoscopy at 3- and 12-months post-TURBT
Intermediate risk (i.e., low-grade pTaG1 tumours over 3 cm, multifocal or recurrent, and G2 tumours)	Cystoscopy at 3-, 6-, 9- and 18-months post-TURBT, then yearly for 5 years
High risk (i.e., high-grade pTa or pT1G3; pT1G2 tumours, or CIS)	Cystoscopy every 3 months for 2 years; 6 monthly for 2 years, then yearly

CIS, carcinoma-in-situ; *TURBT,* transurethral resection of bladder tumour.

small recurrences and new primaries; all tend to be labelled as 'recurrences'.

Follow-up for nonmuscle invasive bladder cancer (T_a, T_1) involves regular 'check' flexible cystoscopies under local anaesthesia. The frequency and duration of check cystoscopy is dictated by whether the tumour is low, medium or high risk (refer to National Institute for Health and Care Excellence guidelines), and is shown in Box 36.3. Urine cytology may also be used for both screening of normal individuals with haematuria or those with risk factors for cancer (i.e., smokers, high occupational risk) and for bladder cancer surveillance.

Recurrent lesions are managed in the same way as the initial lesion, that is, according to the stage of bladder wall invasion. The exception is when the initial treatment involved radiotherapy. For these patients, cure of recurrent cancer is improbable and palliative surgery ranging from TURBT to total cystectomy may be necessary to treat tumour recurrence or intractable problems, such as severe haemorrhage.

37

Stone Disease of the Urinary Tract

Introduction

Stones may occur in all parts of the urinary tract, including the pelvicalyceal system of the kidney, the ureter, the bladder and sometimes even the urethra. Stones most commonly provoke symptoms caused by obstruction or by predisposing to urinary tract infections.

Upper tract calculi are much more common than bladder calculi and the incidence is rising. Stones range from the uncommon **staghorn calculus**, which fills the pelvicalyceal system, to small stones developing in the pelvicalyceal system that can migrate and obstruct the ureter. Acute ureteric obstruction causes severe pain and presents as the surgical emergency **ureteric colic**. Most stone disease is, however, asymptomatic or else presents nonurgently to the outpatient clinic.

Stone disease (urolithiasis) in childhood is now rare in developed countries. The peak incidence occurs between 20 and 50

years of age, and declines slowly thereafter (Fig. 37.1). The life time risk of urolithiasis is 10% to 15% in Western countries and up to 25% in the Middle East. Males are affected nearly twice as often as females. There is also a high incidence of recurrent stones; if preventative measures are not used, the risk is around 10% at 1 year, 33% at 5 years and 50% at 10 years.

Pathophysiology of Stone Disease

Stones are often formed from a mixture of chemical substances and minerals (e.g., calcium and oxalate), when their concentration exceeds their solubility in urine. Intermittent periods of **supersaturation** caused by dehydration, medical conditions or following meals, can lead to the earliest phase of crystal formation (**nucleation**). Crystals coalesce into groups (**aggregation**), and act as nucleus for further stone formation. Promoters of stone formation are low urine volume, low urine pH, calcium, sodium, oxalate, and urate. Lack of crystallisation inhibitors in the urine also plays a role in stone formation. Inhibitors of stone formation include citrate, magnesium, Tamm-Horsfall protein and glycosaminoglycans. Table 37.1 provides a simple classification showing the relative frequency of stone types and their important clinical characteristics and aetiology. Calcium is present in over 80%, as oxalate or phosphate compounds or both. The aetiology of stone disease is multifactorial in most cases.

Predisposing Factors for Stone Disease

A specific predisposing factor can be detected in some cases. These include chronic infection, urinary stasis and foreign bodies, and are summarised in Box 37.1.

Calcium-Containing Stones

In patients with calcium-containing stones, specific underlying abnormalities are rarely discovered. Some patients excrete excessive calcium (**idiopathic hypercalciuria**) without being hypercalcaemic; in these, there may be increased intestinal absorption of calcium leading to increased urinary excretion.

Stones Caused by Excessive Urinary Excretion of a Stone Constituent

A minority of patients have an underlying disorder responsible for excessive urinary excretion of the main constituent of the stone. Examples include **hyperparathyroidism** (calcium), hyperoxaluria (oxalate), **gout** (uric acid), **cystinuria** (cystine stones) and **xanthinuria** (xanthine stones).

Clinical Features of Stone Disease

The clinical problem of discrete urinary stones should not be confused with calcification of the renal parenchyma, which can be a feature of tuberculosis and medullary sponge kidney. These and similar diseases can usually be diagnosed by their characteristic x-ray appearance.

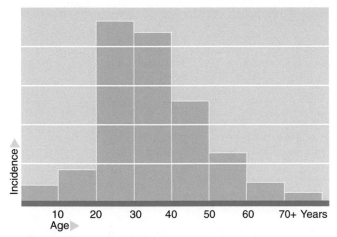

• **Fig. 37.1** Relative Incidence of Stone Disease by Age in Developed Countries.

The clinical presentation of stones depends on the size, morphology and site of the stone(s). Many cause no symptoms but represent a potentially serious problem. Other stones produce marked pathological effects, which present with acute or chronic

---

• BOX 37.1 Predisposing Factors in Stone Formation

- Stasis of urine, particularly when associated with infection—for example, congenital abnormalities, hydronephrosis, chronic obstruction (e.g., benign prostatic hyperplasia, neurogenic bladder)
- Chronic urinary infection (urea-splitting organisms, e.g., *Proteus* cause alkaline urine and the development of magnesium–ammonium–phosphate stones, typically the 'staghorn' calculi of the renal pelvis
- Excess urinary excretion of stone-forming substances—for example, idiopathic hypercalciuria (calcium stones), hyperparathyroidism (calcium stones), hyperoxaluria (oxalate stones), gout (uric acid stones), cystinuria (cystine stones), xanthinuria (xanthine stones)
- Foreign bodies—for example, fragments of catheter tubing, self-inserted artefacts, parasites (schistosome ova), fragments of diseased tissue (e.g., renal papillary necrosis)
- Dietary—for example, high animal protein intake and high salt diet
- Obesity—associated with lower urinary pH, which can promote uric acid stones
- Dehydration—lower volume, concentrated urine encourages crystallisation
- Bowel or digestive disorders—can affect absorption of calcium and water
- Family or personal history of stones
- Prolonged immobility—leads to skeletal decalcification and increased serum calcium levels

---

TABLE 37.1	Chemical Composition, Clinical Features and Aetiology of Urinary Tract Stones		
Chemical Composition	**%**	**Clinical Features**	**Aetiology**
Calcium oxalate	70%–80%	Three types of stone are described: — small smooth 'hemp-seed' stones — small irregular 'mulberry' stones — small spiculated 'jack' stones	Most cases are idiopathic; predisposing factors include urinary stasis, infection and foreign bodies Some are caused by metabolic disorders, which lead to excess urinary excretion of calcium or oxalate: — hyperparathyroidism — hyperoxaluria (rare inherited disorder)
Mixed calcium oxalate and phosphate stones	10%	As earlier	Some are caused by disorders associated with hypercalcaemia, for example, sarcoidosis, multiple metastases, multiple myeloma, milk-alkali syndrome, overtreatment with vitamin D
Pure calcium phosphate stones	1%	As earlier	Some of these patients excrete abnormally large amounts of calcium, possibly as a result of increased absorption (idiopathic hypercalciuria but without hypercalcaemia)
Magnesium ammonium phosphate (struvite/ infection stones)	10%–15%	Typically large 'staghorn' calculi of pelvicalyceal system and some bladder stones	Chronic infection with organisms capable of producing urease, typically *Proteus*. Urease splits urea, forming ammonia if the urine is alkaline
Uric acid	5%–10%	Stones tend to absorb yellow and brown pigments. Pure stones are radiolucent	Occur in primary gout and hyperuricaemia following chemotherapy for leukaemias or myeloproliferative disorders. Childhood urate bladder stones occur in some developing countries when urine pH is low
Cystine or xanthine	1%	Excess urinary excretion of cystine or xanthine. Pure stones are radiolucent	Autosomal recessive inherited disorders

symptoms or are discovered incidentally on investigation of unrelated symptoms. The presentation of urinary tract stones is summarised in Box 37.2.

Obstruction of Urinary Flow

Pelvicalyceal Obstruction

Obstruction of renal calyces causes local urinary obstruction (**hydrocalyx**) and can lead to chronic or recurrent loin pain. Similar pain may also be caused by chronic, incomplete obstruction of the pelviureteric junction (PUJ) or ureter. The result is **hydronephrosis**, that is, dilatation of the renal pelvis, both intrarenal and extrarenal. Severe obstruction may lead to progressive renal parenchymal damage and impaired renal function; the patient may develop renal failure if both kidneys are affected.

Passage of Stones Into the Ureter

If small renal stones pass into the ureter, there are several possible outcomes:

- Stones may pass to the bladder, then exit via the urethra, causing minor symptoms. The patient may intermittently pass this out whole, as 'gravel' or 'sand' (see Fig. 37.2) and experience dysuria and sometimes haematuria.
- Stones may pass into the bladder and act as a nidus for the formation of a larger bladder stone. Bladder stones contribute to lower urinary tract symptoms and infection.
- A stone may impact in the ureter causing chronic partial obstruction and eventually hydroureter. This presents typically as loin pain but, surprisingly, may be asymptomatic.
- A stone may impact in the ureter, causing sudden obstruction. The patient experiences extremely severe, unilateral colicky pain (**ureteric colic**) radiating from loin to groin or tip of the penis. There is often loin tenderness caused by renal distension. The pain is caused by waves of ureteric peristalsis and at the peak of the pain, the patient writhes in agony.

> **• BOX 37.2 Presentation of Stones in the Urinary Tract**
>
> - Incidental finding on x-ray or computed tomography (CT)
> - Loin pain
> - Ureteric colic
> - Painful passage of small stones via urethra
> - Symptoms of infection (cystitis, pyelonephritis)
> - Haematuria
> - Impaired renal function
>
> Urinary tract stones produce their injurious effects in three main ways:
> - by obstructing urinary flow;
> - by predisposing to infection;
> - by causing local tissue irritation and damage.

CASE HISTORY

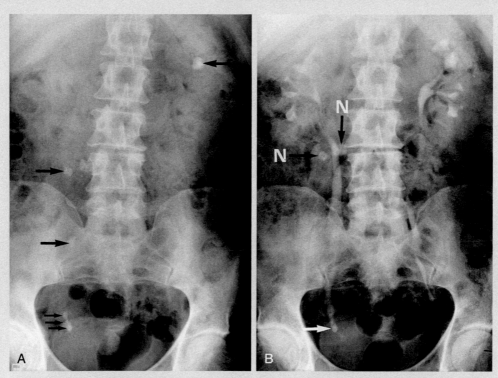

• Fig. 37.2 Recurrent Urinary Tract Stones. This man aged 40 years had a 2-year history of passing small stones and 'gravel' in the urine. **(A)** Plain abdominal x-ray showing what appear to be several stones *(arrowed)* in the right ureter and in the upper pole of the left kidney. **(B)** Intravenous urogram (IVU) of the same patient showing partial obstruction at the lower end of the right ureter *(arrowed)*; note that two of the radiopaque objects on the right side lie outside the area of contrast and thus probably represent calcified mesenteric lymph nodes *(N)* rather than ureteric stones; metabolic studies showed that this patient has idiopathic hypercalciuria. CT is now routinely used to diagnose stones and has replaced IVU.

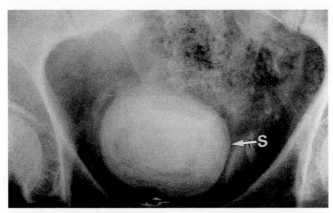

• **Fig. 37.3** Bladder Stone. Plain x-ray showing a massive bladder stone (S) in an 85-year-old man with benign prostatic hypertrophy and recurrent urinary tract infections; such stones are rare nowadays.

Predisposition to Infection

Stones predispose to infection by causing urinary stasis, by preventing proper 'flushing' of the tract and by providing niches in which bacteria multiply. Pelvicalyceal or ureteric stones can cause **acute pyelonephritis** and occasionally a **perinephric abscess**. Bladder stones predispose to cystitis and ascending infections (Fig. 37.3).

Local Irritation and Tissue Damage

Stones may present as a result of their irritant effects on local tissues. Simple inflammation may cause bleeding and present as **haematuria**. Chronic inflammation may lead to fibrosis; if this occurs at a narrow part of the tract, typically the PUJ or ureter, a **stricture** may form. Prolonged irritation of the bladder mucosa by stones may cause **squamous metaplasia** and eventually **squamous carcinoma**.

Investigation and Management of Suspected Urinary Tract Stones

Approach to Investigation

When investigating a patient with urinary tract stones, the objectives are:
• to confirm a stone is present;
• to locate the stone(s);
• to evaluate any deleterious effects of the stone(s) on renal function and urinary tract morphology;
• to identify any structural disorders of the urinary tract acting as local predisposing factors;
• to identify any metabolic predisposing factors.

Methods of Investigation

In general, the objectives can be met by performing the following investigations. For convenience, they are conducted concurrently:
• Urine dipstick testing followed by microscopy, culture and sensitivities if evidence of infection.
• Tests of renal function, that is, plasma urea, electrolytes and creatinine levels.
• A 'KUB' (kidney, ureter, bladder) plain abdominal x-ray. Around 90% of stones are radiopaque because they contain calcium. Urate stones are radiolucent.

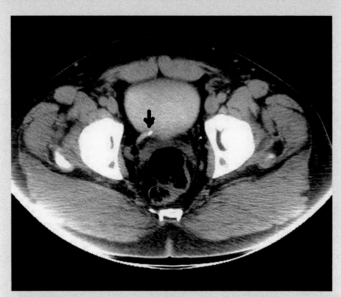

• **Fig. 37.4** Computed Tomography (CT) Imaging in Ureteric Colic. This 37-year-old man presented with right ureteric colic. The CT scan shows a stone at the vesicoureteric junction, with a column of secreted contrast held up in the proximal ureter.

• BOX 37.3 Indications for Removal of Urinary Tract Stones

• Obstruction of urinary flow
• Infection
• Persistent, recurrent or severe pain
• Stones likely to cause future obstruction or infection
• Small 'metabolic' stones likely to grow rapidly in size
• In patients where colic could be disastrous, for example, airline or military pilots
• Patients with a solitary kidney

• Computed tomography (CT) imaging of the abdomen and pelvis. In developed countries, this has become the standard modality for diagnosing loin pain and renal tract stones (Fig. 37.4).
• Intravenous urography (IVU). This consists of a preinjection KUB and further films at 5 to 20 minutes after injection of radiopaque contrast and after micturition. Fig. 37.2 shows an IVU with the effects of stone obstruction.

RENAL ULTRASONOGRAPHY

• This demonstrates hydronephrosis and renal stones.
• Biochemical analysis of any recovered stones.
• Tests for metabolic disorders (for recurrent stones), that is, serum calcium, phosphate, and, uric acid; 24-hour urinary excretion of calcium, uric acid, oxalate and cystine.

Indications for Stone Removal (Box 37.3)

The finding of a urinary tract stone is not an automatic indication for its removal or destruction. The exception is in airline or military pilots, in whom ureteric colic could prove disastrous. The usual indications for stone removal are summarised in Box 37.3.

Small stones in the pelvicalyceal system often remain unchanged and asymptomatic for many years and can safely be monitored by annual radiography. Stones of 5 mm diameter or less often pass right through the tract, although in doing so, they may produce severe but short-lived symptoms of ureteric colic, haematuria or dysuria. **Medical expulsive therapy** (i.e., tamsulosin alpha blocker medication) is less commonly used, as it does not significantly accelerate stone passage, though it may assist with pain relief.

Methods of Stone Removal

Stones can be removed by endoscopic methods, percutaneously or very rarely by open surgery. The choice of technique depends on the size, nature and site of the stone, the availability of expertise and special equipment, and whether there is a need to correct congenital or acquired structural abnormalities.

Cystoscopic Techniques

Cystoscopic methods are suitable for most small to moderate sized **bladder stones.** One options is to use a stone punch (lithotrite) to break the stone into small fragments (**litholapaxy**) under direct cystoscopic vision (Fig. 37.5A), then evacuating the fragments using an Ellik evacuator. An alternative method is to use an irrigating cystoscope with holmium laser fibre to fragment stones; advantages include reduced bleeding and better surgical views.

A rigid **ureteroscope** can be used to examine the entire length of the ureter and assist with **ureteric stone** removal (see Figs 37.5B and Fig. 37.6A), as well as to apply energy via **holmium laser** directly onto the surface of a stone to destroy it. **Flexible ureteroscopes** (see Fig. 37.5C) allow access to the renal pelvis and calyces, so stone fragmentation can be achieved using a fine holmium laser fibre. Stone fragments can be captured and removed using forceps or basket devices, such as a nitinol 'Zero Tip' basket (see Fig. 37.5D).

A **ureteric stent** is placed after repeated instrumentation of the ureter to assist drainage. If an impacted stone is causing complete ureteric obstruction and leading to marked proximal dilatation, or if there is infection (i.e., infected obstructed kidney), a ureteric stent or percutaneous nephrostomy tube should be inserted above the stone without delay (Fig. 37.7) to preserve renal function.

Open Surgical Methods

Open surgery was often necessary before the advent of current minimal access methods of removing or destroying stones. For the pelvicalyceal system, **pyelolithotomy** was performed; for the ureter, **ureterolithotomy**; and for some large bladder stones, **cystolithotomy** is still required. Open or laparoscopic surgery is now only used when minimally invasive techniques are not available or have failed, where stones are difficult to access (i.e., calculus in a calyceal diverticulum with a narrow or obliterated neck) and for larger stone burden in some cases. If elective correction of an anatomical abnormality predisposing to stone formation is being performed, then open stone removal is indicated at the same operation. Examples are PUJ obstruction or ureteric stricture.

Percutaneous Techniques of Stone Removal

Direct percutaneous access to the renal pelvis can be obtained using radiological (fluoroscopic) or ultrasound guidance. **Percutaneous nephrolithotomy** or PCNL is used to remove larger stones (>2 cm) from the kidney by the creation of a track from the skin, via the loin into the pelvicalyceal system. Progressively, larger dilators are passed, and a sheath is left in the track, which allows insertion of a nephroscope and other instruments. Small stones can be retrieved using a basket or a steerable grasping tool. Larger stones can be broken into fragments with

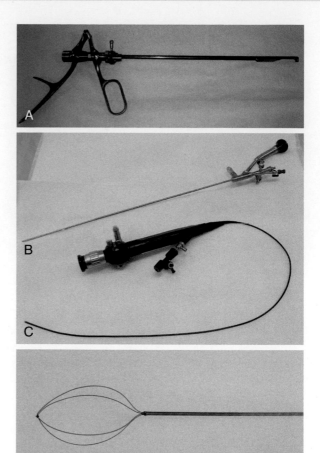

• **Fig. 37.5** Instruments for urinary stone removal **(A)** Straight stone punch (lithotrite) for bladder stones. A telescope fits through the centre of the lithotrite, allowing a direct view as the stones are crushed between the jaws, with an outer irrigating sheath over both components. **(B)** Fine rigid ureteroscope. Used for the treatment of ureteric stones. **(C)** Flexible uretero-renoscope. Used to access and treat small stones in the pelvicalyceal system of the kidney. **(D)** Zero Tip **nitinol basket**. In a closed position, this is inserted through a channel in the ureteroscope, and advanced just beyond the stone. The basket is opened, pulled down to capture and then closed around the stone, and the whole instrument and basket is withdrawn back down to the bladder (where the stone can be washed out) or removed via the urethra, where the stone is collected for analysis.

laser (which are retrieved with a basket or forceps), or with an ultrasonic **lithoclast** probe, which can also remove the debris of stone destruction using suction (see Fig. 37.6B). Pneumatic (or ballistic) lithotripsy probes can also be used and residual fragments removed with forceps. A nephrostomy is often left temporarily as a drain postoperatively, but once removed the track closes spontaneously after a short period.

Noninvasive Stone Removal Technique (Fig. 37.6C)

Extracorporeal shock wave lithotripsy is a noninvasive method of destroying stones using externally applied shock waves, which pass into the patient to shatter the stone. The ultrasound beam is focused on the stone by ultrasound or x-ray. Stone fragments are passed out in the urine and may cause ureteric colic or ureteric obstruction.

Management of Acute Ureteric Colic

Most patients with ureteric colic are seen urgently by a General Practitioner or brought straight to the accident and emergency department. Nonsteroidal anti-inflammatory drugs (NSAIDs)

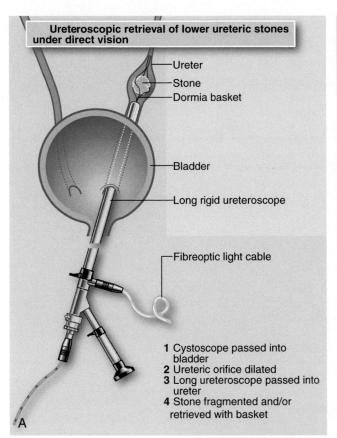

Ureteroscopic retrieval of lower ureteric stones under direct vision

Ureter
Stone
Dormia basket

Bladder

Long rigid ureteroscope

Fibreoptic light cable

1 Cystoscope passed into bladder
2 Ureteric orifice dilated
3 Long ureteroscope passed into ureter
4 Stone fragmented and/or retrieved with basket

A

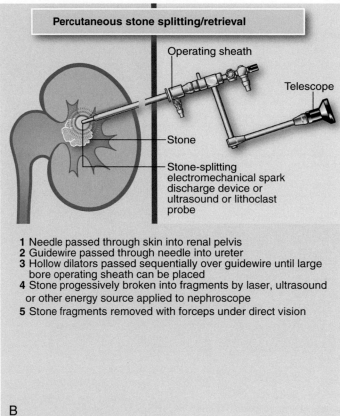

Percutaneous stone splitting/retrieval

Operating sheath

Telescope

Stone

Stone-splitting electromechanical spark discharge device or ultrasound or lithoclast probe

1 Needle passed through skin into renal pelvis
2 Guidewire passed through needle into ureter
3 Hollow dilators passed sequentially over guidewire until large bore operating sheath can be placed
4 Stone progessively broken into fragments by laser, ultrasound or other energy source applied to nephroscope
5 Stone fragments removed with forceps under direct vision

B

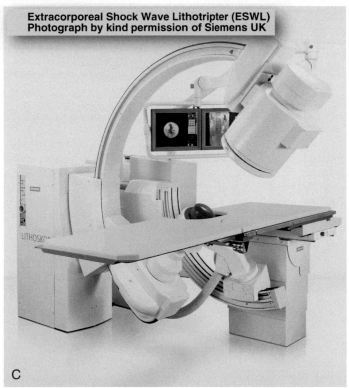

**Extracorporeal Shock Wave Lithotripter (ESWL)
Photograph by kind permission of Siemens UK**

C

• **Fig. 37.6** Current Methods of Urinary Tract Stone Removal.

given as suppositories are very effective as first-line drugs to settle the pain. Opioids could be used if severe pain failed to settle or if NSAIDs were contraindicated; pethidine is avoided owing to the risk of vomiting. The patient may have become pain-free by the time of first examination, but the pain history is usually diagnostic. Occasionally, ureteric colic is less severe but more persistent, in which case, it may mimic other acute abdominal conditions. It is essential during assessment to exclude other important differential diagnoses, such as a ruptured aortic aneurysm in older patients, appendicitis, pyelonephritis or diverticulitis.

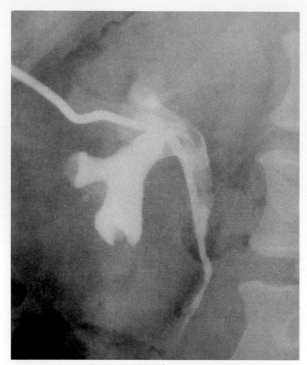

• **Fig. 37.7** Percutaneously Placed Nephrostomy Drainage Tube. A ureteric stone caused complete ureteric obstruction and the patient suffered continuing pain and developed a fever. Urgent drainage was required to prevent renal damage from a combination of obstruction and infection.

Many patients settle with a single analgesic dose but two or three doses may be required. In most cases, the stone gradually passes down the ureter and into the bladder. Each stage of movement may be accompanied by an attack of colic. If a stone is retrieved, it should be chemically analysed. If there is **complete obstruction** of the ureter, or infection above an obstructing stone, urgent intervention is usually required to prevent renal damage. Immediate treatment may involve placing a percutaneous nephrostomy tube to drain the renal pelvis under local anaesthesia (see Fig. 37.7), placing a ureteric stent alongside the stone to allow drainage, or removing the stone endoscopically. After nephrostomy or stent placement, the stone sometimes passes spontaneously, but more often further treatment is required. In cases with persistent pain not needing immediate intervention, plain abdominal x-rays usually record changes in the stone's position. Very large stones may have to be surgically removed. If a stone appears to be small enough to pass spontaneously, yet fails to progress, the patient can safely be allowed home, provided criteria for urgent intervention are not fulfilled. The patient can be reviewed after a week or two with a plain abdominal x-ray and a decision taken then about any need for intervention.

Investigation of Ureteric Colic

Urine dipstick testing is useful to exclude infection and to investigate for haematuria. An acute sudden onset of ureteric colic is associated with **microscopic haematuria** in most, but patients presenting after several days of colic are less likely to show a positive result, so a clear test does not exclude a stone. Blood tests of renal function, calcium and uric acid levels should be performed. A noncontrast CT scan (or an IVU) should then be performed urgently to confirm or refute the diagnosis (see Fig. 37.4). CT is rapid and will diagnose most stones. It can demonstrate alternative causes for flank pain and is now the gold standard investigation. Rare indinavir drug-related stones are not visible on CT. If a stone is identified, a plain KUB x-ray will show whether the stone is radiopaque, and if so, the patient can be monitored with x-ray for stone migration.

Characteristic radiological features of acute ureteric obstruction on CT or IVU are:
• **Delay** of all phases of contrast passage through the kidney and collecting system on the affected side; the more severe the obstruction, the longer the delay. If there appears to be no excretion on IVU, further films are taken every few hours for up to 24 hours; usually contrast will eventually pass into the system, demonstrating the site of obstruction.
• **Dilatation** of the collecting system above the point of obstruction.

Ureteric Stones in Pregnancy

Flank pain in pregnancy can be difficult to assess. Ultrasound is the safest modality to use, but is not accurate for diagnosing ureteric stones. Pregnant women develop a physiological bilateral hydronephrosis, as gestation advances, owing to the effects of progesterone and pressure on the ureters from the gravid uterus (the right kidney is usually more dilated than the left). Because of ureteric dilatation, most ureteric stones can be expected to pass, and management is largely about good pain relief, unless there are worrying features, such as infection or renal impairment. In the few with persisting severe pain, insertion of a ureteric stent or nephrostomy is required, or more rarely, ureteroscopic removal of the stone. The risk of encrustation of stents and nephrostomies is higher in pregnancy and these devices need to be exchanged regularly until definitive treatment can be performed after delivery.

Long-Term Management of Urological Stone Disease

Management of Metabolic Abnormalities

Whist most **calcium oxalate stones** are idiopathic (i.e., cause unknown), a variety of metabolic problems involving excessive excretion of substances in the urine (hypercalciuria, hyperoxaluria, hyperuricosuria), coupled with deficiencies of other constituents (hypomagnesiuria, hypocitraturia) are known to contribute. These abnormalities can be identified on '24-urine collection' analysis. **Hypercalciuria** associated with a raised serum calcium level should prompt a serum parathyroid hormone test to investigate for hyperparathyroidism. This would require surgical correction with parathyroidectomy. Hypercalciuria with a normal serum calcium level is called *idiopathic hypercalciuria*. Treatment includes good fluid intake, low salt diet, potassium citrate and thiazide drugs.

Excessive oxalate excretion in the urine (**hyperoxaluria**) is caused by increased hepatic production (rare), increased bowel absorption or excessive dietary intake. General advice is to reduce intake of oxalate rich foods, such as nuts and chocolate and drinks, such as tea and coffee.

Hyperuricosuria (excessive urinary excretion of uric acid) can lead to the formation of uric acid stones and uric acid crystals, which can act as a nidus for calcium oxalate stone formation. **Uric acid stones** are seen in patients with gout and myeloproliferative disorders or can be idiopathic. Treatment is with good fluid intake and dietary purine reduction. Increasing the urine pH to more alkaline levels promotes the solubility of uric acid and is worthwhile. Patients can be prescribed allopurinol, if these measures fail to work.

Cystine stones are rare (1%), occur only in patients with cystinuria, and are considered at high risk of recurrence. Prevention is with a high fluid intake, low salt diet, maintaining urine pH >7.5 (keeping it alkaline with sodium bicarbonate or potassium citrate to improve the solubility of cystine), with the addition of the drug, tiopronin, in select cases.

Long-Term Follow Up of Patients With Urinary Tract Stones

For many patients, a symptomatic urinary tract stone manifests as an isolated episode with no apparent predisposing cause. Long-term follow-up for these patients is not usually needed. Patients with stones that do not need removing, or with recurrent stones, can be offered follow up with ultrasound or regular plain abdominal x-rays. Stones that enlarge during follow up, that cause symptoms or obstruct, need removing. Any patient with stone disease should be advised to increase fluid intake. Dietary advice based on stone composition may also help. Drinking excessive fluids during a bout of ureteric colic is misguided and is likely to cause increased pain. Patients with recurrent stones should undertake metabolic screening with serum blood testing for calcium, phosphate and uric acid levels, and analysis of two 24-hour urine collections (including calcium, oxalate, phosphate, citrate, electrolyte and uric acid levels).

38

Urinary Tract Infections

Introduction

Urinary tract infections (UTIs) are a common problem in surgery. They may be responsible for urinary tract symptoms presenting to a clinician for diagnosis or for abdominal pain that is not obviously urological. More often, UTIs are a secondary problem. They can occur after operation, particularly if a urinary catheter has been used, or may complicate surgical disorders of the urinary tract, such as tumours or stones. Most infections are caused by common bacteria of faecal origin—*Escherichia coli* being the most prevalent.

UTIs may also be caused by unusual organisms, in particular *Mycobacterium tuberculosis*. On a worldwide basis, other organisms are more important causes of infection, notably the trematode *Schistosoma*. One variety causes severe bladder disease in some developing countries.

Urethral infections are commonly caused by sexually transmitted infections with organisms, such as gonococci and *Chlamydia*. A late result of gonorrhoea in males may be a fibrous **urethral stricture**. Urethral strictures are covered in this chapter, although they can also be idiopathic or related to trauma.

Bacterial Infections of the Lower Urinary Tract

Pathophysiology of Lower Urinary Tract Infections

Common UTIs caused by gram-negative organisms involve the **bladder**, the **upper tract** (kidney, pelvicalyceal system and ureter) or both. The bladder is infected most often, with females being particularly susceptible. Half of all females are affected at some time. Infection rate rises with increasing age, and there is increased risk in low oestrogen states and during pregnancy. In females, the infecting organisms enter via the urethra, which is only 4 cm long. Organisms easily spread from perineal skin, particularly during sexual intercourse.

Normally, the bladder is flushed clean by the frequent passage of newly produced urine, preventing multiplication of bacteria. Stasis—such as incomplete bladder emptying, dehydration or immobility—interferes with this mechanism and predisposes to infection. Urethral instrumentation greatly predisposes to infection in either gender.

Clinical Features of Lower Urinary Tract Infections

Typical symptoms of bladder infection are **dysuria**, **frequency**, **urgency** and a sensation of **incomplete bladder emptying**. The term *cystitis* is often used by patients to mean symptoms in this list, however, bacterial infection is not always the cause. Cystitis can also be related to inflammation, or as a result of other bladder irritants, such as ketamine misuse, intravesical instillation of bladder cancer therapies (Mitomycin C and Bacillus Calmette-Guerin therapy), and pelvic radiotherapy. Even when infection is present, symptoms may be trivial or absent, making diagnosis difficult. Abdominal pain may be the only symptom, so most patients with abdominal pain should have urine tested as a matter of course.

There may be no localising symptoms in the elderly or the very young, and the patient may be nonspecifically unwell. In any ill patient in these age groups, urine must be sent for examination before antibiotics are given. Recurrent fever in a child can result from urinary infection. A sudden onset of **enuresis** or **urinary incontinence**

- Dysuria with frequency and urgency of micturition (very common)
- Lower abdominal pain (common)
- Unexpected development of incontinence (common in older frail people)
- Development of enuresis (bed-wetting) in a previously 'dry' child
- Nonspecific ill-health in previously well infants or older people (including pyrexia of unknown origin and systemic sepsis)
- Haematuria (haemorrhagic cystitis)—this requires reassessment after urinary tract infection treatment

in children or the elderly should also suggest bladder infection. Presentations of bladder infection are summarised in Box 38.1.

Bacteriological Diagnosis of Lower Urinary Tract Infections

UTI is confirmed by examining a 'midstream' specimen of urine (MSU). If the specimen cannot be examined quickly, it should be refrigerated or it rapidly loses its diagnostic value. The main point of care test is urine dipstick analysis. If urine dipstick is positive for the presence of nitrites and leukocytes and/or there is high suspicion of infection, the specimen is examined microscopically for white blood cells ('pus cells') and bacteria, and cultured to identify the organism and determine antibiotic sensitivity. A proven infection is defined as more than 100,000 (10^5) organisms per mL, however, it is recognised that patients can have symptomatic infection at lower bacterial counts (not always picked up on urine culture) and careful patient assessment is also crucial in making the diagnosis. Enteric organisms are almost always responsible, the usual culprits being *E. coli*, *Proteus* spp., *Enterococcus faecalis* and *Pseudomonas* (the last in debilitated or catheterised patients). *Staphylococcus saprophyticus* is an important cause of uncomplicated bladder infection in young sexually active females.

Significant pus cells without bacterial growth (sterile pyuria) most often result from patients taking antibiotics. If not, a stone, tumour, prostatitis or tuberculosis must be suspected and investigated. Infection often causes visible or nonvisible haematuria, but only warrants investigation if it persists after treating the infection.

Some females experience symptoms typical of urinary infection but no evidence of bacterial infection of urine is found despite multiple MSUs. Careful assessment will help differentiate between a low grade or chronic UTI, which has not been detected with standard urine culture and other potential causes (i.e., inflammatory cystitis caused by chemical irritation or bladder pain syndrome/interstitial cystitis).

Further Investigation

The role of investigation is to identify any possible nidus of infection. Urinary tract ultrasound can look for evidence of obstruction and urinary stasis (such as large bladder residuals or hydronephrosis) and renal, ureteric or bladder stones. Cystoscopy has a role in the investigation of recurrent infection particularly if associated with haematuria, persisting urinary frequency and urgency, bladder pain, and in men.

Management of Bladder Infections

Antibiotic therapy is the treatment for bacterial bladder infection, chosen on a 'best-guess' (or empirical) basis if treatment is urgent, and changed if necessary, once culture results are available.

Patients who have had UTIs should be encouraged to increase fluid intake. This is often effective with early or mild symptoms and probably allows mild infections to resolve without drugs.

In **pregnancy**, ureters and renal pelvis dilate under the effect of progesterone and become more susceptible to infection caused by urinary stasis. Where bladder infection is suspected, significant bacterial growth should be treated with appropriate antibiotics, whether or not the patient is symptomatic. This is because of the risk of infection ascending to upper tracts (pyelonephritis) and the increased risk of preterm labour and intrauterine growth retardation with UTI in pregnancy. The antibiotic must be safe for use in pregnancy and nonteratogenic, and adjusted according to completed weeks of pregnancy (i.e., trimethoprim must be avoided in the first trimester as it can deplete folate, which can affect fetal neural tube development). Standard texts, such as the *British National Formulary* should be consulted on prescribing in pregnancy.

Recurrent Bladder Infections

Recurrent infections are defined as two UTIs in 6 months or three in 12 months. Patients at increased risk include:
- older patients (in particular women) with further increased risk if institutionalised;
- young and middle-aged women of reproductive age;
- patients with urinary tract abnormalities predisposing to infection (such as bladder outlet obstruction or incomplete bladder emptying leading to high post void residuals or bladder stones);
- presence of an indwelling catheter.

Prevention of Recurrent Urinary Tract Infection

Treat any reversible factors and remove any nidus of infection (i.e., treat bladder outlet obstruction, remove bladder stones, drain large bladder residuals with intermittent self-catheterisation in bladder underactivity).

General measures are to ensure a good oral intake of fluid and optimise bladder emptying (i.e., treat benign prostatic enlargement with alpha blocker medication, offer surgical corrections or intermittent self-catheterisation for bladder underactivity). In females, advise emptying the bladder soon after intercourse; avoid perfumed soaps in perineum, which can strip away the protective natural lactobacilli commensal organisms; start topical oestrogen therapy in postmenopausal women (please note contraindications include a history of breast or uterine cancer).

Antibiotic prophylaxis can be provided as a one-off preventative treatment after sexual intercourse, if this is a trigger; alternatively, a full antibiotic course can be taken on demand at the first signs of infection (self-start), or a low-dose antibiotic given nightly for 3 to 6 months.

Other preventative measures include a course of methenamine hippurate tablets (Hiprex). This has broad-spectrum antibacterial effects because of its conversion to formaldehyde in the urine, which is bacteriostatic, and hence inhibits bacterial growth, with the advantage of avoiding antibiotic resistance. Whilst methenamine cannot treat an active infection, it is a useful alternative prophylactic agent.

Alternative Treatments for Recurrent Urinary Tract Infections
Bladder instillation therapy can be considered where infections persist despite optimal medical management. The aim is to enhance the natural lining of the bladder and make it more robust to infections with glycosaminoglycan replacements, such as sodium hyaluronate and chondroitin sulphate, either alone or

in combination. These are administered into the bladder via an in-and-out catheter and left for around 1 hour. Courses of treatment are usually weekly for 6 weeks and then monthly for 6 months, if benefit has been proven.

Antibiotic Resistance

Bacteria, which are not susceptible to concentrations of an antibiotic in the urine (or serum), are termed *resistant*. Such resistance can be intrinsic (via selection of a resistant mutation) or genetically transferred between bacteria by R plasmids. Gram-negative bacteria that produce extended spectrum β-lactamases (ESBL) are often multidrug resistant and result in complicated infections that require specific (and sometimes nonstandard) antibiotic treatment and patient isolation to avoid spread to others. Complicated UTIs are also caused by gram-positive cocci, such as methicillin-resistant *Staphylococcus aureus* (MRSA). To avoid resistance, it is advisable to avoid starting antibiotics if there is no clinical evidence of an infection (exceptions include asymptomatic bacteriuria in pregnancy and before urological intervention), and local microbiology guidelines should be followed.

Upper Urinary Tract Infections

Pathophysiology of Upper Urinary Tract Infections

Infections of the pelvicalyceal system and renal parenchyma (**acute pyelonephritis**) arise by upward extension of a lower tract infection or via the bloodstream (haematogenous). **Ascending infections** are most common when there is an abnormality causing ureteric reflux or stasis, such as ureteric obstruction, abnormal peristalsis (as in megaureter) and congenital incompetence of the cystoureteric antireflux mechanism. During pregnancy, ureters dilate under hormonal influences and this increases the risk of upper UTIs.

With upper tract stasis, infection can be haematogenous. Common causes are stones in the renal pelvis or pelviureteric junction obstruction. In these, lower tract infection is a secondary phenomenon. Factors initiating renal infections are often unknown, but preexisting renal damage is a strong predisposing factor.

Pathological examination of an acutely infected kidney shows extensive neutrophilic infiltration of renal parenchyma, often with small abscesses. Usually only one kidney is involved and the causative organisms originate in the gastrointestinal tract, as in other UTIs.

Clinical Features of Upper Urinary Tract Infections

The classic clinical features of acute pyelonephritis are unilateral loin pain and tenderness (Box 38.2). The patient is generally unwell with systemic features of infection, that is, pyrexia and tachycardia. The urine is usually cloudy and there may be typical symptoms of bladder infection. Often the symptoms and signs are less specific, with unilateral abdominal pain or discomfort that may be mistaken for early acute appendicitis, unless the urine is examined. Pyelonephritis may present without localising signs, especially in infants and the elderly, who may be more unwell and even develop signs of systemic sepsis.

> **• BOX 38.2 Presenting Features of Acute Pyelonephritis**
>
> - Unilateral loin pain and tenderness
> - Poorly localised abdominal pain and discomfort
> - Dysuria plus cloudy, strong-smelling urine
> - Haematuria
> - Pyrexia and tachycardia
> - Systemic sepsis (especially young children and older people), often without urinary symptoms

Management of Upper Urinary Tract Infections

Diagnosis is based on clinical symptoms, signs and urine examination. Blood is also taken for culture when there are systemic signs of infection. Treatment is with antibiotics, initially on a 'best-guess' (empirical) basis, based on local microbiological advice. Dosage and route of administration depend on the severity of the illness; severe cases are treated with intravenous antibiotics.

Imaging is necessary to rule out obstruction (an infected obstructed kidney is a urological emergency and requires drainage) and to search for predisposing factors. This is usually ultrasonography in the acute setting, or computed tomography (CT), if there is suspicion of a renal colic. In children, depending on age, response to antibiotic therapy and whether it is deemed to be an atypical or recurrent infection, further investigation may include a contrast micturating cystogram and/or a radionuclide scintigram (dimercaptosuccinic acid [DMSA] or mercaptoacetylglycine [MAG 3] renogram) to identify evidence of renal scarring, reduced function or ureteric reflux (see Ch. 51).

Complications of Acute Pyelonephritis (See Figs 38.1 and 38.2)

Pyonephrosis

Severe infections may be complicated by pelviureteric outlet obstruction, resulting in accumulation of pus in the renal pelvis. If untreated, this destroys the renal parenchyma. Treatment involves surgical or percutaneous drainage followed by correction of the obstruction.

Perinephric Abscess

In severe infections, sometimes in the presence of a large 'staghorn' calculus, the accumulating pus may discharge through the renal capsule into surrounding fat, resulting in a perinephric abscess (see Fig. 38.2). This presents as a slowly expanding loin mass, often with persisting low-grade local and systemic symptoms. Urine investigation will reveal pyuria, whilst ultrasound and radiology will show a nonfunctioning renal mass containing fluid-filled areas. A large renal calculus may also be seen. A perinephric abscess sometimes develops as a result of **haematogenous infection** of a traumatic perinephric haematoma. The treatment of perinephric abscess is drainage.

Xanthogranulomatous Pyelonephritis

This is a severe renal infection, commonly associated with renal obstruction or stones, presenting with pain, fever and haematuria, and can result in destruction of renal tissue. Initial treatment is with intravenous antibiotics. On CT, appearances can be mistaken for renal cell carcinoma, which often prompts a nephrectomy. When the infection is treated, DMSA renogram can assess the renal function, and a 'simple' nephrectomy can be offered for a nonfunctioning kidney.

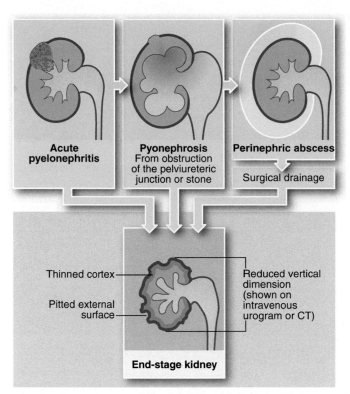

• **Fig. 38.1** Consequences of Untreated Renal Infection. *CT,* Computed tomography.

Emphysematous Pyelonephritis

This is an uncommon but severe acute necrotising condition, characterised by pain and fever, with loculi of gas seen in the kidney on CT scan (see Fig. 38.3). Predisposing factors are diabetes and renal stones. Patients are septic and require resuscitation, intravenous antibiotics, percutaneous drainage of the kidney, and control of blood sugars under the care of an intensive care unit. The mortality rate is around 25%.

Urinary Tract Infection in the Catheterised Patient

Even with the best of care, almost all catheterised patients eventually develop bacteriuria. To minimise the risk of generating antibiotic-resistant bacteria, antibiotic treatment should be used only if there are systemic signs of infection.

Genitourinary Tuberculosis

Pathophysiology of Genitourinary Tuberculosis

About 4% of patients with tuberculosis have genitourinary involvement. Mycobacteria reach the kidney or epididymis via the bloodstream, causing typical centrally caseating granulomatous lesions, which may later calcify. From the kidney, direct spread can occur to ureter (causing a fibrous stricture) or to bladder. Tuberculosis of the bladder usually begins around a ureteric opening and spreads to cause patchy ulceration of the bladder wall, and later fibrotic contraction. Young adults are more commonly affected and there is an increased incidence among patients with acquired immune deficiency syndrome (AIDS).

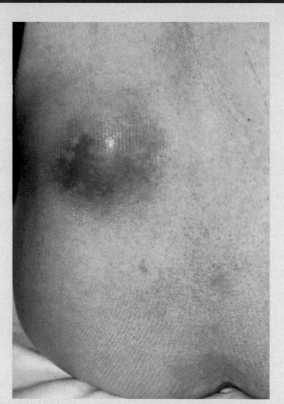

• **Fig. 38.2** Perinephric Abscess. This woman of 55 years presented with a 3-week history of left loin pain and 48 hours of rigors. The photograph shows a large abscess surrounding the left kidney, 'pointing' in the posterior loin. A plain abdominal film showed a staghorn calculus in the kidney and isotope studies showed no function in that kidney. The abscess was drained percutaneously and she was treated with antibiotics. The kidney was later removed.

Clinical Features and Investigation of Genitourinary Tuberculosis

Urinary tract tuberculosis is often asymptomatic and is diagnosed during investigation of 'sterile pyuria', although painless urinary frequency, nocturia and haematuria are sometimes present. Systemic features may also be present, including weight loss, night sweats and respiratory symptoms if the lungs are affected.

When tuberculosis is suspected, three early morning urine (EMU) specimens are sent to the laboratory to be stained and cultured for tubercle bacilli (also known as *acid-fast bacilli* [AFB]). The entire volume of the first urine passed in the morning is collected and centrifuged to concentrate the small number of organisms. Culture usually takes 6 to 8 weeks, but unfortunately a negative result does not exclude tuberculosis. Polymerase chain reaction (PCR) techniques of analysing urine are now quicker and reliable alternative methods to make the diagnosis.

If there is a red patch around a ureteric orifice at cystoscopy, this can be biopsied and examined histologically for caseating granulomas and stained for tuberculosis organisms, thus accelerating the diagnostic process. Blood is tested for anaemia, lymphocytosis and elevation of the erythrocyte sedimentation rate (ESR), and for biochemical indicators of renal function. A chest x-ray is taken to search for pulmonary disease. Renal calcification may be seen on plain abdominal x-ray, while CT urography may show renal abnormalities or ureteric strictures.

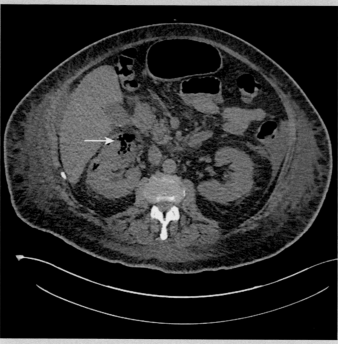

• **Fig. 38.3** A 65-year-old poorly controlled diabetic woman presented acutely to the emergency department with high fevers, rigors and right loin pain after failing to respond to a course of antibiotics prescribed by her General Practitioner. Noncontrast axial computed tomography image demonstrates air in the right kidney consistent with a diagnosis of emphysematous pyelonephritis (the *white arrow* points to the air locules seen as black patches).

Management of Genitourinary Tuberculosis

Drug therapy is the mainstay of treatment, as for pulmonary tuberculosis, with agents chosen according to the local prevalence of particular strains, and the results of culture and sensitivities. Surgery may be required later to treat ureteric strictures or a contracted bladder, or to excise damaged kidney tissue (partial or total nephrectomy). For ureteric tuberculosis, corticosteroids are usually given along with antituberculous therapy to reduce the risk of stricture formation. Plasma urea and creatinine should be monitored during the usual 6 months of therapy, and signs of upper tract dilatation sought with periodic ultrasound examinations.

Schistosomiasis

Schistosomiasis (bilharzia) is the most important parasitic disease of the urinary tract worldwide. It causes chronic inflammatory lesions in the bladder that lead to severe fibrotic damage. Schistosomiasis also predisposes to stone formation and squamous carcinoma of the bladder.

Three *Schistosoma* species, *S. haematobium*, *S. mansoni* and *S. japonicum*, have a wide tropical distribution and are important human pathogens. The most destructive bladder disease is caused by *S. haematobium*, which is endemic to tropical and North Africa (particularly the Nile valley), and is also in some Middle Eastern and southern European countries. Treatment with **praziquantel** has dramatically reduced the reservoir of infection and the incidence of cases in Egypt, but therapy is relatively expensive and hence it still remains an endemic problem in several other countries.

The schistosome has a sophisticated life cycle that depends on poor sanitation. Humans (the main definitive host) are infected by working or bathing in contaminated water. The free-swimming adult forms (**cercaria**) penetrate the skin and pass through the venous circulation and lungs to the systemic arterial circulation, which disseminates them throughout the body. In the portal veins, male and female worms mate. The females, crammed with fertilised ova, find their way, via mesenteric veins to the venous plexuses of the pelvic viscera, notably the bladder, where ova are released. Aided by lytic enzymes, the ova then pass through the bladder wall into the urine and thence to the external environment. They then complete their life cycle, via an intermediate host, a freshwater snail.

Clinical Presentations of Schistosomiasis

Initial skin penetration may cause mild local inflammation or cercarial dermatitis ('swimmer's itch'), in previously exposed individuals. Active schistosomiasis manifests from 2 to 12 weeks. The phase of haematogenous spread may cause a spectrum of systemic symptoms including general malaise, low-grade pyrexia and eosinophilia. This is also referred to as *Katayama fever*. About 12 weeks after infestation, ova invading the bladder mucosa cause local inflammation, and manifests as frequency, dysuria and haematuria at the end of micturition. In some, the early symptoms may be trivial and may pass unnoticed.

The main bladder damage caused by schistosomiasis is caused by an intense chronic inflammatory reaction to dead ova, which

- Skin rash at site of cercarial penetration
- Low-grade systemic illness with eosinophilia
- Urinary frequency and terminal haematuria

Later Sequelae
- Chronic inflammation of the bladder
- Bladder fibrosis and contracture
- Bladder stones
- Squamous cell carcinoma (two-thirds of carcinomas) or urothelial cell carcinoma (one-third) of the bladder

Idiopathic (Unknown)
Inflammation
- Secondary to gonococcal urethritis
- Balanitis xerotica obliterans (BXO)

Trauma
- Perineal or pelvic trauma
- Iatrogenic (catheters; bladder outlet surgery)

have become sequestered in the urothelium. Granulomatous 'pseudotubercles' develop around each ovum and later become fibrotic and calcified. Heavy or recurrent infestations result in a variety of destructive lesions including **ulcers**, **papillomata**, **cysts**, **giant granulomata** and **severe bladder contracture**. All predispose to secondary bacterial infection and bladder stones. Squamous metaplasia is common and strongly predisposes to **carcinoma**: two-thirds of these are squamous cell and one-third urothelial carcinoma. The clinical features of urinary schistosomiasis are summarised in Box 38.3.

Management of Schistosomiasis

Bladder or ureteric calcification is almost diagnostic of schistosomiasis. Diagnosis is confirmed by microscopy of midday urine for ova or more reliably by cystoscopic biopsy of bladder lesions. Serological tests may also be of value in travellers from the developed world without previous exposure.

Treatment is with the drug **praziquantel** given in two oral doses of 20 mg/kg body weight on 1 day, 6 hours apart. Surgery is occasionally needed later to correct or palliate residual lower urinary tract deformities.

About 5% of the world's population is affected by schistosomiasis and prevention must be the cornerstone of disease control. Effective treatment of affected individuals substantially reduces the pool of infection and the number of new cases, but better sanitation and clean water supplies are essential. Ironically, the rapid expansion of water conservation and irrigation schemes has spread the disease to previously unaffected populations.

Urethral Infections and Strictures

Urethral Infections

Infections of the urethra (urethritis) are commonly related to sexually transmitted diseases. The most frequent are **gonorrhoea** and **chlamydial** infections. The acute condition usually presents with urethral discharge and dysuria. The surgical importance of urethritis, particularly gonococcal, is that it may lead, months or years later, to fibrous stricturing of the urethra. Fortunately, these strictures are becoming less common, as effective antibiotic therapy is more readily available. However, in recent years, multiantibiotic-resistant strains have begun to emerge, particularly in the Far East.

The standard tests for diagnosis now involve molecular amplification (e.g., PCR). which can be done on urethral swabs and first-catch urine samples.

Urethral Stricture

Urethral stricture disease may result from inflammation or infection. It is more commonly seen in men, and rare in women. Narrowing of the urethra results from scar formation in the spongy erectile tissues surrounding the urethra, via a process termed **spongiofibrosis**. Aetiological factors are listed in Box 38.4. Inflammation of the urethra leading to fibrosis can result from **iatrogenic trauma**, such as traumatic urethral catheterisation or cystoscopy. The risk associated with bladder outlet procedures, such as transurethral resection and holmium laser enucleation of the prostate, is around 5%. A few strictures result from urethral tearing or rupture following displaced pelvic fractures. These usually require open surgical reconstruction.

Urethral strictures are described according to their anatomy; the posterior urethra includes the prostatic and membranous parts, the anterior urethra contains the bulbar and penile urethra, and most distal components are the fossa navicularis (urethra within the glans penis) and the external urethral meatus (Figs 38.4 and 38.5).

The characteristic symptom of urethral stricture is a progressive decrease in urinary stream, which may result in acute urinary retention; in this scenario, it may not be possible to place a urethral catheter and the patient will need a suprapubic catheter insertion. If the patient is voiding, but has developed chronic urinary retention, there may be frequency and urgency, symptomatic of bladder outlet obstruction. Diagnosis is made by direct inspection using a cystourethroscope or by urethrography.

Strictures may be short, elongated or multiple. Initial surgical options are stretching of the scar tissues (**urethral dilatation**) or with tight strictures in the bulbar urethra, to cut the stricture longitudinally with a urethrotome, under direct urethroscopic vision (**optical urethrotomy**). The risk of recurrence with these techniques is around 50%. Recurrent or complex strictures are suitable for open surgical treatment (**urethroplasty**). Short bulbar strictures can be widened by reconfiguring the urethra (nontransecting anastomotic urethroplasty); or the strictured urethral segment is excised (transected) and an end-to-end anastomosis performed. For longer strictures in both the midpenile and bulbar urethra, the stricture is opened (stricturotomy) and an inlay of graft tissue from the mouth (buccal mucosa) can be inserted to widen the urethral lumen. For distal penile urethral strictures, the urethra is opened up from the external urethral

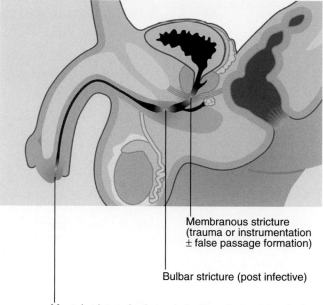

Membranous stricture
(trauma or instrumentation
± false passage formation)

Bulbar stricture (post infective)

Meatal stricture (catheter, balanitis or instrumentation)

• **Fig. 38.4** Common Sites of Urethral Strictures.

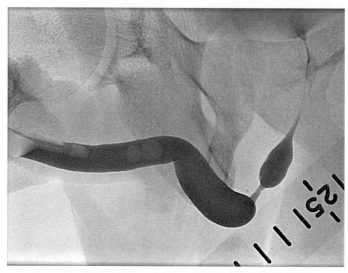

• **Fig. 38.5** Retrograde Urethrogram. A fine catheter is placed in the distal urethra, contrast injected into the urethra and oblique views are imaged. This demonstrates a 1-cm bulbar urethral stricture in a 30-year-old male with poor flow, straining to void and incomplete bladder emptying.

meatus to healthy tissue, slightly beyond the stricture, the scar tissue is excised, and graft tissue is sutured onto the underlying tissues as a replacement 'urethral plate'. This is left open to heal for around 3 months (with the patient passing urine from the meatus, which is now more proximal on the penile shaft), until the urethra (and penis) is closed (or retubularised) in a second operation.

Urethral strictures cause lifelong disability, and many can be avoided by extreme care of the urethra during catheterisation and urethral instrumentation. As a general rule, the urethra should not be catheterised or interfered with unless absolutely essential. Any catheter or other urological instrument should be placed gently and with minimal force or else under direct vision.

39

Congenital Disorders and Diseases Secondarily Involving the Urinary Tract

Congenital Urinary Tract Disorders

Introduction

Serious congenital disorders of the kidneys and urinary tract nearly all present at birth or in early childhood (see Ch. 51). The exception is **polycystic kidney**, which presents more commonly in adulthood. Less common abnormalities of the upper tract may interfere with normal flow dynamics and predispose to infection, for example, duplex systems or medullary sponge kidney. Asymptomatic abnormalities, such as unilateral renal agenesis, renal cysts or horseshoe kidney, may be discovered incidentally during investigation or during surgery. With advancing age, a large proportion of the population develops benign renal cysts; these are usually of no clinical consequence. A summary of congenital disorders that present after childhood is given in Table 39.1.

Polycystic Kidneys

Adult polycystic kidney disease is characterised by bilateral multiple cysts of renal parenchyma (Fig. 39.1). The cysts slowly expand, compressing the parenchyma, and may disrupt local control of blood pressure and eventually impair renal function. Polycystic kidneys have four main variants:

- A rare infantile form also affecting the liver; affected children often die young (autosomal recessive polycystic kidney disease).
- A serious adult form manifesting in middle age with hypertension or progressive renal failure (autosomal dominant polycystic kidney disease or ADPKD). It is the commonest cause of inherited renal failure. Kidneys can appear normal on ultrasound scanning up to about the age of 20 years.
- A less serious adult form usually found incidentally in later life, with almost normal renal function. Patients are usually hypertensive.
- Acquired disease seen in patients with end-stage renal failure undergoing dialysis.

Thus adult (autosomal dominant) polycystic kidney may present with **hypertension** or progressive **chronic renal failure**. The enlarged kidneys may cause loin pain or be discovered incidentally on abdominal examination. These kidneys are vulnerable to even minor trauma, and **haematuria** and urinary tract infections are common presentations. Patients can also have multiple cysts in the liver and sometimes in the pancreas. They present with massive abdominal swelling caused by gross liver enlargement. In addition, there is a risk of cerebral Circle of Willis berry aneurysms, which can result in subarachnoid haemorrhage, and also renal tumours (adenomas). There is no specific treatment for polycystic kidney disease, and despite good conservative management, about 50% will eventually require dialysis or renal transplantation.

Medullary Sponge Kidney

This is caused by cyst-like dilatation (**ectasia**) of the renal medulla collecting ducts and may affect one or both kidneys. Cysts tend to calcify, giving a characteristic radiographic appearance of streaky linear calcification of renal papillae (see Fig. 39.2). On excretion pyelography (intravenous urogram [IVU]), tubular ectasia can be demonstrated as a 'flare' in the

TABLE 39.1	**Congenital Abnormalities of the Urinary System Presenting After Childhood**
Nature of Abnormality	**Presentation**
Kidney	
Medullary Sponge Kidney	
Cystic dilatation of collecting ducts of one or more medullary pyramid (the subunits of the medulla) in one or both kidneys	May be found incidentally or during investigations for urinary infection. Cysts tend to become calcified and have characteristic x-ray appearance
Adult Polycystic Kidney	
Autosomal dominant disorder with multiple cysts throughout the parenchyma	Usually presents after age 30 years with chronic renal failure, hypertension, haematuria or recurrent urinary tract infections
Renal Cysts	
Can be simple or complex	Often an incidental finding. May present with loin swelling or pain
Horseshoe Kidney	
Fusion of lower poles of kidneys preventing normal developmental ascent	Often found incidentally, but may cause hydronephrosis because of pelviureteric obstruction
Ectopic kidneys and abnormalities of rotation	
Because of failure of developmental ascent	Found incidentally or during investigation of complications, such as pelviureteric obstruction
Pelvicalyceal System and Ureters	
Ureterocoele	
Cystic dilatation of intravesical part of ureter commonly associated with stenosis of ureteric orifice	Incidental finding or may cause infection or symptoms of obstruction. Commonly associated with a duplex kidney
Duplex Systems	
Partial or complete duplication of a ureter	Often an incidental finding or cause of recurrent infection or loin pain caused by reflux or obstruction
Bladder and Urethra	
Urachal Abnormalities	
Cyst, sinus, abscess, secondary malignancy	Cysts and sinuses may present in adulthood as a result of persistence of urachal remnants. Adenocarcinoma sometimes develops in the urachal remnant

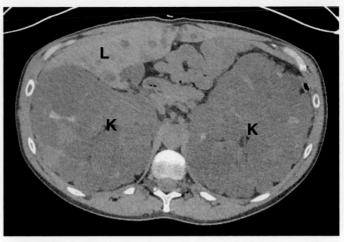

• **Fig. 39.1** Polycystic Kidneys. Computed tomography scan from a 50-year-old woman with hypertension, renal impairment and microscopic haematuria; both kidneys *(K)* are significantly expanded in size by multiple parenchymal cysts. Note also the liver *(L)* cysts.

managed with good fluid intake, a diet low in salt and animal protein, plus thiazide diuretics, if needed.

CASE HISTORY

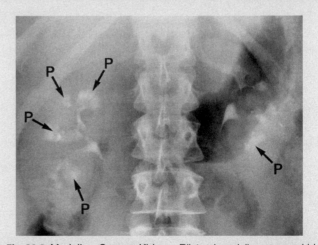

• **Fig. 39.2** Medullary Sponge Kidney. Bilateral medullary sponge kidney on an intravenous urogram from a 55-year-old woman with recurrent urinary tract infections; the renal papillae *(P)* has a typical 'flared' appearance and retains contrast because of the dilated collecting ducts. No radiopacity was visible on the control film, although it can be seen in a considerable proportion of cases because of calcification in the ectatic ducts of the papillae.

renal papilla (like 'bristles on a brush'). Most are asymptomatic, however marked degrees of medullary sponge kidney predispose to recurrent infection, haematuria and stone formation because of intrarenal urinary stasis and ureteric colic. Patients rarely present before adulthood. Minor degrees are often discovered on IVU or computed tomography (CT), but are not causing symptoms. Up to half of patients will have excessive urinary excretion of calcium (hypercalciuria), which should be

Duplex Systems

The urinary collecting system may be duplicated to a greater or lesser extent. Duplication is usually complete proximally, in the pelvicalyceal system and kidney, but may be incomplete distally. A complete (or total) duplication has two ureters draining into the bladder separately;

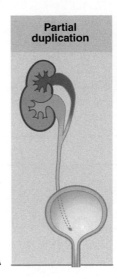
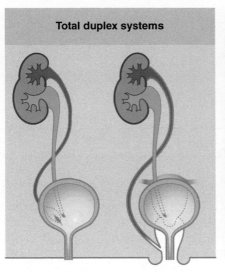
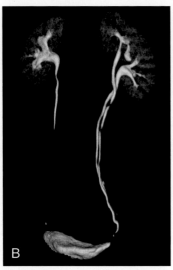

• **Fig. 39.3** Duplex Systems. **(A)** In a partial duplex system *(left)*, the ureters join and enter the bladder as one entity. In a total duplex, the ureters enter the bladder separately *(centre left)*; the upper renal moiety ureteric orifice is below and medial to the orifice of the lower renal moiety ureter, and is prone to stenosis, resulting in a ureterocoele (dilated distal ureter). Occasionally, the upper moiety ureter can insert ectopically into the urethra or vagina *(centre right)*, causing persistent urinary incontinence. **(B)** Reformatted coronal computed tomography image of a left sided total renal duplex system with ureters entering the bladder separately

in an incomplete (or partial) duplication, both join to enter the bladder, as a single ureter. Lesser duplications are usually asymptomatic and discovered by chance on imaging. Complete duplex ureter is relatively common and may result in renal damage from infection, reflux or obstruction (Fig. 39.3). The ureter draining the **upper renal pole** (upper moiety) joins the bladder ectopically, **below** and **medial** to the orifice of the lower pole ureter (Weigert-Meyer rule). The orifice can become stenosed causing obstruction. This causes back pressure on the kidney and sometimes, distal ureteric dilatation, known as a **ureterocoele**. Rarely, it can insert ectopically into the lower urethra or vagina, resulting in continuous incontinence.

The ureter draining the **lower renal moiety** has a shorter tunnel, as it travels through the bladder wall and can have a defective distal antireflux mechanism, predisposing to vesicoureteric reflux, infection and renal parenchymal damage.

Renal Cysts

Isolated renal parenchymal cysts are a common developmental abnormality and although rarely symptomatic, can be found in a fair proportion of the population in later life. They are usually recognised incidentally during imaging. Their importance lies in distinguishing them from solid tumours and hydatid cysts, which is usually easy with ultrasonography or enhanced CT scanning. Renal cysts can be simple or complex (containing blood, calcification or solid components), and are categorized by the Bosniak classification, according to their features on contrast enhanced CT. Simple or benign cysts are type 1 and 2, and can occasionally enlarge to cause pain or swelling. For these, aspiration alone is of no value, as the cysts rapidly refill. If intervention is required, cysts should be deroofed laparoscopically (in contrast to the treatment of polycystic disease). Complex cysts classified as Bosniak type 3 and 4 are malignant and require partial or total nephrectomy.

Horseshoe Kidney

This abnormality is caused by embryological fusion of the two developing kidneys at their lower poles. Normal renal ascent

in fetal life is prevented by the inferior mesenteric artery at the abdominal aorta, so the isthmus of the kidney comes to lie across the aorta, at the third or fourth lumbar vertebral level. Horseshoe kidney is usually asymptomatic and a chance finding on imaging (Fig. 39.4). Symptoms may occur however, because of complications caused by poor drainage, infection, stones and hydronephrosis, caused by pelviureteric junction obstruction.

Renal Ectopia and Other Renal Abnormalities

Other renal abnormalities may be found incidentally. These include ectopic kidneys (Fig. 39.5), rotational abnormalities, unilateral agenesis, aplasia or hyperplasia. These abnormalities may confuse the diagnosis of the condition being investigated and can sometimes result in surgical difficulties, for example, pelvic kidney mistaken for an ovarian tumour; note that transplanted kidneys are usually deliberately sited in the iliac fossa.

Urachal Abnormalities (Fig. 39.6)

During fetal development, the urogenital sinus communicates with the allantois, via the urachus. Occasionally, this tract persists as a **fistula** between bladder and umbilicus. Sometimes the fistula does not open until adulthood. Similarly, a remnant may form a blind urachal **sinus** that opens at the umbilicus or result in a urachal **cyst**, in the lower abdominal midline. These structural abnormalities may then become infected. Very rarely, an **adenocarcinoma** develops in a urachal remnant in the bladder vault or elsewhere.

Diseases Secondarily Involving the Urinary Tract

Introduction

Abdominal disorders, such as tumours, inflammatory bowel disease, aneurysms and retroperitoneal fibrosis may

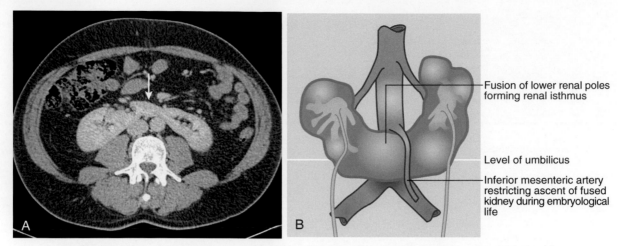

• **Fig. 39.4** Horseshoe Kidney. Horseshoe kidney shown on computed tomography; the pelvicalyceal systems are oriented anteriorly and converge in the midline at the isthmus (shown by the *arrow*). In this anomaly, the renal pelvis and ureter is more medially placed than normal and the whole renal mass lies much lower than normal because of restriction from the interior mesenteric artery.

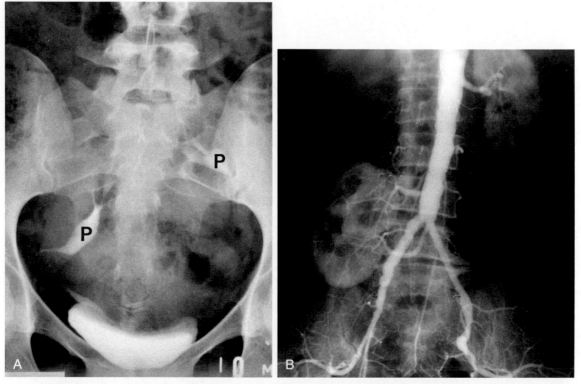

• **Fig. 39.5** Ectopic Kidneys. **(A)** A 48-year-old woman with recurrent urinary tract infections; intravenous urogram shows abnormal pelvicalyceal systems *(P)* of bilateral pelvic kidneys. **(B)** Right pelvic kidney discovered incidentally during arteriography for severe claudication. Its blood supply can be seen to arise from the distal aorta and iliac artery. The patient needed an aortofemoral bypass, but when faced with the technical difficulties, agreed to conservative management of her claudication

secondarily involve the urinary tract, as may iatrogenic (surgical) damage. Any of these may affect the urinary tract by obstructing one or both ureters. Bowel tumour or diverticular disease can result in a fistula between bowel and urinary tract. Obstruction of one ureter alone may not be symptomatic, although it may cause loin pain or predispose to infection; bilateral involvement usually presents with acute or chronic renal insufficiency.

Tumours and Inflammatory Causes

Of tumours outside the urinary tract, advanced **carcinoma of the uterine cervix** most commonly produces bilateral ureteric obstruction, because of its close relationship to the lower ureters. This cancer may also ulcerate anteriorly into the bladder, causing a **vesicovaginal fistula**, resulting in continuous urinary incontinence. This anatomical closeness of the ureters makes them vulnerable to compression

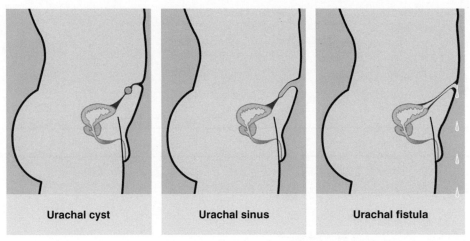

• **Fig. 39.6** Urachal Abnormalities.

from a pelvic mass and at risk of injury during pelvic surgery, even an uncomplicated hysterectomy. Abdominal, vaginal and laparoscopic-assisted hysterectomy can be associated with damage to the ureter, causing stenosis and hydronephrosis, urinary leak (urinoma) or a ureterovaginal fistula. An iatrogenic vesicovaginal fistula can also be produced. Carcinoma of the ascending or rectosigmoid colon itself rarely obstructs the right or left ureter, respectively; most ureteric damage in relation to large bowel cancer results from colectomy operations.

Inflammatory disease that involves bowel serosa may extend to involve ureters and bladder and cause possible fistula formation. This is important in **Crohn disease** and **diverticular disease**. A fistula between bowel and urinary tract (colovesical fistula) presents as recurrent urinary infection, often with pneumaturia or faecuria.

An expanding abdominal mass can compress one or both ureters and cause symptoms from partial obstruction; sometimes, **aorto-iliac aneurysms** are responsible. An 'inflammatory' aneurysm near a ureter is likely to cause obstruction. This variant occurs in about 5% of aortic aneurysms. The cause is unknown, but the effect is to produce retroperitoneal fibrosis across the anterior surface of the aneurysm. A common cause of ureteric dilatation is **pregnancy**, in which bilateral dilatation of the pelvicalyceal systems and ureters (hydronephroureterosis) results from the effects of progesterone and compression from the gravid uterus, when it enlarges. The main significance of bilateral ureteric dilatation in pregnancy is predisposition to upper renal tract infection. Thus significant bacteriuria in pregnancy, symptomatic or not, should be treated with antibiotics. Retention of urine can be caused by a pelvic mass, such as a pregnancy of around 14 weeks or an ovarian lesion of similar size.

Retroperitoneal Fibrosis

This relatively uncommon condition is characterised by progressive, intense fibrosis of the connective tissue, lying posterior to the peritoneal cavity. Most are idiopathic (cause unknown). Recognised aetiologies include inflammatory aneurysms, retroperitoneal spread of malignant disease, immunoglobulin G4 disease, drugs (methysergide, beta-blockers), radiation and inflammatory bowel disease. Retroperitoneal fibrosis sometimes causes hypertension via its effect on the kidneys.

Retroperitoneal fibrosis compresses both ureters, causing bilateral hydronephrosis and eventually renal failure. It can also be associated with inferior vena cava obstruction. Diagnosis is usually made on IVU or CT scanning, which shows bilateral hydronephrosis (Fig. 39.7). The fibrotic process also draws the ureters closer together in the midline. The erythrocyte sedimentation rate (ESR) is characteristically elevated.

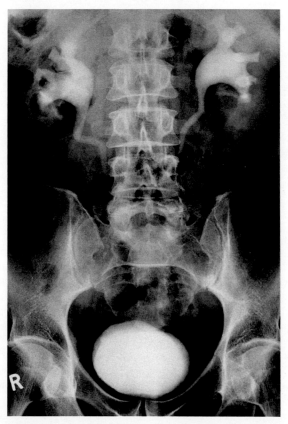

• **Fig. 39.7** Retroperitoneal Fibrosis. This man of 62 years presented with back pain. The intravenous urogram shows bilateral hydronephrosis caused by ureteric compression; note how the ureters are tapered and characteristically drawn medially by the fibrotic process

Treatment usually involves a trial of high-dose steroids and insertion of **double-J stents** to maintain upper tract function, whilst awaiting improvement. Surprisingly, ureters compressed by retroperitoneal fibrosis can usually be catheterised with ease. If medical treatment fails, the next step is usually dissection of the ureters from the retroperitoneal tissue (**ureterolysis**), which are either wrapped in omentum or resited within the peritoneal cavity in an attempt to prevent recurrent obstruction. A biopsy of the retroperitoneal tissue should be taken to exclude malignancy and confirm the diagnosis. If obstruction recurs, corticosteroid therapy may suppress the condition. Aortic grafting is indicated if a substantial aneurysm is present.

40

Pathophysiology, Clinical Features and Diagnosis of Vascular Disease Affecting the Limbs

CHAPTER OUTLINE

Introduction

The term 'peripheral arterial disease' (PAD) is often used to mean obstructive ('obliterative') disease of major lower limb arteries, causing ischaemia. However, a range of vascular disorders can cause symptoms in upper and lower limbs, including any disease of arteries, veins or lymphatics outside the heart. This chapter concentrates on lower limb vascular-related problems as they are much more common. Upper limb symptoms are outlined in Table 40.5 (p. 514).

Patients with vascular limb disorders may present to any medical specialty and some require urgent action, for example, acute limb ischaemia or a symptomatic abdominal aortic aneurysm. Thus all clinicians need to understand the principles of diagnosis and the scope and timing of treatment. This chapter covers the **pathophysiology** of limb vascular insufficiency, plus the details of **history taking** and **examining patients** with suspected vascular disease, and the process of reaching a broad, 'first stage' diagnosis.

Vascular Insufficiency of the Limb (Table 40.1)

Arterial insufficiency and venous insufficiency are common and may be either acute or chronic. Vascular disorders of the lower limb are caused mainly by atherosclerosis, arterial thromboembolism, aneurysms, complications of diabetes, and thrombotic and varicose disorders of the venous system. Some patients have arterial and venous conditions together.

Arterial insufficiency means inadequate arterial blood supply to a limb that can occur over hours or days (acute) or over months or years (chronic). Acute arterial insufficiency is frequently caused by an embolism, often of cardiogenic origin, that lodges at a bifurcation of a normal artery. The lack of collaterals means that the ischaemia is often severe and limb threatening. Acute limb ischaemia can also be caused by in situ thrombosis of an atherosclerotic plaque in a lower limb artery, or much less commonly, by thrombosis of a popliteal aneurysm (Table 40.2) or an aortic dissection extending into the lower limb vessels.

Symptoms and Signs in the Limb

Taking an accurate history is key to the diagnosis of lower limb vascular problems. This must include an assessment of major risk factors (Table 40.3). Detailed history taking is covered in Table 40.4 and examination in Fig. 40.1. In a suspected vascular case, the student or doctor tries to decide if the problem is arterial, venous or lymphatic, or has some other cause.

The principal symptoms and signs of vascular disease are pain, changes in skin texture, colour and temperature, tissue loss including ulceration, and swelling. The upper limb is affected by a largely different range of disorders with signs and symptoms (Table 40.5).

Pain

Most limb pain is caused by musculoskeletal disorders, such as arthritis or by trauma rather than vascular disease. Where lower limb peripheral ischaemia is the working diagnosis, a full cardiovascular workup is needed (see Table 40.4 and Fig. 40.1).
- **Lower limb**—patients may have itching and aching with varicose veins, or have exercise-related muscular cramp-like pain or severe and constant pain, initially in the toes and foot, caused by obliterative arterial disease. Where the history is short (<2 weeks), acute ischaemia may be the cause.
- **Upper limb**—vascular-related pain is uncommon. Aching and swelling may be caused by subclavian or axillary vein thrombosis. Claudication is rare and acute ischaemia is usually because

TABLE 40.1 Pathophysiology of Arterial and Venous Insufficiency—the Clinical Consequences of Vascular Diseases Affecting the Lower Limb[a]

Basic Disease	Pathophysiological Process	Clinical Manifestations
Atherosclerosis and Embolism Causing Ischaemia		
Atherosclerotic narrowing of large distributing arteries	Arterial supply inadequate to supply muscles during exercise Arterial supply inadequate even at rest, with relative ischaemia of all tissues. Risk of pressure ulceration. Healing severely impaired Limb is critically ischaemic; risk of limb necrosis in 6–8 hours unless urgently revascularised Thrombotic occlusion of atherosclerotic artery; clinical features as acute critical ischaemia	**Intermittent claudication**—muscle pain on walking, quickly relieved by rest **Chronic severe ischaemia**—rest pain in foot, worse at night. Onset chronic over weeks or months. Skin pale/red/purple **Acute-on-chronic ischaemia**—sudden onset (within 2 weeks) of acute ischaemia in patient with a previous history of chronic ischaemia
Embolism from heart Mitral stenosis with left atrial thrombus; atrial fibrillation; endocarditis; recent MI **Embolism from an aortic aneurysm**	Masses of thrombus detach and impact at arterial bifurcations, occluding flow	**Acute severe ischaemia** of upper or lower limb, brain or intestine.
Diabetes Mellitus		
The 'diabetic foot' (imprecisely known as the *neuroischaemic foot*)	Accelerated atherosclerosis and neuropathy. Loss of sensation predisposes to injury and ulceration and failure to heal because of ischaemia	Foot lesions (often painless)—deep ulceration in pressure areas, necrotic toes. Assume atherosclerotic ischaemia unless foot pulses palpable. Infection spreads rapidly, with potential limb-threatening necrosis and systemic sepsis. Needs early and vigorous treatment
	Lesions often complicated by pyogenic infection	Response to infection impaired in diabetics
Venous Disorders		
Thromboembolism **Acute deep venous thrombosis (DVT)** May be complicated by **pulmonary embolism**	Spontaneous thrombosis in deep veins of calf or thigh; may propagate to iliofemoral veins Obstructs venous return causing swelling and warmth. Venous gangrene in extreme cases, which requires early treatment often with thrombolysis.	**Pain and swelling of calf and ankle**, often with calf tenderness, but often asymptomatic without clinical signs. Thigh swollen if iliofemoral veins thrombosed. Associated with risk factors, particularly immobility. Leg usually blueish or normal colour
Chronic venous insufficiency Postthrombotic limb and venous eczema	Late complication of DVT Spontaneous recanalisation of occluded veins damages valves causing incompetence (reflux) and local venous hypertension Similar clinical features to those in gross superficial venous insufficiency in varicose veins	**Chronic brawny oedema** of leg often with narrow ankle because of lipodermatosclerosis ('champagne bottle leg'). Skin atrophic, scaly and pigmented and gaiter area above ankle vulnerable to chronic ulceration after minor trauma

[a]Aneurysms are covered in Chapter 42 and varicose veins and thrombophlebitis in Chapter 43.

MI, Myocardial infarction.

TABLE 40.2 Symptoms and Signs of Popliteal Aneurysm—different clinical consequences of a similar underlying disorder

Clinical Presentation	Pathophysiology
Asymptomatic—pulsatile swelling in popliteal fossa discovered by patient, by chance or during examination of patient with vascular problem	Often part of multianeurysmal disease
	Examine for other aneurysms— contralateral popliteal fossa, abdomen, femoral arteries
Acute ischaemia	Thrombosis of aneurysm or distal embolisation of clot from within aneurysm
Chronic ischaemia	Gradual occlusion of aneurysm or arterial runoff by thrombus or atherosclerosis. Similar symptoms to those in atherosclerotic disease
Apparent deep venous thrombosis (DVT)—swelling, cyanosis of leg	Large aneurysmal swelling occludes popliteal veins. May lead to DVT
Rupture of aneurysm	Sudden pain and swelling behind knee; swelling and pain in leg—often misdiagnosed as a DVT; occasionally evidence of distal ischaemia

TABLE 40.3	Preliminary Assessment of the Vascular Patient for Obvious Risk Factors	
Factors to Assess First	**Significance**
Major Risk Factors for Arterial Disease—'Gasd'	
Gender	Men affected by atherosclerosis and aneurysms 10 years earlier than women
Age	Peripheral atherosclerosis rare below 55 years—most common age 60–70 years. DVT unlikely below 20 years
Smoking cigarettes	Risk of atherosclerosis proportional to 'pack-years' smoked; PVD unlikely in people who have never smoked
Diabetes (especially type 2)	Premature and accelerated atherosclerosis, predominantly more distally in limb. 25% of PAD patients are diabetic compared with 2%–3% of general population Peripheral neuropathies (sensory, motor and autonomic) Reduced resistance to infection
Other Risk Factors	
Hypertension	Predisposes to atherosclerosis, stroke and aneurysm expansion
Hypercholesterolaemia and hypertriglyceridaemia	Risk factors for atherosclerosis. Some inherited types have major adverse effects
Obesity and sedentary lifestyle	Difficult to quantify but likely to be significant factors

DVT, Deep venous thrombosis; *PAD,* peripheral arterial disease; *PVD,* peripheral vascular disease.

of embolism. **Thoracic outlet syndrome** is also rare. The brachial plexus may be compressed as it passes between the clavicle and first rib (or extra cervical rib) causing nerve root symptoms. Even less commonly, the condition may cause arterial or venous obstruction at the thoracic outlet.

Intermittent Claudication

Chronic lower limb arterial insufficiency usually presents as muscular pain on walking. The history is characteristic: pain begins at a reproducible distance, is worse walking uphill and increases if walking continues; the patient usually begins to **limp**, accounting for the name 'intermittent claudication' (Latin: *claudicare* to limp), and the patient is forced to stop. Symptoms usually predominate in one limb. The pain subsides within a minute or two of stopping and recurs at the same walking distance. Pain is almost always in the calf, whatever level the arterial obstruction, but may extend into thigh or even buttock in aortoiliac obstruction. If associated with impotence, this is known as *Leriche syndrome*.

After a thorough history, only **cauda equina claudication** or **pseudo claudication** might be mistaken for 'true' claudication. This is caused by compression of the cauda equina in the spinal canal by central disc protrusion or canal stenosis. Lower limb pain is also brought on by exercise, but there are important differences—Table 40.6.

Chronic Ischaemic Rest Pain

With more severe arterial obstruction, ischaemic pain occurs when the patient is in bed or even when sitting. Termed **rest pain**, this is usually felt in the skin and soft tissues of the foot and is very severe and burning. It occurs mostly at night because gravity assistance to arterial supply is lost, cardiac output falls at rest, and skin vessels dilate with warmth. The pain is characteristically relieved by hanging the leg out of bed or even walking around and is not fully relieved by any analgesics. Often, patients end up sleeping in a chair, causing lower limb oedema. Patients often present after tolerating this severe pain for several weeks. Only 10% of claudicants progress to rest pain.

TABLE 40.4	History Taking in Suspected Limb Arterial or Venous Disease	
History of Presenting Complaint	
Limb Symptoms	**Important Features of the History**
Symptoms and signs Pain Changes in skin texture Changes in skin colour (including gangrene) Changes in skin temperature Ulceration and tissue loss Swelling Loss of sensation	**Detailed history of each symptom:** **Where?** Upper/lower limb; one or both; which part of the limb; precipitating/relieving factors; extent of changes **When?** When did it start; sudden or gradual onset; progress—getting worse or better; worse during day or night **Initiating factors?** Preceding activity or event, for example, trauma/excess exercise **Exacerbating factors?** For example, exercise/posture **Relieving factors?** For example, hanging leg out of bed/elevation/analgesics **Nature of symptoms?** Severity; periodicity, that is, continuous or intermittent **Pain?** Site/severity/timing/precipitants/onset/radiation **Impact of symptoms?** What is the patient prevented from doing (working/walking/sleeping/sitting comfortably) **Disability?** For example, impaired grip; heavy arm **Recent trauma to limb?** For example, fracture and treatment, dislocation, soft tissue trauma
Past Medical History	**Important Features of the History**
General cardiovascular history **Peripheral vascular disease**	Venous or arterial thromboses; bleeding tendency
Arterial	Intermittent claudication; previous limb surgery—bypass operations; angioplasty; arterial thrombosis
Venous	Varicose veins/previous surgery; thrombophlebitis; DVT or pulmonary embolism; arm swelling; trauma + immobilisation, for example, lower limb fracture/treatment/ligament injury (predisposing to silent DVT)
Related history	In claudication—back problems and surgery (possible cauda equina claudication) Cervical rib; hypothyroidism Preexisting lymphatic disorder of limb (e.g., primary lymphoedema)

TABLE 40.4	History Taking in Suspected Limb Arterial or Venous Disease—cont'd
History of Presenting Complaint	
Cardiac Disease	
Manifestations	Ischaemic heart disease; (angina, MI) Heart failure (chronic lower bilateral limb oedema) Hypertension; valvular disease; arrhythmias
Interventions	Medication/thrombolysis Coronary angiography/angioplasty /pacemaker Coronary stent (type and length of dual antiplatelet therapy required) Cardiac surgery, for example, CABG; valve surgery, TAVI (transcatheter aortic valve implantation)
Cerebrovascular Disease	
Manifestation	Ischaemic/haemorrhagic stroke; transient ischaemic attacks (TIAs)
Interventions	Medication; carotid artery surgery/stent
Renal failure	Acute or chronic renal failure ± dialysis
Rheumatological disease	Collagen/vascular disease: Raynaud; rheumatoid disease Systemic sclerosis/scleroderma; other connective tissue disorders; vasculitis
Miscellaneous contributing factors	
Lower limb paresis or deformity	Predisposes to pressure ulcers: stroke or congenital spinal problems, for example, spina bifida
Haematological disorders	Thrombophilias, for example, thrombocythaemia, factor V Leiden mutation, antithrombin III, protein C or S deficiency; polycythaemia vera
Drug History	
Is patient taking:	Antihypertensives (ACE inhibitors, beta-blockers, calcium-channel blockers, diuretics); antiplatelet drugs (aspirin, clopidogrel, etc.) Anticoagulants (e.g., warfarin, DOAC—direct oral anticoagulant); a statin
Social History	
Smoking	Smoker/ex-smoker/passive smoker; how many pack-years
Exercise	Physically fit; regular exercise
Employment	Do symptoms impact on work; how does occupation impact on symptoms. Effect of claudication symptoms on quality of life is main indication for treatment
Family History	
Hereditary cardiovascular disease?	Cardiac, peripheral arterial disease, aneurysm, arterial or venous thrombosis

ACE, Angiotensin-converting enzyme; *CABG,* coronary artery bypass grafting; *DVT,* deep venous thrombosis; *MI,* myocardial infarction.

There may also be skin changes or tissue loss, such as gangrene and ulceration (see later). The term **critical ischaemia** implies that loss of part of the limb is inevitable unless it is revascularised. Beware of the trap in **diabetic patients** with neuropathy—**severe ischaemia may be painless**. Disruption of small vessel autonomic control may mean a severely ischaemic foot is warm and red (often referred to as a *sunset foot*) rather than cold and white or blue. In the absence of palpable pulses, imaging will help determine the severity of the ischaemia.

Acute Critical Ischaemia

This is of sudden onset, associated with severe pain similar to rest pain. However, if peripheral blood flow is very low, pain may be absent in the distal, most severely affected area, which becomes numb or has diminished sensation (paraesthesia) because of nerve ischaemia. Muscle paralysis is marked in severe ischaemia, as is

muscle pain on moving the foot. It is vital to recognise acute arterial insufficiency quickly, as without timely treatment, it rapidly progresses to irreversible necrosis.

The cardinal clinical features of acute critical ischaemia are:

- **Pain**—severe but variable in intensity, affecting distal part of limb.
- **Pallor**—the ischaemic area is initially white but later becomes mottled (marbling) because of stagnation of deoxygenated blood. If this blanches on pressure, the limb is still viable. If the mottling does not blanch (fixed staining) then the limb is nonviable.
- **Pulselessness**— foot pulses are absent and popliteal and femoral pulses may be lost, depending on level of arterial occlusion.
- **'Perishing' coldness**—most extreme at foot (or hand).
- **Paraesthesia** (reduced sensation) or **anaesthesia** of the periphery. This only occurs if ischaemia is severe.

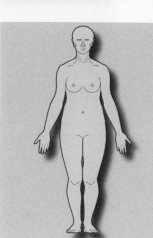

GENERAL VASCULAR EXAMINATION

INSPECT

Breathless?

Can patient lie flat? (exclude orthopnoea)

Skin / mucous membranes — pallor / cyanosis

JVP — elevated in cardiac failure

PALPATE

Abdomen
For abdominal aortic aneurysm

Pulses
Radial — for rate and rhythm
Carotid — for pulse volume and wave form

Ankles
For bilateral pitting oedema as evidence of cardiac failure

AUSCULTATE

Heart sounds
Heart murmurs / signs of cardiac failure

Arterial bruits
Abdominal aorta, carotids, subclavians, renals and femorals

Lung bases
Crepitations as evidence of cardiac failure

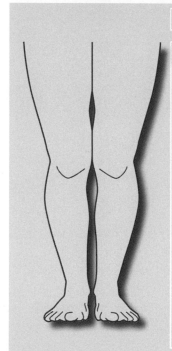

VASCULAR EXAMINATION OF LIMBS

INSPECT

Take down any dressings

Is active limb and hand / foot movement normal (motor activity)

Colour change or pigmentation — white / red / blue / black

Previous amputation of digits

Surgical scars e.g., bypass graft

Always inspect for ulceration between toes and under heels

Trophic (nutritional) changes i.e., tissue loss / gangrene/ ulceration
— are surrounding tissues involved (e.g., bone)
— ulcer — site, size, shape / shallow or deep / granulation tissue or slough at the base / pus or discharge

PALPATE

Skin temperature
Use back of hand; compare similar parts of both limbs

Capillary refill
Press big toe; refill should be less than 2 seconds

Peripheral pulses
Femorals, popliteals, dorsalis pedis and posterior tibials — is pulse palpable / how strong (-,+,++) / possible aneurysm

Neurological examination
In possible neurological ulcers, test vibration sense (tuning fork)

AUSCULTATE

Arterial bruits
Abdominal aorta, carotids, subclavians, renals and femorals

• **Fig. 40.1** Examination of the Vascular Patient. *JVP,* Jugular venous pressure.

TABLE 40.5	Summary of Signs and Symptoms of Vascular Disease of the Upper Limb	
Sign or Symptom	Underlying Disorder	Other Clinical Features
Swelling of Arm and/or Forearm		
	Axillary vein thrombosis/Paget Schroetter syndrome Predisposing causes: Unaccustomed use of arm overhead, for example, decorating Excess weight lifting Cervical rib or congenital bands obstructing vein Too narrow a space between first rib and clavicle	Blueness and heaviness of arm; later, prominent collateral veins over deltopectoral area. Symptoms usually abate spontaneously but early thrombolysis worth considering
Colour Change		
Acute whiteness or blueness	Embolism (causes as lower limb) Trauma to brachial artery, for example, supracondylar fracture	Acute ischaemia—hand cold, painful, loss of sensation and motor function

TABLE 40.5	Summary of Signs and Symptoms of Vascular Disease of the Upper Limb—cont'd	
Sign or Symptom	**Underlying Disorder**	**Other Clinical Features**
White finger(s)	Raynaud disease (common): fingers go white then turn blue then red, often in response to cold. Because of vasospasm—pathogenesis unknown	Recurrent symptoms especially in cold weather May lead to atrophy of finger tips but rarely major tissue loss
	Secondary Raynaud phenomenon (rare); underlying disorders include: Limited cutaneous scleroderma (CREST) Mixed connective tissue disease Sjögren syndrome Systemic lupus erythematosus Hand-arm vibration syndrome (HAVS) from use of vibrating tools	As Raynaud disease
Red painful fingers	Reflex sympathetic dystrophy posttrauma following fracture, especially forearm	Pain, redness, disability in arm
Pain		
Vascular	Substantial subclavian arterial narrowing. Rarely symptomatic because of excellent upper limb collaterals	Muscle pain on exercise—arm 'claudication'. Low systolic pressure
	Acute ischaemia—most commonly embolism of cardiac thrombus; sometimes acute-on-chronic thrombosis (see acute ischaemia earlier)	Acute pain of vascular origin plus other features of ischaemia—pulselessness, pallor, paralysis, loss of sensation
Neurovascular	Thoracic outlet syndrome—95% neurological symptoms, 5% arterial—lower trunk symptoms affecting C8/T1 most common. Rare and difficult to diagnose	Chronic pain—usually musculoskeletal but may be because of thoracic outlet syndrome

CREST, Calcinosis, Raynaud phenomenon, esophageal dysmotility, sclerodactyly and telangiectasia.

TABLE 40.6	Comparison Between Cauda Equina Claudication and Arterial Claudication
Arterial Insufficiency	**Cauda Equina Syndrome**
History	
'Fixed' claudication distance	'Variable' claudication distance
Pain exacerbated by walking uphill	Pain often absent when walking uphill; often better when cycling
No history of low back problems	History of low back problems
Pain disappears after 1–2 minutes rest	Pain takes 15–30 minutes to subside
Examination	
Absent peripheral pulses and low ankle pressure in affected limb	Pulses usually present and ankle pressure normal
No evidence of a lower motor neurone (LMN) lesion	Evidence of an LMN lesion, such as diminished or absent lower limb tendon reflexes
Duplex ultrasound scan or arteriography shows arterial obstruction	CT or MRI scanning of the spinal canal is diagnostic, demonstrating a narrow spinal canal or disc protrusions impacting on the cauda equina

CT, Computed tomography; *MRI*, magnetic resonance imaging.

- **Paralysis** of calf muscles. The patient is unable to flex or extend toes or ankle. This only occurs if ischaemia is extreme. Pain may disappear at this stage.

(As an *aide-mémoire*, these features are known as the six Ps: **P**ain, **P**allor, **P**ulselessness, **P**erishing coldness, **P**araesthesia,

Paralysis. Not all are present all of the time; anaesthesia and paralysis are dire prognostic features and indicate that revascularisation is required immediately.)

Deep Venous Thrombosis (Acute Venous Insufficiency)

In symptomatic deep venous thrombosis (DVT), swelling and heaviness are the usual presenting symptoms, but pain is always less severe than in severe ischaemia. Physical examination usually distinguishes readily between the conditions. In DVT, the limb is warm not cold, pulses are detectable (by palpation or Doppler flow detector) and there is no colour change (except in very severe cases). Swelling is often a feature of DVT, but not in acute arterial ischaemia.

Skin Changes

Changes in **skin texture**, **colour**, **pigmentation** or **temperature** (and their distribution) help to distinguish between limb vascular disorders. In chronic conditions, the epidermis and dermis may become atrophic because of deficient oxygenation and nutrition; these are termed **trophic changes**.

In arterial insufficiency, whatever level the obstruction, the trophic effects are most evident at the periphery, that is, the foot and toes or hand. In contrast, the changes caused by chronic venous insufficiency are most severe around the medial ankle above the malleolus (the 'gaiter area'), almost never on the foot. Evidence of chronic venous disease includes venous eczema and haemosiderin deposition, progressing to lipodermatosclerosis (cutaneous fat around the ankle becomes thinned and indurated [hardened] by fibrosis) and the characteristic 'champagne bottle' leg (marked sclerosis and narrowing at the ankle with oedema above—see Fig. 43.1C).

Changes in Skin Colour and Temperature (Table 40.7)

Many people, particularly the elderly, suffer from cold feet in cold weather; if both feet are pale or blueish when cold but are painless

TABLE 40.7	Interpretation of Colour and Temperature Change in Limbs	
Colour of Limb	**Signs**	**Interpretation**
White (see also Buerger test, Fig. 40.4)	If cold with pulses	Physiological or vasospastic disorder/small vessel disease
	If cold without pulses	Acute ischaemia
	Asymptomatic	Constricted venules
Blue or cyanotic	Painful, absent pulses	Acute or chronic ischaemia
	Swollen	DVT/dependency
Red	Intact skin, warm	Cellulitis or the diabetic ischaemic trap (see earlier)
	Superficial gaiter area ulceration, little pain	Chronic venous insufficiency
	Ulceration in foot or ankle plus severe pain; cold with absent pulses	Severe ischaemia
Brown	In gaiter area ± ulcer	Chronic venous insufficiency
Black	Toes or distal foot	Necrosis or gangrene
Temperature	**Other Signs**	**Interpretation**
Cold	White (compare other limb)	See 'white' earlier
Warm or hot	Swollen	DVT
	Indurated, oedematous skin	Cellulitis
	Ulcerated distally in diabetic + absent foot pulses	The diabetic ischaemic trap—do an arteriogram
	Always hot—patient puts feet in fridge to cool them	Erythromelalgia; unknown aetiology

DVT, Deep venous thrombosis.

with normal pulses, this is normal. If pathological, the cause may be caused by a **vasospastic disorder**, such as Raynaud disease, although this more commonly affects the hands.

Colour Change in Venous Thrombosis

Noticeable colour change is unusual in DVT, but massive pelvic vein thrombosis may cause changes sometimes mistaken for arterial occlusion. Massive thrombosis was once more common, especially during late pregnancy. The condition was known as **white leg of pregnancy** or **phlegmasia alba dolens**. The whole lower limb is painful, pale and massively swollen. In contrast to arterial occlusion, the limb is warm and pulses are detectable despite the oedema. A more serious variant is **blue leg** or **phlegmasia caerulea dolens**, which represents incipient venous infarction.

Blue Toes. In severe claudication or rest pain, the onset of dusky skin in the foot suggests developing tissue necrosis (**pregangrene**). If finger pressure is applied to the skin, the rate of colour return gives some indication of skin perfusion (capillary refill). However, many elderly people with few symptoms have a slow refill time; these rarely have arterial disease and this can easily be excluded by Doppler ankle pressures.

Black Toes. Necrosis in chronic ischaemia may be patchy and localised, if there is a developed collateral circulation (see Fig. 40.2). Such necrosis is usually confined to toes or part of the forefoot. The necrotic area slowly becomes hard, black and mummified (**dry gangrene**) and may eventually separate spontaneously from viable tissue. However, there is a risk that the necrotic area becomes infected. The tissue then becomes boggy and ulcerated and the infection and gangrene spread proximally, particularly in diabetics. This **wet gangrene** requires urgent treatment, often with a combination of revascularisation and amputation.

Redness. Skin redness indicates oxygenated blood is present in capillaries and implies there is no venous congestion or obstruction. With ischaemia, there is reactive dilatation of the microvasculature to hypoxia, a physiological attempt to extract the maximum oxygen from whatever blood is reaching the area. Thus severely ischaemic skin may feel cool but, paradoxically, be red—the 'sunset foot'.

Buerger's test for severe ischaemia (Fig. 40.3) involves high elevation of the leg for a minute or two. If peripheral arterial pressure is inadequate to overcome gravity, the entire foot becomes white. When the leg is hung down, it gradually becomes blueish-red as blood flow returns. This test is easily misinterpreted—even in the normal limb, the foot will blanch somewhat with elevation.

Inflammatory dilatation of the microcirculation causes redness, and the skin is warm and slightly swollen because of enhanced blood flow. An example is low-grade bacterial **cellulitis**, which may be seen in diabetes or chronic venous insufficiency or may arise spontaneously. Note that if a severely ischaemic limb becomes infected, the usual signs of inflammation may not develop and the extent of infection may be underestimated. If blood supply is later restored, signs of inflammation appear.

Abnormal Pigmentation

Brown pigmentation around the gaiter area is often caused by superficial or deep **chronic venous insufficiency** because of gross reflux in veins or a **post-thrombotic limb**. In the latter, the valves of the deep vein have been disrupted by the initial inflammation associated with the thrombus, with subsequent organisation and recanalisation of the deep vein(s). Valves thus become incompetent and allow **deep venous reflux**. This limits the effectiveness of the calf muscle pump and leads to chronic venous insufficiency. In gross superficial or deep venous reflux, standing causes venous stagnation, increased venous pressure in the leg (**venous hypertension**) and chronic leg swelling. Red cells extravasate into the tissues and form haemosiderin deposits, which cause brown pigmentation. This, accompanied by dry, scaly, atrophic skin, is described as **varicose** or **venous eczema** (see Fig. 40.4).

Lower Limb Ulceration (Box 40.1)

Chronic ulceration is common, particularly in the elderly. These ulcers are usually managed initially by General Practitioners and community nurses, with more difficult cases referred to a dermatologist or vascular surgeon. About 70% are venous—a complication of varicose veins or a late complication of DVT. Most of

CASE HISTORY

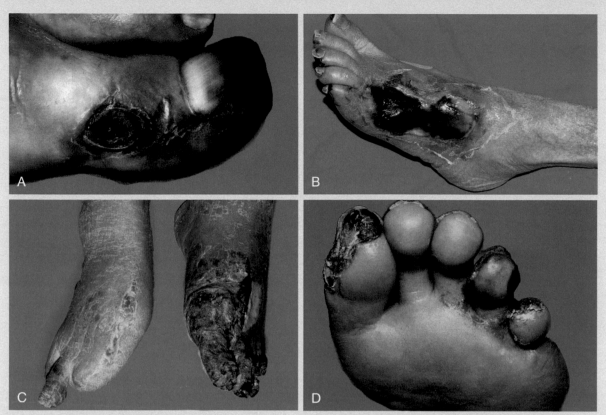

• **Fig. 40.2** Necrosis from Severe Ischaemia. **(A)** Sudden thrombosis of an atherosclerotic superficial femoral artery ('acute-on-chronic' occlusion) led to acute ischaemia, manifesting as rest pain and necrosis of big toe. **(B)** Embolism of thrombus from left atrium into femoral artery led to severe ischaemia and necrosis of skin within 6 hours. Embolectomy was performed as early as possible. The photograph shows the resulting acute ischaemic ulcer of dorsum of foot. **(C)** Left foot shows signs of severe chronic ischaemia with dry gangrene. Right foot has healed following successful femoropopliteal bypass grafting and local amputation. **(D)** Typical patchy distal necrosis following spontaneous embolism of thrombus from within an abdominal aortic aneurysm.

the rest are caused by arterial insufficiency or diabetic neuroischaemia and a few by vasculitis or ulcerating tumours. In developed countries, infection rarely plays a primary role but various tropical ulcers and tuberculosis are important causes in developing countries. Intractable cases may be because of several factors, for example, local trauma, diabetic neuropathy and obliterative atherosclerosis.

Effective treatment depends on clinical evaluation of the patient's general condition first, then the following factors:
- history of the origin and evolution of the ulcer
- the site of the ulcer
- the characteristics of the ulcer
- the nature of the surrounding tissues
- relevant regional findings

History of the Ulcer

Details of the initial skin lesion and how it occurred may provide clues. **Minor trauma** or an insect bite may initiate it, but failure to heal can usually be attributed to abnormal skin nutrition. The common causes include chronic venous insufficiency, arterial ischaemia and diabetic neuropathy. The ulcer often begins insidiously, with minor breakdown in a patch of atrophic skin. In venous insufficiency, the leg is often oedematous and the skin may 'weep' serous fluid.

The ulcer duration, its healing, and recurrences or change in extent or distribution give further clues. **Ischaemic ulcers** present early because pain becomes intolerable (except in diabetics with coexisting neuropathy and ischaemia)—Table 40.8. In contrast, post-thrombotic and varicose ulcers are not severely painful and fluctuate between healing and breakdown. Very rarely, squamous carcinoma develops in a longstanding ulcer and is recognised by proliferative change at the ulcer margin. These are sometimes known as **Marjolin ulcers** and more frequently follow burns, which failed to heal (Fig. 40.5). Primary skin malignancies on the leg may ulcerate, but these usually begin as a cutaneous lump.

If the patient has claudication or rest pain, this suggests an ischaemic cause (Fig. 40.6). Neuropathic or mixed diabetic ulcers tend to be painless because of sensory neuropathy (which may be the main predisposing cause). Neuropathic changes to motor nerves affect small muscles of the foot, altering its shape and pressure areas, and autonomic dysfunction results in dryness, both predisposing to ulceration. A history or strong suspicion of previous DVT makes venous insufficiency the likely cause.

Site of the Ulcer

Postthrombotic and varicose ulcers typically arise just above the medial malleolus and may extend circumferentially (Fig. 40.7). They rarely occur elsewhere. Diabetic neuropathic ulcers always

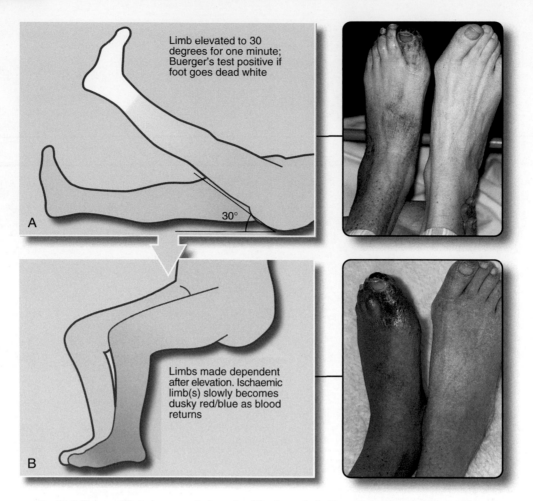

Limb elevated to 30 degrees for one minute; Buerger's test positive if foot goes dead white

A 30°

Limbs made dependent after elevation. Ischaemic limb(s) slowly becomes dusky red/blue as blood returns

B

• **Fig. 40.3** Buerger Test. In severe ischaemia of the lower limb, Buerger test is only truly positive when limbs are severely ischaemic. This 78-year-old man had severe ischaemia of both legs with the left being critically ischaemic. **(A)** In the first stage, one or both feet are elevated. Both feet go pale but the right is white. The left big toe is seen to be necrotic distally. **(B)** In the second stage, with dependency, both feet go blueish red, most marked on the left.

occur on the foot either as pressure-related ulcers on the sole beneath metatarsal heads or at other bony prominences; these include the toes, the ball of the great toe and the malleoli (see Fig. 41.8, p. 531), but ischaemia must always be excluded first.

Arterial ulcers may occur anywhere below midcalf. **Pressure ulcers** occur mainly in debilitated, elderly or unconscious patients, especially at the heel (see Fig. 12.8). Even a few minutes resting on a hard casualty trolley or operating table may initiate necrosis in an ischaemic limb. Pressure ulcers usually begin as a circumscribed patch of discolouration, becoming necrotic and later ulcerating. The heels of vulnerable patients should be nursed carefully and regularly inspected to avoid this. Treatment of pressure ulcers is difficult and prolonged and it is best to prevent them.

Characteristics of the Ulcer

Most ulcers are shallow, involving only skin and subcutaneous fat. Diabetic ulcers tend to penetrate deeply into the foot, where there is necrotic and infected tissue and often osteomyelitis. The base of any ulcer usually contains slough and fibrin, but granulation tissue may be visible beneath. Slough should not be removed unless arterial insufficiency can be excluded. If there is proliferating tissue in the ulcer, this should be biopsied.

The edge of most chronic lower limb ulcers slopes towards the base, with no diagnostic features, although epithelial proliferation growing inwards from the edge suggests healing. Diabetic foot ulcers have a characteristic 'punched-out' edge with abrupt transition from normal skin to the necrotic crater. On the sole, diabetic ulcers have a hyperkeratinised edge in response to excess pressure during walking caused by foot distortion and loss of sensation. Malignant ulcers may have a raised margin.

Nature of the Surrounding Tissues

The surrounding tissues indicate the background on which the ulcer has formed. These include colour, for example, chronic venous pigmentation, texture, for example, induration, and perfusion (shown by temperature, blanching response, venous filling and Buerger test), as well as swelling.

Regional Features

Regional examination should search for diagnostic clues, for example, peripheral pulses, inguinal lymphadenopathy (infection or malignancy), varicose veins and deep or superficial venous thrombosis.

CASE HISTORY

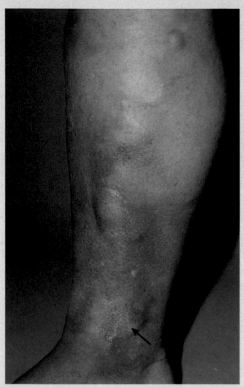

• **Fig. 40.4** Skin Changes of Chronic Venous Insufficiency. This 53-year-old woman suffered a deep vein thrombosis during her second pregnancy many years earlier. The leg is pigmented around the ankle and this tissue is woody on palpation (lipodermatosclerosis). The scar of a healed varicose ulcer is seen above the medial malleolus (arrowed).

• BOX 40.1 Causes of Chronic Leg Ulcers

- Chronic venous insufficiency
  - Previous deep venous thrombosis (postthrombotic limb)
  - Varicose veins (superficial venous insufficiency)
  - Combined deep and superficial insufficiency
  - Congenital reflux—defective deep vein valves
- Chronic arterial insufficiency
- Diabetic neuropathy (often called *neuroischaemia*) or other sensory neuropathies
- Pressure sores
- Vasculitis, for example, in rheumatoid disease and other collagen diseases
- Tropical ulcers involving bacterial or fungal infections, tuberculous ulcers. Ulcers common on feet of surfers—likely combination of trauma and infection
- Malignant tumours (Marjolin transformation of a chronic ulcer, lymphoma, basal cell carcinoma (BCC), squamous cell carcinoma (SCC), malignant melanoma)

Limb Swelling

Lower limb swelling may be unilateral or bilateral. The causes are summarised in Table 40.9. If bilateral, this suggests a 'central' cause, such as heart failure. Systemic causes, and conditions listed under 'sluggish venous return' cause bilateral swelling. Unilateral swelling is more likely to present to a surgeon. The other causes usually produce swelling of only one limb. Most causes of unilateral swelling are chronic and painless, except for acute DVT and cellulitis.

TABLE 40.8	Main Characteristics of Ischaemic Versus Venous Ulcers	
	Ischaemic Ulcer	**Venous Ulcer**
Pain	Yes, unless neuropathic	Minimal; not intolerable
Duration	Less than 6 weeks	Often months or years
Past history	Cardiac ischaemia/ coronary artery bypass graft common	DVT; severe varicose veins
Limb Signs		
Swelling	Not swollen unless patient has been sleeping in a chair to relieve pain	Usually nonpitting plus pitting oedema unless effective bandaging in place
Temperature	Usually cold	Usually normal or warm
Pulses	Absent; low Doppler pressure	Present; normal Doppler pressure

DVT, Deep venous thrombosis.

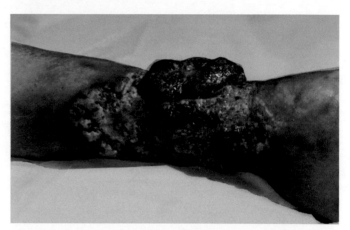

• **Fig. 40.5** Squamous Carcinoma Developing in a Chronic Venous Ulcer. This very rare transformation, sometimes known as Marjolin ulcer, followed 34 years of continuous venous ulceration. The leg was amputated below the knee and the patient cured.

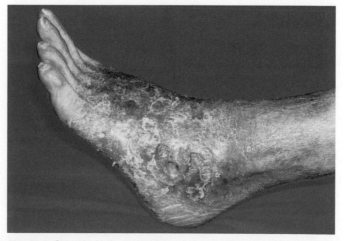

• **Fig. 40.6** Chronic Ischaemic Ulcers. This elderly man had intolerable pain in his foot, worse at night for 7 weeks. Note the foot is red and there are multiple ulcers over the lateral malleolus.

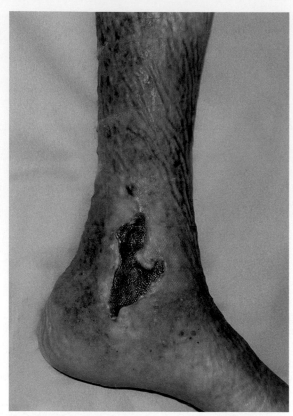

• **Fig. 40.7** Venous (Varicose) Ulcer. This longstanding ulcer is typical of venous ulceration by its site, the medial gaiter area of the ankle, its relative painlessness and the presence of venous eczema surrounding it. The visible corrugations in the skin above the ulcer are caused by four-layer compression bandaging—the first-line treatment for venous ulceration.

TABLE 40.9	Causes of Swelling of the Lower Limbs

Unilateral Swelling	Bilateral Swelling
A. Local Causes	
	'Sluggish venous return', for example, immobility, pregnancy, prolonged sitting in a chair, inefficient calf muscle pump (e.g., paralysis because of polio or hemiplegia)
	Lymphatic obstruction by filariasis (in tropical Africa and Asia)
Chronic venous insufficiency	
Destruction of valves in deep venous system following venous thrombosis (postthrombotic limb)—superficial venous reflux	May be bilateral
Congenital lymphatic aplasia or hypoplasia, for example, Milroy disease	May be bilateral
Acute obstruction of venous return, for example, deep venous thrombosis/ extrinsic pelvic compression (by tumour or May-Thurner syndrome—abnormal compression by left iliac artery)	
Chronic cellulitis (usually streptococcal)	
B. Regional Causes	
	Left ventricular failure
	Venous obstruction by pelvic mass, for example, advanced pregnancy, ovarian cyst, pelvic malignancy
	Lymphatic obstruction by malignant involvement of inguinal or more proximal nodes, or after block dissection or radiotherapy
	Lymphatic obstruction by filariasis (tropical disease)
	Inferior venal caval obstruction
C. Systemic Causes	
	Congestive or right-sided cardiac failure
	Hypoalbuminaemia, for example, malnutrition, nephrotic syndrome
	Fluid overload

41

Managing Lower Limb Arterial Insufficiency, the Diabetic Foot and Major Amputations

Introduction

The specialty of **vascular surgery** has evolved over the last 60 or so years, with a move towards more noninvasive imaging and greater use of endovascular revascularisation.

Peripheral atherosclerosis is well recognised as a marker for coronary and cerebrovascular atherosclerosis (approximately 30% 5-year mortality in intermittent claudication and 50% in patients with critical limb ischaemia), and best medical therapy (antiplatelet agent, statins, optimal blood pressure treatment and diabetic control, smoking cessation, exercise) is often more important than dealing with the leg problem in claudicants.

Chronic lower limb arterial insufficiency can cause mild to severe intermittent claudication or when more advanced, rest pain/ulceration/distal gangrene. It can also be asymptomatic or picked up on screening (e.g., for diabetic foot).

Chronic Lower Limb Ischaemia

Intermittent Claudication

Symptoms

Intermittent claudication is the usual presentation of lower limb peripheral arterial disease (PAD). It more often affects men and is present in 5% of the male population over 65 years. The patient experiences cramping pain in leg muscles on walking, which is relieved by rest. The calf is involved first because the superficial femoral artery is the most commonly affected with atherosclerosis. If arterial disease is mainly more proximal (i.e., iliac artery), the pain may ascend to the thigh or the buttock if walking continues. The distance before onset of pain is remarkably reproducible and is reduced by walking uphill.

Symptom onset is usually insidious and often attributed to musculoskeletal causes. The patient seeks medical advice only when symptoms have lasted a few months without improving. Risk factors for intermittent claudication are the same as any atherosclerotic disease, and patients often also have ischaemic heart disease (angina, previous myocardial infarction [MI], coronary artery bypass grafting [CABG]) or cerebrovascular disease (previous stroke or transient ischaemic attack). Intermittent claudication is about twice as common in diabetic patients as in nondiabetics. Nearly all have smoked cigarettes at some stage. The severity of PAD increases with the number of cigarettes smoked, with heavy smokers having a fourfold risk of claudication. Even one cigarette a day has been shown a significant risk factor for atherosclerosis, as is passive smoking. Nonsmokers affected invariably have other risk factors; most are hypertensive, who have a 2.5- to fourfold age-adjusted risk of developing PAD, depending on gender. The presence of coexisting risk factors increases the risk exponentially, particularly cigarette smoking. Polycythaemia is a rarer causative factor. There is also some evidence of genetic prothrombotic disorders clustering in male relatives of men with PAD.

Physical Signs of Intermittent Claudication

Peripheral pulses are usually absent or reduced on the affected side but local examination is otherwise unremarkable. The dorsalis pedis, posterior tibial and popliteal pulses are almost invariably absent; the femoral pulse is weak or absent in about 30%. Trophic (nutritional) skin changes are rarely present. General systematic examination should seek other signs of atherosclerosis likely to bear on management and prognosis.

Natural History of Intermittent Claudication

The Fate of the Leg

The clinical course of intermittent claudication is largely benign. Three-quarters of patients either stay the same or spontaneously improve their walking distance. Only 2% with claudication later progress to major amputation. Continued smoking increases the risk of needing reconstructive surgery or major amputation. Patients with diabetes have a higher risk of major amputation in part because of significant distal vessel atherosclerosis.

The Fate of the Patient

Lower limb PAD is a marker of systemic atherosclerosis. The severity of PAD (as estimated by ankle brachial pressure index, ABPI) is associated with increasing coronary artery disease and overall mortality rate. Some 10% of claudicants have a nonfatal cardiovascular event (MI or stroke) within 5 years and the 5-year mortality rate is 30%, with three quarters being cardiovascular events. Smoking increases mortality amongst claudicants by 1.5 to 3.0 times.

Severe Ischaemia

Severe lower limb ischaemia most commonly presents in patients who are generally older and less physically active than typical claudicants.

The first manifestations of severe ischaemia develop in the foot (most distal from the heart) and can include:
- intolerable rest pain initially at night, later becoming continuous during the day;
- trophic skin changes—atrophic shiny red skin of the leg; ischaemic ulcers between toes, in foot pressure areas or on the leg;
- patchy necrosis of the toes or skin of the foot;
- positive Buerger test;
- failure of trivial injuries to heal;
- extreme vulnerability of feet to pressure sores.

If untreated, a very small proportion improve and lose their pain, but most continue with intolerable pain or progress to necrosis. Once the deep tissues of the foot become necrotic, local defences are overwhelmed and infection spreads widely in vulnerable ischaemic tissue, especially in diabetics. This causes wet gangrene and, ultimately, death from sepsis and multiorgan dysfunction. This sequence rarely runs its course since rest pain is so severe and signs of sepsis so obvious that vascular reconstruction or amputation becomes unavoidable.

Critical Ischaemia

Critical ischaemia occurs when arterial insufficiency is so severe that it threatens the viability of foot or leg. This is formally defined by a European consensus document as follows: persistently recurring rest pain requiring regular analgesia for more than 2 weeks, or ulceration or gangrene affecting the foot, plus an ankle systolic pressure of less than 50 mmHg (*Note*: in diabetics, absent ankle

pulses on palpation replace pressure, as calcification may give falsely high pressure readings).

Managing Lower Limb Ischaemia

Investigation of Chronic Lower Limb Arterial Insufficiency

How far to investigate a patient with symptomatic ischaemia depends on the clinical picture (claudication vs. critical ischaemia) and, in claudication, whether it seriously impairs quality of life. Note that patient-reported claudication distance is unreliable and is not alone an indication for treatment. All patients with critical limb ischaemia should be considered for revascularisation.

Ankle Systolic Pressure and the Ankle Brachial Pressure Index

Patients with claudication should have resting ankle systolic pressures measured in clinic to confirm the diagnosis. Pressure is measured using a **Doppler ultrasound flow detector** (see Fig. 5.8, p. 67). Normal pressure is slightly above brachial systolic, whilst patients with claudication usually range between 50 and 120 mmHg. Results are often expressed as a ratio, the **ABPI**, with normal values from 0.9 to 1.2. Note that Doppler pressures can be misleading; experience is needed in taking and interpreting measurements, and radical treatment should not be based on random pressure measurements. Values may be spuriously elevated in diabetics owing to calcification in the arterial media which prevents cuff compression. In nonclassical exercise-induced leg pain or those with a good history of claudication, but normal resting ABPI, a treadmill test with pre- and postexercise pressure or ABPI helps the diagnosis. A drop in ankle pressure after exercise gives an indication of arterial disease severity and the recovery rate an indication of collateral compensation.

Duplex Ultrasonography

This combines greyscale ultrasound imaging (GSUS) and colour Doppler flow estimation. GSUS allows estimation of plaque narrowing and colour Doppler allows estimation of flow velocities, which increase in areas of stenosis. These methods provide a 'road map' of atherosclerosis in the arterial tree and are usually performed in a vascular laboratory by specialist ultrasonographers. It is noninvasive and does not require intravenous contrast media. There is a high degree of operator dependency in the results. Other noninvasive imaging modalities include computed tomography (CT) and magnetic resonance (MR) angiography.

Arteriography (See Ch. 5)

Arteriography should be reserved for patients thought to require angioplasty or reconstructive surgery. It maps the arterial system (Fig. 41.1), showing sites and severity of stenoses and occlusions, the quality of inflow (arteries feeding the area of concern) and the runoff (arteries beyond the main obstruction, Fig. 41.2). Arteriography is sometimes used wrongly by nonspecialists to assess chronic arterial insufficiency, but it does not measure blood flow to the tissues or dynamic circulatory responses to exercise; it helps only with the mechanics of revascularisation. Traditional arteriography was performed via direct arterial puncture, but carries risks of vessel trauma, and high doses of contrast aggravate chronic renal impairment. It is being replaced by less invasive CT and MR angiography, which use lower doses of intravenous contrast.

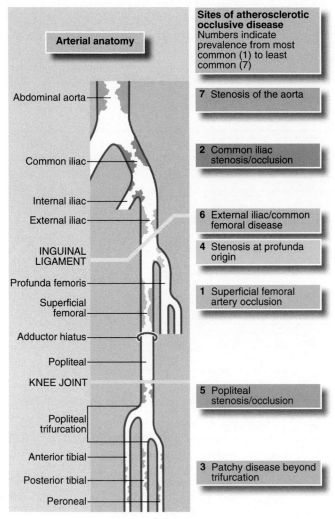

Arterial anatomy

Abdominal aorta

Common iliac

Internal iliac

External iliac

INGUINAL LIGAMENT

Profunda femoris

Superficial femoral

Adductor hiatus

Popliteal

KNEE JOINT

Popliteal trifurcation

Anterior tibial

Posterior tibial

Peroneal

Sites of atherosclerotic occlusive disease
Numbers indicate prevalence from most common (1) to least common (7)

7 Stenosis of the aorta

2 Common iliac stenosis/occlusion

6 External iliac/common femoral disease

4 Stenosis at profunda origin

1 Superficial femoral artery occlusion

5 Popliteal stenosis/occlusion

3 Patchy disease beyond trifurcation

• **Fig. 41.1** Typical Patterns of Lower Limb Arterial Disease.

Approach to Management of Chronic Lower Limb Arterial Insufficiency

Treatment options range from conservative or 'expectant' treatment for most, to reconstructive procedures for the few with severe ischaemia. Treatments are summarised in Box 41.1.

Conservative Management

In intermittent claudication, management starts with **lifestyle measures**, such as stopping smoking, attention to diet (reduced sugar and fat, more fruit and vegetables, weight reduction) and regular systematic exercise. Cigarette smoking is the most powerful primary risk factor in causing atherosclerosis (after genetic disorders) and a secondary risk factor in causing deterioration, as well as causing occlusions or stenoses of angioplasty or graft after reconstruction. Symptoms are more likely to resolve (by collateral development) if the patient stops smoking. Giving up is difficult, as nicotine is highly addictive, but smoking cessation programmes can help, as well as pharmacological aids, such as vaping, nicotine replacement therapy, bupropion (Zyban) and varenicline (Champix). All family members need to give up together to improve motivation.

Medical management is important, with blood pressure control and regular antiplatelet agents (usually aspirin or clopidogrel) and a statin (even if cholesterol levels are normal). These measures

aim to reduce mortality by treating systemic atherosclerosis, as well as encourage collateral vessels to develop. Treatment with the phosphodiesterase inhibitor, **cilostazol**, provides a small increase in walking distance but has significant side-effects.

The degree of handicap in claudication is assessed clinically by careful history-taking and perhaps by walking with the patient. There is a marked trend towards conservative treatment these days, now that we know many patients recover function and that this recovery is more durable than intervention. The choice of active treatment depends on the handicap, the patient's willingness to give up smoking, the potential for treating the pattern of atherosclerosis and the patient's overall preference. Severe and critical ischaemia are clear indications for revascularisation (or amputation), since the symptoms cannot be tolerated in the long term.

Mild to Moderate Claudication

Most patients are optimally treated with best medical management and lifestyle advice. Symptoms can improve over 6 to 18 months, especially if the patient stops smoking, exercises regularly and loses excess weight. Simple advice to walk more slowly and use a walking stick often greatly extends the claudication distance. Supervised exercise programmes produce a sustained increase in walking distance but need to continue for at least 3 months to show benefit—there is often a problem with compliance. These programmes are not yet offered nationally in the National Health Service.

Disabling Claudication

Disabling claudication usually requires treatment unless the patient is too unfit even for angiography. Symptoms may include severe exercise restriction in younger patients or markedly worsening symptoms, especially if proximal arterial obstruction is the cause (shown by absent femoral pulses), which is often easily treated by angioplasty. Reconstructive surgery is sometimes needed.

Techniques of Revascularisation for Chronic Arterial Insufficiency

Percutaneous Transluminal Angioplasty

Percutaneous transluminal angioplasty (PTA) involves cannulating an artery (usually the common femoral, but occasionally the brachial), introducing a guidewire into the remote artery and advancing it to lie across the stenosis. A balloon catheter is passed over the wire and into position (Fig. 41.3) and the balloon inflated to a high pressure (5–10 atmospheres), crushing the atheroma into the arterial wall to relieve the obstruction. Success is very operator-dependent and also depends upon the site, length and nature of the diseased artery. PTA is most effective for isolated short stenoses in iliac arteries. With increasing experience, longer stenoses and occlusions in smaller vessels can be tackled, avoiding the need for major surgery. Increasingly, **stents** are used within the superficial femoral artery to help maintain patency. PTA is less successful for distal calf arteries. Angioplasty often provides symptom improvement for a few years but disease progression (and failure to modify lifestyle) is a limiting factor.

Arterial Reconstructive Surgery

Arterial reconstructive surgery began in the 1950s with open removal of atheromatous plaques and thrombus from the aorta and iliac arteries. This is known as **thromboendarterectomy**, and is technically difficult, bloody and time-consuming and

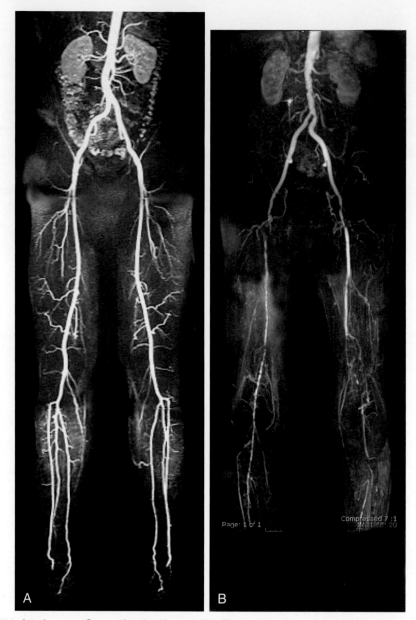

• **Fig. 41.2** Arteriograms Comparing the Normal With Typical Patterns of Arterial Obstruction Affecting the Lower Limbs. **(A)** This magnetic resonance angiogram is entirely normal, showing smooth, regular arterial walls, all branches intact and three normal infrainguinal arteries below knee on each side. **(B)** This composite subtraction arteriogram was performed because the patient suffered bilateral severe claudication. The aorta is irregular and narrowed by atherosclerosis from above the renal arteries to the bifurcation. The common, internal and proximal external iliacs are normal and smooth, but the right external iliac is occluded and the left stenosed. Both profunda femoris arteries are occluded. The superficial femoral arteries are both diseased and occluded distally. On the left side, collaterals are visible around the knee area. The infrageniculate vessels are diseased on both sides, with stenoses and occlusions. Reconstruction would have been extensive, difficult and risky, and hence conservative management alone was undertaken, in the absence of rest pain or tissue loss.

was soon replaced by bypass grafting, except for carotid and femoral endarterectomy, which remains the standard procedures for stenosis and for isolated common femoral artery occlusions.

Arterial bypass grafting was first developed during the Korean War to treat arterial trauma, using homografts from human cadavers. The initial results were excellent but grafts eventually suffered from aneurysmal dilatation and rupture. This led to the introduction of synthetic graft materials for large arteries, now available

in a variety of shapes, sizes and types of cloth. Knitted polyester (Dacron) is the most popular and is the standard material for aortoiliac obstruction. Many grafts are now sealed with gelatine or other proteins to minimise porosity. For smaller arteries, autologous **long (great) saphenous vein** (LSV) from the leg is the best conduit, provided it is large enough (usually > 3 mm in diameter) and not damaged by thrombosis. Vein is also inherently resistant to infection, a useful attribute when treating infected lower limb wounds and ulcers.

> ### • BOX 41.1 Treatment Options for Chronic Lower Limb Ischaemia
>
> **Mild to Moderate Claudication**
> - No active treatment except advice to stop smoking, exercise regularly, take statin and aspirin, lose weight
> - Endovascular management
>
> **Disabling Claudication**
> - Endovascular management
> - Reconstructive arterial surgery
>
> **Critical Ischaemia**
> - Intravenous drug therapies, such as prostacyclin
> - Lumbar sympathectomy (surgical or by phenol injection)
> - Balloon angioplasty
> - Reconstructive arterial surgery
> - Amputation (below, through or above knee)
> - Palliative care including appropriate analgesia

Recognition that conservative management of claudication is often as good as intervention, and the availability and success of angioplasty has meant that surgical reconstruction is now sparingly used and is largely reserved for severely ischaemic limbs, or when angioplasty is unsuitable or unsuccessful.

The most common procedures are synthetic 'trouser' grafting for aortoiliac (suprainguinal) disease and femoropopliteal grafting using saphenous vein for infrainguinal disease (Figs. 41.4 and 41.5). However, a range of other bypasses and endarterectomy techniques sometimes have to be used to cope with nonstandard disease.

Aortoiliac Disease

The usual surgical procedure is a Dacron trouser or 'Y' graft (see Fig. 41.4), anastomosed to the side of the aorta below the renal arteries and to both common femorals below the inguinal ligament (aortobifemoral graft). This is a major operation, needing a laparotomy to access and cross-clamp the aorta and carries a mortality risk reaching 5%. In patients with critical ischaemia, but poor physiological reserve, legs can be revascularised using **extra-anatomic synthetic grafts**, with a lower operative risk. Examples include a **cross-over graft** to supply blood from one femoral artery to the other or an **axillobifemoral graft**, supplying blood from one axillary artery to both femorals, tunnelling the graft subcutaneously along the lateral chest and abdominal wall.

Femoropopliteal Disease

The superficial femoral artery is the most commonly stenosed or occluded peripheral artery. If endovascular intervention is unsuitable, **femoropopliteal bypass grafting** is used ideally using an autogenous vein graft. The long (great) saphenous vein (LSV) is dissected from groin to knee, its tributaries ligated and then reversed proximal to distal so the valves do not obstruct flow. An end-to-side anastomosis is performed at each end. If the LSV is unsuitable (i.e., diseased, of small diameter or previously removed for CABG), the LSV from the other leg or veins from the arm can be used. An alternative technique leaves the vein in situ and destroys the valves with a **valvulotome** (see Fig. 41.5). As the vein tapers from proximal to distal, this allows bypasses to tibial, dorsalis pedis artery or smaller foot arteries for distal disease. These

infrapopliteal or femorodistal grafts are used only for severe ischaemia rather than claudication because of the higher risk of graft occlusion.

Synthetic materials (e.g., polytetrafluoroethylene or Dacron) are much less satisfactory; these have lower long-term patency, particularly when crossing the knee joint, and are more prone to infection.

Complications of Arterial Surgery

These are summarised in Box 41.2.

Other Therapies for Arterial Insufficiency

Intravenous and Intraarterial Drug Therapies

Drug therapy has no substantial effect in relieving claudication or severe ischaemia but recent research has examined gene therapy and local stimulation of angiogenesis (new blood vessel formation) in patients with critical limb ischaemia. However, outcomes are not yet robust enough to use clinically.

Sympathectomy

Blood flow in the skin (but not muscle) is controlled by the sympathetic nervous system. Thus early rest pain affecting the skin may sometimes be relieved by sympathetic blockade even if the overall arterial supply is inadequate. It is not beneficial in claudication.

Sympathectomy can be performed by excision of part of the lumbar sympathetic chain or, more commonly, by translumbar injection of 6% aqueous phenol. **Chemical sympathectomy** is performed under local anaesthesia with radiographic control. Only about 15% of patients obtain sufficient relief to avoid reconstructive operation or amputation and there is no way of selecting those likely to benefit; sympathectomy is certain to fail in the presence of tissue loss (gangrene) and is most likely to succeed in early rest pain. It may also help heal ulcers, where moderate ischaemia coexists with chronic venous insufficiency.

Acute Lower Limb Ischaemia

Pathophysiology

The lower (or upper) limb can become acutely ischaemic from **embolism** or **thrombosis**.

Embolism

A large embolus impacting in a major distributing artery causes the distal blood supply to cease abruptly; since the distal arteries are not usually atherosclerotic in these patients, collateral networks have not developed and ischaemia is all the more severe. Most large emboli originate in the heart, as a result of **atrial fibrillation** or **mitral stenosis** or both (left atrial thrombus), or of **MI** (mural thrombus). Emboli usually impact at branching points, where the lumen abruptly narrows. Common sites are the aortic bifurcation (**saddle embolus**), the common femoral bifurcation and the popliteal trifurcation. Aortic or popliteal aneurysms can be a source of embolism if thrombus accumulated in the sac travels distally (Figs 41.6 and 41.7).

Thrombosis

Thrombotic causes include acute occlusion of a narrowed artery, a previous bypass graft or angioplasty site, and less commonly, thrombosis of a **popliteal aneurysm**. Occasionally, **widespread thrombosis** occurs in normal arteries, causing acute ischaemia. This was a complication of early high oestrogen oral contraceptives and can be a complication of **blood disorders**,

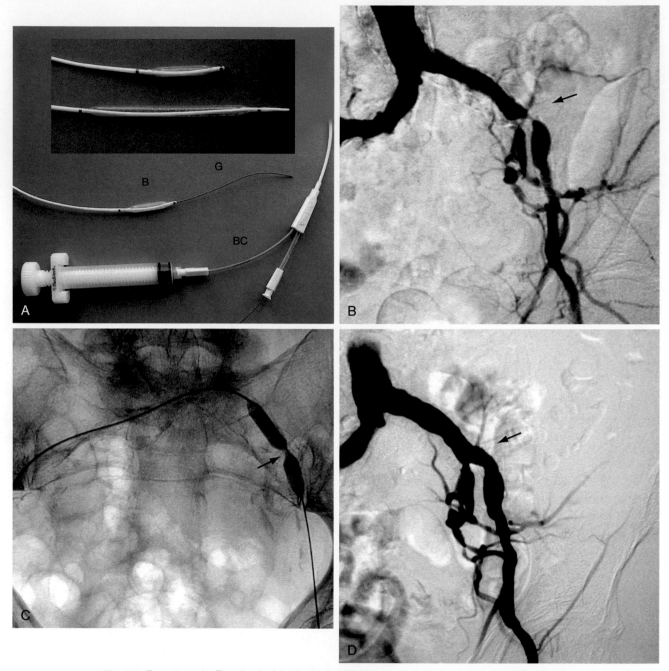

• **Fig. 41.3** Percutaneous Transluminal Angioplasty. **(A)** Balloon angioplasty equipment. This catheter is used for balloon dilatation of arterial stenosis. First, an artery some distance from the stenosis (usually the femoral) is punctured with a needle. A flexible guidewire *(G)* is passed through the needle, along the artery and manipulated across the stenosis. The catheter is then threaded over the guidewire until the distal balloon *(B)* (which is designed to only be inflated to a predetermined diameter) lies within the stenosis. The balloon is then inflated to high pressure, using a special syringe attached to the balloon channel *(BC)*. Note the radioopaque markers at each end of the balloon to allow it to be sited radiographically. **(B)** Arteriogram showing a tight stenosis at the distal end of the left common iliac artery *(arrowed)*. **(C)** Catheter access proved impossible via the left femoral artery, so a guidewire was passed from the right femoral, over the bifurcation and across the stenosis. An angioplasty balloon catheter was then guided across the stenosis. As it was inflated, the 'waist' caused by the arterial stenosis became clearly visible *(arrowed)*. With further inflation to 4 atmospheres pressure, the waist disappeared. **(D)** Appearance of the arteries postangioplasty. This procedure was completed in under an hour, on a day-case basis, under local anaesthesia and proved durable over several years.

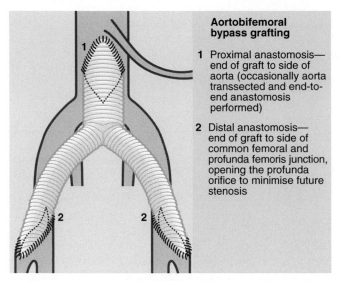

Aortobifemoral bypass grafting

1 Proximal anastomosis—end of graft to side of aorta (occasionally aorta transsected and end-to-end anastomosis performed)

2 Distal anastomosis—end of graft to side of common femoral and profunda femoris junction, opening the profunda orifice to minimise future stenosis

• **Fig. 41.4** Aortobifemoral Bypass for Aortoiliac Disease Using a Trouser or 'Y' Graft. A Dacron bifurcation graft or prosthesis is used to bypass the aortoiliac segment when it is occluded or stenosed, or to replace it when aorta and iliacs are aneurysmal. In the latter case, the distal anastomoses are to the iliac arteries not the femorals so as to maintain pelvic perfusion.

including polycythaemia vera, thrombocythaemia or leukaemias, in nephrotic syndrome or in hyperosmolar hyperglycaemic states in diabetics.

Acute thrombotic occlusion causes catastrophic results when it occurs in critical sites, namely the popliteal artery (with few useful collaterals), the external iliac/common femoral arterial trunk (the axial blood supply of the limb) or the profunda femoris (if the superficial femoral artery is already occluded).

If an essential distributing artery, narrowed by atherosclerosis becomes obstructed by thrombosis or by rupture of an atherosclerotic plaque (**acute-on-chronic occlusion**) acute ischaemia may develop. The clinical presentation is often less severe because collaterals have developed to maintain distal circulation. This may allow time for less urgent investigation and management.

Clinical Features of Acute Lower Limb Ischaemia (Box 41.3)

The condition usually presents as a sudden onset of pain, coldness and pallor, extending from the foot for a variable distance up the leg. If the blood supply is completely cut off, nerve ischaemia causes **loss of sensation**, and then muscle **paralysis**, after an hour or two (the **six Ps**—see Ch. 40). Acute severe arterial occlusion must be recognised quickly, as limb viability is in immediate danger and urgent steps are needed to revascularise it. Unfortunately, this urgency is not always appreciated by the patient, nursing staff or inexperienced doctors (often in internal medicine or geriatrics). Even with successful revascularisation, ischaemic changes may already be irreversible and with late intervention, there is a serious risk of muscle necrosis and permanent nerve injury from **reperfusion injury** and/or **compartment syndrome** (see Ch. 17).

Later, tissue ischaemia becomes obvious, when the affected area becomes mottled, dusky blue and discoloured. If the mottling still blanches, then the limb may still be saved, but worsening ischaemia leads to fixed mottling and skin blistering; this is now irreversible and limb loss inevitable. These changes always involve the foot and may extend proximally (though rarely above the knee). At this stage, the upper limit of necrosis is usually well demarcated from proximal viable tissue.

Principles of Managing the Acutely Ischaemic Limb

Management should be carefully planned at the outset. The window of opportunity before necrosis is short and delay or procrastination increases morbidity or mortality. Treatment is best carried out by cooperation between vascular surgical and radiological specialists, so the full range of appropriate and timely treatment can be offered. As a first step, the patient should be anticoagulated with a bolus dose of 5000 U of **intravenous heparin** to prevent propagation of thrombus proximal and distal to the occlusion. If the diagnosis is later confirmed as embolism, oral anticoagulation is usually continued after surgery.

Thrombosis or Embolism?

Distinguishing clinically between thrombosis and embolism is unreliable, although the history may provide clues. Evidence of mitral stenosis, an arrhythmia or recent MI suggests embolism, whereas a history of claudication or a prothrombotic blood disorder points to thrombosis. Examining the affected limb may not help distinguish but the other limb provides evidence of the state of peripheral arteries. If it is well perfused with good pulses and normal ankle pressure, then embolism is more likely. If there is arterial disease, then in situ thrombosis is more likely; the severity of ischaemia may also be less profound. The popliteal fossa must always be palpated to exclude a **thrombosed popliteal aneurysm**. A large **saddle embolus** lodging at the aortic bifurcation often presents with severe ischaemia of both limbs, extending into the proximal leg and thigh. This can be fatal, partly from the severity of ischaemia, but also from intense reperfusion injury once limbs have been revascularised. Very rarely, a spontaneous aortic dissection can cause severe bilateral acute limb ischaemia.

If clinical signs are strongly in favour of embolism, immediate surgical embolectomy can be undertaken with on-table **arteriography** if necessary. If there is doubt, urgent duplex scanning or angiography (usually CT angiography 'out of hours') is available, a definitive diagnosis can be rapidly determined and the best intervention delivered. This may be radiological rather than surgical.

In acute ischaemia, the speed of treatment is the key to success. Any patient with sensory loss affecting more than just the toes, especially with evidence of muscle weakness, requires immediate treatment with embolectomy, thrombectomy or bypass graft (see Figs. 41.4 and 41.5). In limbs that have been profoundly ischaemic, **fasciotomies** at the time are often required to prevent compartment syndrome. Thrombolysis is now rarely undertaken, except for unblocking a thrombosed bypass graft in a patient whose foot is predicted to remain viable for at least 12 hours.

Embolectomy

Embolectomy is often performed under local anaesthesia but the patient and theatre should be prepared for general anesthaesia, just in case; full monitoring should be applied. The patient has usually been anticoagulated with heparin. A groin incision exposes the femoral artery bifurcation, the vessels are all temporarily clamped and an incision (**arteriotomy**), made in the common femoral artery (see Fig. 41.7), which may reveal the obstructing clot. A **Fogarty balloon catheter** is then passed gently into each main vessel in turn, proximally first, then distally for 10 cm or so, the balloon is inflated gently and the catheter drawn back to sweep out any obstructing clot. This is repeated 10 cm further each time, until the distal limit is reached. The operation is successful if clot is retrieved and blood flows ('**back-bleeding**') from each vessel,

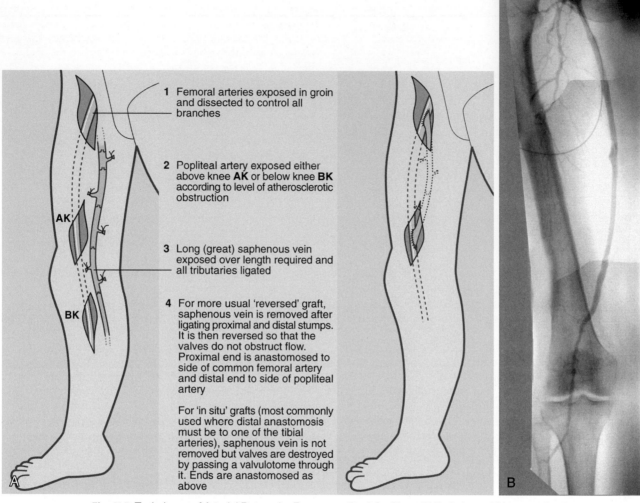

1 Femoral arteries exposed in groin and dissected to control all branches

2 Popliteal artery exposed either above knee **AK** or below knee **BK** according to level of atherosclerotic obstruction

3 Long (great) saphenous vein exposed over length required and all tributaries ligated

4 For more usual 'reversed' graft, saphenous vein is removed after ligating proximal and distal stumps. It is then reversed so that the valves do not obstruct flow. Proximal end is anastomosed to side of common femoral artery and distal end to side of popliteal artery

For 'in situ' grafts (most commonly used where distal anastomosis must be to one of the tibial arteries), saphenous vein is not removed but valves are destroyed by passing a valvulotome through it. Ends are anastomosed as above

• **Fig. 41.5** Techniques of Arterial Bypass by Femoropopliteal Grafting. (A) Technique of femoropopliteal grafting. (B) Composite arteriogram showing patent femoropopliteal bypass after operation.

as it is unclamped. If the embolectomy catheter will not pass easily, this usually indicates acute-on-chronic thrombosis. Immediate arteriography and surgical treatment are required, as delay carries a high rate of limb loss and death.

The Diabetic Foot

The evolving epidemic of diabetes means that managing diabetic foot problems will become an increasing part of the surgical workload. Treatment should be delivered by a multidisciplinary diabetic team (vascular surgeon, diabetologist and diabetic nurse, podiatrist, orthopaedic surgeon and orthotist).

Pathophysiology of the Diabetic Foot

Diabetic patients are prone to serious ulceration and infection of the feet. The underlying disorder is neuropathy, obliterative atherosclerosis or both together. Type 2 diabetic patients are at greater risk than type 1, but remember, **there is no such thing as mild diabetes**. All diabetic patients should be screened for potential complications of diabetes.

Several factors may contribute to diabetic foot problems:
- **Neuropathy.** Microangiopathy in combination with metabolic toxicity from sorbitol and advanced glycation end-

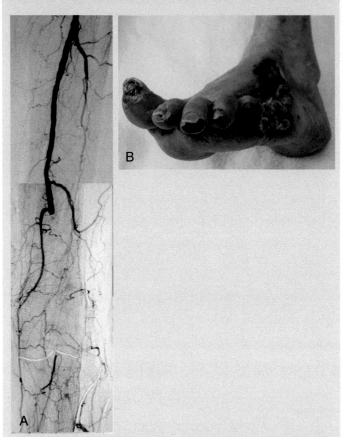

• **Fig. 41.6** Embolic Occlusion of Popliteal Arteries. **(A)** Angiogram showing the thigh and upper leg arteries in a woman of 70 years who presented with rest pain for 48 hours and necrosis of the dorsum of her foot and black toe tips for 24 hours. The left popliteal is occluded with a sharp cut-off typical of embolism. The patient was in atrial fibrillation and the likely source of the embolus was the left atrium. She underwent a successful embolectomy, but because of the delay, a below-knee fasciotomy was performed to prevent compartment syndrome. **(B)** The foot ulcer 3 weeks after revascularisation. The ulcer gradually healed completely.

products probably causes peripheral neuropathies affecting motor, sensory and autonomic nerves. Affected **motor nerves** supply the small muscles of the foot and the consequent unmodified traction of the calf muscles distorts the morphology and weight-bearing characteristics of the foot. **Sensory neuropathy** lessens pain sensation and hence awareness of potential injury from ill-fitting footwear and foreign bodies in shoes. Damaged **autonomic nerves** disrupt vascular control and cause loss of sweating. Ulceration and infection in neuropathic feet are often painless and hence are often neglected by the patient.

• **Arteriovenous communications.** These open beneath the skin, perhaps diverting nutrient flow away from it. Damaged tissue thus heals poorly and is vulnerable to infection, even if the injury or pressure damage is minor. This may also explain why an ischaemic diabetic foot can be warm and pink.

• **Arterioles.** In a few cases, these become narrowed and restrict capillary perfusion.

• **Impaired intermediary tissue metabolism** and a glucose-rich tissue environment. Both of these favour bacterial growth and spreading infection.

• **Obliterative atherosclerosis.** Diabetics have a markedly increased predisposition to arterial insufficiency. Although 1% to 5% of the general population have diabetes, 25% of patients with lower limb ischaemia have diabetes. Atherosclerotic disease in diabetic patients follows the usual pattern (although often more distal), but tends to develop at a younger age.

Identifying the Causes of Diabetic Foot Problems

Diabetic foot problems may be identified as primarily neuropathic or primarily atherosclerotic, but most have elements of both. The term '*neuroischaemic*' foot is sometimes used but is not clinically precise. Typically, the **neuropathic foot** is painless, red and warm with strong pulses, whereas the **atherosclerotic foot** without neuropathy is pale, painful, cold and pulseless. However, when both occur together, **the diabetic trap** is that the limb can be seriously ischaemic yet painless, warm and pink. If the foot is neuropathic and pulseless, only **arteriography** or duplex scanning will properly demonstrate the arterial insufficiency.

Patients most at risk of neuropathic foot complications are elderly, poorly controlled, type 2 diabetics and younger patients with longstanding type 1 diabetes. Similarly, patients with diabetic renal or retinal complications have an increased risk of foot problems. Recognising the **'at-risk' foot**, that is, the neuropathic foot, before trouble strikes is fundamental, as virtually all neuropathic foot complications can be prevented with proper education, regular inspection and chiropody (podiatry). This is best managed by a dedicated diabetic nurse (Box 41.4).

Management of atherosclerotic ischaemia is similar in diabetic and nondiabetic patients. For mixed disease, the arterial insufficiency must nearly always be treated first, if there is to be any hope of healing.

Clinical Presentations of Diabetic Foot Complications

Foot complications of diabetic neuropathy present in four main ways (see Fig. 41.8):

• **Painless, deeply penetrating ulcers.** These usually develop in pressure areas caused by distortion of foot morphology, often beneath the first or fifth metatarsal head. The infecting organism is usually *Staphylococcus aureus*. Infection and necrosis spread through the plantar spaces and along tendon sheaths. Infection and local venous thrombosis appear to be the predominant factors causing tissue destruction. Osteomyelitis is a common consequence and is difficult to treat.

• **Chronic ulceration of pressure points** and sites of minor injury. Skin perfusion is otherwise adequate.

• **Extensive spreading skin necrosis** originating in an ulcer and caused by superficial or deep infection. This develops very rapidly and spreads proximally, threatening limb and life.

• **Painless necrosis of individual toes.** These first turn blue, then later become black and mummified, and may eventually be shed spontaneously. This usually occurs in mixed neuropathy and atherosclerosis and the management hinges on whether local amputations will heal or whether arterial reconstruction is needed.

Management of Neuropathic Foot Complications
Control of Infection

After excluding ischaemia, control of infection is the first priority in managing the diabetic foot. Minor foot lesions must

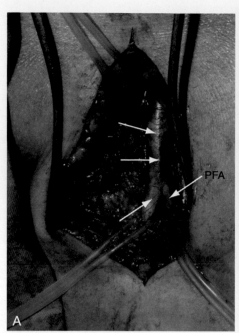
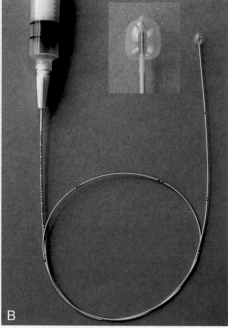
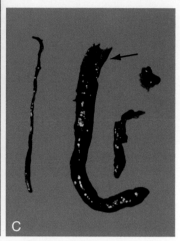

• **Fig. 41.7** Femoral Artery Embolectomy. **(A)** Surgical exposure of the femoral artery bifurcation, usually performed under local infiltration anaesthesia (but with full monitoring). The common femoral artery *(CFA)*, the profunda femoris *(PFA)* and the superficial femoral artery *(SFA)* are dissected cleanly and silicone slings placed around each artery. A transverse arteriotomy is made just proximal to the bifurcation (position *arrowed*). **(B)** A Fogarty balloon catheter is passed distally, the balloon is gently inflated and the catheter withdrawn to extract embolic and thrombotic material. This is performed in stages, until the catheter can be passed to ankle level and back-bleeding occurs. **(C)** Embolic material removed at operation from the superficial femoral artery and beyond using a Fogarty catheter. Note the paler embolic material *(arrowed)* and the darker thrombus propagated beyond it.

• **BOX 41.3** **Clinical Features of Acute Severe Lower Limb Ischaemia**

Risk Factors Predisposing to Embolism or Thrombosis

- Presence of a prothrombotic disorder
- Recent chest pain or other evidence of myocardial infarction
- History of rheumatic heart disease
- History or finding of atrial fibrillation
- Previous arterial thromboembolism
- History of intermittent claudication or other symptoms of atherosclerosis
- Polycythaemia vera (prone to intravascular thrombosis)
- Popliteal aneurysm in contralateral limb (possible thrombosis or embolism in affected limb)
- Aortic aneurysm (possible source of embolism)
  Recent temporary/permanent cessation of anticoagulation

Symptoms Suggesting Acute Lower Limb Ischaemia

- Sudden onset of continuous pain, usually in one periphery. *Note:* may be painless in diabetic neuropathy
- Sudden and persistent coldness, usually in one periphery
- Sudden numbness or paraesthesia, usually in one periphery

Signs of Acute Lower Limb Ischaemia

- Pallor or blueness of the periphery; in late cases, the fixed pigmentation of necrosis or skin blistering
- Unexpected coldness of the peripheral part of one or (less commonly) both legs
- Absent lower limb pulses (particularly if known to have been present before)
- Poor peripheral capillary return after pressure blanching
- Progressive paralysis and foot drop (late sign)
- Ankle pulses undetectable by Doppler or very low ankle systolic pressure

---

• **BOX 41.4** **The Problem of the Diabetic Foot**

'Diabetic Gangrene Is not Heaven-Sent but Earth-Born' (Joslin 1934)

- There is no such thing as 'mild' diabetes; all diabetics are potentially at risk
- Four out of five patients with diabetic foot problems have type 2 diabetes
- Foot problems are responsible for 47% of days spent in hospital by diabetics
- Diabetic foot problems are responsible for 12% of all hospital admissions in (internal) medicine
- In diabetics with new foot ulcers, 90% have peripheral neuropathy (compared with 20% in a diabetic control group), whereas only 14% have peripheral arterial disease compared with 10% in controls (Miami 1983–1984)
- Patients with diabetic foot problems are incapacitated for an average of 16 weeks
- Diabetic foot problems are largely preventable
- Care and prevention of diabetic foot problems require specialist surveillance and management by a dedicated team; foot ulceration in diabetics represents a failure of medical management

---

always be taken seriously and treated early with **oral antibiotics (including cover for anaerobes)** and frequent local cleansing and dressing.

If there is any sign of spreading infection or systemic involvement (i.e., pyrexia, tachycardia or loss of diabetic control), the patient should be admitted to hospital for intensive treatment, including parenteral antibiotics, elevation, excision of necrotic

CASE HISTORY

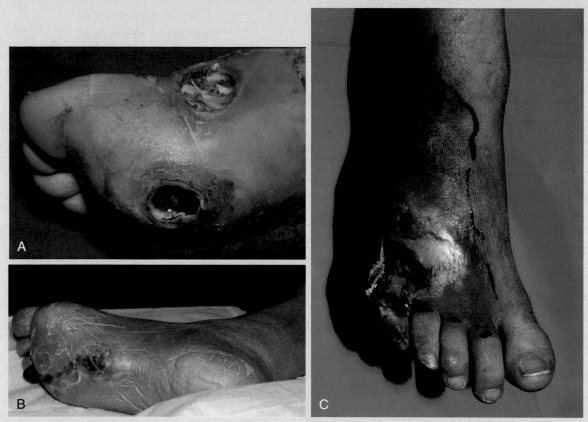

• **Fig. 41.8** Foot Complications of Diabetes. **(A)** Chronic penetrating ulcers in a 60-year-old man with maturity-onset diabetes. He had no evidence of major vessel disease, but had signs of neuropathy. The deep ulcer beneath the head of the first metatarsal is characteristically surrounded with a thick keratin margin, and the ulcer on the medial side of the foot has an exposed tendon in its base. **(B)** This patient has a combination of neuropathy and arterial insufficiency. This foot was painless despite spreading necrosis and a collection of pus in the sole of the foot. He underwent femoropopliteal bypass and local excision of dead tissue and healing was eventually complete. **(C)** This man of 34 years presented with a neglected infection in his foot. He had severe neuropathy, but no arterial disease. The entire dorsum of his foot was necrotic and he had to undergo a primary below-knee amputation. This complication would have been entirely avoidable had he sought and received treatment earlier.

tissue and attention to blood glucose control. Pus in superficial or deep tissues is a medical emergency and requires immediate drainage. This can be difficult to diagnose clinically and foot imaging with MR imaging (MRI) is required. Specialist management of blood sugar is often required, as it is often grossly elevated.

Removal of Necrotic Tissue

Surgery may involve anything from simple **desloughing** of an ulcer to major amputation (Fig. 41.9). If performed correctly, these result in complete and rapid healing. If good foot care is available, amputation of more than single toes is rarely required. Before debridement, arterial inflow must be assessed and the foot revascularised if necessary, before debridement or digital amputation to maximise the chances of wound healing.

Osteomyelitis occurs in up to 20% with a diabetes-related foot ulcer. Diagnosis is clinical, if an ulcer can be probed down to bone, or else radiological (plain x-ray or MRI). Treatment consists of long-term antibiotics guided by culture (often parenteral), with a success rate of around 80%, or surgical excision. There is no current consensus on optimal treatment but prolonged antibiotics can increase the risk of *Clostridium difficile* and emergence of multidrug-resistant organisms.

Prevention of the Diabetic Foot

All clinicians dealing with diabetics should place the highest priority on prevention. All patients should be screened for peripheral neuropathy and those at risk given detailed advice on self-care and high-quality chiropody or podiatry. Foot ulceration occurs in about 15% of patients with diabetes and precedes 84% of all diabetes-related lower leg amputations; it **can** be prevented. Careful attention should be given to footwear to correct abnormal pressure patterns. Special insoles or special shoes may need to be made by an orthotist or surgical fitter. Careful follow-up and regular monitoring by a diabetic specialist nurse or clinic can successfully anticipate and prevent dire trouble.

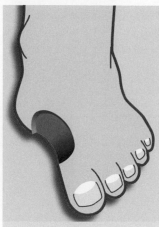

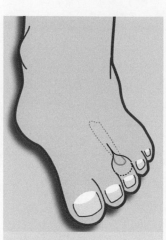

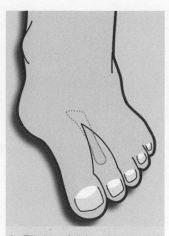

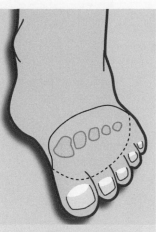

1 Excision of all necrotic tissue from ulcer, which is left to granulate

2 Digit amputation using racquet-shaped incision; toe is removed with both phalangeal bones and cartilage is nibbled from metatarsal (shaded)

3 Filleting of digit and metatarsal if infection has spread more deeply. A cake-slice is taken out of the foot and the wound left unsutured to heal by granulation (see (b))

4 Transmetatarsal amputation

A

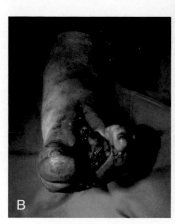

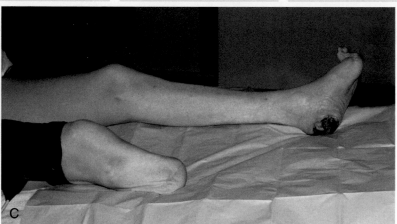

B   C

• **Fig. 41.9** Operations on the Diabetic Foot. **(A)** Types of local amputation. **(B)** This patient had a neuropathic ulcer and necrotic toes, but no arterial disease. The second and third metatarsals have been excised, together with all the necrotic tissue, in a 'cake slice' procedure. The wound was left open to heal by secondary intention, eventually giving a remarkably good functional result. **(C)** This elderly man suffered from a combination of neuropathy and obliterative atherosclerosis. He was blind as a result of diabetic retinopathy. The right leg was eventually amputated below knee because of spreading infection, but the left was saved by angioplasty of stenoses in the iliac and superficial femoral arteries, together with local surgery to remove necrotic tissue. Note the typical 'clawed foot' and distorted sole of motor neuropathy. Note also that the great toe has already been amputated. The heel has not yet been debrided.

Lower Limb Amputation

Strenuous efforts should be made to preserve ischaemic limbs by reconstructive surgery or interventional radiology. This is because the functional results of successful revascularisation are far better than even the best major amputation. Mobility with artificial limbs is always disappointing, especially in the elderly or infirm. However, amputation cannot be avoided in patients where revascularisation is technically impossible (particularly in diffuse distal arterial disease), or if there is substantial tissue necrosis and a functionally useless foot, or deep spreading infection.

Level of Amputation

Two principles guide the level of amputation (Fig. 41.10):
• The amputation must be made through healthy tissue. If not, there is a high risk of wound breakdown and chronic ulceration, requiring further amputation at a higher level. When amputation is for (uncorrected) peripheral ischaemia, it is almost always necessary to amputate at midtibial level or above to ensure healing.
• The choice of amputation level must take into account the fitting of a prosthetic limb. For this purpose, the midtibia (**below-knee**) and lower femoral levels (**above-knee**) are preferred. If the knee joint can be saved, the functional success of a prosthesis is much better. With improved prostheses, through-knee amputation is possible but healing rates are poor; most surgeons and prosthetists prefer above-knee to through-knee amputation, as it has a better healing rate and easier prosthetics.

The traditional 'guillotine' amputation of the battlefield simply sliced off the limb, leaving the wound to heal by secondary intention. This reduced the risk of fatal gas gangrene or tetanus, but the outcome for fitting a prosthetic limb was poor. There

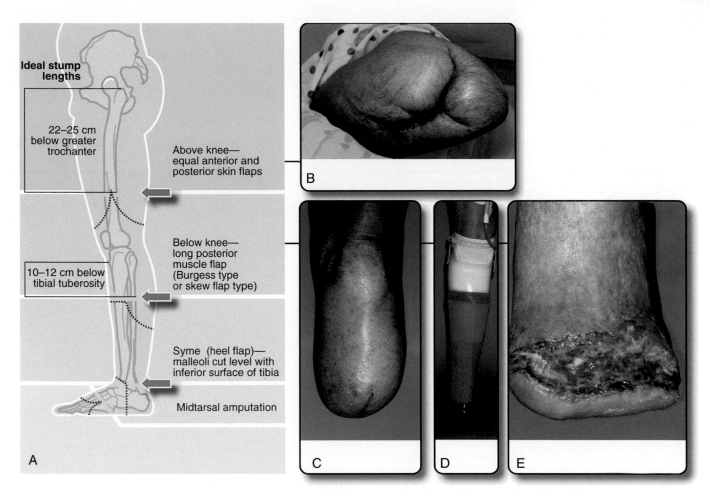

• **Fig. 41.10** Lower Limb Amputations. **(A)** Sites of election for lower limb amputations. **(B)** Above-knee stump in a diabetic patient. Unfortunately, the original above-knee wound broke down and necrotic muscle had to be excised. The wound was left open and had nearly healed by secondary intention 2 months later. **(C)** A well-healed below-knee stump at 6 weeks. The operation used a long posterior muscle flap and equal length 'skew' skin flaps. **(D)** The same patient fitted with a modular below-knee prosthesis retained by a close-fitting socket and a small strap above the knee. Note the urinary catheter. **(E)** Breakdown of below-knee stump because of inadequate arterial blood supply.

have been huge developments in amputation techniques over the years, particularly in the use of **myoplastic flaps**. For below-knee amputations, a long posterior flap of muscle and skin is wrapped forward over the amputated bone and sutured in place. This results in more reliable healing and a suitably shaped and cushioned stump. A variation, the Robinson **'skew flap'**, uses a long posterior muscle flap but equal skin flaps. The healing rate is no better but the stump is better shaped for earlier prosthetic fitting. With these techniques and in experienced hands, 70% or more of below-knee amputations for ischaemia will eventually

heal, even without revascularisation, preserving the knee joint and allowing reasonable walking. Modern below-knee prostheses are **modular** in construction and weight is borne mainly on the patellar tendon.

For above-knee amputations, myoplastic flaps are used, in which the bony amputation level is proximal to the muscle/skin amputation level. This allows the muscles to be sutured over the exposed bone end. Short anterior and posterior skin flaps are then closed over the muscle.

42

Aneurysms and Other Peripheral Arterial Disorders

Aneurysms (Table 42.1)

Pathology of Aneurysms

An aneurysm is defined as a localised area of pathological arterial dilatation. For the abdominal aorta, an anteroposterior diameter of ≥3 cm is generally accepted as defining an aneurysm. In some patients with aneurysmal disease, all major arteries are wider (arteriomegaly) and one or more becomes truly aneurysmal. Aneurysms of the abdominal aorta and the iliac, femoral and popliteal arteries are often branded 'atherosclerotic' but the primary disorder is **degeneration of the elastin and collagen** of the arterial wall. Atherosclerosis that can be found within aneurysms is not causative; it is likely that the two pathologies share risk factors. Aneurysms are relatively uncommon; found mainly in males over 70 years of age, they are even less common in women, in whom they present about 10 years later. At least a quarter of patients have more than one aneurysm.

Degenerative aneurysms are usually **fusiform**, slowly expanding in diameter. As it enlarges, the vessel wall thins, expansion accelerates and the risk of rupture increases. Most abdominal aortic aneurysms (AAAs) involve only the infrarenal aorta; some extend distally to involve common iliac arteries; sometimes there are separate aneurysms of internal iliac arteries (Fig. 42.1). A few extend proximally to become **thoracoabdominal aneurysms**.

Clinical Presentation of Aneurysms (See Table 42.1)

Aortoiliac aneurysms are often found **incidentally**. The patient may notice a pulsatile abdominal mass or a pulsatile mass may be discovered on abdominal examination. An aneurysm may also be noticed incidentally on radiological investigation—as calcification on a plain abdominal x-ray, as an obvious aneurysm on computed tomography (CT) or, most commonly, on ultrasound scanning for obstructive urinary symptoms (see Fig. 42.2). More recently in the United Kingdom, a national AAA screening programme has been implemented, with the aim of offering all men an abdominal aortic ultrasound scan on reaching 65 years.

Despite screening, a proportion of cases that reach surgeons present because of symptoms of retroperitoneal **leakage or rupture**. This carries a very high mortality. Several studies have shown that the total community and hospital mortality after rupture is more than 75%, whereas elective treatment can have a mortality rate of less than 5%. **Pain** is the most common symptom of a leaking aneurysm. The patient often gives a history of transient or persistent **cardiovascular collapse** (fainting, hypotension), which should alert clinicians to the probable diagnosis. The clinical picture ranges from an 'acute abdomen' to abdominal or back pain of up to a week's duration, and the diagnosis is usually confirmed by finding a pulsatile abdominal mass. Sometimes the symptoms can mimic renal colic or back pain, so an AAA must be excluded in all older men presenting with such symptoms. Intraperitoneal rupture and often extraperitoneal rupture are rapidly fatal and can be an unrecognised cause of **sudden death** in the elderly, with the cause often attributed to myocardial infarction.

Femoral and popliteal aneurysms are relatively uncommon and usually present as pulsatile masses. The larger they become, the more likely complications are to ensue. Femoral aneurysms

TABLE 42.1	Clinical Presentation and Pathophysiology of Aortic, Iliac, Femoral and Popliteal Aneurysms	
Clinical Presentation		**Pathophysiology**
Asymptomatic—discovered incidentally as pulsatile mass in abdomen, groin or popliteal fossa, on abdominal x-ray, CT or ultrasound scan		Progressive aneurysmal dilatation. May be self-limiting if hypertension and smoking controlled
Symptomatic—abdominal or back pain with tender aneurysm. Needs urgent surgery		Rapidly expanding aneurysms cause pressure on adjacent structures
Sudden death—acute, usually fatal, cardiovascular collapse. Often misdiagnosed as myocardial infarction		Sudden rupture of aneurysm only detected at autopsy or in the dissection room (or not at all)
Leaking/ruptured aneurysm—ill-defined back or abdominal pain often simulating ureteric colic or other abdominal emergency. Diagnostic if accompanied by transient collapse. Sometimes a history of recent similar episodes. Pulsatile abdominal mass palpable in 50%		Dilatation and thinning of the wall of an aneurysm leading to leakage of blood into retroperitoneal tissues—usually leads to catastrophic rupture within hours
Symptoms and signs of **acute severe leg ischaemia**; often pulsatile popliteal aneurysm on contralateral side		Sudden thrombotic occlusion of aneurysmal popliteal artery
Complete arterial occlusion—sudden distal ischaemia affecting lower limb caused by embolism of thrombus from within aneurysm		Thrombotic occlusion of popliteal artery
Screening—discovered on population screening or opportunistic screening for aneurysm		

CT, Computed tomography.

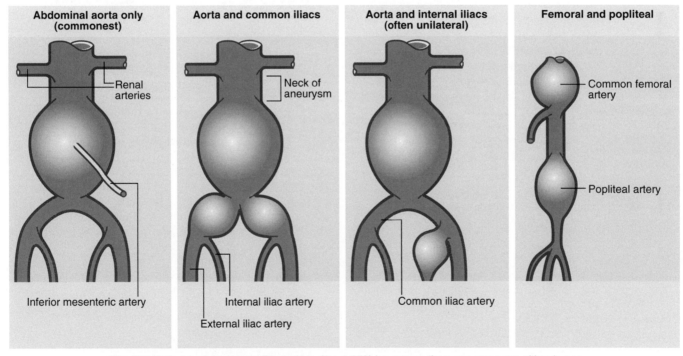

• **Fig. 42.1** Patterns of Aneurysm Formation. About 25% have more than one aneurysm either in continuity (common iliac, internal iliac, thoracoabdominal) or not (femoral 10%; popliteal 20%; thoracic 5%). Abdominal aortic aneurysms rarely extend above the renal arteries. External iliacs are never aneurysmal.

occasionally rupture causing pain and massive swelling in the groin. Popliteal aneurysms are liable to undergo thrombosis or embolise, causing an **acutely ischaemic leg** (Table 40.2). A thrombosed popliteal aneurysm carries a 50% risk of limb loss. In any patient presenting with an acutely ischaemic leg, it is vital to exclude this diagnosis as successful treatment will require extensive surgery (often a bypass graft). Popliteal aneurysms can occasionally rupture and cause a variety of other presentations listed in Table 40.2.

Principles of Management of Aneurysms

Indications for Operation (Box 42.1)

For **asymptomatic** aneurysms, the risk of rupture increases almost exponentially as the aneurysm dilates. Most vascular surgeons would consider operating on abdominal or thoracic aortic aneurysms of 5 to 5.5 cm or more, or those that expand more than 0.5 cm a year; 6 cm is generally considered to be critical, since 40% of such aneurysms can be expected to rupture over the following 2 years.

CASE HISTORIES

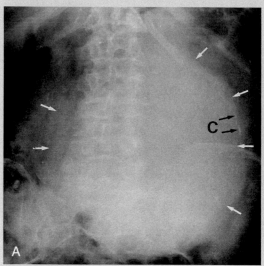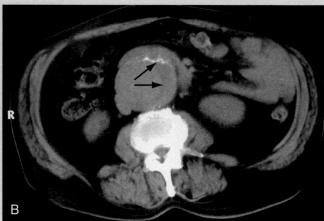

• **Fig. 42.2** Abdominal Aortic Aneurysm (AAA). **(A** and **B)** This very obese 64-year-old man complained of continuous aching back pain for 2 weeks. **(A)** Plain abdominal x-ray showing huge abdominal aneurysm (outlined by *arrows*). Note calcification *(C)* along its left-hand aspect. **(B)** Computed tomography scan of a different patient with a 6-cm AAA. The thrombus lining the wall can clearly be seen *(arrowed)*. Calcification is visible in the anterior wall where the third part of the duodenum is closely applied to it. Rarely, a primary aortoduodenal fistula develops at this point.

• BOX 42.1 **Indications for Operating on Abdominal Aortic Aneurysms**

- **Leaking or ruptured aneurysms**—if patient's state and general fitness permit
- **Symptomatic aneurysms**—aneurysms causing pain (particularly if tender), ureteric obstruction or embolism
- **Expanding aneurysms**—aneurysms that enlarge at a rate of more than 0.5 cm in 1 year
- **Size**—most arterial surgeons now recommend operation on aneurysms of 5.5 cm diameter or greater, or any saccular aneurysm

---

If there are **symptoms**, such as back pain or abdominal pain, or signs of tenderness that can be attributed to the aneurysm, imminent rupture must be assumed and urgent operation performed.

A **leaking or ruptured** AAA is a surgical emergency. Less than half the patients reach hospital alive, and only about half of those undergoing surgery survive. The majority of patients die of shock before reaching the operating theatre or else of myocardial infarction or acute renal failure after operation. The true mortality of rupture is thus more than 75%. On the other hand, the mortality after elective operation or endovascular repair (endovascular aortic repair [EVAR], see p. 538) for aneurysm can be less than 5%. Thus the decision to operate electively on a known aneurysm depends on the estimated risk of rupture versus the risk of elective intervention. Indications for operation are summarised in Box 42.1.

Investigation of Aneurysms (See Fig. 42.2)

Nonruptured Abdominal Aortic Aneurysm

For asymptomatic aneurysms considered too small to warrant operation, ultrasonography is used for periodic **monitoring**, with referral to a surgeon once the size reaches an index diameter (usually 5 or 5.5 cm) or is seen to expand more than 0.5 cm in a year.

Where elective operation is planned, CT scanning is used to show the relationship of the aneurysm to the renal arteries; the 5% of cases, where the aneurysm extends above the renal arteries, require a **thoracoabdominal** operative approach and the operation carries a greater risk. CT can also show if iliac arteries are aneurysmal and if the aneurysm is **inflammatory** (i.e., has a thick layer of inflammatory tissue on its anterior surface that makes surgery technically difficult). Representative CT slices are usually taken through the chest to ensure the thoracic aorta is not aneurysmal; if there is a **thoracic aneurysm**, the management plan will have to accommodate it, according to size and position. If an aneurysm patient requiring surgery also has evidence of lower limb **ischaemia**, some form of arteriography is usually necessary, in case a combined reconstruction is required.

Leaking or Ruptured Abdominal Aortic Aneurysm

Any patient with a suspected leaking or ruptured AAA should be treated as a true surgical emergency, but not necessarily by immediate transfer to the nearest operating theatre. There is good evidence that the survival rate increases when ruptured AAAs are treated by a specialist team of surgeons and anaesthetists, and this may mean transfer to a vascular centre. Overaggressive blood pressure resuscitation of the hypotensive patient may convert a stable, contained leak into a free rupture, and many clinicians support the use of **permissive hypotension** to facilitate transfer (see Ch. 15), that is, not treating relative hypotension, whilst the patient remains conscious and free from cardiac symptoms. This principle has increased the time available for transfer and/or further investigation.

Provided the patient with a leaking AAA is not demonstrating signs of gross cardiovascular instability, a CT scan can be valuable in planning treatment by demonstrating how the aneurysm relates to renal and visceral arteries and showing any secondary

TABLE 42.2 Comparison of Conventional and Endovascular Therapy for Aortic Aneurysm		
	Conventional Surgery	**Endovascular Therapy**
Mortality related to procedure	Approximately 3%–5%	1.7%
Length of hospital stay	7–14 days	1–2 days
ITU/HDU care needed	Likely	Unlikely
Anatomical constraints	Distance between AAA and renal arteries can be less than 15 mm	Needs 10–15 mm of relatively normal aorta below renals
Past medical history	More difficult with previous surgery or peritonitis	Unaffected by previous abdominal surgery
Follow up	Discharge at 3 months. Rescan after 5–7 years. Reintervention unlikely	Frequent CT and ultrasound for life. Reintervention rates high but improving

AAA, Abdominal aortic aneurysm; *CT*, computed tomography; *HDU*, high-dependency unit; *ITU*, intensive treatment unit.

CASE HISTORY

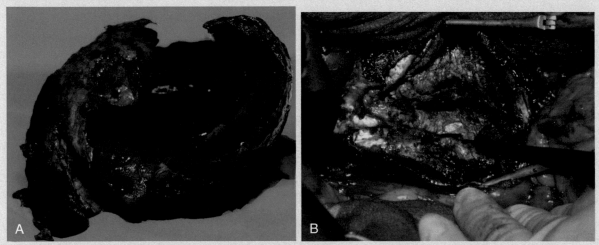

• **Fig. 42.3** Abdominal Aortic Aneurysm. **(A)** A 70-year-old asymptomatic man in whom a pulsatile abdominal mass was an incidental finding. This cast of thrombus was removed from within the aortic aneurysm at operation; note the false lumen and concentric lamellae of thrombus progressively laid down, as the aneurysm expanded over many months. **(B)** This shows the aneurysm sac opened at operation on a different patient, who had complained of chronic back pain. The posterior wall of the aorta is completely deficient in part and the anterior longitudinal ligament is visible in its base.

iliac aneurysms; sometimes other abdominal pathology is shown that influences the decision to operate, for example, liver metastases. In units equipped to undertake emergency EVAR (see later), CT can show whether this is possible.

Principles of Aneurysm Surgery

The dilated aneurysmal segment is surgically corrected by means of a graft. Over recent years, there has been a trend towards treating AAAs using minimally invasive stent-graft placement (EVAR) via the femoral artery. Many patients still, however, undergo open surgery. The indications and relative merits of each technique are shown in Table 42.2. **Tube grafts** or **bifurcation grafts** of synthetic material (usually Dacron) are used for aortoiliac and femoral aneurysms, whilst **autogenous saphenous vein** is preferred for popliteal aneurysms.

Open Abdominal Aortic Aneurysm Surgery (Fig. 42.3)

For abdominal aneurysms, the standard open approach is a long midline or a transverse abdominal incision. The aorta is usually reached via the peritoneal cavity or sometimes via an extraperitoneal approach. The patient is usually anticoagulated perioperatively, with intravenous heparin, to prevent distal thrombosis, and the iliac arteries and the infrarenal aorta are clamped (Fig. 42.4). The aneurysm is incised longitudinally and any clot within it removed. Bleeding lumbar arteries opening into the posterior aortic wall are closed with sutures.

Proximally, the graft is sutured just above the upper limit of the aneurysm to (relatively) normal aortic wall within the aneurysmal sac, and to the native aorta, at the bifurcation within the sac distally. Sometimes a bifurcated ('trouser') graft is used in aortoiliac aneurysmal disease, with the distal graft ends sutured to an area of normal iliac artery. The aneurysm sac is left in situ and later closed around the graft. This is known as *inlay grafting*: it allows separation of the graft from the intestine, reducing the risk of an aortointestinal fistula arising later from the graft anastomoses.

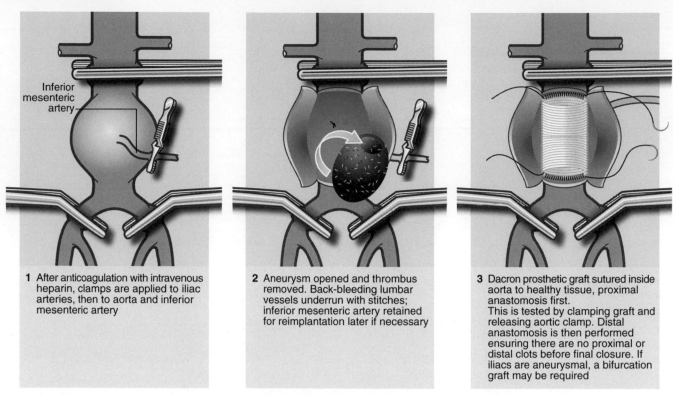

1 After anticoagulation with intravenous heparin, clamps are applied to iliac arteries, then to aorta and inferior mesenteric artery

2 Aneurysm opened and thrombus removed. Back-bleeding lumbar vessels underrun with stitches; inferior mesenteric artery retained for reimplantation later if necessary

3 Dacron prosthetic graft sutured inside aorta to healthy tissue, proximal anastomosis first.
This is tested by clamping graft and releasing aortic clamp. Distal anastomosis is then performed ensuring there are no proximal or distal clots before final closure. If iliacs are aneurysmal, a bifurcation graft may be required

• **Fig. 42.4** Technique of open Abdominal Aortic Aneurysm Surgery.

Endovascular Aneurysm Repair (Fig. 42.5)

EVAR is a minimally invasive technique using combined stent-grafts. In the United Kingdom, the National Institute for Care and Health Excellence has approved it, but recommends that clinicians ensure patients fully understand the long-term uncertainties and potential complications, including endovascular leaks, the possibility of secondary intervention and the need for lifelong follow up.

Most cases are performed under general anaesthesia, but many can be done under local anaesthesia. The procedure is performed in an operating theatre using a mobile x-ray image intensifier or in a specialist endovascular suite. The **stent-graft** consists of a self-expanding metal framework with a nonporous cloth covering; it is supplied in a constrained state within a sheath, which measures around 8 mm in diameter. When in situ, the main body of the device resembles a pair of trousers with one short leg.

Short transverse incisions are used to access common femoral arteries in the groin, but the procedure can also be performed totally percutaneously, without groin incisions, and using specially made closure devices for the arteriotomies, at the end of the procedure. The main device is passed into one femoral artery and guided proximally using radiological guidance to its position below the renal arteries. An angiogram checks the device can release below the renals. The constraining mechanism is then removed and the stent opens and expands against the vessel wall. The contralateral femoral artery is then exposed and a guidewire passed proximally to enter the main graft body, through the short leg. The second limb of the stent-graft is then completed by passing another covered stent over the guidewire and securing it into the main graft body and the iliac artery. After completion, the device looks like a complete pair of trousers and extends from the renal arteries to the common iliacs.

Other Applications of Endovascular Aortic Repair

Open surgical repair of **thoracic aneurysms** carries a mortality of 10% to 20% and a high morbidity, but many can be repaired by EVAR using just two small groin incisions. Even **ruptured aneurysms** (abdominal or thoracic) can often be repaired using this technique, often using local anaesthesia. **Incomplete traumatic aortic transsections** have also been successfully treated with endovascular therapy. Advances continue to be made in EVAR technology so that more complex cases can be managed via this route, including the use of custom-made fenestrated EVAR grafts (FEVAR). These allow juxta- and suprarenal aneurysms to be treated, by creating windows in the EVAR, through which stents can be placed into renal and mesenteric arteries.

Upper Limb Problems (See Table 40.5, P. 514)

Upper Limb Ischaemia

Ischaemia of the upper limb is rare. This is because atherosclerosis is less common here and also because there is a rich collateral blood supply via scapular anastomoses that can bypass subclavian occlusive disease. Upper limb ischaemia usually occurs when the subclavian is compressed at the thoracic outlet or when emboli obstruct the brachial or more distal arteries. Occasionally, vasospastic disorders, such as severe Raynaud disease cause digital ischaemia. Embolic disease here has similar causes, presentation and treatment to embolism affecting the lower limbs (see Ch. 41 p. 525).

Thoracic Outlet Compression

The subclavian artery and vein and brachial plexus pass through the space between the first rib and clavicle. If this becomes unduly

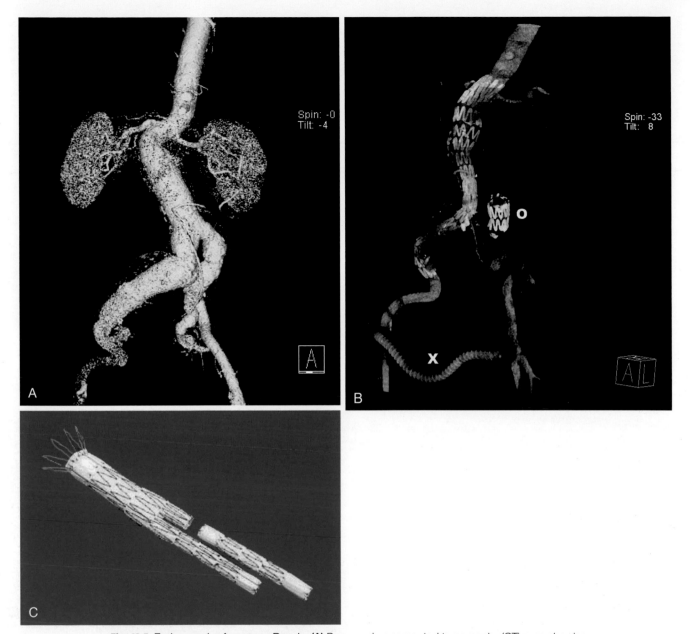

• **Fig. 42.5** Endovascular Aneurysm Repair. **(A)** Preprocedure computed tomography (CT) scan showing lumen of aortoiliac aneurysm, suprarenal aorta and kidneys. On this view, the much larger diameter of the aneurysmal aortic wall is not visible. **(B)** Postprocedure CT scan showing the stent-graft in position extending from the right common iliac to just above the renal arteries. In this case, there were technical problems placing a bifurcation graft and so the left common iliac origin was deliberately blocked with an occluding stent *(O)* and the left lower limb was revascularised with a crossover femorofemoral graft *(X)*. **(C)** Typical two-piece stent graft. Note the body and one limb are in one piece and the other limb is fitted afterwards. Note also the retaining wires at the proximal end.

narrow, neurological or arterial symptoms may appear; either can be part of **thoracic outlet syndrome**. Neurological symptoms are much more frequent but either variety of thoracic outlet syndrome is rare. Congenital causes include upward pressure exerted by a **cervical rib** lying above the first rib, or by fibrous bands. The gap may be encroached upon by acquired causes, including a healed clavicular fracture, excess muscle development in weight lifters or other unknown means.

Neurological symptoms of thoracic outlet syndrome usually cause deficits in the T1 nerve root distribution (wasting and weakness of small muscles of hand; paraesthesia of inner forearm and hand). Symptoms of arterial compression include upper limb 'claudication' in people who habitually work with

arms above their heads, as the artery becomes more compressed in this posture. In longstanding cases of subclavian artery compression, the artery, beyond the stenosis, may become dilated into an aneurysm (**poststenotic dilatation**), which may collect thrombus. This can later embolise into the brachial artery causing acute ischaemia.

Occasionally, arterial compression is diagnosed by finding a lower blood pressure in the affected arm, and this varies with arm posture; obstruction can be confirmed by duplex ultrasonography or arteriography. Most cases are not so straightforward. Overall, the diagnosis of these syndromes is difficult and is best performed in specialist centres with input from neurologists, surgeons, radiologists and physiotherapists.

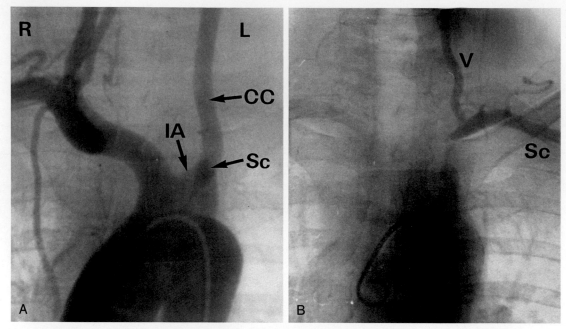

• **Fig. 42.6** Subclavian Steal Syndrome. Subtraction angiograms from a 55-year-old house-painter, who complained of dizziness when painting walls and ceilings. **(A)** Aortic arch (with 'pigtail' arteriogram catheter visible) showing normal right innominate artery, with its subclavian and common carotid branches. On the left, the arterial anatomy is anomalous, with the common carotid *(CC)* arising from a left innominate artery *(IA)*, rather than direct from the aorta (a 'bovine arch'). The left subclavian artery *(Sc)* appears to be occluded beyond a short stump. **(B)** X-ray exposure taken 4 seconds later; the aortic arch and its branches are now clear of contrast, but contrast has appeared in the left vertebral artery *(V)*, flowing downwards from the circle of Willis. This has flowed onwards to fill the left subclavian artery *(Sc)* retrogradely. Thus there is complete obstruction of a segment of the left subclavian artery proximal to the origin of the vertebral artery, and the vertebral artery now supplies the left upper limb at the expense of the cerebral circulation. This results in episodes of transient cerebral ischaemia, at times of high vascular demand from the left upper limb.

Operative intervention is becoming less common as conservative management improves. If indicated, treatment is by excising a cervical rib if present and/or excising the first rib, and dividing any obstructing bands. A poststenotic subclavian aneurysm should be resected and replaced with a graft.

Subclavian Steal Syndrome

This unusual syndrome is caused by stenosis or occlusion of the subclavian artery proximal to the vertebral artery origin. In consequence, the subclavian is fed by retrograde flow from the vertebral artery via the carotids and circle of Willis. This situation remains asymptomatic until there is excessive demand by the upper limb, when blood becomes diverted ('stolen') from the cerebral circulation, causing transient cerebral ischaemia. Fig. 42.6 illustrates a classic example. Treatment is by angioplasty or stenting of the subclavian disease or more rarely by bypass with a graft, however these treatments carry a risk of stroke.

Extracranial Cerebral Arterial Insufficiency

Strokes are common worldwide and about 1 million occur each year in the United Kingdom. Extracranial atherosclerosis is common and is probably responsible for at least 10% of cases. The **common carotid bifurcation** is the area most affected by atherosclerosis, but can affect the distal internal carotid in the **carotid siphon**. Vertebral arteries are the next most commonly affected extracranial arteries. Less frequently, the orifices of the **great vessels** become obstructed, where they branch from the aortic arch.

Atherosclerotic strokes are often heralded by a transient ischaemic attack (TIA) or a minor stroke. This recovers spontaneously without serious disability, but is a 'red flag' symptom, as the risk of recurrent stroke in recently symptomatic patients with severe carotid stenosis is as high as 28%, over the course of the next 2 years.

Carotid Artery Insufficiency

Pathophysiology of Carotid Artery Disease

Carotid artery disease often results in **stenosis**, with cerebral blood flow becoming impaired when luminal narrowing exceeds about 70% (see Fig. 42.7). Cerebral autoregulation of blood flow is able to compensate up to this point. Rough atherosclerotic plaques without gross narrowing may also be a source of **platelet emboli**. Small emboli may cause **TIAs** (including transient blindness, known as **amaurosis fugax**), with symptoms lasting less than 24 hours. In contrast, large emboli or embolism into critical areas cause major strokes and risk permanent brain damage. **Asymptomatic** stenoses may be discovered on investigation of **carotid bruits** or as part of general investigation before major arterial surgery elsewhere.

CASE HISTORIES

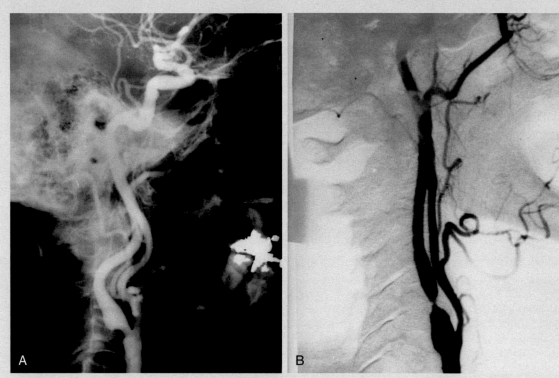

• **Fig. 42.7** Carotid Artery Disease. **(A)** This 71-year-old man suffered two transient episodes of left hemiparesis in 1 week (transient ischaemic attacks, TIAs). Carotid angiography shows a localised 50% stenosis of the internal carotid artery, just distal to the common carotid bifurcation; this degree of stenosis alone would not explain the symptoms. Note the typical poststenotic dilatation immediately beyond the stenosis. The rest of the cerebral arterial system appears normal. At operation, an ulcerated atheromatous plaque was found, which was undoubtedly the source of the emboli that caused the TIAs. Endarterectomy was performed and the patient has been entirely well since. Studies in the United States of America and Europe have shown surgery is definitely better than medical management in patients with a 70% or greater stenosis. **(B)** Subtraction film from a carotid angiogram in a different patient. This shows a 90% stenosis in the internal carotid artery, which is haemodynamically significant, causing cerebral ischaemia

Investigation of Suspected Carotid Artery Disease

A minority suffering TIAs or stroke are found to have a **bruit** on carotid auscultation. However, this does not indicate the extent of narrowing; a significant stenosis may be silent, as of course is complete occlusion.

Patients with strokes and TIAs should be investigated urgently for carotid stenosis by noninvasive means, ideally in a dedicated clinic. The preferred method is **duplex Doppler scanning**, which allows simultaneous imaging of carotid arteries and measurement of blood flow velocity. A measured rise in velocity allows the degree of stenosis to be estimated. In high-grade stenosis in symptomatic disease (i.e., over 50%), surgical intervention is the preferred treatment. With skilled duplex examination, many surgeons feel that conventional **carotid angiography** is no longer necessary or desirable, particularly as this invasive technique carries a risk of stroke. Some centres now use magnetic resonance angiography as a less invasive form of imaging, but it can overestimate the degree of stenosis.

Treatment of Carotid Artery Disease

Medical Versus Surgical or Radiological Intervention

The choice of treatment for symptomatic carotid artery stenosis consists of **medical** antiplatelet therapy (with aspirin 75–150 mg or clopidogrel 75 mg daily), surgical **endarterectomy** (i.e., removing the obstructing disease and thrombus) or, latterly,

minimally invasive **stenting**. Carotid endarterectomy enjoyed an enormous uncontrolled vogue in the 1970s and 1980s for TIAs, completed stroke and asymptomatic carotid stenosis, particularly in the United States of America, but the role of surgery became much clearer after major randomised studies from Europe and the United States of America in 1998. These showed that surgery only reduced stroke rate better than medical therapy in patients with stenosis, greater than 70%. In these high-grade stenoses, surgery reduced the annual stroke rate from about 6% in the 'medical' group to about 2% to 3%.

Recent studies show that patients with 50% or greater stenosis may benefit from surgery. Certainly, for patients suffering repeated symptoms but with lesser stenosis, cogent arguments can be made for intervention. Current risks of surgery include a stroke risk of about 2% and a myocardial infarction risk of between 1% and 2%. Unfortunately, surgery does not reduce long-term mortality from carotid artery disease even in high-grade stenosis. The mortality rate of about 5% per annum over 5 years is comparable in medically and surgically treated patients, taking the operative mortality of 2% to 3% into account.

Acute Symptoms

There is good evidence that any symptoms referable to potential carotid disease, even a minor TIA, should be investigated urgently. This is because carotid endarterectomy most effectively prevents threatened or future strokes, if performed within 2 weeks of the herald symptoms. This benefit halves if patients are left untreated for 6 weeks or longer.

Asymptomatic Carotid Stenosis

The role of surgery in patients with **asymptomatic** carotid disease remains controversial. Recent trials indicate that even in the hands of surgeons with low complication rates, 15 asymptomatic stenoses need to be treated to prevent a single stroke. The figure for symptomatic disease is about six operations. There is also good evidence that the advent of best medical therapy (antiplatelet treatments, statins, strict blood pressure control and smoking cessation) has further reduced the risk of stroke in asymptomatic carotid disease.

Technique of Endarterectomy

Currently, about 2000 carotid endarterectomies are performed annually in the United Kingdom. At present, seven males are treated for stenosis for every three females. The usual operation is **endarterectomy** and may be under general or local anaesthesia (studies have found no clinical differences with regard to anaesthetic technique used). The carotid bifurcation is incised longitudinally after clamping the carotid arteries and anticoagulating the patient. A temporary **shunt** is commonly used to maintain cerebral perfusion, with one end of the shunt in the common carotid below the stenosis and the other in the internal carotid above it, bypassing the operation site. The stenotic plaque is then dissected out and the carotid closed by direct suture (if the artery is large) or more often patched using vein or synthetic material to maintain the diameter. Carotid surgery carries an appreciable risk of mortality or cerebral complications, such as stroke (2%–3%), which needs to be taken into account, when auditing individual results, and when comparing patients treated medically or surgically.

Carotid Angioplasty and Stenting

Angioplasty with stenting is well established for treating peripheral and coronary artery disease, but is relatively novel for carotid stenosis. Potential advantages include the lack of a neck incision, lower rates of haematoma formation and cranial nerve damage, and shorter hospital stays, but **disadvantages** include the higher risk of embolism during the procedure and possibly a higher rate of late restenosis. Recent meta-analysis suggests stenting causes more strokes in the short term, whilst endarterectomy risks cranial nerve injury and a higher cardiac event rate. Current practice in the United Kingdom is to perform surgical endarterectomy as first-line treatment, with stenting reserved for patients who have undergone previous endarterectomy, had radiotherapy to the neck and for those unfit for open surgery.

The technique of stenting involves passing a guidewire from the femoral artery to the area of stenosis. A filter or basket at the end of the guidewire is opened, like an umbrella, to catch debris to prevent it embolising to the brain and causing a stroke. A balloon-tipped catheter is then fed over the guidewire to the target area and inflated to a high pressure to compress the plaque into the wall. The balloon is withdrawn and a self-expanding stent is guided to the area and released. The filter and balloon catheter are finally removed.

Arterial Insufficiency in Other Organs

Mesenteric Ischaemia

Blood supply to portions of the bowel may be compromised in four main ways:

- **Strangulation.** This is a mechanical problem presenting as bowel obstruction described in detail in Chapter 19, p. 298. It may be the result of a **hernia** (see Ch. 32), **volvulus** of small or

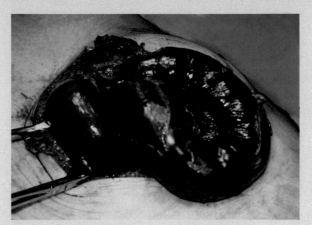

• **Fig. 42.8** Acute Mesenteric Ischaemia. This woman of 77 years presented with moderate abdominal pain and circulatory collapse requiring vigorous resuscitation. She was in atrial fibrillation and was acidotic. Mesenteric embolism was suspected and was confirmed at operation. Unfortunately, as often happens, the entire midgut territory, between a point 20 cm along the jejunum to the midtransverse colon was necrotic and no beneficial procedure was possible.

large bowel, or **fibrous bands** resulting from previous surgery (see Ch. 12, p. 182).
- **Acute thrombotic or embolic obstruction** (see Fig. 42.8). This is analogous to acute thrombosis or embolism of the lower limb described in Chapter 41. The cause is usually superior mesenteric artery occlusion and the condition presents as an 'acute abdomen' (see Ch. 19).
- **Transient ischaemia.** This presents as inflammation of the bowel characterised by abdominal pain and rectal bleeding. The condition is known as **ischaemic colitis** and is discussed at the end of Chapter 29.
- **Chronic mesenteric artery insufficiency.** This rare condition presents with gross weight loss and abdominal pain following eating; it is analogous to intermittent claudication, caused by lower limb arterial insufficiency.

Chronic Mesenteric Ischaemia

The rare condition of chronic mesenteric ischaemia or '**gut claudication**' occurs when the visceral blood supply is restricted to a point, where it becomes inadequate during active digestion, but remains adequate at rest. This occurs when there is gross atherosclerotic narrowing of all three main mesenteric vessels (coeliac, superior mesenteric and inferior mesenteric arteries). These patients present with severe epigastric pain on eating, which causes '**fear of food**'. There is always **gross weight loss** and sometimes an epigastric bruit can be heard on auscultation.

Diagnosis is by arteriography with lateral views showing the origins of the three main vessels or CT angiography. Treatment is by stenting or surgical reconstruction of the origins of one or more mesenteric arteries.

Renal Ischaemia

Renal Artery Stenosis

Pathophysiology of Renal Artery Stenosis

This relatively uncommon condition arises in two main ways. In children and younger adults, the cause is **fibromuscular**

hyperplasia. In older patients, **atherosclerosis** is the usual cause. Renal artery stenosis may present with hypertension (ischaemia of kidneys causes poor perfusion, activating the renin–angiotensin system) or functional renal impairment. It is sometimes discovered incidentally on urography as a nonfunctioning or poorly functioning kidney.

Treatment

Fibromuscular hyperplasia responds well to balloon dilatation, which often results in blood pressure returning to normal. Atherosclerotic disease may be treatable by angioplasty or reconstructive surgery, but randomised trials have shown no real improvement in blood pressure control or renal function. Renal artery stenosis needs to be recognised in patients having aortic reconstructive surgery, whether for occlusive or aneurysmal disease. This is because hypotension during the operation may initiate thrombotic occlusion of narrowed renal arteries and cause kidney failure. These stenoses may need to be treated before operation by angioplasty, or by reconstruction at the time of the aortic operation.

Complications of Arterial Surgery

Specific complications are summarised in Box 41.2 (p. 528). Local complications include **haemorrhage**, **embolism**, **thrombosis**, **graft infection** and **false aneurysm** formation.

Systemic Complications of Arterial Surgery

Patients undergoing arterial surgery are subject to the usual complications of major surgery. In addition, they invariably have **generalised atherosclerotic arteriopathy**, rendering them vulnerable to serious or fatal cardiovascular complications. Patients with obliterative disease are more likely to have serious cardiac disease than those with aneurysms. For aortic and other major arterial operations, prolonged general anaesthesia, **aortic clamping** and heavy operative blood loss place extra stress on a compromised cardiovascular system.

Common systemic complications include myocardial infarction, cardiac failure, acute arrhythmias, strokes, renal failure and intestinal ischaemia. To minimise the risk, preparation for elective arterial surgery should include thorough preoperative cardiovascular assessment and sometimes treatment of cardiac abnormalities. Preexisting medical conditions, such as cardiac failure or hypertension should be stabilised, under expert advice. Patients also require intensive monitoring during and after operation. Perioperatively, this usually includes central venous and peripheral arterial catheterisation for accurate pressure measurements. For patients with severe myocardial disease, transoesophageal ultrasound helps estimate cardiac output and guide fluid replacement. These and other high-risk patients should be closely monitored during the early postoperative period in an intensive care or high-dependency unit, so that complications can be recognised and treated early.

Local Complications of Arterial Surgery (Fig. 42.9)

Haemorrhage

During surgical access to affected arteries, nearby veins are vulnerable to tearing even when great care is taken in dissection. For example, iliac veins cross deep to the iliac arteries and are often adherent to them. Venous tears are more alarming than arterial ones because veins are very thin-walled, friable and difficult to

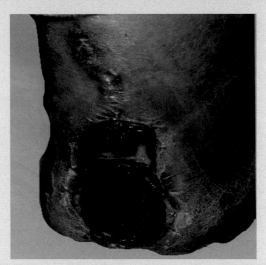

CASE HISTORY

• **Fig. 42.9** Complication of Arterial Surgery. This patient was admitted to hospital with a ruptured aneurysm. He suffered arterial thrombosis of the lower limb during operation, and a thrombectomy to relieve it, left him with an ischaemic foot. Poor attention to heel pressure relief during the early postoperative period led to this heel necrosis, which took several months to heal.

repair. They are often inaccessible and thus lacerations can be difficult to identify and control; such tears often result in massive blood loss.

Completing a satisfactory arterial anastomosis is demanding under the best of conditions, but it is made even more difficult, if there are friable diseased vessels and calcified atherosclerotic plaques, as is so often the case. In the high-pressure arterial system, any defect is quickly revealed and blood sprays everywhere once clamps are released. Fortunately the arterial system can be remarkably forgiving and small leaks are quickly plugged by platelets if swabs are held in place for a few minutes. If blood loss is massive (10–25 units), platelets and coagulation factors are consumed and haemostasis is progressively impaired (**consumption coagulopathy**). Standard blood transfusions are of little help except as volume replacement, since stored blood lacks functioning platelets and clotting factors. In a deteriorating situation (and preferably in anticipation of it), expert haematological advice to infuse **platelet concentrates, cryoprecipitate (contains fibrinogen)** and **fresh frozen plasma**, for example, provides the main answer. Where bleeding is difficult to control by sutures or packing, **organic-based glues** can be helpful in sealing bleeding areas. Patients are usually heparinised perioperatively before the arteries are clamped to prevent distal thrombosis. This does not usually interfere with haemostasis, but if necessary, the effect can be reversed by injecting **protamine**.

There is a trend for the standard use of **cell-saving devices** intraoperatively, to cope with anticipated heavy blood loss. These enable the patient's spilled blood to be collected, washed, concentrated and reinfused, minimising the use of stored blood. Inevitably, clotting factors are lost in the process.

Early postoperative haemorrhage is uncommon provided adequate haemostasis is achieved before completing the operation and closing the wound. When bleeding does occur, it usually results from a pinhole leak at the anastomosis or a slipped ligature. Haemorrhage is manifest by generalised signs of **hypovolaemia**, by progressive abdominal distension or, in the lower limb, by swelling beneath the wound. Postoperative haemorrhage occasionally stops spontaneously following transfusion of blood and clotting factors, but if blood loss continues, further operation must not be delayed.

Embolism

In aneurysm surgery, embolism is usually caused by dislodging fresh or organised thrombus from within the aneurysmal sac. It is largely preventable by clamping the outflow vessels before the aneurysm is manipulated. Large emboli that lodge in femoral vessels can be retrieved with a Fogarty balloon catheter, but the more common case of fragmented distal embolism may cause infarction of digits or even the whole foot ('**trash foot**'). Infarction caused by this distal embolism is irreversible and usually necessitates amputation later. If embolism occurs during **carotid** artery dissection under general anaesthesia, the event is not usually apparent until the patient wakes up and is found to have suffered a stroke. Under local anaesthesia, embolic events may be immediately detectable.

Thrombosis

Thrombosis of reconstructed vessels is a major potential problem in arterial surgery. It rapidly leads to profound distal ischaemia and results in limb loss unless urgently corrected.

Sluggish flow leads to thrombosis and may arise for a variety of technical reasons as follows:

- unrecognised stenosis or occlusion proximal or distal to the reconstruction causing poor inflow or runoff;
- faulty anastomotic technique causing stenosis or partial luminal obstruction;
- dissection of the layers of the distal vessel wall resulting in a loose flap of tunica intima and media, which acts as a 'flap valve' occluding the lumen;
- twisting or kinking of a graft;
- in situ thrombosis during arterial clamping.

Thrombosis usually occurs in the first few hours after operation and becomes evident by deteriorating colour, temperature and pulses of the affected limb from the satisfactory state achieved at operation. Urgent reoperation is usually required. Judicious use of preoperative antiplatelet agents and/or inhibitors of the coagulation system can help prevent this complication. It is good practice to spend time at the end of the operation, ensuring satisfactory flow in the reconstruction and good peripheral perfusion, as well as securing haemostasis. This can avoid the need for reoperation for a thrombosed graft or to arrest haemorrhage in the middle of the night.

Graft Infection

Infection of a synthetic graft is uncommon but can be a devastating complication. It can occur in the early postoperative period or at any time months or years later. The infecting organisms are usually from the patient's own intestine or skin, depending on the site of the graft. Infection is minimised by avoiding opening bowel, meticulous asepsis and haemostasis, and perioperative antibiotic cover. Antibiotics are normally given intravenously at anaesthetic induction and over the next 24 hours. A combination of gentamicin and flucloxacillin is usually suitable; where methicillin-resistant *Staphylococcus aureus* is prevalent, specific agents, such as vancomycin are used as well according to local protocols. In addition, protein-coated Dacron grafts can be soaked in an antistaphylococcal antibiotic before placement, for example, rifampicin or else antibacterial silver impregnated grafts used.

Graft infection should be suspected if there is recurrent pyrexia and malaise or a persistently discharging wound sinus; occasionally, the wound breaks down, exposing the infected graft. Major graft infection, particularly when involving an anastomosis, has a bleak prognosis even when treated, the eventual outcome often being death from sepsis, or anastomotic breakdown with catastrophic bleeding. Standard treatment is to restore the distal circulation with an **extra-anatomic graft** (e.g., axillobifemoral), which bypasses the infected area, and remove the infected graft. Some units advocate use of the role of superficial femoral vein as a replacement conduit in the treatment of aortic graft infections. In early graft infection without anastomotic breakdown, prolonged graft irrigation with antibiotics can be successful on its own.

False Aneurysm Formation

A false aneurysm is the result of a slow anastomotic leak or a leak from an arterial puncture (e.g., a femoral artery puncture for coronary artery stenting) that is confined by surrounding tissues. A slowly expanding blood-filled cavity results, which can eventually rupture or undergo thrombosis. A false aneurysm usually presents as a palpable pulsatile mass. False aneurysms following a femoral artery puncture can be observed (if <2 cm diameter, they can thrombose of their own accord), treated percutaneously with injection of thrombin, or repaired surgically. Patients are often taking dual antiplatelet therapy and have advanced coronary artery disease, the reason for the angiogram in the first place.

False aneurysms can also occur at an anastomosis (usually between a synthetic graft and artery). They used to be more common because of gradual breakdown of silk suture materials, but can still occur, sometimes as a consequence of low-grade infection. They often require surgical reconstruction.

Occasionally, a false aneurysm at an upper anastomosis of a graft with the abdominal aorta leaks into the overlying duodenum. This produces an **aortoduodenal fistula** and presents with major haematemesis. Aortoduodenal fistula may also result from graft infection.

Long-Term Follow Up After Arterial Surgery

All patients with obliterative atherosclerotic disease are liable to disease progression and new ischaemic events. In fact, the risk of sudden cardiovascular death in claudication patients is the same as someone who has suffered a nonfatal myocardial infarction. Ideally, patients should be on 'best medical treatment' for atherosclerosis, that is, a statin, aspirin or clopidogrel, blood pressure control and, if diabetic, tight control of blood sugar. Effective advice regarding smoking cessation and exercise should be given.

Most patients are followed up long term after surgery or angioplasty to monitor deterioration, to detect new disease and to enable timely intervention if needed. Femoropopliteal vein grafts can be examined at intervals using duplex Doppler scanning. Such **graft surveillance** can detect early graft stenoses, enabling them to be treated and the graft preserved, although the efficacy of this is not proven. Aneurysm patients after open operation, on the other hand, can be discharged from regular follow up, 3 months after operation if there are no complications, but should be rescanned by ultrasound at 5-yearly intervals for new aneurysms (see Fig. 42.10). Stent-graft follow up needs to be more rigorous as the devices are not as securely fixed as conventional grafts sewn in place. EVAR patients generally undergo CT scanning every 6 months to a year to look for leaks around the graft (**endoleaks**), but as devices have become more reliable there is a move towards 6-monthly ultrasound scans.

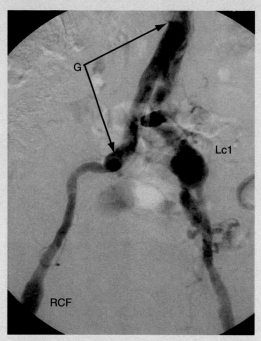

• **Fig. 42.10** Late Formation of New Aneurysm After Aneurysm Surgery. This arteriogram was performed for claudication, 10 years after a trouser or 'Y' graft for abdominal aortic aneurysm. The trouser graft *(G)* is opacified and a new aneurysm has appeared in the left common iliac artery *(LCI)*, beyond the graft. A small aneurysm is also seen in the right common femoral *(RCF)*. Neither was large enough to require surgery but periodic follow up was continued using ultrasound. Obliterative disease responsible for the claudication was found in the superficial femoral arteries distal to this film.

43

Venous Disorders of the Lower Limb

Venous Thrombosis and the Post-thrombotic Limb

Anatomy of the Lower Limb Venous System

Blood is drained from the lower limb via two separate systems. The **deep venous system** drains the deep tissues of the foot and muscles of the lower leg and thigh. These deep veins lie within the mass of lower limb muscles and include the large **soleal venous sinuses**. Muscle contraction during walking and other exercise pumps blood back towards the heart against gravity (**the muscle pump**). Reverse flow is prevented by valves in the system.

The skin and other tissues, superficial to the deep fascia, drain into the **superficial system** with two main vessels, the **long (great) saphenous vein** and the **short (small) saphenous vein**. The long saphenous vein (LSV) receives tributaries from the anteromedial aspect of the limb (and lower anterior abdominal wall), and penetrates the fascia lata in the groin to drain into the (deep) femoral vein (see Fig. 43.3). The short saphenous vein (SSV) drains the posterior part of the leg and passes through the deep fascia into the popliteal vein of the deep venous system. There is a network of interconnecting superficial veins that drain blood from the limb, if LSVs or SSVs are removed or ablated. The superficial system has no muscle pump to aid venous return, but the valves normally prevent retrograde flow, particularly at saphenofemoral and saphenopopliteal junctions. Several **perforating veins** drain superficial blood into the deep system; valves on these normally ensure

one-way flow. Most perforators lie medially on the calf above the ankle, but there is a fairly constant '**Hunterian perforator**' in the medial midthigh.

Presentation and Consequences of Venous Thrombosis

Thromboembolic disease and its consequences are common and include acute deep vein thrombosis (DVT), pulmonary embolism and superficial thrombophlebitis ('phlebitis'). Deep venous thrombosis most commonly occurs as a complication of major surgery, lower limb fractures, myocardial infarction or other severe illness. About one-third of DVTs present with no apparent cause, though many of these patients have a detectable **prothrombotic state**. The risk factors, clinical presentations and management of acute DVT and pulmonary embolism are discussed in Chapter 12.

Deep venous thrombosis is an acute local problem, and often causes major **long-term limb complications,** but has the added risk of pulmonary embolism. The affected extremity is known as a **post-thrombotic limb** or, less accurately, a **postphlebitic limb**. Often patients present with a post-thrombotic limb without a symptomatic or diagnosed DVT previously, though many have had major surgery or lower limb fractures.

Pathophysiology of Post-thrombotic Problems

Following a DVT, the clot gradually undergoes **inflammation**, **organisation** and then **recanalisation** of the vein. During this process, valves are often damaged and become incompetent. This is because valve cusps fail to meet and interrupt the column of blood, allowing blood to reflux back downwards, causing increased pressure distally. This is **chronic deep venous insufficiency** and can take months or years to develop.

In the normal adult limb, ankle venous pressure while standing is about 125 cm of water. This falls markedly during walking as a result of the calf pump and valve function. In the post-thrombotic limb, where blood refluxes or veins remain occluded, ankle venous pressure remains high during walking. This leads secondarily to valve incompetence in perforating veins. Blood is forced out into the superficial system, causing local venous hypertension, disrupting normal vascular dynamics in skin and subcutaneous tissues. This may impair skin

TABLE 43.1 Summary of Lower Limb Venous Disorders

Basic Disease	Pathophysiological Process	Clinical Manifestations
Varicose veins—incompetent valves in veins connecting deep and superficial venous systems; often begins with saphenofemoral valve incompetence	Failure of muscle pump means blood is forced from deep venous system to superficial system through incompetent valves causing slowly progressive tortuous dilatation of superficial veins Venous hypertension may cause chronic skin changes and sometimes ulceration. Women more often affected than men; varicosities often first appear during pregnancy	Slowly progressive development of prominent purple, dilated, tortuous superficial veins. Patient often complains of aching, especially after long period of standing. Patients may be distressed by cosmetic appearance or, if there is a family history, fear of progression or ulceration. Pain relieved by elevation. Dilated vessels are vulnerable to trauma and may bleed profusely
Superficial venous thrombosis (i.e., thrombophlebitis)—usually occurs in tortuous dilated varicose veins; more common in pregnancy. Occasionally, affects normal veins in **thrombophlebitis migrans** occurring in patients with visceral malignancy	Spontaneous thrombosis in superficial veins; excites an inflammatory response in the vessel wall and surrounding tissues	Rapid onset of acute, highly localised pain and tenderness, associated with varicose veins. Overlying skin red and oedematous; underlying veins hard and nodular. Infection is not a feature so antibiotic treatment is illogical. Treatment is with nonsteroidal anti-inflammatories. Occasionally, ligation of the superficial vein at its junction with the deep vein is required to prevent thrombus propagating into the deep venous system
Deep venous thrombosis—predisposed to by previous deep vein thrombosis, pregnancy, oestrogen therapy, major surgery, trauma, obesity, abdominal or pelvic malignancy, immobility, a thrombophilia and increasing age. Long haul flying can be a factor, may be complicated by pulmonary embolism	Thrombosis in deep venous system of calf; may propagate proximally into iliofemoral veins. Can obstruct venous return in both short and long term Spontaneous recanalisation may cause deep vein valvular incompetence, that is, chronic venous insufficiency, and local swelling. Late complication is postthrombotic venous hypertension. This obstructs capillary flow and inhibits metabolic exchange; leakage of red cells causes subcutaneous deposition of haemosiderin Combined effects cause atrophy of skin and subcutaneous fat, fibrosis, poor healing and predisposition to ulceration	Classic acute presentation is pain and swelling of calf and ankle with calf tenderness but is often asymptomatic. Dorsiflexion may cause pain (Homans sign). Leg usually warm and normal in colour, but pulses may be impalpable because of oedema. If iliofemoral veins involved, thigh also swollen. Late complication is post-thrombotic limb with chronic brawny oedema and narrow ankle because of lipodermatosclerosis. Skin atrophic, scaly and pigmented (varicose/venous eczema). Skin above medial malleolus most vulnerable to chronic ulceration after minor trauma

---

• BOX 43.1 Signs of a Gross Post-thrombotic Limb

- Chronic lower leg **swelling** with brawny oedema
- **Varicose veins** with incompetent perforating veins
- Inflammation and haemosiderin **pigmentation** in the area above the medial malleolus (the 'gaiter' area) and other parts of the lower half of the leg. This is known as **varicose** or **venous eczema** and may be complicated by low-grade cellulitis
- Active or healed venous **ulceration** above the medial malleolus
- **Lipodermatosclerosis** around the ankle (replacement of soft subcutaneous fat with firm collagenous scar tissue). This causes the 'champagne-bottle leg' with oedema above and a narrow atrophic ankle below

• BOX 43.2 Initial Examination of Varicose Veins

- **Severity**—examine the extent and severity of varicose veins with the patient standing. Many patients attend with unsightly 'spider veins', which are not varicose. Others attend for advice because they are worried they will develop ulcers ('like my mother').
- **Skin changes**—examine the leg for swelling, ulcers and varicose eczema. If present, could indicate a post-thrombotic limb.
- **Long or short saphenous**—examine the distribution of varicose veins. Are there varicosities above knee, indicating probable saphenofemoral incompetence? Could these be short saphenous system varicosities, that is, posterolateral calf veins feeding towards popliteal fossa, where short saphenous may be palpable?

---

vitality and healing ability. Characteristic local signs of a gross post-thrombotic limb are listed in Box 43.1 (also see Fig. 43.1).

The following factors contribute to the clinical features:

- Venous stagnation restricts arterial replenishment of capillary blood.
- Arteriovenous shunts beneath the affected skin divert blood away from dermal capillaries.
- Venous hypertension causes dilatation of local venules and the capillary network, allowing plasma proteins to leak into the interstitial spaces. Fibrin polymerises forming **pericapillary cuffs**, which may interfere with metabolic exchange between blood and tissues.

Investigation of Venous Insufficiency

Chronic venous insufficiency usually presents with a chronically swollen limb and/or typical skin changes of venous insufficiency around the ankle, and sometimes with ankle ulceration. This may be caused by superficial or deep venous reflux (post-thrombotic or congenital absence of valves) or a combination of both.

The diagnostic pathway depends on responses to the following questions:

- Is the condition venous in origin? This is suggested by a history of DVT, prolonged bed rest in the past or lower limb fractures, or a finding of varicose veins or a '**champagne-bottle**' leg (i.e., proximal limb swelling caused by oedema and distal

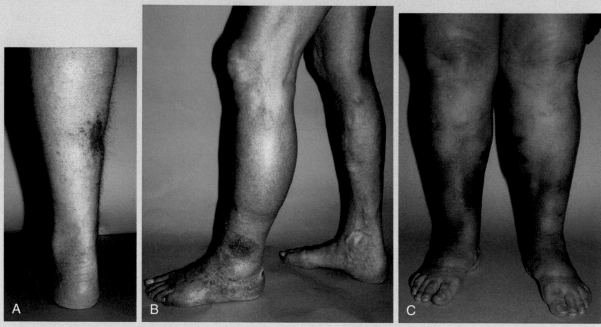

• **Fig. 43.1** Post-thrombotic Limbs and Venous Eczema. (A) Healed venous ulcer showing local loss of subcutaneous fat and surrounding pigmentation. (B) Man of 66 years with no history of deep vein thrombosis showing marked swelling of the left leg with pigmentation in the lateral gaiter area representing venous eczema. The right leg has moderate varicose veins; the blue discolouration around both ankles is an age change, caused by dilated venules and is of no clinical consequence. On colour duplex ultrasound examination, there was evidence of deep venous thrombotic damage in the left leg. (C) Bilateral post-thrombotic limbs in a woman of 57 years with gross venous eczema, fat atrophy, signs of healed venous ulceration and varicose veins.

narrowing caused by fat atrophy and fibrosis). If the condition is not venous, another cause of ulceration and swelling should be sought.

- If it is venous, is there superficial (see Fig. 43.2) or deep venous insufficiency, or a combination of both?
- If a combination, how much is caused by superficial venous insufficiency and therefore likely to respond to surgery (unlike deep venous reflux).

Patients should undergo **colour-flow duplex Doppler ultrasound** investigation, now the 'gold standard'. This can give detailed information on the presence and severity of reflux in deep and superficial veins, as well as determining whether there is venous obstruction. Functional detail will also be gleaned about the superficial system to enable targeted and appropriate treatment.

Management of Post-thrombotic Problems

The main post-thrombotic problems requiring active treatment are chronic venous ulcers and acute cellulitis.

Venous Ulcers

Ulcers may develop spontaneously but are more commonly initiated by minor trauma, which fails to heal, often complicated by secondary infection. Most venous ulcers can be healed by nonoperative methods, provided treatment is applied skilfully. Even if operative treatment is needed, conservative measures are used to prepare the limb. These include reducing swelling by multilayer compression bandaging, removing necrotic tissue from the ulcer base and controlling cellulitis.

The systolic arterial pressure in the leg should be measured relative to the upper limb (i.e., ankle–brachial pressure index [ABPI]—see Ch. 41). If the ABPI is <0.8, the arterial circulation may be inadequate; it should be assessed and necessary treatment instigated before compression therapy as: (1) poor arterial supply may be part of the reason for nonhealing of an ulcer, and (2) compression bandaging with low arterial pressure will make ulceration worse.

Properly applied support and compression of skin and superficial tissues is the mainstay of treatment, provided initially by elastic bandages and when healed, by correctly fitting graduated compression stockings. In both cases, the aim is for pressure to be greatest at the ankle (up to 40 mmHg), reducing progressively up the limb. Great care must be taken that pressure does not cause ischaemia, or abrasions over tendons or bony prominences. Most venous ulcers can be healed rapidly whilst keeping the patient ambulatory by competent four-layer bandaging, avoiding the need for hospital care unless complications occur or skin grafting is required.

Spreading cellulitis should be treated with systemic antibiotics. Infection confined to the ulcer may be treated by saline soaks and perhaps excision of dead tissue; antiseptics are avoided, as they may retard granulation tissue production and epithelialisation. Local antibiotics have no place in the management of ulcers.

Venous surgery may be indicated if there is superficial venous incompetence. Varicose veins should be primarily treated by endovenous means if possible or ligated, unless there is gross deep venous incompetence. Effective treatment of superficial venous reflux reduces the healing time for ulcers and halves the recurrence rate. Surgical

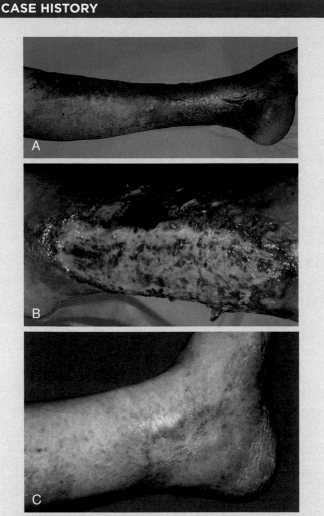

• **Fig. 43.2** Venous Ulceration. **(A)** Post-thrombotic limb with marked venous pigmentation and a chronic ulcer, which heals and breaks down periodically. **(B)** Chronic venous ulcer in a post-thrombotic limb. The ulcer is virtually circumferential and represents a serious management problem. **(C)** Chronic ulcer that healed several years before, following a Cockett operation, an open procedure for subfascial ligation of perforators, the scar of which is visible. This operation and endoscopic variations in the subfascial endoscopic surgery procedure are rarely performed nowadays.

disruption or ligation of incompetent perforating veins is of doubtful value, even if performed by subfascial endoscopic surgery. Intractable or large ulcers may require skin grafting once the ulcer base is clean. Deep venous reflux is treated conservatively with compression therapy, as there are no surgical options that deliver long-term success.

Long-Term Care and Prevention

As soon as a post-thrombotic limb is recognised, the patient should use graduated compression stockings and take care to avoid even minor trauma, especially to the gaiter area above the medial malleolus. Flaking and dryness of the skin should be treated with a moisturiser.

For minor venous insufficiency, well-fitting class I **elastic stockings** or tights provide suitable support. In more severe insufficiency, class II or III compression stockings may reverse tissue damage or arrest its progress. They also provide protection from minor trauma. Ideally, they should be worn at all times except

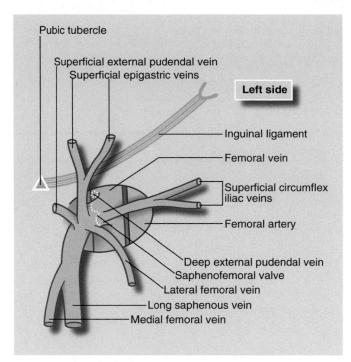

• **Fig. 43.3** Saphenofemoral Junction—Anatomy.

in bed. Correctly fitted stockings are vital; proximal constricting bands impair venous return and stockings sometimes need to be custom made. Effective elastic support will often be required for life, but may not prevent further episodes of cellulitis or ulceration.

Axillary Vein Thrombosis

Axillary vein thrombosis is uncommon and is the upper limb equivalent of DVT. It usually presents with a sudden onset of swelling of hand, forearm and arm, and aching pain in the whole arm. The limb often has a bluish tinge and sensation is preserved. The cause can be primary or secondary. A primary presentation often has no detectable cause but may be associated with visceral malignancy (**thrombophlebitis migrans**), or a thrombotic predisposition. **Paget–Schroetter** syndrome is also referred to as *effort-induced thrombosis*. It usually occurs in younger people as a result of external compression of the subclavian vein between first rib and clavicle. The space may be congenitally narrow or physical activity, such as weight lifting may cause muscle hypertrophy or local trauma. Treatment options include anticoagulation to prevent propagation of thrombus and to encourage spontaneous clot lysis, or **thrombolysis** to restore vessel patency. Following successful lysis, patients may benefit from surgical excision of the first rib via an axillary or supraclavicular approach to prevent further compression.

Secondary causes include long-term venous catheters, commonly used in renal dialysis, and patients requiring long-term venous access for chemotherapy or parenteral nutrition. Catheter problems are usually managed with formal anticoagulation.

Varicose Veins

Varicose veins are dilated, tortuous and prominent superficial veins in the lower limb (see Fig. 43.5). Varicose veins are common worldwide, being present in about 20% of people aged 20 years, increasing to 80% at 60 years. Nevertheless, only about 12% have symptoms or develop complications.

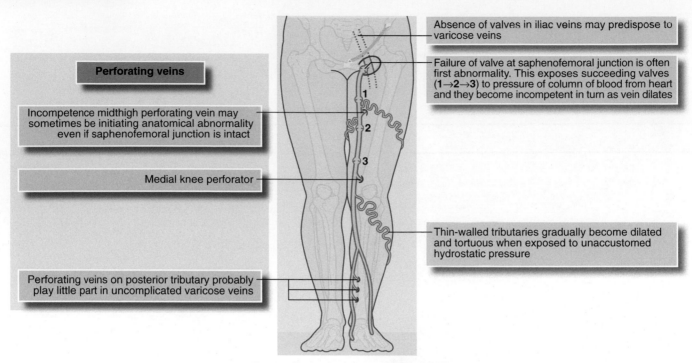

Perforating veins

Incompetence midthigh perforating vein may sometimes be initiating anatomical abnormality even if saphenofemoral junction is intact

Medial knee perforator

Perforating veins on posterior tributary probably play little part in uncomplicated varicose veins

Absence of valves in iliac veins may predispose to varicose veins

Failure of valve at saphenofemoral junction is often first abnormality. This exposes succeeding valves (1→2→3) to pressure of column of blood from heart and they become incompetent in turn as vein dilates

Thin-walled tributaries gradually become dilated and tortuous when exposed to unaccustomed hydrostatic pressure

• **Fig. 43.4** Pathophysiology of Varicose Veins.

Pathophysiology of Varicose Veins (Fig. 43.4)

Abnormal communication between deep and superficial venous systems is crucial in the development of varicose veins. The process probably begins with failure of the valve at the saphenofemoral junction, leading to an uninterrupted column of blood from the heart, which progressively dilates superficial veins down the limb (Fig. 43.5A). Varicose veins usually develop slowly over 10 to 20 years, so surgical treatment is rarely urgent. The long saphenous system is involved in about 90% and the short saphenous in 25% (some have both systems involved).

Women are affected about six times more often than men, with most developing during or soon after a second or third pregnancy. An important factor is probably the high level of progesterone, causing changes in collagen structure (which may not fully recover), as well as smooth muscle relaxation. Pressure on the pelvic veins by the enlarging uterus may contribute by restricting venous return.

Hereditary factors appear to play a part in some patients, especially in men and in those who develop varicosities in their teens. Predisposing anatomical factors may include congenital absence of valves in iliac veins or abnormal vein wall elasticity. DVT plays little part in causing varicose veins. Rarely, multiple congenital arteriovenous fistulae (**Klippel–Trenaunay** and other syndromes) cause gross varicose veins. In these patients, there is gigantism of the lower limb and often venous ulceration (see Ch. 46). A technique of examining varicose veins is shown in Fig. 43.6.

Symptoms and Signs of Varicose Veins

The most common complaints related to varicose veins are:
- aching legs, usually after standing all day;
- poor cosmetic appearance, especially in summer when the legs are exposed;
- fear of future leg ulcers ('like my mother had');

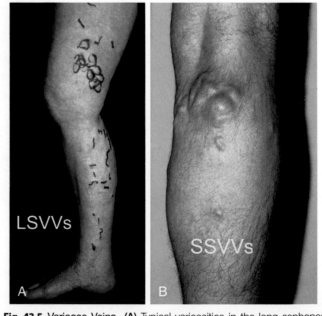

• **Fig. 43.5** Varicose Veins. **(A)** Typical varicosities in the long saphenous territory (*LSVVs*) evident both above and below knee and most prominent on the medial side of the limb. The indelible black markings were made immediately before surgery by the operating surgeon with the patient standing. **(B)** Typical short saphenous varicosities (*SSVVs*), which do not extend above the knee. These veins could not be controlled with an above-knee tourniquet and there was gross reflux evident on hand-held Doppler examination, confirmed on colour duplex Doppler scanning. The saphenopopliteal junction (SPJ) has a variable position and should be marked before surgery using ultrasound so the surgeon knows where to site the incision.

- bleeding or worry about varicosities bleeding, particularly if traumatised;
- varicose eczema or ulcers;
- ankle oedema;
- recurrent superficial thrombophlebitis.

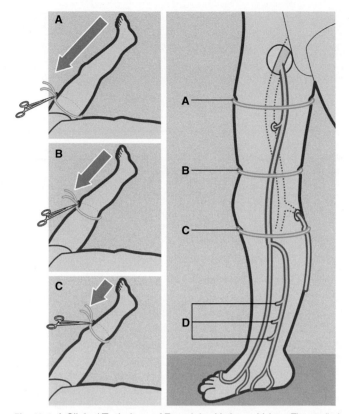

• **Fig. 43.6** A Clinical Technique of Examining Varicose Veins. Elevate limb and ensure veins are emptied by massaging distal to proximal. Apply tourniquet tightly around upper thigh *(A)* then stand patient up. Does tourniquet prevent veins filling and removing it cause rapid filling from above? If so, main communication is at the saphenofemoral junction. If veins fill rapidly with tourniquet in place, repeat the test with tourniquet above the knee *(B)*. If this controls filling, then main communication is midthigh perforator. If this tourniquet fails to control filling, repeat below knee *(C)*. If this controls filling, communication is likely to be short saphenopopliteal or medial knee perforator incompetence. If no tourniquet controls filling, communication is probably by one or more distal perforating veins, often post-thrombotic in origin *(D)*. Note that 80% of varicose veins involve the long saphenous system, sometimes with short saphenous incompetence as well.

Investigation of Varicose Veins

Traditional investigation of varicose veins includes clinical examination and tourniquet techniques (see Fig. 43.6). As a screening investigation in clinic, hand-held ultrasound Doppler allows assessment of reflux at saphenofemoral (SFJ) and saphenopopliteal junctions (SPJ) and within the LSVs and SSVs. The probe is placed over either junction, the calf is pressed and the examiner can hear if there is significant reflux outwards through the junction. Formal duplex scanning is now advocated for all cases where intervention is planned. This gives accurate assessment of superficial and deep systems, determining anatomical areas of reflux and allowing appraisal for endovenous therapy.

Management of Varicose Veins

Most patients with longstanding varicose veins do not have venous complications. For these, surgical treatment is not usually necessary, but advice can be given to elevate the legs when sitting and to wear supporting elastic stockings when standing for long periods.

Indications for Surgical Treatment of Varicose Veins

The main indications are **aching legs** after standing, relieved by elevation or when in bed at night (particularly with unilateral ankle oedema),

haemorrhage from a varicose vein, **superficial thrombophlebitis** and **venous skin changes** caused by superficial venous insufficiency. All of these can be treated with support bandages or stockings, but endovenous treatment or surgery is often preferable and more permanent.

Injection sclerotherapy (e.g., Fegan technique) is used for treating small cosmetically unattractive varicose veins below the knee, but is unsuitable for major varicosities, particularly in the thigh. This type of injection sclerotherapy and surgery for varicose veins is shown in Fig. 43.7.

Endovenous Treatment of Varicose Veins

Newer endovenous treatments of main trunk varicose veins (i.e., LSV and SSV) have been introduced. These aim to ablate the main incompetent superficial vein using **foam sclerotherapy**, or **laser** or **radiofrequency ablation**. All can be performed under local anaesthesia without a groin incision, using ultrasound to give accurate guidance, and give a quicker return to normal activities.

Foam sclerotherapy involves injecting a sclerosant into a vein (e.g., sodium tetradecyl sulphate or polidocanol). It is first mixed with air or a physiological gas, such as carbon dioxide in a syringe to create foam. Foaming increases the surface area of the sclerosant and ensures it displaces the blood, allowing it to act directly on the vein wall. For catheter ablation, the distal truncal vein is located by ultrasound and cannulated, using a Seldinger technique to place a sheath into the vein. A laser fibre or a radiofrequency catheter is positioned just distal to the SFJ or SPJ, using ultrasound guidance. Before treatment, a tumescent mixture of local anaesthetic and normal saline is injected around the length of the vein for analgesia and to act as a heat sink. The vein is then heated internally by drawing the laser fibre or the ablation catheter along its length.

Results of all heat delivered treatments appear at least comparable with surgery, but longer term evaluation is in progress. Foam sclerotherapy is less effective for the treatment of truncal varicosities, but does have a role in the treatment of recurrent varicose veins.

Perioperative Management of the Patient Having Varicose Vein Surgery

When performing open surgery, varicose veins must be marked out indelibly on the legs before operation, ideally by the surgeon doing the operation. The patient must stand first, often for some minutes, to allow veins to fill, and marking performed in this position. Most surgeons mark all prominent veins that are visible or palpable. Extra marks are often added for areas needing special surgical attention, such as suspected perforating veins. Duplex scanning is often used to assist marking of perforators or of the **SPJ**, well known to have a variable anatomy.

Patients with a history of deep or superficial venous thrombosis should be prescribed **low-dose subcutaneous heparin,** as should those with other risk factors for DVT, especially obese patients. The first dose should be given 1 to 2 hours before operation.

Immediately after operation, the whole leg is bandaged firmly with an elastic bandage. The patient should then be mobilised and encouraged to walk about. All dressings can be removed 24 to 48 hours later, and the bandage exchanged for a graduated elastic stocking (class 2), which should stay on for a minimum of 2 weeks. On return home, patients should be encouraged to be active, walking several times a day for at least the first 2 weeks. The legs should be elevated when sitting, and the patient should get up and walk around about every half hour. All these measures are designed to discourage venous stagnation and venous thrombosis. Most patients can drive a car 24 hours after operation and return to work after a week. The patient should be warned that the legs will be bruised when bandages are removed.

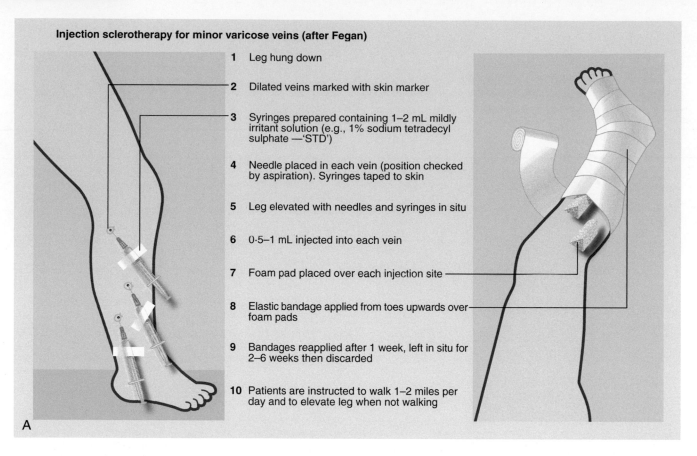

Injection sclerotherapy for minor varicose veins (after Fegan)

1 Leg hung down

2 Dilated veins marked with skin marker

3 Syringes prepared containing 1–2 mL mildly irritant solution (e.g., 1% sodium tetradecyl sulphate —'STD')

4 Needle placed in each vein (position checked by aspiration). Syringes taped to skin

5 Leg elevated with needles and syringes in situ

6 0.5–1 mL injected into each vein

7 Foam pad placed over each injection site

8 Elastic bandage applied from toes upwards over foam pads

9 Bandages reapplied after 1 week, left in situ for 2–6 weeks then discarded

10 Patients are instructed to walk 1–2 miles per day and to elevate leg when not walking

A

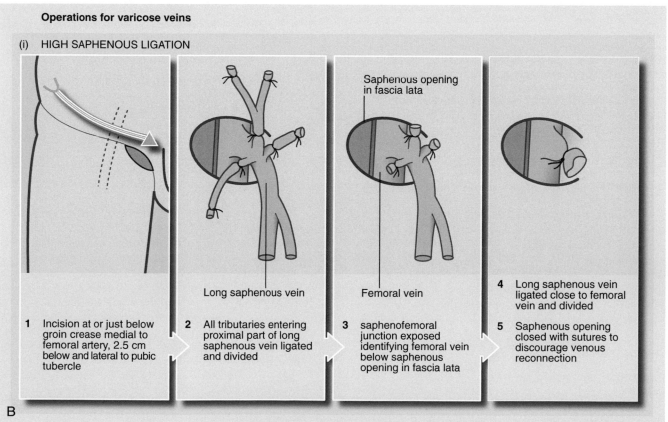

Operations for varicose veins

(i) HIGH SAPHENOUS LIGATION

Saphenous opening in fascia lata

Long saphenous vein

Femoral vein

4 Long saphenous vein ligated close to femoral vein and divided

1 Incision at or just below groin crease medial to femoral artery, 2.5 cm below and lateral to pubic tubercle

2 All tributaries entering proximal part of long saphenous vein ligated and divided

3 saphenofemoral junction exposed identifying femoral vein below saphenous opening in fascia lata

5 Saphenous opening closed with sutures to discourage venous reconnection

B

• **Fig. 43.7** (A) Treatment of varicose veins. (B) Surgical treatment of varicose veins.

Operations for varicose veins

(ii) LONG SAPHENOUS STRIP

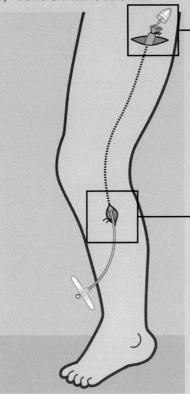

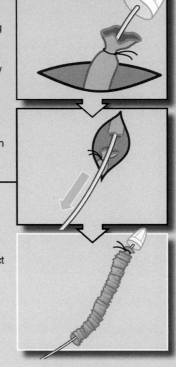

1. The stripper is a long flexible wire with a bullet-shaped knob on the 'business' end. The entry vein (proximal or distal, according to choice) is prepared as shown and the narrow end of the stripper passed down or up the long saphenous vein until it can be brought out to the surface within 15 cm below knee, not to the ankle as was done in the past

2. Stripping is usually downward. The vein is ligated to the wire at the bullet end and the narrow end is pulled smoothly and firmly, tearing off tributaries and any perforators on the way, emerging with the complete vein bunched up on the stripper

3. The wounds are closed and the limb firmly bandaged to minimise subcutaneous bleeding. Patients should be warned to expect postoperative bruising

(iii) AVULSION OF VARICOSITIES

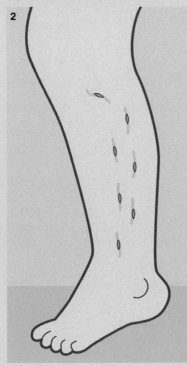

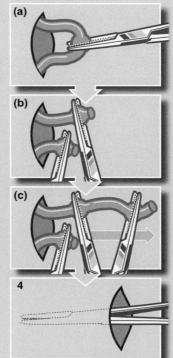

1. Before operation, all varicosities are marked by the surgeon with the patient standing, using an indelible spirit based fibre-tipped pen

2. Very small incisions are made over the marks in a longitudinal direction, or transverse around the knee. As much vein as possible is pulled out ('nick and pick') as follows:

   (a) Vein grasped with artery forceps or special vein hook

   (b) Second forceps applied and vein divided

   (c) One end is drawn out of wound gently and further traction applied by means of another forceps

3. The vein will eventually break and bleeding is controlled by finger pressure. The process is repeated for the other end of vein

4. Forceps can be passed subcutaneously to retrieve nearby varices thus reducing the number of incisions required

5. Each wound is left open or closed neatly with 'steristrips' or a fine suture, and nonadherent gauze applied to each one. The limb is bandaged firmly from the foot to the upper thigh using crepe

B

• **Fig. 43.7, cont'd**

44

Cardiac Surgery

Introduction and Cardiopulmonary Bypass

Surgery of the heart has long fascinated surgeons, but only a very limited range of cardiac procedures was possible until cardiopulmonary bypass was first successfully used in 1953. For the first time, the systemic circulation could be sustained artificially with the heart and lungs bypassed. The emptied heart could be manipulated and lung ventilation discontinued, giving optimal conditions for operating on the heart.

For more than half a century, most open heart surgery has been carried out via a median sternotomy incision using cardiopulmonary bypass. The heart is arrested by clamping the ascending aorta just proximal to where the aortic cannula returns arterial blood from the bypass machine to the patient (Fig. 44.1), and flushing of the isolated aortic root with a cold (4°C–12°C) high-potassium cardioplegic solution (Table 44.1). The combination of cooling and diastolic arrest of the heart provides a certain degree of protection to the ischaemic myocardium, and a bloodless operating field.

Several problems may arise when blood is exposed to artificial surfaces in a cardiopulmonary bypass machine:
- Activation of the clotting cascade could result in **intravascular coagulation.** This is prevented by anticoagulating with high-dose heparin (300 IU/kg), which is later reversed with **protamine sulphate**, after coming off cardiopulmonary bypass.
- Clotting factors and platelets are consumed in the extracorporeal circuit (mainly within the oxygenator), leading to a coagulopathy and bleeding diathesis. Blood products may be required to reverse this.
- Activation of the complement cascade and other inflammatory mediators may result in systemic inflammatory response syndrome after bypass.

In keeping with the move towards minimally invasive surgery, coronary artery bypass grafting (CABG) and various valvular procedures can now be performed on the beating heart without using cardiopulmonary bypass, that is, 'off-pump', avoiding the potential side effects of cardiopulmonary bypass.

Assessing Risk in Cardiac Surgery

The complexity of cardiac surgery makes it potentially risky. In the United Kingdom, all cardiac surgical units have to undertake prospective audit including risk assessment and submit data to the **National Institute for Cardiovascular Outcomes Research**, a national cardiac audit programme focusing on quality improvement. Individual surgeon's outcomes are published online, allowing suitable standards to be developed and maintained and to help inform patient choice.

Several scoring systems have been devised to take patient factors into account, to predict the risk of morbidity and mortality for an individual undergoing a particular operation, a process called **risk stratification**. These systems generally take account of the surgical procedure, its urgency and preexisting comorbidities. Online calculators for Society of Thoracic Surgeons score and for EuroSCORE II are the latest tools and are based on actual outcomes in large numbers of the patients recently operated upon.

Congenital Cardiac Disease

Types of Congenital Heart Disease

Congenital heart disease occurs in about 2 per 1000 live births and falls into two main groups: those with and those without cyanosis.

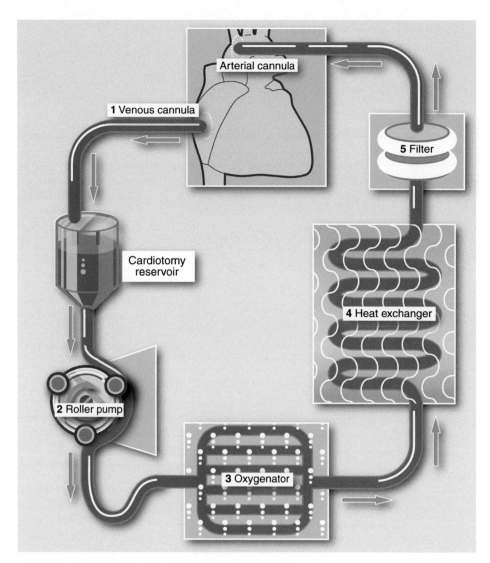

- **Fig. 44.1** The Standard Circuit for Cardiopulmonary Bypass.
1. Systemic venous blood from the right atrium (or from the superior and inferior vena cavae) is siphoned by gravity into a reservoir via a venous cannula.
2. Venous blood from the reservoir enters a roller pump.
3. Blood is pumped under pressure through a membrane oxygenator.
4. Oxygenated blood then passes through a heat exchanger to cool or rewarm the blood as necessary.
5. The oxygenated and temperature-controlled blood finally passes through an arterial filter and is returned to the systemic arterial circulation, usually via the ascending aorta. Note: if the right-sided heart chambers need to be opened for surgical access (e.g., for atrial septal defect repair), the superior and inferior vena cavae are individually cannulated and snared, to prevent air from entering the venous circuit and locking the gravity siphon.

TABLE 44.1	Constituents of a Typical Infusate for Cold Cardioplegia (St Thomas Solution)
Constituent	**Quantity**
Sodium chloride	110.0 mmol/L
Potassium chloride	16.0 mmol/L
Magnesium chloride	16.0 mmol/L
Calcium chloride	1.2 mmol/L
Sodium bicarbonate	10.0 mmol/L
Procaine	16.0 mmol/L

Cyanotic Heart Disease

Cyanotic heart disease exists when there is mixing of systemic arterial and venous blood through a predominantly **right-to-left shunt** in the heart. The most common examples are:
- **Tetralogy of Fallot**—the four features are ventricular septal defect (VSD), pulmonary stenosis, right ventricular hypertrophy and an aorta, which overrides the ventricular septum, receiving blood from both ventricles.
- **Transposition of the great arteries**—the pulmonary artery arises from the left ventricle and the aorta from the right ventricle.
- **Tricuspid atresia**—absence of a functional tricuspid valve.
- **Truncus arteriosus**—the pulmonary artery and aorta fail to develop separately.

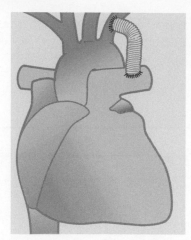

• **Fig. 44.2** Palliation of Tetralogy of Fallot With a Modified Blalock–Taussig Shunt.

- **Total anomalous pulmonary venous drainage**—pulmonary venous blood drains into the right side of the heart.
- **Eisenmenger syndrome**—increased pulmonary blood flow caused by a left-to-right shunt from birth eventually results in severe pulmonary hypertension in later life and spontaneous reversal of the intracardiac shunt to become right-to-left.

Acyanotic Heart Disease

Acyanotic congenital heart disease may involve:

- A shunt from left to right sides of the heart (e.g., via an atrial or VSD) or a ductus arteriosus, which persists in its antenatal patent state (Patent Ductus Arteriosus [PDA]).
- Failed or incomplete embryological development of parts of the heart or great vessels without shunting, for example, coarctation of the aorta.

Management of Congenital Heart Disease

In the past, palliation was often all that could be offered, sometimes followed by a corrective operation when the child was larger. Nowadays, corrective procedures are usually offered at the outset, as operations have become more routine, myocardial protection is more predictable and operative risks are lower.

Palliating Congenital Cardiac Disorders

When pulmonary blood flow is **reduced** (as in tricuspid atresia, tetralogy of Fallot or pulmonary artery stenosis), palliation aims to increase pulmonary flow by creating a shunt between the systemic arterial circulation and the pulmonary artery (Fig. 44.2).

When pulmonary blood flow is **too great** (e.g., VSD or truncus arteriosus), the aim is to reduce the pulmonary flow by artificially narrowing the main pulmonary artery using external banding.

Correcting Congenital Cardiac Disorders

Surgical correction of congenital heart disease is based on accurately identifying the lesion or lesions, then performing procedures, which restore the normal flow and functioning of the heart. Correction may be straightforward (e.g., PDA closure; resection of coarctation; VSD repair) or highly complex (e.g., total correction of Fallot tetralogy; correction of anomalous pulmonary venous drainage). These are high-risk procedures and should only be performed in specialist paediatric cardiac surgical units with audited and published outcomes.

Acquired Heart Disease

The types of acquired heart disease are listed in Table 44.2.

Coronary Artery Disease (See Table 44.3 for Clinical Presentations)

Pathophysiology

Coronary artery disease (ischaemic heart disease) is nearly always atherosclerotic, with subintimal thickening caused by deposition of cholesterol-containing lipids, plus hyperplasia of media smooth muscle cells, which migrate into the subintimal area. Together, these changes reduce the luminal diameter. Since resistance to flow is proportional to the fourth power of the radius (Poiseuille Law), a small change in cross-sectional area causes a dramatic reduction in coronary blood flow. When assessed on angiography, a 50% reduction in coronary artery diameter shown in two planes is regarded as significant. A more reliable method to determine whether a coronary artery stenosis is significant is to use a pressure wire to measure the fractional flow reserve, under conditions of maximal myocardial hyperaemia.

Acute coronary ischaemia is usually brought on by thrombosis of already narrowed coronary arteries, in some cases precipitated by rupture of atherosclerotic plaques.

The worldwide distribution of coronary atherosclerosis is predominantly a disease of developed countries. Men are at greater risk than women, with 45% of men over 65 years having some manifestation of it. Areas of historically high incidence include Scotland and Finland. The rates in some countries, notably the United States of America and much of Europe, have been falling dramatically in recent years, largely as a result of reduced cigarette smoking, control of hypertension, use of statins and perhaps changes in diet and exercise.

Risk factors for coronary atheroma (and atherosclerosis elsewhere) include unfavourable cholesterol and lipid profiles (often hereditary), cigarette smoking, diabetes, hypertension, obesity and a sedentary lifestyle (and perhaps a life of severe unrelieved stress and lack of control). The presentations of coronary heart disease are outlined in Table 44.3.

Control of Predisposing Factors

The first step in treatment is to advice the patient to modify risk factors known to contribute to disease progression. There are two purposes: if progression can be arrested, physiological development of collateral blood supply can proceed, which may make intervention unnecessary. Secondly, occlusion of any form of revascularisation is more likely if risk factors, particularly cigarette smoking, continue. On average, patients who continue to smoke gain **no benefit** from CABG. Nothing can yet be done about hereditary factors, but smoking, obesity and inactivity can be tackled. The benefits of lowering blood lipid levels are well established. Statins are widely used for this, but have other beneficial effects including reducing arterial wall inflammation.

Management of Coronary Artery Disease

Coronary artery disease can be managed conservatively ('medical management'), by interventions, using percutaneous techniques or surgical revascularisation, that is, CABG. The anatomy of the coronary arteries is shown in Fig. 44.3.

TABLE 44.2 Types of Acquired Heart Disease

Type	Pathophysiology	Clinical Presentation
Ischaemic heart disease	Usually caused by coronary atherosclerosis and rarely, by spasm, embolism or trauma	a. Reversible ischaemia presenting as angina b. Painless or silent ischaemia discovered incidentally c. Myocardial infarction

Valvular Heart Disease, Affecting Aortic, Mitral, Tricuspid or Pulmonary Valves	1. Congenital valve disorders (e.g., bicuspid aortic valve) predisposing the valve to later malfunction, degeneration or disease
	2. Rheumatic valvular heart disease—mitral valve most common; also affects aortic valve (occasionally follows rheumatic fever, causing thickening and tethering of leaflets, shortening of mitral valve chordae and valve calcification)
	3. Secondary involvement of valves caused by disruption of nearby structures:
	  • aortic dissection involving the aortic valve
	  • myocardial infarction involving the papillary muscles
	  • myocardial ischaemia leading to scarring and contraction of the papillary muscles
	  • autoimmune disorders, for example, Libman–Sacks endocarditis
	  • 'metabolic' defects, for example, Marfan syndrome
	4. Infective endocarditis, usually on diseased valves
		a. Disordered valve function
		  • valve stenosis restricts blood flow
		  • valvular incompetence causes reflux of blood
		b. Disordered valve function Accumulation of 'vegetations' or thrombus, which may embolise into the peripheral arterial tree
		c. Infection of vegetations or thrombus (bacterial endocarditis)
		  • systemic symptoms (fever, anorexia, weight loss)
		  • deteriorating valve function
		  • infected systemic embolism to brain, kidneys, etc.

Disease Affecting the Great Arteries		
Aorta Pulmonary artery	1. Aortic dissection within the media resulting from atherosclerosis or cystic medial necrosis 2. Aneurysm (connective tissue degeneration, syphilis, trauma, infection) 3. Traumatic transsection	a. Acute severe chest pain b. Acute severe hypovolaemic shock with collapse or sudden death
	Peripheral deep venous thrombosis detaches and passes through the heart to impact in the pulmonary arteries	a. Acute occlusion by pulmonary embolism—may be silent, symptomatic or 'massive' and fatal b. Recurrent embolism may cause pulmonary hypertension
Pericardial disease	1. Pericardial constriction (scarring or tumour)	Signs of constrictive pericarditis: systemic venous congestion with hepatomegaly and ascites; often atrial fibrillation
	2. Pericardial effusion	Retrosternal pressure; muffled heart sounds; cardiac tamponade if acute and severe

TABLE 44.3 Presentation of Coronary Artery Disease

Presentation	Secondary Effects	Clinical Effects
Ischaemic damage discovered incidentally in an asymptomatic patient	Potential risk of further MIs; developing complications of ischaemic heart disease (IHD); increased risk when performing an unrelated operation	Found incidentally, for example, on electrocardiogram
A past history of myocardial infarction (MI)	Risk of further MIs; complications of IHD; risk during unrelated operation	History of typical pain (but note that 25% of MIs are painless)
Angina pectoris	Mortality/morbidity risks of unrelated operations increased	Typical pain brought on by exercise, anxiety or excitement
Complications of MI	1. Rupture of part of the heart	Rupture of external wall of left ventricle Septal rupture causing a ventricular septal defect Papillary muscle rupture causing mitral or tricuspid regurgitation
	2. Fibrosis or scarring following MI	Generalised fibrosis may cause cardiac failure through loss of contractile myocardium Localised fibrosis of an infarcted ventricular wall may cause a **ventricular aneurysm** Discrete fibrosis near a valve may cause tethering of a mitral leaflet resulting in mitral regurgitation Mural scars may disrupt the conducting system causing ventricular arrhythmias
	3. Mural thrombus may accumulate on a subendocardial infarct as an early response to injury	Thrombus may detach and cause systemic arterial embolism, for example, to brain, lower limb or superior mesenteric artery; usually an early complication of MI (1–6 weeks)
	4. Sudden death - usually caused by ventricular arrhythmia	

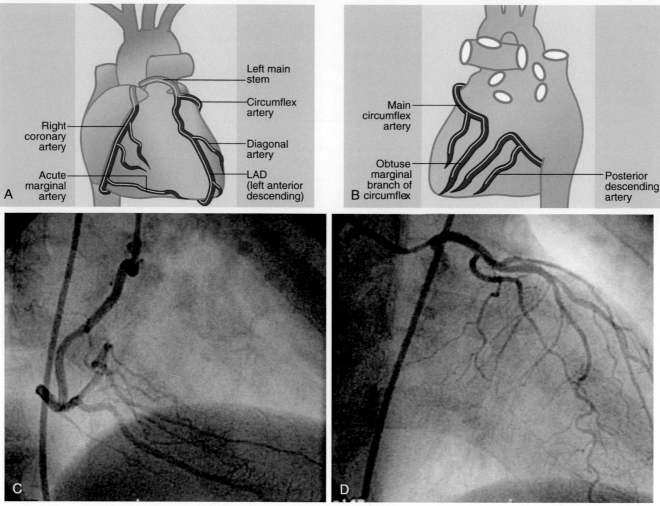

• **Fig. 44.3** Anatomy of the Coronary Arteries. **(A)** Anterior view of coronary arteries. **(B)** Posterior view of coronary arteries. **(C and D)** Selective coronary angiography (AP views as in **A**). **(C)** Normal right coronary artery; **(D)** normal left coronary artery.

Percutaneous Coronary Interventions

Percutaneous techniques to dilate stenoses or recanalise occluded coronary arteries have progressed since the early 1980s; these are performed by interventional cardiologists and if performed rapidly enough after an acute coronary occlusion, can save lives and minimise myocardial damage. The mainstay of treatment is **percutaneous transluminal coronary (balloon) angioplasty (PTCA)** and insertion of intracoronary artery **stents**. Stents are expensive, particularly drug-eluting stents (e.g., sirolimus or paclitaxel coated stents) aimed at minimising in-stent restenosis. In selected patients with noncomplex coronary lesions, large-scale randomised studies have shown equivalent medium-term survival when compared with CABG, albeit with a greater need for reintervention.

When performed expertly, these techniques cause little disruption to the patient's life and recovery is rapid. However, set against this, there remains a definite early failure rate and a substantial medium-term restenosis rate (30% for bare-metal stents and about 10%–15% for drug-eluting stents, at 6 months). In addition, the patient has to be prepared to undergo an emergency operation if things should go wrong during angioplasty. With improving medium-term results, the main indication for PTCA is for emergency revascularistion and for first-time intervention for relieving symptomatic single or double coronary artery stenoses.

Coronary Artery Bypass Grafting

CABG is usually indicated in two categories of patient:

1. Those with chronic stable angina not relieved by medical therapy or who are intolerant of it. This is by far the largest group. Most are operated upon electively, but increasingly, patients admitted to hospital with acute coronary syndrome or crescendo angina are kept in for urgent or emergency surgery.
2. Patients in categories believed to have a better prognosis after surgery than with medical therapy.

Studies in the United States of America and Europe suggest improved survival after surgery is likely in patients with the following morphological characteristics:

- Stenosis of the left main stem coronary artery (before it bifurcates into anterior descending and circumflex arteries).
- Triple-vessel disease (i.e., disease of the right coronary, the left anterior descending and the circumflex arterial systems) plus impaired left ventricular contractility.
- Two-vessel disease, which includes a proximal stenosis in the left anterior descending coronary artery.

The results of CABG are encouraging, with 85% to 90% relieved of angina, without need for medication. A further 5% are substantially improved but require antianginal drug therapy.

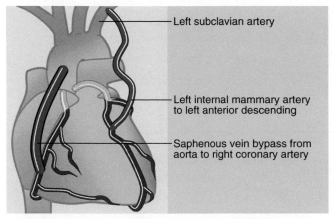

- Left subclavian artery

- Left internal mammary artery to left anterior descending

- Saphenous vein bypass from aorta to right coronary artery

• **Fig. 44.4** Methods of Coronary Artery Bypass Grafting. Note that an explanted autogenous radial artery may be used as a bypass graft instead of saphenous vein.

Surgical Technique (Fig. 44.4)

The aim of CABG is to bypass occlusive disease and provide a new source of blood flow into the distal coronary arteries. Occlusive disease is usually in the proximal third of the epicardial coronary arteries. This fortunate morphology enables the distal end of bypass grafts to be anastomosed to patent recipient arteries, beyond the point of disease. Saphenous veins are used as conduits to bypass the coronary lesion, from the ascending aorta to the distal coronary artery; for lesions of the left anterior descending artery, the preference is to mobilise the nearby left internal mammary artery to form a bypass graft.

Prosthetic materials give poor results for CABG and are rarely used. Early conduits were exclusively reversed autologous great saphenous vein. However, long-term patency is poor, with 50% to 70% occluding within 10 years of surgery. Long-term patency is better when the left internal mammary artery is grafted onto the left anterior descending coronary artery (see Fig. 44.4). This graft seems to be resistant to occlusion (>90% patency at 10 years) and is the current choice for this site. The great saphenous vein is used most commonly for grafts to other coronary vessels. Other arteries used for CABG including radial, right gastroepiploic and inferior epigastric.

In elective patients, CABG surgery has a 2% chance of stroke (especially with a previous history of stroke) and an overall mortality risk close to 1%. Mortality rates for CABG are higher in patients with heart failure and those requiring emergency operations. The risk also increases with age.

To minimise the potentially damaging effects of cardiopulmonary bypass noted earlier, and also the cognitive deficit that probably follows all such operations, there has been a vogue for revascularising 'off-pump'. Operating conditions are more demanding, which may adversely affect the accuracy of anastomoses and increase the occlusion rate. Surgeons are also more inclined to overlook diseased arteries that are harder to reach, resulting in incomplete revascularisation. So far, randomised studies comparing CABG on-pump and off-pump have failed to demonstrate benefit for the off-pump approach.

Other Types of Surgery for Ischaemic Heart Disease

Other forms of surgery in addition to CABG may be required for complications of myocardial infarction. These carry a higher risk than isolated CABG surgery and include:

- Excision of a left ventricular aneurysm—mortality about 5%.
- Replacement or repair of a leaking mitral valve as a result of ischaemia—mortality 5% to 8%.

- Surgical identification and ablation of a ventricular arrhythmic focus—mortality 10% to 15%.
- Emergency repair of a postmyocardial infarction ventricular septal rupture—mortality 20% to 40%.
- Post-CABG heart failure necessitating ventricular support (intraaortic balloon pump) or cardiac transplantation—mortality about 10% at 1 year.

Valvular Heart Disease

Valvular heart disease manifests with symptoms or signs of **stenosis**, causing restricted blood flow across the valve, or **regurgitation** where the valve becomes incompetent, allowing blood to leak through the valve when closed. There is a trend towards preserving and repairing the native valve whenever possible; however, if the native valve is too diseased (e.g., senile calcific aortic valve stenosis), valve replacement remains the standard of care.

Aortic Valve Disease

Aortic stenosis is most commonly caused by so-called senile degeneration and calcification of a normal tricuspid aortic valve, affecting 2% to 4% of patients in their sixth to eighth decades. Bicuspid aortic valves are the most common valvular anomaly, affecting 1% to 2% of the general population, and may degenerate in the fourth to fifth decade of life. Aortic valve regurgitation may result from aortic leaflet abnormality (e.g., leaflet prolapse or perforation) and/or abnormal dilatation of the aortic valve annulus, a condition known as **annuloaortic ectasia**.

Severely stenotic aortic valves are usually treated by resection and replacement with a prosthetic valve. Some regurgitant valves are repaired, but long-term durability is uncertain. A recent treatment for patients with aortic valve stenosis unfit for aortic valve replacement (AVR) is a catheter technique via the left ventricular apex or femoral artery. It involves balloon dilatation of the stenotic valve and insertion of a stent-mounted prosthetic valve into the space. This transcatheter aortic valve insertion (TAVI) technique is less invasive than surgical AVR. Greater than 80% of TAVIs are performed via a transfemoral route, using local anaesthesia under conscious sedation. In patients who are too frail to undergo TAVI, a simple balloon aortic valvuloplasty may provide short-term palliation of symptoms.

Mitral Valve Disease

Mitral stenosis following rheumatic fever can be successfully treated by **valvotomy** (separation of fused valve leaflets), if performed before calcification makes the leaflets immobile. Techniques include percutaneous transseptal balloon dilatation of the stenosed valve and direct **open valvotomy** under cardiopulmonary bypass.

In regurgitant valvular disease, surgical valve repair is possible in most patients but has been most successful for myxomatous or degenerate regurgitation. This conservative technique has a lower perioperative risk than valve replacement and better preserves left ventricular function. Thus the overall functional result may be better than valve replacement. Repair techniques may also be used for diseased tricuspid or aortic valves. Only where valvotomy or repair is inappropriate or has failed are valves replaced.

Valve Prostheses (Fig. 44.5)

The leaflets of prosthetic heart valves are constructed from artificial material or biological tissue. Various types of prosthetic valves are available (see Fig. 44.5). The mechanical demands on prosthetic

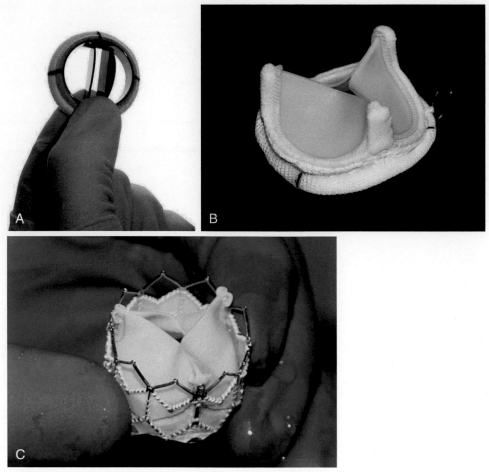

• **Fig. 44.5** Prosthetic Valves. Three commonly used prosthetic heart valves are shown here. **(A)** A St. Jude bileaflet mechanical valve—used in 90% of patients requiring a mechanical prosthesis. Lifelong anticoagulation is mandatory for all patients receiving mechanical valve prosthesis. **(B)** An Edwards Magna Ease bovine pericardial stent mounted bioprosthesis. **(C)** An Edwards SAPIEN transcatheter bioprosthetic valve.

heart valves are extreme. They must provide minimal restriction to blood flow when open, yet prevent reflux when closed; they must be biocompatible, nonthrombogenic, resistant to infection and, most demanding of all, capable of opening and closing 70 times a minute for many years without mechanical failure. Modern mechanical valves are durable but thrombogenic and generally require lifelong anticoagulation, which carries its own risk with a mortality of about 2% over 5 years. Even with effective anticoagulation, there is still a small risk of valve thrombosis and embolisation.

Replacement tissue valves may be **homografts** (human) or **xenografts** (animal origin). Xenografts are most commonly made from bovine pericardium or porcine heart valves. In general, tissue valves are less thrombogenic (anticoagulation not necessary) but less durable. However, in patients over 60 years given an aortic bioprosthesis, 90% or more are free from structural valve degeneration at 10 years. Homograft valves may be more resistant to degeneration and are preferred for young patients.

Infection of valve prostheses is devastating but fortunately rare. The risk is probably lowest for homograft valves. Prosthetic valve endocarditis carries a very high mortality and needs protracted antibiotic treatment, often requiring explantation (removal) of the infected prosthesis.

Indications for Valve Surgery

Valvular heart surgery is most successful when carried out at the right time, namely when risks of surgery are least, potential benefits greatest and before irreversible ventricular dysfunction has occurred.

In aortic or mitral valve stenosis, surgery is indicated when patients become symptomatic. In aortic or mitral regurgitation, surgical intervention is best when there is left ventricular systolic dysfunction or dilatation in an asymptomatic patient.

Pericardial Disease

Pericardial inflammation may result in constriction of the pericardium and cardiac compression. Worldwide, this occurs most commonly in tuberculosis, but may also occur in autoimmune conditions, such as rheumatoid arthritis, following pericardial trauma or mediastinal radiotherapy. Pericardial constriction impairs filling of the cardiac chambers causing equalisation of diastolic pressures in all four chambers of the heart. Clinical signs are those of pulmonary and systemic venous congestion, together with a low cardiac output. Surgical treatment involves excision of the entire pericardium.

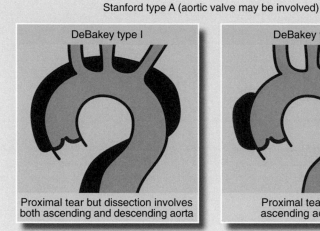
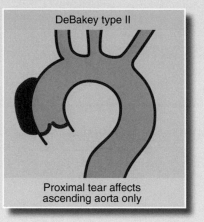
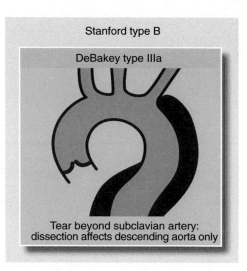

Stanford type A (aortic valve may be involved)

DeBakey type I

Proximal tear but dissection involves both ascending and descending aorta

DeBakey type II

Proximal tear affects ascending aorta only

Stanford type B

DeBakey type IIIa

Tear beyond subclavian artery: dissection affects descending aorta only

• **Fig. 44.6** Thoracic Aortic Dissection.

Disease of the Thoracic Aorta

Aortic Dissection

In aortic dissection, a breach in the luminal surface allows blood to leak out and split the media, then flow along a false lumen for variable distances proximally and/or distally. The dissection flap may occlude any aortic branch and disrupt the aortic valve. The likely aetiology is degeneration of elastin and collagen in the media. Dissection occurs most often in the ascending aorta (65%), but also in the aortic arch (10%), or the descending thoracic aorta, just distal to the ligamentum arteriosum (20%). Risks factors include age >65 years, uncontrolled high blood pressure, smoking, aortic aneurysm and congenital conditions, such as Marfan syndrome and bicuspid aortic valve. Patients present with sudden, severe tearing chest pain, which radiates to the back. The diagnosis can be confirmed on contrast-enhanced computed tomography or echocardiography.

Dissection is classified according to the part affected; the most widely used method is the **Stanford classification**. Type A indicates that only the ascending aorta is involved, while type B is when any other part of the thoracic aorta is affected. An alternative classification method is that of DeBakey (Fig. 44.6).

Without surgery, Stanford type A dissection carries an 80% mortality in the first month; with surgical management, this falls to less than 20%. The operation involves resecting the ascending aorta and replacing it with a synthetic vascular graft. If the dissection reaches the aortic valve, it is likely to be disrupted, causing acute severe regurgitation and perhaps occluding the coronary artery origins. In these cases, the valve will need resuspending or replacing.

Uncomplicated type B dissections have a 20% mortality at 30 days, and the outcome is similar whether surgically or medically managed. Medical management is by control of pain and blood pressure. Surgery is required in type B dissections complicated by aortic rupture, occlusion of vital branches, progressive dissection or, later, by aneurysm formation. The introduction of endoluminal stent graft for treatment of descending aortic conditions has made open surgery much less common. Note that abdominal aortic aneurysms occur years later in about 50% after thoracic dissection.

Thoracic Aneurysms

Aneurysmal dilatation of the thoracic aorta may occur in the ascending part (Fig. 44.7), the arch or the descending part.

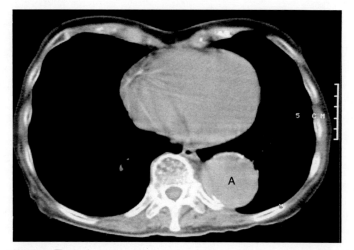

• **Fig. 44.7** Thoracic aortic aneurysm computed tomography scan of chest showing a 5-cm aneurysm of the descending thoracic aorta *(A)*.

There is a risk of rupture and surgical intervention is usually recommended when the aneurysm reaches ≥55 mm diameter; however, for those with a bicuspid aortic valve, the threshold is ≥50 mm and for patients with Marfan syndrome, the threshold is ≥45 mm. Surgery on the descending thoracic aorta, particularly when there is thoracoabdominal disease, threatens the main blood supply of the spinal cord (the artery of Adamkiewicz at about T10), so that paraplegia complicates 10% to 30% of these operations. There is an increasing trend towards endoluminal stent-grafting for appropriate thoracic aneurysms and this is associated with lower morbidity and mortality.

Trauma to the Thoracic Aorta

This may result from blunt or sharp injury. Blunt trauma is usually associated with severe deceleration as occurs in head-on impact in road traffic collisions. The common injury is a partial or complete transection of the aorta at the junction between the arch and the descending aorta, close to the ligamentum arteriosum. Complete transection with free rupture is rapidly fatal; partial transection with an intact adventitia and a contained haematoma is liable to rupture at any time and must be diagnosed to enable early emergency treatment. There is a trend towards treating these with intraluminal stent grafts via the femoral artery. Late aneurysm formation may also occur in those patients who survive an untreated occult aortic transection.

Pulmonary Embolism

Emergency surgical removal of a massive pulmonary embolism has become increasingly rare with the introduction of effective thrombolytic agents. Emergency pulmonary embolectomy is still indicated for failed thrombolysis or where thrombolytic therapy might carry unacceptable risks, for example, after recent surgery or during pregnancy. The operation is carried out under cardiopulmonary bypass.

In 2% to 4% of patients with acute pulmonary embolism, the embolic material does not resolve. Instead, they become organised into fibrous plugs, which progressively obliterate the pulmonary vasculature, causing **chronic thromboembolic pulmonary hypertension**. Life expectancy is substantially shortened when the mean pulmonary artery pressure exceeds 30 mmHg. Pulmonary endarterectomy is a highly specialised operation, whereby surgeons systematically dissect and remove all the obstructing material inside the pulmonary arteries, well into the segmental and subsegmental levels (Fig. 44.8). A successful operation can be curative, normalising pulmonary artery pressures, providing symptomatic relief and restoring normal life expectancy.

Advanced Heart Failure

Heart failure is a clinical syndrome of symptoms and signs caused by structural or functional abnormalities of the heart. In the United Kingdom, it affects 900,000 people and the prevalence is rising because of the ageing population and improved survival of patients with ischaemic heart disease. The majority of heart failure patients are elderly and the average age at first diagnosis is 76 years.

Patients with heart failure are medically managed with a combination of diuretics, beta-blockers, angiotensin converting enzyme inhibitors or angiotensin II receptor blockers, aldosterone antagonists and vasodilators. Patients with cardiac dyssynchrony may benefit from biventricular pacing to resynchronise cardiac contractions; insertion of an automated implantable cardioverter defibrillator has been shown to improve survival in those at risk of sudden death from ventricular arrhythmias. Prognosis of heart failure is poor and despite the aforementioned therapies, 30% to 40% of patients diagnosed with heart failure die within a year.

Surgical Therapy for Heart Failure

Heart failure patients with reversible ischaemic myocardium may be treated by percutaneous coronary interventions or high-risk conventional CABG. Structural abnormalities of the heart, such as valvular lesions and ventricular aneurysms may be corrected surgically. Selected patients with heart failure that is refractory to conventional treatments may benefit from more advanced heart failure therapies, such as heart transplant and mechanical circulatory support.

Heart Transplantation

The first human heart transplant was carried out in Cape Town by Christian Barnard in 1967. To date, over 140,000 heart transplants have been carried out worldwide, mostly in North America and in Europe. The commonest indications are dilated and ischemic cardiomyopathies. To be eligible, potential recipients must not have other comorbidities that potentially limit their life expectancy or increase their likelihood of developing adverse events posttransplant. Lifelong immunosuppression is required and these are accompanied with a spectrum of significant side effects. Nevertheless, the best centres can now achieve 1-, 5- and 10-year survivals of 90%, 80% and 70%, respectively, with dramatically improved quality of life and life expectancy for selected patients with refractory heart failure.

Mechanical Circulatory Support

The greatest limitation to heart transplantation is the severe shortage of suitable donor organs. Some patients with advanced heart failure deteriorate rapidly and die before a suitable donor heart becomes available. Artificial blood pumps can provide mechanical circulatory support to maintain adequate cardiac output and perfusion to the rest of the body, keeping the patient alive, until a suitable heart becomes available, a process called *bridging to transplantation*. These range from temporary blood pumps that can be inserted percutaneously to longer-term devices that are implanted surgically. Implantable left ventricular assist devices (LVADs) usually drain blood from the failing left ventricle and return it to the ascending aorta. The implanted LVAD is connected to an external controller and rechargeable batteries via a percutaneous driveline, providing flow of up to 10 L/min (Fig. 44.9). Medium-term survival rates on LVAD therapy have been improving and are currently 85% and 70% at 1- and 2-years, respectively. This has led to the use of implantable LVADs as a permanent therapy in selected patients with advanced heart failure, a process that is sometimes called 'destination therapy'. With continued improvements in LVAD technology, their usage can be expected to grow in the future.

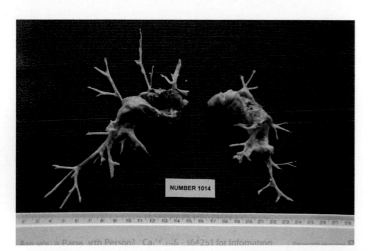

• **Fig. 44.8** A pulmonary endarterectomy specimen removed from a patient with chronic thromboembolic pulmonary hypertension. It consists of laminated thrombi in the main pulmonary arteries and a fibrous cast of the segmental and subsegmental pulmonary artery branches from organised thrombi.

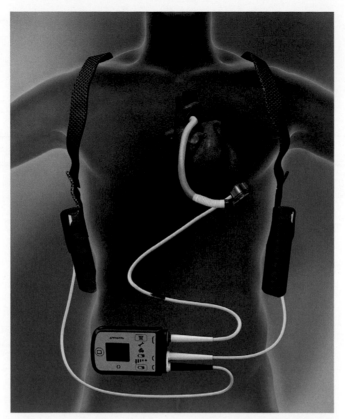

• **Fig. 44.9** The HeartMate 3 Implantable Left Ventricular Assist Device (LVAD). The inflow cannula drains blood from the left ventricular apex and the centrifugal pump returns blood to the ascending aorta via an outflow graft; the implanted LVAD is connected to a wearable external controller and rechargeable batteries via a percutaneous driveline. (Courtesy Abbott Laboratories, Illinois, United States.)

45

Disorders of the Breast

CHAPTER OUTLINE

Introduction to Breast Disease

Virtually every woman with a breast lump, breast pain or discharge from the nipple fears she has cancer. The anxiety results from the unknown course of the disease, the threat of mutilation and the fear of dying. This has often prevented women from seeking medical advice, but publicity about self-examination and screening (see Ch. 6) and the potential benefits of early treatment has encouraged earlier presentation.

Anxiety may be heightened by friends' or relatives' experiences of breast cancer or a recent 'celebrity diagnosis'; for this reason, reassuring the 'worried well' is important. The effects of breast surgery on attractiveness and femininity must be considered; breast care nurses can provide psychological support throughout investigation and treatment.

Rates of referral to breast clinics have increased, reflecting easier access, widespread breast screening and public awareness of breast cancer. Despite the fears of those referred, in the United Kingdom less than 15% prove to have cancer. The rest include benign breast conditions and others within the normal range of anatomy and physiology (Box 45.1).

Anatomy of the Female Breast

The breast consists of 15 to 20 lobes containing lobules linked by ductules that combine to form ducts. The glandular tissue is supported by fibrous tissue connected by Astley Cooper ligaments and lies over pectoralis major and minor. It is supplied by branches of the axillary and internal mammary arteries. Lymph drains primarily to the axillary nodes.

Symptoms and Signs of Breast Disease

Patients may present with symptoms or signs (Fig. 45.1). Two-thirds complain of a discrete lump or lumpiness.

Special Points in History Taking

A detailed history can provide important clues to the pathology of a breast problem. Age alters the probability of different breast disorders (Fig. 45.2); in particular, the risk of malignancy rises with age. The **duration of symptoms** should be established at the outset; cancers are usually slow-growing, whilst cysts can appear rapidly, sometimes almost overnight. Benign conditions, such as fibroadenosis and fibroadenoma may present with lumps that **fluctuate with the menstrual cycle** or have decreased in size since first noticed. They are also more likely to be **painful and tender** than a malignant lesion.

A **previous history** of breast conditions, particularly malignancy, cysts or fibrocystic change, can be an indicator of the nature of a current breast problem. Aside from high risk predisposing germline gene mutations, the greatest single risk factor for breast cancer is a previous history of the condition, however long ago (1% risk per year)—Box 45.2. There is some evidence that patients with recurrent benign breast disorders are at greater risk of cancer. If cancer is confirmed, it is important

• BOX 45.1 Types of Breast Disease of Surgical Importance

Malignant Neoplasms
- Ductal adenocarcinoma
- Lobular adenocarcinoma
- Sarcoma
- Metastasis from other tissues

Benign Tumour-like Lesions
- Fibroadenoma
- Intraduct papilloma
- Lipoma

Disordered Physiological Responses of Breast Tissue (Abnormalities of Normal Development and Involution, ANDI)
- Fibroadenosis (also known as *fibrocystic disease, benign mammary dysplasia* and *chronic mastitis*)

Mammary Duct Ectasia
- Chronic periductal inflammatory reaction caused by retained duct secretions

Infections
- Cellulitis and breast abscess
- Subareolar abscesses in mammary duct ectasia

to establish the patient's menopausal status as this influences future treatment decisions. If this is unclear, serum follicle-stimulating hormone and oestradiol levels should be measured.

Trauma from seatbelt injuries is common and patients should be asked whether bruising of the breast was followed by the appearance of a lump.

Drug history, particularly of the oral contraceptive pill (OCP) or hormone replacement therapy (HRT), should be recorded, including the type, duration and how recently the drug has been used. These drugs modulate the hormonal environment of breast tissue and tend to increase the risk of breast cancer. Other hormone-related risk factors for cancer include late age at first full-term pregnancy, lower parity (number of pregnancies), early age of menarche and late age of menopause. Enquiry should be made about a **family history** of breast or ovarian cancer, including number of first- and second-degree relatives, age of onset and bilaterality. Some families have mutations in the tumour suppressor genes *BRCA1, BRCA2, PALB2* and others, which can strongly predispose to breast and other cancers. Increasing alcohol consumption is fuelling a rise in the incidence of breast cancer.

Examination of the Breasts

There are several accepted methods for examining the breasts; one is shown in Fig. 45.3. All areas of the breast must be examined, with particular attention to the axillary tail and retroareolar regions. Breast examination involves six distinct manoeuvres:
- observation with the patient sitting up;
- observation with the patient raising and lowering her arms;
- examination of the nipples;
- systematic palpation of each breast;
- palpation of axilla and supraclavicular fossa;
- general examination for signs of distant metastases.
    During inspection, the signs to be looked for are listed in Fig. 45.1.

Palpation may be done **circumferentially** using the flat of one hand, starting at the nipple then moving in progressively larger circles; **radially** from the nipple outwards, like the spokes of a wheel; or by **sectors**, examining each quadrant in turn. Axillary lymph nodes are palpated, whilst the examiner's other hand supports the patient's arm (see Fig. 45.3G and H). This helps relax the muscles and aids assessment of the nodal groups (**medial, lateral, anterior, posterior and apical**). Note that clinical assessment of axillary nodes is unreliable, with a 30% false positive and a 30% false negative rate.

A history of **nipple discharge** can often be confirmed by pressure over the appropriate sector near the areola. Discharges not obviously blood-stained should be tested for blood using urinalysis dipsticks. In all cases, a smear preparation should be examined for cytological abnormalities.

Lumps

The differential diagnosis of a discrete breast mass is:
- cyst
- fibroadenoma
- focus of fibrocystic change or fibroadenosis
- fat necrosis (rare)
- carcinoma

During the examination, the patient needs to point out any lump she is worried about. The normal breast has a wide range of textures, from soft through nodular, to hard, so the texture of the rest of the breast must be taken into account. When a lump is found, its characteristics should be defined (Box 45.3), in particular whether it is discrete or dominant or whether it is an area of nodularity or 'thickening'. If there is a discrete mass, does it appear benign or suspicious for malignancy? (Characteristic signs of cancer are shown in Fig. 45.4). Note that even for breast specialists, clinical examination has a low sensitivity (i.e., ability to detect real abnormalities) of 65% to 80%. In one clinical evaluation system, increasing levels of suspicion are graded E1 to E5; an E3 designation may prompt a core biopsy even if radiological findings are not suspicious. Only 3% of breast cancers occur under the age of 30 years but a discrete lump in a patient over 65 years is a cancer until proved otherwise.

Skin tethering (as opposed to direct infiltration) can be a subtle sign and is accentuated by raising the arms to put the breast suspensory ligaments under tension. Deep fixation can be assessed by checking the mobility of the lump over pectoralis major with the muscle relaxed and then tensed.

Paget Disease of the Nipple

Some patients with breast carcinoma present with eczema-like reddening and thickening of the skin of the nipple and areola, together with fissuring and ulceration. This is more common in the elderly and is known as *Paget disease of the nipple* (see Fig. 45.10).

Investigation of Breast Disorders

'One-stop' clinics allow rapid and comprehensive preliminary assessment. **Triple assessment** includes clinical examination, breast imaging and biopsy (when indicated) on the same day. This has an overall accuracy of 99.6%, when performed by experienced personnel, meaning the chances of missing a cancer are less than 1%; patients shown not to have cancer can usually be discharged. If there is a clinically suspicious lump and needle biopsy is negative or equivocal, diagnostic **excision biopsy** should be performed. The discrete lump is completely excised and examined histologically.

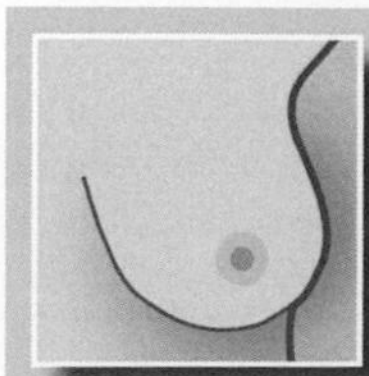

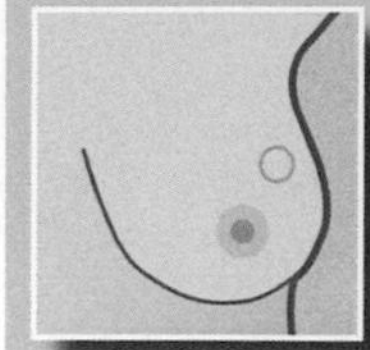

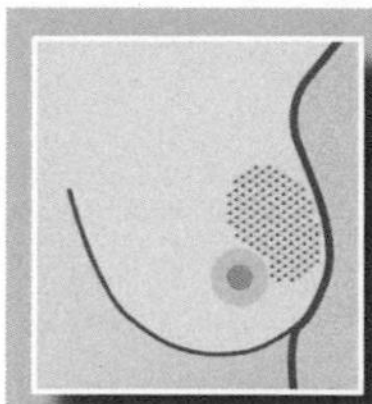

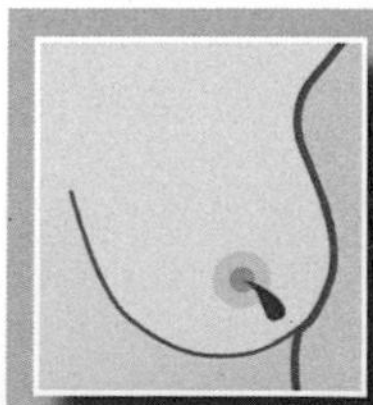

SYMPTOM OR SIGN	CLINICAL SIGNIFICANCE
1. Pain	
Varying with menstrual cycle	Suggests a physiological cause such as premenstrual syndrome or fibroadenosis. Both are responsive to treatment
Independent of menstrual cycle	Not diagnostic but may occur in carcinoma, fibroadenosis or infection
2. Lump in the breast	
Hard lump **Refer urgently if ≥ 30 yrs**	A discrete mobile lump with a smooth surface is most likely to be a fibroadenoma or a fibroadenotic cyst. An ill-defined margin and any suggestion of tethering to superficial or deep structures strongly suggest carcinoma but are sometimes caused by noninfective inflammation or fat necrosis
Firm, poorly defined lump or lumpiness **Refer urgently if:** **≥30 yrs with lump ± pain** **≥30 yrs with lump ± axillary node** **Refer non-urgently if:** **<30 yrs with lump ± pain**	Suggests fibroadenosis, especially if outline is difficult to distinguish from normal breast tissue or if the breast is generally lumpy. Risk of malignancy small but see referral guidelines opposite
Soft lump	Usually a lipoma or occasionally a lax cyst
3. Skin changes in the breast **Refer urgently if changes suggest cancer**	
Skin dimpling or tethering	Sometimes a subtle sign but highly suggestive of carcinoma
Visible lump	Cyst, carcinoma or phylloides tumour. Cysts can appear with alarming speed
Peau d'orange (appearance of orange peel)	Over a lump, this is virtually pathognomonic of carcinoma. It is caused by tumour invasion of dermal lymphatics causing dermal oedema. However, it may occur over an infective lesion
Redness	Usually infection, especially if skin is hot. Sometimes a feature of mammary duct ectasia. Beware inflammatory carcinoma
Ulceration	Neglected carcinoma in the elderly (often slow-growing)
4. Nipple disorders	
Recent inversion or change in shape **Refer urgently ≥50 yrs and only one nipple affected**	Suggests a fibrosing underlying lesion such as a carcinoma or mammary duct ectasia but can be malignancy
'Eczema' (rash involving nipple or areola, or both) **Refer urgently ≥50 yrs and only one nipple affected**	If unilateral and persistent, this is the classic sign of Paget disease of the nipple, a presentation of breast cancer
Nipple discharge	
Milky	Pregnancy or hyperprolactinaemia
Clear	Physiological
Green	Perimenopausal, duct ectasia, fibroadenotic cyst
Blood-stained	Possible carcinoma or intraduct papilloma
Refer if ≥50 yrs and symptoms affecting one nipple	May be a sign of benign disease

• **Fig. 45.1** Symptoms and Signs of Breast Disease (see also Figs 45.3 and 45.4.) UK National Institute for Care and Health Excellence guidelines for urgent and nonurgent referral to a specialist are indicated on a pink background.

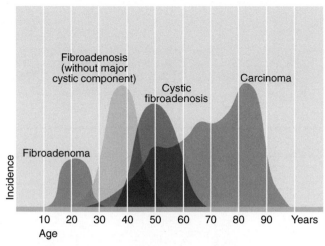

• **Fig. 45.2** Age Incidence of Common Breast Disorders.

• BOX 45.2   Risk Factors for Breast Cancer

- Increasing age
- Family history (number of first- and second-degree relatives, their age of onset and bilaterality, known *BRCA1/BRCA2* mutations)
- Previous history of breast cancer or carcinoma-in-situ
- Early age of menarche (age <12 years)
- Late age of menopause (age >55 years)
- Late age at first full-term pregnancy (age <20 years protective)
- Nulliparity
- Previous breast biopsies showing nonmalignant abnormalities
- Hormonal therapy—oral contraceptive pill or hormone replacement therapy
- Radiation at a young age (mantle irradiation for lymphomas, atomic bomb survivors)
- See also http://www.cancerresearchuk.org/about-cancer/breast-cancer/risks-causes/risk-factors

---

Imaging

Mammography (breast radiography) is an important method of radiological assessment of the breasts. In women over 40 years, it has a sensitivity of 88% for carcinoma. It is less sensitive in younger women because the breast tissue is denser, and is rarely performed below 35 years.

During mammography, the breast is compressed firmly in the machine. This spreads the tissue to an even thickness to give correct exposure for all the breast tissue to make it easier to detect any mass lesion. Radiological views are taken in two directions, mediolateral oblique and craniocaudal. Localised compression views can reduce the problem of superimposed structures simulating a mass. Focused magnified views can better display any abnormal area. Full digital mammography, which permits post-processing enhancement of the image, has nearly replaced film mammography.

Features looked for on a mammogram include:

- the presence of a mass lesion
- microcalcification
- architectural distortion
- asymmetry
- skin thickening
- lymph nodes

A typical carcinoma appears as a **spiculated** mass lesion (dense centre with radiating lines), which may have malignant-type fine linear or granular microcalcification (Fig. 45.5). Fine granular microcalcification within a spiculate lesion is virtually pathognomonic of cancer. Tumours as small as 2 to 3 mm are sometimes detectable radiologically, long before they become palpable.

Benign-type microcalcification is coarse and 'chunky' (Fig. 45.6). Fine branching microcalcification is characteristic of **ductal carcinoma-in-situ (DCIS)**. Architectural distortion and asymmetry are subtle radiological signs, but should be viewed with suspicion.

Ultrasound has long been used to distinguish solid lesions from cysts and has a specificity of 100% for this. Modern B-mode ultrasound demonstrates breast anatomy in great detail and is complementary to mammography. Benign lesions can be distinguished from malignancy with a sensitivity for cancer of at least 85%. Ultrasound can accurately measure the size of a cancer (Fig. 45.7) and can guide percutaneous needle biopsies and cyst aspiration (Fig. 45.8).

The strength of breast imaging comes from performing mammography and ultrasound together, as the physical characteristics tested by the two techniques are different. The information acquired by mammography results from attenuation of the x-ray beam through breast structures, whilst ultrasound tests the reflectivity of a pulsed ultrasound beam (of about 12 mHz), caused by subtle attenuation changes at tissue interfaces within the breast.

Biopsy

Most palpable and all nonpalpable image-detected masses are biopsied under image guidance, as are suspicious areas of calcification. **Fine-needle aspiration cytology (FNAC)** specimens are rarely used for tissue diagnosis now (Box 45.4). FNAC has a sensitivity of 95% for detecting malignancy, but cannot distinguish between in situ and invasive cancers. By contrast, **core biopsy** has a sensitivity of 98%. The tissue architecture is preserved so that invasion can be confidently diagnosed on histology and tumours can be pathologically graded. After core biopsy, patients need to return later for the results as the pathology has to be read after the specimen has been fixed. This has the advantage that any bad news can be broken in a phased manner. If needle biopsy is negative or equivocal, a discrete lump should be completely excised with a wide margin of apparently normal breast tissue and the specimen examined histologically. This procedure, **excision biopsy,** can also form the first step in controlling local disease.

Eczematous lesions suspicious for Paget disease of the nipple can be 'punch' biopsied under local anaesthesia in the clinic.

Breast Cancer

Introduction

In Western societies, breast cancer is the leading cause of death in European women. About 1 in 8 to 10 women will develop breast cancer (i.e., a lifetime risk of ~10%–12%) and ~1 in 18 will die from it. In the United Kingdom, more than 50,000 new cases are diagnosed annually and ~12,000 women die each year. Worldwide, there are about half a million deaths from breast cancer each year, but despite this increasing global incidence, mortality rates have gradually fallen with earlier diagnosis and improved treatments, including advances in hormonal and targeted therapy. Around 27% of cases in the United Kingdom are preventable.

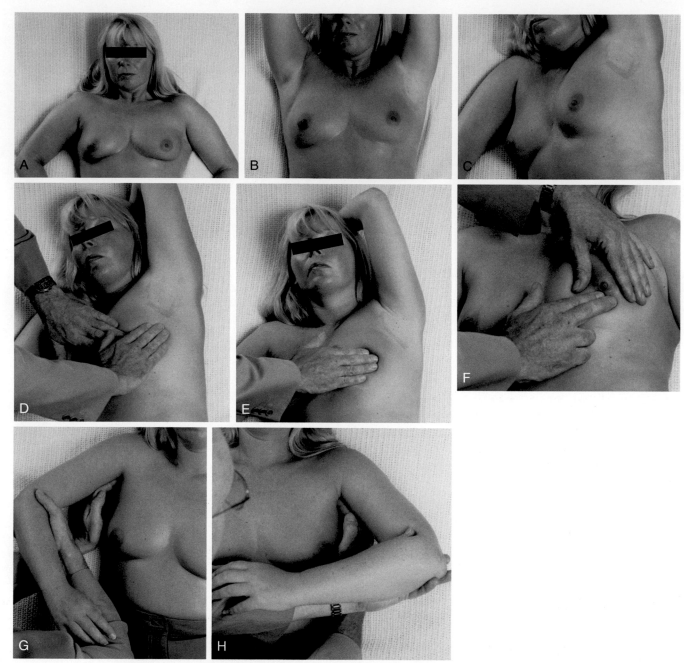

• **Fig. 45.3** Technique of Breast Examination. Inspection: the breasts should be inspected for asymmetry, skin tethering and dimpling and changes in colour. This should be performed with the patient sitting comfortably, pressing hands on hips **(A)**, lifting arms in the air **(B)**, and pressing hands on top of the head. Palpation: the patient should sit on an examination couch as shown in **(C)**, with the backrest at about 45 degrees and rolled slightly to the contralateral side. The arm on the side to be examined should be elevated and the head rested on the pillow. The effect of these manoeuvres is to spread the breast over a greater area of the chest wall. The flat of the right hand is used to palpate the breast circumferentially by quadrants **(D–F)**. The central part of the breast and the axillary tail must also be palpated. If there is a history of nipple discharge, the areola is pressed in different areas **(F)** to identify the duct from which it emanates and therefore the segment involved. Finally, the axillary lymph nodes are palpated as shown in **(G)** and **(H)**. The right axilla is palpated with the left hand **(G)** and the left axilla is palpated with the right hand **(H)**. It is important to relax the axillary muscles by supporting the weight of the patient's arm as shown. The fingers of the examining hand are firmly held in a curve, pressed high into the apex of the axilla against the chest wall and drawn downwards. The hand will then 'ride over' any enlarged axillary nodes.

Risk Factors

Age

Age is a major risk factor. Incidence rates rise from about 25 years, more steeply between 40 and 55 years, with a slight levelling off until about 70 years. After that, another fairly steep rise continues into old age (see Fig. 45.2). Breast cancer is the commonest cause of death in women aged between 40 and 50 years.

• BOX 45.3 **Clinical Characteristics of a Breast Lump**

- Solitary or multiple
- Size—in centimetres
- Location—quadrant of breast or clock face
- Contour—smooth and round/ovoid (likely to be benign) or firm/hard (probable malignancy)
- Mobility—mobile (likely to be benign) or fixed (probable malignancy)
- Associated changes—skin/nipple retraction, skin tethering, bloody nipple discharge, erythema
- Axillary lymphadenopathy—enlarged and mobile or enlarged and fixed

---

Genetic Factors

The aetiology of breast cancer is multifactorial, with genetic factors being relatively more important in premenopausal women and environmental factors more so after the menopause. These play a small role in calculating the risk of breast cancer, but the risk is greater in women with a strong family history (two first-degree relatives, bilateral breast cancer or diagnosis before the age of 50 years). Such a family history accounts for 10% of cancers, with half caused by genetic mutations, mainly *BRCA1* (17q21) and *BRCA2* (13q41) genes, which are transmitted in an autosomal dominant fashion. A mutation in either of these leads to an 80% to 90% lifetime risk of developing the disease. The same mutations are also strongly linked to ovarian and other cancers. Women with a *BRCA* mutation should be counselled about their individual risk of breast and ovarian cancer and the treatment options (ranging from surveillance to risk-reducing bilateral mastectomies, which reduce the cancer risk by more than 90%, and oophorectomy).

Hormonal Factors

Growth of most breast cancers is promoted by oestrogens, hence reproductive physiology and behaviour influence cancer risk. It

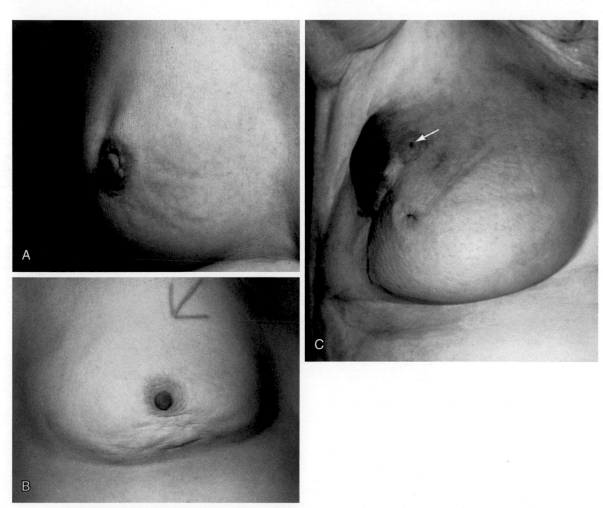

• **Fig. 45.4** Carcinoma of the Breast. **(A)** and **(B)** Characteristic skin dimpling over breast carcinomas. This may be a subtle sign and only be visible in tangential light. **(C)** Nipple retraction and widespread 'peau d'orange' resulting from a large central breast carcinoma. Peau d'orange is caused by a combination of cutaneous infiltration by tumour and skin oedema (and occasionally by infection). Locally advanced breast cancer may cause distortion of the breast. The colour change and ulceration are uncommonly seen and only occur in neglected cases. Note also the puncture wound of a core biopsy *(arrowed)*. There was no obvious axillary node enlargement.

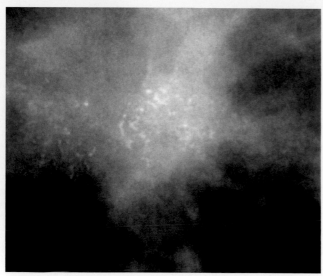

• **Fig. 45.5** Carcinoma of the Breast on Mammography. This 58-year-old woman presented with a 2-week history of a nontender lump in the left breast. Clinical examination confirmed a hard irregular mass without skin dimpling, and a palpable left axillary node. Enlarged view of the carcinoma showing typical malignant-type microcalcification. This contrasts with the coarser calcification occurring in benign breast conditions (see Fig. 45.6C).

has long been known that nulliparous women are at greater risk: Ramazzini commented in 1703 that breast cancer was common in Catholic nuns, who as 'Vestalis Virgines' were prone to 'horrendis mammarium canceris'.

The interval between menarche and menopause is the **oestrogen window** and is an estimate of cumulative exposure to endogenous oestrogen; the longer the interval, the higher the cancer risk. Women who begin menses before the age of 12 years, or start the menopause after 55 years are at an increased risk. A natural or a 'medical' menopause under 40 years reduces cancer risk by two-thirds. Nulliparity and a late age at first pregnancy increase risk and a first full-term pregnancy under 20 years halves the risk compared with one between 30 and 35 years or nulliparity, although the risk is still small.

Prolonged use of the **OCP** increases the risk of breast cancer by 20% and combined HRT for more than 10 years also increases the risk, although this falls when HRT is stopped.

Social and Geographic Factors

Breast cancer is more common in the Western world and in women in higher socioeconomic classes. Obese women are at a higher risk, possibly caused by conversion of androgens to oestrogen in adipose tissue. Consuming more than three units of alcohol a day increases the risk by 50%.

Epidemiology

Breast cancer is not a new disease; it was recognised by the ancient Egyptians and mastectomy was certainly performed in Roman times. Nowadays, breast cancer is predominantly a disease of Western society, but most differences in incidence are more likely environmental than genetic. The disease is uncommon in Japan, but Japanese immigrants to the United States of America acquire local incidence rates within two generations.

Breast cancer rates are rising fastest in Asiatic countries that have adopted Western lifestyles. The rise is most likely caused by

changes in reproductive practice, including deferring childbirth until past 30 years of age, smaller families, and prolonged use of the OCP.

Environmental Factors

Exposure to irradiation in the teenage years may initiate some breast cancers, which are then promoted by other factors years later. Female survivors of the atomic bombs of Hiroshima and Nagasaki have a high risk of developing breast cancer, as do those who have received mantle irradiation for Hodgkin disease. Surprisingly, no link has been shown between smoking and breast cancer.

Pathology

Tumour Types

Almost all breast cancers are adenocarcinomas and arise from the terminal duct/lobular unit. Over 85% originate from the ductal component and are designated invasive **ductal carcinomas** of 'no special type' (Fig. 45.9). About 8% arise from the lobules and are known as **lobular carcinomas**. These are similar in behaviour and prognosis to ductal carcinomas, but can be difficult to see on mammography and often present late. Microscopically, these tumours are characterised by linear arrangements of cells, so-called 'Indian filing' (see Fig. 45.9B). A few invasive carcinomas have ductal and lobular features and are termed *mixed tumours*.

The remaining 12% to 15% of cancers are known as **special types** (tubular, mucinous, medullary and micropapillary carcinomas). Special types are well differentiated and generally have a better prognosis. At diagnosis, oestrogen receptor (ER) and progesterone receptor (PR) status is determined by immunohistochemistry, and human epidermal growth factor receptor (HER)2 amplification status is determined by immunohistochemistry and/or in situ hybridisation. Increasingly, genetic/genomic assays are being used to further subclassify breast cancers, to guide prognosis and optimise treatment.

In-Situ Carcinoma

Breast cancers can develop from an in situ or noninvasive precursor known as **ductal carcinoma-in-situ** or **DCIS**. These are primarily detected through breast screening programmes as suspicious microcalcifications. Post-mortem studies suggest there is only a 20% chance of DCIS progressing to invasive cancer. DCIS ranges from low to high grade, and higher-grade lesions are more likely to progress if untreated.

Paget Disease of the Nipple

In Paget disease, the epidermis becomes infiltrated by neoplastic cells arising from an underlying ductal carcinoma. These reach the surface by intra-epithelial spread along mammary ducts (Fig. 45.10).

Inflammatory Carcinoma

Inflammatory carcinoma may be difficult to distinguish from infective conditions of the breast. It often develops without a palpable mass, and can be misdiagnosed as cellulitis. It should be suspected in older women with inflammation that does not respond to antibiotics. Mammography and ultrasound are helpful in establishing the diagnosis although appearances can be similar as a breast abscess often contains necrotic debris simulating a solid mass on imaging. Chronic mastitis during pregnancy may mask an underlying inflammatory carcinoma and delay diagnosis.

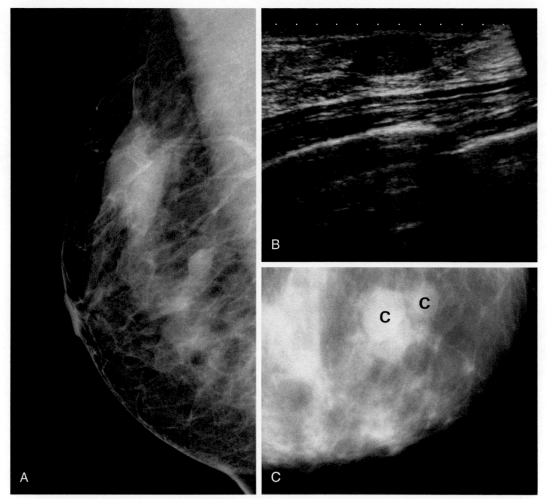

• **Fig. 45.6** Fibroadenoma of the Breast. This 35-year-old patient presented with a 3-month history of a lump in the upper aspect of the left breast, which was slightly tender at the time of menstruation. Clinical examination revealed a smooth round mobile mass, which was firm and very mobile. **(A)** This mammogram shows simple lobulated mass lesion in the upper part of the breast with a well-defined border. These appearances are suggestive of a benign lesion (in this case a fibroadenoma). **(B)** This image shows the ultrasound appearances of the lesion in **(A)**; it is a well-defined solid lesion with regular internal echoes and no posterior enhancement (compare with Fig. 45.8B). The lesion is 'broad' rather than 'tall' and is typical of a fibroadenoma. **(C)** An enlarged mammographic view of a different fibroadenoma in an older woman showing the much coarser calcification *(C)* associated with benign breast lesions compared with carcinoma.

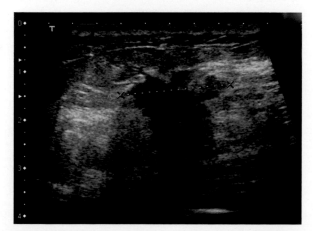

• **Fig. 45.7** Carcinoma of the Breast on Ultrasound. Ultrasound scan of the patient shown in Fig. 45.5. This shows a hypoechoic mass lesion extending the width of the *blue dotted line*. It has an irregular border and some internal echoes. The lesion is characteristically 'tall', that is, deep, and there is acoustic shadowing deep to the lesion. This image should be contrasted with the appearances of a benign fibroadenoma (see Fig. 45.6B).

Tumour Grade

Breast carcinomas are graded histologically I–III according to degree of differentiation. Higher grade tumours tend to infiltrate blood and lymphatic vessels which increases the chance of lymph node and haematogenous metastases, and thus have a worse prognosis. Unfortunately, grade III tumours are more common in premenopausal women. Also, the larger the tumour, the worse the grade tends to be.

Natural History of Breast Cancer

Estimates of tumour doubling times suggest that many cancers have been present for 4–6 years before diagnosis. Individual breast cancers vary greatly in their behaviour. Some women present with advanced metastatic disease, others refuse treatment and live for many years, and yet others relapse 20 years or more after apparently successful treatment. Breast cancer tends to be more aggressive in young women and many have an early relapse after treatment. Once a metastatic relapse has been diagnosed, the median survival is 2–3 years, although this is improving owing to advances in systemic treatments.

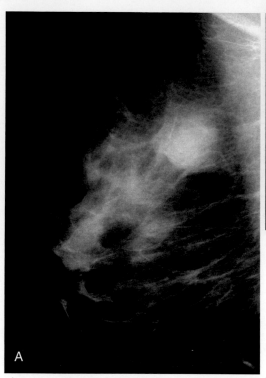
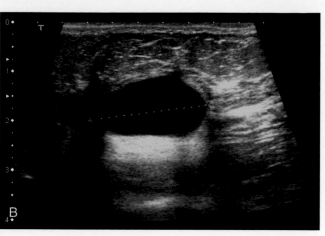

• **Fig. 45.8** Breast Cyst. This 42-year-old woman presented with a tender lump in the superior aspect of the right breast. There was a previous history of breast cysts. Examination revealed a smooth, round and slightly fluctuant mass. **(A)** Mediolateral oblique view mammogram showing a well-defined lesion with circumscribed margins in the upper part of the breast. The appearances are of a benign lesion. **(B)** Complementary ultrasound examination reveals an anechoic mass with sharp, well-defined margins and posterior acoustic enhancement. This is diagnostic of a simple cyst.

• **BOX 45.4** **Reporting Categories for Fine-Needle Aspiration Cytology**

C1—inadequate specimen
C2—benign
C3—suspicious but probably benign
C4—suspicious and probably malignant
C5—malignant

There are two main theories about the biological dissemination of breast cancer. **Halsted** proposed in the 1880s that cancer spreads sequentially from a focus in the breast to regional lymph nodes and then into the bloodstream to produce haematogenous metastases. Thus, distant spread occurs only after lymph nodes have been invaded and their filtration capacity overwhelmed. On this basis, locoregional control by radical mastectomy and/or radiotherapy would cure most patients. By contrast, **Bernard Fisher's** research between 1957 and 1970 challenged Halsted's concept (which mandated radical surgery) with evidence that breast cancer might already be systemic long before the primary is detectable. Furthermore, disseminated cancer cells could potentially metastasise throughout life and it is these that ultimately determine the patient's fate (Fig. 45.11).

In practice, both theories appear to apply in different situations, and breast cancers may show either biological behaviour. Poorly differentiated cancers in younger women are more likely to have distant micrometastases at the time of diagnosis and carry a higher chance of recurrence and death; hence screening to detect the primary would be less beneficial. Conversely, cancers in older patients often have lower metastatic potential even when locally

advanced and screening may detect them before systemic spread when they remain potentially curable.

Principles of Management of Breast Cancer (Boxes 45.5 and 45.6)

The overall prognosis for breast cancer patients has not changed substantially over the past few decades, but the duration of disease-free survival and, to a lesser extent, the survival rates for advanced disease have improved. Over the past 20 years, 10-year survival has increased from 55% to >75% and 20-year survival from 44% to >64%. Some of this improvement is caused by earlier detection causing **lead-time bias**, but most of it is caused by improved adjuvant therapy which acts on metastases as well as the primary, and better treatments for advanced disease. Ideally, investigation and treatment should be performed in specialist units that see >150 cases of early breast cancer per year.

Whilst the aim of treatment is generally cure, in practice, prolonging the disease-free survival or optimal management of metastatic disease may be a more realistic goal. Treatments have been evaluated in randomised trials and national and international guidelines for treatment have been formulated from these (see, for example, the ESMO and NCCN guidelines). For patients with advanced disease, palliation is the main objective, with particular emphasis on optimising quality of life, alongside its prolongation.

Staging

Once a diagnosis of cancer has been made, the disease should be staged to define the extent of spread. Staging begins with triple assessment of the breast and axilla (see earlier, p. 566). If there is no evidence of axillary nodal or distant involvement and the

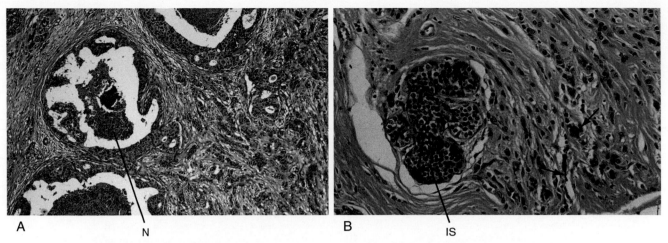

A N   B IS

• **Fig. 45.9** Breast Adenocarcinoma—Histopathology. **(A)** Ducts to the left of the picture contain highly atypical epithelium, with central necrosis *(N)*, a type of in situ ductal carcinoma also known as *comedocarcinoma*. On the right of this micrograph is invasive ductal carcinoma composed of many small glandular structures, diffusely invading breast tissue. **(B)** In situ *(IS)* and invasive lobular carcinoma. Malignant cells tend to be less atypical than in ductal carcinoma and do not form glands, but often invade in 'single-file' *(arrowed)*. Intracellular mucin is also characteristic of this variant of breast carcinoma

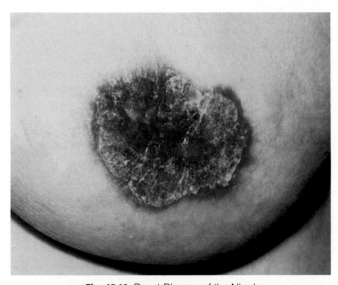

• **Fig. 45.10** Paget Disease of the Nipple.

cancer is amenable to surgery, no further investigations are performed. Clinical signs that may preclude initial surgery are peau d'orange and inflammatory cancer, fixation to the chest wall and distant metastatic disease. These may be indications for **neoadjuvant** chemotherapy, that is, in advance of surgery.

If there is evidence of axillary disease, a tumour ≥5cm, aggressive histopathological factors, or suspicious blood test results (such as deranged liver function or elevated ALP), the heightened risk of metastatic spread mandates a CT chest and abdomen and a bone scan to investigate this. FDP PET/CT scanning is used in some cases to clarify staging.

Prognostic Status

The TNM system (Fig. 45.12 and Table 45.1) classifies cancer according to the size of the primary **T**umour, the pathological **N**odal status and the presence or absence of distant **M**etastases. TNM grading is used to stage breast patients into four categories (see Table 45.1) and this correlates well with observed rates of

relative survival at 5 years: ~99% for stage I, ~88% for stage II, ~55% for stage III and 15% for stage IV tumours. In addition to this traditional staging system, the Nottingham Prognostic Index (see Table 45.3), Adjuvant! Online (http://www.adjuvantonline.com), and the PREDICT score, are widely used to prognosticate and guide treatment decisions.

Other factors used to assess prognosis are hormone receptor (ER and PR) status, HER2 status, histological type, and Ki67 score (an indirect measure of proliferation rates within the tumour). Genomic analysis has identified different subtypes of breast cancer with distinct behaviours (e.g., luminal A/B, HER2-positive nonluminal, and basal-like). Clinicopathological surrogates to identify which genomic subset to which an individual cancer is likely to belong (based on integration of the aforementioned information) is increasingly important for guiding prognosis and treatment. A large study of a 21 tumour gene expression assay (Oncotype DX) in ER-positive 'early' breast cancers (about 50% of those diagnosed) showed that 70% could avoid chemotherapy when its use is guided by the 21 gene recurrence score to identify those at low risk for metastatic disease. The expense of such testing make access to it inequitable across the globe.

Note that as a result of screening, the proportion of small tumours detected has increased, but it is uncertain whether this brings an overall survival advantage.

Locoregional Treatment

The purpose of locoregional treatment is to control disease in the breast, chest wall and axillary lymph nodes. For patients with small tumours of favourable grade and some screen-detected lesions, locoregional treatment alone is potentially curative. These treatments involve surgery or radiotherapy or a combination of the two. Complete removal of the breast (**mastectomy**) was the standard operation for invasive breast cancer, but over the past 30 years, **breast conservation surgery** has become more prevalent. Each patient with breast cancer is best discussed at a multidisciplinary team meeting involving surgeon, radiologist, histopathologist and others, and recommendations regarding surgery and further treatment are made (including any role for systemic neoadjuvant treatments to allow breast conservation surgery to proceed).

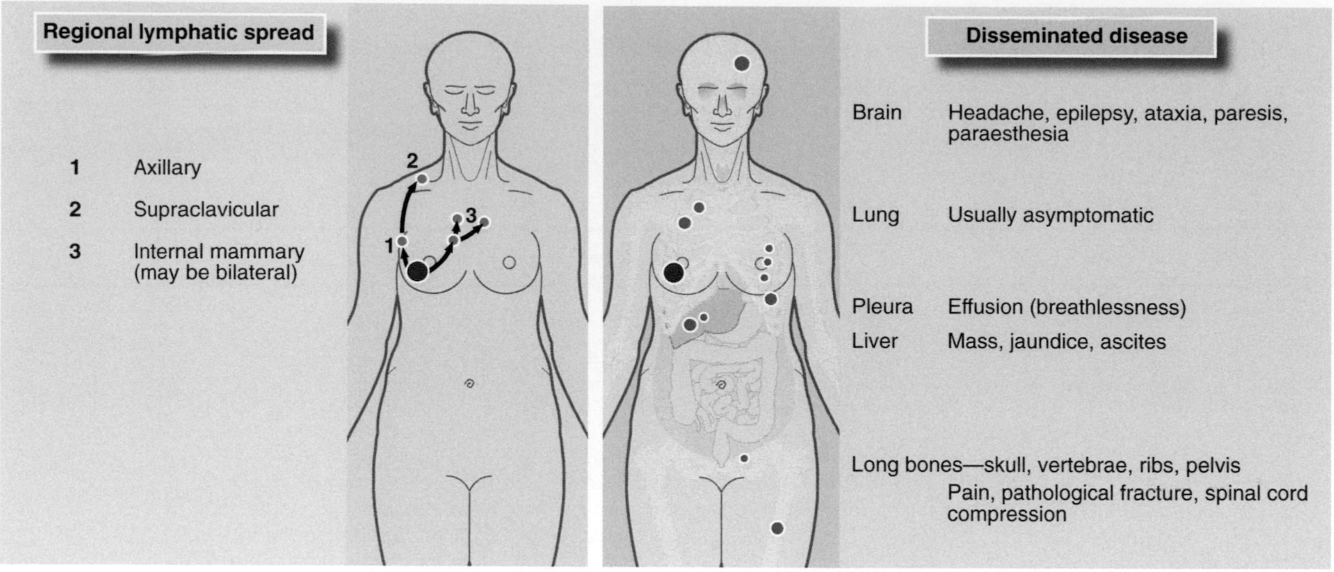

Regional lymphatic spread		Disseminated disease	
1	Axillary	Brain	Headache, epilepsy, ataxia, paresis, paraesthesia
2	Supraclavicular	Lung	Usually asymptomatic
3	Internal mammary (may be bilateral)	Pleura	Effusion (breathlessness)
		Liver	Mass, jaundice, ascites
		Long bones—skull, vertebrae, ribs, pelvis	Pain, pathological fracture, spinal cord compression

• **Fig. 45.11** Common Sites of Spread of Breast Carcinoma.

• **BOX 45.5** **Principles of Management of Breast Cancer**

- Establish the diagnosis
- Control disease in the affected breast and chest wall
- Prevent and treat local and regional disease in early breast cancer
- Control advanced and disseminated disease

• **BOX 45.6** **Primary Treatment for Breast Cancer**

Note that surgery and radiotherapy constitute locoregional treatment.

Surgery
- Mastectomy (radical, modified radical, simple)
- Breast conservation (lumpectomy, wide local excision, quadrantectomy)

Radiotherapy
- Breast radiotherapy (postbreast conservation surgery)
- Chest wall (postmastectomy)

Systemic Therapy
- Hormonal therapy
- Chemotherapy
- Biological therapy

Breast Conservation Surgery

Most newly diagnosed breast cancers in Europe can be treated with breast conservation surgery. This involves removing the tumour with a margin of surrounding breast tissue, followed by radiotherapy to the breast to minimise local recurrence; several long-term clinical trials have shown that overall survival is comparable with mastectomy. Despite this, some patients still opt for mastectomy, even if suitable for conservation surgery, and patient choice is an important part of the decision-making process. In parts of the world where radiotherapy is unavailable or is feared, mastectomy remains the treatment of choice.

Selection criteria for conservative surgery are shown in Box 45.7. **Wide local excision** aims to remove the tumour with a 1-cm macroscopic margin of normal breast tissue. Skin is not usually excised unless there is tethering. It is possible to remove up to 20% of the breast volume and still achieve a reasonable cosmetic result. For impalpable tumours, excision can be directed by ultrasound-guided skin marking over the cancer or insertion of a hooked wire, under mammography. A **quadrantectomy** is sometimes performed, which removes the tumour within a quadrant-shaped resection. However, this yields a poor cosmetic result.

Patients undergoing breast conservation surgery generally report better body image and sexual functioning than those undergoing mastectomy, but levels of anxiety and depression are similar.

Mastectomy

Mastectomy techniques have changed since the operation was first introduced. The **radical mastectomy** was devised by William Halsted in the 1880s in the United States of America. This operation involved removal of the breast, axillary lymph nodes and pectoralis major and minor muscles.

Patey later devised a less mutilating operation, in which the pectoralis major was preserved, but pectoralis minor was removed to facilitate lymph node clearance (**modified radical mastectomy**). Modern practice now preserves both pectoralis muscles and this **simple mastectomy** is now standard for invasive breast cancer. The cosmetic effects of mastectomy are of great psychological importance to patients and their families. Careful attention to this can alleviate distress and improve acceptance of disfigurement. Preoperative counselling by breast care nurses prepares the patient for treatment and after mastectomy, patients who do not undergo reconstruction, can be fitted with a life-like breast prosthesis incorporated into the cup of a bra. Risk reducing mastectomy can be offered to very high-risk women (e.g., *BRCA1/2* mutation carriers, where risk of cancer and related mortality can be reduced by 90% to 95%). Increasingly, women with breast cancer are opting for bilateral mastectomy, even when breast conservation is possible, to reduce the risk of developing a second primary cancer.

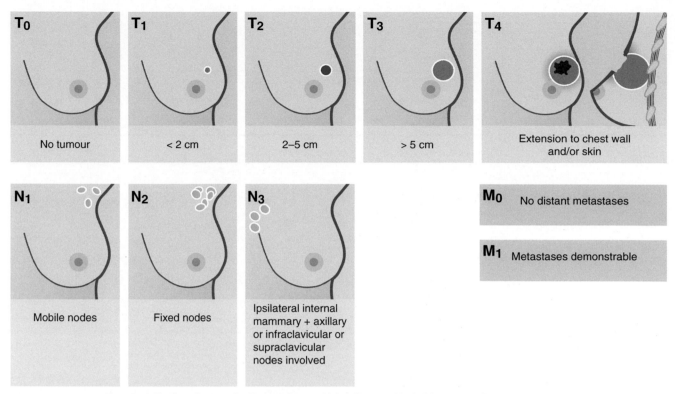

• **Fig. 45.12** Staging System for Breast Cancer Using Tumour Node Metastasis (TNM) Classification (2017).

TABLE 45.1	American Joint Committee on Cancer (AJCC) Staging System Based on TNM Status (8th Edition 2017)		
T Status	**N Status**	**M Status**	**AJCC Stage**
Tis (in situ)	N_0	M_0	Stage 0
T_1	N_0	M_0	Stage IA
T_0	$N_{1(mi)}$	M_0	Stage 1B
T_1	$N_{1(mi)}$	M_0	Stage 1B
T_0	N_1	M_0	Stage IIA
T_1	N_1	M_0	Stage IIA
T_2	N_0	M_0	Stage IIA
T_2	N_1	M_0	Stage IIB
T_3	N_0	M_0	Stage IIB
T_1	N_2	M_0	Stage IIIA
T_2	N_2	M_0	Stage IIIA
T_3	N_1	M_0	Stage IIIA
T_3	N_2	M_0	Stage IIIA
T_4	N_0	M_0	Stage IIIB
T_4	N_1	M_0	Stage IIIB
T_4	N_2	M_0	Stage IIIB
any T	N_3	M_0	Stage IIIC
any T	any N	M_1	Stage IV

TNM, Tumour Node Metastasis.

• **BOX 45.7** Selection Criteria for Breast Conservation Surgery

- Single lesion clinically and mammographically
- Tumour not larger than 3 cm (4 cm in larger breast)
- No extensive in situ component
- Tumours more than 2 cm away from nipple/areola
- Lesion of lower histological grade
- No extensive nodal involvement
- Adequate response to neoadjuvant systemic treatment based on aforementioned parameters

Reconstructive Surgery

Patients having a mastectomy can now be offered breast reconstruction, either immediate or delayed. The aim is to restore the natural breast shape, reestablish symmetry and create a nipple-areolar complex. With **immediate reconstruction**, a **skin-sparing mastectomy** is first performed, removing all of the breast tissue via a periareolar incision. The simplest reconstruction option is with an implant or tissue expander, placed deep to the pectoralis muscle. Expanders are gradually inflated and later exchanged for a permanent implant. This is a relatively quick operation compared with tissue transfer techniques, with no donor site morbidity, but it is difficult to recreate larger, ptotic breasts with implants.

The second option to recreate the breast is to use a myocutaneous flap, using skin, fat and muscle (if necessary). Tissue can be taken from the abdominal wall ('TRAM'—transverse rectus abdominis myocutaneous flap, or 'DIEP'—deep inferior epigastric perforator flap), or from the back ('LD'—latissimus dorsi flap) or from the buttock and inner thigh (Fig. 45.13). All of these can be augmented by implants. Tissue transfer produces a more natural-feeling and moving breast, but the operation takes a lot longer and there is substantial donor site morbidity. Most patients

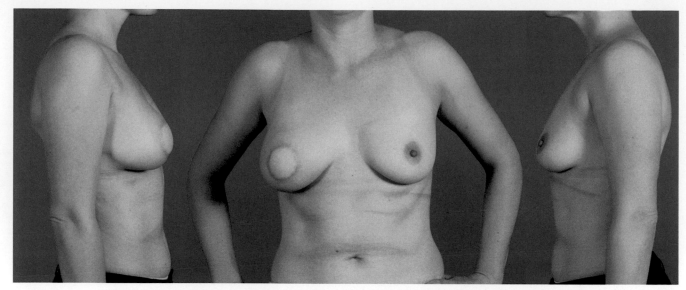

• **Fig. 45.13** Breast Reconstruction Following Skin-Sparing Mastectomy Using Latissimus Dorsi Flap and Silicone Implant. Via a circumareolar incision, the entire breast tissue, including the nipple–areolar complex is excised and the axillary node dissection performed. The latissimus dorsi muscle is mobilised as a pedicle flap, together with an ellipse of overlying skin, and tunnelled anteriorly to lie in the breast cavity. Excess skin is trimmed from the flap to leave a circular disc to replace the excised nipple. A silicone implant is sandwiched between the latissimus dorsi and pectoralis muscles to provide bulk and reshape the breast.

need additional procedures to augment or reduce the contralateral breast for symmetry and to create a new nipple. Immediate reconstruction aims to improve psychological well-being, but the effects of postoperative radiotherapy on the implant and reconstruction must be considered. Sometimes reconstruction is delayed because of the need for adjuvant chemoradiotherapy, where wound healing problems could delay the treatment.

Axillary Surgery

Axillary nodal status is the most important prognostic factor in breast cancer. Only 25% of patients present with involved lymph nodes and performing a clearance on every patient causes unnecessary morbidity and is no longer necessary unless nodes are involved. Axillary ultrasound at the time of initial assessment is now standard practice. If suspicious nodes are located, a core biopsy or aspiration cytology specimen is taken. If this is positive for metastasis, the patient can then be offered a primary axillary clearance, so only one axillary procedure is necessary. If the biopsy is negative, the patient is offered a sentinel node biopsy.

Sentinel Node Biopsy

Lymphatic spread nearly always follows a predictable pattern, with a sentinel node the first to be affected, so the standard diagnostic procedure is now **sentinel lymph node biopsy** (Fig. 45.14). This node is identified using both a radioactive isotope bound to albumin, injected next to the tumour 12 hours before surgery, and a blue dye injected into the periareolar area at the start of surgery. Radioactivity is detected at surgery and the visibly blue nodes are excised and examined by the pathologist. This can be done by immediate frozen section, and if the nodes are positive, an axillary clearance can be completed.

By detecting positive axillary nodes, sentinel node biopsy has significantly reduced the morbidity associated with axillary surgery for 75% of patients.

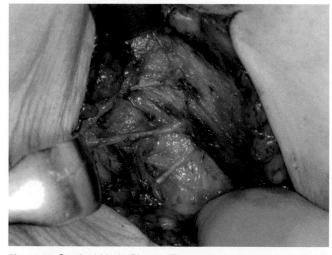

• **Fig. 45.14** Sentinel Node Biopsy. The sentinel node is usually the first axillary node to receive lymphatic drainage from the tumour. Before operation, a blue dye and a radiotracer are injected into subareolar area, and at operation the sentinel node is identified visually and by using a device to detect radioactivity.

Axillary Clearance

Axillary surgery is performed both to fully stage the axilla and to treat proven axillary disease to improve local control and prevent recurrence. However, the indications for, and the extent of axillary surgery remain controversial, and the significance of small numbers of positive nodes and micrometastatic (0.2–2 mm) disease is unclear. If axillary surgery is indicated, techniques need to keep the morbidity low to minimise lymphoedema and reduced shoulder function. Lymphoedema affects ~25% of women following axillary clearance, rising to ~40% when combined with axillary radiotherapy.

TABLE 45.2	Clinicopathological Subclassification of Breast Cancer	
Subtype of Cancer	**Pathological Features**
Luminal A-like	ER+, HER2-, Ki67$_{low}$, PR$_{high}$
Luminal B-like (HER2-negative)	ER+, HER2-, Ki67$_{high}$, PR$_{low}$
Luminal B-like (HER2-positive)	ER+, HER2+
HER2 overexpressing	ER-, HER2+, PR-
Basal-like	ER-, PR-, HER2-

ER, Oestrogen receptor; *HER2*, human epidermal growth factor receptor 2; *PR*, progesterone receptor.

The **surgical levels** of axillary nodes are defined in relation to the pectoralis minor muscle. Most nodes are level I, below its lower edge. Level II is at the level of the muscle and level III is above it. Malignant cells generally progress from level I to level II to level III, with 'skip' metastases in only about 3% (i.e., involving higher levels without lower levels).

Most surgeons accept a level II clearance, as optimising local control and staging; level III clearance causes higher morbidity, with no survival benefit, and should be performed only if higher nodes are suspicious.

Radiotherapy

Radiotherapy to the breast is mandatory after breast conserving surgery. It improves the 10-year risk of locoregional or distant relapse by ~15%. Treatment is by external beam irradiation (40–50 Gy over 3 or 5 weeks); patients with larger tumours or with a narrow margin of normal tissue in the excised specimen may receive a localised booster dose of 12 to 16 Gy; this can halve the local relapse risk.

Radiotherapy is also given to the 25% or so of patients who, after mastectomy, are shown to have large, poorly differentiated tumours with lymphovascular invasion and four or more involved nodes (and increasingly to those with fewer involved nodes). In general, the supraclavicular nodes and the internal mammary chain are also irradiated. Postmastectomy radiotherapy reduces local recurrence by up to 50% and is believed to improve survival by about 10%, but it also increases the risk of arm lymphoedema.

Adjuvant Systemic Treatment

The low cure rate for apparently early breast cancer is caused by occult metastatic spread. The aim of systemic therapy is to delay or prevent metastases. Important changes have been made to recommendations for systemic therapy in recent years, improving disease-free and overall survival outcomes and reducing the morbidity of overtreating patients at low risk for recurrence. This is a complex field, and treatment decisions take into account an increasing array of variables, from traditional staging and pathology to molecular and genetic biomarkers. For example, patients in the best prognostic group are unlikely to have micrometastases and do not generally require adjuvant systemic chemotherapy. For the rest, the choice of adjuvant therapies (or none) involves detailed discussion between patient and doctor about the balance of benefit and side-effects. Table 45.2 summarises current thinking about how to classify tumours from a histopathological perspective, to guide adjuvant systemic therapies. As discussed earlier,

web-based systems are widely used internationally, to estimate the benefits and side-effects of different therapies in individual patients and the likely risk of cancer-related mortality or relapse without adjuvant therapy. Data are entered about the patient and their cancer (age, tumour size, nodal involvement, histological grade, ER/HER2 status, etc.) and estimates are then printed as graphs and texts to inform consultations. These should be used alongside evolving evidence to provide up-to-date recommendations, taking into account the patient's general fitness, comorbidities and preferences. Treatment should ideally commence 2 to 6 weeks following surgery. The most important principles are: (1) all luminal cancers (ER-positive cancers) should be treated with endocrine therapy; (2) most luminal A cancers carry low risk for relapse and most can avoid cytotoxic chemotherapy; and (3) HER2-positive cancers should be treated with a plan incorporating trastuzumab.

Endocrine Therapy

Endocrine therapy for breast cancer includes selective ER modulators, such as tamoxifen, aromatase inhibitors (AIs), such as letrozole and anastrozole, and ovarian ablation. This therapy is recommended in all patients with invasive breast cancer, in whom at least 1% of the tumour cells express the ER; the type of recommended treatment depends on the patient's menopausal status.

For premenopausal patients, where endogenous oestrogens are made by the ovaries and by peripheral conversion of androgens, tamoxifen is used for 5 to 10 years. Any added benefit from ovarian suppression (e.g., by gonadotropin-releasing hormone agonists or oophorectomy) remains controversial, but is used in selected cases. Note that many patients are premenopausal at diagnosis, then become postmenopausal during the adjuvant treatment period so treatment plans must be modified in the context of current menopausal status. Symptoms of oestrogen withdrawal can be severe and there are advantages in treating patients with an AI at some point during the adjuvant period. For postmenopausal patients, either AIs or tamoxifen are used for at least 5 years.

Tamoxifen is a selective ER modulator that blocks the peripheral action of oestrogen in the breast by binding to the receptor. The main side effects are menopausal symptoms, such as vaginal dryness and hot flushes. In addition, the drug carries moderately increased risks of thromboembolism, endometrial cancer and visual disturbances. Treatment of ER-positive cancers with tamoxifen for 5 years reduces the risk of death from breast cancer by at least 20% to 30%. Tamoxifen has similar benefits in pre- and postmenopausal women, and its action is additive to that of chemotherapy, where appropriate.

Aromatase inhibitors (AIs) prevent oestrogen synthesis in peripheral adipose tissues by blocking the conversion of androgens to oestrogen by the enzyme aromatase. AIs significantly reduce peripheral oestrogen levels and block intratumoural synthesis of oestrogen. They can only be prescribed in postmenopausal women, or in the context of pharmacological ovarian suppression.

AIs decrease the risk of cancer recurrence and have fewer side-effects than tamoxifen, but carry an increased risk of osteoporosis and fractures. **Bisphosphonates** should be discussed in patients undergoing endocrine therapy—in addition to maintenance of bone health, they can prolong disease-specific survival.

In general, hormonal therapy has been shown to reduce the risk of local and distant recurrences, as well as the risk of a contralateral breast cancer, and significantly improves breast cancer survival. Tamoxifen is also recommended in patients treated for ER-positive DCIS, where it reduces recurrences (invasive and noninvasive) and second primary cancers. Primary endocrine therapy can also sometimes be used alone in the neoadjuvant setting, particularly in carefully selected postmenopausal patients.

Patients who are elderly and unsuitable for surgery with ER+ tumours can be treated with primary endocrine therapy to slow disease progression.

Adjuvant Chemotherapy

Several cycles of systemic adjuvant chemotherapy (around 12–24 weeks), using combination regimens, improves the survival of certain groups of patients: generally this is recommended for triple negative breast cancers (ER-negative, PR-negative and HER2-negative), most HER2-positive breast cancers, and high risk luminal cancers—see earlier for how recommendations are made regarding chemotherapy. Some of the benefit results from chemotherapy-induced ovarian ablation (in premenopausal women).

Short-term toxicities of chemotherapy depend on the type of agent and include neutropenia, nausea, vomiting, alopecia, mucositis, gastrointestinal disturbances, neuropathy, and cardiotoxicity. Long-term complications include premature ovarian failure and induction of early menopause. There are many combination chemotherapy regimens available, and most involve sequential use of both anthracyclines and taxanes; these regimens reduce mortality by around one-third. These have superseded CMF chemotherapy (cyclophosphamide, methotrexate and 5-fluorouracil), which was used for many years.

Neoadjuvant chemotherapy, that is, given before surgery, is generally used in young women with large, high-grade tumours. One advantage is that the response of the cancer to treatment can be assessed directly. Neoadjuvant chemotherapy can also be used to downsize large tumours, so that breast-conserving surgery might be possible. Where a full course of neoadjuvant chemotherapy has been given, there is no need for adjuvant treatment after surgery.

Biological Therapies

Antibody-based therapies can be used alone or combined with hormonal and cytotoxic therapies. **Trastuzumab (Herceptin)** is a humanised monoclonal antibody to the HER2/ErbB2 transmembrane receptor, which is overexpressed in 15% to 25% of breast cancers. This indicates an intrinsically poor prognosis reversible by HER2-directed treatments. Trastuzumab is recommended for the adjuvant treatment of HER2-positive breast cancers, with nodal involvement, as well as for node-negative tumours, where the primary tumour size is at least 1 cm. When used along with chemotherapy, trastuzumab decreases the recurrence risk by around one half in HER2-positive cancers compared with chemotherapy alone. Trastuzumab is currently given after surgery and chemotherapy at 3-weekly intervals for 1 year, although recent data suggests that 6 months of treatment is sufficient, which reduces cardiotoxicity, the major side effect of trastuzumab. Regular echocardiography is required for patients receiving trastuzumab.

For HER2-positive cancers requiring neoadjuvant treatment, the combination of trastuzumab and another HER2-directed antibody therapy (pertuzumab), improves pathological complete response rates and disease-free survival when combined with chemotherapy.

Control of Advanced and Disseminated Disease (Figs 45.15–45.18)

About two-thirds of breast cancer patients now survive for at least 20 years, but many eventually succumb to micrometastatic disease, later progressing to clinically evident metastases. Once

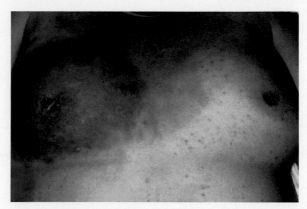

• **Fig. 45.15** Advanced Breast Cancer. This 60-year-old woman had been aware of a lump in her right breast for over a year before she could be persuaded to seek treatment. The whole breast is involved and malignancy has spread through the skin widely across the chest wall. Palliative treatment was given with radiotherapy and tamoxifen.

metastases have appeared, treatment is palliative, but very worthwhile prolongation of life and improved quality of life can often be achieved. The commonest sites for metastases are bones, liver, lung and brain. **Bone metastases** are more likely in postmenopausal women with well-differentiated, ER-positive tumours. More than 90% of patients with metastatic disease have bone lesions. These are usually lytic and commonly affect ribs and vertebrae. They can be very painful and lead to pathological fractures (see Fig. 45.17). Fortunately, they often respond to palliative radiotherapy or systemic treatments. **Lobular carcinoma** can metastasise to unusual sites, such as skin (see Fig. 45.18) and gastrointestinal tract.

Locally advanced breast cancer (stage III disease) often involves most of the breast tissue (see Fig. 45.15). The skin becomes infiltrated (peau d'orange or inflammatory cancer, where dermal lymphatics are involved), and eventually ulcerates; the tumour can invade the chest wall. Ultimately, much of the chest wall may become involved, when it is known as **carcinoma en cuirasse**. Locally advanced disease of breast and axilla may initially be inoperable, but neoadjuvant hormonal or chemotherapy can downsize the cancer, so that a **toilet mastectomy** can be performed. Radiotherapy alone can be used for palliation of advanced skin, breast, chest wall and lymph node disease.

Stage IV (metastatic cancer) remains incurable, but significant benefits are provided by supportive interventions and systemic treatment. Recurrent **pleural effusions** result from **pulmonary metastases** (see Fig. 45.16) and are managed with aspiration or pleurodesis (obliterating the pleural cavity by instilling tetracycline or bleomycin) or performing surgical pleurectomy. **Ascites** occurs secondary to **liver** involvement, and patients can present with nausea, anorexia, weight loss and jaundice. **Lymphangitis carcinomatosa** (widespread dissemination in skin or lung lymphatics) and fulminant liver metastases may occur in the terminal stage of the disease. **Brain metastases** can present with headaches and neurological symptoms, caused by a rise in intracranial pressure—aside from steroids, which reduce peritumoural oedema, radiotherapy can also be used, either to the whole brain or as radiosurgery, depending on the location and bulk of disease. Neurosurgery is also used in selected cases.

For inoperable or advanced disease, the same principles of treatment apply as per adjuvant approaches, and again depend on the ER, PR and HER2 status of the tumour. Many different types of cytotoxic chemotherapy can be used (usually as monotherapies

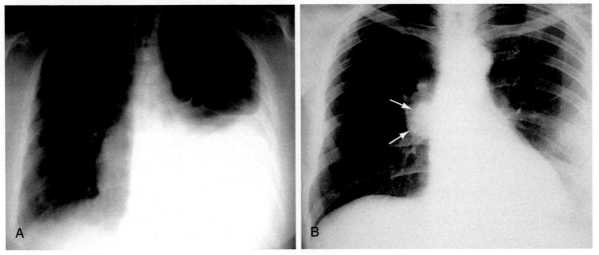

• **Fig. 45.16** Chest Manifestations of Metastatic Breast Carcinoma. **(A)** This 38-year-old woman had undergone a right mastectomy for ductal carcinoma 7 years before and presented with increasing short-ness of breath. This chest x-ray shows a large left pleural effusion confirmed on cytology to be malignant. It was palliated by drainage and pleurodesis. **(B)** A different patient who had been treated 5 years before for lobular carcinoma of the breast. She presented with a chronic nonproductive cough and was found to have a mass of lymph nodes at the right hilum *(arrowed)* and a right recurrent laryngeal nerve palsy caused by invasion in the region of the carina.

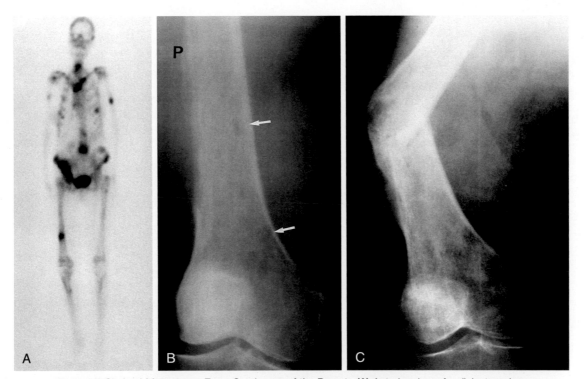

• **Fig. 45.17** Skeletal Metastases From Carcinoma of the Breast. **(A)** Anterior view of radioisotope bone scan of a 48-year-old woman complaining of pain in the neck and right hip. She had undergone a mastec-tomy for carcinoma 8 years previously. The scan shows large metastatic deposits in the lower cervical and lumbar spine, right pelvis, right femur and left humerus, as well as several smaller deposits in the ribs and elsewhere in the skeleton. **(B)** X-ray of the lower femur in a 79-year-old woman presenting with a fungating breast carcinoma and pain in the left knee. The x-ray shows radiolucencies *(arrowed)* in the distal femur and elevation of the periosteum *(P)* medially, indicating bony metastasis. Radiotherapy was arranged to alleviate the symptoms. **(C)** Some weeks later, despite treatment, the patient returned with this pathological fracture of the femur.

in contrast to the adjuvant setting). Several classes of endocrine therapies are now approved in the metastatic setting for hormone receptor-positive breast cancer, and can be used sequentially. The standard first-line treatment for advanced HER2-positive disease is the combination of chemotherapy with trastuzumab and pertuzumab. Newer agents are beginning to transform the care of patients with advanced breast cancer. Cyclin-dependant kinase 4/6 inhibitors (such as palbociclib) can be combined with hormonal treatment, leading to substantial improvements in progress-free survival. Polyadenosine diphosphate ribose inhibitors, which exploit intrinsic deficiencies in deoxynucleic acid repair mechanisms within certain breast cancers, such as those with *BRCA* mutations, are also now approved (e.g., olaparib provides 3 months more progression-free survival than chemotherapy). Sadly, current treatments remain palliative—they help prolong life and control or delay symptoms. Bisphosphonates are an important adjunctive therapy in the context of bony disease or endocrine treatment.

Long-Term Follow Up

Women who have had one breast cancer have a 15% lifetime risk of developing a second cancer in the other breast. The risk is higher if the original lesion was a lobular carcinoma. Breast tissue in these women may have an increased susceptibility to cancer, or else breast cancer may have arisen at the same time in multiple foci. Thus patients with breast cancer should be followed up clinically and by mammography for 5 years after initial treatment, before returning to a screening programme (if within the screening age group). There is no evidence that more prolonged follow up improves outcomes.

Life Expectancy and Prognosis

When long-term survival curves have been examined statistically, there is no evidence of 'cure' in the normally accepted sense (Fig. 45.19), although a 'personal cure' is achieved in about 50% of patients, who die from some other disease. Micrometastatic foci can remain dormant for 35 years or more before becoming active again for unknown reasons, leading to progressive metastatic disease and death. Locoregional relapse often occurs within the first 5 years, but distant disease tends to occur much later.

Breast cancer survival estimates from prognostic scoring systems are meaningful only for about 10 years, and as estimates are based on group analyses, they are of doubtful relevance for any individual. As discussed earlier, a commonly used tool is the Nottingham Prognostic Index, which divides patients into four prognostic groups (Table 45.3), although recent advances in prognostication mean that such estimates are becoming outmoded.

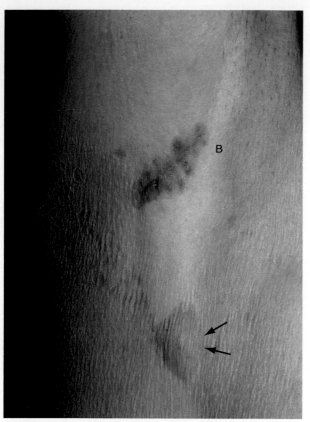

• **Fig. 45.18** Skin Secondaries Following Simple Mastectomy and Radiotherapy. This patient presented with painless, slightly elevated nodules in the skin below the axilla, 3 years after treatment for lobular carcinoma of the breast. In this photograph, the arm is elevated and one skin secondary can just be made out *(arrowed)*; the site of excision biopsy of another is seen at *(B)*.

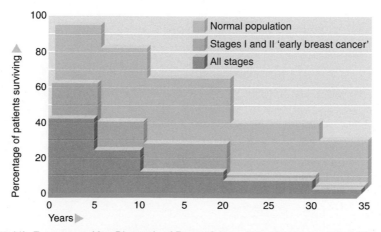

• **Fig. 45.19** Life Expectancy After Diagnosis of Breast Cancer (After Brinkley and Haybittle). Note that 5- and 10-year survival has improved in recent years, as a result of better diagnosis and treatment, but it is uncertain if long-term survival will also improve.

TABLE 45.3	Nottingham Prognostic Index (NPI) for Breast Cancer[a]	
Nottingham Prognostic Group	NPI Score	Cancer-Specific 10-Year Survival
Excellent	≤2.4	96%
Good	>2.4 and ≤3.4	93%
Moderate	>3.4 and <5.4	78%
Poor	>5.4	44%

[a]The NPI is calculated as follows: 0.2 × tumour size in cm + histological grade (1–3) + lymph node status (node negative scores 1; one to three positive nodes scores 2, and three or more positive nodes scores 3)

Benign Breast Disorders

Most patients referred to breast clinics are found to have benign breast conditions. These include fibrocystic change or fibroadenosis (the most common), fibroadenoma, duct papilloma, fat necrosis, breast infections and mammary duct ectasia.

Abnormalities of Normal Development and Involution (ANDI)

Pathology

In women of reproductive age, breast tissue is constantly undergoing physiological changes in response to circulating hormones. This can produce a spectrum of proliferative and regressive changes in the breast parenchyma including distortion and overgrowth of the main structural components—the ducts, lobules and fibrous tissue. The concept of 'abnormalities of normal development and involution (ANDI)' thus encompasses a variety of clinicopathological features, which histologically include fibrosis, adenosis, apocrine metaplasia, epithelial hyperplasia and macro- and microcyst formation.

These changes together result in areas of general or focal **nodularity** associated with varying degrees of pain and tenderness. The term **fibrocystic change** or **fibroadenosis** has historically been applied to this condition. The main components are cyst formation, epitheliosis, fibrosis and proliferation of lobular acini, known as **adenosis**. Fibrosis may occur within areas of adenosis, splitting acini; this is known as **sclerosing adenosis**. Several of these features are often present within a single lesion, or in different areas of the same or the contralateral breast.

By definition, the hyperplastic element in ANDI is not histologically atypical and there is no increased risk of malignancy in this complex of benign breast changes.

Clinical Presentation and Management

Fibrocystic change (fibroadenosis) presents as either a single lump or areas of lumpiness, which are painful and tender premenstrually, that is, cyclically (Fig. 45.20). These changes may be difficult to distinguish clinically from carcinoma, and florid fibrocystic change can mask a cancer both clinically and radiologically. Fibrocystic change is most common between the ages of 35 and 45 years.

Cyst formation is more prevalent over the age of 40 years and in perimenopausal women. Cysts may present symptomatically as single or occasionally multiple lumps. Cysts develop from lobules and are fluid-filled spaces. **Microcysts** are part of the involutionary process and may coalesce to produce a larger cyst, which presents as a smooth, round palpable lump. Larger cysts may be tense, tender and fluctuant, with the texture of a table tennis ball. Cysts can usually be diagnosed clinically and are readily confirmed with ultrasonography; they are usually recognisable on a mammogram. Simple cysts can be aspirated under ultrasound control or freehand. Provided the cyst fluid is not blood-stained, there is no residual lump postaspiration and there are no sonographically suspicious features, patients can be discharged without further follow up, although cysts can recur or new cysts develop (Fig. 45.21). Cysts are uncommon over the age of 60 years, unless the patient is taking HRT. Under these circumstances, it is important to exclude an intracystic papilloma, intracystic carcinoma or a cystic carcinoma.

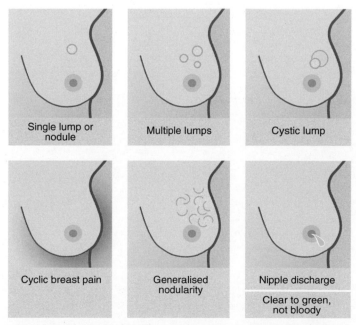

Single lump or nodule; Multiple lumps; Cystic lump; Cyclic breast pain; Generalised nodularity; Nipple discharge — Clear to green, not bloody

• **Fig. 45.20** Clinical Presentation of Fibroadenosis (Fibrocystic Change).

Managing Fibrocystic Change

Once the patient has been reassured she does not have cancer, the symptoms of pain and tenderness associated with fibrocystic change can be treated. **Gamolenic acid** in high doses may relieve cyclic symptoms in some women, but has to be used for a minimum of 3 months to see results. More than 90% of patients with mild to moderate breast pain can be satisfactorily managed with reassurance and simple analgesia. For those with moderate to severe cyclic pain, danazol or bromocriptine offers relief in 70% of women, but both these drugs have substantial side-effects, which reduce compliance. Danazol inhibits pituitary gonadotrophin secretion and has androgenic side-effects of acne and hirsutism. Bromocriptine inhibits pituitary prolactin release and can produce dizziness.

Fibroadenoma

Pathology

A fibroadenoma is a localised form of ANDI rather than a benign tumour. This lesion arises from a single lobule and is composed of epithelial and fibrous components (Fig. 45.22). Fibroadenomas undergo involution in the perimenopausal years but can persist into old age and become calcified.

Clinical Presentation and Management

Fibroadenomas are most common between the ages of 15 and 30 years and thus occur in a younger group than fibroadenosis. They

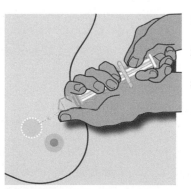

1 Fluid should not be blood-stained

2 Lump should disappear

3 Cyst should not recur

• **Fig. 45.21** Cyst Aspiration and Criteria for Exclusion of Cancer Associated With a Cyst.

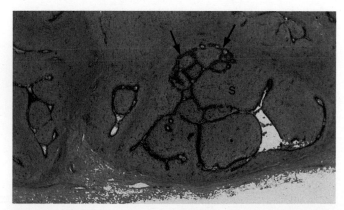

• **Fig. 45.22** Fibroadenoma—Histopathology. This benign lesion shows proliferation of both glands *(arrowed)* and stroma *(S)*. In the variant illustrated, gland lumina are compressed by stroma. Fibroadenoma typically has a histologically well-defined edge.

present as a single rounded mass, which is smooth, firm and highly mobile. Smaller lesions are sometimes described as **breast mice**, since they slip away from beneath the palpating fingers. Fibroadenomas are occasionally multiple and bilateral and are more frequent in an Afro-Caribbean population. Larger fibroadenomas should be distinguished from benign **phyllodes tumours**, which have similar features clinically, radiologically and on core biopsy. Where suspicion of phyllodes exists or a fibroadenoma is enlarging, excision biopsy is indicated, otherwise the lesions regress spontaneously in 85% to 90% and do not require excision. Confirmatory tissue biopsy is unnecessary below 25 years, but is advisable over this age.

Duct Papilloma

Intraductal papillomas are localised areas of epithelial proliferation. They are villous lesions composed of a fibrovascular core covered by a double layer of epithelium. They usually occur as solitary lesions in the main lactiferous ducts close to the nipple, but multiple papillomas can occur more peripherally. Papillomas are not premalignant (Fig. 45.23). They present as spontaneous blood-stained or clear watery nipple discharge, often from a single duct; a retroareolar mass may be palpable. These lesions are best imaged with ultrasound and the diagnosis confirmed on core biopsy. Papillomas are treated by excision of the affected duct (microdochectomy) or a group of ducts (wedge resection). If the causative lesion cannot be found at operation, a subareolar excision of all the ducts may be necessary.

Traumatic Fat Necrosis

Trauma to the breast, either accidental or surgical, can produce an area of fat necrosis that can mimic carcinoma clinically and radiologically. There is an initial acute inflammatory response, which can persist, provoking chronic inflammation and a fibrotic reaction. This gives a hard irregular lump, which may have skin dimpling. Mammography may show a stellate area of distortion with calcification. Core biopsy distinguishes fat necrosis from carcinoma.

Infections of the Breast

Breast infection is occasionally seen in neonates, but is commonest in premenopausal women. **Lactational mastitis** usually occurs during the first 3 months of breast feeding and can lead

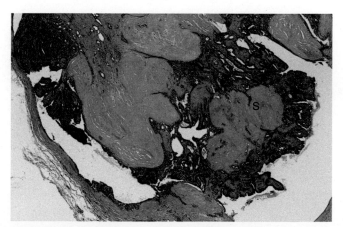

• **Fig. 45.23** Duct Papilloma. This is essentially a localised form of epitheliosis. Papilloma in a larger duct must be distinguished from papillary carcinoma, which lacks the well-defined stromal cores *(S)*. Both lesions can present with blood-stained nipple discharge.

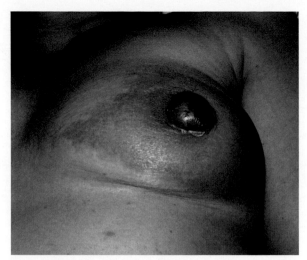

• **Fig. 45.24** Breast Abscess. This woman of 40 years presented with a neglected left breast abscess a few weeks after ceasing breast feeding. The abscess was drained at open operation, but had destroyed much of the breast tissue. The organism was *Staphylococcus aureus* as is commonly the case.

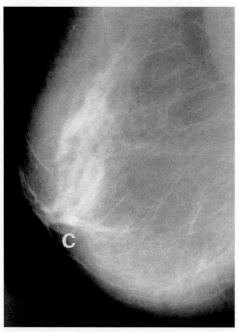

• **Fig. 45.25** Mammary Duct Ectasia. Radiopaque mass of dilated ducts with no features of malignancy. Large duct calcification *(C)* is also seen. Note the skin indentation caused by fibrosis. Clinically, this condition can be mistaken for carcinoma.

to septicaemia. Risk factors include a cracked nipple and poor feeding technique, causing milk stasis. The organism responsible is almost always *Staphylococcus aureus*. Patients present with pain, swelling and erythema. Treatment is with empirical antibiotics (such as flucloxacillin), together with continued feeding or milk expression. If the patient becomes septic, she may need intravenous antibiotics. If an abscess develops (Fig. 45.24), this should be drained with repeated ultrasound-guided aspiration, until resolution. Surgery is only indicated if the skin is threatened or necrotic. In this case, a small stab incision is made, and the abscess cavity is flushed until all the pus is drained.

Nonlactational mastitis is mainly periductal, with active inflammation in nondilated ducts, and should not be confused with duct ectasia. It is treated with broad-spectrum antibiotics with anaerobic cover (such as co-amoxiclav), and either aspiration or incision and drainage, although this risks a mammary duct fistula.

The diagnosis of an abscess is usually obvious, with local signs of acute inflammation, a tachycardia and fever. The affected segment of the breast is tender, red and warm. If the infection is inadequately treated, the abscess becomes fluctuant and eventually 'points' to the surface and discharges.

The early cellulitic phase is reversible if treated with appropriate antibiotics. Flucloxacillin is usually the antibiotic of choice on an empirical basis, but progress must be closely followed. The need for surgical drainage has declined in recent years because of prompt and appropriate antibiotic treatment, sometimes aided by needle aspiration.

Duct Ectasia

Mammary duct ectasia refers to dilatation and shortening of the major lactiferous ducts. It is a common involutional change appearing around the menopause. It presents with spontaneous cream, yellow or green nipple discharge, a palpable subareolar mass or nipple inversion. Plasma cells are a characteristic feature on histology; this may be described as **plasma cell mastitis**. Ducts can calcify and be seen on a mammogram (Fig. 45.25). Duct ectasia should be managed conservatively, unless radiological findings

are suspicious for malignancy. Persistent discharge can be treated by subtotal or total nipple duct excision.

Male Breast Disorders

The two main breast conditions in males are gynaecomastia and cancer.

Gynaecomastia (Fig. 45.26)

Gynaecomastia is a benign proliferation of the male breast, which feels like a rubbery firm mass extending concentrically from the nipple. It results from an imbalance of oestrogens and androgens acting on the breast. Primary gynaecomastia is physiological and occurs in three phases: **infantile** gynaecomastia is present at birth in response to oestrogens crossing the placenta and resolves spontaneously over several weeks. In **puberty**, the condition is bilateral in 50% to 60%; the mechanism is unknown but most resolve spontaneously. **Senescent** gynaecomastia peaks at 50 to 69 years of age and is more likely in obese men.

Secondary gynaecomastia is either caused by medication or is pathological:
- **Medication**—drugs include spironolactone, digoxin, ranitidine, calcium-channel blockers, together with anabolic steroids and cannabis use. Hormonal treatment for prostate cancer can also cause gynaecomastia.
- **Pathological**—alcoholic cirrhosis interferes with the metabolism of oestrogens and decreases free testosterone and some testicular germ cell tumours may secrete oestrogens. Other predisposing illnesses include chronic renal failure, diabetes and hypogonadism.

Adults with gynaecomastia should undergo triple assessment and have blood tested for prolactin, luteinising hormone, oestrogen, testosterone and human chorionic gonadotropin to exclude

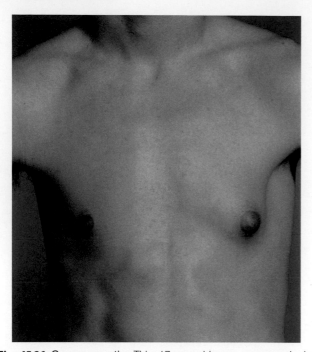

• **Fig. 45.26** Gynaecomastia. This 17-year-old was concerned about excess breast development on the left side. The breast tissue was removed via a subareolar incision.

hypogonadism and testicular tumours. Most men can then be reassured without treatment. Surgery is usually performed in younger males for cosmetic purposes.

Male Breast Cancer

Between 0.5% and 1% of breast cancers occur in males, who are an average of 10 years older than women at presentation. Male breast cancer is more common in carriers of *BRCA2* mutations and in states of hyperoestrogenism, such as liver disease and Klinefelter syndrome. The patient may present late because the diagnosis has not been considered. Mastectomy is the usual surgical option and tamoxifen is prescribed for ER-positive tumours (80%–90% are ER-positive). Stage for stage, the prognosis is similar for breast cancer in men and women; male breast cancer tends to behave like postmenopausal disease in women. The same principles for treatment of female breast cancer should be applied to cases in males.

46

Disorders of the Skin

Introduction

Only a few skin disorders are surgically important, including unsightly lesions, lumps and potentially malignant lesions. These are often referred to surgeons for excision or for definitive management following biopsy. **Lower limb ulcers** in the West are usually venous, arterial or diabetic neural and/or ischaemic in origin (see Chs 41 and 43). Leg ulcers in the tropics often have a bacterial origin. Ulceration is also a characteristic of malignant skin lesions.

Surgical skin disorders are often referred to a dermatologist, but still comprise about 15% of new general surgical outpatient referrals. Many require only excision biopsy under local anaesthesia. Others are referred for advice after a lesion has been excised by a family practitioner.

Most skin malignancies are ideally managed by a multidisciplinary team (MDT) of surgeons, dermatologists, oncologists, pathologists and sometimes radiologists and specialist nurses.

A small proportion of skin lesions have a potentially sinister course, notably malignant melanoma (MM). These comprise around 5% of skin cancers in the United Kingdom but account for most skin cancer deaths (75%). The incidence of all skin cancers (melanoma, basal cell carcinoma [BCC] and squamous cell carcinomas [SCCs]) and their premalignant stages increases with sun exposure and is highest in fair skinned people. The frequency of all skin cancers is rising in the West with increasing foreign travel, and in sunny countries like Australia, they have reached epidemic proportions.

Finally, the nails, which are specialised skin appendages, pose surgical problems in the form of infected **ingrowing toenails** and **onychogryphosis**. The rare **subungual melanoma** is an important diagnosis, which must not be missed.

Overview of the Skin

The skin is the largest organ in the body and its main functions are **protection, regulation and sensation**. The skin protects against mechanical forces, such as pressure and abrasion; ultraviolet light and heat; and acts as a barrier against pathogens. Regulation functions include temperature (via vasodilatation and constriction, and sweating), metabolism of vitamin D and preventing fluid losses, whilst sensation include touch, pressure, itch and pain.

Structure of Normal Skin (Fig. 46.1)

The skin has three main strata, the epidermis (the protective waterproofing layer), the dermis and the hypodermis:

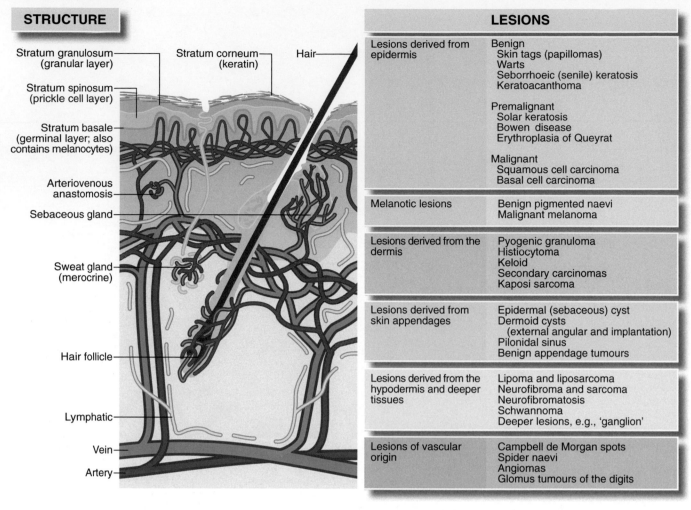

STRUCTURE		LESIONS	

Stratum granulosum (granular layer)	Stratum corneum (keratin) Hair	Lesions derived from epidermis	Benign
			  Skin tags (papillomas)
			  Warts
			  Seborrhoeic (senile) keratosis
			  Keratoacanthoma
			
			Premalignant
			  Solar keratosis
			  Bowen disease
			  Erythroplasia of Queyrat
			
			Malignant
			  Squamous cell carcinoma
			  Basal cell carcinoma

• **Fig. 46.1** Structure of the Skin and Lesions of Surgical Importance.

- The epidermis has four layers—from the base outwards: basal, prickle-cell, granular and keratin layers. Cell division normally occurs only in the basal layer.
- The **dermis** consists of **papillary** and **reticular layers**, separated by a vascular (middermal) plexus. The dermis contains keratinocytes and collagen and elastin fibres produced by fibroblasts, and also ground substance composed mainly of glycosaminoglycans.
- The deepest layer is the **hypodermis**, consisting of loose fibrofatty tissue and containing skin appendages—sweat glands (mainly eccrine), apocrine glands (sweat glands in armpits, groins and around nipples), hair follicles and associated sebaceous glands. The skin is generally mobile over deeper structures, because the hypodermis is only loosely connected to the superficial fascia, but is tightly bound to fascia in the palms, the soles of the feet and the scalp.

Collagen in the deeper reticular layer provides much of the skin's strength, while the elastin contributes to its elasticity. Both layers are well vascularised and rich in nerve endings. The orientation of collagen and elastin fibres in the dermis determines lines of skin tension known as **Langer lines**. These are surgically important because incisions parallel to them heal with minimal scarring.

Signs and Symptoms of Skin Disorders

As the incidence of skin cancers continues to rise in all adult age groups, the numbers of patients referred with skin lesions also increases. Patients may be concerned by changing appearances of a lesion, such as size, shape or colour; or changes in its behaviour, such as pain, bleeding or ulceration. Assessing any new skin lesion begins with a clinical history and examination, to formulate a differential diagnosis and management plan.

History

Pertinent questions about the skin lesion include:
- How long has the lesion been present?
- How is it changing?
- Is it getting bigger?
- Is any size increase slow or rapid?
- Is it itchy?
- Is it painful?
- Is there any bleeding or other discharge?
- Is there any change in colour?

Past history includes any previous skin lesions, surgery or trauma to the affected area. Previous skin cancer makes this diagnosis more likely, whilst surgery or trauma can lead to implantation cysts, keloid scarring or a chronic inflammatory response to a foreign body. The history should also seek disorders predisposing to infection or causing immunosuppression. Previous radiotherapy can increase the risk of skin cancer.

Family history can direct the diagnosis towards rarer genetic disorders, such as neurofibromatosis, Muir-Torre and tuberous sclerosis. There may also be a genetic link in some melanomas.

Social history should include occupational details (environmental exposures to carcinogens increase the risk of BCC and SCC). The sun exposure history can be clarified by questions about work, living abroad or frequent sunny holidays. Previous service in the armed forces may have included deployment to tropical climates. When dealing with suspected melanomas in particular, a history of childhood sunburn is important. Chronic ulcers may be contracted during foreign travel or after injury, and with chronic nonhealing wounds and burns, there is a small risk of malignant transformation.

Drug history—immunosuppressive therapies may be relevant

Clinical Examination

The lesion should be examined in detail with an A–E Assessment:
- **A**symmetry
- **B**order
- **C**olour
- **D**iameter
- **E**levation/evolution

Other characteristics, including consistency, mobility and tenderness, should also be assessed and documented (Table 46.1). A top to toe examination should then be carried out, searching for other similar lesions, lymphadenopathy or sources of primary malignancy elsewhere that has metastasised to skin. The glabrous (nonhairy) surfaces of hands and feet and the nails should be examined for melanotic lesions.

The lesion in question should ideally be photographed and **dermoscopy** performed to examine it in detail, assessing its pigmentation and vascularity and seeking features of malignancy. If skin malignancy is suspected, regional lymph node basins should be examined.

Principles of Managing Skin Lesions

Many skin lesions can be diagnosed from the history and clinical examination alone. If there is concern about malignancy, a biopsy should be performed. Incision and excision biopsy techniques are illustrated in Chapter 10, p. 14, and Box 46.1 summarises surgical options for skin conditions.

An excision biopsy takes an ellipse of skin with a 2-mm or so margin of normal tissue and an underlying cuff of fat. The ellipse should be placed along natural skin tension lines to enable the skin edges to be readily opposed. All excised lesions should be sent for histological evaluation. For large lesions, an incisional biopsy can be taken or, if facilities allow, the lesion can be excised and a dressing placed on the wound awaiting histological confirmation of clearance.

Following the diagnosis, management may involve other members of a MDT as well as deciding on long-term follow up.

Lesions Originating in the Epidermis

Benign Epidermal Lesions

Skin Tags

Skin tags or squamous papillomas are small benign polypoid lesions consisting of loose connective tissue covered by epithelium. They are common in adults and occur particularly on the trunk, face, neck, axillae and groins. Although benign, they can be irritated by clothing or jewellery and cause bleeding. Nonsurgical management includes cryotherapy (freezing) or tying a thread around the base and so the tag becomes ischaemic and falls off. A surgical approach is narrow-margin excision under local anaesthesia.

Warts

Warts are small, virus-induced epidermal lesions (frequently caused by human papillomavirus or HPV), which present as epidermal thickening with hyperplasia and hyperkeratosis, plus enlarging dermal papillae known as *papillomatosis*. Morphology varies with location. The **common wart** (verruca vulgaris), is a papilliferous lesion up to 1 cm across, most often found on the fingers and back of the hands. Warts are often multiple in children, and can occur on the face, where the lesions are often less keratotic and have a smoother, more dome-like shape. They are often called *juvenile* or *plane warts* (verruca plana juvenilis). Lesions on the sole of the foot, **plantar warts** (verruca plantaris), become very keratotic and flattened by pressure. They may extend deeply into the foot and cause pain. Warts may also occur on the genitalia, perineum and perianal area. These originate from HPV infection and are usually spread by sexual contact. Genital warts sometimes grow large and are then known as **condylomata accuminata**.

Warts are common in immune-suppressed patients. They can grow and regress spontaneously over months and years. Most are managed conservatively with topical antiviral creams or ointments. If inadequate, other measures include cryotherapy, laser treatment or surgical excision. National Institute for Care and Health Excellence (NICE) guidance also considers that photodynamic treatment may be of benefit.

Seborrhoeic Keratosis

Seborrhoeic keratoses (**seborrhoeic warts**) or basal cell papillomas, are very common in older patients and arise primarily on the torso and neck. The patient may present with multiple different sized lesions, with varying pigmentation. Lesions appear waxy and raised with a 'stuck on' appearance and keratotic plugs on the surface (Fig. 46.2).

Histologically, there are several types, which can be classified as acanthotic, hyperkeratotic, clonal, reticulated or irritated. Owing to the superficial nature of the lesion, they can be 'scraped off' with a curette or scalpel under local anaesthesia. Alternatively, they can be treated with cryotherapy, electrocautery or laser.

Keratoacanthoma

Keratoacanthoma (KA) is an epithelial tumour that can present as a nodular skin lesion with well-defined, raised edges and an irregular central crater containing keratotic debris. Previously considered completely benign, pathologists are moving

TABLE 46.1   Symptoms and Signs of Skin Disorders

Symptoms and Signs	Diagnostic Significance
1. Lump in or on the skin Size, shape and surface features revealed by inspection—is the lesion smooth-surfaced, irregular, exophytic (i.e., projecting out of the surface)?	Epidermal lesions (such as warts) usually have a surface abnormality but deeper lesions are usually covered by normal epidermis. A punctum suggests the abnormality arises from an epidermal appendage, for example, epidermal (sebaceous) cyst
Depth within the skin Superficial and deep attachments Which tissue is the swelling derived from?	Tends to reflect the layer from which lesion is derived and therefore the range of differential diagnosis (i.e., epidermis, dermis, hypodermis or deeper)
Character of the margin Discreteness, tethering to surrounding tissues, three-dimensional shape	A regular shaped, discrete lesion is most likely cystic or encapsulated (e.g., benign tumour). Deep tethering implies origin from deeper structures (e.g., ganglion). Immobility of overlying epidermis suggests a lesion derived from skin appendage (e.g., epidermal cyst)
Consistency Soft, firm, hard, 'indurated', rubbery	Soft lesions are usually lipomas or fluid-filled cysts. Most cysts are fluctuant unless filled by semisolid material (e.g., epidermal cysts), or the cyst is tense (e.g., small ganglion) Malignant lesions tend to be hard and irregular ('indurated') with an ill-defined margin caused by invasion of surrounding tissue Bony-hard lesions are either mineralised (e.g., gouty tophi) or consist of bone (e.g., exostoses)
Pulsatility	Pulsatility is usually transmitted from an underlying artery, which may simply be tortuous or may be abnormal (e.g., aneurysm or arteriovenous fistula)
Emptying and refilling	Vascular lesions (e.g., venous malformations or haemangiomas) empty or blanch on pressure and then refill
Transilluminability	Lesions filled with clear fluid, such as cysts 'light up' when transilluminated
Temperature	Excessive warmth implies acute inflammation, for example, pilonidal abscess
2. Pain, tenderness and discomfort	These symptoms often indicate acute inflammation. Pain also develops if a noninflammatory lesion becomes inflamed or infected (e.g., inflamed epidermal cyst). Malignant lesions are usually painless
3. Ulceration (i.e., loss of epidermal integrity with an inflamed base formed by dermis or deeper tissues)	Malignant lesions and keratoacanthomas tend to ulcerate as a result of central necrosis. Surface breakdown also occurs in arterial or venous insufficiency (e.g., ischaemic leg ulcers), chronic infection (e.g., tuberculosis or tropical ulcers) or trauma, particularly in an insensate foot
Character of the ulcer margin	Benign ulcers—the margin is only slightly raised by inflammatory oedema. The base lies below the level of normal skin Malignant ulcers—these begin as a solid mass of proliferating epidermal cells, then the centre eventually becomes necrotic and breaks down. The margin is typically elevated 'rolled' and indurated by tumour growth and invasion
Behaviour of the ulcer	Malignant ulcers expand inexorably (though often slowly), but may go through cycles of breakdown and healing (often with bleeding)
4. Colour and pigmentation *Normal colour*	If a lesion is covered by normal-coloured skin, then the lesion must lie deeply in the skin (e.g., epidermal cyst) or deep to the skin (e.g., ganglion)
Red or purple	Redness implies increased arterial vascularity, which is most common in inflammatory conditions, like furuncles. Vascular abnormalities which contain a high proportion of arterial blood, such as Campbell de Morgan spots or strawberry naevi are also red, whereas venous disorders, such as port-wine stain are darker. Vascular lesions blanch on pressure and must be distinguished from purpura or haematoma, which does not
Deeply pigmented	Benign naevi (moles) and their malignant counterpart, malignant melanomas, are nearly always pigmented. Other lesions, such as warts, papillomata or seborrhoeic keratoses may become pigmented secondarily. Hairy pigmented moles are almost never malignant. Rarely, malignant melanomas may be nonpigmented (amelanotic). New darkening of a pigmented lesion should be viewed with suspicion, as it may indicate malignant change
5. Rapidly developing lesion	Keratoacanthoma, warts and pyogenic granuloma may all develop rapidly and eventually regress spontaneously. When fully developed, these conditions may be difficult to distinguish from malignancy. Spontaneous regression marks the lesion as benign
6. Multiple, recurrent and spreading lesions	In certain rare syndromes, multiple similar lesions develop over a period. Examples include neurofibromatosis and recurrent lipomata in Dercum disease. Prolonged or intense sun exposure predisposes a large area of skin to malignant change. Viral warts may appear in crops. Malignant melanoma may spread diffusely (superficial spreading melanoma) or produce satellite lesions via dermal lymphatics
7. Site of the lesion	Some skin lesions arise much more commonly in certain areas of the body. The reason may be anatomical (e.g., pilonidal sinus, external angular dermoid or multiple pilar cysts of the scalp) or because of exposure to sun (e.g., solar keratoses or basal cell carcinomas of hands and face)
8. Age when lesion noticed	Congenital vascular abnormalities, such as strawberry naevus or port-wine stain may be present at birth. Benign pigmented naevi (moles) may be detectable at birth, but only begin to enlarge and darken after the age of 2 years

Principles of Management of 'Surgical' Skin Lesions

Simple excision or other physical methods, for example, electrocautery, laser therapy or cryotherapy—for small, obviously innocent lesions.

Excision biopsy—if there is any risk of malignancy or the clinical diagnosis is doubtful (only for small lesions).

Incisional biopsy—for large lesions, where only a representative section is removed. Definitive therapy is then planned according to the histology.

Wide local excision with or without skin grafting—for malignant melanomas and sometimes for other large malignant lesions.

Radiotherapy—an alternative to excision for basal cell carcinoma and primary squamous cell lesions. Also sometimes used if regional lymph nodes are involved in squamous cell carcinoma.

Topical chemotherapy—with 5-fluorouracil cream (or other agents) for certain skin malignancies.

Photodynamic therapy—for certain skin malignancies. Malignant cells absorb a photosensitising chemical, which reacts with light of a particular wavelength applied locally to destroy the cells.

Surgical lymph node clearance—if nodes are involved by malignant melanoma or squamous carcinoma.

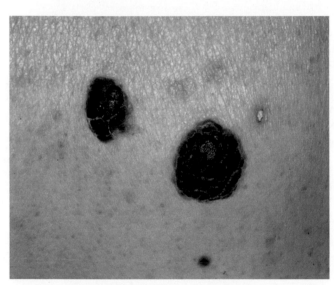

• **Fig. 46.2** Seborrhoeic Keratoses.

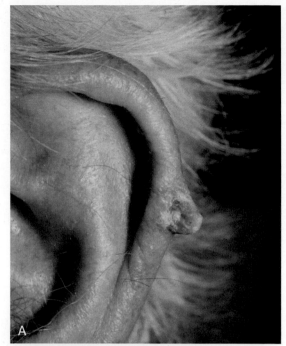

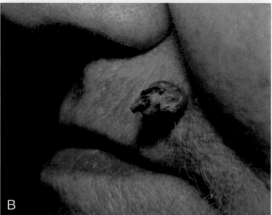

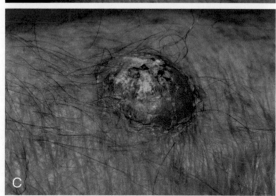

• **Fig. 46.3** Keratin Horn and Keratoacanthoma. **(A)** Keratin horn on the pinna of an elderly man. If untreated, these can grow large. **(B)** This alarming looking lesion is a benign keratoacanthoma. The central keratin plug is characteristic. Resolution is spontaneous after a few weeks. **(C)** Similar lesion on the back of the hand. Squamous and basal cell carcinoma need to be excluded.

towards considering them a form of low-grade SCC. They typically have a rapid acute growth phase, and then regress spontaneously over a few weeks. When seen during the growth phase, it can be clinically difficult to distinguish from an SCC, and it is a brave surgeon who opts to wait for the lesion to involute.

If the lesion is regressing, watching and waiting is acceptable, but one should have a low threshold for biopsy if there is diagnostic uncertainty. It can be difficult to distinguish even histologically between KA and well-differentiated SCC, and these cases should be managed as for SCC.

Keratin (cutaneous) horns may look similar but rarely regress (Fig. 46.3). They tend to arise in older people.

Pigmented Lesions

Melanocytes are derived from the neural crest during embryological development and are located in the basal layer of the epidermis. They synthesise melanin and distribute it to nearby epidermal cells, where it is responsible for skin colour. A localised collection of melanocytes confined to the epidermis is known as a *freckle* or *lentigo*. If a cluster of normal melanocytes enters the dermis, this is known as a ***naevus*** (plural naevi).

Naevi can be classified into **naevus cell naevi** (subdivided into congenital, acquired or special naevi), and **melanocytic naevi**, which may be epidermal or dermal.

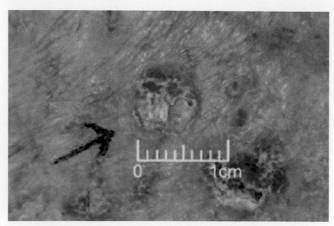

• **Fig. 46.4** Clinical Appearance of Actinic (Solar) Keratosis.

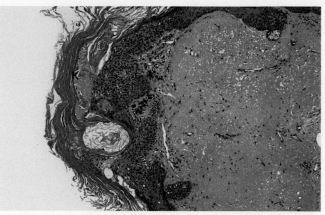

• **Fig. 46.5** Solar Keratosis—Histopathology. Occurring in sun-exposed areas, this lesion typically shows thickening of the keratin layer *(K)*. Epidermal cells can show a range of atypia, which may amount to squamous cell carcinoma-in-situ. The dermis shows severe solar damage.

Congenital naevus cell naevi are either *giant* (projected to be reach >20 cm in adulthood) or **nongiant congenital melanocytic naevi**. Giant naevi used to be considered at risk of malignant transformation, and young children were offered excisional surgery. However, this risk has proved relatively low. So operation is not offered for risk reduction, but the lesion is monitored for changes in appearance or new symptoms, such as bleeding in any area of it. In this case, a biopsy of the troublesome area should be performed.

Acquired naevus cell naevi are of three main types—junctional, compound and intradermal. These are rare in infancy and can appear up to the age of about 50 years. New naevi that develop after the age of 50 should be considered suspicious. The pigmentation of acquired naevi can change with age but the pattern remains the same.

Special naevus cell naevi include **Spitz, atypical** and **halo naevi**. Spitz naevi tend to occur in young adults, and clinically, can appear similar to melanomas. Excision biopsy is recommended to make or confirm the diagnosis.

Epidermal Melanocytic Naevi

A **lentigo** (plural = lentigines) is a flat pigmented lesion. All, except freckles, maintain their pigmentation in the absence of sun exposure. There are several types including simple lentigo, café-au-lait patches and Becker naevi, all of which are benign. However, **lentigo maligna** is a premalignant lesion containing abnormal melanocytes confined to the epidermis (and is a precursor of lentigo MM). Lentigenes are different from freckles (ephelis) in that they contain increased numbers of melanocytes and show hyperplasia, whereas freckles just have increased melanin. **Solar lentigo** are commonly referred to as 'liver spots' and occur on the face and hands of older patients.

Dermal Melanocytic Naevi

This category includes Mongolian blue spots, naevi of Ota and Ito (typically present at birth) and blue naevi, which tend to appear in childhood or young adulthood. They are all characterised by melanocytes in the dermis and thus present with bluish pigmentation. They are thought to result from failure of normal melanocyte migration from the embryonic neural crest to the epidermal basal layer.

Premalignant Skin Lesions

Actinic Keratosis (Solar/Senile Keratosis)

Actinic keratoses (AK) are flat, well-demarcated, brown, scaly or crusty lesions with an erythematous base (Fig. 46.4). They bleed easily, if traumatised or scratched, and are frequently found as multiple patches on sun-exposed surfaces, such as the face, neck and upper limb. On histology, there is hyperkeratosis and acanthosis, with a variable degree of dysplastic change and abnormal mitotic activity deep in the epidermis (Fig. 46.5). Although these features suggest malignant transformation, the basal layer remains intact, thus AK is managed as a premalignant condition, predisposing to squamous carcinoma. However, not all actinic keratotic patches will progress to a malignancy.

Squamous Carcinoma-In-Situ

These lesions look similar to AK, but histology shows dysplastic changes extending the full thickness from basal layer to the surface, yet without invasion. The lesion is termed carcinoma-in-situ, also known as *Bowen disease* (Fig. 46.6). The aetiology is cumulative sun exposure and though it typically occurs on sun-exposed sites, it can occur on other parts of the body. Eczema unresponsive to topical treatments could be Bowen disease and thus a biopsy should be performed.

When Bowen disease occurs on the glans penis, it is known as **erythroplasia of Queyrat**.

Management of Squamous Carcinoma-In-Situ

Conservative management includes advice on limiting sun exposure and using sun screen skin protection. Patient choice may be to watch and wait with regular follow-up for possible invasive SCC, but medical treatment with topical 5-fluorouracil or imiquimod cream is possible, either alone or in combination. Alternative options include cryotherapy, curettage or excision.

Lentigo Maligna

Lentigo maligna are slowly-growing lesions confined to the epidermis (also known as *melanoma-in-situ*), which can transform to become invasive MM. Lesions have an indeterminate edge even under dermatoscope evaluation and can have varying pigmentation across their width. These are best managed by surgical excision, taking a 5-mm margin of healthy tissue to reduce the risk of local recurrence. A large resulting defect may need reconstructing with a skin graft or flap, depending on the site of the lesion.

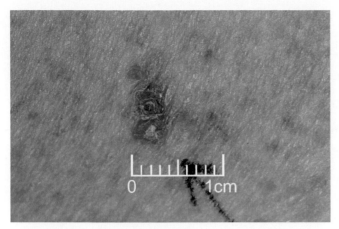

• **Fig. 46.6** Squamous Carcinoma-In-Situ or Bowen Disease.

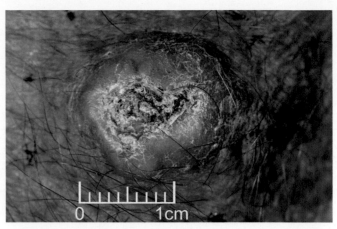

• **Fig. 46.7** Keratocanthoma—like squamous cell carcinoma (SCC).

Malignant Skin Conditions

Squamous Cell Carcinoma

Cutaneous SCCs (cSCCs) occur anywhere on the skin, particularly in areas repeatedly exposed to ultraviolet light, and usually in older age groups. Historically, cSCCs developed in skin chronically exposed to industrial carcinogens, such as arsenic or chromium compounds, soot, tar, pitch or mineral oils. Examples include carcinoma of the scrotum in chimney sweeps in the 19th century, with soot as a predisposing factor, whilst smokers are at risk for developing SCCs on the lips.

Chronic inflammation in chronic nonhealing burn wounds, osteomyelitis sinuses or longstanding ulcers predisposes to SCC. These SCCs are termed **Marjolin ulcers** and tend to have a worse prognosis. Other risk factors for cSCCs include long-term immunosuppression, such as therapeutic in transplant patients and in those with leukaemias and lymphomas.

cSCC can present clinically as an enlarging painless ulcer with a rolled, indurated (hardened) margin. In other cases, lesions can have an exophytic (outward growing, proliferative) cauliflower-like appearance with areas of ulceration, bleeding or serous exudation. cSCCs can invade deeper tissues and metastasise, so it is important to determine whether the lesion is fixed to underlying structures, such as bone or cartilage and to examine the regional lymph nodes for spread.

Several histological subtypes are described. Microscopically, there is invasion of dysplastic keratinocytes (with varying differentiation) throughout the stratum basale to the dermis. The cells tend to form concentric layers, giving the appearance of keratin pearls. On dermoscopy examination, there may be glomerular or irregular vascular patterns and areas of erosion and ulceration. Clinically and even histologically, well-differentiated cSCCs can appear similar to KA (Fig. 46.7).

Cutaneous SCCs are graded using **Broder ratio** of differentiated to undifferentiated cells, and staged using Tumour Node Metastasis (TNM) classification. Lesions with poorly differentiated cells on histology, or perineural or perivascular invasion are more likely to recur and metastasise. Cutaneous SCCs are thus classified as low-risk or high-risk, according to the risk of recurrence and metastasis. High-risk cSCCs tend to have the following characteristics:

• Size—diameter >2 cm
• Site—ear, lip, central face, non-sun-exposed sites, within chronic wounds
• Patient immunosuppressed
• Histological features—tumour thickness >4 mm, poorly differentiated histology, or with invasion of the subcutaneous tissue, nerves and blood vessels

Management of Cutaneous Squamous Cell Carcinoma

Surgical excision is appropriate in most cases, with the margin width determined following a biopsy, and discussion at a specialist skin cancer MDT. In low risk tumours (<2 cm), a 4-mm peripheral margin is usually sufficient. In larger or high-risk lesions, a 6-mm peripheral margin is needed. If the lesion is large and has an indistinct border, **Mohs micrographic surgery** (MMS) can be carried out to preserve more normal tissue in cosmetically sensitive areas, such as around the eyes or nose, or in cases of recurrence, where the lesion edge is ill-defined. The principle is to take smaller margins with the initial lesion, rapidly freezing the lesion for immediate histology and depending upon the presence of remaining tumour, for further margins to be excised as necessary. This process is repeated until clear margins are obtained.

In cosmetically sensitive areas, such as the lip, radiotherapy alone is an option. For smaller, well-defined low risk lesions, alternative options include cryotherapy, curettage and cautery.

There is evidence to show that 75% of local recurrences and metastatic disease will be detected within the first 2 years, and up to 95% in the first 5 years, thus recommended follow up of cSCC is generally 3- to 4-monthly for the first 2 years, then 6-monthly for a further 3 years to a total of 5 years. This may vary according to specific tumour factors.

Basal Cell Carcinoma

BCCs are slow growing locally invasive malignant epidermal tumours that occur predominantly in sun exposed areas of the head, neck and limbs (80%) and most frequently over the age of 40 years (85%). Most BCCs arise on the upper part of the face (Fig. 46.8), although any area of skin can be involved. Most patients present early because lesions are so visible. In immunosuppressed patients, there is a greater risk of multiple BCCs and recurrences.

BCCs can be broadly categorised into low-risk (e.g., nodular, superficial) and high-risk (e.g., morpheic [ill defined and spreading laterally], infiltrative) although 26 histopathological types have been described. Lesions commonly present as pearly-white nodules with a rolled edge and a central ulceration or crust, often with arborising blood vessels. Although they are surface lesions, they have the potential to erode into underlying tissues, such as cartilage and bone if neglected (Fig. 46.9). A very small percentage of BCCs metastasise, although this is rare. Histologically, the central tumour cells have basophilic nuclei and small amounts of cytoplasm, whilst the peripheral cells are arranged in a palisade pattern reminiscent of normal basal cells.

Management of Basal Cell Carcinomas

Several options are available and depend upon risk status of the BCC and patient factors. Risk is deemed to be high in lesions of greater size (>2 cm) or poorly defined edges; if the lesion is a recurrence; or on biopsy is shown to have perineural or perivascular invasion or is of an infiltrative or morphoeic subtype. Other high-risk factors include immunosuppressed patients, or if lesions are located on the central face or ears.

Surgical treatment of BCC is excision with a margin width determined by the lesion size and definition of its edges. In 95%, a BCC with a well-defined margin and smaller than 2 cm can be cleared using a 4- to 5-mm peripheral margin and a deep cuff of fat. In larger BCCs with ill-defined margins, a 13- to 15-mm peripheral margin is needed to achieve the same percentage of clearance. Alternatively, Moh's micrographic surgery (MMS) can be carried out.

Low risk, small lesions can be treated by cryotherapy or topical chemotherapy with 5-fluorouracil or imiquimod cream, though a biopsy may be needed to confirm histological subtype to help assess risk. Other alternatives include local radiotherapy, curettage combined with electrocautery, carbon dioxide laser or Photo Dynamic Therapy (PDT). PDT is useful for superficial BCCs and uses a topical photosensitising agent (Methyl Amino-Levulinate [MAL]-cream) and light therapy. The lesion is first curetted, then MAL cream is applied and left to absorb for up to 3 hours, then it is exposed to red light with a wavelength of 630 nm. This causes oxygen free radicals to be created, aiming to selectively target tumour cells, while leaving normal cells unharmed. This procedure leaves minimal scarring and can give an excellent cosmetic result.

In patients with inoperable BCC, or patients with large BCCs who do not want to have complex surgery, another option is oral vismodegib, a targeted therapy for part of the *hedgehog signalling pathway*.

Follow-up of BCCs depends on the perceived risk of recurrence and whether there have been previous lesions or recurrences. For most solitary BCC managed appropriately, self-checking (with written instructions) and referral back to the general practitioner for monitoring is sufficient in most cases.

Malignant Melanoma (Fig. 46.10)

In 2015 MM was the fifth most common cancer in the United Kingdom and accounted for 4% of skin cancers. The incidence rose by 128% over the previous 20 years and is projected to increase further over the next 20 years. Most subtypes of MM are predominately found in fair-skinned patients with a history of substantial sun exposure, although the **acral lentiginous subtype** is found in darker-skinned people. MM is the result of malignant transformation of melanocytes and there are several histological subtypes. Identifying a melanoma early gives a better prognostic outcome.

Risk Factors

Short periods of intense sun exposure leading to blistering sunburn appear to be more important risk factors for MM than the cumulative sun exposure leading to other skin malignancies. Unaccustomed exposure to strong sunlight can suppress immunological responses generally and, most likely, immunological tumour surveillance. This might explain MMs on areas of skin not generally exposed to sun, such as the soles of the feet and anal canal.

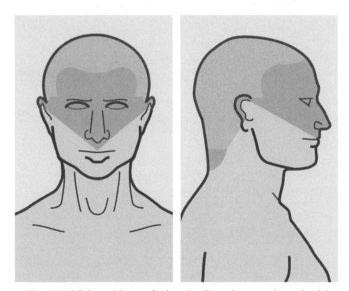

• **Fig. 46.8** Highest risk area for basal cell carcinomas shown in pink.

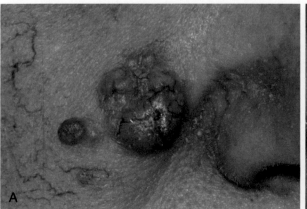
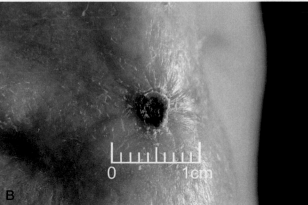

• **Fig. 46.9** **(A)** Nodular basal cell carcinoma with a rolled pearly edge. **(B)** Nodular basal cell carcinoma with central ulceration.

Other risk factors include **previous history** of melanoma and premalignant lesions (congenital melanotic naevi), sunbed use, family history of MM or atypical moles, large numbers of naevi and Fitzpatrick skin phototypes 1 and 2 (i.e., fair-skinned people with a tendency to burn easily in the sun). Patients with evident risk factors for melanoma can be referred to specialist clinics for counselling, mole mapping and training on self-examination of naevi.

Clinical Features of Malignant Melanoma

Most MMs have variations in pigmentation—a mixture of black, dark brown and pink—and can be flat or nodular lesions, which may bleed or ulcerate (Fig. 46.11). If a preexisting or new mole enlarges, darkens, bleeds or becomes inflamed, ulcerated or itchy, it must be regarded with great suspicion. Any new naevi in a patient over the age of 50 years should also be treated as suspicious. New pink lesions in individuals with skin phototypes

CASE HISTORIES

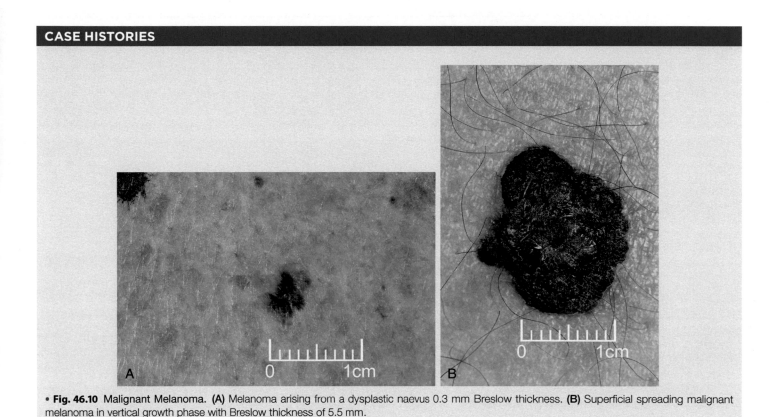

• **Fig. 46.10** Malignant Melanoma. **(A)** Melanoma arising from a dysplastic naevus 0.3 mm Breslow thickness. **(B)** Superficial spreading malignant melanoma in vertical growth phase with Breslow thickness of 5.5 mm.

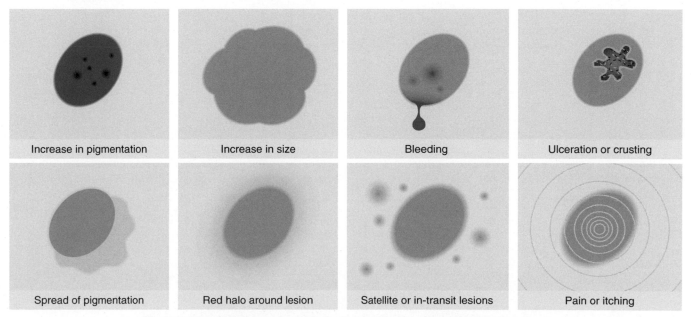

Increase in pigmentation   Increase in size   Bleeding   Ulceration or crusting

Spread of pigmentation   Red halo around lesion   Satellite or in-transit lesions   Pain or itching

• **Fig. 46.11** Clinical Features in a Pigmented Lesion That Suggest Malignant Melanoma.

TABLE 46.2	Risk of Regional and Distant Metastasis in Malignant Melanoma According to Breslow Thickness		
Tumour Thickness	Risk of Regional Metastases	Risk of Distant Metastases	10-Year Survival Without Nodal or Distant Metastases
Less than 1 mm	3%–5%	3%–5%	95%
1–4 mm	25%–60%	10%–20%	60%–75%
More than 4 mm	>60%	70%	45%

1 and 2 should be suspected of being amelanotic melanomas. **Superficial spreading melanoma** can be mistaken for a pigmented seborrhoeic keratosis and can bleed with trauma (see Fig. 46.2). Lateral spread of melanomas in dermal lymphatics may produce **satellite lesions** around the primary nodule, and **'in-transit'** lesions along the course of lymphatic drainage. Haematogenous spread occurs later and can involve lung, liver, bone, brain and other tissues.

Melanoma Subtypes

The presentation of melanoma depends on its subtype. The most common are **superficial spreading** and **nodular**, but other variants include amelanotic, lentigo maligna melanoma and acral lentiginous types. Rarer subtypes are sometimes seen in specialist clinics.

Superficial spreading melanoma is the most common form of melanoma. It usually presents as a broadening pigmented macule owing to the initial epidermal radial growth phase, and later can become thicker and more nodular during the vertical growth phase.

Nodular melanoma is the second most common form. These lesions are defined by a greater vertical growth phase and are considered more invasive; they appear not to spread superficially. Five percent of nodular melanomas are amelanotic.

Lentigo maligna melanoma arises from lentigo maligna, when the abnormal melanocytes have invaded the dermis. It is typically seen on the face.

Acral lentiginous melanoma occurs on the palms or soles or under the nails and can appear as a 'smudge' of pigmentation. They are the most common form of melanoma in non-white people (also refer to subungual melanoma on p. 602).

Amelanotic melanoma is a rarer form often missed in its early stages because it is clinically similar to common benign skin lesions. A new pink area within an existing naevus may reflect the neovascularisation of a neoplasm and thus warrants investigation.

Desmoplastic melanoma of desmoplastic-spindling stroma is a rare subtype that presents as a thickening and scar-like lesion, and is often but not always nonpigmented. These are often found on the head and neck of elderly men rather than women.

Mucosal melanoma is rare and can occur on any mucosal surface from mouth to anus, pharynx, paranasal sinuses or vagina. Mucosal melanomas often behave aggressively, in part because of late diagnosis owing to nonvisible locations. Risk factors include viral infections such as human immunodeficiency virus (HIV), and chemical and physical irritants.

Ocular melanoma arises from uveal melanocytes and is the most common ocular malignancy. It can affect the iris, ciliary body and posterior uvea. Most are thought to be sporadic, but there is a higher prevalence in skin phototype 1 individuals.

Prognostic Factors

When diagnosed in stage 1 (<1 mm thickness ± ulceration), survival rates at 5 years are 100%. This drops to 80% to 90% for stage 2 (1–2 mm thickness ± ulceration), 50% for stage 3 (2–4 mm thickness ± ulceration) and 10% to 25% for stage 4 (>4 mm thickness ± ulceration). Early diagnosis is key in survival. Features that can affect the prognosis include the site, tumour thickness on histological examination and the presence of ulceration. **Breslow thickness** is the measurement from stratum granulosum to the deepest point of tumour invasion, and has proved more accurate in prognostication than the older Clark level of invasion. Tumour thickness correlates with the likelihood of regional and distant metastases (Table 46.2). Other factors affecting prognosis include the mitotic index of the lesion, lymphovascular or perineural invasion, the presence of 'satellite lesions' around the primary or 'in-transit' lesions between the primary and draining lymph nodes. Lymph node metastases at the time of primary diagnosis is associated with a poorer outcome.

Management of Malignant Melanoma

A formal excision biopsy needs to be carried out to establish the diagnosis. The lesion should be excised with a 2-mm margin and a cuff of subcutaneous fat. For lesions in large or a cosmetically-sensitive areas, an incisional biopsy of the most suspicious area may be appropriate, or else the lesion can be excised completely and subjected to frozen section histology to confirm complete excision.

The histopathologist will comment on microscopic features recommended in the Royal College of Pathology datasets. These include the Breslow thickness, the Clark level of dermal invasion, the presence of ulceration, the mitotic rate, and the presence of lymphovascular and perineural invasion.

Overall surgical management is guided by histological reports of the primary excision. Melanomas are staged using the TNM system, incorporating the Breslow thickness, nodal involvement and evidence of other metastases.

Once MM has been diagnosed, surgical management involves **wide local excision** of the primary site, with the width determined by the Breslow thickness. The aim is to give optimum local control by removing micrometastases in the surrounding tissue.

Sentinel lymph node biopsy (SLNB) should be considered for tumours over 0.8 mm thick, and discussed with the patient. This aims to remove the first draining lymph node and identify microscopic spread within it. The node is identified in a way similar to breast cancer, by combined preoperative injection of radioactive tracer to the primary site and intraoperative lymphoscintigraphy, plus intraoperative injection of a blue dye. The Multicenter Selective Lymphadenectomy Trial

1 (MSLT-1) concluded that SLN status is the most important prognostic indicator of recurrence and survival in patients with intermediate thickness melanomas. The patient needs to understand that this is a diagnostic test, which gives good prognostic information, and it may give a survival benefit to some patients.

If the sentinel lymph node is positive, computed tomography (CT) scans may be performed to exclude distant disease. Traditionally, SLN+ patients were offered completion lymphadenectomy, but this carried substantial morbidity, such as seroma, infection, poor wound healing and lymphoedema. In 2018 the MSLT-2 trial found no difference in melanoma-specific survival in SLN+ patients having completion lymphadenectomy. Hence the current trend for SLN+ patients is for radiological surveillance, managing recurrences if and when they present.

Chemotherapy can be used alone for metastatic disease but gives poor results. However, improving understanding of the genetics and molecular biology of melanoma has led to recent development of targeted therapies. These include immunomodulatory medications, such as ipilimumab (a monoclonal antibody that prevents downregulation of T-cell activation, facilitating an immune response to malignant cells), and vemurafenib (a *BRAF* signal transduction inhibitor). Occasional complete cures of widespread disease have been reported with these newer agents and further work is urgently in progress.

Follow-up for melanoma patients depends on staging. Most patients are reviewed 3-monthly for 3 years, then 6-monthly to complete 5 years of follow-up. More advanced stage melanomas are followed up for 10 years, with annual follow-ups after 5 years. Patients are taught how to self-check likely lymph node regions of potential spread, and regular CT surveillance is often carried out on those with stage III disease.

Recurrent melanomas are managed with surgical or medical treatment, as advised by the specialist MDT. In locoregional recurrences, treatment options include surgically excising solitary lesions or electrochemotherapy (systemic chemotherapy plus short bursts of electrical energy to render cells permeable to it). Isolated limb infusion/perfusion chemotherapy may be offered in extensive limb disease, and targeted immunotherapy may be beneficial in systemic disease, depending on the melanoma's specific mutations (e.g., *BRAF*).

Merkel Cell Carcinoma

Merkel Cell Carcinoma is a rare and aggressive skin tumour of neural crest origin and is increasing in incidence. Risk factors include sun exposure, previous lymphoma and Merkel cell polyomavirus. The lesion presents as a firm and painless bluish-red nodule up to 5 cm in diameter; up to 80% develop lymph node metastases. Merkel cell carcinomas usually occur on the head and neck in elderly males. Treatment is usually wide local excision, and as the tumours are radiosensitive, radiotherapy to the primary site and regional lymph node basin.

Lesions Originating in the Dermis

Benign Dermal Lesions

Dermal lesions can arise from any skin appendages and over 80 different adnexal tumours are described. They are classified by the appendage from which they are derived.

Dermatofibroma

Dermatofibromas, also known as **histiocytomas**, are common painless skin lesions occurring mainly on the limbs, and are formed of an overgrowth of fibrous tissue in the dermis. Lesions present as firm nodules up to 1 cm in diameter and vary from pink to deep reddish-brown. They are mobile with the skin and have no deep attachments. Management is typically surgical excision.

Sebaceous Gland Lesions

Sebaceous gland hyperplasia can present as small yellowish papules and typically occur on the face. One example is a rhinophyma of the nose. Management may include shave excision, carbon dioxide laser or dermabrasion.

The sebaceous naevus of Jadassohn, often found on the scalp soon after birth, is a benign hair follicle tumour and a type of epidermal naevus, which presents as a smooth hairless patch of yellow-orange pigmentation. Although benign, there is a risk of malignant change (to BCC), and hence excision is warranted. This is often performed before the patient reaches adulthood.

Sebaceous adenomas present as solitary pink or yellow nodules on the head and neck in the elderly. Clinically these lesions are often mistaken for BCCs. In a younger person presenting with a sebaceous adenoma on the torso, the lesion should be excised and sent for immunohistochemistry diagnosis, owing to an association with Lynch syndrome and colon cancer.

Pilar Lesions

Pilar or trichilemmal cysts arise from the hair root sheath and can be large and numerous. Multiple cysts are less common on the face or neck than on the scalp. Pilar cysts range from a few mm to many cm in diameter but grow very slowly. They can readily be excised under local anaesthesia. Other benign lesions with hair follicle differentiation include trichoepithelioma, trichofolliculoma, trichoblastoma and trichilemmoma. If multiple trichilemmomas (small warty papules commonly on the face) are present, this can be diagnostic for Cowen disease, with a high risk of breast, endometrial and thyroid carcinoma.

Sweat Gland Lesions

Sweat glands can be of eccrine or apocrine differentiation. Benign lesions include poromas, syringoma, cylindromas and hidrocystomas.

Cysts

Epidermoid Cysts

These are far the most common superficial skin cysts and are often incorrectly described as 'sebaceous cysts'. Usually solitary, they may be found anywhere on the body (except the palms or soles), most commonly on the scalp, trunk, face and neck. They range up to several cm in diameter. Epidermoid cysts are smooth and rounded, covered by normal epidermis and usually have a visible punctum (a small opening that connects the cyst to the overlying epidermis). On palpation, they are a firm subcutaneous swelling. They originate in skin, so are attached to it, but are mobile over deeper tissues. Multiple small epidermoid cysts sometimes develop on the scrotal skin or areola and can cause embarrassment.

Histologically, an epidermal cyst has a stratified squamous lining epithelium and is filled with keratin and sebum, produced by the sebaceous gland, hence their common name of sebaceous cysts. Removal must include excision of the punctum and the entire cyst sac, without disrupting the sac itself. Recurrence is likely if remnants of the cyst are left.

Dermoid Cysts

Dermoid cysts are congenital lesions arising from differentiation of epithelial remnants left behind at lines of embryological fusion. They are usually found in the midline of the scalp, neck and lower jaw and at the outer angle of the eyebrow (external angular dermoid). Some midline facial dermoid cysts communicate with deeper structures, and these need imaging to exclude an intracranial extension. Treatment is by careful excision, including underlying tracts (if present), which may need more extensive surgery. True dermoid cysts are similar histologically to epidermal cysts, being lined by keratinising squamous epithelium. They can contain hair, sebaceous glands and other ectodermal structures, as well as keratin. Although present from birth, they may not become evident until the child grows.

Implantation Cysts

These small keratin-filled cysts arise from epidermal fragments implanted in the dermis by (minor) penetrating injuries, most often under a scar of a previous laceration. Though not derived from epidermal appendages, they are histologically similar to epidermoid cysts, but may contain small foreign bodies.

Surgical Management of Cutaneous Cysts (Also See Chapter 10)

Cysts need removing mainly because of recurrent inflammation and infection. In the acute inflammatory phase, the options for management include incision and drainage, or antibacterial therapies. Surgical excision of the cyst should not be undertaken when infected or inflamed, as identifying planes is difficult, and there is a real risk of incomplete excision and recurrence.

Miscellaneous Lesions

Keloid Scars

Keloids are formed by deposition of excessive collagen in the dermis during wound healing. The result is an elevated nodular lesion covered by normal epidermis, which can be tender, itchy or cause a burning sensation. Anyone can develop a keloid scar following even minor trauma to the skin, however they are more common in people with darker skin, and at certain sites of the body (e.g., the ear and presternal areas).

Treatments are nonsurgical or surgical and include compression and silicone dressings, topical and intralesional steroids, or intralesional excision. Often a single modality of treatment results in recurrence, so multimodality treatment is preferred (e.g., a keloid scar of the ear may be managed by intralesional excision followed by compression with a custom-made pressure clip). In extreme cases, excising the scar followed by low-dose radiotherapy may suppress further keloid.

Malignant Dermal Lesions

Cutaneous Sarcomas

Malignant fibrous histiocytoma are rare aggressive tumours. Ten percent present as firm nodules in subcutaneous tissue, most often in the thighs and upper limbs of older patients. These lesions are treated with surgical excision or MMS. Adjuvant radiotherapy is often used owing to the risk of recurrence.

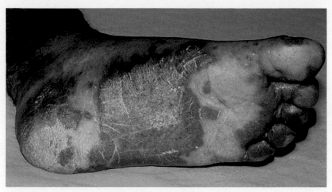

• **Fig. 46.12** Kaposi Sarcoma.

Atypical fibroxanthoma is a superficial form of malignant fibrous histiocytoma that presents with firm nodules in the dermis. These are also more common in older patients on the head and neck. These lesions are also treated with wide local excision but do not have the same risk of recurrence.

Dermatofibrosarcoma protuberans is a rare slowly growing tumour originating in the dermis. It can be locally aggressive, invading into soft tissues and bone. It initially presents as a firm red nodule or plaque, usually on the torso or proximal limbs, and often in young adults. Surgical excision with a wide margin of 2 to 4 cm down to and including fascia was traditionally used, but Mohs surgery gives lower recurrence rates. The tyrosine kinase inhibitor, imatinib, can be used for inoperable, metastatic or recurrent disease.

Secondary (Metastatic) Carcinoma

With skin metastases, there is usually a history of treated malignancy elsewhere. Metastatic tumour deposits often present as small hard painless skin nodules, which are usually located in the dermis and covered by normal epidermis. Visceral malignancy, for example, pancreatic or colon cancer, can present with a metastasis at the umbilicus (Sister Joseph nodule). Carcinomas of breast, stomach, uterus, lungs, large bowel and kidneys can also metastasise to skin. Occasionally, biopsy of a mysterious skin lesion leads to a diagnosis of occult malignancy. Management depends on the primary diagnosis, but the prognosis is usually poor. Treatment is palliative, or by local excision, radiotherapy or chemotherapy, depending on the severity of symptoms and the size, number and location of secondaries.

Kaposi Sarcoma

There are four variants of Kaposi sarcoma (KS): HIV-related, classic, transplant and endemic. All are associated with human herpes virus 8 and frequently affect the skin and mouth. Lesions appear as painless, bluish-red to brown nodules or plaques, which may progress and merge to form a single larger lesion (Fig. 46.12). Excision biopsy confirms the diagnosis. KSs are characterised by proliferating dysplastic fibroblasts accompanied by chronic inflammation, endothelial proliferation and haemorrhage. Treatment depends upon the subtype. The classical type usually does not need treatment, but larger lesions respond to radiotherapy, cryotherapy or excision. Endemic KS is in many cases caused by undiagnosed HIV and is treated with antiretroviral therapy similarly to HIV-related KS. Transplant KS needs to be treated quickly by reducing or changing immunosuppressants. If this is not successful, it may require radiotherapy and chemotherapy.

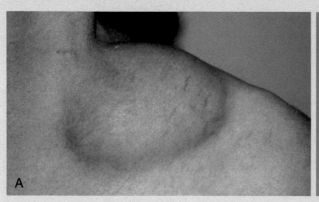
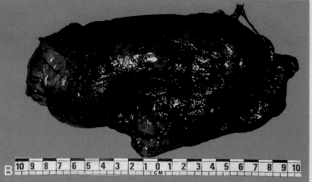

• **Fig. 46.13** Lipoma. **(A)** Large soft lipoma overlying the supraclavicular fossa in a 46-year-old woman. This is a common site for lipomas. It had been present for many years but had recently started to enlarge. **(B)** The surgical specimen. Note that it is larger than its clinical appearance would suggest.

Lesions of the Hypodermis and Deeper Tissues

Lipoma and Liposarcoma

Lipomas are benign tumours of fat and can occur anywhere fat is normally present, though most frequently in the hypodermis of trunk and limbs (Fig. 46.13). Lipomas have a soft consistency and vary greatly in size. They consist of a multilobular mass of fatty tissue with thin fibrous septa. A tenuous fibrous capsule usually defines the lesion clearly from surrounding tissue. Lipoma cells are histologically indistinguishable from normal adipocytes. Lesions are excised if they cause compression symptoms or for cosmetic reasons.

If there is concern about potentially sinister features, such as pain, diameter greater than 5 cm, rapid growth or location deep to the fascia, the lump should be investigated to exclude sarcoma. Sarcomas arise from mesenchymal tissues, which form connective tissues, such as muscle, bone and fat. **Liposarcoma** is a rare malignant tumour of fat cells (though still the second most common sarcoma). It usually occurs in adults and is a soft tissue sarcoma with five histological subtypes. Initial imaging is usually with ultrasound, but magnetic resonance imaging scanning with gadolinium contrast gives a definitive image. CT scanning can identify solid, mixed or pseudocystic patterns of tissue, and can assess for metastatic disease. Diagnosis is confirmed by biopsy and treatment involves specialist centres and a MDT approach. Surgical excision and sometimes radiotherapy aims to achieve local control. Systemic control may include chemotherapy. Follow-up depends on the type and grade and is tailored according to the risk of recurrence.

Neurofibroma, Neurofibromatosis and Schwannoma

Neurofibromas are benign nonencapsulated tumours arising from nonmyelinated Schwann cells that make up the sheaths of peripheral nerve cells, or from fibroblasts. Neurofibromas may be dermal or plexiform subtypes, and plexiform can be subdivided into nodular or diffuse. Neurofibromas may present in the skin as solitary sessile or pedunculated lesions near peripheral nerves.

Neurofibromatosis has two main forms; both can be autosomal dominant inherited conditions, via a gene on chromosome 17, although 50% arise spontaneously by mutation. Type 1 neurofibromatosis, also known as **von Recklinghausen disease**, is

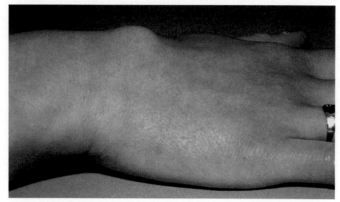

• **Fig. 46.14** Ganglion. This ganglion is in a common site, the dorsum of the hand.

characterised by the presence of more than two of the following: multiple neurofibromas, axillary and/or inguinal freckling, more than six café-au-lait spots (coffee-coloured skin patches), more than two Lisch nodules (iris hamartomas) and optic glioma. Associated features in type 1 include hypertension, scoliosis and learning difficulties. People with neurofibromatosis type 1 have a 10% lifetime chance of developing a malignant peripheral nerve sheath tumour, within a plexiform neurofibroma. Neurofibromas can be numerous and cause pain by nerve compression and may require excision.

Neurofibromatosis type 2 is known as *central neurofibromatosis* and often presents as bilateral vestibular schwannomas.

Schwannomas are benign encapsulated tumours arising from Schwann cells supporting peripheral nerves. They present as firm, nodular lesions tethered to a nerve. Pressure on the nerve may cause pain in its distribution. Treatment is by careful excision, attempting to preserve the affected nerve, using an operating microscope and microsurgical manipulation.

Ganglia

Ganglia are mucin-filled cysts attached to joint capsules or tendon sheath. They present as firm, immobile lumps, which can be painful (Fig. 46.14). They are most common at the wrist, dorsum of the hand and around the ankle. The skin is normal and mobile. It may be possible to transilluminate a ganglion. Historical treatment was a sharp blow with a heavy book (often the family bible), which would dissipate the cyst contents into the tissues, but recurrence

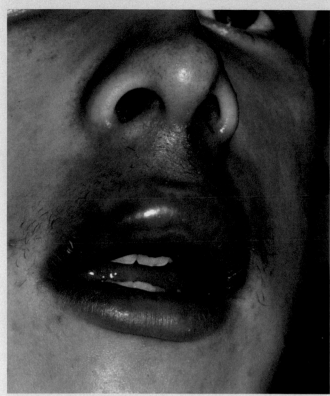

• **Fig. 46.15** Acute Cellulitis of Upper Lip. This 18-year-old presented with 4 days of increasing swelling and pain affecting the upper lip following 'picking' of an acne spot. This infection lies in the 'danger triangle' involving the nose and upper lip, where serious infection can be complicated by cavernous sinus thrombosis. This patient responded rapidly to intensive antibiotic therapy. The organism proved to be *Streptococcus pyogenes*.

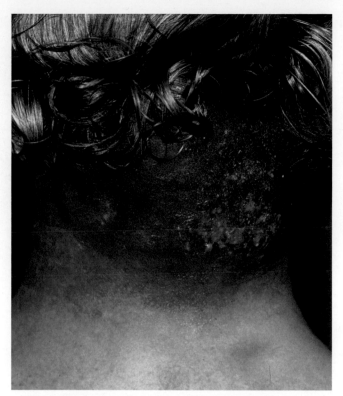

• **Fig. 46.16** Carbuncle on Back (Nape) of Neck.

rates were high. If not interfering with function, ganglia can be left alone and reassurance given; they sometimes resolve spontaneously. Needle aspiration can give temporary symptomatic relief, and surgical excision is possible but recurrence is common.

Inflammatory and Infective Lesions

Furuncle (Boil) and Carbuncle

A **furuncle** is a staphylococcal abscess that develops in a hair follicle in the dermis. Small lesions can be easily treated with topical fusidic acid. Diabetes can be a predisposing factor. The lesion enlarges rapidly and eventually 'points' at the surface, spontaneously discharging pus. In larger lesions, the centre can contain a core of necrotic tissue. Once pus has discharged, the lesion heals spontaneously but a necrotic core may need excising to speed healing. Drainage may be encouraged with poultices, such as magnesium sulphate paste. Furuncles are most common in young men with acne, especially on the face, back and lower limbs. Axillary furuncles are common in middle-aged women and tend to recur. Surgical treatment may be needed if a chronic abscess develops. A furuncle may be a source of sepsis, especially in uncontrolled diabetes. **Cavernous sinus thrombosis** is a rare but very serious (and often fatal) complication of a furuncle on the lateral aspect of the nose/infraorbital area. This area drains into the cavernous sinus via the facial vein and inferior ophthalmic veins (Fig. 46.15).

A **carbuncle**, also staphylococcal, is larger than a furuncle and consists of a honeycomb of abscesses, often draining (inadequately) via multiple sinuses. The back (nape) of the neck is the usual site (Fig. 46.16); here the skin is tightly bound by interlacing bundles of fibrous tissue. Carbuncles are more likely to occur in diabetics, and may bring diabetes to light. Treatment is with antistaphylococcal antibiotics, such as flucloxacillin as early as possible. The aim is to minimise pus formation and necrosis that would lead to skin loss and delay healing. If pus has formed, thorough desloughing and drainage of the abscesses is required, usually leaving wounds open to heal by secondary intention.

Necrotising Fasciitis

This serious and alarming condition is usually a complication of surgery or traumatic wounds and is covered in Chapters 3 and 17.

Lesions of Vascular Origin

Vascular anomalies are currently classified according to the 2018 International Society for the Study of Vascular Anomalies, and are broadly classified into tumours (which can be benign, borderline or locally aggressive, or malignant—Table 46.3), and malformations (Table 46.4). **Angioma** is a term given to a lesion of endothelial cell origin arising from the vascular or lymphatic vessel wall.

Pyogenic Granuloma

Pyogenic granulomas are benign lesions that arise following irritation, hormonal changes or trauma, although the actual cause is not known. There is overgrowth of highly vascularised and friable tissue, resulting in profuse bleeding (Fig. 46.17). Pyogenic granulomas appear as red fleshy nodules that may be polypoid. They usually develop over about a week and can be variously managed with cautery, curettage, excision or laser surgery.

TABLE 46.3 Vascular Anomalies

Benign	Locally Aggressive or Borderline	Malignant
Infantile Haemangioma	Kaposiform Hemangioendothelioma	Angiosarcoma
Congenital Haemangioma	Retiform Hemangioendothelioma	Epitheliod Haemangioendothelioma
Tufted Angioma	Dabska Tumour	
Spindle-cell Haemangioma	Composite Haemangioendothelioma	
Epithelioid Haemangioma	Kaposi Sarcoma	
Pyogenic Granuloma	Polymorphous Hemangioendothelioma	
Others	Others	

TABLE 46.4 Vascular Malformations and Associated Clinical Syndromes

Simple	Combined	Malformations of Major Named Vessels	Associated With Other Syndromes
Capillary Malformation (CM)	CVM, CLM	Also known as *Channel type* or *Truncal* Vascular Malfor- mations	Klippel-Trenaunay Syndrome
Lymphatic Malformation (LM)	LVM, CLVM		Parkes-Weber Syndrome
Venous Malformation (VM)	CAVM	Described by what is 'affected' (lymphatics, veins or	Sturge-Weber Syndrome
Arteriovenous Malformation (AVM)	CLAVM	arteries) or the 'anomalies of' (origin, course, number,	CLOVES Syndrome
Arteriovenous Fistula (AVF)		length, diameter, etc.)	

Combinations are created as follows:
- CM + VM (CVM)
- LM + VM (LVM)
- CM + LM + VM (CLVM)
- CM + AVM + VM (CAVM)
- CM + LM + AVM + VM (CLAVM).

For example: Klippel-Trenaunay syndrome is a combined capillary lymphaticovenous malformation (CM + VM +/- LM + limb overgrowth); Parkes-Weber syndrome is a combined capillary arteriovenous malformation (CM + AVF + limb overgrowth). **CLOVES** syndrome is **C**ongenital **L**ipomatous **O**vergrowth, **V**ascular Malformations, **E**pidermal nevi and **S**coliosis/skeletal/spinal anomalies, and is a rare condition, with a subgroup also having AVMs around the spinal cord.

CASE HISTORY

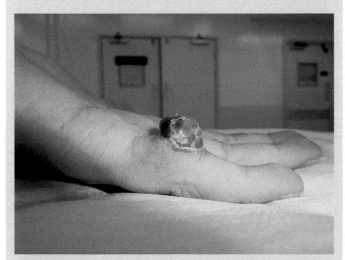

• **Fig. 46.17** Pyogenic Granuloma. This man of 29 years suffered a minor penetrating injury to his forearm from a piece of sharp metal. The wound did not heal normally but produced this friable proliferative lesion. The appearance is typical of a pyogenic granuloma, composed largely of granulation tissue. It was removed by curettage under local anaesthesia and healing afterwards was uninterrupted.

Infantile Haemangioma

Infantile haemangiomas are benign vascular tumours, also known as **strawberry naevi**, which appears in the first few months of life. They present initially as bright-red fleshy lesions, which go through three phases: the lesion grows for up to a year in the **proliferating** phase. There is then a **static** phase, before the **involuting** phase, which occurs over several years, where the lesion becomes less vivid and regresses. The skin then appears normal but some are left with loose thin skin. Large haemangiomas can cause obstruction, for example, ocular (disrupting visual development), oral (risk of airway compromise) or aural (can lead to conductive deafness). Other complications can include infection and high cardiac output in very large lesions. Lesions at risk of causing occlusion or bleeding, can be treated with oral beta-blockers, such as propranolol. Recent treatments include intralesional steroids and laser ablation. Surgical excision may leave a disfiguring scar and risks recurrence. Watch and wait observation is the mainstay of management for most cases, with surgery only indicated to deal with redundant skin after involution.

Campbell De Morgan Spots

These small, bright-red spots on the trunk, usually in older patients are also known as *cherry haemangiomas*. These highly localised capillary proliferations blanch when compressed and then refill and do not need treatment.

Glomus Tumour (Glomangioma)

This is an uncommon benign tumour derived from glomus bodies (small arteriovenous communications found normally in fingers and often beneath the nails, although sometimes in the gastrointestinal or respiratory tract). Lesions usually present as small (1–3 mm) red nodules, which are exquisitely tender to the touch or with changes in temperature. Treatment is by surgical excision and specimens should be sent for histological evaluation. as they can have malignant features.

Vascular Malformations

Vascular malformations are not tumours. Malformations can be capillary, venous, arterial, lymphatic or mixed origin. They can be classified into high or low flow lesions, and can be associated with syndromes (see Table 46.4). They arise from a development anomaly and are present from birth. They do not regress, and often grow progressively.

Spider Naevi

Spider naevi are small red lesions consisting of an enlarged central arteriole from which radiate dilated capillaries. Also termed *spider angiomas*, they can be isolated lesions found in normal people but are more common in patients with thyroid and chronic liver disease, or in pregnancy when levels of oestrogen are high. These lesions can sometimes regress and treatment is not usually necessary. Laser therapy is an option for aesthetic management, but there is a risk of recurrence.

Capillary Malformations

'**Port-wine stains**' can occur anywhere, but can cause cosmetic distress when on the face, neck and/or scalp. They are present from birth and remain unchanged throughout life. Lesions are flat or slightly elevated and reddish-blue, with an asymmetrical outline and range up to many centimetres in diameter. Trauma may cause bleeding or ulceration. Treatment options include laser therapy, such as the pulse dye laser tuned to the frequency of haemoglobin. Covering cosmetics remain the best advice for most.

Port-wine stains can be associated with other conditions. For example, one located over the ophthalmic division of the trigeminal nerve could indicate the presence of Sturge-Weber syndrome, a neurocutaneous condition accompanied by facial capillary malformations ± cerebral and ocular vascular malformations.

Klippel–Trenaunay syndrome is a combined capillary-lymphaticovenous malformation also characterised by varicose veins and bone and soft tissue hypertrophy, involving one or more limb and may include the pelvis.

Lesions Derived From Skin Appendages

Benign Appendage Tumours

Cylindroma

This is the most common appendage tumour and is derived from sweat glands. Diagnosis is usually made only on histological examination of an excised nondescript skin lump.

Pilonidal Sinus and Abscess are described in Chapter 30.

Disorders of the Nails

Ingrowing Toenail

Pathophysiology

An ingrowing toenail (Fig. 46.18) occurs when the distal edge of the nail persistently cuts into the adjacent nail fold. The problem almost always affects the great toe. In effect, there is a laceration, which cannot heal because of the presence of a foreign body (the toenail). Superimposed infection by local bacterial and fungal flora complicates the picture. The combination of acute inflammation and attempts at repair produces exuberant granulation tissue around the laceration, plus inflammatory swelling. Swelling aggravates trauma caused by the nail edge.

Ingrowing toenail is mainly confined to teenagers and young adults, particularly males. It probably results from a combination of inadequate hygiene, unsuitable footwear, cutting the nails too short at the corners and the macerating effect of sweat on the skin. High levels of circulating testosterone in adolescence may be an aetiological factor.

Management

The main objective of treatment is to prevent persistent trauma by the nail edge. Surgical operations result in a week or more of discomfort and immobility, so conservative treatment should be tried first.

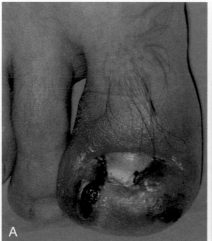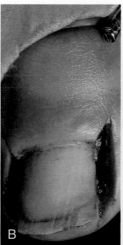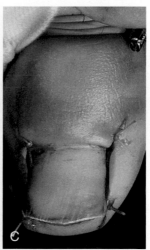

• **Fig. 46.18** Ingrowing Toenail. **(A)** Inflamed ingrowing toenail affecting medial and lateral sides. There is a great amount of hypertrophy, making suitable footwear hard to find. **(B)** and **(C)** A different patient undergoing wedge resection and phenolisation of both sides of the nail. Note the use of a tourniquet.

Conservative Treatment

In all cases, simple conservative measures include regular bathing, frequent changes of socks (which should be cotton), avoiding tight or narrow shoes and avoiding trauma to the toe when inflamed, for example, from kicking a football.

For an inflamed ingrowing toenail, foot soaks in warm saline should be carried out twice daily for at least 10 minutes. Surgical spirit applied twice daily may also help. Once inflammation is settling, a useful further measure is to pack a small pledget of cotton wool beneath the nail corner to lift it out of the laceration. At the same time, the nail fold can be pushed away by packing an elongated pledget between nail fold and nail edge. These tiny packs can be left in place for days but need to be expanded as the nail corner rises away from its bed. Loose fitting footwear should be worn.

Conservative measures often succeed even in severe cases but demand perseverance. Systemic antibiotics should be used only if infection is spreading; topical antibiotics are of little use.

Surgical Treatment

Urgent surgical treatment involves avulsing the whole nail, or removing one side of it. This immediately removes the 'foreign body' and permits rapid resolution. For recurrent ingrowing toenails, particularly if abnormal nail morphology is a factor, part of the nail bed is best removed. Popular procedures are illustrated in Fig. 46.19. Operations are usually performed under local anaesthesia using a ring block and tourniquet. Local anaesthetic incorporating a vasoconstrictor, such as adrenaline (epinephrine) must *never* be used in digits, because of the risk of ischaemic necrosis.

Onychogryphosis

Onychogryphosis ('ram's horn nail') (Fig. 46.20) is a gross abnormality of nail growth. It affects the great toenail, which becomes thickened and distorted, so nail cutting with ordinary nail scissors becomes impossible. Onychogryphosis is usually seen only in elderly patients and probably results from previous nail bed trauma. The condition usually presents when it interferes with wearing shoes. A chiropodist (podiatrist) can treat onychogryphosis with

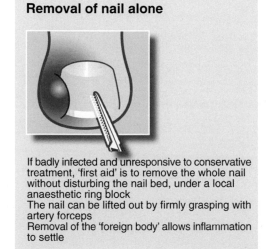
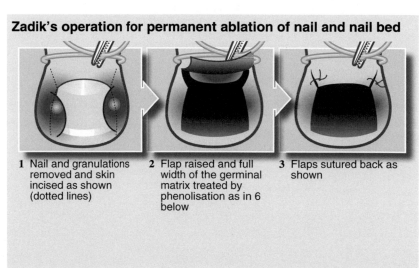
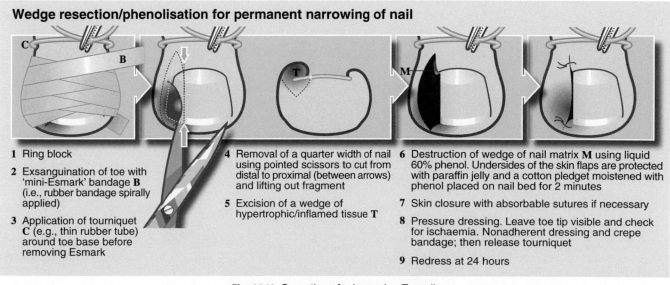

• **Fig. 46.19** Operations for Ingrowing Toenail.

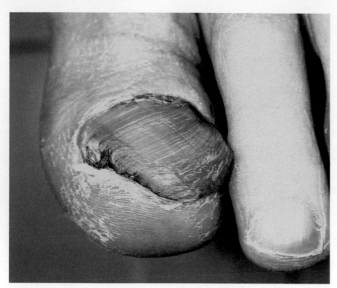

• **Fig. 46.20** Onychogryphosis. Moderate degree of nail thickening and 'heaping up'.

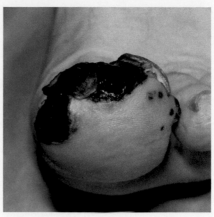

• **Fig. 46.21** Subungual Malignant Melanoma. Aggressive malignant melanoma arising from beneath the nail of the first toe. Note the large main lesion and the satellite lesions nearby. This patient died of melanomatosis 1 year after this picture was taken.

grinding instruments, at regular intervals. Surgical removal of the nail and ablation of the bed is sometimes performed.

Subungual Melanoma

MMs sometimes develop beneath finger or toenails (Fig. 46.21). They are difficult to diagnose—historically such melanomas in less obvious areas have a reputation for aggressive behaviour, but this may be because of late diagnosis. Melanoma under finger or toenails can easily be mistaken for old subungual haematomas, but these migrate distally as the nail plate grows whereas melanoma does not. Nail melanomas often present early as a changing pigmented nail streak or **longitudinal melanonychia**. Features suggesting melanoma include widening of the pigmentation band, nail distortion or pigmentation becoming more proximal. Advanced melanoma presents as destruction of the nail bed, which is replaced by an ulcerating growth. Any suspicious lesion under the nail should be biopsied to avoid the disaster of missing a potentially curable MM.

47

Lumps in the Head and Neck and Salivary Calculi

CHAPTER OUTLINE

Introduction

Neck lumps are common and may be related to disorders of the mouth, throat or skin. Infection in the cervical region can cause difficulty swallowing (dysphagia) and put the airway at risk. Referrals are often made to exclude malignancy, whilst some are for surgical treatment of a metabolic disorder, such as thyrotoxicosis or hyperparathyroidism. There is a large overlap with specialties in this area, notably ear, nose and throat (ENT), oral and maxillofacial surgery, plastic surgery and dermatology.

Thyroid swellings may be confused with other anterior neck swellings, so head and neck examination must include the thyroid area, described in Chapter 49.

In hospitals, mouth problems are managed by oral and maxillofacial surgeons, but patients often obtain advice first from other clinicians, particularly in emergency departments. As such, it is important they understand the presentation of oral and dental disease and appreciate the necessary management (see also Ch. 48).

History and Examination in the Head and Neck

Many different tissues are concentrated here, so there is a profusion of conditions causing lumps. Box 47.1 provides a simple classification.

Special Points in the History and Examination

As always, the history provides important clues to the diagnosis. The patient's age, the rate of growth of the lump and symptoms, such as pain, discharge or swelling related to eating ('mealtime syndrome') may point to the diagnosis.

Most lumps are best examined with the patient sitting, so the examiner can palpate from in front and behind. The examiner should establish the **characteristics of the lump** (Box 47.2) and determine how it relates to overlying or underlying structures. For example, a lump in the cheek may originate in skin, parotid, buccinator muscle, oral mucosa or parotid duct. In clinical examinations, it is useful to describe the characteristics as if to someone who cannot see the patient.

With a lump or swelling, the whole of scalp, back of neck and skin behind and in the ears should be examined. Head and neck lymph nodes must be palpated. A simple method considers nodes lying in two planes, horizontal and vertical (Fig. 47.1), which can be examined systematically. For lumps in the lower half of the face or submandibular region, the **oral cavity** should be examined to exclude salivary gland lesions, oral malignancies or sources of infection, such as a dental abscess. For lumps in the parotid region, the integrity of the **facial nerve** should be tested since malignant tumours often cause neurological deficits. If the presenting complaint is **lymph node enlargement**, nasendoscopy of upper airways and pharynx may be necessary to exclude primary tumours or infected lesions.

Examination of the Oral Cavity

For many doctors, asking the patient to open the mouth represents the entire oral examination; however, the simple but thorough technique illustrated in Fig. 47.2A–D, will enable most significant lesions to be seen without special instruments.

First, the patient should remove dentures. Then lips and their mucosal lining, and the lining of cheeks and gums are inspected. To do this, the lips are retracted by the examiner's gloved fingers or a wooden spatula and the mouth illuminated with a pen torch. Teeth are inspected for obvious decay and gum inflammation. A flap of gum over a partially erupted lower wisdom tooth can cause painful inflammation (see Fig. 48.6).

If parotid disease is suspected, the duct papilla opposite the upper second molar should be identified and palpated. If the patient has dentures or irregular teeth, inspect for papillary scarring causing obstruction. The palate is best examined if the patient tilts the head backwards. Finally, the tongue and floor of the mouth are inspected for mucosal lesions. To assist, the patient first protrudes, then elevates the tongue before finally pushing the tongue towards the left and right cheeks.

Lumps in the floor of the mouth, submandibular area and cheeks should be palpated **bimanually** as shown in Fig. 47.2D. Lumps in these areas are often mobile and tend to move away from examining fingers.

Tumours of Salivary Glands

There are three pairs of major salivary glands, **parotid**, **submandibular** and **sublingual**. The parotid produces serous (watery) saliva, the submandibular a mixed seromucous saliva and the sublingual a more mucous secretion. The parotid and submandibular glands each drain into the mouth via long ducts, whereas the sublingual drains via multiple small ducts into the floor of the mouth, sometimes via the submandibular duct.

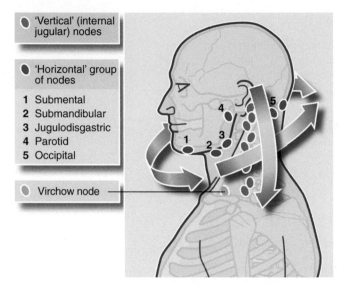

'Vertical' (internal jugular) nodes

'Horizontal' group of nodes

1 Submental
2 Submandibular
3 Jugulodigastric
4 Parotid
5 Occipital

Virchow node

• **Fig. 47.1** Simple Technique for Palpating Head and Neck Lymph Nodes.

Surgical disorders of major salivary glands include benign and malignant tumours, stones, bacterial and viral infections and rare autoimmune disorders, all of which present as salivary gland lumps. The oral mucosa also contains numerous small 'minor' salivary glands, which can undergo neoplastic change or form retention cysts.

Salivary Gland Tumours

Pleomorphic Adenoma

Pleomorphic adenoma presents as slow growing, painless lumps (Fig. 47.3). Most are in the parotid, some in the submandibular gland and a few are in minor salivary glands. Pleomorphic adenoma is the most common lump in the parotid and by far the most common salivary gland neoplasm. Eighty percent of parotid tumours are benign and of these, 80% are pleomorphic adenomas. They present in middle age or later, and both sexes are equally affected.

Pleomorphic adenomas are derived from salivary gland epithelium and are benign but show variable differentiation. The name comes from the varied histological appearance. Columns and islands of neoplastic epithelial cells are separated by myxomatous connective tissue stroma, often with areas resembling immature cartilage. Some without myxomatous tissue are described as **monomorphic**.

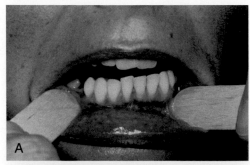
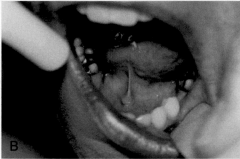
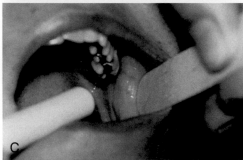
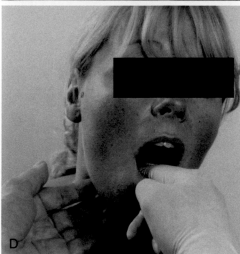

• **Fig. 47.2** Technique of Oral Examination. Teeth, gums and buccal sulci can be inspected by retracting the lips with wooden spatulas or fingers **(A)**. The palate is inspected by tilting the patient's head back and retracting the lips, and the floor of the mouth, and movements of the tongue examined as shown in **(B)**. The parotid papilla is demonstrated in **(C)**. Finally, bimanual palpation of the submandibular area, including the course of the submandibular duct, is performed with a gloved finger inside the mouth, as shown in **(D)**.

Pleomorphic adenomas have a well-defined but thin capsule over a nodular surface, which is important when attempting removal, as there is a risk of incomplete excision and consequent

recurrence. They also have a 1% year-on-year risk of malignant change (carcinoma-ex-pleomorphic adenoma).

Most parotid tumours occur in the superficial part, external to the plane of the facial nerve. Occasionally, they occur in the deep part in intimate association with the facial nerve. In either case, the tumour can extend between the nerve branches, but being benign, it does not invade the nerve to cause facial palsy. Facial nerve damage is a risk during excision, especially of deeper lesions. Patients should be warned of this possibility before operation.

If an older patient has a slowly growing solid parotid lump without facial palsy, it is best to assume it is a pleomorphic adenoma or Warthin tumour (adenolymphoma). Definitive diagnosis can usually be made by ultrasonography and core biopsy or by fine-needle aspiration cytology and confirmed histologically after excision. If malignancy is suspected, computed tomography scanning may be needed.

Treatment

Treatment is by excision. For superficial lesions, the standard operation has long been a **superficial or partial superficial parotidectomy** to excise all glandular tissue superficial to the facial nerve. This is effectively a facial nerve dissection. Nowadays, many surgeons perform **extracapsular dissection** of the lump alone and in benign disease, this cures the problem and carries a lower risk of side-effects, particularly facial nerve damage and **Frey syndrome** of gustatory sweating (see later). Recurrence is uncommon with either procedure. For deeper lesions, an attempt should be made to excise the entire lesion, carefully identifying and preserving the facial nerve branches.

Complications of Parotid Surgery

The main complication is facial nerve injury. Damage to the temporal or zygomatic branches may impair closure of the eye, leading to corneal drying and damage. Mandibular branch damage causes weakness at the angle of the mouth leading to oral incontinence and a lopsided smile. Nerve damage may also complicate submandibular gland excision: the mandibular branch of the facial nerve is vulnerable if the incision is sited too high. The lingual and hypoglossal nerves lie close to the deep surface of the gland; injury causes unilateral tongue wasting and numbness, respectively.

Salivary fistula is an occasional complication following parotid surgery, causing saliva to leak onto the face at mealtimes. The fistula usually resolves spontaneously after several weeks.

Frey syndrome is a late complication of superficial parotidectomy in 25% or more cases, but is virtually unknown after extracapsular dissection. It probably results from divided parasympathetic secretomotor fibres regenerating in the skin, where they assume control of sweat gland activity. Facial sweating occurs in response to salivatory stimuli; known as **gustatory sweating**, this can be embarrassing. It can be managed by use of fragrance-free antiperspirants or injection of botulinum toxin.

Adenolymphoma (Warthin Tumour)

This unusual benign lesion constitutes less than 10% of salivary neoplasms, and occurs almost exclusively in the parotid. They usually arise after middle age and there is a male predominance and a strong association with cigarette smoking. They sometimes occur bilaterally (up to 10%), at the same time or at different times.

Histologically, the tumour is composed of large glandular acini. The epithelium is embedded in dense lymphoid tissue with lymphoid follicles. Histogenesis is not understood, but the glandular part may be hamartomatous salivary duct tissue within a normal parotid lymph node.

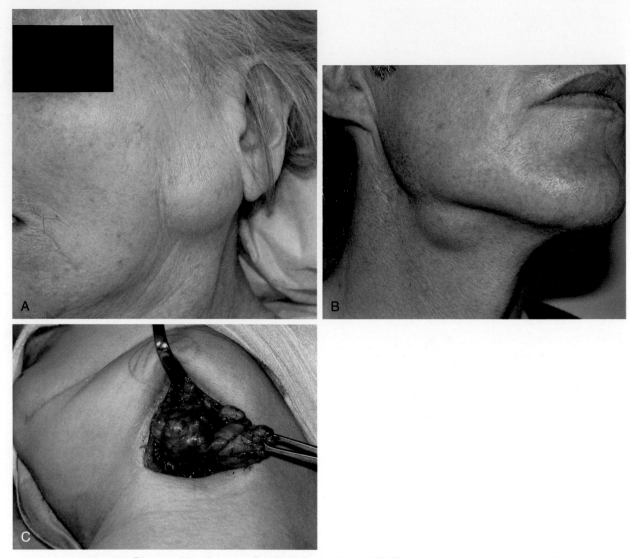

• **Fig. 47.3** Pleomorphic adenoma of major salivary glands. **(A)** Sizable preauricular lesion in the left parotid glandin an older female patient. **(B)** this man presented with a firm mass within the right submandibular gland. **(C)** intra-operative picture of a 14 year old female with a pleomorphic adenoma arising from the anterior pole of the left submandibular gland.

Adenolymphomas are benign. They present as a parotid lump, clinically indistinguishable from pleomorphic adenoma. The diagnosis can usually be made by core biopsy or sometimes fine-needle aspiration cytology, then they are either enucleated or left alone. Adenolymphomas do not recur, but a satellite lesion may enlarge and present as another tumour.

Malignant Primary Salivary Tumours

Malignant tumours are rare in major salivary glands, but seen more frequently in minor salivary glands scattered throughout the oral mucosa. With parotid lumps, facial nerve weakness is diagnostic of malignancy. Primary malignant tumours include **adenocystic carcinomas, mucoepidermoid tumours, acinic cell carcinomas** and **squamous cell carcinomas**. In Australia, a frequently seen parotid tumour is malignant melanoma invading from skin. Overall, the commonest parotid malignancy is metastatic squamous carcinoma to lymph nodes from a cutaneous scalp primary.

Adenoid cystic carcinomas have a characteristic cribriform (sieve-like) microscopic appearance, with small spaces in a tightly packed tumour cell mass. These are highly invasive with early regional and systemic metastasis. Treatment involves radical surgery, which sometimes necessitates sacrifice of the facial nerve. Unfortunately, recurrence is very common and may occur as long as 15 years after apparently successful eradication. The tumours are unresponsive to radiotherapy and prognosis is almost generally poor.

Secondary Tumours in Salivary Glands

Lymph nodes within the parotid may become involved by metastases from face or scalp cancers. Similarly, secondaries from the mouth may develop in submandibular gland nodes. Finding a parotid or submandibular lump should therefore prompt a search for a primary locally, including the pharynx. Lymphomas, particularly arising from mucosal-associated lymphoid tissue, also sometimes affect lymph nodes within salivary glands.

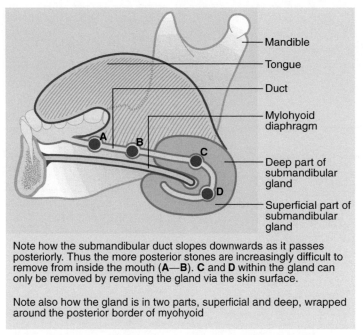

Note how the submandibular duct slopes downwards as it passes posteriorly. Thus the more posterior stones are increasingly difficult to remove from inside the mouth (**A—B**). **C** and **D** within the gland can only be removed by removing the gland via the skin surface.

Note also how the gland is in two parts, superficial and deep, wrapped around the posterior border of myohyoid

• **Fig. 47.4** Submandibular Gland and Duct Showing Common Sites for Stones.

Salivary Gland Stone Disease (Sialolithiasis)

Pathophysiology

The submandibular gland and duct are prone to form calcified stones (calculi), which obstruct salivary outflow and predispose to infection. Calculi also occur in the parotid duct but much less commonly. The aetiology is unknown, but the submandibular gland may be vulnerable because of its more viscid secretion and elongated duct.

Stones are not the only cause of obstruction causing gland swelling. In parotid and submandibular glands, duct orifice trauma may cause stenosis and salivary stasis.

Submandibular stones may be found anywhere along Wharton duct (Fig. 47.4), including its course within the gland. Stones vary from millimetres to a centimetre or more in diameter. Those in the distal duct tend to have an elongated 'date stone' shape (Fig. 47.5A).

Clinical Features

Salivary calculi rarely cause complete obstruction and the patient usually experiences intermittent swelling or pain with or just before eating when salivary flow is high ('mealtime syndrome'). The swelling then subsides over the next hour or so. Acidic foods such as lemon juice stimulate rapid salivary flow, and can be used as a test in clinic. Pain is not usually a prominent feature; rather, patients describe a sensation of fullness. Salivary calculi occasionally present with acute or chronic bacterial infection (**sialadenitis**). Secondary infection in the obstructed system leads to rapidly worsening symptoms and even spreading cellulitis of the floor of the mouth (**Ludwig angina**, Fig. 47.6).

Anatomically, the submandibular gland wraps around the posterior edge of the mylohyoid muscle medial to the body of the mandible, so there is little to see externally. In symptomatic stone disease, bimanual submandibular palpation usually confirms the gland is enlarged and firm. This involves a gloved finger palpating the floor of the mouth and the other hand below the jaw; any swelling can be felt between the two. This is the only clinical way to assess the gland size and may also palpate a stone in the duct. Palpation is performed from the back towards the front of the mouth to avoid displacing a mobile stone backwards into the gland. On intraoral examination, a stone may be visible if impacted at the duct orifice.

Management of Salivary Calculi

Plain x-rays demonstrate most calculi. For the submandibular gland and duct, an **occlusal film** held between the teeth shows the floor of the mouth, and a lateral oblique gives a second viewpoint. For the parotid, anteroposterior and lateral views are often used. Contrast radiography of the ducts (**sialography**) is sometimes indicated if the history suggests stone disease, yet no stone is palpable or visible on plain x-ray. Ultrasound is also very useful. Sialography (see Fig. 47.7) requires cannulation of the salivary duct, which may reveal a stenosis of the orifice and may relieve symptoms temporarily. Stenosis alone of any part of the duct may produce symptoms similar to calculus obstruction.

The anterior two-thirds of the submandibular duct lie in the floor of the mouth and calculi here are removed via an intraoral (see Fig. 47.5A) approach. Immediately before operation, the stone should be confirmed to be present by palpation or x-ray. Operation may be performed under local or general anaesthesia. A longitudinal incision is made in the duct over the stone and the stone lifted out. If the stone is impalpable, the duct is incised from the orifice backwards and the stone removed with forceps. The incision is not sutured but left open to improve salivary drainage. Stones can also be removed endoscopically or destroyed by lithotripsy.

Stones can lie within the gland and may be multiple (see Fig. 47.5C–E). The usual treatment is to excise the entire

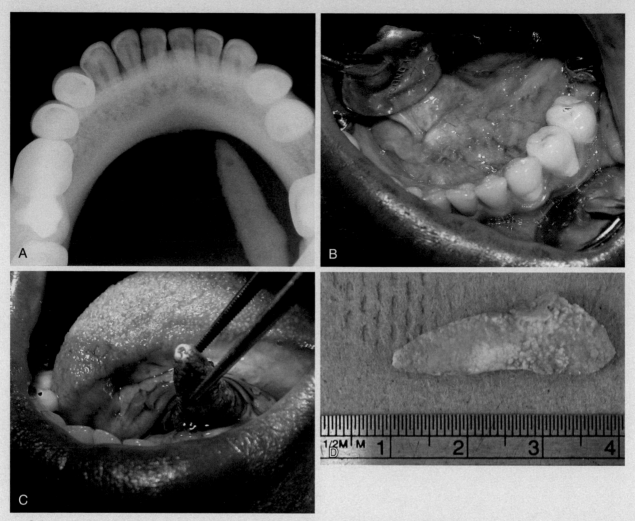

• **Fig. 47.5** Submandibular duct calculus. **(A)** Lower occlusal view shows a lrge stone in the anterior floor of mouthwhich was confirmed on clinical inspection **(B)** including bimanual examination. This young lady underwent removal of the stone under local anaesthetic **(C)** producing a 3cm **(D)** stone!

submandibular gland via an incision below the mandible, placed to avoid damaging the mandibular branch of the facial nerve. The hypoglossal and lingual nerves are also nearby and must be preserved.

Parotid duct stenosis may respond to dilatation and attention to the dentition if causing trauma. If this fails, ductoplasty can be performed, although this is often unsuccessful.

Inflammatory Disorders of Salivary Glands

The salivary glands are subject to infection by viruses (such as mumps) and by bacteria. Mumps is rare outside childhood and young adulthood, is usually bilateral, and resolves spontaneously. It is rarely a surgical problem unless secondary bacterial infection occurs. The glands may also be affected by autoimmune disorders, such as **Sjögren syndrome**.

Acute Bacterial Sialadenitis

Acute parotitis was once common in postoperative patients because of dehydration and poor oral hygiene, but is now rare because of intravenous fluids and nursing attention to mouth care. It now usually occurs in elderly, dehydrated or debilitated patients, or in children, arising from a suppurating lymph node within the parotid capsule. Dehydration and reduced salivary flow encourage ascending infection with resident oral flora, usually *Streptococcus viridans* or pneumococci. The result is a painful, unilateral swelling and **trismus** (limited mouth opening), pyrexia and tachycardia. The parotid is tender and diffusely enlarged and a purulent discharge may ooze (or can be 'milked') from the duct orifice.

Bacterial sialadenitis should be treated promptly with antibiotics. If a parotid abscess has formed, external surgical drainage may be necessary.

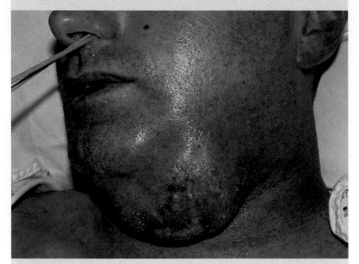

• **Fig. 47.6 Ludwig angina.** This middle aged man presented with fever and potential airway compromise due to bilateral severe infection either side of the mylohyoid muscle in the floor of mouth. In his case, this was due to dental infection. This septic episode was resolved with incision and drainage of the neck abscess and removal of the causative tooth. He required an awake fibre-optic intubation hence the topical local anaesthetic agent being applied to the left nostril.

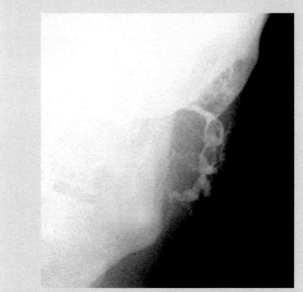

• **Fig. 47.7 Parotid Sialography Showing Stones.** This man of 58 years complained of intermittent swelling in the region of the left parotid gland, relieved on occasions by discharge of pus into the mouth. Contrast was injected into the orifice of the left parotid gland to outline the duct structure. The main duct is dilated and contains filling defects diagnosed as stones. This is an unusual finding as stones are much more common in the submandibular gland.

Chronic Sialadenitis

Prolonged calculus obstruction of a major salivary gland causes chronic inflammation. Glandular secretory elements progressively atrophy and are replaced by fibrous and adipose tissue. The duct system becomes dilated, fibrotic and infiltrated by chronic inflammatory cells. Chronic sialadenitis and salivary calculi usually involve the submandibular gland. The gland is swollen and there may be purulent duct discharge. The swelling is aggravated by eating. Treatment is by removing the duct obstruction; antibiotics may also be necessary. Glandular function may become irreversibly damaged, and the gland may require removal, although this is challenging because of fibrosis.

Recurrent Sialadenitis

This uncommon condition may occur at any age and usually affects the parotid. One or both glands are subject to recurrent attacks of painful swelling. The cause is low-grade bacterial infection usually without duct obstruction. Recurrent attacks cause chronic swelling. Sialography shows dilatation of the duct system with terminal sacculation described as **sialectasis**. The cause is often a ductal orifice stenosis, or stenoses proximally along the duct of unknown origin.

Immediate treatment includes antibiotics, chosen after culture of parotid duct discharge, as well as attention to oral hygiene. **Ductoplasty** to open the duct orifice is often successful. If sialography shows remote duct stenoses, these can sometimes be dilated using balloons similar to angioplasty devices.

Autoimmune Salivary Gland Disorders

The salivary glands occasionally become involved in a chronic inflammatory process characterised by diffuse lymphoid infiltration and fibrosis. This is part of various poorly understood autoimmune disorders, which also involve lachrymal glands and mucous glands of mouth and upper respiratory tract. The parotid and submandibular glands become diffusely and symmetrically enlarged, and salivary production is curtailed. The resulting dry mouth (**xerostomia**) causes discomfort and dysphagia and predisposes to rampant dental caries. Diminished lachrymal secretion results in **keratoconjunctivitis sicca** affecting the eyes.

In isolation, the condition is known as **primary Sjögren syndrome**. It may also occur in rheumatoid arthritis and other connective tissue disorders where it is known as *secondary Sjögren syndrome*.

Salivary Retention Cysts

Large retention cysts sometimes develop in the floor of the mouth. A cyst of the sublingual gland can reach several centimetres across and is known as a **ranula** ('little frog'). The ranula typically appears as a blue-grey dome-shaped swelling beneath the tongue. It may burst spontaneously, discharging its contents and collapsing, but typically recurs. The condition is painless but occupies space in the mouth. Excision is difficult because of the tenuous lining and because of the proximity to vital structures in the floor of the mouth; incomplete removal leads to recurrence. The usual treatment is excision of the sublingual gland, although **marsupialisation** is an option, that is, deroofing the cyst, so that it opens into the floor of the mouth. Ranulas may present as a lump in the neck, a so-called plunging ranula, where a portion of the gland herniates through the mylohyoid muscle of the floor of the mouth.

Lymph Node Disorders of the Head and Neck

Patients are often referred to a surgeon for biopsy of an enlarged cervical lymph node, often with no other symptoms or signs. **Isolated lymph node enlargement** may be caused by local disease

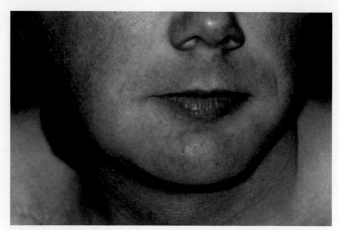

• **Fig. 47.8** Suppurating Lymph Node in the Neck. This patient presented with a suppurating node in the neck which required external drainage. The primary site of sepsis was a dental abscess on a lower molar tooth.

CASE HISTORY

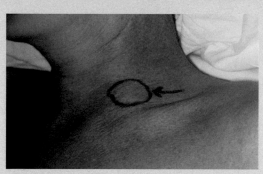

• **Fig. 47.9** Virchow Node. This 48-year-old woman noticed a painless lump in the left side of her neck. She had also lost a substantial amount of weight and had a poor appetite. Node biopsy revealed malignant adenocarcinoma cells and endoscopy showed that an advanced carcinoma of stomach was the cause. Palpation of a malignant node in this site is known as Troisier sign, after the French physician who diagnosed gastric cancer in himself.

in its field of drainage. Examples of local disorders include tonsillitis or dental infection, tonsillar tuberculosis or a malignant oral or oropharyngeal tumour. Nodes draining a bacterial infection may themselves suppurate, sometimes after the primary disorder has disappeared (Fig. 47.8). Enlarged nodes may be part of a **systemic lymphadenopathy** caused by glandular fever, lymphoma or human immunodeficiency virus. Thus any patient presenting with an enlarged lymph node requires general examination, as well as of the head, neck and mouth. The latter often includes endoscopy of the pharyngeal area, usually by head and neck, maxillofacial or ENT surgeons.

General clinical examination includes palpation of axillary and inguinal lymph nodes, liver and spleen. A chest x-ray may show enlarged thoracic nodes. If node biopsy is necessary, a fine-needle aspiration or core biopsy under ultrasound control may suffice, although some pathologists are unhappy with needle biopsies in lymphoma. If excision biopsy is required, this should be performed under general anaesthesia if practicable, since the operation is often unexpectedly troublesome because nodes are intimately related to vital structures and preoperative palpation often underestimates the size and extent of node involvement.

Cervical Tuberculosis

Tuberculosis involving the cervical glands (**scrofula**) was once common in Western countries, with the infection acquired by drinking milk from cattle infected with bovine tuberculosis. Cervical tuberculosis is now very rare in developed countries, but may be seen in recent immigrants. The primary infection occurs in the tonsils but presents with secondary involvement of cervical nodes, which become progressively enlarged and matted. In advanced cases, liquefaction of caseous material forms **cold abscesses**. If untreated, these eventually drain spontaneously onto the neck and leave disfiguring scars.

In the past, surgery was often required to drain and remove the affected glands. With modern chemotherapy, this is rarely necessary and surgery is confined to diagnostic excision biopsy.

Lymphomas

An enlarged cervical lymph node is a common presentation of non-Hodgkin lymphoma or Hodgkin disease. The disease is often at an early stage without other clinical symptoms or signs. The diagnosis is made by histological examination of a biopsy specimen.

Secondary (Metastatic) Tumours

Cervical lymph node metastases may originate from primary cancers in the head or neck, chest or abdomen. An enlarged node may be the first indication of a cancer or represent a recurrence following treatment.

Head and neck cancers usually metastasise initially to nodes in the submandibular region and upper anterior triangle, although disease lower in the neck at presentation is not unusual. The following head and neck tumours commonly metastasise to cervical lymph nodes:

- squamous carcinoma or melanoma of the skin of neck, face, scalp and ear;
- squamous carcinoma of mouth and tongue;
- squamous carcinoma of nasopharynx, oropharynx, larynx and paranasal sinuses. Note the primary tumour may be exceedingly small;
- Adenoid cystic carcinoma of major or accessory salivary glands;
- papillary (and occasionally medullary) carcinomas of the thyroid.

In contrast, tumours from the chest or abdomen usually metastasise to the lower part of the posterior triangle, particularly to **Virchow node** (Fig. 47.9), lying deeply in the angle between sternocleidomastoid and clavicle on the left side.

Miscellaneous Causes of a Lump in the Neck

Congenital Cysts and Sinuses

A variety of congenital cystic lesions occur in the head and neck and some may have an external sinus opening. All are uncommon except in clinical 'short-case' examinations! They can be subdivided into thyroglossal cysts, branchial cysts, fusion-line dermoid cysts, preauricular cysts and sinuses, and cystic hygromas (now termed *lymphatic malformations*). All are true epithelial cysts

CASE HISTORY

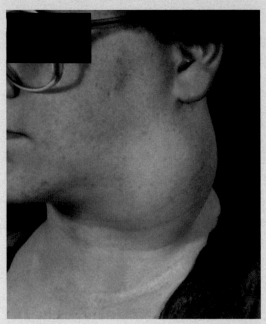

• **Fig. 47.10** Branchial Cyst. This 30-year-old woman reported the sudden appearance of this large swelling in her neck associated with moderate pain over the previous week. The swelling was nontender and fluctuant. Ultrasound confirmed it contained fluid. It was aspirated several times but failed to resolve and was eventually excised. It is not known why branchial cysts often come to attention so suddenly.

except for cystic hygroma, which is a hamartomatous lymphatic or lymphovascular malformation.

Branchial Cysts, Sinuses and Fistulae

The embryological origin of these is disputed, but they probably arise from remnants of the second pharyngeal pouch or branchial cleft. **Branchial cysts** usually present in early adulthood but sometimes later (see Fig. 47.10). Such late presentation is unusual for congenital lesions generally. The patient typically complains of a painless swelling in the side of the neck, which varies in size. Some present with a sudden painful red swelling caused by inflammation or infection of a previously unnoticed cyst.

The lump lies anterior and deep to the sternocleidomastoid, at the junction of its upper third and lower two-thirds. It protrudes into the anterior triangle of the neck and is soft and fluctuant. Provided it is not inflamed, the cyst usually transilluminates. Treatment is by surgical excision; percutaneous drainage is rarely permanent. Inflamed cysts may require urgent drainage.

Branchial sinus or fistula present as a discharging sinus near the lower end of the anterior border of the sternocleidomastoid.

A **sinus** ends blindly on the lateral pharyngeal wall, whereas a **fistula** communicates with the oropharynx near the tonsillar fossa. Surgical excision may be required.

Fusion-Line Dermoid Cysts

Dermoid cysts of congenital origin arise from epithelial remnants along lines of embryological fusion in the head and neck. The most common are **external angular dermoids**, cystic swellings at the outer aspect of the supraorbital ridge usually noticed soon after birth. These cysts are tense and firm and do not transilluminate because of their thick keratinous contents. They are deeply fixed and immobile. External angular dermoids are usually removed for cosmetic reasons during childhood.

Midline dermoid cysts are described as teratoid cysts because they contain a mixture of ectodermal, mesodermal and endodermal elements (e.g., nails and teeth, glands, blood vessels). Rarely, dermoid cysts can arise in the midline of the head or neck, usually during the first year of life. They should be removed surgically.

Preauricular Cysts and Sinuses

Small cysts and sinuses may arise from developmental abnormalities of the first and second branchial arches that form the external ear. They become evident in early childhood, lying anterior to the tragus of the ear and present as a small lump or a tiny discharging sinus that occasionally becomes infected. There may be an obvious associated auricular abnormality. Treatment is usually by surgical excision.

Cystic Hygromas (Lymphatic Malformations)

Cystic hygromas are not true cysts but lymphatic or lymphovascular hamartomas, which form multilocular cyst-like spaces. They may be huge and disfiguring lesions present at birth. Smaller lesions may present in older children or adolescents as a painless lump in the neck, below the angle of the mandible, and are soft and fluctuant and highly transilluminable. Surgical excision may be difficult, as they often extend deeply into cervical and orofacial tissues. Injection of sclerosants, such as bleomycin are gaining popularity.

Actinomycosis

Actinomycosis is a rare infection of the cervicofacial region caused by *Actinomyces israelii*, an anaerobic gram-positive bacterium, with a filamentous growth pattern similar to fungal mycelia. Actinomycosis is a chronic granulomatous infection, which if untreated eventually forms multilocular abscesses that drain to the skin via multiple sinuses.

Actinomycosis is treated with a prolonged course (4–6 weeks) of high-dose penicillin. If necessary, the abscess network is surgically explored and drained. Actinomycosis also occurs in the ileocaecal area, gaining access from appendiceal perforation. Rarely, the infection is encountered in the pelvis, complicating intrauterine contraceptive devices.

48

Disorders of the Mouth

CHAPTER OUTLINE

Disorders of the Oral Cavity (Excluding Salivary Calculi)

The mouth should be examined in a systematic way after removal of dentures, taking note of the condition of the teeth and oral soft tissues. Teeth are straightforward to identify: they are either upper or lower and then left or right; they are then numbered from the midline backwards from 1 to 8. In this way, they can then be used as signposts to oral lesions, for example, 'the cheek lining adjacent to the upper left fifth tooth'.

The main oral disorders are **dental caries** (tooth decay) and its sequelae, inflammation of the gums and supporting bone (**periodontal disease**), **tumours** and premalignant conditions of mucosa (leukoplakia and squamous carcinoma) and **disorders of the minor salivary glands**, such as retention cysts. The main symptoms and signs are summarised in Box 48.1. Salivary gland disorders are covered in Chapter 47.

Dental Caries

Pathophysiology and Clinical Features

In developed countries, dental caries (tooth decay) is a common bacterial disorder. First, the surface enamel of the tooth is breached by the demineralising action of lactic acid generated by commensal oral bacteria, as a by-product of carbohydrate metabolism, particularly of refined sugars. The most vulnerable sites for decay are just below the contact points of adjacent tooth crowns and the pits and fissures on the biting (occlusal) surface of molars and premolars. These sites are relatively inaccessible to natural oral cleansing mechanisms and to tooth brushing.

Once enamel is breached, proteolytic bacteria enter the less calcified **dentine** beneath and cause progressive destruction. The enamel remains intact until the dentine is undermined and the enamel fractures. Thus dental caries may be well advanced but invisible, even to a dental mirror and probe, and detectable only on x-ray. The decay process is asymptomatic until close enough to the tooth pulp to cause inflammation and pain. Eventually, there is swelling of the pulp leading to autoinfarction and pulpal death. The pathological process and corresponding symptoms are outlined in Fig. 48.1.

Once the pulp is necrotic, bacteria move into the space and multiply, then spread to the periapical region forming an apical **abscess**. This leads to painful oral and facial swelling, and if untreated, eventually drains into the mouth or occasionally onto the face, as a discharging sinus. However, the initiating cause, the necrotic pulp, remains, so a chronic abscess flares up intermittently or continues with a persistent discharge.

The pain of dental caries is usually well recognised as a 'toothache', but is often poorly localised and can cause nonspecific facial pain. In the upper jaw, it may simulate sinusitis. Dental caries should always be considered before rarer diagnoses. A surprising amount of dental caries, even with periapical infection, is asymptomatic.

Management of Dental Caries

Provided the dental pulp has not been invaded by infection, a dentist can usually drill out the carious enamel and dentine and restore it (Fig. 48.2) with synthetic resin, silver amalgam or gold, with a sedative insulating lining below. Once the pulp is involved, the necrotic tissue must be removed by **endodontic treatment**, and the pulp cavity filled; this is 'root filling' (see Fig. 48.2). The tooth can often be preserved in this way.

Management of Dental Abscesses

A periapical abscess is the most common late manifestation of caries seen by general practitioners or casualty officers. Primary treatment, as for other abscesses, is drainage of pus. Extracting the offending tooth is most effective, but if the patient wishes to preserve the tooth, draining the abscess via the root canal, then root filling it later is an alternative. Patients with periapical abscesses should be referred to a dentist.

Large acute abscesses 'pointing' within the mouth can be drained by incising at the site of greatest fluctuation. Oral penicillin should be prescribed for spreading infection. Antibiotics have no part in managing toothache, unless there is swelling

Symptoms and Signs of Oral Disease and Their Main Causes

- **Pain**—dental caries and its sequelae, acute gingival inflammation, such as pericoronitis and Vincent infection (acute ulcerative gingivitis)
- **Bleeding**—chronic gingival inflammation
- **Halitosis**—dental caries and chronic periodontal disease
- **White lesions**—epithelial dysplasia (leukoplakia), lichen planus and candidal infection
- **Oral ulceration**—aphthous ulcers, squamous carcinoma, retained tooth roots, chronic tooth or denture trauma, and rare epidermal disorders (e.g., lichen planus or Behçet syndrome)
- **Discharging sinuses**—periapical tooth abscess ('gum boil')
- **Bony lumps in the jaws**—fibrous dysplasia, tumours, cysts, ectopic teeth
- **Salivary glands and duct-related lumps**—retention cysts, submandibular duct stones, tumours

or other signs of an acute abscess. A dental abscess occasionally presents on the face but usually settles with extraction of the offending tooth. Dental abscesses are rarely complicated by osteomyelitis, unless there are medical comorbidities that put the patient at increased risk.

Tooth Extraction and Postextraction Problems

Medical practitioners are rarely required to extract teeth except in isolated places. Caries prevention with fluoride toothpaste and modern restorative and endodontic techniques have made extraction much less common. Patients, however, often attend General Practitioners or accident departments after tooth removal, with bleeding, pain or swelling.

Bleeding Tooth Socket After Extraction

A small amount of blood mixed with saliva can mimic significant haemorrhage. A normal socket should be filled with firm clot with minimal ooze at the gingival margin. This is aggravated if the anxious patient disturbs the clot by rinsing or 'exploring' the socket with the tongue. Aspirin may also promote bleeding. If there is bleeding, the extraction site should be inspected after careful suctioning.

Oozing or minor bleeding is easily controlled by the patient biting on a folded gauze swab and maintaining pressure for 10 to 15 minutes. Persistent bleeding can usually be controlled by adrenaline-containing local anaesthetic before inserting sutures through the gingival margins across the socket (Fig. 48.3), then biting on a dry gauze pad. Absorbable polyglactin sutures are preferred, as they do not leave irritating sharp ends and dissolve in 5 to 10 days. If bleeding continues after these simple measures, the patient should be investigated for a coagulation or platelet abnormality.

Pain After Tooth Extraction

Moderate pain is a normal consequence of tooth extraction and this is managed with simple analgesics. Removal of lower molar teeth may cause **trismus** (spasm of the muscles of mastication), causing limitation of jaw movements. Increasing pain appearing several days after extraction may be caused by a superficial osteitis of exposed socket bone because of loss of the organised clot. This condition, known as a **dry socket**, is intensely painful and requires dental treatment. The role of antibiotic therapy is unclear.

Swelling After Tooth Extraction

Soft tissue swelling is uncommon after extraction, with the exception of surgically removed teeth, especially lower third molars ('wisdom teeth'). Extraction of these, often causes swelling around the angle of the mandible, with trismus and pain. This represents a normal inflammatory response plus interstitial haemorrhage rather than infection. The swelling subsides within a week or so and does not warrant antibiotic therapy.

Inflammation of the Periodontal Tissues

Gingivitis and Periodontitis

Teeth arise from bony **alveolar ridges** in both jaws. A thin layer of **cementum** (a bone-like material) on the root surface connects to the alveolar bone via a tough **periodontal membrane or ligament**. The **attached gingiva** or gum is bound to the underlying alveolar bone and normally forms a tight cuff around the tooth neck, protecting alveolar bone from bacteria and trauma. The **gingival crevice** extends down to the cementoenamel junction, where the tough stratified oral epithelium becomes a thin vulnerable layer.

If oral hygiene is inadequate, commensal slime-forming bacteria colonise the gingival margin and form a white gelatinous **plaque** (Fig. 48.4). Bacterial toxins from the plaque then cause gingival inflammation or **marginal gingivitis**. This appears as swelling and redness of the gums and bleeding during tooth brushing. If allowed to persist, plaque adherent to the tooth becomes mineralised and forms **calculus**, which cannot be removed by tooth brushing alone.

Fig. 48.5 shows gingivitis causes eversion of the gingival margin. This encourages more plaque and calculus to form and results in greater gum trauma from food, both leading to more inflammation. If untreated, inflammation extends to deeper tissues causing progressive resorption of alveolar bone and destruction of periodontal membrane, known as **periodontitis**. By this stage, the gingiva is thickened and inflamed with a purulent discharge. This explains the old term 'pyorrhoea' or flowing of pus. Despite this, the patient is remarkably pain free, although **halitosis** may be notable.

As periodontitis progresses, more alveolar bone is destroyed and gums recede. The root surface becomes exposed to view, giving rise to the expression 'long in the tooth'. Teeth gradually become more mobile until they fall out or can be extracted with the fingers! Periodontal disease is an insidious process typically seen in adulthood. It was once thought to be inevitable with advancing age, but is almost entirely preventable. In adults, **periodontitis** is the leading cause of tooth loss. Inflammatory destruction of alveolar bone leads to resorption of the mandible and maxilla leading to loss of vertical facial height and makes it difficult to construct satisfactory dentures for many of these patients, owing to a lack of remaining alveolar ridge.

Sometimes an acute **periodontal abscess** may complicate periodontitis.

Management of Gingivitis and Periodontitis

Gingivitis and periodontitis is preventable by thorough and regular tooth brushing and use of interdental cleaning aids, such as dental floss. Gingivitis is reversible by improving mouth care, and whilst periodontitis can be arrested, loss of periodontal attachment is very difficult to recover. During the early stages of improved oral hygiene, bleeding increases through brushing inflamed tissues but soon subsides as the plaque load is reduced.

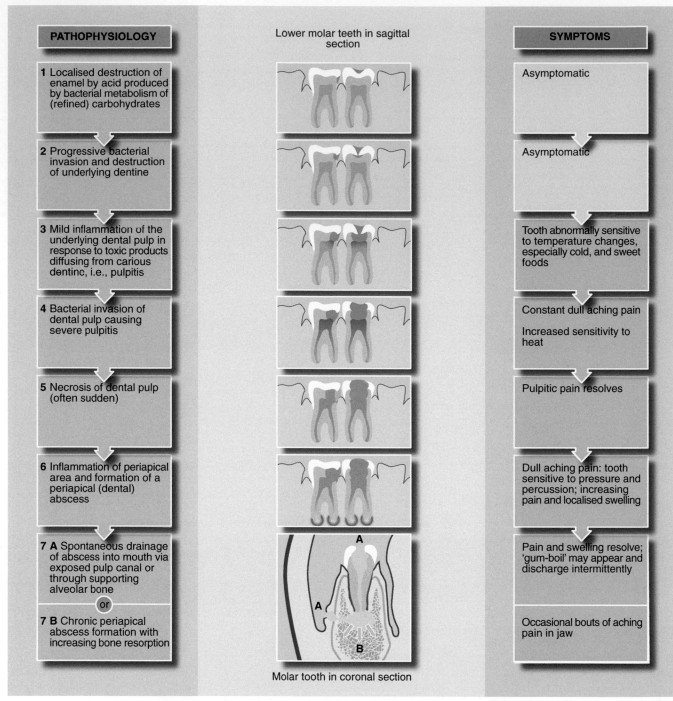

• **Fig. 48.1** Pathophysiology and Symptoms of Dental Caries and Its Sequelae.

Once established, periodontitis requires meticulous daily oral hygiene after thorough cleaning of plaque and calculus. Lost bone is not replaced, and the gingival contour remains abnormal, making effective oral hygiene difficult. Surgical recontouring of the gingiva and underlying bone (**gingivoplasty**) may be appropriate. Antibiotics play no part in treating chronic gingivitis or periodontitis. Antibiotics are useful for acute gingival conditions, such as pericoronitis and Vincent infection (**acute ulcerative gingivitis**).

Pericoronitis

Pericoronitis is inflammation around the crown of a partially erupted tooth, usually because of infection. This can occur with any tooth, but is particularly associated with the third molars (wisdom teeth), especially when they are impacted against the second molar or the ramus of the mandible, so that eruption is prevented (see Fig. 48.6). There is a space around the crown of the partially erupted tooth with a flap (**operculum**) of gum overlying the crown, preventing clearance of food and plaque debris (see Fig. 48.6B) which, in turn, leads to acute infection. Unchecked, this infection can spread into the deep tissue planes of the neck including the parapharyngeal space.

The patient complains of severe, poorly localised pain near the mandibular angle. Pain is aggravated by chewing because the

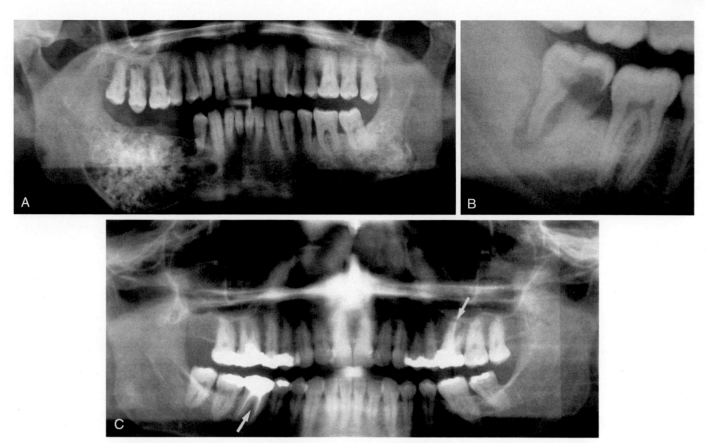

• **Fig. 48.2** Various jaw and dental findings on X-ray. (A) Fibrous dysplasia affecting the lower jaw. (B) Carious molar resulting in an apical abscess. (C) This oral pantomograph film shows silver amalgam restorations for caries in posterior teeth (shown as *white radiopacities*) and synthetic resin restorations in front teeth (relative radiolucencies in the upper incisors). In addition, the upper left first molar and the lower right first molar *(arrowed)* have radiopaque root canal fillings, necessitated by dental caries invading the pulp.

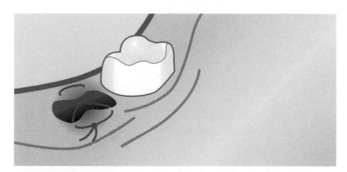

• **Fig. 48.3** Suture Technique for Arresting Bleeding from a Tooth Socket. A 'figure of eight' suture occludes bleeding gum edge on alveolar bone. The patient should bite for at least 10 minutes on a folded swab after suture to encourage clotting.

opposing tooth bites on the swollen gingival flap. On examination, the pericoronal tissues of the affected tooth are red and swollen, with a purulent discharge from beneath the flap. Oral examination may be difficult because of trismus. Externally, the submandibular and upper cervical lymph nodes are enlarged and tender.

Management of Pericoronitis

Pericoronitis progressing to cellulitis, with incipient abscess formation, caused by mixed organisms, is usually sensitive to penicillin or metronidazole. It is treated by irrigating beneath the flap with hydrogen peroxide or chlorhexidine and mouth washes several times daily with warm salty water. Rapid relief is obtained by removing the upper wisdom tooth, if it impinges on the flap. Oral phenoxymethylpenicillin (penicillin V) and metronidazole are given if the patient is systemically unwell. If attacks are recurrent, the lower wisdom tooth may be removed surgically.

Acute Ulcerative Gingivitis (Vincent Infection)

This is an acute inflammatory condition with necrotising ulceration of the gingival margin. It is caused by a mixture of gram-negative organisms, which are normal oral commensals. The most prominent are *Fusobacterium fusiformis*, *Borrelia vincentii* and *Bacteroides melaninogenicus*. Acute ulcerative gingivitis most commonly occurs in young adults who 'burn the candle at both ends' and become run down. Poor oral hygiene, pericoronitis and smoking may contribute. Acute ulcerative gingivitis is now uncommon, but was widespread in the First World War when it gained the name '**trench mouth**'.

There is an abrupt onset of gingival pain and bleeding, accompanied by a foul, often metallic taste and marked halitosis. Cervical nodes are enlarged and tender, and there may be fever, malaise and anorexia. Oral examination reveals characteristic ragged ulceration

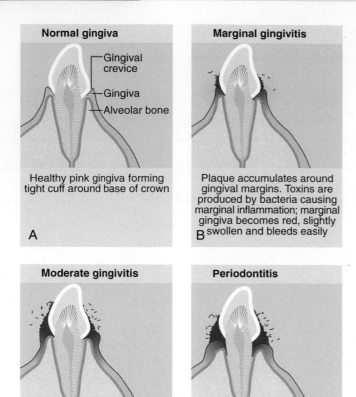

Normal gingiva

- Gingival crevice
- Gingiva
- Alveolar bone

Healthy pink gingiva forming tight cuff around base of crown

A

Marginal gingivitis

Plaque accumulates around gingival margins. Toxins are produced by bacteria causing marginal inflammation; marginal gingiva becomes red, slightly swollen and bleeds easily

B

Moderate gingivitis

More severe gingival inflammation: loss of tight protective cuff of gingiva allows accumulation of bacterial plaque and calculus in gingival crevice

C

Periodontitis

The inflammation involves the supporting alveolar bone, which is progressively resorbed so that adequate tooth support is eventually lost

D

• **Fig. 48.4** Pathogenesis of Periodontal Disease.

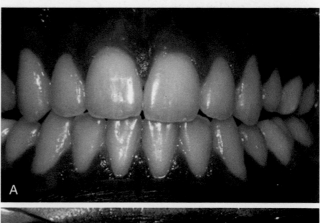

A

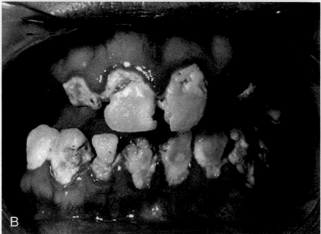

B

• **Fig. 48.5** Gingivitis and Periodontitis. **(A)** Normal healthy gingivae. **(B)** Chronic gingivitis showing accumulated plaque and calculus around the gingival margins. At this stage, no alveolar bone has been destroyed and the inflammatory process is potentially reversible. Many of these teeth had to be extracted however, because of rampant caries.

of the gingiva, especially between the teeth. In severe cases, the pharyngeal mucosa becomes inflamed and ulcerated (**Vincent angina**). Acute ulcerative gingivitis is easily distinguished from **herpetic gingivostomatitis**, as the former is confined to the gingival margin, whereas herpetic ulcers are scattered all over the oral mucosa.

Management of Acute Ulcerative Gingivitis
Vincent infection rapidly responds to metronidazole or penicillin, usually with full recovery of gingival morphology. Tooth brushing is necessary, but painful during an attack, and the mouth should be frequently rinsed with warm water or weak hydrogen peroxide to keep it clean. Afterwards, careful attention to oral hygiene usually prevents recurrence.

Tumours of the Oral Mucosa

Pathophysiology and Aetiology
The oral cavity and tongue are lined by stratified squamous epithelium. Oral squamous cell carcinoma (SCC) accounts for about 3% of all malignancies, and is the most common cancer on the Asian subcontinent. Like their skin counterparts, these usually occur in older people, though this trend is changing, possibly as

a result of human papillomavirus (HPV)-induced SCC. Men are affected twice as often as women, but in HPV cancers, the ratio is more even.

Tobacco, in any of its forms, is the greatest risk factor for mouth cancer and alcohol is another important precursor. Together, smoking and alcohol are synergistic in the aetiology of mouth cancer. The ventral and lateral tongue and floor of mouth are the highest risk sites in the West. Cancer of the lower lip also occurs and in some cases is because of ultraviolet exposure from sunlight.

In India, Sri Lanka, Papua New Guinea and other countries, the habit of chewing *paan,* a stimulant package of betel leaf, areka nut, and sometimes cured tobacco and slaked lime, causes a very high incidence of both oral cancer and submucous fibrosis, which results in trismus and is itself premalignant.

Leukoplakia is a premalignant dysplasia found in 50% of patients with oral carcinoma.

Clinical Features of Oral Cancer
Oral cancer usually presents as a red or red and white oral swelling with an irregular surface, which steadily enlarges. If it outgrows its own blood supply, the central area will ulcerate leaving a craggy, palpably firm mass. Mouth cancer is typically painless in the early stages, until it involves local nerves directly or becomes

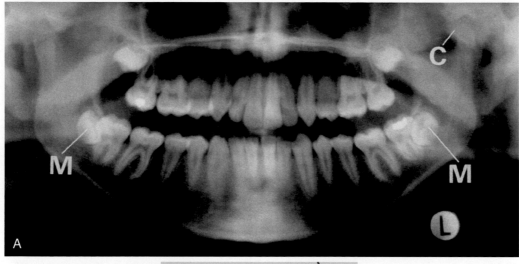

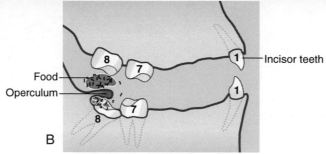

• **Fig. 48.6** Impacted Lower Third Molars and Pericoronitis. **(A)** This orthopantomagram radiograph of a 16-year-old girl shows the whole lower jaw 'opened out'. Both lower third molars *(M)* are seen to be angled towards the second molars and impacted against them. The roots are not fully formed and there is little chance of these teeth erupting normally. These were an incidental finding, the x-rays having been taken to demonstrate a fracture of the neck of the left mandibular condyle *(C)*. **(B)** shows the mechanism of pericoronitis.

secondarily infected (Fig. 48.7B and C). Cancer of the tongue, for example, may cause pain referred to the ear or pharynx via the lingual nerve or chorda tympani.

Oral SCC invades locally and usually metastasises initially to submandibular and upper cervical lymph nodes. Even small tumours can cause metastases. Tumours can interfere with speech, mastication and swallowing and are particularly distressing symptoms. Distant metastases are rare in the absence of neck nodes.

Management of Oral Cancer

Nonhealing oral ulcers should undergo biopsy to exclude malignancy.

Oral cancers are excised with at least a 1-cm margin of normal tissue. If the resultant defect is large, complex reconstructive surgery may be required. Involved lymph nodes are removed by neck dissection, whilst preserving vital structures, such as the accessory nerve and jugular vein, where possible.

Oropharyngeal cancers (for example, tongue base) can be effectively treated with radiotherapy or chemoradiotherapy. Radiotherapy is via external beam and brachytherapy (radioactive implants) is now rarely used. Intensity modulated radiotherapy has reduced

the damage to salivary gland tissue, which previously lead to xerostomia. It also spares other essential structures, such as the spinal cord.

Cancer of the lip has the best prognosis. The crude 5-year survival rate of oral cancer is around 50%, with small tumours having the best prognosis. Regional node involvement reduces the chance of cure by half.

Leukoplakia

Leukoplakia means 'white plaque', and describes white patches on oral mucosa, which cannot readily be scraped off (Fig. 48.7A). This distinguishes them from candidal infections. White plaques may be caused by friction, smokers keratosis, oral lichen planus or a number of other rarer conditions, but the main importance of leukoplakia is that it may represent epithelial dysplasia or even carcinoma-in-situ.

The cheeks and tongue are most often affected, although dysplastic patches may develop anywhere on oral mucosa. An innocent white line is often seen along the inside of the cheek known as *linea alba*, which corresponds to the biting surfaces of the teeth and is caused by friction.

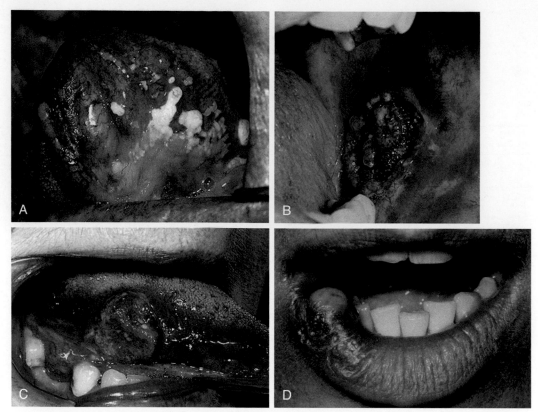

• **Fig. 48.7** Premalignant and Malignant Conditions of the Mouth. (A) Leukoplakia under tongue. (B) Ulcerating squamous cell carcinoma (SCC) of the cheek. (C) Ulcerating SCC of the tongue. (D) SCC of the lip. This man of 60 years had smoked a pipe most of his life. He tended to keep the pipe constantly in his mouth, while he worked. He presented with a nonhealing ulcer of the lip, proven to be a well-differentiated SCC on biopsy. A wedge resection of the lip was performed and produced a cure.

Severe or extensive leukoplakia should be referred for specialist maxillofacial opinion and biopsy. Areas of severe dysplasia may require laser excision and ablation.

Epulis

An epulis is a benign, localised gingival swelling. Two types are recognised: fibrous epulis and giant cell epulis.

A **fibrous epulis** is simply a benign fibrous tissue tumour arising from periodontal membrane or nearby periosteum. It forms a smooth, firm, slowly growing lump, covered with normal gingiva. A fibrous epulis usually emerges between two teeth, which may be pushed apart by pressure. Treatment is by excision with curettage of the base to prevent recurrence (Fig. 48.8).

A **giant cell epulis** arises in a similar location but grows much faster. It forms an irregular red fleshy mass, which ulcerates and bleeds. The lesion consists of numerous giant cells in a vascular stroma, which may invade local bone. Treatment involves extracting associated teeth and excising and curetting bone to avoid recurrence (see Fig. 48.8).

Pyogenic granulomas may occur on gums or oral mucosa of the lips. They look like pyogenic granulomas of skin and often occur in pregnancy (see Ch. 46, p. 598).

Miscellaneous Disorders Causing Intraoral Swelling

Retention Cysts of Accessory Salivary Glands

The oral mucosa contains numerous minor salivary glands. Small retention cysts develop as a result of gland or ductal trauma. Most retention cysts are smaller than 1 cm in diameter. They commonly occur in the lower lip mucosa, where they are irritating and are repeatedly traumatised. These cysts are blue-grey and are soft to palpation. They may rupture spontaneously, but typically reform. Most retention cysts can usually be removed under local anaesthesia. Swellings in the upper lip have a higher risk of neoplasia and should be biopsied.

Tumours of Accessory Salivary Glands

Tumours occasionally arise in minor salivary glands. These are often malignant **adenocystic or mucoepidermoid carcinomas**. They present as small, firm lumps in the oral mucosa, upper lip or hard and soft palate, and are often discovered before invading deeply or metastasising. Treatment is by wide excision and the prognosis may be poor; it depends on grade and stage.

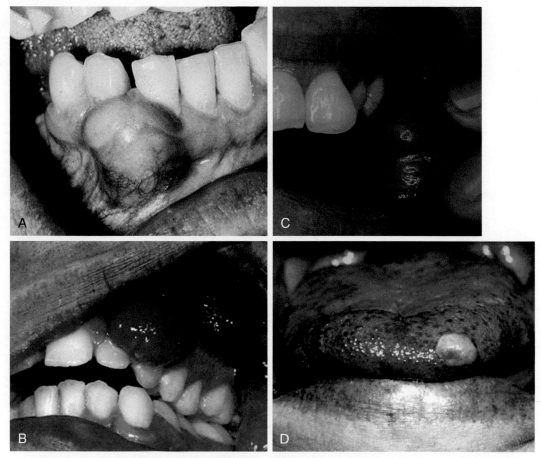

• **Fig. 48.8** Lumps and Bumps Around the Mouth. **(A)** Fibrous epulis. This can be seen to be moving the nearby tooth out of alignment. **(B)** Giant cell epulis. Both of these are in typical interdental location. The fibrous epulis is the same colour as the gum, while the giant cell epulis is a deeper red. **(C)** Fibroepithelial polyp inside cheek. These lesions are common and are probably initiated by minor biting trauma to the cheek or lip. They are often inadvertently chewed upon and gradually become larger. Excision is usually straightforward. **(D)** Pyogenic granuloma of the tongue. These are probably initiated by injury and maintained by an excessive healing response. They can occur on the gum or anywhere else in the mouth.

Bony Exostoses

Local outgrowths of jaw bones are common and produce an intraoral lump, which may be suspicious of neoplasia to the uninitiated doctor. The common site is the middle of the hard palate, known as a **torus palatinus**. A similar exostosis, usually bilateral, occurs on the lingual (tongue) side of the mandible, opposite premolar teeth and is known as **torus mandibularis** (Fig. 48.9).

These lesions are bony hard and are covered by normal oral mucosa. Excision is rarely needed unless there are problems in wearing a denture.

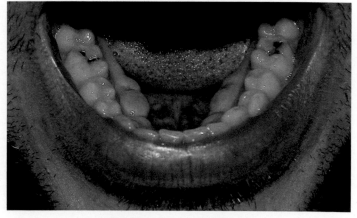

• **Fig. 48.9** Torus Mandibularis.

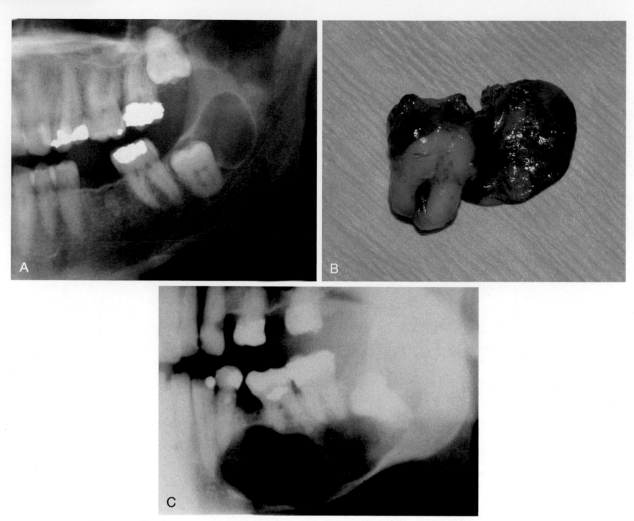

• **Fig. 48.10** Dentigerous cyst and residual dental cyst. **(A)** Dentigerous cyst associated with an unerupted third molar (wisdom tooth). This arose from cystic enlargement of the follicle surrounding developing crown of the tooth **(B)** surgical specimen following removal. **(C)** Large residual dental or apical cyst originally arising from an apical area on the lower left second premolar which had a been extracted some time before due to chronic periapical infection.

Cysts and Tumours of the Jaws

Cysts and tumours of odontogenic origin arise in the jaws. They arise from tooth-forming epithelium and may be developmental or acquired. Fig. 48.10B shows a mandibular dentigerous cyst around the crown of an unerupted third molar.

They are uncommon and can usually be diagnosed radiologically. The jaws are occasionally the site of benign or malignant bone tumours, such as osteosarcoma. They can also be affected by metastatic tumours from breast or prostate. Bony growth disorders, such as fibrous dysplasia and Paget disease may also affect the jaw.

49

Disorders of the Thyroid, Parathyroid and Adrenal Glands

CHAPTER OUTLINE

Introduction

Patients with thyroid disorders most often present to the surgeon with a **neck lump**, which may be asymptomatic or it may cause symptoms or cosmetic deformity. A thyroid enlargement is generically known as a **goitre**, from the Latin for throat *guttur*, and increasingly, patients are being referred with nodule(s) detected by ultrasound, whilst investigating unrelated neck symptoms. Enlargement may be a discrete lump or an enlargement of the whole gland; in any case, the priority is to exclude malignancy. Most patients are clinically and biochemically euthyroid (i.e., have normal hormone levels). Some may be **hyperthyroid** (thyrotoxic) and are referred for surgery because medical treatment has failed and radioisotope treatment is unsuitable.

Patients with **parathyroid disease** may present with symptomatic hypercalcaemia or asymptomatic biochemically detected hypercalcaemia caused by excess parathormone (**hyperparathyroidism**). The cause may be a solitary adenoma, multigland hyperplasia or rarely, carcinoma. Primary hyperparathyroidism (pHPT) can be cured only by surgery.

Adrenal disease may present as an asymptomatic adrenal mass found during cross-sectional imaging; such 'incidentalomas' are found in around 4% of adult computed tomography (CT) scans. Symptomatic adrenal masses manifest with clinical features of hormonal excess, which vary with the cell of origin of the tumour.

Thyroid Disorders

Pathophysiological and clinical features of the various disorders are summarised in Table 49.1, except for thyroid malignancy, outlined later in Table 49.3.

Clinical Presentations of Thyroid Disease in Surgical Practice

Diffuse or Generalised Enlargement of the Thyroid

Most large thyroid swellings in developed countries are **sporadic colloid goitres**, that is, multinodular or diffuse hyperplasia. Multinodular goitres (MNGs) are the more common. They grow slowly and may eventually develop dominant nodules with functional autonomy (i.e., toxic nodules in older people).

Iodine deficiency is the usual cause of *endemic* goitres, often found in isolated mountainous regions, such as Himalayan Nepal. These are preventable by adding iodine to the diet. These endemic goitres are usually soft and composed of hyperplastic nodules. They may be symmetrical and can be enormous (Fig. 49.1). Although unsightly, endemic goitres cause surprisingly few symptoms and the patient is usually euthyroid.

Anaplastic carcinoma causes hard fixed thyroid swellings, usually in elderly patients. There are usually symptoms of invasion, such as **hoarseness** (recurrent laryngeal nerve invasion), and **stridor** caused by tracheal invasion (Fig. 49.2). The uncommon thyroid **lymphoma** presents with diffuse enlargement and needs to be distinguished from anaplastic cancer.

In **Graves disease** (GD, primary hyperthyroidism), there is usually smooth mild thyroid enlargement. In **Hashimoto** thyroiditis, the gland is moderately enlarged, firm and finely nodular.

TABLE 49.1 Benign Diseases of the Thyroid

Disease	Pathophysiology	Clinical Features and Treatment
Inflammatory and Autoimmune Disorders		
Autoimmune thyroiditis (AIT) or Hashimoto thyroiditis *(common)*	Diffuse lymphocytic infiltration. Over a period of years, follicles progressively destroyed producing atrophy and fibrosis. Antithyroid autoantibodies may be elevated (e.g., anti-TPO/anti-TG). Associated with other autoimmune disorders for example, pernicious anaemia/gastritis	Presents in adulthood with mild/moderate diffuse goitre or no goitre. Thyroid may be tender initially thyrotoxic/euthyroid phase followed by hypothyroidism. Females>>males NB **thyroid lymphoma** develops almost exclusively on background of autoimmune thyroiditis **Treatment** Reassurance. Thyroxine supplements for overt hypothyroidism
Autoimmune diffuse toxic goitre or Graves disease *(fairly common)*	Stimulation of thyrocytes by thyroid receptor antibodies (TRAbs) causing hyperthyroidism	Main presenting features are of thyrotoxicosis ± eye disease Diffuse goitre of variable size ± thyroid bruit. Infiltration of periorbital tissues causing Graves eye disease **Treatment** Antithyroid drugs Radioiodine ablation Surgery (total thyroidectomy) ± treatment of eye disease
Acute inflammatory thyroiditis or de Quervain thyroiditis *(uncommon)*	Granulomatous thyroiditis with probable viral aetiology	Prodromal viral illness is common. Exquisitely tender thyroid with moderate goitre. May be thyrotoxic in initial phase. Lasts weeks to months. May recur **Treatment** Self-limiting; supportive management with NSAIDs or aspirin Steroids occasionally given for prolonged local symptoms
Fibrotic thyroiditis or Riedel woody goitre *(rare)*	Dense fibrosis of the thyroid gland ± surrounding tissues. Aetiology uncertain but possibly autoimmune	Extremely hard, 'woody' thyroid. May cause compressive symptoms. May occur in conjunction with other fibrotic conditions, for example, retroperitoneal fibrosis or sclerosing cholangitis **Treatment** Distinguish from malignancy for example, anaplastic cancer by core or open biopsy Surgical resection of isthmus if airway compromise
Acute suppurative thyroiditis	Bacterial or fungal infection	Tender thyroid with systemic illness **Treatment** FNA to confirm diagnosis Antibiotics/antifungals
Postpartum thyroiditis	Possible autoimmune aetiology	Initial thyrotoxic phase followed by hypothyroid phase which persists long term in ~25% **Treatment** Beta-blockade in thyrotoxic phase. Thyroxine may be required for hypothyroidism
Hyperplastic and Metabolic Disorders		
Simple nontoxic colloid goitre *(very common)*	Benign, diffuse or multinodular hyperplasia of thyroid follicles. Cause is unknown but possibly minor abnormality of thyroid hormone synthesis	Diffuse or sporadic multinodular thyroid enlargement or single 'adenomatous' nodule or cyst. Patient clinically euthyroid and all thyroid function tests normal. Affects females much more than males
Endemic goitre *(very rare in United Kingdom)*	Diffuse hyperplasia of thyroid follicles because of dietary iodine deficiency or goitrogenic foods. Endemic in inland, developing countries, especially in mountainous areas	Diffuse, often massive thyroid enlargement, which may later become nodular. T4 is low or normal and TSH tends to be elevated
Drug-induced goitre *(uncommon)*	Diffuse thyroid hyperplasia secondary to interference with thyroid hormone synthesis. Drugs causing this are antithyroid drugs used in therapy (e.g., carbimazole) or others like lithium and aminoglutethimide	Diffuse thyroid enlargement. Patient usually euthyroid. Can be prevented by using replacement dose of T4 concurrently with blocking drugs ('block and replace')
Dyshormonogenesis *(very uncommon)*	Diffuse thyroid hyperplasia caused by a variety of uncommon genetic (recessive) defects affecting thyroid hormone synthesis	Presents at birth or in childhood with thyroid enlargement and severe hypothyroidism (cretinism). In developed countries, these defects are usually diagnosed at birth by neonatal screening tests before any goitre has developed
Physiological *(common)*	Diffuse thyroid hyperplasia often associated with pregnancy and puberty	Mild diffuse thyroid enlargement. Patient euthyroid

FNA, Fine needle aspiration; *NSAIDs*, nonsteroidal anti-inflammatory drugs; *T4*, thyroxine; *TG*, thyroglobulin; *TPO*, thyroid peroxidase; *TSH*, thyroid stimulating hormone.

TABLE 49.2	Causes of Goitre
Type of Goitre	**Example**
Simple euthyroid goitre (sporadic/endemic)	Diffuse goitre Multinodular goitre
Toxic goitre	Diffuse autoimmune (Graves) Toxic multinodular (Plummer) Solitary toxic nodule
Thyroiditis	Autoimmune (Hashimoto) Subacute (de Quervain) Fibrotic (Riedel)
Neoplasia	Adenoma Carcinoma (primary/metastasis)
Other	Amyloidosis Chronic bacterial infection (tuberculosis/ syphilis) Actinomycosis

Solitary Thyroid Nodule

Solitary thyroid nodules on clinical examination are common but half prove to be multinodular on imaging. The clinical appearances of MNG are shown in Fig. 49.3. A solitary nodule is usually idiopathic hyperplasia and if discrete, is a **thyroid adenoma**. **Thyroid cysts** are fairly common and adenomas and cysts both fall within the description **simple or multinodular colloid goitre**.

Small nodules are found incidentally—noticed when the patient swallows, or on ultrasonography. Only 5% of true solitary nodules are malignant but this rises substantially in patients with a history of neck irradiation. Fallout from the Chernobyl nuclear meltdown caused many thyroid cancers in children exposed under the age of 14 years. Thyroid cancer risk is higher in nodules at the extremes of age, more particular in childhood. Malignancy needs to be excluded in any solitary nodule, with fine-needle aspiration cytology (FNAC) as the investigation of choice.

Other Features Associated With Thyroid Enlargement

A new area of enlargement in an existing goitre may result from haemorrhage into a cyst or nodule (this appears rapidly), growth of a hyperplastic nodule or a developing carcinoma. If enlargement extends into the anterior mediastinum behind the sternum (see Fig. 49.6), this **retrosternal goitre** may compress or displace the trachea, causing **stridor**, often obvious only with the neck in certain positions, such as sleeping on one side. Hoarseness or stridor may also result from malignant invasion of the recurrent laryngeal nerve or trachea. Vocal cord palsy causes dysphonia (speech abnormalities) and should prompt vocal cord examination with fibreoptic nasendoscopy in the clinic.

Pain and tenderness are uncommon presenting features but characterise the rare infective **de Quervain thyroiditis**. Sometimes the thyroid is painful and tender in Hashimoto thyroiditis.

Hyperthyroidism

Thyrotoxicosis is the term for the clinical syndrome of hypermetabolism resulting from an excess of thyroid hormones, thyroxine (T4) ± triiodothyronine (T3). The clinical manifestations are summarised in Box 49.1 (also Fig. 49.4). Mild hyperthyroidism may occur in the early stages of Hashimoto thyroiditis, burning out later with the patient becoming hypothyroid. A solitary adenomatous nodule may produce excess hormone causing hyperthyroidism and is known as a **toxic** or **hot nodule**.

Hypothyroidism

Hypothyroidism is a deficiency of thyroid hormones resulting from inadequate synthesis and is usually because of autoimmune thyroiditis, primary gland atrophy or following treatment for thyrotoxicosis. Hypothyroidism is a complication in up to 25% of cases after subtotal thyroidectomy (now less commonly performed), after radioiodine therapy for thyrotoxicosis, and is inevitable after total thyroidectomy. Hypothyroidism is more common in women of advancing age and should be considered in surgical patients presenting with constipation. It has also been implicated in spontaneous aortic thrombosis in middle-aged women.

Special Points in Examining a Thyroid Swelling

The patient should be seated in a chair with space to palpate from behind and have a glass of water available to swallow (Fig. 49.5). General examination should look for signs of hyperthyroidism (as listed in Box 49.1) and for specific signs of Graves eye disease (see Fig. 49.4) (exophthalmos and ophthalmoplegia). Next, the front of the neck is inspected, while the patient swallows; the characteristic rise of a thyroid swelling results from its investment in **pretracheal fascia** attached to the larynx above. A normal thyroid is not visible even on swallowing and is not normally palpable.

The thyroid area is next palpated from behind. This is best for examining the size, shape and consistency of the gland. It also allows the lower edge of a swelling to be palpated to identify retrosternal extension. The thyroid lobes wrap around the larynx and lie deep to the strap and sternomastoid muscles, which tend to conceal thyroid enlargement and make it tricky to examine the whole gland. Thyroid tenderness may indicate thyroiditis; a diffuse and smoothly enlarged gland suggests a benign process, such as endemic, multinodular or physiological goitre. A clinically solitary or dominant nodule or firmness, irregularity of margins, fixity and/or dysphonia may indicate malignancy. Most retrosternal goitres arise in continuity with a large component in the neck, whilst others may be predominantly substernal.

The jugular chain of **lymph nodes** should be palpated for metastases. In thyrotoxicosis, auscultation may reveal a **bruit** of increased vascularity.

If there is suspicion of recurrent laryngeal nerve palsy because of **hoarseness**, laryngoscopy should be performed, especially if surgery is contemplated.

Approach to Investigation of a Thyroid Mass

The questions during investigation are summarised in Box 49.2 and described in detail later. Patients after neck radiotherapy should be considered at high risk of thyroid carcinoma.

General Thyroid Status

First establish whether the patient is **euthyroid**, **hyperthyroid** or **hypothyroid**. Initially, this is clinical but plasma thyroid stimulating hormone (TSH) level is low in hyperthyroidism and elevated in hypothyroidism. Most laboratories measure just the TSH level

TABLE 49.3	Malignant Diseases of the Thyroid	
Condition (Relative Frequency in Developed Countries)	Pathophysiology	Clinical Features and Treatment
Papillary thyroid cancer (PTC) *(relatively common—85% of thyroid malignancies, more in children)*	Pathogenesis—activation of the *RET* protooncogene (rearranged during transfection) in 20% to 70% Forms complex branching structure with a fibrous stroma (papillary pattern) and psammoma (sand grain) bodies. Variable degree of dysplasia. Tends to be multifocal and locally invasive Commonly metastasises to cervical nodes even with small tumours, but distant metastases rare	All age groups affected but more common in young/ middle-aged women Prognosis may be predicted using classifications, such as 'AMES' (age, metastases, extent, completeness of surgery). With appropriate treatment, only 10% die of their disease Surgery: hemi or total thyroidectomy and lymphadenectomy for known nodal spread or prophylactically in high-risk tumours Radioiodine therapy for all high-risk patients plus TSH suppression with high-dose thyroxine
Follicular thyroid cancer *(relatively uncommon—10% of thyroid malignancies)*	Tumour forms a well-developed follicular pattern reminiscent of normal thyroid. In general, well differentiated but metastasis is usually distant, for example, lungs and bone	Older age group affected Diagnosis: FNAC only identifies follicular nature but histology (possibly diagnostic hemithyroidectomy) needed to determine benign or malignant Prognosis less favourable than PTC, mainly because older age-group affected Surgery: extent depends on tumour characteristics with lymphadenectomy only if evident nodal spread is demonstrated Radioiodine ablation, TSH suppression and follow-up as for papillary carcinoma Inoperable differentiated cancer may be treated with targeted agents (e.g., the tyrosine kinase inhibitor Sorafenib)
Hürthle cell carcinoma *(uncommon)*	Prognosis: similar to an aggressive papillary carcinoma	Surgery: total thyroidectomy and central compartment lymphadenectomy
Anaplastic carcinoma *(uncommon)*	Dedifferentiated, aggressive variant of papillary or follicular carcinoma, rapidly spreading beyond confines of gland	Affects patients older than 60 years. Presents with a rapid appearance of a goitre Diagnosis: likely to require core biopsy Prognosis: very poor: survival >3 months is unusual Treatment: combination therapy with surgery, external beam radiotherapy and chemotherapy may help
Medullary thyroid cancer *(very uncommon)*	Aetiology: sporadic or part of MEN2 syndrome. Spreads via lymphatics	Surgery is the mainstay of treatment, as radioiodine not taken up Prognosis: intermediate between differentiated and anaplastic cancers
Lymphoma *(uncommon)*	Almost always a history of autoimmune thyroiditis	Chemoradiotherapy can be curative in localised disease
Thyroid metastases from elsewhere *(rare)*	Renal, breast, uterine or melanoma	Surgery: thyroidectomy may be appropriate Liaison with the team looking after the primary

FNAC, Fine-needle aspiration cytology; *MEN2,* multiple endocrine neoplasia type 2; *TSH,* thyroid stimulating hormone.

initially but estimations of free T4 (fT4) may follow. If the patient is clinically hyperthyroid, but the fT4 is normal, elevated T3 levels are likely and can be measured.

Thyroid autoantibodies are assayed if autoimmune disease or lymphoma is possible (lymphoma usually occurs on a background of Hashimoto thyroiditis). Hashimoto is characterised by elevated antithyroid peroxidase antibodies. If **medullary thyroid carcinoma** (MTC) is suspected, calcitonin level should be checked and if elevated, plasma or urinary metanephrines measured because MTC can be associated with phaeochromocytoma in multiple endocrine neoplasia type II syndrome (MEN 2).

Morphology of the Gland

Imaging is next performed to assess the morphology of the thyroid and to guide FNAC. It can also detect retrosternal extension. Core biopsy for histology is not required except in suspected lymphoma or anaplastic thyroid cancer. Ultrasound is recommended by the British Thyroid Association to classify thyroid nodules. Ultrasound features suggesting malignancy include hypoechoicity, microcalcification and irregular margins (all 80%–90% sensitive), nodules that are 'taller than wide' and those with central vascularity. Ultrasound also has excellent sensitivity and specificity in detecting cervical lymphadenopathy when staging thyroid malignancy, particularly in the lateral compartment, and can guide FNAC of nodes.

CT scanning of neck and thoracic outlet is used in:
- apparent tracheal displacement or compression;
- assessing the extent of retrosternal goitres;
- detecting lymph node and distant metastases if malignancy is suspected.

Tissue Diagnosis

The gold standard for investigating possible malignancy in solitary and dominant thyroid nodules is FNAC. Ultrasound guidance reduces the false negative and nondiagnostic rate

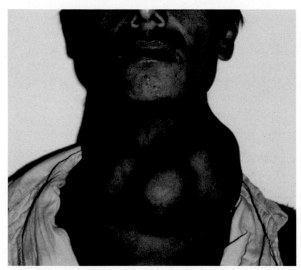

• **Fig. 49.1** Endemic Goitre. This condition, caused by iodine deficiency, is extremely common in isolated mountain regions. The thyroid can reach an enormous size, yet the patient suffers only minimal symptoms and is usually euthyroid. This typical example in a Nepalese man is only of moderate size by local standards.

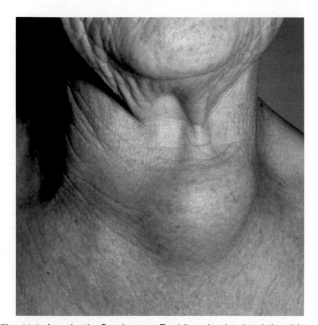

• **Fig. 49.2** Anaplastic Carcinoma. Rapidly enlarging hard thyroid mass in an elderly woman. The mass was firmly tethered to strap muscles and deeper structures. Treatment was purely palliative, as this tumour does not respond to treatment.

compared to 'freehand' FNAC and in the United Kingdom, cytology is reported using the 'Thy' classification. If a **colloid nodule** is diagnosed, excision is needed only for compressive symptoms or less commonly for cosmetic deformity. Obviously malignant lesions usually require surgery. These include **papillary**, **medullary** and early **anaplastic carcinomas**. Most **lymphomas** are inadequately sampled by FNAC or core biopsy and may need open incision biopsy. **Follicular carcinomas** cannot be distinguished cytologically from **benign follicular adenomas**; both display sheets of follicular cells, so lesions with this appearance should be removed, although only 20% will be malignant.

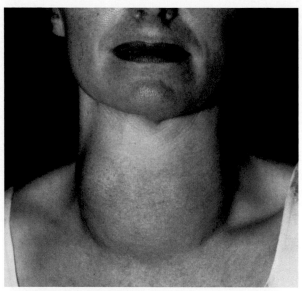

• **Fig. 49.3** Multinodular Goitre. Longstanding multinodular goitre in a woman of 40 years, with a strong family history of thyroid disorders. The thyroid is multinodular on palpation, and on ultrasound there are multiple nodules of various sizes, plus some small cysts. Any change in a multinodular goitre may herald malignancy.

• **BOX 49.1** **Clinical Manifestations of Thyrotoxicosis**

Metabolic—heat intolerance, increased appetite with weight loss, diarrhoea, menorrhagia
Cardiovascular—palpitations, tachycardia even while asleep, atrial fibrillation
Neuropsychiatric—hyperkinesis, insomnia, emotional instability, tremor, proximal myopathy
Ocular—exophthalmos including proptosis, lid retraction and eventually ophthalmoplegia
Cutaneous—pretibial myxoedema

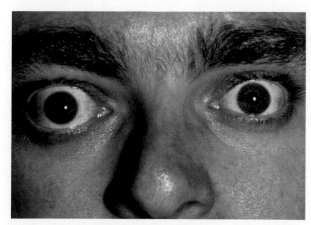

• **Fig. 49.4** Hyperthyroidism. Exophthalmic eye signs of hyperthyroidism in 43-year-old man with 6-month history of hyperthyroidism. His family had noticed his increasingly staring eyes. He had proptosis and lid lag.

Functional Activity of Glandular Tissue

Radionuclide (iodide) imaging proved unreliable at predicting malignancy and its current role is in characterising the cause of thyrotoxicosis (Fig. 49.7): GD shows even uptake across the gland, whereas toxic MNG shows patchy uptake. In solitary toxic

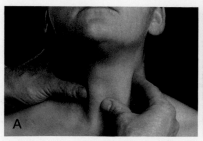
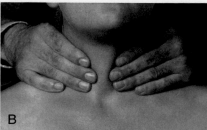
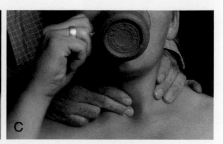

• **Fig. 49.5** Examination of the Thyroid Gland. The patient should be sitting upright in a chair with room for the examiner to approach from behind. **(A)** Gentle palpation from the front with slight sideways pressure from the left hand whilst palpating with the right. This is repeated for the right side of the gland. **(B)** General palpation of the gland from behind. Is there enlargement? Is it a single nodule or multinodular? How big is it? **(C)** Palpation of the gland while the patient swallows. Does the gland rise with swallowing? Is there retrosternal extension?

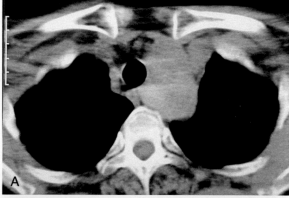

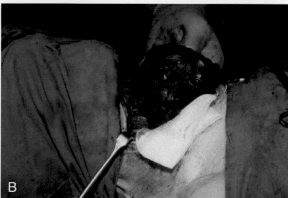

• **Fig. 49.6** Retrosternal Goitre. This 38-year-old woman had suffered stridor at night for several months. On palpation, the thyroid was not particularly large but the trachea was markedly deviated (see Fig. 49.8). **(A)** Computed tomography scan at the level of the clavicles, showing enlargement of the left side of the thyroid gland, with moderate deviation, but no compression of the trachea. **(B)** At operation, this huge retrosternal extension was drawn up out of the anterior mediastinum. As this was a multinodular goitre, a total thyroidectomy was performed. Histopathology confirmed a benign multinodular goitre.

adenoma (which is rarely malignant), the nodule is intensely avid, while the rest of the gland uptake is suppressed. Viral thyroiditis is characterised by no uptake and a blank film. Isotope scanning can also identify and localise **ectopic thyroid tissue** (in the tongue or along the course of the thyroglossal duct), **retrosternal extension** of a thyroid swelling and **metastases** of functioning thyroid carcinomas, provided the thyroid has previously been removed or ablated.

• **BOX 49.2** **Principles of Investigation of a Thyroid Mass**

General thyroid status—thyroid function tests and thyroid autoantibodies
Morphology of the gland, that is, size, shape and physical consistency, effects upon surrounding structures—ultrasound, plain x-rays of thoracic outlet, computed tomography scanning
Tissue diagnosis—fine needle aspiration cytology or needle biopsy, incision or excision biopsy

---

Specific Clinical Problems of the Thyroid and Their Management

Multinodular Goitre

With benign multinodular goitre, surgery is only indicated to relieve compressive symptoms; large nodule size is not of itself an indication. Most retrosternal goitres can be removed via a broad neck incision though sternotomy is occasionally required.

Hyperthyroidism (Thyrotoxicosis)

Two percent of women and 0.2% of men in the United Kingdom have hyperthyroidism. Untreated, it causes weight loss, anxiety, tachycardia, palpitations and increased risk of cardiovascular-related death. Most are caused by Graves' disease, some by toxic multinodular goitre and a few by toxic adenoma. Graves' disease is an autoimmune condition in which antibodies stimulate TSH receptors, causing excess thyroid hormone synthesis; secretion becomes independent of pituitary feedback. Thyroid hypertrophy results in a mild diffuse goitre. Eye manifestations occur in up to 50% including proptosis, exophthalmos and a staring appearance, which arise from autoimmune involvement of periorbital muscle, fat and skin causing retroorbital oedema. These can produce symptoms of diplopia, pain, visual deterioration (because of optic nerve compression and stretching) and rarely, corneal scarring from extreme dryness. The diagnosis of Graves' disease is usually suspected clinically and confirmed by thyroid autoantibody titres: thyroid receptor antibody (TRAb) is elevated in 80% to 90% of patients with Graves.

Hashimoto thyroiditis may produce transient hyperthyroidism. If in doubt, the aetiology of hyperthyroidism can be determined by radioisotope scanning. Carcinoma is very rarely found in hyperthyroid patients.

Treatment of Hyperthyroidism

There are three options: antithyroid drugs, radioiodine destruction of functioning thyroid tissue and thyroidectomy.

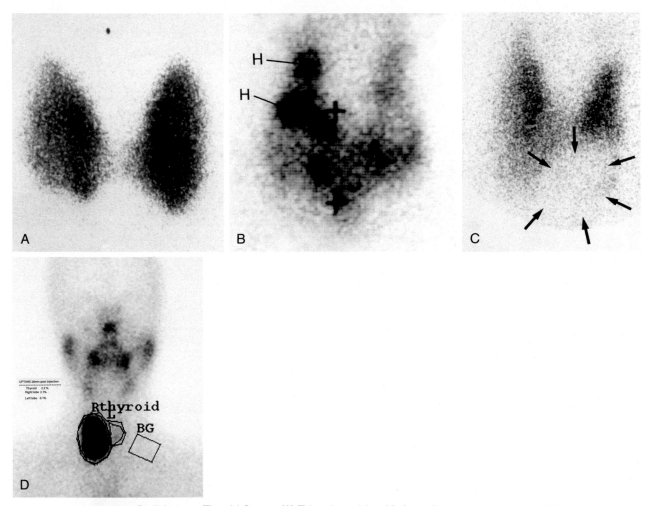

• **Fig. 49.7** Radioisotope Thyroid Scans. **(A)** This enlarged thyroid shows homogeneous tracer uptake typical of a simple colloid goitre. **(B)** Heterogeneous tracer uptake in a multinodular colloid goitre. The dark areas *(H)* are 'hot nodules'; to maintain the euthyroid state, the rest of the gland exhibits diminished uptake. The *(+)* signs indicate the positions of the thyroid cartilage and the suprasternal notch. **(C)** Solitary 'cold' thyroid nodule. The area of low uptake (outline *arrowed*) at the lower left pole of the thyroid corresponds with a palpable nodule. In the case of a solid lesion (as confirmed by ultrasound), a cold nodule may indicate malignancy. **(D)** Solitary 'hot' thyroid nodule. The area of high uptake in the lower part of the right lobe corresponds to a palpable mass. This patient was hyperthyroid and the lesion could be described as a 'toxic nodule'. Activity of the rest of the gland is suppressed by pituitary-mediated negative feedback from the high serum thyroxine level. The rectangle marked *(BG)* measures the background radiation to quantify the thyroid uptake.

Antithyroid drugs are the first line in Europe except in the elderly and unfit, whereas radioiodine is preferred as an early treatment in the United States of America. Patients with arrhythmias, angina or osteoporosis are usually treated with radioiodine from the outset. Antithyroid drugs can cause hypothyroidism, which is avoidable by using a 'block and replace' regimen (concurrent antithyroid drug and T4). Carbimazole is favoured in the United Kingdom, with propylthiouracil used in pregnancy (as it crosses the placenta less readily) or as second line if carbimazole causes side effects. Beta-adrenergic blockers, such as **propranolol**, rapidly control the distressing and dangerous effects of thyrotoxicosis and are useful in extremely toxic patients, until antithyroid drugs take effect, or if a patient needs to be stabilised urgently before thyroidectomy. In those treated surgically, recurrence is rare after total thyroidectomy. All groups report 95% satisfaction, with no differences in quality of life between the groups.

Radioactive Iodide Therapy

Iodine-131 (I-131) ablation is safe and has been used for nearly 75 years with no evidence of later malignancy, as a relatively low radiation dose is used. Absolute contraindications are pregnancy and breast-feeding and active Graves eye disease. Up to 60% of patients develop hypothyroidism within a year of treatment and close monitoring of thyroid function tests is mandatory. Radioactive iodine is given by mouth as capsules or solution, in doses 100 times higher than for diagnostic scanning. Beta particle emission destroys the most active thyroid tissue over a period of weeks or months. Antithyroid drugs usually need to continue until radioiodine achieves its greatest effect. After treatment, gamma rays are emitted from the patient's body and may be absorbed by others nearby, so relative isolation is necessary at first. Patients should avoid pregnancy for 6 months afterwards.

Many units now aim to make patients hypothyroid within 6 months and routinely provide levothyroxine replacement.

Toxic multinodular disease and toxic adenoma also respond to radioiodine. Radioiodine may make thyrotoxic ophthalmopathy worse, whereas antithyroid drugs and surgery do not affect its course. Surgery is generally preferred in Graves patients with ophthalmopathy.

Surgical Management

Surgery for thyrotoxicosis may be indicated:

- When a quick and effective cure is desired that avoids long-term drug therapy. It is often the best treatment for Graves disease, particularly in younger patients in whom the disease is unlikely to burn itself out for years.
- If there is poor control by antithyroid drugs or relapse after initial successful treatment.
- In toxic MNG, where response to drug treatment is unpredictable; surgery also deals with the cosmetic deformity.
- In toxic solitary nodules ('hot nodules'), which are best excised to allow suppressed normal thyroid to recover.
- In active Graves eye disease, or another contraindication to I-131, plus intolerance or poor compliance with antithyroid drugs.
- If there are large goitres or possible malignant thyroid nodules.

Total thyroidectomy is the gold standard; subtotal thyroidectomy is now a historical operation, given the risk of recurrence. Proper preparation for surgery involves rendering the patient euthyroid, or at least achieving cardiovascular stability, using antithyroid drugs, beta-blockade and/or saturation of the gland with iodine. Lugol iodine or potassium iodide are effective, but surgery must be done within 14 days or rebound toxicity may occur. For all thyroid operations, preoperative assessment usually includes **laryngoscopy**, to demonstrate normal vocal cord function, should there be a question of operative damage later. There may be a more subtle change in voice quality after thyroidectomy, sometimes because of external laryngeal nerve damage. Patients should be warned of this, especially if they are singers or politicians!

At operation, a transverse collar incision along a skin crease gives the best cosmetic result. Meticulous care is required in ligating the terminal branches of the **inferior thyroid artery** (after identifying the recurrent laryngeal nerve) and the **upper pole vessels**. Primary or postoperative haemorrhage is a serious complication, causing laryngeal oedema and airway compromise. To avoid suffocation from a postoperative bleed, instruments for emergency reopening of the wound should be kept at the patient's bedside after operation. The potential complications of thyroidectomy are summarised in Box 49.3.

Thyroid Malignancies (See Table 49.3)

Thyroid cancer is the most common endocrine malignancy with 3500 new diagnoses a year in the United Kingdom. Nevertheless, overall thyroid malignancies represent less than 1% of all malignant tumours. Overall mortality from thyroid cancer is relatively low (380 deaths per annum in the United Kingdom) with 80% of patients expected to survive 10 years. However, thyroid cancer has a huge range of aggressiveness from indolent microscopic papillary cancers to wildfire anaplastic cancer in older patients, amongst the most aggressive cancers known.

Classification

Thyroid cancers are classified by cell type of origin as primary or secondary, and grouped according to level of differentiation. Cell types involved are **thyrocytes** (giving rise to papillary, follicular,

---

• BOX 49.3 Complications of Thyroidectomy

Complications During Operation

- Haemorrhage—uncommon.
- Recurrent laryngeal nerve injury—may result from traction or heat (and be potentially reversible) or from division (rare). Bilateral nerve damage presents as laryngeal obstruction after tracheal extubation and may necessitate tracheostomy. Unilateral damage causes hoarseness and a weak voice and impairs coughing.
- Inadvertent damage to other structures—tracheal or oesophageal perforation or damage to laryngeal muscles or nerves.

Early Postoperative Complications (Within the First 12 Hours)

- Major haemorrhage—can be devastating if rapid, leading to venous congestion, laryngeal oedema and airway embarrassment. Risk highest in first 24 hours and in patients with Graves disease or after nodal dissection. Risk may be reduced by nursing patients in a semi-sitting position. The fear of haematoma is the main argument against day case thyroidectomy.
- Early hypocalcaemia—transient postoperative hypocalcaemia (<2 mmol/L) because of compromise of the parathyroids is common: 25%–40%. Permanent hypoparathyroidism occurs in 1%–3%. Profound hypocalcaemia causes hyperexcitability with initial perioral and fingertip paraesthesia. May progress to tetanic contractures, seizures and death if untreated. Oral calcium ± activated vitamin D are sufficient in most cases if commenced early; IV calcium should be avoided. Serum calcium and PTH should be measured at least once in the 24 hours postoperative.
- Mediastinal haemorrhage (rare)—presents with hypovolaemic shock.
- Thyrotoxic crisis (rare but may occur after surgery in Graves disease)—presents with abrupt onset of extreme agitation and confusion, hyperpyrexia, profuse sweating and rapid tachycardia or other arrhythmia. Requires emergency beta-blockade, IV hydrocortisone and potassium iodide. The mortality of thyrotoxic crisis is 10%—from coma, pulmonary oedema or circulatory collapse. It is rare if the patient has been rendered euthyroid by drug treatment before operation.
- Tracheomalacia (rare)—removal of a longstanding lesion compressing the trachea may lead to tracheal collapse and stridor.

Later Postoperative Complications

- Hypoparathyroidism—persistent hypocalcaemia because of inadvertent parathyroid damage. Presents with muscle cramps, paraesthesia and tetany within 36 hours of operation. Treatment is with calcium and vitamin D analogues.
- Unilateral recurrent laryngeal nerve damage—presents with hoarse voice and defective cough.
- External laryngeal nerve damage—changes the quality of the voice.

Long-term Complications

- Hypothyroidism—often overlooked because it develops insidiously. Features are loss of energy, weight gain, depression and intellectual deterioration and intolerance of cold weather.
- Recurrent thyrotoxicosis—insufficient gland removed. Rare in total thyroidectomy.

IV, Intravenous; *PTH,* parathyroid hormone.

Hürthle cell and anaplastic carcinomas), **parafollicular C cells** (medullary thyroid cancer) and **lymphocytes** (lymphoma). Metastatic spread occasionally occurs to the thyroid from renal, breast or uterine carcinoma or melanoma. Differentiated thyroid cancers (papillary and follicular) show typical features of their parent cell type, with low metastatic potential, and carry the best prognosis. Undifferentiated cancers have the worst prognosis and medullary cancer carries an intermediate prognosis.

In most thyroid cancers, no aetiological factor is identified, but known risk factors for primary thyroid malignancy are:

- Age—malignancy rates in thyroid nodules are twice as high under 30 years or over 60 years compared with 30 to 60 years.
- Gender—malignancy is three times as common in females, but a thyroid nodule in a man is twice as likely to be malignant.
- Radiation exposure—evidence comes from survivors of nuclear bombs (Hiroshima and Nagasaki in 1945) and accidents (Chernobyl in 1986). The risk is highest if exposure occurs under 14 years and with concurrent iodine deficiency.
- Inherited disorders—medullary cancer may arise in multiple endocrine neoplasia (MEN) 2. Papillary and follicular cancers also have familial variants.

Treatment of Thyroid Cancer

Treatment of differentiated cancers has three elements: surgery (thyroidectomy ± lymph node dissection), radioiodine ablation and TSH suppression. For medullary cancer, treatment is surgery (with no role for I-131 or TSH-suppression), plus chemotherapy in metastatic disease. Anaplastic cancer is best managed with a combination of surgery, external beam radiation and chemotherapy but outcomes are poor.

Papillary Carcinoma

Papillary carcinoma constitutes two-thirds of thyroid malignancies in adults and nearly all in children. Females are affected three times more than males and the peak incidence is 30 to 45 years. Epithelial dysplasia ranges between apparently benign and obviously malignant, but most tumours grow slowly. Papillary carcinomas are microscopically multicentric in about 80% and about one-third affect both lobes—important in planning treatment.

Metastasis is to central and later lateral cervical **lymph nodes** and only rarely to distant sites, such as lung or bone. Lymph nodes are involved in about 40% (90% in children) at presentation. Node enlargement is often the presenting feature; histology is so close to normal that this used to be known as **lateral aberrant thyroid**. The prognosis is the best of all thyroid carcinomas, with only about 10% dying of it by 10 years (of remote metastases); it is remarkable that survival is hardly prejudiced by node metastases. The prognosis is even better for 'papillary thyroid microcarcinoma', defined as a single tumour less than 1 cm in diameter.

Management

The standard management is **total thyroidectomy** because of the high probability of other foci in the gland (Fig. 49.8). Macroscopically involved cervical nodes are removed at the same operation. Total thyroidectomy also permits the use of radioiodine for the destruction of microscopic local lymph node or distant metastatic disease. A further advantage is that plasma thyroglobulin can then be used as a **tumour marker** to detect recurrent disease. After treatment, oral T4 replacement is always necessary at levels that keep TSH close to zero, to minimise the risk of stimulating any residual malignant cells. Tumour recurrence in cervical nodes is treated by excision and even this does not adversely affect prognosis. Since papillary carcinomas progress so slowly and only about 15% develop macroscopic contralateral lobe recurrence, there is a trend towards hemithyroidectomy, if the primary tumour is small and there are no detectable nodules.

Follicular Carcinoma

Follicular carcinoma is another differentiated thyroid cancer. Histologically, neoplastic cells form a well-developed **follicular pattern**, impossible to distinguish from benign adenomatous hyperplasia on FNAC. The diagnosis can be challenging, even on histology of the surgical specimen, unless there is evident capsular or vascular invasion. Unlike papillary carcinoma, multicentricity is uncommon. The peak incidence is 40 to 50 years, older than papillary carcinoma, but it is three times commoner in women. In general, follicular carcinoma grows slowly and metastasises late. In contrast to papillary carcinoma, metastasis occurs via the bloodstream to lungs, bone and other remote sites rather than local nodes.

Since follicular carcinoma is rarely multicentric, management depends on local invasion. A tumour with only microinvasion of the capsule has a very good prognosis and only requires removal of the tumour-containing lobe. If there is gross capsular or vascular invasion (or known remote metastases), total thyroidectomy is performed to enhance the radioiodine uptake of metastases for diagnosis or for treatment with high-dose radioiodine. Prognosis for the primary can be predicted by the degree of capsular and vascular invasion. Without invasion, 10-year survival is close to 100%, but falls to about 30%, with extensive local invasion.

Anaplastic Carcinoma

Anaplastic carcinoma is an extremely aggressive disease almost exclusively in the elderly, with an appalling prognosis. Most patients die within a year of diagnosis. Anaplastic carcinoma consists of sheets of very poorly differentiated cells, which proliferate rapidly, producing a diffuse, hard thyroid enlargement. The tumour soon invades surrounding structures, causing tracheal and oesophageal obstruction and recurrent laryngeal nerve damage. There is also early dissemination to regional lymph nodes and haematogenous spread to lungs, skeleton and brain.

Anaplastic carcinomas respond poorly to radiotherapy and chemotherapy. The distressing symptoms of tracheal obstruction can sometimes be relieved by placing a luminal tracheal stent.

Medullary Carcinoma

This uncommon malignancy arises from parafollicular or C-cells. The tumour usually secretes abnormal quantities of **calcitonin**, used as a marker of tumour recurrence after excision. Tumours may also secrete other peptides and amines, such as **serotonin** and **adrenocorticotropic hormone** (**ACTH**)-like peptide. Medullary carcinoma usually arises sporadically, but may be transmitted genetically in **MEN 2**. This is an autosomal dominant trait, with 50% penetrance, and is associated with other APUD cell tumours, particularly **adrenal phaeochromocytoma** and **parathyroid adenomas**. Thus patients with medullary carcinoma should be tested for these before surgery, as a phaeochromocytoma would take operative precedence.

Medullary carcinoma grows relatively slowly, metastasising first to regional lymph nodes and later to lungs, bone, liver and elsewhere. The tumour does not take up radioiodine and is resistant to radiotherapy; hence an aggressive surgical approach is required. Standard treatment is total thyroidectomy and clearance of involved anterior cervical and superior mediastinal lymph nodes. In the absence of metastases, surgery is often curative, but in cases with nodal involvement, 10-year survival falls to 50%. During follow up, calcitonin levels are monitored and raised levels indicate tumour recurrence.

Thyroid Lymphoma

Thyroid lymphomas are rare and usually arise in preexisting autoimmune (Hashimoto) thyroiditis. Most are non-Hodgkin lymphomas. Diagnosis requires core needle biopsy or more likely,

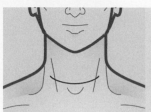

- GA and positioning using head ring, shoulder bolster and semirecumbent position
- Local anaesthetic infiltrated along the wound before skin incision
- 'Collar' incision made one finger's breadth below cricoid cartilage
- Vessels may be ligated or using an energy device

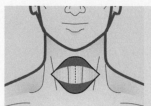

- Platysma divided transversely and subplatysmal flaps created using diathermy
- Vertical incision in midline between strap muscles which are retracted laterally on side of interest. Division of the head of sternothyroid

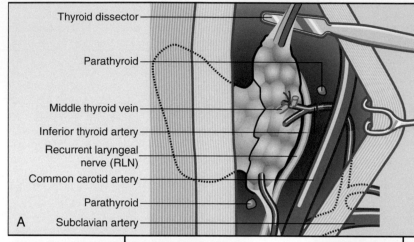

Thyroid dissector
Parathyroid
Middle thyroid vein
Inferior thyroid artery
Recurrent laryngeal nerve (RLN)
Common carotid artery
Parathyroid
A Subclavian artery

- Retract thyroid lobe medially, dissect down to common carotid artery and divide middle thyroid vein
- Retract superior pole inferomedially and ligate vessels supplying superior pole close to gland. External branch of superior laryngeal nerve should be sought and preserved
- Identify recurrent laryngeal nerve (RLN) in tracheooesophageal groove; usually lies posterior to inferior thyroid artery
- Identify and preserve parathyroid glands: in 90%, the superior lies within 1 cm of where the inferior thyroid artery and RLN cross and the inferior lies near the lower pole of thyroid anterior to the RLN
- Ligate inferior thyroid artery ligated close to gland taking care to avoid the RLN
- Ligate veins draining inferior lobe
- Trace RLN carefully to where it enters the larynx; the lobe may then be freed from attachments to trachea
- One lobe may be removed by dividing the isthmus. For total thyroidectomy the process is repeated for the contralateral lobe
- Haemostasis must be checked carefully: the anaesthetist should increase blood pressure to above normal and elevate the venous pressure by tilting head down and increasing the intrathoracic pressure with a Valsalva manoeuvre

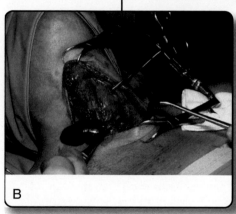

B

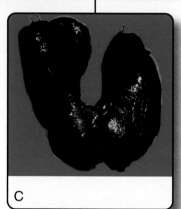

C

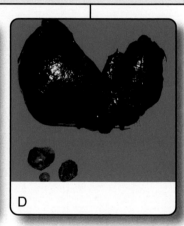

D

• **Fig. 49.8 Thyroid Operations.** Thyroidectomy technique. **(A)** The drawings show the standard neck exploration approach to thyroid (and parathyroid) operations, and the structures at particular danger—the recurrent laryngeal nerve and parathyroid glands. In the photographs, **(B)** shows neck exploration for hyperparathyroidism. A collar incision has been made and upper and lower flaps are held apart with the specially designed retractors. A single large parathyroid adenoma is clearly visible. **(C)** Subtotal thyroidectomy specimen after operation for hyperthyroidism. **(D)** Total thyroidectomy specimen with lymph nodes after an operation for right-sided medullary carcinoma.

open biopsy as FNA is inadequate. Treatment is with radiotherapy, and survival depends on whether spread has extended beyond the thyroid capsule. For lesions within the capsule, 5-year survival is 85%, falling to 40% with local spread.

Goitres and Thyroid Nodules

Several hyperplastic and metabolic disorders cause diffuse or nodular thyroid enlargement (see Tables 49.1 and 49.2).

Idiopathic Nontoxic Hyperplasia

In developed countries, most goitres referred to surgeons are simple idiopathic hyperplasia of thyroid follicles. The condition probably begins with diffuse micronodular enlargement; later nodules become heterogeneously enlarged to form a **multinodular colloid goitre**. Within the same spectrum, are **solitary**

hyperplastic nodules (often adenomas) and **thyroid cysts**, which are large colloid-filled follicles or else contain straw-coloured fluid.

Secretory activity within the gland is patchy, explaining the distribution of radioiodine uptake on scanning, but hormone secretion is usually within the euthyroid range. Diffuse or multinodular idiopathic goitres develop slowly and may cause little trouble.

The reasons patients are referred to surgeons with thyroid enlargement are:
- A localised lump has appeared in the thyroid region. This may be a solitary adenomatous nodule, part of an asymmetrical multinodular or multicystic enlargement, a cyst or, in 5%, thyroid cancer.
- A preexisting multinodular goitre has undergone rapid asymmetric change.
- The patient has become hyperthyroid.

- The patient has developed stridor from tracheal compression because of enlargement of a retrosternal extension.
- A goitre has become so large as to be cosmetically unacceptable.

Surgical Management of Goitre

Indications for thyroid surgery are:
- proven malignancy or a solitary or dominant nodule suspected of malignancy
- a retrosternal thyroid causing compression
- thyrotoxicosis (Graves disease, toxic MNG or toxic adenoma)
- cosmetic deformity

In principle, only enough thyroid tissue is removed to achieve the objective, but in MNG, recurrence is likely and optimal treatment is total thyroidectomy, with lifetime T4 replacement.

Patients presenting for cosmetic reasons, with moderate thyroid enlargement, have often been treated with T4, but this is ineffective. Thyroid cysts are diagnosed as fluid-filled lesions on ultrasound or by aspiration. Fluid cytology should be performed to exclude malignancy. Large or recurrent cysts are best treated surgically.

Technical Points

- Thyroid surgery is usually performed under general anaesthesia
- Vessels may be ligated or sealed using bipolar diathermy, Ligasure or Harmonic scalpel
- The optimal skin incision is centred one finger's breadth below the cricoid cartilage
- Injury to the recurrent laryngeal nerve (RLN), external branch of the superior laryngeal nerve and parathyroid glands can best be avoided by visualising them clearly and preserving their blood supply and the parathyroid venous drainage
- The recurrent laryngeal nerve is vulnerable to injury directly before it is identified, and from traction or heat from energy devices, even after visualisation
- Haemostasis must be meticulous to avoid what can become airway-compromising haemorrhage

Complications of Thyroid Surgery

- Injury to the recurrent laryngeal nerve
- Transient hypocalcaemia
- Permanent hypoparathyroidism
- Haematoma
- Injury to the external superior laryngeal nerve
- Wound infection
- Hypothyroidism (unavoidable in total thyroidectomy)
- Thyrotoxicosis (if insufficient tissue is removed)

Postoperative Hypocalcaemia

Transient hypocalcaemia (<2 mmol/L), caused by parathyroid compromise is common, occurring in 25% to 40%. This persists as permanent hypoparathyroidism in 1% to 3% in the best hands. Profound hypocalcaemia disrupts neuromuscular signalling, causing hyperexcitability, first manifest as perioral and fingertip paraesthesia. Untreated, this can progress to tetanic contractures, seizures and death. Oral calcium ± activated vitamin D are sufficient in almost all cases if begun early; intravenous (IV) calcium should be avoided. Serum calcium and parathyroid hormone (PTH) should be measured in the 24 hours postoperative, oral supplements given and blood tests repeated to monitor improvement.

Congenital Thyroid Disorders

Embryology

The thyroid originates as a midline diverticulum between the first two branchial pouches. Its origin is represented in the adult by the **foramen caecum**, visible at the junction of the anterior two-thirds and the posterior third of the tongue. The thyroid diverticulum forms the **thyroglossal duct**, which extends caudally through the developing tongue. It passes down in relation to the hyoid bone (in front of, through or behind it) to reach its normal position below the larynx. By this time, it has become a bilobed structure, with the lobes connected by a narrow central **isthmus**. The thyroglossal duct later atrophies. The calcitonin-secreting C-cells originate from the **ultimobranchial body** of the fifth pouch.

Thyroglossal Cyst and 'Fistula'

Part of the thyroglossal duct may persist and become cystic. Thyroglossal cysts presents in children and occasionally adolescents as a smooth, rounded, midline swelling in the neck. Most thyroglossal cysts occur below the hyoid, or rarely in the submental region. A diagnostic feature is that the cyst rises when the patient swallows or protrudes the tongue. Most thyroglossal cysts are asymptomatic but are prone to inflammation causing pain and swelling. If an inflamed cyst is drained, it may become an intermittently discharging **sinus**, often incorrectly described as a **thyroglossal fistula** (Fig. 49.9).

Thyroglossal cysts are usually excised along with the thyroglossal tract, up to the base of the tongue. This requires removing the middle third of the hyoid (**Sistrunk operation**). A persistent sinus or a recurrent cyst is likely to complicate incomplete excision.

Ectopic Thyroid Tissue

An ectopic thyroid is a rare congenital abnormality resulting from interruption of normal descent. It may present like a thyroglossal cyst or as a lump in the tongue. As this may be the patient's only thyroid tissue, isotope scanning should check if there is thyroid tissue in the normal position before excision.

CASE HISTORY

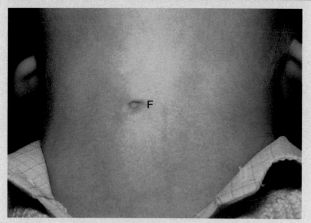

• **Fig. 49.9 Thyroglossal 'Fistula'.** This photograph shows the front of the neck in a 14-year-old boy. An attempt had been made to remove a thyroglossal cyst several years previously. The inevitable result of incomplete surgical removal was an intermittently discharging fistula (*F*) in the midline of the neck.

Disorders of Parathyroid Glands

Anatomy

Parathyroids have the most variable position of any organ. Healthy glands are 2 to 7 mm long and weigh 35 to 40 mg and are a distinctive tan brown. The parathyroids are usually four (two superior and two inferior) distributed around the thyroid, but 6% have one or more supernumerary glands. Ninety percent of superior glands can be found within 1 cm of the intersection of recurrent laryngeal nerve and inferior thyroid artery, whereas inferior glands are much more variable.

Hyperparathyroidism

Hyperparathyroidism is characterised by elevated serum calcium and inappropriately raised (unsuppressed) serum PTH. The most common form is primary hyperparathyroidism (pHPT) and usually occurs in adults. Many cases remain undetected but greater use of serum calcium estimations mean that patients rarely present with florid sequelae of pHPT. Estimates suggest that about 1% of the adult population has pHPT. Most cases are discovered incidentally or during investigation for nonspecific symptoms. **Secondary hyperparathyroidism** (sHPT) may result from vitamin D deficiency or renal failure, or less common causes, such as malabsorption because of crohn or coeliac disease, or hypermagnesaemia.

Symptoms and Signs

Patients are usually referred to the surgeon after hypercalcaemia is discovered, whilst investigating musculoskeletal pain or recurrent urinary tract calculi, or else is found by chance on measuring calcium blood levels for other reasons. Classic features include bone pain, urinary tract stones, abdominal pain (caused by peptic ulcer or recurrent pancreatitis), and mental changes, such as confusion, depression or even psychosis. These can be remembered by the aide mémoire: **bones, stones, abdominal groans** and **psychic moans**. Many apparently asymptomatic patients turn out to have suffered nonspecific neurocognitive symptoms, including fatigue and malaise, or have signs of hypertension.

Most pHPT is sporadic, but risk factors include neck irradiation, long-term lithium medication or MEN 1 and 2a, which tend to present younger. In MEN 1, pHPT may be associated with pancreatic islet cell tumours secreting insulin or gastrin or pituitary tumours, and in MEN 2, medullary carcinoma of the thyroid and/or phaeochromocytomas. In sporadic disease, the cause of pHPT is a single adenoma in up to 90%, with the rest caused by multiple gland disease, mainly hyperplasia.

Raised plasma calcium eventually causes systemic problems or loss of bone density. From Fig. 49.10, it is paradoxical that urinary tract calculi are common in hyperparathyroidism, since parathormone *reduces* urinary calcium excretion. The probable reason is that phosphaturia leads to increased urinary alkalinity, predisposing to calcium salt precipitation.

Control of Plasma Calcium (See Fig. 49.10)
Physiology

Plasma calcium level is maintained within a very narrow range by the combined effects of parathormone and vitamin D and a complex feedback loop involving levels of serum calcium, vitamin D and calcitonin. Parathormone secretion rate is governed directly by the plasma concentration of ionised calcium. If parathormone is overproduced, this raises plasma calcium and causes

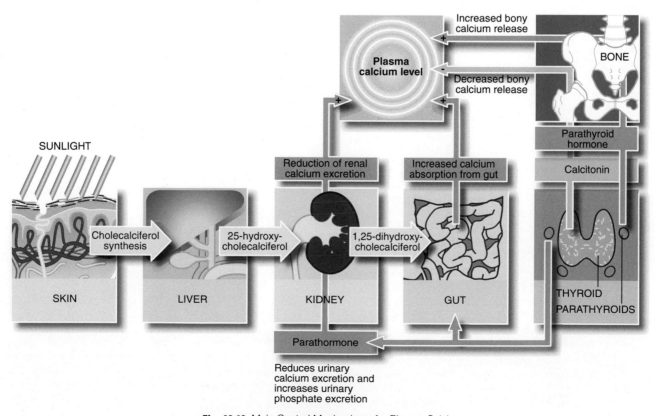

• **Fig. 49.10** Main Control Mechanisms for Plasma Calcium.

phosphaturia, thereby decreasing serum phosphate. Parathormone acts on the renal system, gastrointestinal tract and bone to increase serum calcium as follows:

Renal
- Enhances renal tubular reabsorption of calcium and diminishes reabsorption of phosphate, thereby increasing the renal clearance of phosphate
- Activates 25-hydroxy vitamin D into 1,25-dihydroxy vitamin D

Bone
- Mobilises calcium stores via osteoblasts (fast phase in hours) and osteoclasts (slow phase in days)

Gastrointestinal Tract
- In the presence of activated vitamin D from renal tract, promotes calcium absorption from small intestine

Types of Hyperparathyroidism
Hyperparathyroidism is classified by origin as follows:

Primary Hyperparathyroidism
a. Single Parathyroid Adenoma. The most common cause of pHPT, found in 80%+ of cases. One gland becomes replaced by a benign neoplasm, secreting parathormone in excessive amounts. Secretion by the other parathyroids is suppressed.

b. Diffuse Parathyroid Hyperplasia. Uncommon. The secretory cells of two or more of the glands undergo idiopathic hyperplasia.

c. Parathyroid Carcinoma. This is extremely rare (1% of pHPT) and involves only one gland. These are often palpable and cause gross elevation of plasma calcium.

Secondary and Tertiary Hyperparathyroidism
In **sHPT**, there is an abnormal chronic stimulus to parathormone production, most often in chronic renal failure (including nearly all patients on dialysis), but also in vitamin D deficiency. Glands undergo **diffuse hyperplasia**. These patients develop osteomalacia and osteitis fibrosa cystica, as well as ectopic calcification around joints and in arteries.

After renal transplantation, hyperparathyroidism may persist if the hypertrophied parathyroid glands fail to regress. Autonomous oversecretion continues, with normal or even elevated serum calcium levels. This is called tertiary hyperparathyroidism and has clinical effects similar to sHPT.

Malignant Hypercalcaemia
The other common cause of hypercalcaemia is malignant disease. This is because of secretion of **parathormone-related protein (PTH-rP)** in 70%, and in the rest, to widespread bone destruction from **lytic bone metastases**. Tumours that secrete PTH-rP include squamous cell carcinoma of lung, renal cell carcinoma and bladder cancer. Tumours causing hypercalcaemia by bone destruction include breast cancer, leukaemias and multiple myeloma.

Management of Primary Hyperparathyroidism
Surgery is the only definitive cure. Current indications include all patients with symptomatic disease or proven end-organ damage.

Imaging Before Surgery
Ultrasound can localise a diseased gland or glands but is unreliable for visualising ectopic glands or distinguishing atypical adenomas from thyroid tissue or lymph nodes. Before reoperative surgery, ultrasound can guide preoperative needle aspiration of potential adenomas for parathormone sampling.

Radionuclide tracer imaging: no isotope is specific for parathyroid tissue, but SestaMIBI accumulates in mitochondria in thyroid and parathyroid tissue, but it washes out faster from thyroid, leaving parathyroid visible later. Dual isotopes can also be used, as can three-dimensional images constructed digitally from images at different angles.

Surgical Management
For a well-localised single adenoma, a *focused lateral approach* involves an incision directly over it, otherwise a standard collar incision enables all glands to be explored. In the focused approach, intraoperative PTH can be measured with a rapid analyser after removing the gland, to confirm the operation is complete. A 50% drop at 10 minutes after excision (the 'Miami criterion') is most widely relied upon.

Parathyroid exploration for a gland or glands not identified on preoperative imaging can be exacting and time-consuming, often interrupted by histological examination of frozen section biopsies. Surgical access is the same as for thyroidectomy. The likely anatomical site of each parathyroid is then meticulously explored. Parathyroids have a characteristic yellow-brown colour, but are often difficult to distinguish from thyroid tissue, especially after surgical trauma.

If no individual gland is disproportionately enlarged, the possibility of a missing adenoma in a fifth gland should be considered, in the absence of which, excision of the largest 3/3.5 glands is performed—'subtotal parathyroidectomy'. Total parathyroidectomy with reimplantation of a free graft of parathyroid tissue ('autotransplantation') in a forearm muscle pouch is now a largely obsolete, historical procedure.

The chief adverse outcome is failure to cure the patient of pHPT. The success rate in first time parathyroid surgery depends on patient volume and experience; cure rates of over 95% are expected in a specialist centre.

Complications of parathyroidectomy are similar to thyroid surgery (see Box 49.3, earlier) although the rate of injury to the recurrent laryngeal nerve should be extremely low. Following removal of a single adenoma, temporary hypoparathyroidism may occur, and so plasma calcium must be monitored in the early postoperative period, and treated if low.

Special Cases

Parathyroid Carcinoma
Treatment is en-bloc parathyroidectomy and hemithyroidectomy, plus excision of local lymph nodes; it is often curative. These tumours are not radiosensitive.

Primary Hyperparathyroidism in Pregnancy
pHPT may be unmasked and hypercalcaemia can put mother and foetus at risk of intrauterine growth retardation, miscarriage, preeclampsia, stillbirth and neonatal hypocalcaemic tetany. Most need definitive surgery during the second trimester, ideally in a specialist centre.

Primary Hyperparathyroidism in Known Multiple Endocrine Neoplasia 1
This occurs in 90% and generally presents before the age of 20 years. It is characterised by metachronous multiple gland disease, that is, occurring at different times. Subtotal parathyroidectomy can achieve normocalcaemia for 10 years, in 60% of patients, and is the preferred approach in these young patients.

Secondary and Tertiary Hyperparathyroidism

In **secondary hyperparathyroidism**, the elevated PTH results from an external stimulus to parathyroids. **Tertiary HPT** occurs when hyperfunction becomes autonomous after treating secondary disease. Both are characterised by hypercalcaemia and hyperphosphataemia, profound PTH elevation, bone erosions and in extreme cases, osteitis fibrosis cystica. Common causes are chronic renal failure and in a milder version, chronic vitamin D deficiency.

Symptoms of sHPT include pruritus, bone pain and deformity, neuromuscular and psychiatric symptoms, with weakness and depression, erythropoietin-resistant anaemia and cardiac failure. As both calcium and phosphate become elevated, vascular, and valvular calcification and/or calciphylaxis (necrotic areas of skin caused by calcification in small vessels) may occur.

sHPT is largely manageable with medical measures but refractory symptoms, hyperphosphataemia (a calcium-phosphate product >4 implies urgency) and rising PTH (especially if >100 pmol/L) require parathyroidectomy. Total parathyroidectomy is indicated in patients not undergoing renal transplantation, to prevent recurrence of HPT. sHPT usually resolves after renal transplantation, but tertiary HPT may occur and need emergency parathyroidectomy. Here, residual tissue is a lifeline preventing hypoparathyroidism so subtotal parathyroidectomy is optimum treatment.

Hypoparathyroidism

The most common cause of hypoparathyroidism is surgical removal or devascularisation of parathyroids, during thyroid or parathyroid surgery. Autoimmune hypoparathyroidism also occurs occasionally.

Hypoparathyroidism presents clinically with the effects of hypocalcaemia. A fall in plasma calcium level increases neuromuscular excitability, causing cramps or **tetany** in severe cases. An early symptom is paraesthesia, especially around the lips. After thyroid or parathyroid operations, plasma calcium estimations should be performed the next morning and 24 hours later.

Clinical tests for hypocalcaemia include tapping over the parotid gland. This provokes transient contraction of the facial muscles known as **Chvostek sign**. A further test involves inflating a sphygmomanometer cuff on the upper arm above systolic pressure. This induces carpal spasm within about 3 minutes (*main d'accoucheur* or *obstetrician's hand*).

Early postoperative hypocalcaemia is treated with calcium supplements. Persistent hypocalcaemia is controlled by oral administration of high doses of calcium and vitamin D analogues.

Adrenal Glands

Anatomy and Physiology

The adrenal glands lie in the retroperitoneum above and medial to the kidneys and have a dual embryological derivation reflected in their function and pathologies. The **medulla** is derived from the neural crest, part of the autonomic nervous system, and produces adrenaline, noradrenaline and dopamine. The adult adrenal **cortex** has three distinct layers derived from mesothelium; the outermost *zona glomerulosa* produces aldosterone, the *zona fasciculata*, corticosteroids and the *zona reticularis*, androgens. Neoplasms are classified according to tissue of origin, whether benign or malignant, primary or secondary, and functional or not (i.e., producing an excess of one or more adrenal hormones).

The Adrenal 'Incidentaloma'

An adrenal tumour is detected in about 4% of adults undergoing abdominal cross-sectional imaging. The questions then are whether this could be malignant and whether is it functional.

On CT with IV contrast, features suggesting malignancy are large size (> 4cm = 90% sensitive, 75% specific), irregular border, inhomogeneous density or calcification and delayed washout of contrast.

Patients should be screened for excess cortisol secretion and for phaeochromocytoma. Any with hypertension or unexplained hypokalaemia also need screening for aldosterone excess. If imaging suggests adrenocortical cancer, dehydroepiandrosterone sulphate and sex hormone levels should be checked. If imaging is not suspicious and there is no hormonal excess, patients require no further investigation.

Adrenal Hyperfunction

Phaeochromocytoma

Functioning medullary tumours are rare (~2/100,000) and diagnosis is often delayed because they mimic other pathologies. Typically, patients have intermittent headache, sweating, palpitations and anxiety. Traditionally known as the *ten percent tumour* because 10% are bilateral, 10% malignant, 10% extraadrenal 'paragangliomas', 10% are in children and 10% familial. At least a quarter occur in a germline mutations, such as MEN 2. A firm diagnosis requires elevated catecholamines and an adrenal or extraadrenal tumour on imaging.

Surgery is the only definitive treatment, ideally by laparoscopic or retroperitoneoscopic adrenalectomy. Operation requires prearranged perioperative care by a multidisciplinary team, including an endocrinologist and an anaesthetist with experience. Incremental alpha-blockade is begun (usually with phenoxybenzamine) plus beta-blockade if the patient experiences palpitations. This prevents hypertensive crises caused by gland manipulation that increases catecholamine output, and it prevents profound postoperative hypotension.

Cushing's Syndrome

Cushing's syndrome is characterised by excess cortisol secretion and overt features of hypercortisolaemia, such as facial plethora, buffalo hump, centripetal obesity, proximal myopathy, osteoporosis, diabetes and hypertension. So-called **adrenal Cushing's** results from autonomous ACTH-*independent* secretion of cortisol from an adrenal lesion or lesions. Hypercortisolaemia secondary to ACTH excess may result from a pituitary lesion (Cushing's disease) or ectopic ACTH secretion (most commonly from small cell lung or bronchial neuroendocrine tumour).

Adrenal Cushing's may result from an adenoma, carcinoma or bilateral adrenal hyperplasia and is characterised by cortisol excess and ACTH suppression. Dexamethasone suppression tests are a screening tool and a confirmatory test of the diagnosis. Once diagnosed, adrenal pathology should be sought on abdominal CT scanning. Laparoscopic or retroperitoneoscopic adrenalectomy is the treatment of choice. Patients undergoing adrenalectomy always require postoperative steroid cover because of a suppressed pituitary adrenal axis and a potential life-threatening Addisonian crisis.

Conn's Syndrome

Primary hyperaldosteronism or Conn's syndrome is classically suspected in hypertension plus hypokalaemia. Conn's syndrome is now believed to account for 10% of major hypertension. Note that 10% to 40% Conn's patients are not hypokalaemic. The common causes are an aldosterone-producing adenoma or bilateral adrenal hyperplasia. Treatment depends on the cause, with adrenalectomy recommended in unilateral adenoma. Medical management is currently recommended for bilateral disease.

Adrenal Surgery

The function of any adrenal tumour must be assessed before surgery, to avoid a hypertensive crisis from an unrecognised phaeochromocytoma.

Indications for surgery are:
- Phaeochromocytoma (following optimisation with alpha blockade)
- Cushing's syndrome, with a unilateral adrenal mass
- Cushing's disease, with failure of pituitary surgery (offer bilateral adrenalectomy)
- Malignancy or suspected malignancy

50

Acute Surgical Problems in Children

Introduction

A **neonate** is a newborn less than 28 days old, an **infant** is less than a year, a **child** is 1 to 17 years old and an **adult** is 18 years or older. In the United Kingdom, paediatric clinical practice generally covers children only up to the age of 16 years. Increasingly, those between 13 and 18 years are being managed in adolescent units, where their needs are better met. Many children are treated by general surgeons with a paediatric interest, but surgical problems in infants, major congenital abnormalities and malignant tumours are usually managed in regional centres by specialists. The range of surgical conditions in children differs from adults and also varies between age groups, particularly for emergency presentations. Paediatric emergencies are considered here by age group, that is, **newborn** (the first few days of life, including premature babies), **infants and young children** (up to about 2 years) and **older children** (up to puberty). During puberty, the disorders merge with those of adulthood.

Physiological Differences Between Infants and Adults

Successful paediatric surgical care depends on managing the physiological differences between neonates, infants, children and adults. For example, the **basal metabolic rate** is very high in the newborn, with an oxygen demand of 5 to 8 mL/kg per min. This falls in older children and adults to 2 mL/kg per min. The **blood volume** in a baby is 80 mL per kg body weight, a much higher volume to weight ratio than an adult, but the total blood volume is very small (typically around 250 mL in a full-term newborn infant), so operative technique needs to be meticulous to minimise loss. In an adult, losing 100 mL is negligible, but can be life-threatening to a small child; even small losses need to be accurately measured and replaced during surgery if necessary.

Fluid and Electrolyte Problems

Fluid deficiency and **electrolyte imbalances** occur rapidly because each compartment has such a small fluid volume. In addition, paediatric fluid requirements are relatively greater than adults because the kidneys have a lesser concentrating ability and so obligatory urine output is greater. Faecal fluid losses are higher, particularly under 2 years. In cases of severe diarrhoea, dehydration and electrolyte disturbances develop with frightening speed. Signs of fluid depletion are also different from adults. Young fluid-depleted children are often lethargic or drowsy and may even be comatose. The eyes and anterior fontanelle may be sunken but skin turgor is **not** lost. Tachycardia is usual, but hypotension is a late sign because of compensatory mechanisms. Urine output is likely to be low; normal output should be at least 1 mL per kg body weight per hour.

Blood Glucose

Hypoglycaemia readily occurs because a baby's glycogen stores are meagre; there needs to be a regular supply of glucose by feeding or intravenous (IV) infusion. Adrenergic responses to trauma and stress also increase glucose requirements. Hypoglycaemia is likely to occur if a baby is fasted before surgery, but not given IV dextrose, or when a blood transfusion temporarily replaces IV dextrose. All small children undergoing surgery need close monitoring of blood glucose to prevent hypoglycaemic brain damage.

Temperature Regulation

Temperature regulation in infants is less robust and **hypothermia** is a real hazard. Infants have a relatively large surface area, poor vasomotor control of skin vessels and are unable to generate heat by shivering. These differences are more marked in premature neonates, who are poorly adapted to life outside the uterus. A controlled, heated environment is essential for operating on and nursing newborn infants. For those under 1 kg, the temperature is set between 34.5°C and 35.5°C, and for those over 3 kg, between 31.5°C and 34.5°C. The infant is placed on a heated mattress and all parts of the body kept insulated. IV fluids and skin cleansers are warmed and anaesthetic gases humidified and warmed.

Liver Function

Liver function is immature in the newborn. Physiological jaundice caused by high levels of unconjugated bilirubin is common because the immature liver cannot synthesise the enzyme **glucuronyl transferase**. There is also reduced ability to detoxify analgesic drugs, and many drugs cross the blood–brain barrier more readily and hence are more likely to cause cerebral side effects. Drugs must often be used in greatly reduced doses, after checking a paediatric formulary. A further consequence of liver immaturity is reduced **prothrombin** production. Prophylactic vitamin K should be given after a baby's birth, or intravenously in the perioperative period.

Immunity

Infection can be rapidly fatal in small babies, particularly premature and small-for-dates babies who are likely to have impaired immunological defences. Infection can be minimised by good surgical technique, meticulous haemostasis to avoid haematomas, and prophylactic antibiotics where appropriate. Vigilance for perioperative infection is essential.

Managing Surgery in Infants

Survival of babies undergoing complex surgery has steadily improved as their specific problems have become better understood and managed, with surgeons and paediatricians working together. Examples include: effective **total parenteral nutrition** to prevent babies dying from malnutrition, whilst waiting for paralytic ileus to resolve; and better understanding of how to manage mechanical ventilation. Specialised understanding of fluid and electrolyte balance, drug effects and nutritional demands is necessary for safe pre- and postoperative care of these small patients. The successes of neonatal surgery over the past 30 years have been achieved because of advances in neonatal care.

> ● **BOX 50.1** Main Non-urological Abdominal Emergencies that occur in the Newborn
>
> - Incarcerated or strangulated inguinal hernia
> - Gastrointestinal atresias and stenoses
> - Midgut malrotation with volvulus
> - Anorectal abnormalities
> - Meconium ileus and other problems with meconium
> - Hirschsprung disease
> - Congenital diaphragmatic hernia
> - Deficiencies in the abdominal wall (gastroschisis, exomphalos and ectopia vesicae)
> - Necrotising enterocolitis

Surgical Emergencies in the Neonate

More neonates with congenital abnormalities can be identified before birth because of the widespread use of **antenatal ultrasound** during pregnancy, and improved foetal medicine. This allows for antenatal counselling and timely preparation for postnatal management. The more common abdominal emergencies in the neonate are summarised in Box 50.1.

Intestinal Obstruction

Intestinal obstruction occurs in around 1 in 2000 live births. Most are not detectable antenatally, so vigilance is needed for neonates that do not tolerate feeds. Intrauterine obstruction of the gastrointestinal (GI) tract prevents the foetus from passing amniotic fluid through the GI tract after swallowing. This results in **polyhydramnios**, which may result in premature delivery and prematurity. It is often the only antenatal sign of oesophageal atresia. Intestinal obstruction in neonates presents with a **failure to tolerate feeds**, **vomiting**, **failure to pass meconium,** and in cases of distal obstruction, **abdominal distension.**

Causes of obstruction fall into four main categories (**LIFE**):
- **L**uminal discontinuity (e.g., atresias)
- **I**nspissated (thickened) luminal contents (as seen in meconium ileus)
- **F**ailure of normal intestinal peristalsis (as seen in Hirschsprung disease)
- **E**xternal compression of the bowel (as seen in volvulus or more rarely, abdominal masses)

In infants with high intestinal obstruction, abdominal distension is rare and in lower GI obstruction, distension may be a late sign. Abdominal plain films taken soon after delivery should be interpreted with caution because GI gas patterns are not yet normal; it takes several hours for gas to reach the colon.

The most common causes of upper intestinal obstruction in neonates are **small bowel volvulus** (because of foregut rotational abnormalities) and **duodenal atresia** (particularly in babies with trisomy 21). Distal intestinal obstruction can be caused by inspissated luminal contents in **meconium ileus**, abnormal motility in **Hirschsprung disease** or discontinuity of the bowel in **intestinal atresias** (narrowed segments of bowel). A plain radiograph performed after several hours is fundamental in making a preliminary diagnosis of the level of obstruction (Fig. 50.1). When proximal intestine is obstructed, there may be few dilated loops and a lack of distal intestinal

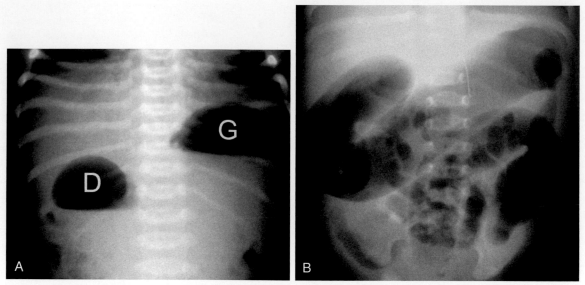

• **Fig. 50.1** Intestinal Obstruction. **(A)** Erect plain abdominal x-ray of a baby with 'high' intestinal obstruction, showing the typical 'double bubble' appearance of gas in the dilated stomach *(G)* and the first part of the duodenum *(D)*. The differential diagnosis includes duodenal atresia, malrotation with volvulus obstructing the duodenum, and a very high jejunal atresia. Fluid levels are seen in this erect film. **(B)** Abdominal x-ray of a baby with a 'low' intestinal obstruction, showing several dilated loops of bowel. The differential diagnosis includes Hirschsprung disease, meconium ileus, and ileal atresia.

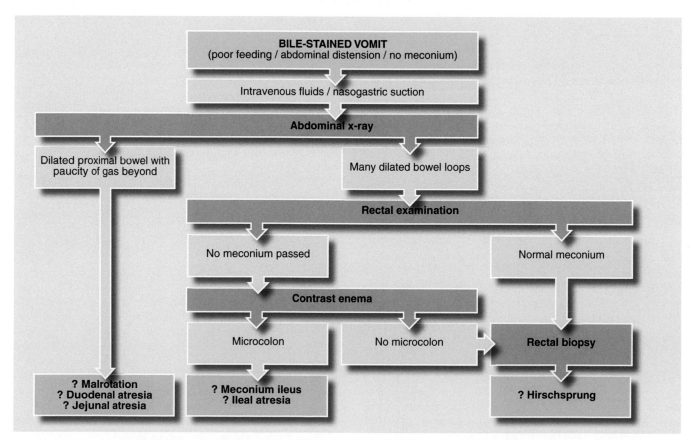

• **Fig. 50.2** Plan for Investigating and Managing Babies With Suspected Intestinal Obstruction.

gas. Conversely, there are often multiple dilated loops in more distal obstruction. Note, however, that the plain radiograph can be normal in volvulus, secondary to malrotation. If this is clinically suspected, an urgent upper GI contrast study can determine whether the duodenojejunal flexure is normally or abnormally positioned. Other causes of intestinal obstruction, such as an anorectal malformations or incarcerated inguinal hernia, can be found on clinical examination without radiology. A plan for investigating babies with suspected intestinal obstruction is outlined in Fig. 50.2.

Gastrointestinal Atresias

Intestinal atresia is complete obliteration or failure to form of a segment of GI tract. These abnormalities are uncommon and complicate around 1:1000 live births. Given there is no continuity of the lumen, the proximal bowel becomes dilated above the obstruction and the distal bowel collapses. Atresias can occur anywhere in the GI tract but are most common in the oesophagus, duodenum, jejunum and ileum.

Oesophageal atresia, duodenal atresia and anorectal malformations are true developmental abnormalities and are frequently associated with other congenital abnormalities, often in predictable patterns. Major cardiac, vertebral or renal anomalies are found in around 40% of babies with oesophageal atresia, and duodenal atresia is common in trisomy 21. In contrast, **small bowel atresias** are believed to result from mesenteric vascular mishaps in utero and are rarely associated with other congenital abnormalities.

Oesophageal Atresia

Oesophageal atresia occurs in between 1 in 2500 to 1 in 5000 live births. It is often seen in combination with 'VACTERL' anomalies, that is, one or more of V—vertebral, A—anorectal, C—cardiac, T—tracheal, E—'esophageal' atresia, R—renal and L—limb abnormalities. In the most common type of oesophageal atresia, the proximal oesophagus ends blindly and there is a fistula between its lower end and the trachea (Fig. 50.3). The other 10% have isolated oesophageal atresia or multiple connections to the trachea.

The diagnosis is suspected before birth, when there is **polyhydramnios** (30% of all cases) or other VACTERL anomalies, or the gastric gas bubble is not seen on a plain radiograph. In infants with oesophageal atresia, aspiration pneumonia and choking episodes can be life threatening so when the diagnosis is suspected, it is vital to check oesophageal continuity before feeding is started.

Once diagnosed, the baby is resuscitated and congenital problems, such as cardiac abnormalities, sought that may impact on the operation. An operation is then performed to correct the oesophageal atresia by anastomosing the two ends and to disconnect the distal oesophagus from the trachea.

In pure atresia without a fistula, there is often a long gap between the ends of the oesophagus. Reconstruction may then involve a sequence of planned operations to bridge the gap.

Duodenal Atresia

Duodenal atresia is found in around 1 in 5000 live births. The obstruction is usually in the second part of the duodenum, distal to the entry point of the common bile duct. Thus the vomiting is bile-stained. The atresia is either complete or there is an incomplete web across the lumen. Complete atresia most commonly presents antenatally with polyhydramnios and after delivery, classically with a '**double bubble**' appearance on plain abdominal radiography, that is, a dilated gastric bubble and proximal duodenum, with no gas distally (see Fig. 50.1A). When incomplete, the presentation is more insidious, with gradually increasing feed intolerance. Oesophageal atresia and duodenal atresia are commonly associated with trisomy 21.

Surgical treatment involves formation of a duodenoduodenostomy, anastomosing the two ends of the discontinuous duodenum.

Small Bowel Atresias

Small bowel atresias are relatively uncommon, with an incidence of 1 in 5000 live births. There are single or multiple atresias causing discontinuity in the bowel lumen. Infants typically present with

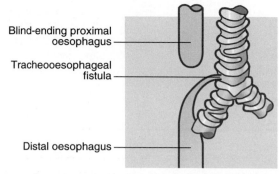

• **Fig. 50.3** Oesophageal Atresia With Tracheo-oesophageal Fistula. This is the most common variant of oesophageal atresia, found in 90% of cases. Air enters the gastrointestinal tract via the fistula and may be seen on plain x-ray. 'Frothy' breathing may occur because the mouth and pharynx are full of saliva.

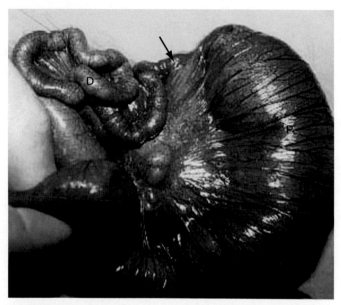

• **Fig. 50.4** Jejunal Atresia. Findings at laparotomy on a neonate presenting with intestinal obstruction. The proximal jejunum (P) is greatly dilated, whilst the distal jejunum is collapsed (D). In between, is an atretic segment without a lumen (arrow). This was resected and the bowel ends joined. The infant thrived soon afterwards.

bile-stained vomiting and failure to pass meconium. Loops of dilated bowel are sometimes visible and palpable on clinical examination, and there are dilated bowel loops with no distal gas on plain x-ray.

Treatment of small bowel atresias is surgical, performing one or multiple intestinal anastomoses to return the bowel to continuity. Fig. 50.4 shows operative findings in jejunal atresia with typically distended proximal jejunum and collapsed distal jejunum.

Midgut Malrotation With Volvulus

During the first trimester, the midgut develops outside the foetal abdominal cavity. Between 10 and 12 weeks' gestation, the midgut undergoes rotation and the duodenum develops its characteristic C-shaped loop by rotating through 270 degrees anticlockwise. The outcome of this intricate arrangement is that the duodenal-jejunal flexure comes to lie to the left of the midline above the pylorus, and the small bowel mesentery develops a broad oblique base, across the posterior abdominal wall, with the caecum lying in the right iliac fossa. When the small bowel mesentery is improperly formed in this way, the bowel has the potential to twist. Children born with malrotation may undergo acute small bowel volvulus at any time, though it occurs most commonly once a child has started feeding and the weight of luminal contents give the bowel the momentum to twist. This obstructs the rotated small bowel and sometimes occludes its blood supply to cause intestinal ischaemia.

A previously well baby presenting with dark green bile-stained vomiting should be assessed urgently and considered to have small bowel volvulus, until proven otherwise. The twisted bowel can untwist spontaneously, so a child may have only a single bile-stained vomit but still be at risk of recurrence. Plain radiography cannot exclude the condition; the gold-standard investigation is an upper-GI contrast study to show where the bowel lies in the abdomen.

At operation, the bowel is untwisted (anticlockwise—'turning back the hands of time'), and warmed by wrapping in warm swabs. *Ladd bands* are then divided and the mesenteric base widened as far as possible. The bowel is then returned to the abdomen, with the duodenum straightened and secured on the right and the caecum on the left. Many surgeons perform an appendicectomy at the same time.

Small bowel volvulus is a serious condition, which, if unrecognised and untreated, often proves fatal or else results in necrosis of much of the small intestine, which then has to be resected. This leads to **short bowel syndrome** and a likely lifelong requirement for parenteral nutrition.

Anorectal Abnormalities

The primitive hindgut forms from the **cloaca** in the first few weeks of intrauterine life. A septum then descends to divide the **anterior compartment** (from which the urinary tract and part of the genital tract are formed) from the **posterior compartment** (which goes on to form the rectum and upper part of the anal canal).

There is a wide spectrum of congenital anorectal disorders and the overall incidence lies between 1 in 2500 and 1 in 3000 live births. Several classifications have been proposed, but the most clinically useful is to group them by whether the large bowel terminates above or below the levator ani. There is usually an abnormal fistulous connection from the end of the bowel; when the malformation is low, the fistula opens onto the skin anterior to the sphincter complex. The perineum must be closely inspected, as sometimes a bead of meconium passes through this fistulous opening, disguising the position of the anus (Fig. 50.5).

In high malformations, there may be a fistula to skin, or a fistulous connection to the vagina in girls or the urinary tract in boys. Urinary tract malformations and lower vertebral anomalies are often associated with anorectal anomalies and should be sought and excluded.

Treatment depends on the level of the distal pouch. In low lesions, the puborectalis muscle is well formed and a relatively simple operation on the perineum may be sufficient. An **anoplasty** is performed to increase the calibre of the fistula and the fistula is moved to open within the sphincter complex. Babies who become unwell, or have **high lesions**, are likely to need a colostomy in the first instance. This rescue procedure allows the baby to feed and empty the bowel. This is followed by complex surgical reconstruction later, involving mobilising the bowel end and reconstructing a sphincter mechanism around it. Long-term faecal continence and bowel and bladder control is imperfect after surgery in many children with high or low anomalies, and careful follow up is needed.

Failure of Passage of Meconium

The date and time of passage of meconium in newborn babies should be recorded. Failure to pass meconium within the first 48

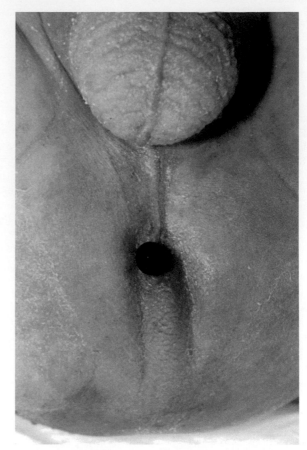

• **Fig. 50.5 Low Imperforate Anus.** This shows an infant's perineum with an anterior fistula through which meconium has passed; the sphincter complex lies posterior to the fistula. The presence of visible meconium makes the diagnosis easy to miss.

hours should alert clinicians to a possible distal obstruction and prompt investigation to exclude serious underlying conditions.

Meconium Ileus

The first few stools in the neonate are called meconium. In meconium ileus, the distal small bowel becomes obstructed by thick, viscid meconium and mucus plugs. About 85% of babies with this condition have **cystic fibrosis** and all babies with meconium ileus should be tested for it. Cystic fibrosis results in abnormal mucus being produced in the lungs, liver, pancreas and small bowel. Pancreatic enzymes, which normally liquefy the meconium, are deficient and the resulting thick meconium can cause intestinal obstruction. The colon and the rectum distal to the obstruction are of a small calibre (microcolon), and this is easily demonstrable on a lower GI contrast study (Fig. 50.6). This investigation is often also therapeutic, as it can chemically loosen the viscid meconium and allow it to pass, thus relieving the obstruction, at least temporarily. In some cases, it may be impossible to relieve the obstruction, even with multiple enemas; there is a risk the colon may perforate causing peritonitis, requiring a laparotomy.

Hirschsprung Disease

Hirschsprung disease is a congenital absence of ganglion cells in the intermyenteric and submucosal plexuses of the distal intestine. The aganglionosis always involves the rectum, extending into the sigmoid in 80% of cases. Less commonly, aganglionosis can affect

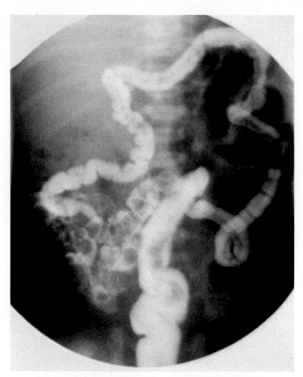

• **Fig. 50.6** Gastrografin Enema in Meconium Ileus. Gastrografin enema x-rays in a baby with meconium ileus, showing the microcolon and the filling defects, caused by abnormal meconium obstructing the distal ileum.

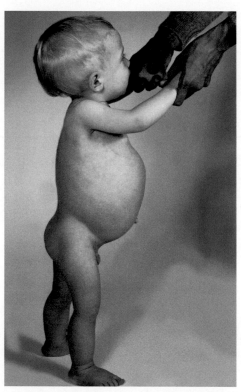

• **Fig. 50.7** Hirschsprung Disease. A historical photograph of a 3-year-old child with neglected Hirschsprung disease demonstrating failure to thrive, with buttock wasting and a dilated abdomen.

the entire colon and reach into the small bowel (long-segment Hirschsprung disease—5% of cases). Aganglionosis results in functional obstruction of the bowel that presents in most cases as a failure to pass meconium. The pathology is continuous, although rarely, 'skip' lesions are described.

The key clinical sign is **abdominal distension** (Fig. 50.7). A rectal examination is often helpful; gentle passage of a rectal thermometer past the anal sphincter often results in an explosive release of air and meconium, partially decompressing the obstruction. Gentle rectal washouts with warm saline can further aid abdominal decompression. Some surgeons like to perform a lower GI contrast study, first to determine the level of the disease by demonstrating dilated bowel above the (collapsed) aganglionic segment.

A formal diagnosis of Hirschsprung disease is made by performing suction rectal biopsies, demonstrating absent ganglion cells in the submucosal plexus and an increase in cholinesterase positive nerves. Initial management is often with formation of a colostomy. In some specialist centres, and in selected cases, a single stage operation is performed at around 6 weeks of age to decompress the bowel, excise the aganglionic segment and perform a 'pull-through' procedure, using intraoperative frozen sections to determine the level of aganglionosis.

Congenital Diaphragmatic Hernia

The diaphragm develops by fusion of the mesodermal primitive septum transversum, the lateral pleuroperitoneal folds and the dorsal mesentery of the embryo at 8 weeks' gestation. The most common type of congenital diaphragmatic hernia is caused by failure of the **pleuroperitoneal canal** to close, resulting in a defect in the posterolateral portion of the diaphragm. The incidence is 1 in 3500 live births and 80% are on the left side. The abdominal viscera are often visible in the chest on antenatal ultrasound. There is

invariably an associated pulmonary hypoplasia (Fig. 50.8), which may be so severe as to be incompatible with life, but will certainly require careful postoperative management.

The diagnosis is usually made antenatally. Overall survival rates are around 50%, but in babies that survive until delivery, this rises to around 90%. Premature birth and the severity of the pulmonary hypoplasia largely determine the prognosis, with right-sided disease, a small thoracic volume and additional cardiac abnormalities giving a worse prognosis.

After birth, the infant is resuscitated and a nasogastric tube passed to decompress the stomach and prevent bowel becoming dilated that would worsen the respiratory status. Assisted ventilation is almost always required to prevent hypoxia and acidosis disrupting cardiovascular function. In some centres, extracorporeal membrane oxygenation is used, but most rely on gentle ventilation.

Surgery is usually delayed until the baby is stable and requiring minimal ventilation. At operation, the diaphragmatic defect is closed. This can be performed open or laparoscopically or even thoracoscopically. There is often bowel malrotation present, which should be assessed at operation and a Ladd procedure performed to prevent later volvulus if appropriate.

Other Causes of Respiratory Problems in the Newborn

Vascular Rings

This rare abnormality is caused by persistence of a double aortic arch or by abnormal configurations of vessels arising from the aortic arch. Either abnormality encircles the trachea and oesophagus resulting in compression. Surgical intervention may be necessary, but children with only mild symptoms may improve spontaneously, as they grow. Older children may present with problems of vomiting, choking or dysphagia, and diagnosis can be taxing.

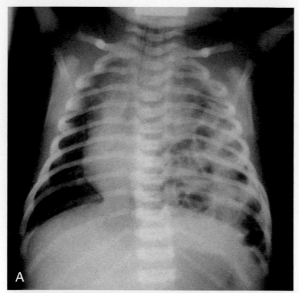

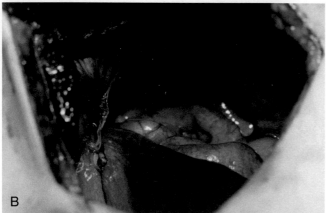

• **Fig. 50.8** Congenital Diaphragmatic Hernia. (A) Plain chest x-ray showing air-containing loops of bowel in the left chest and displacement of the mediastinum to the right. Note the endotracheal tube in place to allow assisted ventilation. (B) An operative picture viewed from the abdomen, showing the pleuroperitoneal canal defect in the diaphragm. Some of the intestine had already been reduced from the thorax.

Congenital Pulmonary Malformations

Congenital cystic lung lesions are traditionally divided into two main groups: **congenital cystic adenomatoid malformations (CCAM)** and **pulmonary sequestrations**. CCAMs result from abnormal development of lung parenchyma and are classified according to the size of the cysts. They are often detected antenatally but computed tomography (CT) scans are used to determine their size and composition after birth. Smaller lesions are usually observed expectantly, as they often remain asymptomatic or can be removed thoracoscopically later in childhood. Symptomatic larger lesions compress normal parenchymal tissue and need fairly urgent surgery. There is a risk of infection or malignant change in persistent CCAM and this must be balanced against the risk of surgery to remove them.

The second group is **pulmonary sequestrations**. These developmental abnormalities of lung tissue are unconnected to normal lung, and are characterised by having their own blood supply, often directly from the aorta. The distinction between these and CCAMs is less clear than previously thought, resulting in the new term **congenital pulmonary malformations** for both. Treatment is dictated by the postnatal clinical course.

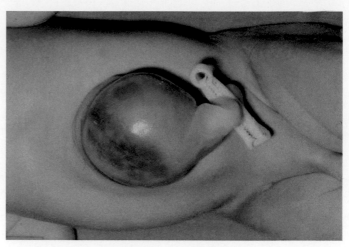

• **Fig. 50.9** Exomphalos.

Congenital Lobar Emphysema

This developmental abnormality affects the upper lobes. Weakness in the wall of a lobar bronchus allows air to enter the lobe, but the bronchus collapses during expiration and distal lung parenchyma continues to gradually expand. This lobar expansion compresses normal lung tissue, leading to deteriorating respiratory capacity. In infants with deteriorating respiratory function, emergency surgical excision of the emphysematous lobe is often necessary.

Abdominal Wall Defects

Major deficiencies on the anterior abdominal wall are usually detected antenatally. Abdominal wall defects are present in up to 1 in 1500 live births, with gastroschisis now more common than exomphalos. Both originate from defects in the abdominal wall so that the bowel and sometimes other viscera lie outside the abdominal cavity. Defects are grouped into two major categories depending upon whether they are covered or uncovered. In **exomphalos**, the viscera are invested with a layer of amnion and peritoneum (Fig. 50.9), whereas in **gastroschisis**, (Fig. 50.10) the contents are uncovered.

CASE HISTORY

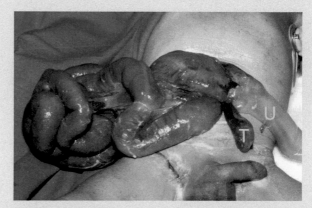

• **Fig. 50.10** Gastroschisis. Gastroschisis in a newborn infant. The defect in the abdominal wall is small, lying to the right of the umbilicus. The intestine has no covering and loops are somewhat matted together by fibrinous adhesions. A testis (T) can be seen lying outside the abdomen on the left. The umbilical cord (U) is also visible.

Exomphalos

In **exomphalos major**, part of the midline abdominal wall is missing. The defect can be very large and presents a surgical challenge to close. Treatment can be delayed or staged, depending on the size of the defect and the general condition of the infant. In **exomphalos minor**, the defect is less than 5 cm in diameter and easier to close. The bowel can usually be reduced and the abdominal wall repaired as a primary surgical procedure.

Up to 50% of infants with exomphalos have one or more other congenital abnormalities, the most common being cardiac problems and neural tube defects. Chromosomal abnormalities or Beckwith-Wiedemann syndrome (gigantism, macroglossia, hypoglycaemia and predisposition to renal tumour formation) can also be present; it is necessary to check blood glucose levels to exclude this diagnosis.

Gastroschisis

This is an abdominal defect characterised by herniation of bowel and sometimes other abdominal viscera through a slit-like defect to the right of the umbilicus. Unlike exomphalos, there are few associated congenital problems, although babies are often small and born prematurely. The defect is usually about 3 cm long and the bowel has no covering membrane (see Fig. 50.10). Exposure to amniotic fluid before birth can cause widespread adhesions and result in a shortening of overall intestinal length.

Management of Abdominal Wall Defects

Once the infant has been resuscitated, it is important to prevent the abdominal wall defect destabilising the delicate physiology of the neonate. To this end, it is important to keep the baby '**warm, pink and sweet**'. In practice this means the bowel should be covered, as soon as possible, with cling-film or a preformed bag to prevent loss of fluid and body heat. Usually babies are actively warmed to prevent hypothermia (**kept warm**) and IV fluids are commenced. The baby is well oxygenated (**kept pink**). A nasogastric tube is placed to prevent intestinal distension and the surgical team is contacted. It is important to look for and to prevent hypoglycaemia (**kept sweet**), in patients with gastroschisis, and more particularly in exomphalos, because of its association with Beckwith-Wiedemann syndrome.

The aim of surgery is to reduce the viscera into the abdomen and to close the abdominal wall. There is often insufficient space in the small abdominal cavity to allow for a one-stage return of the viscera, without compromising ventilation or creating undue pressure on intraabdominal organs. In these cases, it may be necessary to use a **silo bag**, sutured to the edges of the defect and covering the intestine to prevent fluid loss and infection. The bowel is then progressively reduced, over several days, and formal repair of the defect performed, when this process is complete.

Bladder Exstrophy

This is a very rare and complex abnormality present at birth, with bladder mucosa exposed on the abdominal wall, penile epispadias in boys and widening of the symphysis pubis. Treatment involves closing the bladder, urethral, penile and bony defects and repair of the bladder neck, aiming to achieve urinary continence without back-pressure on the kidneys. Initially, the exposed bladder mucosa is covered with cling-film or a silicone dressing to prevent damage to the fragile urothelium, followed by early referral to a specialist centre for continuing management.

Necrotising Enterocolitis

Necrotising enterocolitis is the most common reason for surgical intervention in the neonate. The condition is largely seen in premature infants or those with cardiac abnormalities or with other reasons for poor intestinal perfusion. It is thought that feeding into an intestinal tract, when there is impaired innate immunity, causes damage by bacteria that would not normally cause disease. In a susceptible infant, this then sets up a sequence of bacterial invasion and intestinal damage producing the cardinal feature of the disease, namely gas in the bowel wall on x-ray (pneumatosis intestinalis). There is transmural inflammation of the intestine, which may lead to necrosis and perforation. The condition can affect both small and large bowel and may be part of a more generalised illness with multisystem failure.

The diagnosis can be made on clinical grounds if a neonate has bile-stained vomiting, passage of blood per rectum and abdominal distension (or tenderness); the diagnosis is confirmed when plain radiography shows intramural intestinal gas. Necrotising enterocolitis can progress to bowel necrosis, perforation and generalised peritonitis.

Management involves resuscitation with IV fluids, nasogastric decompression and control of bacteraemia with broad-spectrum antibiotics. Parenteral nutrition is often needed, plus surgical intervention in cases with perforation or those that fail medical management. Unfortunately, mortality remains high.

Abdominal Emergencies in Infants and Young Children

Incarcerated (Acutely Irreducible) Inguinal Hernia

Pathophysiology

The term **incarcerated** implies that a hernia has become acutely irreducible, whereas the term **strangulated** implies there is also impairment of the blood supply to its contents. Strangulation can follow incarceration but is uncommon in young children, unlike in adults (Fig. 50.11).

Incarcerated inguinal hernia is a common cause of acute surgical admission in boys (and sometimes girls) below the age of 2 years, and may occur at any time from birth onwards, especially in premature infants. There is invariably a congenital **patent processus vaginalis**, that is, the hernia is indirect, although an actual hernia may not have been evident before the acute presentation. There is a high incidence of incarceration in premature babies; 40% of hernias in the neonatal period are discovered because they become irreducible and the risk declines as a child becomes older. The high incidence of incarceration in young children is a strong argument for operating upon any hernia in this age group, soon after discovery, with the need greatest in the very young. Beware of using the term incarceration to imply the condition is not urgent; it may be better to designate all acutely irreducible hernias as strangulated to prompt urgent action.

Clinical Features

When a hernia strangulates, it becomes painful, tender and irreducible. Classically, a mother discovers a firm lump in the groin in her crying (usually male) child. He may have vomited, but the

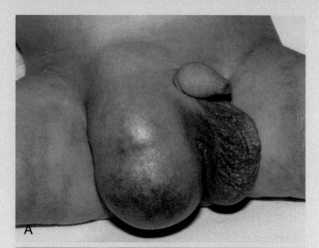

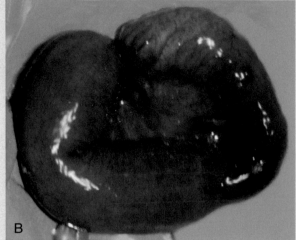

• **Fig. 50.11** Strangulated Inguinal Hernia. (A) Strangulated inguinal hernia in an infant. (B) At operation, an ileal loop trapped in the sac had undergone ischaemic necrosis and had to be resected.

hernia should be drawn towards the opposite, descended testicle, with the external ring held open with the other hand. This results in narrowing of hernial contents, allowing them to pass back through the ring with a satisfying gurgle. Reduction succeeds in about 80% of cases, but competent technique and experience are needed. It is said to be impossible to reduce necrotic bowel in a hernia, but this is untrue, so it is important to carefully monitor a child for clinical deterioration after a difficult reduction, including respiratory rate and oxygen saturation. The hernia must be fully reduced; if there is doubt, or if it proves irreducible, urgent surgery should be performed. Note that failed reduction of an irreducible hernia is associated with a high rate of testicular atrophy (up to 40%).

Congenital Hypertrophic Pyloric Stenosis

Pathophysiology

This common condition of unknown aetiology most commonly presents between 2 weeks and 2 months of age. With the increased use of ultrasound, it is now often diagnosed earlier, particularly in infants with a family history of the condition. It typically presents with a gradual onset of progressive gastric outlet obstruction, with vomiting becoming increasingly forceful, eventually resulting in projectile vomiting. If untreated, this results in dehydration and shock. The underlying cause is marked hypertrophy of the circular muscle in the pyloric region of the stomach, occluding the gastric outlet. The disorder occurs in about 1 in 500 and there is a strong male predominance of around 4 to 1. Hereditary factors clearly play a part, as there is a greatly increased incidence in children with affected relatives. The vomiting caused by pyloric stenosis results in fluid depletion and characteristic electrolyte disturbances, resulting in **hypochloraemic hypokalaemic metabolic alkalosis**.

Clinical Features

Typically, the infant thrives for the first few weeks of life and then begins to vomit after every feed. The vomiting eventually becomes **projectile**, but is not bile-stained. The child is hungry, and in the initial stages of the disease remains well. As the child becomes dehydrated, they may demonstrate poor skin turgor, pallor, delayed capillary refill time, poor perfusion, faltering growth, and then weight loss.

Diagnosis

Persistent vomiting often leads to hospital admission. Ultrasound is reliable in making an early diagnosis and it is also possible to demonstrate pyloric stenosis by performing a test feed. Once the stomach has been emptied with nasogastric decompression, the child is given a small feed of clear fluid or milk. Sometimes, it is possible to see waves of visible gastric peristalsis during the feed and gentle examination of the abdomen allows the clinician to feel a firm olive-like pyloric mass during feeding.

Management

Infants must be adequately rehydrated and have electrolyte and metabolic abnormalities corrected before surgery. The stomach should be emptied by nasogastric tube to reduce the risk of aspiration. Capillary gas samples are taken to demonstrate that electrolyte disturbances and pH have been corrected.

Surgery

The surgical treatment of pyloric stenosis is **pyloromyotomy**. The operation is performed via a supraumbilical incision hidden

diagnosis is usually made before intestinal obstruction becomes established. The child is usually well, with an obvious, irreducible lump in the groin (see Fig. 50.11), sometimes extending into the scrotum. If bowel becomes obstructed, vomiting follows, causing fluid depletion and electrolyte disturbances. The blood supply of the incarcerated segment of intestine may become obstructed (strangulation) causing bowel infarction (see Fig. 50.11B). Pressure on the spermatic cord by the hernia, at the external ring, can cause testicular vascular obstruction, and rapid treatment is needed to prevent testicular infarction and irreversible damage.

Management

There is usually a painful, acutely tender groin swelling. The child is not systemically unwell and the hernia is neither tender nor red. At this stage, it is unlikely that bowel has become infarcted. Emergency surgery is best avoided, except in an unwell child with signs of intestinal obstruction, as the friable hernia sac makes surgery difficult and recurrence likely. Treatment involves manually reducing the hernia, if possible, and performing elective herniotomy 48 hours later, when oedema has resolved. **Active reduction** is by gentle manipulation with the child sedated with IV opiates. The testis and

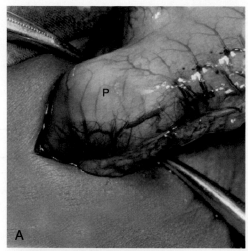

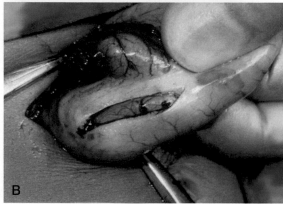

• **Fig. 50.12** Hypertrophic Pyloric Stenosis—Rammstedt Operation. **(A)** A small supraumbilical incision has been made and the stomach and pyloric 'tumour' *(P)* delivered. **(B)** The serosa over the tumour has been incised and the hypertrophic muscle split with forceps. The mucosa is seen bulging through the muscle split.

within the skin crease or laparoscopically. In an open (Rammstedt) operation, the pyloric tumour is 'delivered' into the wound and the outer layer of hypertrophied pyloric muscle incised longitudinally with a scalpel, then split fully with forceps, taking care not to breach the mucosa (Fig. 50.12). This can be checked by blowing a small volume of air down the nasogastric tube and checking for a leak. Postoperative recovery is usually rapid, with full-strength milk feeding started soon after surgery. Some vomiting may occur, but often settles rapidly.

Intussusception

Pathophysiology

Intussusception is an acquired disorder that most commonly occurs in children between the age of 2 months and 2 years. There is a seasonal variation, with increased incidence in the spring and autumn, when certain viruses are more prevalent. The condition arises when a segment of bowel becomes telescoped into bowel immediately distal to it (Fig. 50.13). The lead point that gives rise to the intussuception is usually thickened bowel wall caused by thickened Peyer lymphatic patches. The invaginated segment progressively elongates, as it is propelled distally by the peristaltic action of the gut. **Ileocolic intussusception** is the most common variety requiring surgery. In this, the small bowel is propelled through the ileocaecal valve and often extends into the transverse colon.

Intussusception presents with colicky abdominal pain. It may resolve spontaneously, but if not, it progresses to cause symptoms and signs of intestinal obstruction, with vomiting and dehydration. If the bowel undergoes venous infarction, the child may present with **redcurrant-jelly like stool, bile-stained vomiting, shock** or **peritonitis**.

Intussusception sometimes occurs in older children and adults when the initiating factor is often an abnormal piece of bowel, such as a Meckel diverticulum, bowel polyp, bowel tumour or abnormally enlarged lymphatic tissue (e.g., lymphoma). This is termed a **pathological lead point**.

Clinical Features

Intussusception classically presents with bouts of severe **colicky abdominal pain**. In small children, this is often demonstrated by inconsolable crying, drawing up of the legs, anorexia and vomiting. Occasionally, the child will present with the passage of a small amount of jelly-like blood per rectum (**redcurrant jelly stool**). Vomiting begins later, consistent with distal bowel obstruction, but even without complete obstruction, there may be profound fluid depletion, leading to dehydration and shock. In these children, the most striking feature is one of drowsiness and lethargy in between episodes of screaming.

Diagnosis should be made on clinical grounds. There is often a mass palpable in the upper abdomen. The rectum is empty but may contain a little blood. The right lower quadrant is often scaphoid, that is, hollow *(Dance sign)*. A plain radiograph may show signs of obstruction, but a normal result does not exclude intussusception. A detailed ultrasound examination of the abdomen may demonstrate a classical 'target' sign at the site of intussusception (typically in the upper abdomen). An ileocolic intussusception can be demonstrated by performing an air enema. If air passes all around the colon into the small bowel, this excludes persistent ileocolic intussusception.

Management

Intussusception is a potentially life-threatening surgical emergency. IV access should be secured, as rapid deterioration is possible; passing a nasogastric tube to decompress the stomach is also useful. An ileocolic intussusception can usually be reduced using an air or fluid contrast enema, with carefully controlled pressure, performed under x-ray screening (see Fig. 50.13B). Radiological reduction may not be appropriate if the child is unwell; sometimes features on ultrasound, such as free fluid or avascularity, are relative contraindications to attempting an air enema; in such cases, rapid resuscitation, including administration of broad-spectrum antibiotics is followed by urgent surgery. Patients with evident perforation or peritonitis also need resuscitation and emergency laparotomy.

At operation, the intussusception is reduced by gentle manipulation and the appendix can be removed. If bowel is necrotic, it can sometimes be safely resected (see Fig. 50.13C) and an anastomosis performed, but it is often safer to raise a stoma, proximal to the damaged bowel and a mucous fistula distally, and perform an anastomosis as a second procedure, once the child has recovered.

Swallowed Foreign Bodies

Young children are curious and examine their environment with their mouths. They swallow foreign bodies, such as coins, safety pins and button batteries. This often goes unnoticed with no ill consequences for the child, but some notable exceptions exist. A number of deaths have been reported from swallowing button batteries. If they remain in the GI tract, they set up a constant

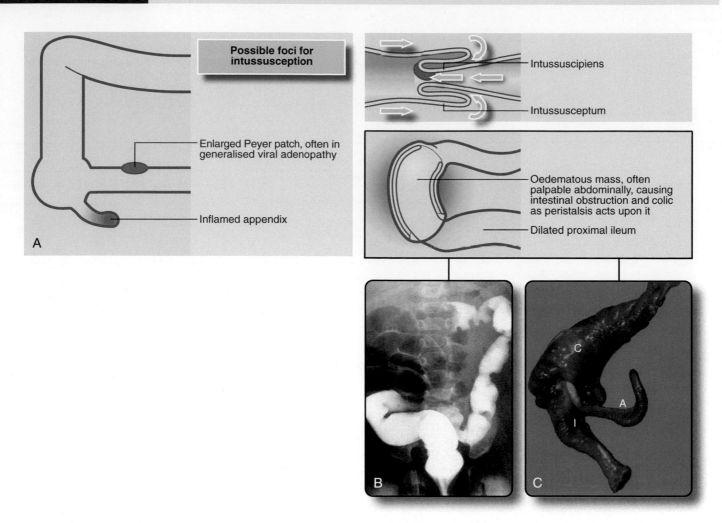

• **Fig. 50.13** Intussusception. **(A)** Mechanism of intussusception. **(B)** This 2-year-old child presented as an emergency with spasms of abdominal pain, having passed 'redcurrant jelly' rectally. This barium enema shows the typical appearance of large bowel obstruction by an intussusception of ileum, which in this case has progressed to the transverse colon. The barium infusion pressure was increased, resulting in hydraulic reduction of the intussusception, which did not recur. **(C)** In this case, neither preoperative barium enema nor manual attempts at reduction were successful so the terminal ileum *(I)* and ascending colon *(C)* were resected. Note the appendix *(A)*.

small electrical current, effectively cooking the bowel they contact. Button batteries should be removed from the stomach, as soon as practicable, by upper GI endoscopy (Fig. 50.14). If they pass beyond the stomach, then GI propulsive agents and laxatives are given and the child is admitted until the battery passes out.

In recent years, some children have come to serious harm after swallowing **multiple magnets**. These are often sold as toys, and if more than one is swallowed, two magnets (or more) may be attracted together and create a fistula between loops of bowel. After swallowing magnets, children generally require admission. If the magnets have not passed by 48 hours, laparotomy may be necessary to remove them and preclude perforation.

Sharp objects longer than 5 cm can cause problems (although this is rare). When possible, these are removed endoscopically from the stomach, if they fail to pass within a few days. Even quite long objects often pass spontaneously during careful monitoring.

Foreign bodies commonly become stuck at the cricopharyngeus, at the lower end of the pharynx or in the lower oesophagus, above the gastrooesophageal junction. All pharyngooesophageal foreign bodies should be removed by endoscopy. Blunt foreign bodies reaching the stomach rarely cause trouble and only require intervention if they obstruct the bowel. This usually occurs at the

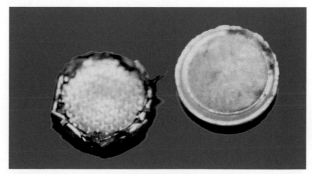

• **Fig. 50.14** Ingested Foreign Bodies—Button Battery. Young children often put small hearing aid-type batteries into their mouths. They are at risk from inhalation and bronchial obstruction, and also from electrical activity burning through the stomach wall. Batteries can be removed without anaesthesia or sedation using a magnet on the end of a nasogastric tube.

ileocaecal valve or sometimes the pylorus. If coins are present in the stomach, parents should inspect the stools for the coins and return with the child if signs of bowel obstruction develop. If the coin has not been found after 2 weeks, a further x-ray is taken and if still present in the stomach, the coin is removed.

- Acute nonspecific abdominal pain
- Acute appendicitis
- Mesenteric adenitis
- Extraabdominal causes

Abdominal Emergencies in Older Children

The Acute Abdomen

Differential Diagnosis (Box 50.2)

From childhood to adolescence, acute abdominal pain is a common cause of admission to hospital. Usually appendicitis is suspected and this condition is described in detail in Chapter 26. The major differential diagnoses are acute nonspecific abdominal pain (which is common), closely followed by mesenteric adenitis (see Box 50.2). Less commonly, acute abdominal pain in this age group is caused by extraabdominal causes such as:

- **lower urinary tract infections** (although urinary symptoms are usually present)
- **basal pneumonia or lower respiratory tract infections**
- **ear, nose or throat infections**
- **torsion of the testis**—this sometimes presents solely with abdominal pain; the external genitalia must always be examined in boys who complain of abdominal pain
- **ovarian pathology**—in postpubertal girls, sometimes an ovarian cyst or a torted ovary can present with abdominal pain, and it is usually wise to perform an ultrasound of the pelvis to look for ovarian pathology
- **meningitis**

Principles of Management

If acute appendicitis is diagnosed when the child is first seen, operation should usually be performed without delay, after the administration of appropriate prophylactic antibiotics and adequate fluid resuscitation. More commonly, the diagnosis of appendicitis is uncertain. In these children, urinary tract infection should be excluded by performing dipstick urinalysis and culture, if urine is positive for leucocytes and nitrite. The child with undifferentiated abdominal pain should be kept under review and re-examined at regular intervals.

Acute Appendicitis (See Also Chapter 26)

Acute appendicitis is uncommon in children less than 2 years. Anorexia is present in almost all appendicitis cases (although some teenage boys continue eating), and vomiting often starts after the onset of pain. Children with appendicitis find that movement or jarring, when driving over bumps in the road, exacerbates the pain and most find they have to bend over when walking. An inflamed appendix descending over the pelvic brim ('pelvic appendix') may cause secondary inflammation of rectum or bladder, causing diarrhoea or urinary symptoms (dipstick testing of urine shows significant leucocytes, but no nitrites).

When assessing suspected appendicitis, a range of other diagnoses must be considered. Mesenteric adenitis (presumably viral in origin) can mimic appendicitis; high fever and widespread lymphadenopathy suggest this as a potential diagnosis. Otitis

media, pharyngeal inflammation, basal pneumonia, testicular torsion or even meningitis can be responsible, particularly in children under 5 years, so general examination must include the ears and throat, the chest, the testes in boys and a search for rashes and neck stiffness.

On examination, the child's breath may be foul (foetor oris), and there may circumoral pallor and signs of dehydration. The child is often pyrexial, but a temperature of more than 38.5°C suggests a cause other than appendicitis, unless there is generalised peritonitis (as in perforated appendicitis). The abdomen is tender in the right iliac fossa, and the cardinal sign is localised involuntary guarding. Perforation can lead to generalised peritonitis, with tenderness and guarding over the whole abdomen. Unlike adults, young children more often present with perforated appendicitis, often with little in the way of a prodromal illness.

A definitive diagnosis of appendicitis often cannot be made on initial assessment of a child with right iliac fossa pain. Investigations are of little help other than to exclude urinary tract infection. The white blood cell count and C-reactive protein may be misleading, as they are raised in other inflammatory conditions. Ultrasound scan by a skilled operator has some positive predictive value, but in general, repeated clinical examination is the mainstay of diagnosis. Investigations should be reserved for those in whom diagnostic uncertainty continues. CT scanning is expensive and the radiation burden in children precludes its general use, but it can be diagnostic in a few selected cases. Laparoscopy gives a precise diagnosis, but requires general anaesthesia and carries a risk of complications; the procedure is best avoided if the appendix is unlikely to be inflamed.

The best way to make a diagnosis of appendicitis in the equivocal case is by **active observation**. The child is admitted and allowed to eat (fasting ameliorates the physical signs and can delay the diagnosis). The child is re-examined several times a day, ideally by the same doctor, including abdominal palpation. By the second or third examination, it is usually apparent whether physical signs are getting better or worse. The argument that active observation risks perforation, pelvic infection and subfertility in girls is not borne out by fact.

The Acute Scrotum

Testicular torsion can occur, when testicular fixation is congenitally abnormal. This predisposes the testis to twisting on its vascular pedicle, which occludes its blood supply. In older children and adults, a 'bell-clapper' deformity, where the testis lies horizontally, predisposes to this **intravaginal** torsion (i.e., within the tunica vaginalis sac).

A diagnosis of torsion must be considered in any male presenting with acute testicular pain, although torsion may present with lower abdominal pain alone. Torsion must not be missed as the torted testis would undergo necrosis in 4 to 6 hours. The predisposition to torsion is usually bilateral and both testes are at risk. Thus, at operation, the nontorted testis should also undergo prophylactic fixation (see Ch. 33).

Where the clinical picture makes torsion possible but unlikely, ultrasound investigation, with Doppler blood flow monitoring, may be reassuring if it shows good blood flow to the testis. However, if torsion is more strongly suspected, ultrasound can delay surgery and may compromise testicular survival. When a diagnosis of torsion cannot be excluded (as is usually the case), the only safe option is to perform urgent surgical exploration. If torsion is present and if the testis is viable, it should be untwisted and fixed to prevent retorsion. The contralateral testis is fixed at the same time, since the abnormal attachment is usually the same on both sides. A nonviable testis should be removed.

Neonates may present with **perinatal torsion**. In these, **extra-vaginal** torsion of the testis, testicular vessels and tunica vaginalis occurs, resulting in a swollen, often nontender hemiscrotum. In many cases, the testis is already necrotic by the time of presentation, but an exploratory operation is performed urgently to remove the dead testis, if necessary, and to secure both sides, if appropriate, because of the small risk of asynchronous torsion in the remaining testis.

Other intrascrotal pathology can mimic testicular torsion including **torsion of a hydatid of Morgagni**, idiopathic scrotal oedema and **epididymitis**. In any of these cases, palpating individual scrotal structures is often impossible because of tenderness and oedema. When palpation is possible, a nontender testis with an acutely tender epididymis (behind the testis) may indicate epididymitis. Very localised tenderness at the upper pole of the testis is sometimes found in torsion of a hydatid of Morgagni. It is then useful to look carefully for a **blue dot**, under the scrotal skin, at the point of maximal tenderness, which confirms the diagnosis. This sign is often lost as scrotal oedema develops. A firm diagnosis of epididymitis is treated with antibiotics after sending a midstream urine sample, while a torted hydatid can be managed conservatively (though it may be diagnosed at surgical exploration and removed).

51

Nonacute Abdominal and Urological Problems in Children

CHAPTER OUTLINE

Introduction

In paediatric surgery, the most important conditions presenting as emergencies are caused by congenital problems presenting in the neonatal period. In contrast to this, nonacute conditions present across the whole age range of childhood. This chapter deals with abdominal and urological problems in children, although it should be remembered that other systems can be affected by disease in childhood. The most common reasons for nonacute surgical referral are hernias and associated problems, abnormalities of testicular descent and foreskin problems. Less often surgeons are asked to manage chronic or recurrent abdominal pain, chronic constipation, rectal bleeding or rectal prolapse. Many of these children present first to a paediatrician and then are referred to a paediatric surgeon.

Importantly, there is a range of urological problems that occur specifically in infancy and childhood. Most of them are unique to young patients, and are dealt with by specialist paediatric surgeons or paediatric urologists, and most significant urinary tract abnormalities are now detected antenatally.

Problems With the Groin and Male Genitalia

Embryology

The indifferent gonad (i.e., ovary or testis) begins to develop at the fifth week in the **gonadal ridge**, part of the mesodermal urogenital ridge that will also form the kidney, ureter and genital ducts, in the male, or uterus and uterine tubes, in the female. At the lower pole of the developing testis, a strand of mesenchyme becomes the cord-like **gubernaculum**. In the eighth week, a prolongation of peritoneum, the **processus vaginalis**, appears beside the gubernaculum (or round ligament), and extends into the labioscrotal fold. The testis then migrates distally along the peritoneal canal.

Hernias and Associated Problems

The processus vaginalis normally closes spontaneously soon after birth. Persistence causes three common problems in boys: patent processus vaginalis (PPV), hydrocoele and inguinal hernia, which may all present as inguinal or scrotal swellings, usually in babies and preschool children (Fig. 51.1).

Patent Processus Vaginalis

This term should be reserved for hydrocoeles communicating with the peritoneal cavity, via a remnant too narrow to admit bowel. Children with these **communicating hydrocoeles** present with scrotal swelling that increases during the day, as peritoneal fluid accumulates, and subsides at night. Treatment is excision of the peritoneal remnant by herniotomy performed after the age of 2 years (see later). Before this age, most settle spontaneously.

Hydrocoele

Non-communicating hydrocoeles are mostly seen in neonates and young babies (Fig. 51.2). The usual type is a scrotal swelling, resulting from incomplete reabsorption of fluid within the tunica

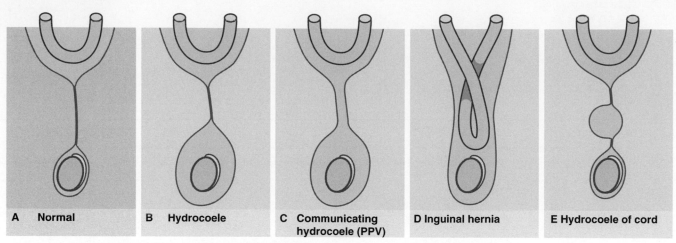

| A Normal | B Hydrocoele | C Communicating hydrocoele (PPV) | D Inguinal hernia | E Hydrocoele of cord |

• **Fig. 51.1** Abnormalities Associated With the Processus Vaginalis. *PPV,* Patent processus vaginalis.

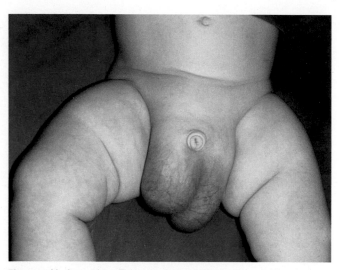

• **Fig. 51.2** Hydrocoeles. This 11-month-old boy had an enlarged scrotum confirmed by transillumination to be the result of hydrocoeles.

vaginalis, after closure of the processus vaginalis. There may be a separate hernia present. These so-called **primary hydrocoeles** sometimes appear following a viral illness. Rarely, a **secondary hydrocoele** results from testicular trauma or torsion, epididymitis or a testicular tumour.

On examination, there is a fluid swelling surrounding a normal testis; the sac transilluminates brightly and the testis can be felt posteriorly (but note that neonatal bowel is thin and may also transilluminate brightly in a hernia), and the examiner's fingers can 'get above' the swelling (i.e., it does not communicate with the groin). Ultrasound investigation can be used to clarify the diagnosis. Hydrocoeles also occur in the spermatic cord (hydrocoele of the cord) or in the round ligament in girls, where they are known as *hydrocoeles of the canal of Nuck.* Most hydrocoeles resolve between 18 and 24 months of age. A hydrocoele persisting beyond the age of 2 years or appearing later may require surgery.

Inguinal Hernia

Inguinal hernias in children arise because the processus vaginalis fails to close after testicular descent; they are true congenital abnormalities. Anatomically, they are the same as indirect inguinal hernias in adults (see Ch. 32), but without a substantial abdominal wall defect. The incidence in infants ranges from 1% to 4.4%, with a male preponderance of 4:1; 98% are indirect. The incidence in **premature neonates** is 30% and the overall incidence is increasing in line with the number of premature neonates surviving.

A hernia usually presents as a lump at the external inguinal ring, when the child cries or strains at stool, but then reduces spontaneously. When seen electively, there is often no abnormality, but most surgeons accept a parent's clear history of a hernia and arrange surgery. With larger defects, a lump is constantly present and expands during crying, and the examiner cannot get above the swelling, that is, the swelling originates in the groin; this is the cardinal feature. The urgency of hernia repair is governed by age; the older, the less likely it will become incarcerated (acutely irreducible). Infants at home should have hernias fixed on the next available operating list. Neonates and preterm infants in hospital should have them fixed before discharge. Older children without episodes of incarceration can have hernias fixed electively.

Inguinal hernias may become **acutely irreducible** and painful, sometimes with obstructive symptoms, such as vomiting (see Ch. 50). In these cases, there is a real risk of testicular necrosis and/or strangulation of the hernia contents, for example, bowel or ovary (see Fig. 50.11). In known hernias, parents should be instructed to bring the child to hospital for urgent surgery if it becomes incarcerated, to prevent these risks.

The standard operation is **inguinal herniotomy**. In babies and children, this involves separating the peritoneal sac from the cord (or round ligament), ligating it at the external ring and removing it. There is rarely any need to perform a repair (herniorrhaphy) (Fig. 51.3). The incidence of an undiagnosed contralateral hernia in boys is between 1:8 and 1:13, but contralateral groin exploration is no longer performed in the United Kingdom.

Femoral Hernia

Femoral hernias are much less common than inguinal hernias in children and are located lower and more medially in the groin. Enlarged lymph nodes can also occur here. Operation includes removing the sac and suturing the medial part of the inguinal ligament to the pectineus fascia, to narrow the femoral canal.

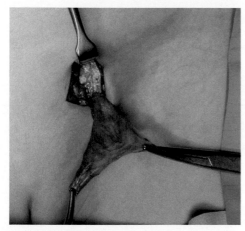

• **Fig. 51.3** Operation for Inguinal Hernia. At operation, the peritoneal sac is being held out before it is excised. No other procedure was necessary in this 4-year-old child. Unusually, the patient was female.

Umbilical Hernia

Many newborn babies have umbilical hernias, particularly if premature (Fig. 51.4), but the defect usually cicatrises and resolves

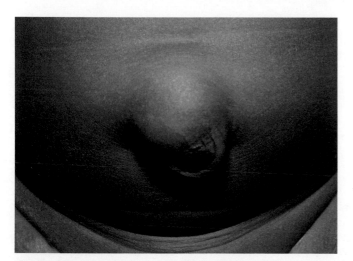

• **Fig. 51.4** Umbilical Hernia in a 14-Month-Old Boy. This was repaired surgically, but smaller ones usually resolve spontaneously.

during the first 2 years of life; they are common in Afro-Caribbean babies, and can run strongly in families. Small umbilical hernias may undergo spontaneous closure up to 4 to 5 years of age. Rarely, they become incarcerated or strangulate. Indications for repair are symptoms and persistence beyond 5 years. The size of the abdominal wall defect should be determined; large defects (>2 cm) are less likely to close spontaneously, although very large swellings appear through small abdominal wall defects likely to close spontaneously. It is important to differentiate umbilical hernias from epigastric hernias, which do not close spontaneously. At operation, a small subumbilical 'smile' incision allows emptying and ligation of the peritoneal sac and placement of a few absorbable repair sutures. The umbilical skin is usually sutured to the repair to restore its normal recessed appearance.

Testicular Maldescent

There are several terms for testes not fully descended into the scrotum, including undescended, maldescended, and cryptorchidism. Most missing testes start along the normal pathway and arrest in the inguinal region (incomplete descent), a few descend to the wrong place (ectopic) and a few are missing altogether (atrophic or absent). Clinically, one or both testes fail to reach the scrotum in 3% of full-term newborn males, with higher rates if premature. Full descent has occurred in most boys by the age of 3 to 6 months, leaving about 1.6% with maldescended testes at 12 months; these rarely descend later, because androgen levels are highest in the first few months and then fall to very low levels until puberty.

The normal mechanism of descent is not fully understood but does occur in two phases. Migration from the gonadal ridge to the internal inguinal ring depends on shortening of the gubernaculum, driven by Leydig cell hormone insulin-like peptide 3. This phase is not androgen-dependent, unlike the second phase of descent, from internal ring to scrotum. A maldescended testis may arrest anywhere on its path of descent. About 20% lie within the abdomen, but 80% lie in the groin area, in the inguinal canal or usually outside the external ring in the **superficial inguinal pouch** or upper scrotum. In addition, 1% of maldescended testes are deflected and lie ectopically. Second phase maldescent can result from the testis being structurally abnormal, rather than any abnormality being caused by maldescent. The common sites of incomplete descent or ectopia are shown in Fig. 51.5.

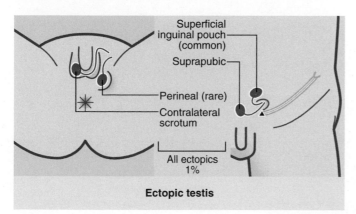

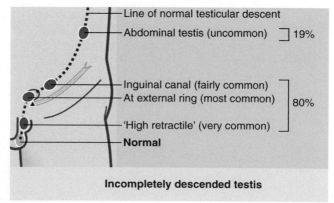

• **Fig. 51.5** Testicular Maldescent.

The main concerns with maldescended testes are the risks of malignancy, subfertility, and torsion or trauma in an abnormal position; cosmetic appearance and potential psychological impact in later life:

- **Neoplasia**—maldescent has up to 10 times the normal risk of testicular malignancy (although the risk is still small); if surgical correction is done sufficiently early, it may reduce this risk, but the principal purpose is so the patient can perform self-examination and report lumps in later life. Long-term follow up after orchidopexy is desirable. Seminomas are the most common tumour (60%) and usually present between 20 and 40 years of age. It is important to inform the parents of the increased risk of malignancy and to reinforce the importance of self-examination in adult life.

- **Subfertility**—maldescended testes exhibit incomplete maturation of seminiferous tubules leading to sperm abnormal in quantity, form or motility. This may be by virtue of being at body temperature instead of at least 1°C cooler in the scrotum. Early orchidopexy, ideally between 6 and 12 months, helps maturation of the tubules and spermatogenesis.

- **Torsion**—incompletely descended testes are abnormally mobile. Torsion of the testis (actually torsion of the spermatic cord), causes strangulation of blood supply, testicular necrosis and later atrophy. Torsion sometimes occurs during **intrauterine life** but may happen at any age. Intrauterine or neonatal torsion occurs proximal to the reflection of the tunica vaginalis (i.e., **extravaginal**). Infarction results in atrophy and loss of the testis, so that at laparoscopy, only blind-ending testicular vessels and vas deferens are found. The condition occurs bilaterally in up to 30%.

- **Psychological**—normal genitalia are important in the development of body image, gender acceptance and personality in adolescence. Orchidopexy at an early age provides reassurance to the child and parents.

Boys should be examined regularly from birth right through school age to identify maldescent and allow timely **orchidopexy**. Periodic examination is needed because unequivocally descended testes can later ascend and parents and doctors should be alert to this possibility. There may be a fibrous band within the processus vaginalis preventing elongation of testicular vessels as the boy grows. The resulting 'stationary' testis appears to ascend, and can no longer be drawn comfortably into the scrotum.

With a history of a missing testis, the chief point is whether the testis is palpable. If palpable at the scrotal neck, it should be gently manipulated into its correct position. If it then stays put, it is **retractile** and needs no treatment, provided it becomes less retractile, as the boy grows. If the testis immediately retracts, it is maldescended and needs treatment.

If the testis is impalpable, investigations should be undertaken to locate it. Laparoscopy is the investigation of choice; the testis may be found intra-abdominally or the cord may be seen entering the deep ring; in either case, the testis is mobilised and placed in the scrotum. Alternatively, a blind-ending spermatic cord may be found indicating the testis is missing, usually as a result of intrauterine torsion. No action is needed if this is unilateral but if bilateral, genetic screening is required and possible hormonal treatment and testicular prostheses.

Surgery for Testicular Maldescent

The optimum age for operation is 6 months to 1 year, so fertility is not compromised. The usual technique of orchidopexy involves mobilising the testis and spermatic cord through a groin incision, separating and excising the processus vaginalis and placing the testis in a subcutaneous pouch, outside the dartos muscle, via a separate scrotal incision. For intra-abdominal testes, the operative technique is a laparoscopic staged Fowler-Stephens procedure. In the first stage, the testis is mobilised by dividing the testicular artery and vein intraabdominally. Six months later the testis is mobilised on the vas with its attendant artery, and delivered into the scrotum laparoscopically. This approach has improved the success rate for intraabdominal testes to almost 90%.

Foreskin Problems

At birth the foreskin (or prepuce) is adherent to the glans penis and undergoes gradual separation between birth and puberty. Parents should not attempt to retract an adherent foreskin as this may provoke fibrosis. Note that some adhesions may perfectly normally persist into adolescence. The prepuce protects the glans from ammoniacal dermatitis when the child is in nappies. By the age of 3 years, the foreskin is retractile in 90%, with only a few persistently nonretractile into adulthood (<1% at age 17 years).

Phimosis

In phimosis, a tight fibrotic ring develops at the end of the foreskin preventing retraction. **Primary phimosis** may cause symptoms of chronic foreskin irritation or 'spraying' on micturition. 'Ballooning' on micturition is just a sign of a nonretractile foreskin and is not necessarily pathological. There is often a history of recent or recurrent **balanoposthitis** (infection beneath the foreskin). Most boys with primary phimosis do not require circumcision; careful attention to hygiene (avoiding forcible retraction) allows the prepuce to retract normally in time. Attempts to dilate the phimosis under anaesthesia are unsuccessful, as this causes further scarring and rapid relapse.

Circumcision may be indicated in cases of recurrent infection particularly in boys with upper renal tract abnormalities or other congenital problems, such as posterior urethral valves, and may help to reduce the incidence of urinary tract infections (UTIs) in these boys. In young men, a non-retractile foreskin may cause sexual problems. For these, the lesser operation of **preputioplasty** may suffice, if the phimosis is not too tight. This involves dividing the tight band longitudinally and suturing it transversely, increasing the meatal calibre to allow easier retraction.

Secondary phimosis is usually caused by **balanitis xerotica obliterans**, which is characterised by a thickened, whitish, fibrotic non-retractile foreskin. Plaques are formed on the deep surface, which adhere to the glans and may cause meatal stenosis. It is more commonly encountered in adult males. In children, the peak incidence is around 8 years and the condition is a definite indication for circumcision.

Paraphimosis

Paraphimosis rarely occurs in children, but may do so if there is an underlying phimosis. The tip of the foreskin forms a tight band and when retracted, becomes trapped in the coronal sulcus behind the glans. The band inhibits venous return and causes swelling of the glans, making return of the prepuce even more difficult. Paraphimosis is painful and requires urgent reduction. This can sometimes be achieved using EMLA cream (local anaesthetic) or a penile block (if tolerated). Manual compression of the glans often allows reduction, but if this fails, general anaesthesia is needed. Sometimes the band needs dividing with a **dorsal slit**. Circumcision is usually performed later, once oedema has settled.

Renal, Vesical and Urethral Abnormalities

About one-third of congenital anomalies affect the genitourinary tract. These include abnormalities of kidney, renal calyces or pelvis and ureters. Anomalies of the bladder and urethra complete the spectrum of paediatric urogenital problems which may present at birth but need long-term follow up, often into adulthood. Around 90% of renal tract abnormalities can now be detected at an antenatal 12- or 20-week scan, allowing parents to be prepared for postnatal management. The most common ones are hypospadias, **pelviureteric junction (PUJ)** obstruction and **vesicoureteric reflux (VUR)**. Renal parenchymal disorders are less common. Some disorders present later, including unilateral renal agenesis, horseshoe kidney and polycystic kidneys (see Table 39.1). Around one in 50 pregnancies is complicated by an antenatally detected urinary tract abnormality.

Renal Dysplasia

Incomplete or abnormal differentiation during development causes renal dysplasia. Dysplasia is classified into **agenesis** (absent), **hypoplastic** (underdeveloped) kidney and **multicystic dysplasia.** Bilateral agenesis is incompatible with life. Unilateral agenesis has an incidence of 1 in 1000 with a male preponderance. The contralateral kidney is usually normal and the disorder is not usually diagnosed until adulthood.

A kidney affected by **multicystic dysplasia** contains many cysts of different sizes. The kidney is non-functional and there is ureteric atresia. Most multicystic kidneys spontaneously involute (atrophy) without complication but nephrectomy is sometimes needed.

In **renal ectopia** (see Fig. 39.5), the kidney lies in an abnormal position in the pelvis, or abdomen. Renal ectopia can be discovered incidentally or associated with other anomalies, such as anorectal malformations.

Abnormal fusion of the developing metanephric masses during the first 2 months of foetal life results in a **horseshoe kidney** (see Fig. 39.4). This may cause hydronephrosis by PUJ obstruction or be discovered incidentally at any age. Skeletal and cardiovascular abnormalities occur in at least a third; girls with Turner syndrome often have a horseshoe kidney.

Neonatal Hydronephrosis

Fetal urinary tract abnormalities occur in about 2% of pregnancies, and hydronephrosis accounts for half. Management depends on severity and whether unilateral or bilateral. Antenatal hydronephrosis may be caused by PUJ obstruction, vesicoureteric junction obstruction or reflux, multicystic kidney, primary obstructive megaureter or posterior urethral valves. The urgency and type of investigation depends on the size of the hydronephrosis. Investigation includes ultrasound, micturating cystography and perhaps isotope renal scans repeated at intervals, to decide if surgery is needed. Early investigation is essential in bilateral severe hydronephrosis, particularly in boys, to exclude bladder outlet obstruction, secondary to posterior urethral valves.

Vesicoureteric Reflux

Any anatomical or functional urinary tract abnormality predisposes to infections. This is particularly true in children, where the commonest predisposing abnormality is VUR, that is, retrograde flow of urine from bladder to kidneys. This exposes the upper tracts to the greater range of pressure variation of the lower tract and to ascending infections. The causes are complex, but in essence, there is a faulty mechanism at the junction of ureter and bladder (vesicoureteric junction), see Box 51.1. Reflux is classified severities ranging from I to V (Table 51.1).

• BOX 51.1 Causes of Vesicoureteric Reflux

Primary (i.e., Maldevelopment of Vesicoureteric Junction)
- Short submucosal tunnel
- Delayed maturity of vesicoureteric junction

Secondary
- Posterior urethral valves
- Duplex system and ureterocoele
- Ectopic ureters
- Congenital megaureters
- Detrusor instability
- Neurogenic bladder
- Surgical procedures to the lower end of the ureter

TABLE 51.1	International Classification of Vesicoureteric Reflux (VUR) and Clinical Classification	
Grade of VUR	International Classification	Clinical Classification
I	Reflux into lower ureter on voiding	Mild nondilating VUR on micturition
II	Reflux into ureter and renal pelvis on voiding but without dilatation	
III	Reflux into the ureter and renal pelvis on voiding with mild dilatation	
IV	Constant reflux with upper tract and ureteric dilatation	Constant severe dilating VUR
V	Constant reflux with blunted calyces and grossly dilated tortuous ureters	

Neonatal VUR is caused by anatomical abnormalities, with both sexes equally affected. Later, the condition appears predominantly in girls, where **voiding disturbances** play a large role. Dysfunctional voiding refers to abnormal storage of urine or an abnormal emptying phase of micturition, presenting with symptoms of urgency, frequency, incontinence and UTIs. A vicious circle may develop, with reflux leading to infection, then bladder overactivity and further dysfunctional voiding. VUR can also be encountered in high pressure bladders in neuropathic patients.

Pathophysiology

In the normal individual, the distal ureter passes obliquely through the bladder wall, which helps to prevent the transmission of intermittent high bladder pressures and avoid reflux of urine into the ureter and kidney. **Primary VUR** is most common and usually results from a minor (often familial) abnormality of ureteric insertion or from ectopic or duplex ureters or congenital megaureter (a peristaltic abnormality). **Secondary VUR** may be caused by bladder outlet obstruction, neuropathic bladder, or surgical procedures to the lower end of the ureter.

Ascending infection of the upper tracts begins with bacteria reaching the bladder, via the urethra. Infected urine refluxes into

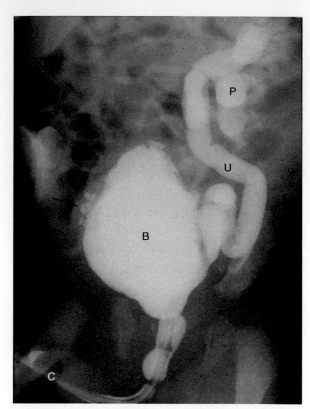

- **Fig. 51.6** Vesicoureteric Reflux. Micturating cystourethrogram in a child with recurrent urinary tract infections. The bladder *(B)* is trabeculated (diverticula *arrowed*). On voiding, the left ureter *(U)* and pelvicalyceal system *(P)* filled with contrast, as a result of severe dilating vesicoureteric reflux. This is defined as grade V reflux. The urethral catheter *(C)* is used to instill contrast into the bladder.

upper tracts, but cannot be cleared effectively from it, infecting the upper tract.

Reflux of sterile urine into the pelvicalyceal system during early childhood probably causes impaired renal development and function, although reflux of infected urine is thought to be most problematic. Mild, nondilating VUR (grades I to III; see Table 51.1) causes little damage, but severe (dilating) VUR (grades IV and V) may cause renal scarring and reflux nephropathy, which may progress to irreversible renal damage if untreated (Fig. 51.6). If both kidneys are involved, this eventually results in renal insufficiency and hypertension. Scarring typically occurs apically in the kidneys. Loss of the normal conical shape of the papillae allows intrarenal reflux, which in the presence of infection, results in pyelonephritis and renal scarring.

Clinical Presentation and Investigation

During antenatal screening, VUR can be detected as urinary tract dilatation. Another common presentation is one or more UTIs at any age. Girls are more prone than boys after the first year, because of a short urethra and its proximity to the anus. Note that infants or young children with urinary infections may not exhibit urinary symptoms or signs; the diagnosis is often made on investigation of vomiting, fever or failure to thrive. Older children typically present with incontinence, frequency or dysuria, or abdominal pain and tenderness (mimicking appendicitis). In **symptomatic UTIs**, the prevalence of VUR is as high as 50% in neonates, and 30% in those aged 2 to 18 years.

In a child with UTI, clinical examination seeks evidence of abnormal external genitalia, spina bifida and impaired perineal innervation (sensation and anal sphincter tone). To demonstrate reflux, the sequential investigations are ultrasound scan, micturating cystography, and isotope scans using dimercaptosuccinic acid (DMSA) and mercaptoacetyltriglycine (MAG3), coupled with indirect radionuclide cystography. Videourodynamics are ideally used if there is evidence of voiding dysfunction to assess bladder function and pressures. **Micturating cystography** should be used only in selected cases (see Fig. 51.6); there is a 1% risk of pyelonephritis and the test is stressful for child and parent. It is the gold standard for demonstrating VUR and excluding posterior urethral valves, but involves instilling contrast into the bladder, via a urinary catheter, which is then removed and x-rays taken during voiding. The radiological grades of severity are shown in Table 51.1 and provide a useful guide to the likelihood of future renal damage. Severe dilating VUR requires **isotope studies**: ^{99m}Tc DMSA, bound to renal tubules, shows differential renal function and scarring within renal parenchyma. In older children, an excretion MAG3 scan and indirect radionuclide cystogram shows differential function, reflux and sites of urinary tract obstruction.

Management of Vesicoureteric Reflux

With no other anatomical abnormalities and an undilated ureter (i.e., grades I and II), there is an 85% chance of resolution of reflux as the child grows. In the meantime, the risk of urinary infection should be minimised by encouraging high fluid intake, avoiding constipation and maintaining perineal hygiene, plus medical management of bladder dysfunction. In selected higher risk cases (history of febrile UTI, age <1 year and higher grades of VUR), continuous prophylactic antibiotics (such as trimethoprim) are given, and the child is followed-up regularly, with serial ultrasound scans and charting growth and development, blood pressure and plasma creatinine. If the child remains well, antibiotics can be stopped once they are toilet trained. If problems persist, further investigation and monitoring is required.

Surgical correction becomes indicated, when there are recurrent infections, deterioration of upper tract function or noncompliance with medical management. Otherwise, surgery is reserved for severe dilated VUR, with complications, and for other obvious anatomical abnormalities. Minimally invasive treatments include injection of Deflux into the submucosa of the ureter, at the junction with the bladder; success rates of up to 90% are possible. Less commonly, operations aim to **reimplant the ureter**, so that a length of it lies deep to the bladder mucosa; this is flattened during voiding, restoring an antireflux mechanism.

Without renal scarring, the child can be discharged from follow up after operation. With unilateral scarring, blood pressure should be monitored lifelong for hypertension. In bilateral scarring, renal function must also be monitored.

Pelviureteric Junction Dysfunction

Pathophysiology

Obstruction at the PUJ may be unilateral or bilateral, and can present any time between birth and the end of the fourth decade. It affects both sexes equally. PUJ dysfunction (most commonly termed *obstruction*) is a congenital condition that manifests as dilatation of the renal pelvis and calyces (**hydronephrosis**) and incomplete or intermittent obstruction of the PUJ. Usually a functional abnormality, there is an aperistaltic segment of ureter that lacks muscle. Aberrant lower pole vessels may cause mechanical obstruction in older children. A normal PUJ prevents urine reflux into the kidney when the ureter contracts, but in PUJ obstruction, urine accumulates and dilates the pelvicalyceal system. This increases pressure in the renal collecting system, which may cause deterioration of renal function. Stasis may also predispose to infection and stone formation.

Clinical Presentation and Diagnosis

PUJ obstruction is now most often diagnosed antenatally. Management is regular postnatal follow up with ultrasound. Those with persistent or progressive hydronephrosis are investigated for VUR, renal function and renal drainage effectiveness, and treated appropriately.

Many with PUJ obstruction go undetected. Others are discovered by chance on ultrasound or urography for an apparently unrelated condition. Symptoms may be intermittent: some patients complain of aching in the renal area; others suffer bouts of severe abdominal or loin pain (renal colic), some with UTI or haematuria (which may be induced by exercise). Symptoms can be exacerbated by drinking large volumes of fluid precipitating a Dietl crisis.

The initial diagnosis is by ultrasound, with detection of a dilated renal pelvis. The next step is to distinguish between static nonobstructive dilatation, with preserved renal function, and genuine PUJ obstruction causing stasis, dilatation and deteriorating function. **Radionuclide diuretic renography (^{99m}Tc MAG3 scan)** is the investigation of choice and in classic PUJ obstruction, gives a characteristic nonexcretion curve.

Indications for operation include a loss of differential renal function >10%, or more commonly an increase in the anterior–posterior diameter of the renal pelvis to >35 mm.

Management

PUJ dysfunction associated with obstructive symptoms, stone formation, recurrent infections or progressive renal impairment, together with an obstructed isotope excretion curve, are indications for intervention. Others include a loss of differential renal function of >10%, or more commonly, an increase in the anterior–posterior diameter of the renal pelvis to >35 mm. Minimal invasive techniques include percutaneous antegrade endopyelotomy and laparoscopic or robotic-assisted laparoscopic pyeloplasty. Standard operations have a high technical success rate and usually prevent deterioration of renal function. If the kidney has less than 10% of total renal function, a nephrectomy may be indicated instead.

Hypospadias and Epispadias

Hypospadias is a common congenital abnormality of penis and urethra. It occurs in 1 in 125 to 300 male births and is increasing in incidence. The distal urethra fails to develop normally, so the urethral meatus lies somewhere along the ventral surface of the penis between glans and perineum (Fig. 51.7). The urethral remnant distal to the meatus is fibrotic, often causing the penis to bend downwards or sideways on erection, known as **chordee**. The more proximal the meatus, the worse the chordee. In addition, the ventral part of the foreskin is absent, giving a hooded appearance. Distal hypospadias is more common, accounting for about 85%, with the urethral opening between glans and the midshaft with minimal chordee.

Surgical correction is a highly specialised procedure performed for function and cosmesis. Functional correction enables the urinary stream (and ejaculate) to be propelled 'straight' out from the end of

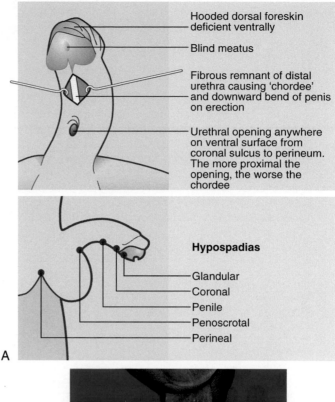

Hooded dorsal foreskin deficient ventrally

Blind meatus

Fibrous remnant of distal urethra causing 'chordee' and downward bend of penis on erection

Urethral opening anywhere on ventral surface from coronal sulcus to perineum. The more proximal the opening, the worse the chordee

Hypospadias

Glandular
Coronal
Penile
Penoscrotal
Perineal

A

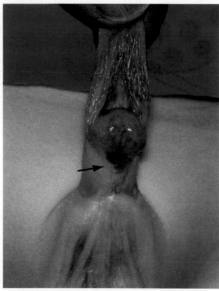

B

• **Fig. 51.7** Hypospadias. **(A)** Hypospadias. **(B)** Distal coronal hypospadias. The urethral meatus is *arrowed* and *(H)* indicates the hooded foreskin. Chordee, a marked downward bend of the penis, was prominent in this case but is not visible here.

the penis (rather than directed towards the floor). Since surgical repair uses the foreskin, circumcision should **never** be carried out without specialist advice. The ideal age for surgery is 6 to 18 months.

Epispadias is rare and may be associated with other genitourinary abnormalities, such as bladder exstrophy. In epispadias, the urethral meatus is on the dorsal aspect of the penis.

Posterior Urethral Valves

Urethral valves are congenital mucosal folds in the posterior urethra of a boy that impede or occlude urinary flow. Antenatal ultrasound screening usually detects the characteristic signs of oligohydramnios, a small thick-walled bladder and bilateral hydronephrosis and hydroureters. If not diagnosed antenatally, complete obstruction becomes apparent soon after birth, although partial obstruction may be overlooked.

Severe oligohydramnios caused by this can be associated with pulmonary hypoplasia, which is incompatible with life. Neonates born with bladder outlet obstruction require urgent assessment. Urethral catheterisation facilitates accurate fluid management in the immediate postnatal period but management of postobstructive diuresis and electrolyte abnormalities can be difficult and is best done in a specialist unit. Ultrasound scan and micturating cystography confirm the diagnosis.

Definitive treatment involves ablating the valves by diathermy or cold-knife, using a paediatric resecting cystoscope. Long-term follow up is imperative, as renal function may deteriorate to the point of renal replacement therapy or transplantation in about 50%. Sometimes a low-capacity, high-pressure bladder persists, requiring drainage or a bladder augmentation procedure.

Abdominal Problems

Chronic and Recurrent Abdominal Pain

Chronic or recurrent abdominal pain is common in children of school age, but no cause is usually discovered and the problem gradually resolves (Box 51.2). Children may be referred to a surgeon if an organic problem seems likely, but psychological factors are common. The common organic cause is constipation, but hydronephrosis, inflammatory bowel disease and gallstones, associated with haemolytic anaemia, are occasional causes.

Chronic Constipation

Chronic constipation is a very common problem in children. It may present as **faecal soiling**, that is, faecal overflow incontinence. A detailed history, including psychosocial factors, may reveal a cause but in most, the aetiology is unknown. The problem should not be neglected as it may lead to lifelong problems. Early constipation usually responds to simple measures, such as a high-fibre diet, increased fluid intake, regular attempts at defaecation, and combinations of osmotic and stimulant laxatives (e.g., lactulose or senna derivative or Movicol).

In severe constipation, it is important to investigate for **cystic fibrosis, hypothyroidism** and **Hirschsprung disease** (Ch. 50, p. 640). If these can be excluded, the child may require an operation, such as anterior resection for redundant nonfunctional rectum, or the creation of a conduit into the colon to allow antegrade enemas (Antegrade Continence Enema or ACE).

• **BOX 51.2** **Organic Causes of Chronic or Recurrent Abdominal Pain in Children**

- Chronic constipation—common
- Lower urinary tract infection—common
- Hydronephrosis—uncommon
- Sickle cell crises—uncommon
- Recurrent appendicitis—rare
- Crohn disease
- Recurrent volvulus of small bowel—rare
- Gallstones—rare, sometimes associated with haemolytic anaemia
- Peptic ulceration—rare

Gastrointestinal Bleeding in Children (see Table 51.2)

Upper Gastrointestinal Bleeding

In neonates, apparent vomiting of blood may result from swallowed maternal blood. In older infants, gastritis may be the cause. Less common causes are bleeding disorders and coagulopathy.

Lower Gastrointestinal Bleeding

Rectal bleeding in neonates is most often caused by anal fissure, necrotising enterocolitis or malrotation with volvulus. Rectal bleeding is a common problem in older infants and children; the causes are summarised in Table 51.2 and include perianal abscess and fistula, anal fissures, large bowel polyps, rectal prolapse and Meckel diverticulum.

Anal Fissure

Anal fissure occurs at any age during infancy and childhood and is probably initiated by straining to pass a large hard stool. This splits the anal mucosa in the midline posteriorly or anteriorly. Anal fissures can also develop after severe diarrhoea. The main symptoms are pain at defaecation and a small amount of bright red blood on the stool or leaking out immediately after defaecation. The condition is readily diagnosed when digital rectal examination is found to be impossible because of extreme tenderness; the posterior end of the fissure may sometimes be seen by parting the buttocks. Treatment is conservative, with medical treatment of constipation and management of painful defaecation. Anal skin tags often develop following healing of an anal fissure.

Polyps

A **juvenile hamartomatous polyp** is a common cause of rectal bleeding. These are nearly always solitary and usually occur in the rectum or sigmoid colon, and a familial predisposition is described (associated with SMAD-4 mutations). Polyps may present with

---

TABLE 51.2	Common Causes of Gastrointestinal Bleeding in Children	
Age	**Upper Gastrointestinal**	**Lower Gastrointestinal**
1–12 months	Oesophagitis Gastritis	Anal fissure Intussusception Necrotising enterocolitis Malrotation with volvulus Perianal abscess and fistula
1–2 years	Peptic ulcer disease associated with: Burns (Curling ulcer) Head trauma (Cushing ulcer) Malignancy Sepsis	Anal fissure Polyps Rectal prolapse Meckel diverticulum Perianal abscess and fistula
2–15 years	Oesophageal and gastric varices Portal hypertension with cirrhosis	Polyps Inflammatory bowel disease Trauma Sexual abuse Gastroenteritis—*Campylobacter* Arteriovenous malformations Miscellaneous lesions

intermittent rectal bleeding in a child, without constipation; as pain on defaecation, without an anal fissure; or by prolapsing through the anus. The polyp may be palpable on digital examination and is confirmed on proctoscopy; it can then be suture ligated and resected. If no polyp is visible, colonoscopy is performed and identified polyps removed by snare. Juvenile polyps are benign (malignancy is rarely described), and they do not recur. **Familial adenomatous polyposis** may present in childhood with rectal bleeding. As described in Chapter 27, polyps of this type inevitably turn malignant from about the age of 16 years.

Rectal Prolapse

Transient rectal prolapse is a common and alarming childhood problem, usually during the first 2 years. The common cause is excessive straining during defaecation. Prolapse may be a presenting feature of cystic fibrosis, because there is less mucus in the bowel and the mucus is thick and sticky. In addition, thick mucus often obstructs exocrine pancreatic secretion, impairing fat digestion. Most prolapses can be gently manipulated back without pain, although they frequently recur unless the stool is kept soft and the child can open the bowels without straining. If the problem is persistent or recurrent, proctoscopy and sigmoidoscopy are indicated. A rectal polyp is occasionally responsible. If simple stool-softening measures fail to prevent recurrence, submucosal injections of hypertonic saline or phenol in oil have been used to induce fibrosis. In the rare event of failure, a subcutaneous circumanal suture may be inserted.

Perianal Abscess

This is common in infants and results from infection of an anal gland, as in adults. The abscess points 1 to 2 cm from the anal verge. Drainage alone would convert this into a **fistula**, so correct treatment involves opening the tract entirely under general anaesthesia, as in adults.

Meckel Diverticulum

A Meckel diverticulum is present in less than 2% of the population. It represents the embryological remnant of the **vitello-intestinal duct**, which joined the foetal midgut and the yolk sac. It is situated on the antimesenteric border of the distal ileum about 60 cm from the ileocaecal junction and is usually asymptomatic.

Meckel diverticula often contain a variety of gut-related tissues. These include **ectopic acid-secreting gastric mucosa**, which may cause inflammation and peptic ulceration. In children below 2 years, this is an important cause of rectal bleeding, which may require transfusion. In older children, the gastric mucosa more often causes chronic occult bleeding leading to iron deficiency anaemia. Much less commonly, **peptic ulceration** results in **perforation**, which presents with signs of peritonitis.

If a Meckel diverticulum is suspected in rectal bleeding, a radionuclide Meckel scan may be positive, but the test has a low negative **predictive value** and a laparoscopy or laparotomy often has to be performed to examine the bowel directly.

A Meckel diverticulum with a narrow neck may become inflamed like appendicitis and cause similar symptoms and signs (see Fig. 26.4, p. 370); the diagnosis is only made at operation. As with appendicitis, the complications are perforation and peritonitis. Meckel diverticulitis is uncommon in children under 10 years.

At operation, the diverticulum should be resected, together with 2 cm of normal ileum on each side, and primary ileoileal anastomosis performed. This is because ectopic gastric mucosa can extend beyond the diverticulum.

Inflammatory Bowel Disease (See Ch. 28 for Adult Disease)

The incidence of Crohn disease in children is increasing and can involve any part of the gastrointestinal tract. Perianal disease is common, with chronic indolent abscesses and fissures. These fissures are often lateral, suggesting the diagnosis. Crohn disease varies greatly in its presentation and this may cause delay in diagnosis. As in adults, there may be a history of recurrent abdominal pain and weight loss. The first presentation in adolescents may be faltering growth or delayed onset of puberty.

Ulcerative colitis presents with diarrhoea, malaise and weight loss; perianal disease and proctitis is uncommon. Management of both conditions is similar to that in adults. A need for surgery is uncommon in childhood and is best managed in a specialist centre.

Abdominal Mass

An abdominal mass is an uncommon reason for surgical referral in children. It may be caused by a malignant embryonal tumour, most often a **nephroblastoma** (Wilms tumour). Other causes include **hydronephrosis** and **posttraumatic pancreatic pseudocyst**.

Nephroblastoma (Wilms Tumour)

Nephroblastoma presents in early childhood, with 80% presenting before the age of 5 years, at a median age of 3.5 years. The tumour arises from embryonal renal tissue in the kidney. Tumours are locally invasive and metastasise to regional nodes, liver, lungs and (less commonly) bone. Often, a large abdominal mass is noticed by the mother as the child is bathed (Fig. 51.8). The mass

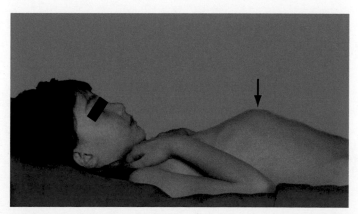

• **Fig. 51.8** Nephroblastoma. This 9-year-old girl presented with a large unilateral mass *(arrowed)*, which was later confirmed to be arising from the left kidney (Wilms tumour or nephroblastoma).

is sometimes so large, as to obscure its site of origin. Less common presenting features include haematuria, classically after trivial trauma, anorexia, weight loss, pyrexia and hypertension. Diagnosis is by clinical examination, and tumour size and characteristics are shown by ultrasonography or computed tomography scan. The diagnosis can be confirmed by Trucut biopsy, where required.

Treatment is by neoadjuvant chemotherapy via a Hickman line followed by surgery (usually a radical nephrectomy with lymph node sampling). In the United Kingdom, all children with Wilms tumour are managed by a multidisciplinary team, using a strict protocol. When surgery was the only treatment, the cure rate was about 10%, but the modern combination of neoadjuvant chemotherapy, surgical resection and sometimes radiotherapy gives a good chance of complete cure, even when distant metastases are present.

Neuroblastoma

This embryonal tumour occurs in early childhood. It is highly malignant and arises from embryonal sympathetic nervous tissue in the adrenal gland or sympathetic chain. Standard treatment is a combination of surgical resection, chemotherapy and radiotherapy, but the prognosis is poor.

Index

Note: Page numbers followed by "f" indicate figures, "t" indicate tables, and "b" indicate boxes.

Subconjunctival haematoma, following head injury, 254–256, 256f
Subdural haematoma, 247–249, 249b
Subfertility, in testicular maldescent, 652
Sublingual salivary gland, 604
Subluxations, 241–243
Submandibular salivary gland, 604, 607f, 608b
Submandibular stones, 607
Subphrenic abscesses, 34, 183, 300, 318
Substance abuse, 6
Subtalar joints, 165
Subungual melanoma, 585, 602, 602f
Succussion splash, acute gastric dilatation, 182
Sucralfate, 327
Sulfasalazine, 114, 395–397
Sulphonylureas, 112
Sunitinib, 194–195
Superficial burns, 268–269
Superficial dermal burns, 268–269
Superficial spreading melanoma, 594
Superficial wound infection, 97
Superior mesenteric artery (SMA), 301
Supplementary nutrition, 28–30
Supralevator abscess, 416
Suprapontine injury, 462
Suprapubic contrast cystography, 468
Suprapubic masses, 290–291
Suprasacral cord conditions, 462–463
Surgeons
 areas of practice, 2
 desirable attributes in, 6b
 general, 2
 iatrogenic disorders, 5
Surgical complications, 170–184, 171b
 acute renal failure, 180–181
 anaesthesia, 170, 171b
 antibiotic-associated colitis, 180
 atelectasis, 175
 cardiovascular, 171b
 caudal anaesthesia, 171b
 colitis, antibiotic-associated, 180
 epidural anaesthesia, 171b
 fluid and electrolyte disturbances, post-surgery, 180
 general, of any operation, 170–174
 general anaesthesia, 171b
 haemorrhage, 172
 hospital acquired pneumonias, 175–176
 impaired healing, 174
 inadvertent trauma, 170–171
 infection, operation site, 172–174
 local anaesthesia, 171b
 pneumonias, 175
 pressure sores, 34–35, 181–182
 prevention, 170
 respiratory, 175–177
 spinal anaesthesia, 171b
 venous thromboembolism, 177–180
Surgical drainage, anorectal abscess, 416
Surgical injury, 172
Surgical misadventure, 5

Surgical sieve, 3–4, 4b
Surgical techniques
 basic, 129–136
 craniotomy, 149–150
 haemostasis principles of, 130–132
 hydrocephalus, 149
 incision, 129–130
 infected tissues, involving, 138–140
 involving infected tissues, 138–140
 laparoscopy, 142–147
 minimal access surgery, 64, 142, 143t–144t
 neurosurgery, 151
 postoperative wound management of, 135–136
Suture fixation rectopexy, 418
Suture needle, types of, 133, 133b
Suturing/surgical repair
 absorbable versus nonabsorbable materials, 132
 gauge of suture material, 133, 133b
 monofilament versus polyfilament sutures, 133
 natural versus synthetic materials, 132–133
 removal of sutures, 136
 skin closure techniques, 135f
 skin edges, methods of approximating, 134f
 staples and other wound closure techniques, 135, 135f
 tension sutures, 174
 type of suture material, 132–135, 132b
 wire sutures, 133
Swabs, bacterial, 39
Sweat gland lesions, 595
Sweating, fluid loss, 23
Swelling
 after tooth extraction, 613
 limbs, 519, 520t
 scrotal, 444
Swinging pyrexia, 32–33
Sympathectomy, 525
Symptoms, of breast disease, 564–565, 566f
Syndrome of inappropriate antidiuretic hormone hypersecretion (SIADH), 150
Synthetic material, 132–133
Syphilis, tertiary gummatous, 446
System failure, clinical audit, 13
Systematic review, versus evidence, 9
Systemic embolism, 67
Systemic inflammatory response syndrome (SIRS)
 clinical conditions leading to, 48–49
 definitions, 48, 48b
 inflammatory fluid, intra-abdominal accumulation, 23
 mediators, 48
 and pancreatitis, 359
 pathophysiology, 48
 preventive factors in at-risk patients, 49
 and septic shock, 52
 surgical aspects, 49
Systemic lymphadenopathy, 609–610
Systemic sepsis, 23, 32–33

Systemic thrombolytic therapy, 179
Systolic blood pressure, 106

T
Tachycardia, 97
 postoperative, 18–19
Tachypnoea, 98
Taeniae coli, 403
Tamoxifen, 577
Tarsal coalition, 159, 159f
Taxanes, 193
Tazobactam, 44
TB. see Tuberculosis
Teeth, vulnerability to damage, 109
Telephone consultation, effective, 8b
Tele-surgery, 145
Temperature regulation, in children, 637
Temporal lobes, brain, 247
Tenesmus, 282, 375, 378
Tennis elbow, 162
Tension pneumothorax, 222t, 425
Tension sutures, 174
Teratomas, 449–450
Terminal disease, obstructive jaundice, 287–288
Terminal ileum, 372
Terminology, surgical, 125b
Tertiary contractions, 338
Tertiary gummatous syphilis, 446
Testes, removal, 480
Testicular atrophy, 438
Testicular cancer
 pathology, 449–450
 recurrence chances, 190
 seminomas, 449
 teratomas, 449–450
Testicular disorders
 cryptorchidism (absent scrotal testis), 451
 lumps, 444
 maldescent, 451, 651–652, 651f
 torsion, 451–452, 647
 trauma, 452
Testicular haematoma, 452
Testicular hydrocoele, 447b
Testicular torsion, 647
Testicular tumours, 448–451, 449f
 classification of, 449b
 clinical features, 450
 fertility and, 450–451
 investigation and treatment, 450–451, 450f, 450b–451b
 semen cryopreservation for, 450–451
 seminomas, 449
 surgery for, 451
 tumour markers, 450
Testis
 inflammation of, 446–447
 torsion of, 451–452, 452f, 452b
Tetanus, 46
Tetanus immune globulin (TIG), 46
Tetracycline, 42
Tetralogy of Fallot, 555, 556f